AF774655

Emergency Department Critical Care

Joseph R. Shiber
Editor

Scott D. Weingart
Consulting Editor

Emergency Department Critical Care

Springer

Editors
Joseph R. Shiber
College of Medicine
University of Florida Health Science Center
Jacksonville, FL
USA

Scott D. Weingart
Resuscitation & Emergency Critical Care
Icahn School of Medicine at Mount Sinai
New York, NY
USA

ISBN 978-3-030-28792-4 ISBN 978-3-030-28794-8 (eBook)
https://doi.org/10.1007/978-3-030-28794-8

© Springer Nature Switzerland AG 2020
This work is subject to copyright. All rights are reserved by the Publisher, whether the whole or part of the material is concerned, specifically the rights of translation, reprinting, reuse of illustrations, recitation, broadcasting, reproduction on microfilms or in any other physical way, and transmission or information storage and retrieval, electronic adaptation, computer software, or by similar or dissimilar methodology now known or hereafter developed.
The use of general descriptive names, registered names, trademarks, service marks, etc. in this publication does not imply, even in the absence of a specific statement, that such names are exempt from the relevant protective laws and regulations and therefore free for general use.
The publisher, the authors and the editors are safe to assume that the advice and information in this book are believed to be true and accurate at the date of publication. Neither the publisher nor the authors or the editors give a warranty, expressed or implied, with respect to the material contained herein or for any errors or omissions that may have been made. The publisher remains neutral with regard to jurisdictional claims in published maps and institutional affiliations.

This Springer imprint is published by the registered company Springer Nature Switzerland AG
The registered company address is: Gewerbestrasse 11, 6330 Cham, Switzerland

Preface

Our goal for this text is to provide a resource for the care of the critically ill and injured patient in the community ED and ICU. Unlike a major academic center that may have all of the necessary resources and specialty consultants on site, the community hospital physician may be required to provide all of the required care themselves for definitive treatment or to stabilize the patient for transport to a referral center.

With that goal in mind, we have created a new book written almost entirely by Emergency Medicine residency-trained physicians with fellowship training in critical care. The only non-critical care-trained authors are Emergency Medicine physicians with additional fellowship training (pediatrics, toxicology, emergency medical systems, etc.). We are proud to include as authors several of the founders of Emergency Medicine Critical Care (EMCC), Drs. Emanuel Rivers and Jay Falk, as well as many of the current group of EM-CC physicians who have taken the baton to lead onward with advancing clinical care, research, and education efforts dealing with Emergency Medicine Critical Care.

This book is a hybrid, just as the authors and the field itself. It is not meant to be a reference textbook on the shelf nor a pocket manual; instead, it is a practical resource for the provider in the ED or ICU with valuable information, critical points, and easy-to-follow diagrams and flowcharts. We are proud to offer this book to residents and fellows as well as practicing attending physicians and believe that it will assist you as you resuscitate and care for the most challenging patients with time-sensitive conditions such as respiratory failure, acute myocardial infarction, multi-trauma with hemorrhagic shock, or sepsis.

Jacksonville, FL, USA — Joseph R. Shiber
New York, NY, USA — Scott D. Weingart

Contents

Contributors

Azeemuddin Ahmed, MD, MBA Department of Emergency Medicine, University of Iowa Carver College of Medicine, Iowa City, IA, USA

Jonathan Auerbach, MD Critical Care Medicine, University of Miami Hospital, Miami, FL, USA

Sara Y. Baker, MD Department of Emergency Medicine, Orlando Regional Medical Center, Orlando, FL, USA

Torben K. Becker, MD, PhD, RDMS, FAWM Department of Emergency Medicine, University of Florida, Gainesville, FL, USA

Morgen Bernius, MD, MS, FACEP, FAAP Department of Emergency Medicine, Medstar Franklin Square Medical Center, Baltimore, MD, USA

Kimberly Boswell, MD University of Maryland School of Medicine, Baltimore, MD, USA

Michael Buscher, MD Critical Care Medicine, Emergency Medicine, Yale New Haven Health, New Haven, CT, USA

Catherine Gogela Carlson, MD Department of Critical Care Medicine, Department of Emergency Medicine, Carolinas Medical Center, Charlotte, NC, USA

Wan-Tsu W. Chang, MD Department of Emergency Medicine, University of Maryland School of Medicine, Baltimore, MD, USA

Nico Chiriboga Division of Pediatric Critical Care, University of Florida, Department of Pediatrics in the College of Medicine, Jacksonville, FL, USA

Neil Christopher, MD Department of Emergency Medicine, Icahn School of Medicine at Mount Sinai, New York, NY, USA

Jason Cohen, DO, FACEP, FCCM Boston MedFlight, Bedford, MA, USA

James Dargin, MD Tufts University School of Medicine, Medical Intensive Care Unit, Boston, MA, USA

Pulmonary and Critical Care Medicine, Lahey Hospital & Medical Center, Burlington, MA, USA

Jennifer H. Edwards, MD Intermountain Healthcare, Murray, UT, USA

Marie-Carmelle Elie, MD, RDMS, FACEP Department of Emergency Medicine, Critical Care, Hospice and Palliative Medicine, University of Florida, Gainesville, FL, USA

Timothy J. Ellender, MD, BSN Department of Emergency Medicine, IU School of Medicine, IU Health-Methodist Hospital, Indianapolis, IN, USA

Jonathan Elmer, MD, MS Departments of Emergency Medicine, Critical Care Medicine and Neurology, University of Pittsburgh School of Medicine, Pittsburgh, PA, USA

Lillian Emlet, MD, MS Critical Care Medicine and Emergency Medicine, University of Pittsburgh Medical Center, Hermitage, PA, USA

Jay L. Falk, MD Department of Emergency Medicine, Orlando Regional Medical Center, Orlando, FL, USA

Emily Fontane, MD Department of Emergency Medicine, Division of Pediatric Emergency Medicine, University of Florida, College of Medicine, Jacksonville, FL, USA

John P. Gaillard, MD Anesthesiology-Critical Care, Emergency Medicine, Internal Medicine-Pulmonary/Critical Care, Wake Forest Baptist Health, Winston-Salem, NC, USA

Jayna Gardner-Gray, MD Department of Emergency Medicine and Division of Pulmonary and Critical Care, Henry Ford Hospital, Wayne State University, Detroit, MI, USA

Munish Goyal, MD, FACEP MedStar Washington Hospital Center, Washington, DC, USA

Emily Gundert, MD Emergency Medicine, UT Southwestern Medical Center, Dallas, TX, USA

Kyle J. Gunnerson, MD Emergency Medicine, Anesthesiology, and Internal Medicine, University of Michigan Health Center, Ann Arbor, MI, USA

Daniel Haase, MD University of Maryland School of Medicine, Baltimore, MD, USA

David Hackenson, MD Emergency Medicine, University of Michigan, Ann Arbor, MI, USA

Alan C. Heffner, MD Department of Internal Medicine, Department of Emergency Medicine, Carolinas Medical Center, Charlotte, NC, USA

Mark Hincapie Division of Pediatric Critical Care to Paediatric Emergency medicine, Jacksonville, FL, USA

Christopher J. Hogan, MD, FACEP Department of Emergency Medicine, Department of Surgery, Division of Trauma/Critical Care, VCU Medical Center, Medical College of Virginia Campus, Richmond, VA, USA

Kami Hu, MD Departments of Medicine and Emergency Medicine, University of Maryland School of Medicine, Baltimore, MD, USA

Gina Hurst, BS, MD Department of Emergency Medicine and Division of Pulmonary and Critical Care, Henry Ford Hospital, Wayne State University, Detroit, MI, USA

Charles Hwang, MD, EMT-T Department of Emergency Medicine, UF Health, Levy County Department of Public Safety, Gainesville, FL, USA

Brad A. Johnson, MD Department of Anesthesiology, University of Iowa Hospital, Iowa City, IA, USA

William A. Knight IV, MD, FACEP, FNCS Emergency Medicine and Neurosurgery, University of Cincinnati, Cincinnati, OH, USA

Natalie P. Kreitzer, MD Emergency Medicine, Neurovascular Emergencies and Neurocritical Care, University of Cincinnati, Cincinnati, OH, USA

Zachary D. Levy, MD Emergency Medicine and Neurosurgery, Zucker School of Medicine at Hofstra/Northwell, Hempstead, NY, USA

Anton Travis Manasco, MD Anesthesiology – Critical Care Medicine, Washington University in St. Louis School of Medicine – Barnes Jewish Hospital, St. Louis, MO, USA

Evie Marcolini, MD, FACEP, FAAEM Departments of Emergency Medicine and Neurology, Divisions of Neurocritical Care and Emergency Neurology and Surgical Critical Care, SkyHealth Critical Care, Yale University School of Medicine, New Haven, CT, USA

Michael T. McCurdy, MD Departments of Medicine and Emergency Medicine, University of Maryland School of Medicine, Baltimore, MD, USA

Fernando Mena, MD, F'AAP Department of Pediatrics, MedStar Franklin Square Medical Center, Rossville, MD, USA

Jay Menaker, MD Program in Trauma, R Adams Cowley Shock Trauma Center, University of Maryland School of Medicine, Baltimore, MD, USA

Nicholas M. Mohr, MD, MS Department of Emergency Medicine, Department of Anesthesia, University of Iowa Carver College of Medicine, Iowa City, IA, USA

Jarrod M. Mosier, MD Department of Emergency Medicine, Department of Medicine, Division of Pulmonary, Allergy, Critical Care, and Sleep, University of Arizona, Tucson, AZ, USA

Rohit Patel, MD, FACS University of Florida Health, Gainesville, FL, USA

Jacqueline Pflaum-Carlson, MD Department of Emergency Medicine and Division of Pulmonary and Critical Care, Henry Ford Hospital, Wayne State University, Detroit, MI, USA

Kabir Rezvankhoo, MD, RDCS New York-Presbyterian Hospital Columbia University Medical Center, New York, NY, USA

Emanuel P. Rivers, MD, MPH Department of Emergency Medicine and Department of Surgery, Henry Ford Hospital, Wayne State University, Detroit, MI, USA

Lauren N. Rodriguez, MD Department of Emergency Medicine, Kaiser Moanalua Medical Center, Honolulu, HI, USA

Michael Schinlever, MD Surgery – Critical Care, Rochester Regional Health, Rochester, NY, USA

Adam B. Schlichting, MD, MPH Department of Emergency Medicine, Department of Internal Medicine, University of Iowa Healthcare, Iowa City, IA, USA

Mark Segal, MD, PhD Department of Medicine, University of Florida Health, Gainesville, FL, USA

Ayan Sen, MD, MSc, FACEP, FCCP Critical Care Medicine, Emergency Medicine, Mayo Clinic College of Medicine, Mayo Clinic Arizona, Phoenix, AZ, USA

Joseph R. Shiber, MD College of Medicine, University of Florida Health Science Center, Jacksonville, FL, USA

Todd L. Slesinger Herbert Wertheim College of Medicine, Florida International University, Miami, FL, USA

Joshua D. Stilley, MD Department of Emergency Medicine, University of Iowa, Iowa City, IA, USA

Amanda F. Tarkowski, MD Department of Emergency Medicine, Orlando Regional Medical Center, Orlando, FL, USA

David A. Wacker, MD, PhD Department of Medicine, University of Minnesota Medical School, Minneapolis, MN, USA

Aimee Wendelsdorf, MD Emergency Medicine and Critical Care Medicine, Presbyterian Hospital, Albuquerque, NM, USA

Brian T. Wessman, MD, FACEP, FCCM Divisions of Critical Care Medicine and Emergency Medicine, Washington University in Saint Louis, School of Medicine, St. Louis, MO, USA

Beranton Whisenant, MD Emergency Department, University of Florida Health – Jacksonville, Jacksonville, FL, USA

Sage P. Whitmore, MD Department of Emergency Medicine, Division of Emergency Critical Care, Ann Arbor, MI, USA

Samantha L. Wood, MD Emergency Department, Maine Medical Center, Portland, ME, USA

Brian J. Wright, MD, MPH Emergency Medicine and Surgery, Stony Brook University School of Medicine, Stony Brook, NY, USA

Qiuping Zhou, DO Emergency Medicine and Cardiothoracic Surgery, Zucker School of Medicine at Hofstra/Northwell, Hempstead, NY, USA

Shock Overview

1

Sara Y. Baker, Amanda F. Tarkowski, and Jay L. Falk

Introduction

Circulatory shock is a clinical syndrome characterized by inadequate tissue perfusion of oxygen and other nutrients, resulting in first reversible and then, if prolonged, irreversible cellular injury. The resulting deficit in tissue oxygenation leads to cellular hypoxia and anaerobic metabolism manifested systemically as lactic acidosis. The magnitude of the oxygen debt correlates with the lactate level, which may be used to quantify the severity of shock [1]. If not interrupted, the cascade of cell death, end-organ damage, and multisystem organ dysfunction can cause significant morbidity and death.

Accordingly, the clinician must recognize the early manifestations of shock, and resuscitation must proceed expeditiously and simultaneously with efforts to identify the specific etiology of the shock state.

Pathophysiology and Monitoring

During the past several decades, understanding the biology of shock at the cellular and subcellular levels has exploded (Fig. 1.1a, b). While an awareness of this complex biology is important, especially in sepsis, the focus of this chapter will be on the clinical issues surrounding oxygen delivery, various methods of recognizing oxygen deficits, and clinical approaches to restoring oxygen delivery and maintaining tissue perfusion.

The presence of hypotension has traditionally been the clinical hallmark of circulatory shock. Current thinking recognizes the fact that patients may remain normotensive despite the presence of systemic hypoperfusion, due to compensatory mechanisms, a situation sometimes referred to as "cryptic shock" [2]. Patients who are hypotensive in the emergency department are at substantially increased risk of end-organ dysfunction and death compared to normotensive patients, even if the hypotension is transient [3].

Adequate perfusion pressure is therefore necessary, but not sufficient to ensure that organs are indeed well perfused. Occasionally, a patient may be hypotensive but NOT in shock (e.g., due to vasodilatation with normal intravascular volume and cardiac output and maintained tissue perfusion); however, the presence of hypotension should garner concern for shock first. Accordingly, monitoring of blood pressure remains a fundamental priority in caring for the critically ill.

Blood pressure may be measured noninvasively by a variety of techniques or directly by the insertion of an arterial catheter. Auscultatory and oscillometric methods rely on vibrations in the arterial wall caused by pulsatile flow through the compressed arterial segments as pressure in the cuff is released. These vibrations are diminished in patients with severe arteriosclerosis,

S. Y. Baker (✉) · A. F. Tarkowski · J. L. Falk
Department of Emergency Medicine, Orlando Regional Medical Center, Orlando, FL, USA

© Springer Nature Switzerland AG 2020

J. R. Shiber, S. D. Weingart (eds.), *Emergency Department Critical Care*,
https://doi.org/10.1007/978-3-030-28794-8_1

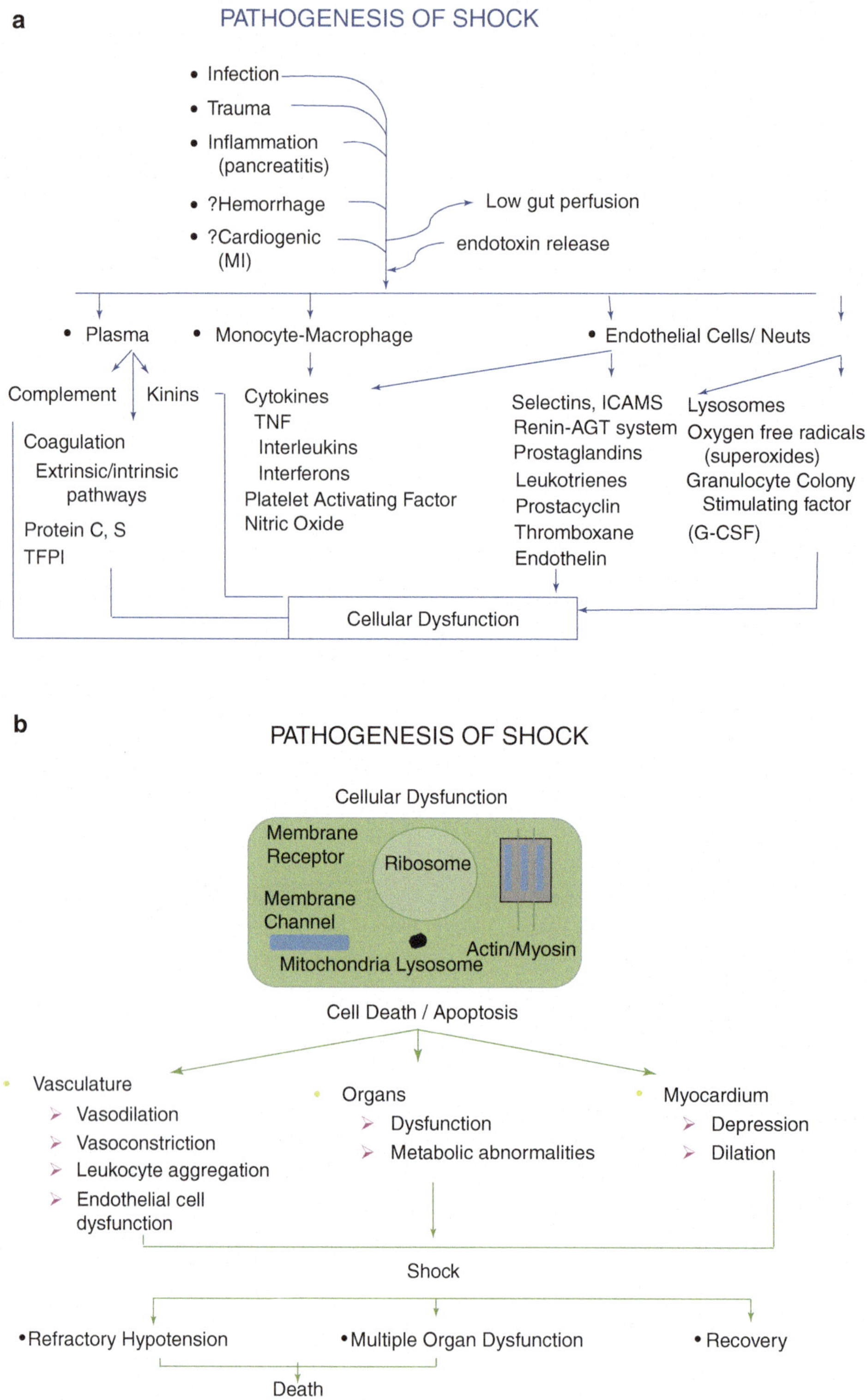

Fig. 1.1 (**a**, **b**) The pathogenesis of shock is complex and involves extensive interactions of various mediators in the plasma, blood, vasculature, and organs, which can lead to apoptosis, refractory hypotension, multiple organ failure, and death if not interrupted. (Courtesy of Dr. Joseph Parrillo)

vasoconstriction, or low flow states. Given that these conditions are prevalent among critically ill patients, placement of an arterial catheter in critically ill patients may be preferable to relying on noninvasive measurements. Indeed, Cohn demonstrated that among patients with low cardiac output and high systemic vascular resistance, cuff pressures grossly underestimated true intra-arterial pressures [4]. More recently, Low et al. confirmed these findings in unstable helicopter transport patients [5]. Arterial lines enable the accurate titration of therapies aimed at maintaining mean arterial pressure (MAP) in the recommended ranges (i.e., MAP >65 mmHg in septic shock and cardiogenic shock patients) [6]. The establishment of an arterial line also enables safe and frequent sampling of arterial blood to measure blood gases and lactate.

Tissue perfusion is determined by several factors, including blood pressure (BP), cardiac output, and vascular tone both at the arteriole and venule levels. Under normal circumstances, 85% of the circulating blood volume is housed in the venous capacitance vessels.

Blood pressure (perfusion pressure) is determined by the interplay between cardiac output (CO) and systemic vascular resistance (SVR) (Fig. 1.2):

$$BP = CO \times SVR$$
$$SV \times HR$$

Physiologic compensatory mechanisms defend against hypotension. During hemorrhage, for example, as blood volume decreases, resulting in decreased stroke volume (SV); heart rate increases, maintaining CO and BP. Further bleeding results in decreased CO, for which the body compensates by increasing SVR to maintain blood pressure. Accordingly, patients may have normal or even elevated blood pressure in the face of substantial systemic hypoperfusion. This makes blood pressure an inadequate monitor of perfusion. Rather than relying on hypotension to define it, shock is best conceptualized as an imbalance between tissue oxygen supply and tissue oxygen demand (Fig. 1.3). Regardless, most authorities recommend maintaining a mean arterial pressure (MAP) of >65 mmHg in patients in shock, which may require the use of vasoactive medications [6].

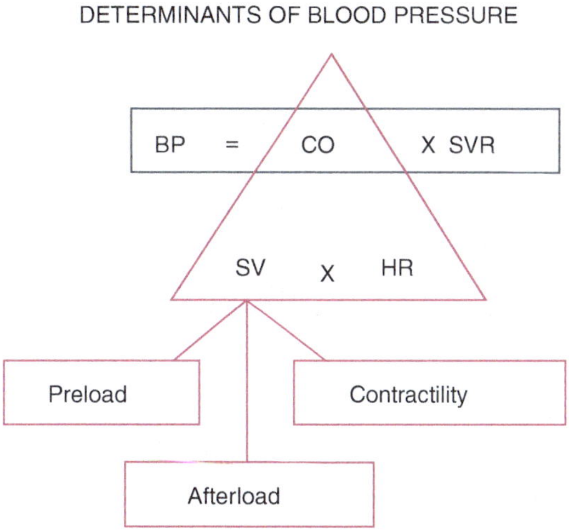

Fig. 1.2 Cardiac output is determined by the product of heart rate and stoke volume (the amount of blood pumped out of the heart with each beat). Stroke volume is affected by the filling of the heart (preload), the pressure against which heart must overcome to eject blood (afterload), and the intrinsic pumping capacity of the heart (contractility)

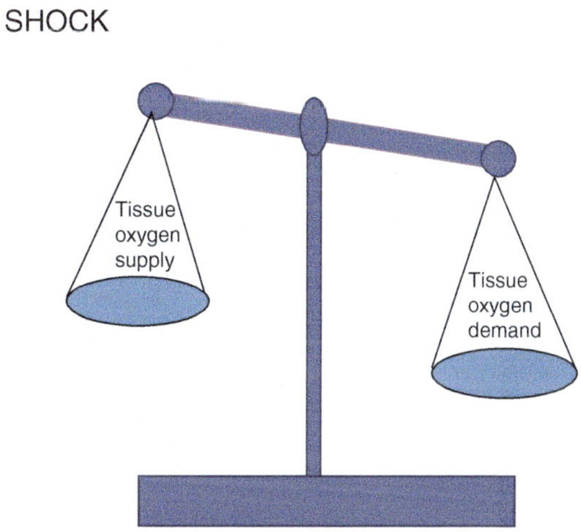

Fig. 1.3 Circulatory shock results from on imbalance between tissue oxygen supply and tissue oxygen demands

In the overwhelming majority of patients in shock, decreased oxygen supply is the primary cause of this imbalance. Factors that increase oxygen demands such as increased work of breathing, fever, seizures, and shivering may tip the scale toward hypoperfusion and should be addressed in these patients.

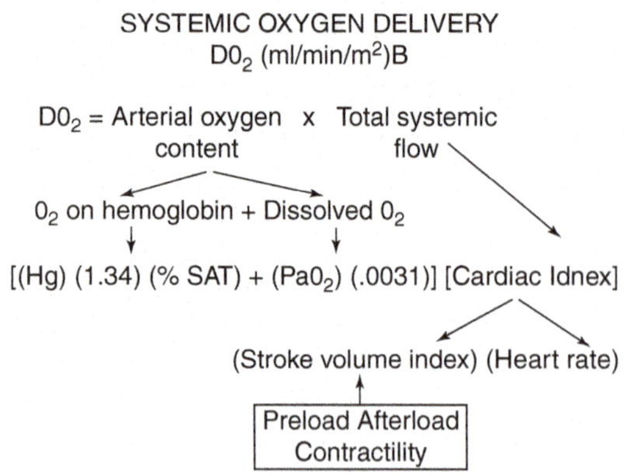

Fig. 1.4 Total systemic oxygen delivery (DO_2), hemoglobin in grams (Hg); 1.34 is a constant that represents the amount of oxygen in cubic centimeters carried on 1 g of Hg when fully saturated; .0031 is the solubility coefficient of oxygen in plasma; Falk et al. [60]

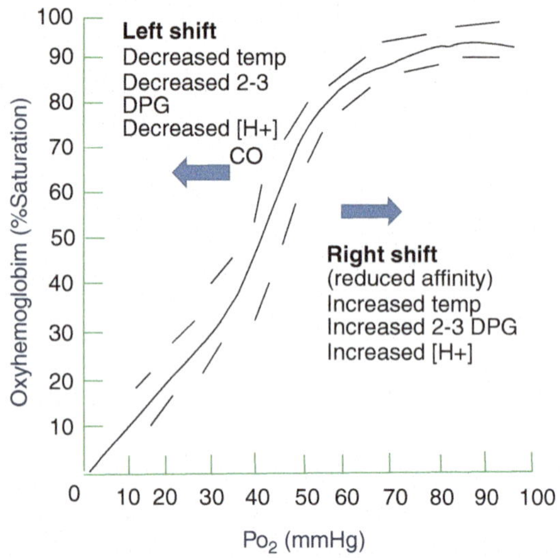

Fig. 1.5 The oxyhemoglobin dissociation curve indicates that at venous levels of PO_2 (40 mmHg), hemoglobin is 75% saturated. When arterial PO_2 falls below 60 mmHg, hemoglobin saturation falls rapidly. At arterial PO_2 levels above 80 mmHg, hemoglobin is nearly fully saturated

To enable intelligent therapeutic intervention in shock patients, clinicians must fully understand the determinants of oxygen delivery. Oxygen delivery (DO_2) is determined by the amount of oxygen contained in the blood (arterial oxygen content) and the total systemic flow (CO) (Fig. 1.4).

Arterial oxygen content comprises oxygen both carried on hemoglobin and dissolved in the plasma. Because the solubility coefficient of oxygen in plasma is very low (0.0031), for clinical purposes, when calculating the oxygen content of blood, the dissolved amount of oxygen is so small that it may be ignored. Conversely, the PaO_2 is critically important because it determines the saturation of hemoglobin (Hgb) (Fig. 1.5).

The PaO_2 should be maintained at 80–85 mmHg, keeping Hgb nearly fully saturated. Interventions aimed at further increasing the PaO_2 do little to increase oxygen delivery because the Hgb is already near full saturation. When the PaO_2 decreases below 60 mmHg, Hgb rapidly desaturates and DO_2 is compromised. When Hgb levels fall, DO_2 may also be compromised. This decrease may be ameliorated by interventions that increase CO or via transfusion of red blood cells. (Transfusions will be discussed further in Chap. 33.)

Manipulating the loading conditions of the heart can increase CO. Fluid resuscitation increases preload, which by the Starling mechanism increases SV and CO. In patients with high SVR, vasodilators can increase SV and CO by decreasing afterload. Inotropic and chronotropic drugs can increase contractility and heart rate to increase CO, but do so at the expense of increasing myocardial oxygen demands.

Optimizing oxygen delivery, therefore, should include respiratory therapy techniques that ensure that hemoglobin is fully saturated. Hemoglobin levels should be maintained with red cell transfusion, and cardiac output should be optimized beginning with the restoration of adequate preload and subsequently with the judicious use of vasoactive medication to maintain both perfusion and perfusion pressure (BP) (Fig. 1.6).

Humans live in a state of oxygen excess, using only 25% of the oxygen delivered to the body each minute. While at rest, this is evidenced by the fact that blood returning to the right heart contains Hgb that is 75% saturated. If illness results in only a modest reduction in oxygen delivery, there is little physiologic impact. As delivery is further reduced, tissues will extract more of the available oxygen and mixed venous saturation will decrease (oxygen extraction ratio increases), maintaining tissue PO_2. As these mechanisms are overwhelmed, tissue PO_2 falls and glucose can no longer be metabolized in the mitochondria in the citric acid (Krebs) cycle. Rather, glucose metabolism is shunted to the cytoplasm. This produces far fewer ATP molecules per moles of glucose metabolized (2 ATP in anaerobic metabolism versus 38 ATP in aerobic metabolism), and the byproduct of this process is lactate (Fig. 1.7).

Lactate has been recognized as a monitor of systemic hypoperfusion in animal models and patients for over 50 years [7]. Arterial lactate concentration remains an excellent tool with which to monitor the presence and severity of oxygen debt in shock patients and its level correlates with the likelihood of survival [8]. (Severe Sepsis and Septic Shock will be discussed further in Chap. 19.)

In classic studies, Weil and Afifi showed that patients in an ICU carried an 80% risk of death when arterial lactate was >10 mm/dl, while that risk was <20% when lactate was <2 mm/dl. Patients with lactates around 5 mm/dl had a 50% mortality rate. More recently, Shapiro and colleagues demonstrated that in patients with serious infections presenting to the emergency department, lactate level could risk stratify patients [9]. Those with arterial lactate levels greater than 4.0 mg/dl had 3-day and 28-day mortality rates of 22.4% and 28.4%, respectively. This mortality rate was significantly higher than among patients with lactates between 2.5 and 3.9 mg/dl (4.6% 3-day mortality and 9.0% 28-day mortality) and those between 0 and 2.4 mg/dl (1.5% 3-day mortality and 4.9% 28-day mortality).

Perhaps, more striking is the ability of lactate to identify patients with systemic hypoperfusion but normal or high blood pressure. Abou-Khalil and Scalea [10] studied seriously injured patients requiring resuscitation and room transfusions at a level one trauma center. At 1 hour into the resus-

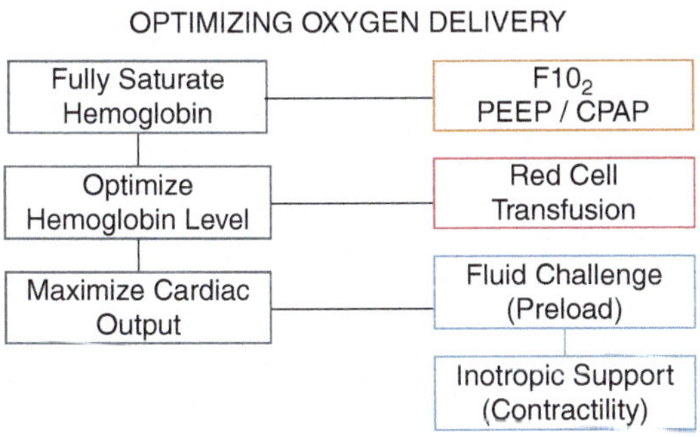

Fig. 1.6 The fraction of inspired oxygen (FIO_2), positive end-expiratory pressure (PEEP), continuous positive airway pressure (CPAP). In the face of systemic hypoperfusion, clinicians can increase oxygen delivery by manipulating the determinants of oxygen delivery in the biologically most cost-effective manner

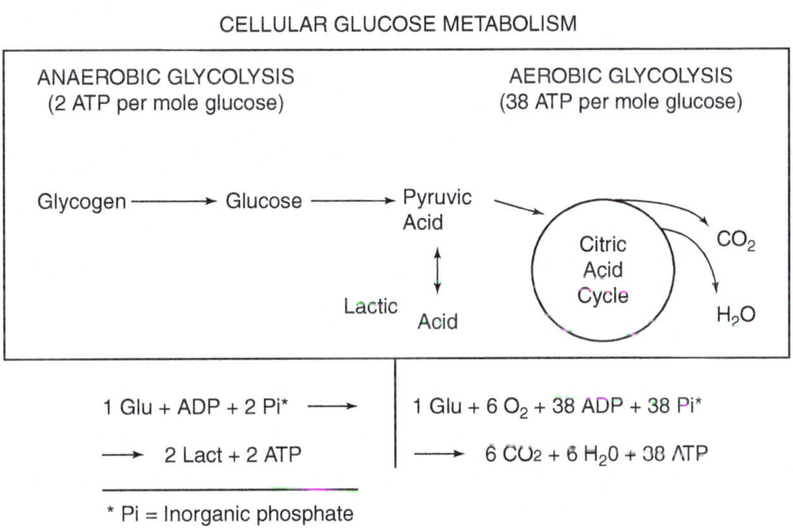

Fig. 1.7 Adenosine triphosphate molecules (ATP), adenosine diphosphate molecules (ADP). In the face of tissue hypoxia, anaerobic metabolism results in fewer moles of ATP produced per mole of glucose metabolized this way. Lactate is a byproduct of anaerobic metabolism

citation, lactate was 7.7 +/− 1.2 mg/dl among patients who died and 4.1 +/− 0.6 mg/dl among survivors (*P* = .001). Mean arterial pressures in both groups were 106 mmHg, and neither BP, HR, CVP, PAWP, Hct, CO nor oxygen consumption was different between the groups. Thus, lactate level was superior to traditional vital signs at identifying patients with hypoperfusion, and higher levels of lactate predicted increased mortality risk.

Similarly, in a subset of septic patients from the Early Goal-Directed Therapy Study (EGDT) reported by Rivers [11], Nguyen found that 23/133 control and 25/130 EGDT patients were normotensive with MAP ≥100 mmHg. At study entry, lactates were 9.6 mm/L and 8.4 mm/L in the control and EGDT groups, respectively. In hospital, mortality was 60.9% in the control group and 20% in the EGDT group. These data substantiate the importance of lactate as an invaluable bedside tool in identifying critically hypoperfused patients [12]. In a study examining lactate levels and survival utilizing data from the Surviving Sepsis Campaign database of 28,150 septic subjects from 218 international sites, Casserly and colleagues demonstrated that elevated lactate levels are highly associated with in hospital mortality. Both hypotensive and normotensive patients who presented with lactate levels greater than 4 mmol/L were demonstrated to have significantly higher risk than those with intermediate levels (2–3 and 3–4 mmo/L) [13].

Peripheral venous lactate may be used as a screening tool that obviates the need for arterial puncture. Younger and Falk [14] demonstrated that peripheral venous lactate was 100% sensitive in predicting arterial hyperlactatemia. Falsely elevated venous lactate levels occasionally occur, most commonly due to specimen-collection issues (e.g., prolonged tourniquet application, long interval between sampling and testing). If concern exists, an arterial sample can be obtained to confirm an elevated venous lactate level, although this is usually not necessary. A normal venous lactate level reliably predicts normal arterial lactate.

Serial lactate measurements can guide ongoing therapeutic interventions. Falk and colleagues demonstrated that patients surviving an episode of septic shock progressively cleared their lactate levels during the first 24 hours following fluid resuscitation, while among patients who expired, lactate levels failed to decrease or increase [15]. Nguyen and colleagues studied septic patients in the emergency setting and determined that mortality was lower among patients with more rapid clearance of lactate. Patients who cleared lactate at a rate greater than or equal to 10% per hour experienced a 60-day mortality rate significantly lower than those who did not [16].

These data suggest that as patients are being resuscitated, serial lactate measurements can be used to help guide resuscitative measures. Therapies can be titrated to maintain lactate clearance at or above 10% per hour. If lactate clearance is slower or if lactate levels are increasing, then further intervention to increase oxygen delivery and decrease oxygen demands is indicated. The choice of intervention should be guided by a firm understanding of the determinants of oxygen delivery. The clinician must choose the intervention that promises the best chance for improving the oxygen delivery/demand balance at the lowest biological cost.

While lactate is an excellent metabolic marker of shock that predicts severity and mortality, it has limitations. It takes time for lactate to accumulate and especially to clear. Regional hypoperfusion (such as the splanchnic bed) may be missed, as blood mixes centrally [17]. Increased sympathetic stimulation may result in increased lactate production without hypoxia at the cellular level. Lactate levels under these circumstances are generally very modest and do not affect the utility of lactate as a monitor. Other causes of elevated lactate are occasionally present; elevated lactate without evidence of systemic hypoperfusion is Type B lactic acidosis. It can be caused by regional hypoperfusion, liver disease, diabetes mellitus (especially with metformin therapy), alcoholism, malignancy, HIV and antiretroviral therapy, thiamine deficiency, mitochondrial dysfunction, poisoning, and other mechanisms. (Type A lactic acidosis refers to lactic acidosis due to systemic hypoperfusion, as discussed earlier.)

Monitoring of mixed venous (SVO_2) or central venous oxygen saturation ($SCVO_2$) may complement lactate monitoring and has the advantage of responding to physiologic changes in real time. In the face of systemic hypoperfusion, tissues will extract more of the available oxygen and venous oxygen saturation will decrease. $SCVO_2$ has been shown to be closely correlated with SVO_2, allowing for either continuous or intermittent sampling of $SCVO_2$ for monitoring purposes without the need to place a pulmonary artery catheter [18].

When SVO_2 or $SCVO_2$ is low, tissue hypoxia is present and measures to increase oxygen delivery are indicated. If this situation occurred acutely, lactate levels may not have had time to increase. It is crucial to understand that normal SVO_2 or $SCVO_2$ does not preclude the presence of hypoperfusion, especially in septic patients. Sepsis can result in disproportionate perfusion of metabolically relatively inactive tissues, such as the skin, while flow is shunted away from critically hypoperfused areas such as the splanchnic bed. Desaturated blood returning from the splanchnic bed and mixing with saturated blood returning from the skin may not show SVO_2 or $SCVO_2$ desaturation [17]. True arteriovenous shunts or "metabolic block" may also contribute to this observation. Under these circumstances, lactate levels will likely be elevated.

Recently, there has been a debate in the literature regarding which shock monitor is preferable as a target for ongoing care during early sepsis therapy. Jones et al. compared lactate and $SCVO_2$ as targets and found no mortality difference between the groups [19]. We would argue that this choice is a false dichotomy. The key issue in caring for these patients is that the clinician must have a firm understanding of the physiology and should use all the available monitoring tools to their best advantage. Venous saturation monitoring and lactate levels should be viewed as complimentary, each providing useful and potentially critical information.

Capnography has emerged as a very useful monitoring tool over the past 25 years. It has been embraced as an essential method to verify endotracheal tube placement in the prehospital and ED settings following the publications by Katz and Falk and Silvestri and colleagues [20, 21]. It has been shown, as well, to be an indicator of the effectiveness of closed chest massage during CPR and the earliest indication that spontaneous circulation has been re-established [22].

Recently, $ETCO_2$ has been used to noninvasively identify patients with metabolic acidosis such as diabetic ketoacidosis [23]. Patients with metabolic acidosis hyperventilate to compensate and would be expected to have low $ETCO_2$, assuming adequate cardiopulmonary reserve. We examined the relationship between $ETCO_2$, lactate, and mortality among patients suspected to be septic. As expected, there was an inverse correlation between lactate and $ETCO_2$. The sickest patients had the highest lactates, the lowest $ETCO_2$, and the highest mortality [24]. Accordingly, we believe a spot $ETCO_2$ may serve as a useful adjunct to SIRS criteria, shock index, and lactate as a rapid, noninvasive screening tool when assessing patients in the emergency department.

Classification of Shock

The Shubin/Weil Classification of Shock, first described in the 1960s, remains a most useful framework for clinicians at the bedside. It recognizes four broad categories of shock: hypovolemic, cardiogenic, obstructive, and distributive (Fig. 1.8). Multiple factors may contribute to the shock state. As the syndrome progresses, common pathways of inflammatory and hormonal mediators are activated, and if unchecked, it results in cellular dysfunction, refractory hypotension, multiple organ dysfunction, and death.

Hypovolemic Shock

Hypovolemic shock is characterized by intravascular volume loss. Acute hemorrhage from trauma, gastrointestinal bleeding, ruptured abdominal aortic aneurysm, ectopic pregnancy, or other causes is the most common etiology of hypovolemic shock. Gastrointestinal disorders

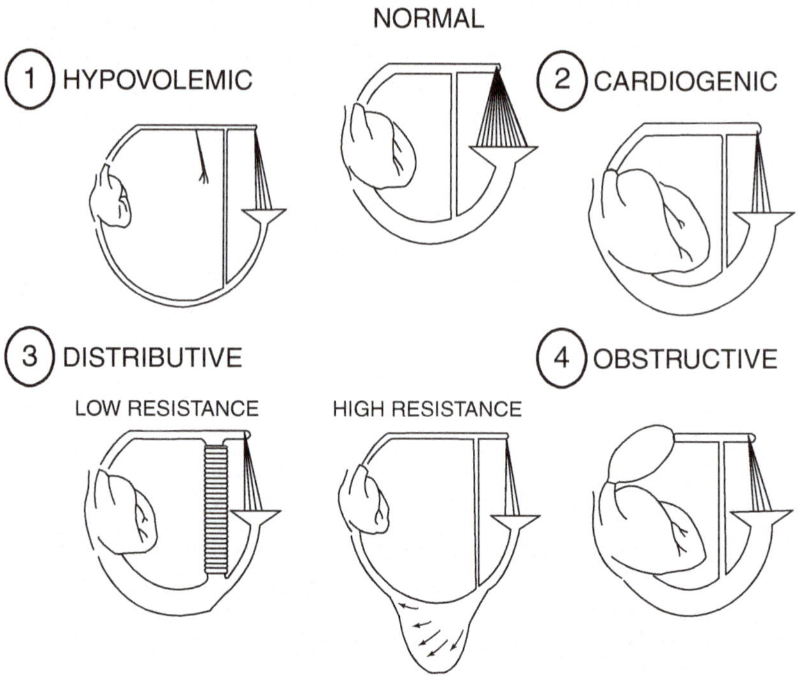

Fig. 1.8 Shubin/Weil classification of shock. The drawings represent components of the circulatory system: the heart, resistance vessels (arteries and arterioles), capacitance vessels (veins), the capillary beds, and arteriovenous shunts. Weil Critical Care Research Institute

that result in substantial fluid losses (i.e., cholera), decreased oral intake, or excessive diuresis as well as third space losses (i.e., pancreatitis) can also cause hypovolemic shock. Insufficient intravascular volume results in decreased preload, decreased cardiac output, and decreased oxygen delivery. Compensatory mechanisms such as tachycardia and arteriolar vasoconstriction may maintain perfusion in some patients for limited periods of time. Patients who are not yet frankly hypotensive may demonstrate postural hypotension, although autonomic dysfunction and medications such as antihypertensive agents, especially among the elderly, may be alternative reasons for this finding. Patients with intra-abdominal bleeding may have paradoxical bradycardia, resulting from vagal stimulation by the irritated peritoneum, most commonly seen in ruptured ectopic pregnancy [25].

Typically, compensatory vasoconstriction produces cool, pale skin and delayed capillary refill. In dehydrated patients, skin and axillae may be dry and the skin may have reduced turgor; in patients with acute hemorrhage, diaphoresis is present. Patients who have hemorrhage may also have pale mucous membranes and conjunctiva. Patients can be in hemorrhagic shock with initial hemoglobin levels that are not dramatically reduced because there has not been sufficient time for transcapillary refill to occur. As asanguineous fluid resuscitation is instituted, hemoglobin level drops dramatically. Recent animal and clinical studies have emphasized the need to stop the bleeding as soon as possible. Pepe and Mattock found that patients with penetrating truncal trauma had improved survival when crystalloid resuscitation was restricted until surgical intervention could be accomplished [26]. Similar findings have been described in patients with gastrointestinal hemorrhage [27]. The notion that restoring blood pressure in hypotensive hemorrhagic shock patients by infusing large volumes of crystalloids may dislodge clots and exacerbate bleeding is supported by animal studies [28]. Accordingly, in hemorrhagic shock patients, the goal of fluid resuscitation should be to achieve an acceptable perfusion pressure (MAP 60–65 mmHg, systolic 100 mmHg; some authors have suggested a systolic goal of 70 mmHg or MAP of 50 mmHg) [26, 29, 30], and once accomplished, crystalloid infusions should be minimized until control of the bleeding is accomplished.

Patients with hypovolemic shock from other fluid losses must have careful monitoring of their electrolytes to correct perturbations in a safe and thoughtful manner. Multiple electrolyte abnormalities may be present in these patients. To avoid the devastating complication of central pontine myelinolysis, hyponatremia must not be corrected too rapidly [31].

Obstructive Shock

Obstructive shock results from an extracardiac process that mechanically obstructs either the filling or emptying of the heart. Stroke volume (SV) is diminished and cardiac output falls. Common etiologies include tension pneumothorax, cardiac tamponade, massive pulmonary embolus, and SVC syndrome. Less common causes are dissecting aortic aneurysm, severe pulmonary hypertension, and constrictive pericarditis. Relieving the obstruction of the circulation is the priority, while other therapies such as fluid administration and vasopressors are temporizing maneuvers.

The presence of diminished breath sounds, tracheal deviation, and distended neck veins in a hypotensive patient are the hallmarks of tension pneumothorax, and immediate needle decompression is indicated. These findings, in a trauma patient, require immediate tube thoracostomy. Muffled heart sounds, distended neck veins, and hypotension with good breath sounds bilaterally suggest cardiac tamponade. (Trauma will be discussed further in Chap. 24.) Immediate bedside echocardiography can demonstrate the effusion as well as tamponade physiology, allowing for immediate bedside pericardiocentesis. Patients with tamponade physiology may maintain their blood pressure through compensatory mechanisms. Jugular venous distention (JVD) may not be present in dehydrated patients until plasma volume is restored with fluid resuscitation.

Massive pulmonary embolism resulting in obstructive shock is a most challenging clinical situation. (Massive PE will be discussed further in Chap. 7.) Historical features suggesting the risk for venous thromboembolic disease (malignancy, travel, recent surgery, etc.) combined with symptoms such as pleuritic chest pain and dyspnea suggest the diagnosis. Syncope may be the only presenting complaint, especially among the elderly. Hypotension, tachycardia, distended neck veins, clear lung fields, and hypoxemia should result in emergent echocardiography. Right ventricular distention with shift of the interventricular septum to the left is diagnostic. Relieving the right ventricular outflow tract obstruction by reducing clot burden is imperative, but exactly how to do that remains controversial [32]. Surgical thrombectomy, catheter retrieval, and local or systemic thrombolysis with or without the use of venoarterial ECMO are techniques that are available in many centers. Maintaining right ventricular perfusion can be accomplished with the liberal use of norepinephrine while avoiding overzealous fluid resuscitation that may exacerbate the over distention of the right ventricle, further compromising left ventricular filling. Intubation may be necessary in these patients, but induction hypotension may impair RV perfusion, and positive-pressure ventilation can increase pulmonary vascular resistance and reduce preload. Accordingly, in patients unstable enough to require intubation, plans for emergent mechanical or pharmacologic embolectomy should be initiated. Central line placement in these patients should anticipate the subsequent need for systemic thrombolysis and/or anticoagulation and should, therefore, be carefully placed by the most experienced operator under ultrasound guidance [32].

In its most advanced stages, obstructive shock may present as a pulseless electrical activity (PEA) cardiac arrest. Accordingly, in patients with PEA arrests, causes of obstructive shock must be sought and treated. Aspiration of as little as 30 mL of pericardial fluid may restore the circulation in patients arresting from tamponade, while a simple needle thoracostomy may do so in patients in PEA arrest from tension pneumothorax.

Cardiogenic Shock

Cardiogenic shock most commonly results from acute myocardial infarction (AMI). When 30–40% of the left ventricular muscle mass is infarcted, the patient may develop cardiogenic shock. This can occur from a single episode or a after a number of smaller infarcts (ischemic cardiomyopathy). The best treatment for cardiogenic shock resulting from AMI is to prevent it by minimizing infarct size through aggressive early intervention. Dramatic progress has been made in this regard by the institution of STEMI alert protocols with reduced door to balloon times [33–36]. (AMI will be discussed further in Chap. 8.) Nonischemic cardiomyopathies (postpartum, viral, infiltrative, etc.) less commonly cause cardiogenic shock. Mechanical causes of cardiogenic shock include acute valvular dysfunction, ventricular septal defects, ruptured ventricular free wall, and blunt cardiac injury. Acute valvular dysfunction can result from slowly progressive syndromes, such as aortic or mitral stenosis, or from abrupt processes, such as severe mitral or tricuspid regurgitation from papillary muscle rupture, or endocarditis. These syndromes are typically associated with characteristic murmurs. Bedside echocardiography is diagnostic and emergent surgical correction is required.

Patients in cardiogenic shock are typically hypotensive and vasoconstricted, cold and clammy, with jugular venous distention (JVD) and pulmonary edema. A subset of patients in cardiogenic shock may be hypovolemic for a variety of reasons. Extravasation of fluid from the vascular space into the pulmonary interstitium (pulmonary edema fluid) may occur as left-sided pressures abruptly increase due to ischemia. Patients may continue to have taken diuretic medications while having been anorexic from ischemia leading up to the event. Accordingly, a modest fluid challenge is warranted in hypotensive AMI patients [37, 38]. Maintaining coronary perfusion pressure is imperative in caring for cardiogenic shock patients, resulting from AMI. Diseased coronary arteries cannot autoregulate, so coronary perfusion is dependent on diastolic pressure. Norepinephrine is the catecholamine agent of choice because it increases blood pressure with less increase in heart rate than agents with more balanced alpha and beta effects (dopamine, epinephrine). Mechanical support with an intra-aortic balloon pump can sustain patients while they await emergent revascularization. Coronary artery bypass surgery has been shown to result in better survival rates than angioplasty in this setting [39]. (CHF and cardiogenic shock will be discussed further in Chap. 12.)

In contradistinction to patients with left ventricular infarcts, patients with right ventricular (RV) infarcts have JVD but clear lungs, and hypotension resulting from decreased left ventricular filling. The electrocardiogram is helpful in evaluating these patients. RV infarcts are most commonly seen in patients with inferior wall MIs. Right-sided chest leads can confirm the diagnosis.

Severe brady or tachydysrhythmias can result in very low cardiac output, mimicking cardiogenic shock. Rapid treatment with transcutaneous electrical pacing, cardioversion, or pharmacotherapy can restore perfusion. (Dysrhythmias will be discussed further in Chap. 9.)

Distributive Shock

Distributive shock is caused by systemic vasodilation, which decreases venous return and preload. In septic shock, vasodilation is often accompanied by leaking capillary membranes, which produces intravascular volume depletion and further decreases preload. Sepsis is the predominant cause of distributive shock. All infective agents can cause the syndrome, but gram-negative and gram-positive bacteria are the predominant pathogens. Distributive shock can also be caused by anaphylaxis, high spinal cord trauma, adrenal insufficiency, and the systemic immune response syndrome (SIRS), resulting from major burns, pancreatitis, or polytrauma.

Distributive shock is typically associated with a compensatory elevation in cardiac output, but this hyperdynamic state requires that intravascular volume be maintained. In severely hypovolemic patients, cardiac output is decreased and resultant vasoconstriction can make them clinically indistinguishable from cardiogenic shock patients. Because capillary leak occurs, patients may have decreased intravascular volume and excessive interstitial fluid (edema). Inflammatory mediators associated with sepsis often produce myocardial depression. Accordingly, patients with distributive shock may have low, normal, or high cardiac output, depending on the interaction among these multiple factors. When cardiac output is high, preferential perfusion of the skin resulting from vasodilation results in these patients typically having warm pink skin ("warm shock"). Patients with neurogenic shock may have inappropriately normal HR or frank bradycardia due to loss of sympathetic cardiac stimulation.

Clinical Assessment

Patients in circulatory shock may demonstrate a variety of vital sign abnormalities. Febrile patients in shock are likely to be septic and should be evaluated carefully for the source of infection. Septic patients may present with hypothermia (<95° F). Noninfectious sources of fever include pulmonary embolism, pancreatitis, and other causes of SIRS.

Bradycardia (typically HR <50) may result in low cardiac output and poor perfusion. Tachycardia may be present as a compensatory mechanism in patients with hypovolemic, distributive, or obstructive shock. Tachydysrhythmias may also result in low cardiac output because ventricular filling is compromised at very rapid heart rates. The clinician must determine if the tachycardia is the primary problem or a compensatory mechanism. Elderly patients frequently present in atrial fibrillation with rapid ventricular response under conditions in which younger patients would have sinus tachycardia. Many patients, especially the elderly, who may have chronotropic incompetence from heart disease, and those who take beta-blockers, calcium-channel blockers, or other medications that limit increases in heart rate may have inappropriately normal heart rates in the face of circulatory shock.

Tachypnea may be the earliest manifestation of sepsis and the most sensitive vital sign abnormality among patients in shock. Sadly, respiratory rate is the one vital sign most likely to be charted incorrectly among hospitalized patients. Normal respiratory rate is 12–16 breaths per minute in adults. Breaths should be counted for a minimum of 30 seconds and reported accurately. Respiratory alkalosis may be an early sign of sepsis, poisoning (Aspirin), and encephalopathy. Tachypnea is an important marker of metabolic acidosis in shock, and $ETCO_2$ measurement may assist in defining the presence of compensatory respiratory alkalosis (low $ETCO_2$). Profound tachypnea with its associated increased work of breathing may also be a source of increased metabolic demands. This has led to the approach of early intubation with controlled mechanical ventilation in shock patients suffering from concurrent respiratory compromise. Reducing the work of breathing can improve systemic perfusion in these patients. Patients with primary pulmonary pathology (pneumonia, pulmonary embolism, COPD exacerbations, asthma, etc.) may, of course, also be tachypneic in the absence of shock. Accordingly, tachypnea is a very sensitive but nonspecific marker of shock.

Low oxygen saturation as measured by pulse oximetry may indicate a pulmonary etiology of shock, such as pneumothorax, pneumonia, or pulmonary embolus. Poor perfusion especially in the cold, vasoconstricted patient in shock or on vasopressors may result in the inability to achieve an adequate pulse oximetry waveform and yield falsely low values. Under these circumstances, arterial blood gas sampling is required.

Physical Examination

Physical examination can provide important clues to the presence of and etiology of shock states. Mild confusion may be an early warning sign of impaired cerebral perfusion. Elderly patients presenting with even subtle mental status changes from baseline should be evaluated for a potential source of infection. Significant shock may be associated with more profound mental status changes, progressing from confusion to delirium to obtundation.

Oliguria (defined as urine output less than 0.5 mg/kg/h) indicates impaired renal perfusion from either intravascular volume depletion, low cardiac output, or shunting of renal blood flow to other vital organs. Urine output is an important monitor of the success of therapeutic interventions and should be monitored closely in all shock patients.

Vasoconstricted patients with cool, clammy, sometimes cyanotic skin often have low cardiac output and increased SVR; vasodilated patients with low SVR (as in distributive shock) may have warm skin. Skin examination should look for evidence of cutaneous abscess, infected joints, decubitus ulcers, and cutaneous signs of endocarditis. Weak or absent pulses indicate poor perfusion.

Auscultation of the heart and lungs may reveal signs of tension pneumothorax (decreased or absent breath sounds unilaterally), pneumonia (crackles), pericardial effusion/tamponade (muffled heart sounds, rubs), heart failure (lung crackles, gallops), or valvular dysfunction (murmurs). Pulmonary edema should raise concern for a cardiogenic cause of shock. Tracheal deviation is a cardinal finding in tension pneumothorax. JVD may be seen in obstructive and cardiogenic shock, while flat neck veins may be present in distributive or hypovolemic shock.

Abdominal and pelvic examinations are crucial in the assessment of shock patients, although the presence of shock may result in less obvious findings than in normally perfused patients. A tender or rigid abdomen indicates the likelihood of a surgical emergency. Bowel perforations, volvulus, intra-abdominal abscesses, appendicitis, ruptured diverticulitis, and pancreatitis may all present this way. Vascular problems, such as ruptured or leaking AAA, or intestinal ischemia must be considered. A rectal examination looking for frank or occult blood should be performed if gastrointestinal bleeding is suspected. Intra-abdominal bleeding from ruptured ectopic pregnancy or retroperitoneal bleeding must be considered in hemorrhagic shock patients without other sources such as gastrointestinal bleeding. Urogenital sources of infection (UTI, gynecologic, Fournier's gangrene, perirectal abscess) should be sought.

In patients with trauma in whom hemorrhagic shock is suspected, careful attention should be paid to abdominal, thoracic, pelvic, and extremity sources of bleeding, as well as hemorrhage from open wounds. Signs of cervical or thoracic spinal trauma may indicate neurogenic shock. (Head and Spinal Cord Injuries will be discussed further in Chap. 23.)

Diagnostic Testing

Laboratory testing routinely includes serum electrolytes, renal function testing, complete blood count, troponin, liver function tests, coagulation profile, and urinalysis. D-dimer may be measured in patients with suspected venous thromboembolism. Amylase and/or lipase should be measured in patients with a suspected intra-abdominal source of infection. Cultures of blood and urine should be obtained in cases of suspected sepsis. Measurements of arterial blood gases provide critical information about oxygenation and acid–base status as well as the presence or absence of carboxyhemoglobin or methemoglobin. Point of care testing that enables very rapid results at the bedside is extraordinarily helpful to the emergency physician when confronted with a critically ill patient. Blood gases, lactate, troponin, sodium, potassium, glucose, and beta HCG are among the most useful available point of care tests.

In critically ill patients, diagnostic imaging should be used liberally. CT scanning of the head, thorax, abdomen, and pelvis has become essential in evaluating critically ill patients, and concerns regarding radiation exposure should not preclude the use of this technology in these patients. The decision of how and when to transport patients away from a resuscitation area for imaging and who should accompany the patient are critical decisions that need to be made by a seasoned clinician in conjunction with nurses and respiratory therapists. Whenever possible, imaging that can be performed at the bedside in the resuscitation area, such as portable x-rays and ultrasound, should be the first option.

Increasingly, bedside ultrasound can assist in the rapid diagnosis of causes of shock; this may be especially useful in patients who are too unstable for other types of imaging:

- FAST: Identify pneumothorax, traumatic cardiac tamponade, and intra-abdominal fluid (which may represent hemorrhage).
- Abdominal/pelvic ultrasound: Recognition of AAA, intraperitoneal/retroperitoneal hemorrhage, ectopic pregnancy.
- Cardiac ultrasound: Identify pericardial effusion and tamponade physiology, estimate preload via IVC measurement, estimate ventricle size and cardiac output, identify RV dilatation associated with massive PE. (Ultrasound will be discussed further in Chap. 35.)

Initial Stabilization

After establishing the ABCs, initial stabilization of the patient suspected to be in shock must proceed rapidly, with the emergency physician orchestrating the priorities in the sequencing of multiple pressing imperatives. While the physical examination primary survey is being conducted, adequate peripheral venous access, electrocardiographic monitoring, noninvasive blood pressure monitoring, and pulse oximetry should be established before bedside chest radiography and 12-lead EKG are attempted. Immediate life threats identified in the primary survey are addressed as they are discovered (i.e., applying pressure to bleeding wounds, tube thoracostomy in tension pneumothorax). As data become available, specific therapies may be initiated, such as emergent cardiac catheterization in STEMI patient or intramuscular epinephrine injection in anaphylactic patients (wheezing, hives, hypotension).

Intravascular Volume Resuscitation

Fluid resuscitation is the mainstay of treatment for most patients in circulatory shock. Fluid resuscitation expands intravascular volume, increases venous return to the heart, and thereby increases preload, resulting in increased stroke volume and cardiac output. This results in increased oxygen delivery, which in hypoperfused (shock) patients will increase oxygen delivery and begin to reverse lactic acidosis (Fig. 1.9). The amount of fluid required varies with the type of shock and individual patient. Patients in septic shock and other forms of distributive shock generally require large volumes of resuscitative fluids. Hemorrhagic shock patients need blood products and should not receive large volumes of asanguineous fluids. Patients in nonhemorrhagic, hypovolemic shock may need substantial fluid resuscitation, but the amounts needed vary considerably from patient to patient, making careful monitoring imperative. Patients with AMI and hypotension, even with pulmonary edema, may benefit from judicious fluid challenge. Patients with obstructive shock should receive emergent mechanical intervention and, generally, should not receive large volumes of resuscitative fluids.

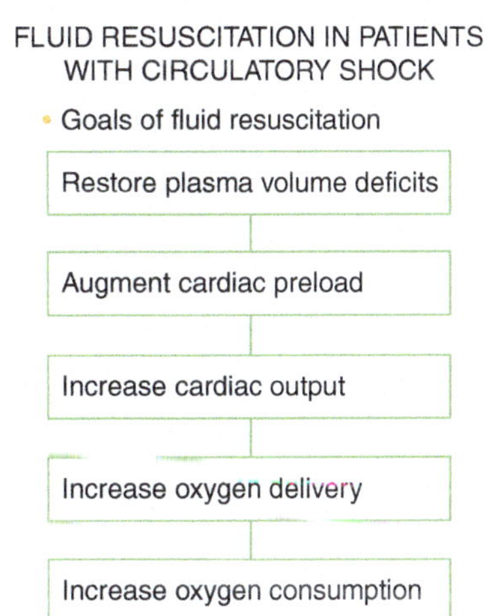

Fig. 1.9 5% dextrose in water (D5W), normal saline (NS), lactated Ringer's solution (LR), albumin (ALB), hydroxyethyl starch (HES), hypertonic saline (HYPER). The figure depicts the impact of infusions of the various fluids on the three fluid compartments in the body

Types of Fluid

Characteristics of resuscitative fluids will determine where they are distributed within the three body compartments (intravascular, interstitial, and intracellular) after infusion into the veins (Fig. 1.10). D5W, lacking any solutes, is distributed throughout the total body water. The intracellular compartment is by far the largest of the three. Accordingly, at the end of an infusion, very little D5W remains in the vascular space. It should not be considered a resuscitative fluid and should not be used for this purpose. Crystalloid fluids, such as normal saline (NS) and lactated Ringer's solution (LR), contain solutes, which are relatively impermeable to the cell membranes. Accordingly, they are distributed only to the vascular and interstitial compartments. Because the interstitial compartment is so much larger than the vascular space, at the end of a 1-L infusion of these isotonic crystalloids, only approximately 200 mL remains in the vascular space. The remainder crosses the vascular membrane and enters the interstitial space. This is why large volume fluid resuscitation with these fluids results in edema formation, with its potential complications. Recent studies indicate that buffered, balanced solutions such as LR may be preferable to NS because NS may result in a hyperchloremic metabolic acidosis when infused in large quantities [40]. Colloid-containing fluids such as 5% albumin (ALB) and 6% hydroxyethyl starch (HES) create oncotic pressure and are retained in the vascular space for longer periods than crystalloids. Under conditions of "leaky capillaries" seen in sepsis and potentially other forms of shock, colloids may also become permeable to the vascular membranes. The starches have been associated with coagulopathies, immune suppression, and AKI with need for RRT and should no longer be used. Hypertonic saline can expand the plasma volume by pulling fluid out of the intracellular and interstitial compartments. This makes them potentially useful in head injured or burned patients where edema can be life threatening.

Although much larger volumes of crystalloid fluids are required to provide the same intravascular volume expansion compared to colloids, they appear to be equally effective, as demonstrated by several studies [41–43]. However, in the SAFE trial [44], subset analysis showed a trend toward improved mortality for septic patients treated with colloids. Enthusiasm for

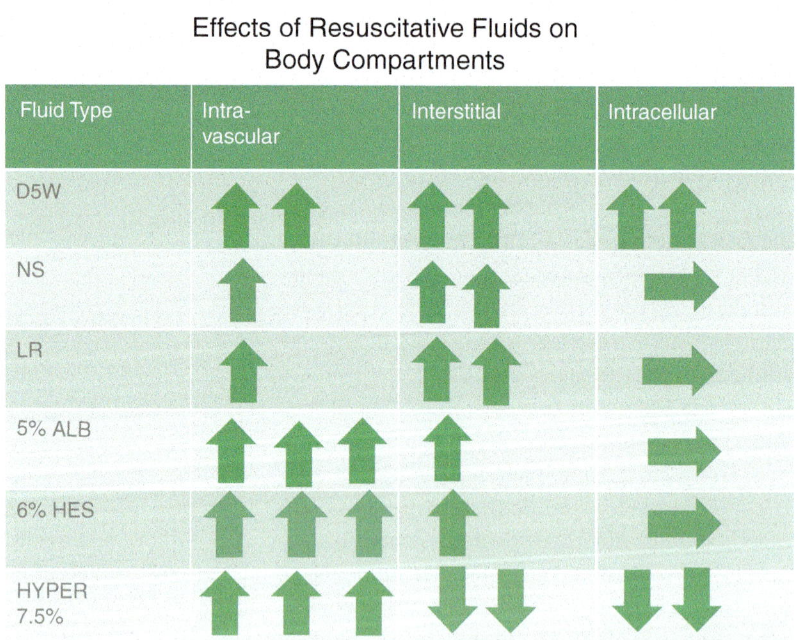

Fig. 1.10 Fluid resuscitation remains the cornerstone for increasing oxygen delivery in shock patients

colloid-containing fluids, especially 5% albumin, is re-emerging in Europe. Hypo-oncotic patients, especially those requiring surgery, are more prone to complications and death. While it has not been definitively established that albumin infusions can reverse this effect, many clinicians infuse albumin-containing fluids to maintain the serum albumin level at 3 mg/dl. Given the lack of proven mortality benefit and the increased expense of albumin, isotonic crystalloid solutions remain the recommended choice for patients in shock. The "colloid/crystalloid" debate rages on.

Goals for Fluid Resuscitation

CVP

The goal of fluid resuscitation is to restore adequate preload to optimize cardiac output (Fig. 1.9). Central venous pressure (CVP) has been used as a tool to estimate preload and guide fluid resuscitation. Multiple studies have demonstrated the lack of correlation between plasma volume and CVP [45]. Nonetheless, a target CVP of 8–12 mmHg has been recommended to optimize fluid administration in septic shock patients and is often used in patients with other types of shock. (Even higher CVPs may be necessary for patients with mechanical ventilation, especially with high PEEP.) It is reasonable to suspect that patients with very low CVP (<4) measurements need additional volume administration, and that patients with very high measurements (>20) are at risk for volume overload. It remains unclear if CVP is routinely useful in patients undergoing fluid resuscitation in shock and if a CVP in the 8–12 mmHg range indicates that further fluid administration will not further increase stroke volume and cardiac output. Additionally, CVP measurement requires placement of a subclavian or internal jugular catheter, which is not without risk.

Fluid Responsiveness

Fluid responsiveness refers to the ability of fluid resuscitation to increase stroke volume and cardiac output and, thereby, improve organ perfusion. Dynamic indices, such as radial artery pulse pressure variation and aortic blood flow peak velocity, may predict fluid responsiveness accurately, with some limitations [46]. These dynamic measurements estimate preload reserve by measuring the variability in predicted stroke volume with respiratory change or estimate stroke volume changes after fluid challenge or simulated fluid challenge by the passive leg-raising maneuver. Ultrasound examination of the vena cava and the presence of collapse during the ventilatory cycle can provide similar data [47]. There is increasing evidence that these dynamic indices are sensitive and specific predictors of fluid responsiveness; however, additional trials are needed before their routine use can be recommended in the management of patients in shock. In addition, many of these methods require a patient to be in sinus rhythm and passively mechanically ventilated, thus limiting widespread use.

Blood Products

For patients with hemorrhage, blood products are the logical choice to replace intravascular volume. In addition to volume expansion (red cells remain in the vascular space as does FFP and platelets), red blood cell transfusion provides additional oxygen-carrying capacity and supports oxygen delivery to tissues. Old banked PRBCs may not effectively carry oxygen until 2,3 DPG is regenerated, which can take many hours. Blood products may also be indicated in patients with preexisting anemia.

In hemorrhagic shock patients, initial resuscitation usually begins with crystalloid administration. For patients with large blood loss, or ongoing bleeding, or those who require more than 30 mL/kg crystalloid, immediate transfusion of packed-red blood cells is indicated. Emergency-release blood may be necessary if cross-matched blood is not yet available.

Patients who receive large amounts of transfused PRBCs are at risk for transfusion related coagulopathy that may worsen hemorrhage.

Early transfusion of FFP and platelets is increasingly recognized as an important component of blood product administration, especially in trauma patients [48, 49]. Evidence for the benefits of massive transfusion protocols, which automatically provide FFP and platelets along with PRBCs, suggests a morbidity and mortality benefit. Patients who are expected to receive >10U PRBCs in 24 hours are good candidates for massive transfusion protocols. (Blood Products will be discussed further in Chap. 33.)

Hemorrhagic shock in trauma represents a special circumstance for clinicians who seek to balance adequate perfusion and tissue oxygenation with limiting ongoing hemorrhage while awaiting operative control. There is evidence to support a strategy that limits initial volume replacement and permits some degree of hypotension (to a systolic BP of 70 mmHg) in some patients until bleeding can be controlled. One prospective trial in patients with penetrating truncal trauma demonstrated survival benefit for patients in whom fluid resuscitation was delayed [26]. Other studies have supported a similar strategy and have shown no evidence of harm associated with permissive hypotension [29, 30]. Patients with coexisting brain injury require adequate cerebral perfusion pressure and are not candidates for permissive hypotension. Results of these limited studies should not be applied to a broad population of trauma patients without further research.

Nonhemorrhagic Shock

There is conflicting evidence on the optimal transfusion threshold for patients with anemia and other (nonhemorrhagic) types of shock. In stable patients, a restrictive transfusion strategy, in which patients do not receive blood products until their hemoglobin is <7 mg/dL, was found to be superior to a more liberal transfusion strategy [50]. RBC transfusion carries risk for infection, SIRS, ARDS, and multiorgan failure and has been associated with increased complications and mortality.

Vasopressors

Vasopressors should be used in patients who cannot maintain MAP (>65) despite adequate volume resuscitation. Norepinephrine has emerged as the vasopressor of choice for the treatment of undifferentiated shock and septic shock patients [51]. (Vasopressors will be discussed further in Chap. 32.)

Norepinephrine acts on alpha-1 and beta-1 receptors, producing potent vasoconstriction and a modest increase in cardiac output. Its vasoconstrictor effect on venous capacitance vessels has the added benefit of moving volume into the active circulation from the venous capacitance bed that ordinarily houses 85% of the circulating blood volume. The chronotropic effect created by beta-1 stimulation is usually modest and may be offset by the reflex bradycardia that occurs in response to increased MAP. Compared to other vasopressor agents such as dopamine and epinephrine, its beta effects are far less prominent. Accordingly, perfusion pressure is improved without the deleterious effects of tachycardia and arrhythmia. Under circumstances in which further increases in cardiac output are required after blood pressure is restored by adequate fluid loading and norepinephrine, an inotropic agent such as dobutamine or milrinone may be added. Because these agents are inotropic vasodilators, careful monitoring of blood pressure is required to be sure that they do not produce hypotension. Under these circumstances, epinephrine alone or added, in small doses, to norepinephrine may accomplish the goals of maintaining perfusion pressure and enhancing contractility. The cost is in increased myocardial oxygen demand and the potential for ischemia.

The physiologic effects of dopamine depend on the dose at which it is administered: at 1–2 mcg/kg/min, it stimulates primarily renal dopamine-1 receptors; at 2–5 mcg/kg/min, it stimulates beta-1 receptors, increasing cardiac output by increasing primarily stroke volume and to a lesser degree, heart rate. At 5–10 mcg/kg/min, it stimulates alpha-1 receptors and produces vasoconstriction and increased SVR. Use of dopamine is primarily limited by the risk for tachycardia and arrhythmia. The ability of low-dose dopamine to convert oliguric renal failure into nonoliguric renal failure has been debunked [52].

Phenylephrine is a purely alpha-adrenergic agent that increases SVR and produces direct vasoconstriction. Reflex bradycardia is common. It is often a second-line agent after norepinephrine. It is available in prefilled syringes and can be given in small bolus doses in critical, time-sensitive situations while preparing a norepinephrine drip [53].

Epinephrine is a potent beta-1 agonist with moderate beta-2 and alpha-1 effects, producing increased inotropy and chronotropy and increased cardiac output. At high doses, predominately alpha-1 effects produce increased SVR. Epinephrine is the preferred agent in anaphylactic shock. Disadvantages include increased splanchnic vasoconstriction and risk for arrhythmia.

Cardiogenic Shock

Norepinephrine is the preferred vasopressor for treating patients in cardiogenic shock with profound hypotension [54]. However, these patients have low cardiac output and intrinsically elevated SVR: Further increases in afterload may limit improvement in cardiac output. This effect may be ameliorated by the concurrent increase in coronary perfusion pressure. Agents with beta-adrenergic activity provide inotropic (and often chronotropic) effects that increase cardiac output; however, this is not desirable in patients with acute ischemia as it increases myocardial work and myocardial oxygen demand. Accordingly, norepinephrine is the first-line agent for patients with severe hypotension to maintain coronary perfusion pressure while arranging for mechanical support and /or revascularization.

Septic Shock

There is evidence to support norepinephrine as the first-line vasopressor in septic shock. In meta-analyses comparing dopamine and norepinephrine in patients with septic shock, increased mortality was seen with dopamine, along with a twofold increase in arrhythmia [55]. Vasopressin may be beneficial when added to norepinephrine or other agents. Some patients with septic shock have myocardial depression and diminished cardiac output: dobutamine may restore cardiac output and improve tissue perfusion and oxygen delivery. Dobutamine may cause peripheral vasodilatation and decreased blood pressure and should be used cautiously. Inotropic therapy is controversial for septic shock patients without clear evidence of myocardial depression. It was used successfully as part of the EGDT algorithm of Rivers et al. [11] when employed in the face of continued evidence of tissue hypoxia after fluids, blood, and vasopressors. More recent trials failed to show mortality benefit to its use in similar, though less critically ill, septic shock patients [56, 57].

Airway Management

Most therapies for shock focus on increasing oxygen delivery to eliminate oxygen debt and anaerobic metabolism. However, many patients in shock have increased work of breathing. Respiratory muscle use can account for significant oxygen consumption, and under these circumstances, perfusion to the diaphragm and other respiratory muscles can rob nutrient flow from other vital organs. Intubation and passive mechanical ventilation (controlled mandatory ventilation) to decrease respiratory muscle work can reduce oxygen demand and improve oxygen debt. Positive-pressure ventilation decreases venous return to the heart. In hypovolemic patients, hypotension and cardiovascular collapse can occur. Appropriate fluid resuscitation prior to intubation can avert this. A low-tidal volume ventilation strategy is recommended for patients in shock with ARDS [58, 59].

Protocol-Directed Therapy

Protocols that combine various physiologic endpoints to guide resuscitation in patients with septic shock have been previously recommended and are commonly used as part of bundled therapy for sepsis. Typically, CVP, MAP, $ScVO_2$, and sometimes UOP and lactate are stepwise targets for fluids and vasoactive agents. Two recent trials were unable to demonstrate a mortality difference between protocolized and standard emergency department care in septic patients [56, 57]. However, in all of the patients, early recognition, attention to adequate volume resuscitation (2 L prior to study entry), and restoration of mean arterial pressure were accomplished. Early antibiotic administration, a most important aspect of care in this group of patients, was also accomplished. The authors did question the need for the routine use of central venous pressure monitoring, $SCVO_2$ monitoring, or ongoing monitoring of lactate. It seems clear that the most important issue is that the physicians directing the care of these patients have a firm understanding of the pathophysiology and current concepts of resuscitation and understand how to monitor the progress of the resuscitative efforts.

References

1. Weil MH, Maafifi AA. Experimental and clinical studies on lactate and pyruvate as indicators of the severity of acute circulatory failure (shock). Circulation. 1970;41:989–1001.
2. Puskarich MA, Trzeciak S, Shapiro NI, Heffner AC, Kline JA, Jones AE, Emergency Medicine Shock Research Network (EMSHOCKNET). Outcomes of patients undergoing early sepsis resuscitation for cryptic shock compared with overt shock. Resuscitation. 2011;82:1289–93.
3. Vorwerk C, Florence L, Gray L, Goss C, Fudge T, Coats TJ. Hypotension on arrival in the emergency department: a predictor of in-hospital mortality. Ann Emerg Med. 2008;51:476.
4. Cohn JN. Blood pressure measurement in shock. JAMA. 1967;199:118–22.
5. Low RB, Martin D. Accuracy of blood pressure measurements made aboard helicopters. Ann Emerg Med. 1988;17:604–12.
6. Dellinger RP, Levy MM, Rhodes A, Annane D, Gerlach H, Opal SM, et al. Surviving Sepsis Campaign: international guidelines for management of severe sepsis and septic shock, 2012. Intensive Care Med. 2013;39(2):165–228.
7. Broder G, Weil MG. Excess Lactate: an index of reversibility of shock in human patients. Science. 1964;43:1457. Weil MH, Afifi AA. Experimental and clinical studies on lactate and pyruvate as indicators of the severity of acute circulatory failure. Circulation. 1970;61:989–1002.
8. Nichol AD, Egi M, Pettila V, Bellomo R, French C, Hart G, et al. Relative hyperlactatemia and hospital mortality in critically ill patients: a retrospective multi-centre study. Crit Care. 2010;14:R25.
9. Shapiro NI, Howell MD, Talmor D, Nathanson LA, Lisbon A, Wolfe RE, et al. Serum lactate as a predictor of mortality in emergency department patients with infection. Ann Emerg Med. 2005;45:524–8.
10. Abou-Khalil B, Scalea TM, Trooskin SZ, Henry SM, Hitchcock R. Hemodynamic responses to shock in young trauma patients: need for invasive monitoring. Crit Care Med. 1994;22:633–9.
11. Rivers E, Nguyen B, Havstad S, Ressler J, Muzzin A, Knoblich B, et al. Early goal-directed therapy in the treatment of severe sepsis and septic shock. N Engl J Med. 2001;345(19):1368–77.
12. Donnino MW, Nguyen B, Jacobsen G, Tomlanovich M, Rivers E. Cryptic septic shock: a sub-analysis of early, goal-directed therapy. Chest. 2003;124(4_MeetingAbstracts):90S.
13. Casserly B, Phillips GS, Schorr C, Dellinger RP, Townsend SR, Osborn TM, et al. Lactate measurements in sepsis-induced tissue hypoperfusion: results from the surviving sepsis campaign database*. Crit Care Med. 2015;43(3):567–73.
14. Younger JG, Falk JL, Rothrock SG. Relationship between arterial and peripheral venous lactate levels. Acad Emerg Med. 1996;3:730–4.
15. Falk JL, Rackow EC, Levy JL, Astiz ME, Weil MH. Delayed lactate clearance in patients with circulatory shock. Acute Care. 1985;16:212–5.
16. Nguyen HB, Rivers EP, Knoblich BP. Early lactate clearance is associated with improved outcome in severe sepsis and septic shock. Crit Care Med. 2004;32:1637–42.
17. Fiddian-Green RG. Should measurements of tissue pH and Po_2 be included in the routine monitoring of intensive are unit patients? Crit Care Med. 1991;19:141–3.
18. Reinhart K, Rudolph T, Bredle DL, Hannemann L, Cain SM. Comparison of central-venous to mixed-venous oxygen saturation during changes in oxygen supply/demand. Chest. 1989;95(6):1216–21.
19. Jones AE, Shapiro NI, Trzeciak S, Arnold RC, Claremont HA, Kline JA, Emergency Medicine Shock Research Network (EMShockNet) Investigators. Lactate clearance vs central venous oxygen saturation as goals of early sepsis therapy: a randomized clinical trial. JAMA. 2010;303:739–46.
20. Katz SH, Falk JL. Misplaced endotracheal tubes by paramedics in an urban EMS system. Ann Emerg Med. 2001;37:32–7.
21. Silvestri S, Ralls GA, Krauss B, Thundiyil J, Rothrock SG, Senn A, et al. The effectiveness of out-of-hospital use of continuous $ETCO_2$ monitoring on the rate of unrecognized misplaced intuba-

tion within a regional EMS system. Ann Emerg Med. 2005;45:497–503.
22. Falk JL, Rackow EC, Weil MH. End-tidal carbon dioxide concentration during cardiopulmonary resuscitation. N Engl J Med. 1988;318:607–11.
23. Fearon DM, Steele DW. End-tidal carbon dioxide predicts the presence and severity of acidosis in children with diabetes. Acad Emerg Med. 2002;9:1373–8.
24. Hunter CL, Silvestri S, Dean M, Falk JL, Papa L. $ETCO_2$ is associated with mortality and lactate in patients with suspected sepsis. Am J Emerg Med. 2013;31:64–71.
25. Demetriades D, Chan LS, Bhasin P, Berne TV, Ramicone E, Huicochea F, et al. Relative bradycardia in patients with traumatic hypotension. J Trauma. 1998;45:534–9.
26. Bickell WH, Wall MJ, Pepe PE, Martin RR, Ginger VF, Allen MK, et al. Immediate versus delayed fluid resuscitation for hypotensive patients with penetrating torso injuries. N Engl J Med. 1994;331(17):1105–9.
27. Villanueva C, Colomo A, Bosch A, ConcepciÛn M, Hernandez-Gea V, Aracil C, et al. Transfusion strategies for acute upper gastrointestinal bleeding. N Engl J Med. 2013;368(1):11–21.
28. Shaftan GW, Chiu C-J, Grosz CS, Dennis C. The effect of transfusion and of certain hemodynamic factors on the spontaneous control of arterial hemorrhage. J Cardiovasc Surg (Torino). 1964;5:251–6.
29. Dutton RP, Mackenzie CF, Scalea TM. Hypotensive resuscitation during active hemorrhage: impact on in-hospital mortality. J Trauma. 2002;52(6):1141–6.
30. Morrison CA, Carrick MM, Norman MA, Scott BG, Welsh FJ, Tsai P, et al. Hypotensive resuscitation strategy reduces transfusion requirements and severe postoperative coagulopathy in trauma patients with hemorrhagic shock: preliminary results of a randomized controlled trial. J Trauma. 2011;70(3):652–63.
31. Cohen BJ, Jordan MH, Chapin SD, Cape B, Laureno R. Pontine myelinolysis after correction of hyponatremia during burn resuscitation. J Burn Care Rehabil. 1991;12:153–6.
32. Weingart S. Pulmonary embolism treatment options and the PEAC Team with Oren Freidman. EMCrit.org [Internet]. New York: EMCrit. 2014 July 14 [cited 2015 Mar 11]. Available from: http://emcrit.org/podcasts/pulmonary-embolism-treatment-team/.
33. Ohman EM, Califf RM, Topol EJ, Candela R, Abbottsmith C, Ellis S, et al. Consequences of reocclusion after successful reperfusion therapy in acute myocardial infarction. TAMI Study Group. Circulation. 1990;82:781–91.
34. GISSI (Gruppo Italiano per lo Studio della Streptochinasi nell'Infarto miocardico). Effectiveness of intravenous thrombolytic treatment in acute myocardial infarction. Lancet. 1986;i:397–401.
35. The GUSTO Angiographic Investigators. The effects of tissue plasminogen activator, streptokinase, or both on coronary-artery patency, ventricular function, and survival after acute myocardial infarction. N Engl J Med. 1993;329:1615–22. [Erratum, N Engl J Med 1994;330:516].
36. Le May MR, So DY, Dionne R, Glover CA, Froeschl MP, Wells GA, et al. A citywide protocol for primary PCI in ST-segment elevation myocardial infarction. N Engl J Med. 2008;358:231–40.
37. Figueras J, Weil MH. Hypovolemia and hypotension complicating management of acute cardiogenic pulmonary edema. Am J Cardiol. 1979;44(7):1349–55.
38. Adler C, Reuter H, Seck C, Hellmich M, Zobel C. Fluid therapy and acute kidney injury in cardiogenic shock after cardiac arrest. Resuscitation. 2013;84(2):194–9.
39. Hochman JS, Sleeper LA, Webb JG, Sanborn TA, White HD, Talley JD, et al. Early revascularization in acute myocardial infarction complicated by cardiogenic shock. SHOCK Investigators. Should we emergently revascularize occluded coronaries for cardiogenic shock. N Engl J Med. 1999;341(9):625–34.
40. Yunos NM, Bellomo R, Hegarty C, Story D, Ho L, Bailey M. Association between a chloride-liberal vs chloride-restrictive intravenous fluid administration strategy and kidney injury in critically ill adults. JAMA. 2012;308(15):1566–72.
41. Perel P, Roberts I, Ker K. Colloids versus crystalloids for fluid resuscitation in critically ill patients. Cochrane Database Syst Rev. 2013;(2):CD000567.
42. Patel A, Laffan MA, Waheed U, Brett SJ. Randomised trials of human albumin for adults with sepsis: systematic review and meta-analysis with trial sequential analysis of all-cause mortality. BMJ. 2014;349:g4561.
43. Annane D, Siami S, Jaber S, Martin C, Elatrous S, DeclÈre AD, et al. Effects of fluid resuscitation with colloids vs crystalloids on mortality in critically ill patients presenting with hypovolemic shock: the CRISTAL randomized trial. JAMA. 2013;310(17):1809–17.
44. Finfer S, Bellomo R, Boyce N, French J, Myburgh J, Norton R, et al. A comparison of albumin and saline for fluid resuscitation in the intensive care unit. N Engl J Med. 2004;350(22):2247–56.
45. Marik PE, Baram M, Vahid B. Does central venous pressure predict fluid responsiveness? A systematic review of the literature and the tale of seven mares. Chest. 2008;134(1):172–8.
46. Marik PE, Cavallazzi R, Vasu T, Hirani A. Dynamic changes in arterial waveform derived variables and fluid responsiveness in mechanically ventilated patients: a systematic review of the literature. Crit Care Med. 2009;37(9):2642–7.
47. Feissel M, Michard F, Faller JP, Teboul JL. The respiratory variation in inferior vena cava diameter as a guide to fluid therapy. Intensive Care Med. 2004;30(9):1834–7.
48. Johansson PI, Oliveri RS, Ostrowski SR. Hemostatic resuscitation with plasma and platelets in trauma. J Emerg Trauma Shock. 2012;5(2):120–5.
49. Holcomb JB, Wade CE, Michalek JE, Chisholm GB, Zarzabal LA, Schreiber MA, et al. Increased plasma and platelet to red blood cell ratios improves outcome

in 466 massively transfused civilian trauma patients. Ann Surg. 2008;248(3):447–58.
50. HÈbert PC, Wells G, Blajchman MA, Marshall J, Martin C, Pagliarello G, et al. A multicenter, randomized, controlled clinical trial of transfusion requirements in critical care. Transfusion Requirements in Critical Care Investigators, Canadian Critical Care Trials Group. N Engl J Med. 1999;340(6):409–17.
51. Hollenberg SM. Vasoactive drugs in circulatory shock. Am J Respir Crit Care Med. 2011;183(7):847–55. Kellum JA, Pinsky MR. Use of vasopressor agents in critically ill patients. Curr Opin Crit Care. 2002;8(3):236–41.
52. Bellomo R, Chapman M, Finfer S, Hickling K, Myburgh J. Low-dose dopamine in patients with early renal dysfunction: a placebo-controlled randomised trial. Australian and New Zealand Intensive Care Society (ANZICS) Clinical Trials Group. Lancet. 2000;356(9248):2139–43.
53. Weingart S. EMCrit.org [Internet]. New York: EMCrit. 2009 July 10 [cited 2015 Mar 22]. Available from: http://emcrit.org/podcasts/bolus-dose-pressors/.
54. De Backer D, Biston P, Devriendt J, Madl C, Chochrad D, Aldecoa C, et al. Comparison of dopamine and norepinephrine in the treatment of shock. N Engl J Med. 2010;362(9):779–89.
55. De Backer D, Aldecoa C, Njimi H, Vincent JL. Dopamine versus norepinephrine in the treatment of septic shock: a meta-analysis*. Crit Care Med. 2012;40(3):725–30.
56. Yealy DM, Kellum JA, Huang DT, Barnato AE, Weissfeld LA, Pike F, et al. A randomized trial of protocol-based care for early septic shock. N Engl J Med. 2014;370(18):1683–93.
57. Peake SL, Delaney A, Bailey M, Bellomo R, Cameron PA, Cooper DJ, et al. Goal-directed resuscitation for patients with early septic shock. N Engl J Med. 2014;371(16):1496–506.
58. Putensen C, Theuerkauf N, Zinserling J, Wrigge H, Pelosi P. Meta-analysis: ventilation strategies and outcomes of the acute respiratory distress syndrome and acute lung injury. Ann Intern Med. 2009;151(8):566–76.
59. Petrucci N, De Feo C. Lung protective ventilation strategy for the acute respiratory distress syndrome. Cochrane Database Syst Rev. 2013;(2):CD003844.
60. Falk JL, Rackow EC, Astiz M, Weil MH. Fluid resuscitation in shock. J Cardiothorac Anesth. 1988;2(6):33–8. https://doi.org/10.1016/s0888-6296(88)80006-1.

Airway Management

2

John P. Gaillard

Critical Points

- Perform an airway examination that includes a history of any difficulty and a physical examination.
- Decide on the following: awake versus asleep, spontaneously breathing or paralyzed, direct or video (including flexible fiberoptic) laryngoscopy.
- Have the appropriate basic and advanced airway equipment available.
- Have a sedative, a muscle relaxant, and a vasopressor medication available.
- Develop an initial plan and backup plans before proceeding.
- Take a timeout prior to the procedure to ensure everyone understands the procedure.
- The primary goal is to maintain oxygenation. Putting a tube in the trachea is a secondary goal.

Introduction

Airway management (AM) is one of the most high-risk procedures in medicine. If done poorly, patients suffer significant morbidity and mortality. Patients undergoing emergent AM are at a higher risk and complexity due to the urgent nature and impending threat to life. The incidence of a difficult airway is much higher when AM occurs out of the operating room (OR) [1]. The incidence of adverse events, complications, and surgical airways is higher for out of OR AM [2–4]. For these reasons, it is crucial to be skilled in all facets of AM. It is not acceptable to begin managing a patient's airway, only to come to a point at which the patient is not being oxygenated and the clinician is beyond his or her capabilities. For the purposes of this chapter, AM will be discussed in terms of urgent or emergent airway manipulation in critically ill patients in the ED or ICU.

Whenever dealing with AM, it is important to try to identify a potentially difficult airway. A difficult airway has no one specific identifying feature. In the American Society of Anesthesiologists (ASA) Practice Guidelines, a difficult airway is defined "as the clinical situation in which a conventionally trained anesthesiologist experiences difficulty with facemask ventilation of the upper airway, difficulty with tracheal intubation, or both" [5]. In clinical practice, a difficult airway may be classified as one in which there is

J. P. Gaillard (✉)
Anesthesiology-Critical Care, Emergency Medicine, Internal Medicine-Pulmonary/Critical Care, Wake Forest Baptist Health, Winston-Salem, NC, USA
e-mail: jgaillar@wakehealth.edu

© Springer Nature Switzerland AG 2020

J. R. Shiber, S. D. Weingart (eds.), *Emergency Department Critical Care*,
https://doi.org/10.1007/978-3-030-28794-8_2

difficulty with the bag valve mask (BVM), laryngoscopy (either direct (DL) or video (VL)), placing a supraglottic airway device (SGA), or obtaining a surgical airway.

Airway Management Plan

Indications

The three main indications for taking over a patient's airway are: (1) The patient is not able to oxygenate. (2) The patient is not able to ventilate. (3) The patient is not able to protect his or her airway. While these indications are most often cited as the need for AM, there are other indications for securing a patient's airway specifically in emergent situations.

If the patient is unable to tolerate or cooperate for a necessary medical evaluation and treatment, then AM may be indicated. Emergency physicians are familiar with this indication, as a significant number of patients present with an altered mental status due to intoxicants. It may be quite difficult to properly evaluate and treat these patients without using sedating medicines. If these medicines do not work or the patient is a danger to himself or herself or staff members, the only other option may be to heavily sedate the patient and secure the patient's airway.

The anticipated clinical course is another indication for taking over a patient's airway. This indication is more subjective and has more to do with the clinician's gestalt. If a patient is critically ill and his or her condition is likely to deteriorate, then it is advisable to secure the patient's airway. Similar to this indication, AM is indicated whenever a clinician feels that the patient's condition warrants it. If the clinician feels that AM is indicated and is in the patient's best interest, then there should not be any second guessing from other clinicians who are not providing bedside patient's care at that time.

Algorithms

The Anesthesiology Society of America had produced guidelines and an algorithm for difficult airway management for the better part of the last 20 years. The latest version of the guidelines was written by a group of 10 anesthesiologists and 2 methodologists. As the authors state, the guidelines are not meant to be the gold standard. The guidelines do not represent requirements or standards and should be modified or rejected according to the bedside clinician's needs [5].

When approaching AM, it is important for the clinician to develop a treatment algorithm that includes every step along the way until a definitive airway is placed. While there are several algorithms that have been developed by different groups with an interest in airways [5, 6], the bedside clinician should develop an algorithm specific to each patient.

There are several questions that the clinician must answer prior to performing AM on a patient. Each question is a potential branch point in a personalized AM algorithm. Should the patient be awake or asleep? Should the patient be given a muscle relaxant or remain breathing spontaneously? What should be done if there is difficulty with mask ventilation? What should be done if there is difficulty with laryngoscopy? Should DL or VL be the primary mode of laryngoscopy? Should fiberoptic intubation be utilized?

The answer to each of these questions depends on the individual patient and the circumstances for which the patient is being intubated. When the clinician has answered all of these questions, he or she can confidently manage a patient's airway.

Predictors of Difficult Airways

The incidence of a difficult airway in the ED or ICU is not truly known because the incidence of difficulty with mask ventilation or with intubation or both is not truly known. There are several findings associated with a difficult airway, but the discriminatory power of these findings is moderate at best [7]. Because the vast majority of patients are critically ill, the need to place an airway is usually urgent or emergent, which increases the risk and difficulty [8]. There are many different mnemonics that have been developed in an effort to help simplify ways to predict a difficult airway. Evidence is lacking as to whether or not these mnemonics improve outcome [9]. Despite this lack of evidence, it is important to review the different markers of a potentially difficult airway. See Tables 2.1, 2.2, and 2.3 for different findings associated with a difficult airway. Since any AM procedure has the potential to be difficult, it is better to be overcautious than under cautious.

Table 2.1 Conditions associated with difficult intubations due to distortion of neck anatomy

Conditions associated with distortions of neck anatomy	
Cervical collar	Obstructive sleep apnea
Congenital abnormalities	Previous radiation
Foreign bodies	Previous surgery
Infections	Scoliosis
Halo cervical immobilization device	Short neck
Hematoma	Thick neck
Kyphosis	Trauma, including burns
Obesity	Tumors

Table 2.2 Physical findings associated with difficult intubations

Physical attributes associated with difficult airways	
Age 40–60	Mallampati class 3 or 4
Cervical collar or limited neck mobility	Mouth opening (<4 cm)
Facial fractures	Prominent upper incisors
Halo traction device	Receding jaw
Kyphosis	Short neck
Large tongue	Thick neck
Angioedema of lips, tongue, pharynx	Thyromental distance <6 cm

Table 2.3 Medical conditions that are commonly directly associated with difficult intubations

Medical conditions directly associated with difficult airways	
Anaphylaxis	Facial trauma
Ankylosing spondylitis	Foreign body
Angioedema	Obesity
Bleeding abnormalities	Obstructive sleep apnea or snoring
Cerebrovascular accident	Pregnancy
Congenital abnormalities	Radiation therapy
Croup	Rheumatoid arthritis
Diabetes	Actively having a seizure
Down syndrome	Tetanus
Epiglottitis	Previous oral or neck surgery

Awake Versus Asleep

Most intensivists and EM physicians are more comfortable sedating a patient completely for AM. A total sedative is not indicated in all patients. Recall that it is possible to completely anesthetize the airway and keep the patient awake. Awake AM may be indicated in patients who have multiple findings of a potential difficult airway. The ability to maintain oxygenation while setting up for an awake intubation may pose a challenge, but this challenge can often be overcome with noninvasive positive-pressure ventilation (NIPPV) and a mild sedative [10].

Use of Muscle Relaxants

The use of a total sedating medication in addition to a muscle relaxant will often permit the best chances for success [11]. That being said, if a clinician is going to paralyze a patient as part of his or her AM plan, then the clinician must be willing and able to perform a surgical airway. Giving a patient a paralytic medication to facilitate AM is not always indicated. If the risk of giving a paralytic to a patient is greater than the benefit of having the patient paralyzed, then a paralytic should not be used. This point is specifically for the patient that has multiple findings of a predicted difficult airway and limited resources for the bedside clinician. If the clinician does not feel that the patient could be adequately oxygenated with mask ventilation or SGA, then a paralytic should not be used.

The process of rapid sequence intubation (RSI) is commonly used in the ED because of the concern for patients being nonfasted. In RSI, the patient is given a dose of a sedative medication, which is immediately followed by a paralytic agent. Oxygen is maintained on the patient, but no attempts are made to provide mask ventilation. When the patient has become apneic, the patient is intubated. RSI is useful in the ED for several reasons [12]. By paralyzing the patient, optimal intubating conditions are achieved. The patient's gag reflex and ability to cough are taken away. The vocal cords are also paralyzed, which makes placing an endotracheal tube (ETT) into the trachea much easier.

There are times in which paralyzing a patient may be contraindicated. In these situations, the provider may elect to only sedate the patient, also known as facilitated intubation. In these cases, it has been demonstrated that providers have more difficulty, worse visualization of the glottic structures, and lower rates of successfully placing an ETT into the trachea [13].

Delayed sequence intubation (DSI) is another process by which patients may be intubated with the use of paralytics. DSI is a method of improving preoxygenation in agitated patients suffering from hypoxia-induced delirium. Patients who are uncooperative and not able to be adequately preoxygenated are good candidates for DSI. These patients are first given a sedative that will not affect spontaneous breathing or impair the airway reflexes. The patients are then oxygenated with 100% FiO_2 via non-rebreather mask or NIPPV. After a period of appropriate preoxygenation, a paralytic agent is administered [14]. After muscle relaxation, the patient is intubated.

Direct or Video Laryngoscopy

Direct laryngoscopy has been the main method of AM for decades. Drs. Miller and MacIntosh developed their respective blades in the 1940s, and the designs have changed little over the years. DL is the standard method for placing an ETT. That being said, many clinicians are moving to using VL for all AM. Each method has its drawbacks. It is important to realize that one method will not work for every situation, and clinicians should be proficient at both methods. DL specifically is a learned skill that must be continuously practiced or the skill will vanish.

Patient Preparation

Patient preparation is integral to any AM procedure. With adequate preparation, one is able to maximize the chances for success and minimize the risk to the patient. There are several steps that go into fully preparing for taking over a patient's airway, and each step should be completed whenever time allows.

The patient needs to have all appropriate monitors in place and be properly positioned. Depending on the airway examination, positioning the patient may be as easy as pulling him or her toward the head of the bed. Positioning the patient may mean using multiple blankets, pillows, and wedges to align the oral, pharyngeal, and laryngeal axes.

Appropriate medications should be at the bedside. Rescue medications (eg. a vasopressor) should always be immediately available. Depending on the situation, other medication may also be needed. These may include a sedating agent, a muscle relaxant, or medicines to provide topical anesthesia.

Initial and Backup Plan(s)

The primary goal of any AM plan is to maximize oxygenation. For every patient, the clinician should develop an initial AM plan. The clinician should also develop at least one backup plan. These plans need to be patient specific, based on the clinical scenario, the patient examination, any predictors of a difficult airway, and the clinician's experience and gestalt. Not every clinician will develop the same primary plan for the same patient in the same clinical situation. The bedside clinician's judgment is being used for the specific clinical scenario.

Every AM plan should have at least one backup plan. Things do not always go as predicted, so it is important to know what to do if the primary plan fails. It may be necessary to have multiple backup plans. The final common plan for all AM is to place a surgical airway.

Timeout

If time allows, an airway timeout should be taken. The only reason not to take an airway timeout is if there is an emergent situation where it is not possible to oxygenate the patient. An airway timeout is a chance to make sure that the patient is as safe as possible [15]. A timeout allows all personnel involved to

Table 2.4 Complications associated with airway management

Complications of airway management	
Aspiration	Lung barotrauma
Bradycardia	Mainstem bronchus intubation
Cerebral ischemia	Myocardial ischemia
Death	Oral soft-tissue trauma
Dental trauma	Pharyngitis
Dysrhythmias	Pneumonia
Esophageal intubation	Tachycardia
Granuloma formation	Tracheitis
Hypertension	Tracheal ischemia
Hypotension	Tracheal perforation
Hypoxia	Tracheal stenosis
Laryngitis	Vocal cord paralysis
Laryngospasm	

make sure that they are on the same page. The timeout should consist of every person stating his or her name and what job he or she will be performing. The AM team leader should be the person actually manipulating the patient's airway. The leader needs to review with the team the resources needed and make sure that those resources are available. The leader should state the primary and the backup plan(s). Most importantly, if a team member has a question or is uncertain about something, he or she must speak up.

Complications

The most feared complication of AM is patient death. Thankfully, this rarely occurs. Most complications are much less serious. Some common complications are dysrhythmias, mild airway trauma, and pharyngitis. Less common complications include laryngospasm, tracheal stenosis, and dental trauma. For a more complete list, see Table 2.4.

Assessment

Clinical Situation

As in any patient encounter, it is necessary to assess the situation. For AM, the clinician should be able to assess the situation within a matter of seconds. Depending on the clinical scenario, action may need to be taken within seconds to prevent patient morbidity or mortality or there may be time to fully investigate, examine the patient, and prepare for placing an airway.

In emergent conditions, there is little, if any, time to do more than focus on getting an airway into the patient. Since it is rare that these truly emergent conditions exist, it is important to develop a plan ahead of time. These truly emergent conditions are predominantly those in which the patient has no airway and is already severely hypoxic or in cardiac arrest. Other personnel may have already tried multiple interventions. A common example is the patient brought to the ED by EMS where the paramedics have not been able to obtain an airway despite multiple attempts with different techniques and equipment, and the patient is in cardiac arrest because of not having an airway. A surgical airway may be indicated and must be performed emergently in an effort to save the patient's life.

Under ideal conditions, the clinician has time to prepare appropriately. It would be possible to develop an AM plan, including backup plans. There would be plenty of assistance, which may include other people who are knowledgeable about airway management. There is time to adequately position the patient and equipment necessary. Ideally, the patient has an empty stomach. The anatomy would be such that the mouth could be opened wide without difficulty. The airway itself would be widely patent and without obstruction. The neck would have a full range of motion. He or she would be able to be preoxygenated and would have a normal and intact respiratory drive. The patient would have a normal body mass index. The hemodynamics would be normal. The patient coagulation would be normal and intact.

Most cases requiring AM in the ED or ICU are somewhere between emergent and ideal conditions. These urgent situations require expedited action, but there is time to properly evaluate the patient and develop a strategy that will maximize the potential for positive results.

Airway Examination

An airway examination should be performed on any patient to be given conscious sedation or undergo intubation. Even due to the emergent nature of airways in the ED and ICU, it is imperative to still perform an airway examination on patients. The intent of the examination is to uncover any potential findings that may predict difficulty in any of the steps of AM. Any airway has the potential to be a difficult airway. A percentage of difficult airways may proceed to become a failed airway. A failed airway is one in which the clinician is not able to place an airway of any type. In emergent AM, a failed airway often equates to a patient death. In an effort to prevent patient deaths, it is important to prepare and plan and have a broad knowledge of different AM techniques.

From mask ventilation to surgical airways, a correctly performed airway exam will give the provider information about how best to take over control of the patient's airway. The provider should use the findings from the airway exam to develop an AM plan that has the lowest risk to the patient. There is no evidence that performing an airway exam will change the intubation experience or outcome. There is no single finding that has been shown to reliably predict a difficult airway [7]. For this reason, it is important for the clinician to look for any of the findings that have been associated with a difficult airway. It is advised to develop a system so that one performs the examination the same way each time, so that nothing is missed.

One way to start the airway exam is by looking at the patient's overall body habitus. Pay particular attention to the head and neck. Begin at the base of the neck and move cephalad. There is a higher risk of difficulty associated with obese patients or those with short or thick necks. Limited neck mobility is another predictor of difficulty. If the patient has a cervical collar or Halo brace in place, it is important to know if there are actual injuries to the cervical spine or spinal cord or is the collar just for precaution. Patients with scoliosis or kyphosis are often difficult to position, which may lead to difficulty with AM. Tumors, trauma, foreign bodies, or any other abnormal anatomy findings are associated with a difficult airway. See Table 2.1 for further. One feature of the neck examination that is often overlooked is the cricothyroid membrane (CTM). It is important to locate and evaluate the patient's CTM in case there is a need for a nerve block or a surgical airway.

A small chin may be a concerning finding. The thyromental (also known as the hyomental) distance is measured from the thyroid notch to the tip of the mandible with the head extended, the neck in a neutral position, and the mouth closed. A length of 6 cm or greater is a favorable finding for direct laryngoscopy. Another acceptable measurement is three of the patient's finger breadths. The thyrohyoid distance is measured from the thyroid notch to the hyoid bone (or base of mouth if unable to palpate) with the neck extended. A distance of more than two of the patient's finger breadths is favorable.

An upper lip bite test (ULBT), also termed a mandibular protrusion test (MPT), examines the amount of protrusion of the patient's mandible or amount of jaw thrust. Have the patient attempt to bite as much of his or her upper lip as possible with the lower incisors. In class I, the lower incisors can bite the upper lip above the vermillion border, making the mucosa of the upper lip invisible. In class II, the lower incisors can bite the upper lip below the vermillion border. In class III, the patient is not able to bite his or her upper lip with the lower incisors. Class II or III has been demonstrated to predict difficulty with mask ventilation [16]. A class III ULBT is associated with difficult intubation [17].

After the chin, move to the face and mouth. Facial hair may decrease the ability to mask ventilate a patient. It may be necessary to shave the patient. When examining the mouth, the length of the central incisors should be noted as large or protruding incisors or an overbite may indicate a difficult airway. Look for loose teeth, as these may come out during manipulation of the airway and become an obstruction or aspiration risk. Dentures may be beneficial for mask ventilation but may make intubation more difficult. Small interincisor distance and a large or protruding tongue are also concerning findings. A high arched palate is also associated with difficult intubations. See Table 2.2 for further information.

Look specifically at the uvula to ascertain the patient's modified Mallampati classification [18]. With the observer at eye level, the patient holds the head in a neutral position, opens the mouth maximally, and protrudes the tongue without phonating. The airway is classified according to the visible structures. In a class I, the soft palate, fauces, uvula, and tonsillar pillars are visible. In class II, the soft palate, fauces, and uvula are visible. In class III, the soft palate and base of the uvula are visible. In class IV (added by Samsoon and Young [19]), the soft palate is not visible. Mallampati considered those patients with class IV and possibly class III to be difficult to intubate [18, 20]. See Table 2.5 and Fig. 2.1 for further information.

Even in emergent situations, a provider is able to perform an airway exam. The examination does not take long to perform and provides useful information so that an AM plan may be developed that minimizes patient risk.

Table 2.5 The modified Mallampati score which evaluates the ability to view structures in the posterior pharynx

Modified Mallampati classification	
Class I	The soft palate, fauces, uvula, and tonsillar pillars are visible
Class II	The soft palate, fauces, and uvula are visible
Class III	The soft palate and base of the uvula are visible
Class IV	The soft palate is not visible

Anesthetic History

In addition to an airway exam, reviewing a patient's anesthetic and surgical history will provide information regarding previous AM experiences. With the increased use of electronic medical records (EMR), this information has become easier to obtain. If deemed to be a difficult airway, anesthesiology providers will make notation so that future providers will have the ability to prepare ahead of time. Information about any difficulty with mask ventilation or intubation should be in the anesthetic records. In addition to information about the airway, these records may have information about other problems encountered, such as hypotension with induction or information about the doses of medications used.

There is no evidence that the current AM plan must be the same as plans done on the same patient in the past. The clinical scenario and the patient may be significantly different than previous AM encounters. The plan must be developed by the bedside clinician based on the clinical scenario and his or her judgment.

Physical Examination

The purpose of the patient evaluation is to identify any risk factor that is associated with a diffi-

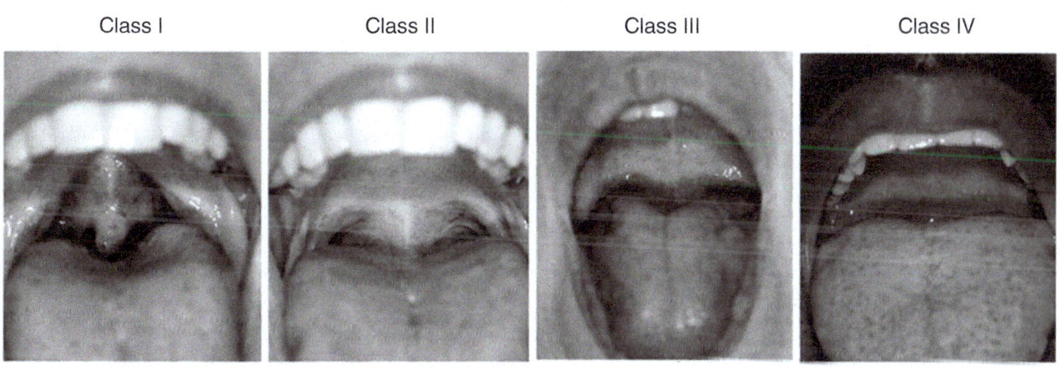

Fig. 2.1 The modified Mallampati classification

cult intubation, so that the provider can prepare his or her intubation plan accordingly. Under ideal circumstances, one would be able to interview the patient to obtain medical history, perform a full physical examination, and then review the patient's medical record for other information, such as electrocardiograms, X-rays, or echocardiograms. When there is ample time, the provider should discuss the details of the intubation procedure and any backup plans with the patient.

In the ICU or the ED, time is limited due to the urgent or emergent patient condition. In these circumstances, the clinician should perform a directed physical examination. The directed physical examination should include an evaluation of the patient's cardiovascular and pulmonary system. It is important to note any abnormal findings. The clinician should develop the AM plan that aims to avoid exacerbating any of these abnormal exam findings. It is also important to perform a directed neurologic exam looking at mental status. It may be necessary to limit sedation in patients with a primary neurologic deficit. Similarly, if there is concern for or a known cervical spine injury, it may be necessary to maintain cervical spine immobilization throughout the AM plan.

In addition to the directed physical examination, it is imperative to review the patient's current vital signs. Hemodynamic instability is commonly seen in patients that require urgent or emergent AM. Many of the medications used will affect the patient's hemodynamics. Laryngoscopy can elevate a patient's intracranial pressure (ICP) significantly. An endotracheal tube that contacts the carina can induce profound bradycardia. When a patient switches from negative-pressure to positive-pressure ventilation, there are significant changes in intrathoracic pressure that will affect hemodynamics. The patient's risk of injury is lower if the provider incorporates the current and predicted vital signs into the AM plan.

Labs and Ancillary Tests

Depending on the patient's condition, there may be time to review potentially pertinent labs or other tests that have been performed. The purpose of reviewing labs and tests is to give the provider more information to formulate an AM plan. Although there is no one lab or ancillary test that must be reviewed, the following studies are often reviewed in an effort to learn more about a patient's clinical status.

An arterial blood gas (ABG) will show the degree of hypoxemia and acidemia. An elevated lactic acid is associated with anaerobic metabolism and may indicate that the patient is in some type of shock. A complete blood count (CBC) would show anemia, which would affect oxygen delivery to the tissues, or thrombocytopenia, which may be, depending on the severity, a risk factor for bleeding. Coagulation studies also provide information about the risk of bleeding during AM. A comprehensive metabolic profile will provide information about the patient's liver function, renal function, and electrolytes, especially the potassium. It is also useful to review cardiac markers to know if the patient has had any cardiac ischemia. All of this information may be helpful in deciding what, if any, medications should be used in the AM plan.

A chest X-ray (CXR) will often provide information about the condition of the patient's lungs. If significant abnormalities are found on the CXR, it will be much more difficult to preoxygenate the patient and maintain high levels of oxygenation during the manipulation of the airway. An electrocardiogram (EKG) may provide information about any conduction abnormalities or active cardiac ischemia. An echocardiogram should provide information about the patient's ejection fraction, right ventricular function, and any valvular abnormalities. All of these tests provide information that is helpful in formulating an appropriate AM plan, so that there is minimal risk for the patient and maximum potential for successful AM without complications.

Medical and Surgical History

As with any other intervention or medical procedure, it is beneficial to know the patient's medical and surgical history. While time may not allow the provider to obtain a full history, it is advantageous to know the immediate history and events leading to why a patient needs AM. In addition to this basic knowledge, the provider should attempt to ascertain if the patient has any medical condition that is commonly associated with a difficult airway. Any medical or surgical condition that distorts the normal anatomy has the potential to make it difficult to place a definitive airway.

There are several medical conditions that are associated with difficult intubations. Obesity is one of the most common medical conditions that is also commonly associated with difficult mask ventilation and difficult laryngoscopy. As the obesity epidemic continues to worsen, the percentage of patients with a difficult airway will increase. See Table 2.3 for a list of medical conditions that are commonly associated directly with a difficult airway. In addition to medical conditions that are directly associated with a difficult airway, it is possible for essentially any severe medical condition to be indirectly related in some way to a difficult AM. The provider's AM plan is limited due to these severe medical conditions because of the significant morbidity and mortality, which is increased when dealing with urgent or emergent AM.

Equipment

There are many different pieces of equipment needed to provide AM. These pieces range from fairly basic to highly advanced, as well as other ancillary items that are equally important but are not specifically for AM. While there is no evidence to support that having every piece of equipment at the bedside will make an airway easier, most clinicians prefer to have all equipment needed for the initial and backup plans readily available. Depending on the situation, this may include an assistant that is also familiar with airway management. The basic equipment used in AM is often what will save a patient's life. The clinician will use any and all of this equipment in preparation for maximum patient oxygenation prior to moving to the advanced equipment that is used for a definitive airway. A list of airway equipment needed for urgent or emergent AM is found in Table 2.6.

Basic

Basic airway equipment is able to provide oxygen to a patient, but it does not provide the patient with a definitive airway. Any person providing patient care should have knowledge in how to use this equipment. Basic airway equipment includes a continuous oxygen source, a bag valve mask (BVM), oral and nasal airways, a positive end-expiratory pressure (PEEP) valve, and suction capabilities. While labeled as basic, this equipment is anything but basic. This equipment is a fall back for any time when it is difficult or impossible to get oxygen into a patient.

A continuous oxygen source allows the provider to maximize a patient's oxygenation status in an effort to prevent desaturation during AM. The patient should be oxygenated with 100% FiO_2 for 3 minutes to achieve maximum oxygenation [21]. This amount of time will also cause nitrogen washout, also known as denitrogenation. During emergent AM, the patient should also be maintained on 100% FiO_2 to fur-

Table 2.6 Airway equipment that may be needed at bedside or readily available for urgent or emergent airway management

Airway equipment for urgent or emergent airway management	
Basic	Advanced
Bag valve mask, self-inflating, with reservoir	Bougie
Facemasks (multiple sizes)	Endotracheal tubes (multiple sizes)
Oral airways (multiple sizes)	Laryngoscope handles
Oxygen source	Laryngoscope curved blades (multiple sizes)
Nasopharyngeal airways (multiple sizes)	Laryngoscope straight blades (multiple sizes)
PEEP valve	Rescue devices
Suction source with Yankauer suction tip	Supraglottic airway devices (multiple sizes)
	Surgical airway kit
	Video laryngoscopy

ther prevent desaturation [22]. The easiest way to do this is by providing 15 lpm 0_2 through a nasal cannula or using a high-flow nasal cannula (HFNC), which can provide up to 60 lpm O_2. Noninvasive positive-pressure ventilation (NIPPV) is another way to maintain continuous oxygenation during AM, but the logistics of using NIPPV make this option less appealing.

An adult BVM (Fig. 2.2) is usually a 1-L bag with a 15-mm standard adapter that allows ventilation via a mask, an SGA, or endotracheal tube. In the ED and ICU, BVMs are usually self-inflating and disposable and have an oxygen reservoir to insure that the BVM delivers the highest oxygen concentration possible. There are different types of the BVMs and not all are self-inflating. Non self-inflating BVMs usually do not have a reservoir and must be connected to an oxygen source to insure that the bag fills up with oxygen. It is important to make sure to have access to smaller BVMs if the patient is significantly smaller than an average adult. Most disposable BVMs come with a mask. Multiple mask sizes should be immediately available to make sure that the mask is adequate for the size of the patient's face.

An oral airway (OPA) (Fig. 2.3) is used to keep the airway open when using a BVM by preventing the tongue from occluding the hypopharynx. There are many different designs that are currently used throughout the world. The OPA should only be used on patients with a depressed gag reflex; otherwise, the patient may vomit and aspirate gastric contents. The correct size of the OPA is determined by measuring from the corner of the mouth to the tragus of the ear. Common sizes for adults are 80, 90, and 100 mm. The OPA is properly positioned when the proximal flange is resting on the patient's lips.

A nasal airway (NPA) (Fig. 2.4) is placed into the nasal passage(s) in an effort to improve the patient's airway and oxygenation. An NPA may be placed in a patient with an intact gag reflex. The correct size of an NPA is determined by mea-

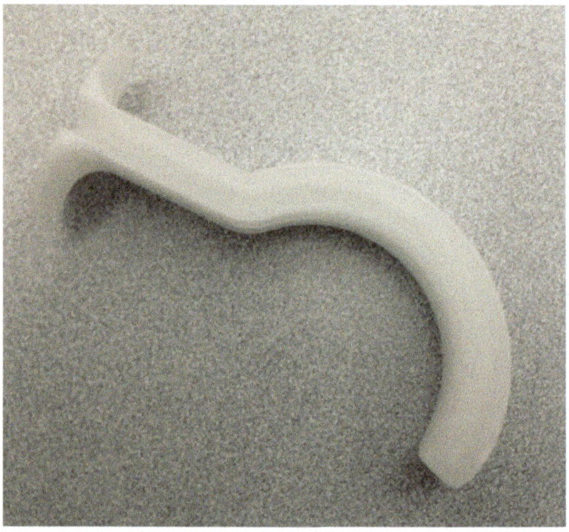

Fig. 2.3 Oropharyngeal airway

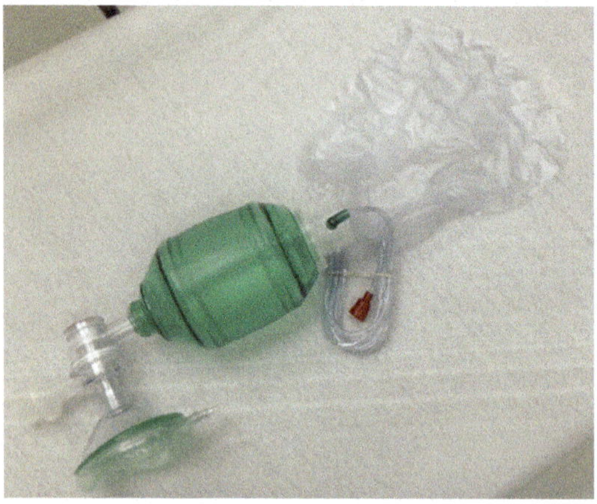

Fig. 2.2 Bag valve mask with facemask and oxygen reservoir

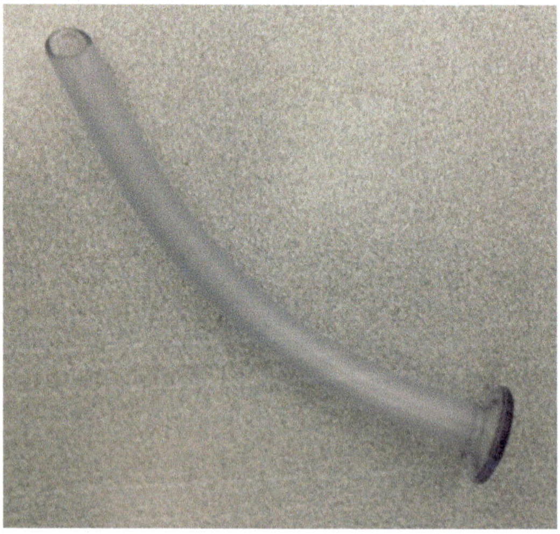

Fig. 2.4 Nasopharyngeal airway

suring from the nasal ala to the corner of the mandible and the size of the largest nare. It is important to use the correct size because if an NPA that is too large is used, it is possible to insert the NPA to the point of stimulating the gag reflex. Common sizes for adults are 5.5–8.5 mm.

A PEEP valve (Fig. 2.5) is beneficial to have immediately available, especially if the patient is severely hypoxic. Similar to PEEP on a ventilator, a PEEP valve attempts to provide end-expiratory pressure in an effort to maintain alveoli open at the end of expiration. By keeping alveoli open, less effort is needed to overcome the resistance of opening a closed alveolus. The end result is an increase in mean airway pressure which equates to improved oxygenation. The provider must be cautious, as a PEEP valve may cause a significant decrease in venous return to the heart, which will be seen clinically as hypotension.

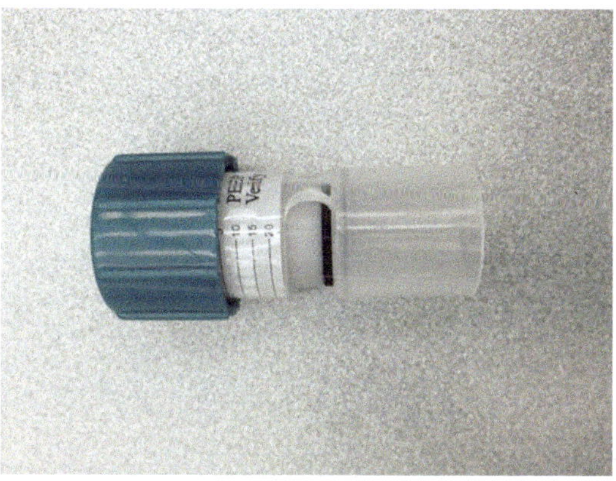

Fig. 2.5 PEEP valve

Finally, suction capabilities are always necessary. It is impossible to accurately predict the amount of secretions or blood in the posterior larynx. Having suction immediately available has the potential to reduce aspiration of contents into the lungs. In clinical situations in which there is copious material in the patient's pharynx, it may be advisable to have more than one suction setup available.

Advanced

A definitive airway is an artificial tube in the trachea. Advanced airway equipment is that which is needed to place a definitive airway. This equipment requires that the provider has advanced training in AM. Advanced equipment includes items for direct and video laryngoscopy, endotracheal tubes, stylets, SGAs, surgical airway placement, and other rescue devices. Equipment options will differ depending on the institution, but the minimal requirement readily available should be equipment for DL, SGAs, rescue stylets, and equipment to obtain a surgical airway.

Laryngoscope handles and blades are needed for direct laryngoscopy. There are many types of straight blades available, including Miller, Wisconsin, and Wis-Hipple (Fig. 2.6). These

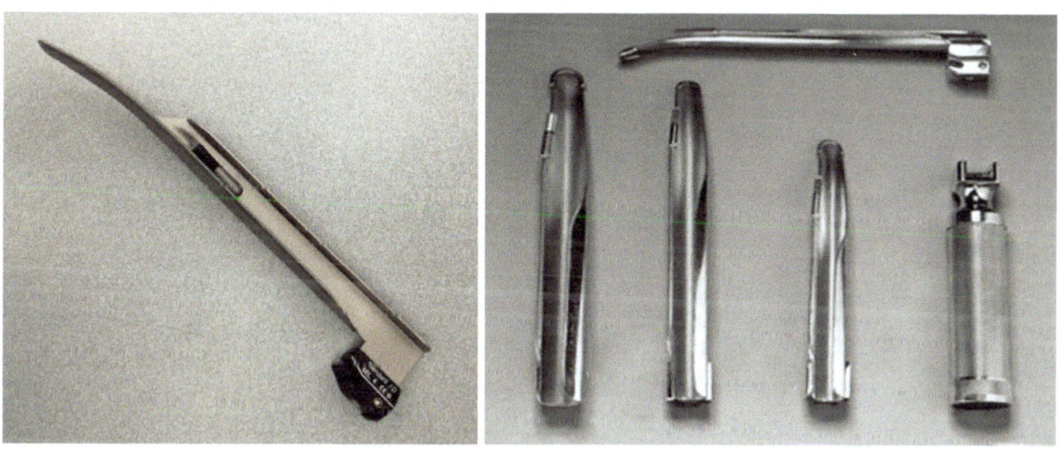

Fig. 2.6 Straight laryngoscope blades. (**a**) Profile view of Miller laryngoscope blade. (**b**) Wis-Hipple laryngoscope blades and handle

blades differ in the size or degree of curvature of the spatula on the end of the blade. The most commonly used curved blades are MacIntosh blades (Fig. 2.7). There are other curved blades available that are modifications of Dr. MacIntosh's original design. All laryngoscope blades come in a variety of sizes. For Miller blades, the smallest size is 00, and the largest size is 4. For MacIntosh blades, the smallest size is 0, and the largest size is 4.

Endotracheal tubes (ETT) also come in a variety of sizes and shapes. For the majority of intubations in the ED or ICU, providers will use ETTs with a gentle curve. In the OR, there are many other designs that may be used depending on the type of surgery (most often otolaryngologic cases). ETT sizes range from 2.5 to 10.0 mm. There is no hard and fast rule about what size ETT to place in adults. Most clinicians prefer to place a 7.5-mm tube so that a bronchoscope may be passed, if the need arises. The ETT size required for a specific patient may be determined from the size of the patient's largest nare or the diameter of his or her fifth digit. There are other factors that must be considered when selecting a size. For example, if the patient is presenting with an inhalation injury or has a history of tracheal stenosis, then smaller ETTs should be prepared. If there is the potential for bronchoscopy, then it may be advantageous to place a larger tube. Although each scenario is different, a good rule of thumb is to use a 7.0–7.5 mm ETT on an adult female and a 7.5–8.0 mm ETT on an adult male.

Stylets are another piece of advanced equipment that should be immediately available for any AM procedure. Malleable stylets are commonly used used to make the ETT into a particular shape. The most common shape used is described as a "J" or a hockey stick. Some VL systems recommend the use of their proprietary rigid stylets. A gum elastic bougie, also known as an Eschmann Stylet, is a rubber or plastic stylet (Fig. 2.8) that is designed to be placed directly into the trachea. The ETT is then positioned into the trachea by using a Seldinger technique over the bougie.

There are many different available SGAs. The first SGA developed for AM is the Combi-Tube. The laryngeal mask airway (LMA) is another

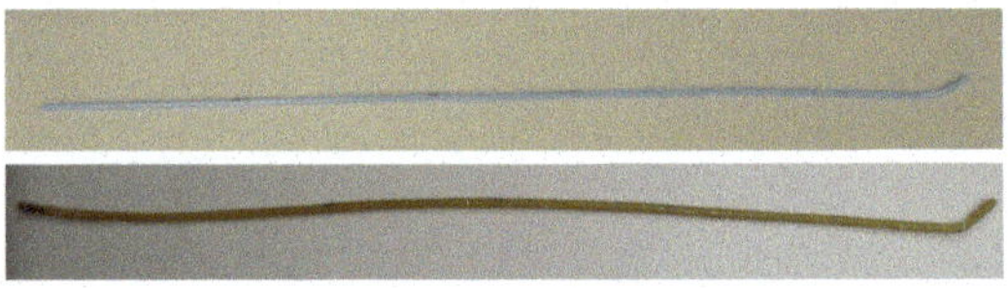

Fig. 2.8 Bougie. (**a**) Disposable plastic stylet. (**b**) Eschmann stylet – Gum elastic bougie

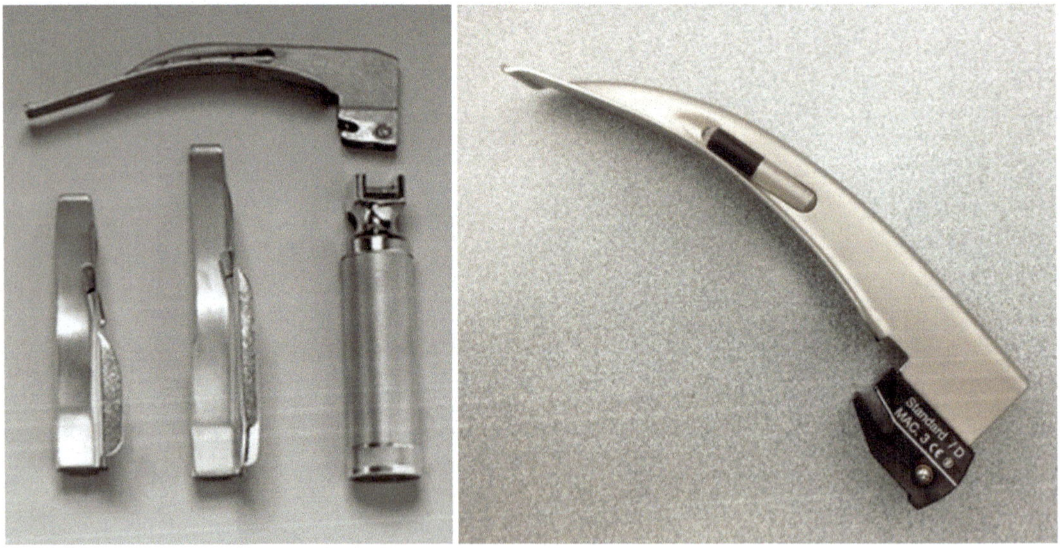

Fig. 2.7 Curved laryngoscope blades. (**a**) MacIntosh laryngoscope blades and handle. (**b**) Profile view of MacIntosh laryngoscope blade

common SGA. The LMA was developed by Dr. Archie Brain. It was first used in 1983 and first available commercially in 1987 [23]. There are now several different versions of LMA available. i-gel, LMA-Fastrach, King Laryngeal Tube, and air-Q are other commonly used SGAs. All SGAs are intended to deliver oxygen to the trachea although no part of the device passes through the vocal cords into the trachea. Some of the devices have supraglottic and infraglottic parts. An ETT may be placed directly into the trachea through some SGAs (known as 2nd generation SGAs).

Medications

Medications will be needed to facilitate AM in the vast majority of cases. The minimum medications that should be immediately available are an induction agent to sedate the patient, a muscle relaxant to take away patient movement and breathing, and a vasopressor to maintain hemodynamics if the patient becomes unstable. Common induction agents include etomidate, fentanyl, ketamine, midazolam, and propofol. These may be used individually or in combination with other medications. Rocuronium and succinylcholine are the most commonly used paralytic medications in the ED or ICU. In a Cochrane Review, rocuronium was found to be "slightly less effective than succinylcholine for creating excellent and acceptable intubating conditions" [24]. Vasopressors that are commonly used as bolus agents include epinephrine, neosynephrine, and vasopressin. These agents plus dopamine and levophed are potential options for a vasopressor administered as a continuous drip. See Table 2.7.

Table 2.7 Medications that are commonly used in urgent or emergent airway management

Medications commonly used in airway management		
Sedation	Paralytic	Vasopressor
Etomidate	Rocuronium	Epinephrine
Fentanyl	Succinylcholine	Ephedrine
Ketamine		Neosynephrine
Midazolam		Vasopressin
Propofol		

If possible, it is important to stabilize a patient's hemodynamics prior to AM. Unstable patients that undergo emergent AM have a high frequency of cardiac arrest in the immediate time period after AM [25]. Even in awake patients, most providers will give an anxiolytic or mild sedative to facilitate ETT placement. There are many different medicines that may be used for different scenarios.

Airway Anesthesia via Topicalization

Most emergency medicine (EM) physicians sedate the vast majority of patients undergoing AM. Having a patient remain awake (or minimally sedated) for AM is not a concept with which most EM physicians are comfortable or have experience [26]. It is unknown how many EM residencies teach how to perform airway nerve blocks or awake intubations. The ability to achieve total airway anesthesia through topicalization and perform an awake intubation is an important skill set for an EM physician to possess. There are many high-risk patients that would benefit from being awake for the AM. Keeping a high-risk patient awake helps reduce the risk of morbidity or mortality.

The nerve blocks commonly performed to achieve total anesthesia of the larynx are the lingual and pharyngeal branches of the glossopharyngeal nerve (GPN), the superior laryngeal nerve (SLN), and the recurrent laryngeal nerve (RLN). The GPN provides innervation to the posterior one third of the tongue and the superior portion of the pharynx. The SLN provides innervation to the inferior portion of the pharynx above the vocal cords. The RLN provides innervation below the vocal cords. To achieve total airway anesthesia, it is necessary to anesthestize all three nerves. Some experts advocate the use of blocks whenever possible, while others advocate that blocks are rarely necessary and that there are alternatives to nerve blocks [27]. The evidence is not clear as to whether one method is better than the other [28–30]. The time to achieve anesthesia by performing the airway blocks is approximately the same as needed to nebulize lidocaine.

To block the GLN, open the patient's mouth and identify the palatopharyngeal fold. A tongue blade or straight laryngoscope blade is inserted and used to move and hold the tongue anteriorly. A small bore, long diameter needle is inserted into the mucosa, and several milliliters (ml) of local anesthetic are injected. A 25-gauge spinal needle and 3 ml of 2% lidocaine is recommended. Take care to aspirate prior to injection so that accidental injection into a vessel does not occur.

To block the SLN, identify the greater cornu of the hyoid bone. After appropriately cleaning the skin, inject a small bore needle just inferior to the greater cornu. Aim the needle medially and anteriorly and inject 3 ml of 2% lidocaine, making sure to aspirate prior to injection.

To block the RLN, a transtracheal block is performed. This is probably the easiest of the blocks. Identify and appropriately clean the CTM. Insert a small bore needle through the membrane into the trachea. Test the location of the needle by aspirating. When air is aspirated, the needle is in the trachea. At this point, inject several milliliters of local anesthetic. Four milliliters of 4% lidocaine is commonly used. The patient will begin coughing, which will disperse the local anesthetic to achieve a greater area of anesthesia.

To anesthetize the larynx without using nerve blocks, nebulized lidocaine has been used for topicalization for many years. Higher concentrations of lidocaine provide anesthesia in a timelier manner. Place 5 ml of 2–4% lidocaine in a nebulizer and have the patient breathe through his or her mouth for approximately 10 minutes or until the nebulizer chamber is empty. This technique is easier than performing the nerve blocks, but the degree of anesthesia is variable. In an effort to improve the degree of anesthesia, the provider may place lidocaine gel or jelly on a tongue blade or OPA and slowly advance it (over several minutes) to the posterior pharynx. The lidocaine gel or jelly will achieve topical anesthesia on the structures with which it comes into contact. Benzocaine is not recommended due to the relative ease of inducing methemoglobinemia.

Nebulized lidocaine may also be used to anesthetize the nasal passages. Lidocaine gel or jelly may be used instead of or in conjunction with nebulized lidocaine. Identify the largest nare and squirt 2–3 ml into it. The solution will slowly make its way down to the posterior pharynx. An alternative to this strategy is to coat an NPA with lidocaine and insert it into the largest nare. After several minutes, the passage should be anesthetized. If planning to nasally intubate a patient, the topical vasoconstrictor, Oxymetazoline, is recommended in an effort to minimize bleeding.

Other Equipment

In addition to the equipment above, there are several pieces of equipment that should be used or be readily available during any AM. Table 2.8 lists the minimum equipment needed. The patient should be connected to a continuous pulse oximeter, a blood pressure cuff that measures every 1–3 minutes, and EKG telemetry. These items should be placed reflexively on any patient who is critically ill. At least one and preferably two working IVs are recommended so that medications and fluid boluses may be given easily. If the patient does not have an IV, intraosseous (IO) access may be an alternative. Some medicines may be given intramuscularly, but the absorption rate is variable and thus not recommended unless there is no other option.

An end-tidal carbon dioxide ($ETCO_2$) device is recommended to help confirm placement of the airway. There are different options available. It is important to give six artificial breaths before a determination about airway placement can be definitively made. $ETCO_2$ devices may not work if a patient has been in cardiac arrest for a prolonged period of time.

Table 2.8 Non-airway equipment that is commonly used during airway management

Non-airway equipment	
Bite block	Magill forceps
Blood pressure cuff	Pulse oximeter
CO_2 detector	Sterile suction catheters
EKG telemetry	Tube securing device
Intravenous or intraosseous access	

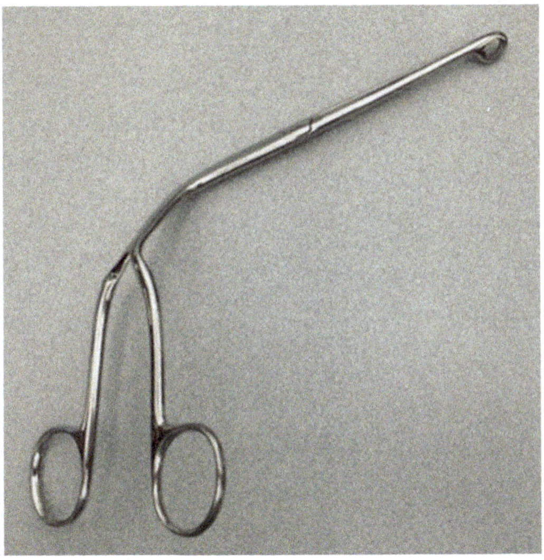

Fig. 2.9 Magill forceps

After an ETT has been placed, it needs to be secured so that the tube does not become accidentally dislodged. Tape may be used to secure the device. Tape is stronger and may prevent inadvertent extubation [31], but a commercially available tube securing device is a better option to prevent skin breakdown [32, 33]. These devices are designed in an effort to minimize tissue necrosis on the face and in the mouth.

Magill forceps (Fig. 2.9) may be needed to retrieve foreign bodies in the airway. Foreign body removal is not common, but when it occurs, it is advantageous to have this piece of equipment. Magill forceps may also be used to help facilitate tube placement into the trachea. These should only be used by providers that have been trained in using Magill forceps, as it is possible to cause trauma to the airway.

Techniques

Mask Ventilation

Mask ventilation is an essential airway skill. Mask ventilation is the initial step used to provide oxygen to a patient requiring AM. Mask ventilation is also the fall back mechanism for providing oxygen to a patient at any point in the AM plan if the patient is hypoxic. If a provider is unable to mask ventilate a patient who is hypoxic and has a poor or nonexistent respiratory drive, then the patient will not likely survive. There are several predictors of difficulty with mask ventilation. See Table 2.9 for further information.

Table 2.9 Predictors of difficult mask ventilation

Predictors of difficult mask ventilation	
Age >57 years old	Edentulous
Beard	Mallampati class III or IV
BMI >30	Snoring history

After the decision has been made to mask ventilate a patient, several steps should occur simultaneously. Adequate resources and personnel should be available. The BVM should be connected to an oxygen source that provides 100% FiO_2 at high flow ~15 L/min. The patient should be properly positioned so that the airway axes are aligned. See Fig. 2.10. The sniffing position or the head-tilt, chin-lift position will allow the best alignment of airway axes. If unable to manipulate the cervical spine due to concern for injury, a jaw thrust maneuver is recommended. In this maneuver, the mandible is elevated by pulling both angles of the mandible anteriorly while maintaining inline stabilization of the cervical spine.

The airway should be opened and a mask placed onto the patient's face such that it completely covers the nose and mouth. The mask cuff should rest between the base of the alveolar ridge and the chin inferiorly, above the bridge of the nose superiorly, and lateral to the nasolabial folds on each side. The provider then pulls the patient's face up into the mask so that the seal is improved. The mask should never be pushed down onto the patient's face, as this may lead to occlusion of the airway or poor oxygenation.

It is possible for a single provider to mask a patient. The provider's nondominant hand is placed on the mask with the thumb and index finger partially encircling the mask connector, similar to an "OK" sign or the letters E and C. The other three fingers are placed under the patient's mandible. It is important to place the fingers on the boney portion of the mandible in an effort to minimize potential injury to the soft tissues. The middle finger is placed beneath the chin. The long

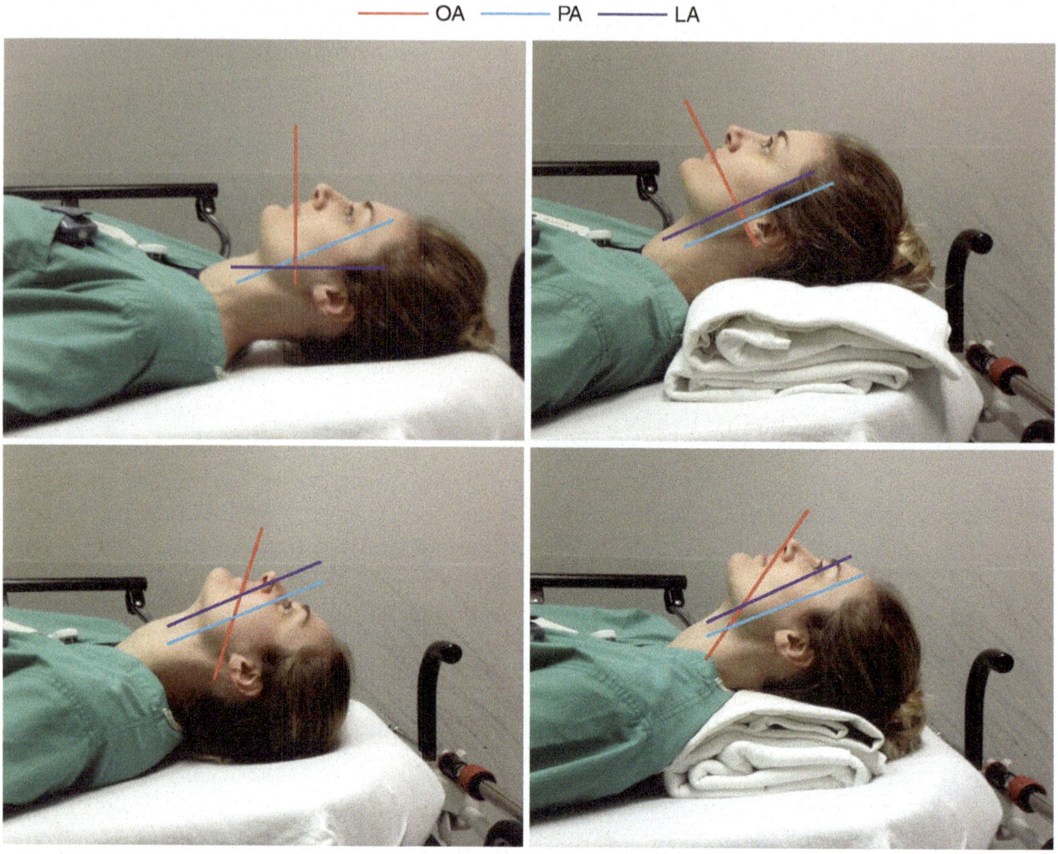

Fig. 2.10 Alignment of the oral axis (OA), pharyngeal axis (PA), and laryngeal axis (LA). (**a**) Head in neutral position. (**b**) Head elevated and neck flexed. (**c**) Head tilted and chin lifted. (**d**) Sniffing position

finger is placed midway between the chin and the angle of the mandible. The little finger is placed under the angle of the mandible. These fingers pull the mandible into the mask in an effort to make a tight seal between the face and the mask. The provider's dominant hand is then used to squeeze the bag to provide positive pressure and oxygen will be forced into the patient's oropharynx, with the goal of proceeding to the lungs.

Whenever possible, a two person, two-handed technique should be utilized. In this technique, it is possible to provide greater air movement [34]. One person's task is to squeeze the bag. The other person's job is to use both hands to achieve an adequate mask seal. There are two options that are commonly used. In the first option, the provider uses both hands to make the "OK" sign or the E and C as described previously. Both hands are used to lift the mandible into the mask. In the second option, the provider places both thumbs on the lateral aspects of the mask and the other fingers under the mandible on the boney portion. The fingers are then used to lift the mandible into the mask.

Cricoid pressure, also known as the Sellick maneuver, may help improve airflow into the trachea. It may also help prevent regurgitation of gastric contents. An assistant applies pressure to the cricoid cartilage in an effort to occlude to esophagus. Dr. Sellick originally recommended 30 Newtons (N) of pressure [35]. Subsequent study has shown that the force needed is between 30 and 40 N (which is the equivalent of 3–4 kg) [36].

When the ability to mask ventilate the patient has been obtained, it is recommended to provide 3 minutes of mask ventilation with 100% FiO_2 for nitrogen washout and fill up oxygen stores

[21]. This denitrogenation will allow the patient to stay on the high portion of the oxygen–hemoglobin dissociation curve longer. How long this effect lasts is unknown, especially in critically ill patients undergoing urgent or emergent AM.

Oropharyngeal Airway

To properly place an OPA, there are two options. Either method is acceptable. The first option is to insert the device with the distal end pointing cephalad and advance the OPA into the mouth. It is important to avoid pushing the tongue into the hypopharynx. Once passed the base of the tongue, rotate the OPA 180° so that the distal end is now pointing caudad. The second option is to use a tongue blade to depress the posterior portion of the tongue and insert the OPA with the distal end already pointing caudad.

Nasopharyngeal Airway

To properly place the NPA, identify the patient's largest nare. Lubricate the tip and shaft of the NPA with lidocaine or a water soluble jelly. Capillary bleeding from the nasal passages is a common complication of NPA insertion. Bleeding is minimized with the use of a lubricating jelly or oxymetazoline, but use caution in patients with severe thrombocytopenia. Insert the NPA into the nare and advance it horizontally along the inferior nasal turbinate. Stop advancing when the flange of the NPA contacts the nare.

Direct Laryngoscopy

Direct laryngoscopy is the hallmark of placing a definitive airway into the trachea. The first recorded successful attempt at DL was done by Alfred Kirstein in Berlin on April 23, 1895 [37]. Since then, there have been many modifications. Today the most commonly used blades are the Miller or the MacIntosh. Robert Miller introduced his design of a straight blade in 1941 [38], and Robert MacIntosh introduced his design in of a curved blade in 1943 [39]. Under emergent conditions, DL has a first pass success rate of 87.4% [40].

Each of the blade designs has a light source at the end of the blade that is powered by batteries in the handle. Most new types of blades are modifications of the design of the original Miller and MacIntosh blades. Fiberoptic versions of the blades are also available. These have the light source in the handle and illumination occurs via the fiberoptic channel on the blade.

To determine the correct size of the blade (either straight or curved), measure from the corner of the mouth to the tragus of the ear and use the blade that most approximates this length. Apply the blade to the handle. There are a variety of different handles available. If time allows, choose the handle that is most comfortable. Once the blade and handle are connected, place the laryngoscope in the left hand.

The patient should be properly positioned and sedate enough so that the gag reflex has been abolished. Taking care to avoid the patient's teeth, the blade is inserted on the right side of the patient's mouth and advanced to the posterior oropharynx. Use the blade to sweep the tongue to the left and then lift up on the blade. It is important for the clinician to avoid using his or her wrist as a fulcrum; otherwise, dental trauma may occur. With the wrist and forearm straight, the laryngoscope is lifted along the handle axis. If unable to visualize the epiglottis, the blade may need to be advanced further and lifted again. Throughout the process, take care to avoid trauma to the structures in the mouth, including the lips.

Once the epiglottis is seen, it is at this point that the two different blades are used differently to obtain a view of the vocal cords. AM clinicians should be equally skilled with either blade. The straight blade tip is used to directly elevate the epiglottis. The curved blade tip is placed in the vallecula at the base of the tongue and then elevates the epiglottis indirectly via the hyoepiglottic ligament. Note that some clinicians advocate using the curved blade to elevate the epiglottis directly. This is an improper use of the blade and may cause harm to the patient.

Instead of a method of slowly advancing the blade while searching for the epiglottis, there is another option for intubation with the straight blade. The straight blade is inserted into the mouth as above and then advanced deep past the oropharynx to the proximal esophagus. The blade is then lifted and slowly withdrawn until the glottis drops into view. The epiglottis may also drop and occlude the view of the glottis. If this occurs, advance the blade so that the tip will be able to directly elevate the glottis.

With the epiglottis lifted out of the way, the glottis should come into view. It is at this point that the Cormack–Lehane view [41] is ascertained. Grade 1 indicates that most of the glottis is seen. Grade 2 indicates that only the base of the vocal cords is seen. More of the glottis may be seen with light pressure on the larynx. A Grade 3 view indicates that only the epiglottis is visualized and no part of the glottis is seen. Grade 4 indicates that no part of the epiglottis is seen, and alternative intubation techniques or equipment may be needed. See Fig. 2.11 for the different Cormack–Lehane views.

If there is difficulty visualizing the vocal cords, it may be necessary to use laryngeal manipulation. A BURP maneuver is commonly attempted. This maneuver involves manipulating the trachea with the provider's right hand by applying a backward, upward, and rightward pressure. Once the best view of the vocal cords is obtained, an assistant takes over holding the trachea in the optimal position.

When the best glottic view has been obtained, the clinician inserts an ETT into the trachea and advances it approximately 1–2 cm beyond the vocal cords. The corresponding ETT depth at the teeth should approximate three times the internal diameter of the ETT. A more correct determination of depth can be obtained by the formula: (body height in cm/5) – 13 [42]. The ETT is held in position manually, and the laryngoscope is withdrawn, taking care not to cause any trauma. The cuff on the ETT is then inflated to a pressure of 20–25 mmHg. Commercial manometers are available to measure the pressure. It is not possible to tell how much pressure is in the cuff by squeezing the pilot balloon manually or by inflating the pilot balloon with a specific amount of air [43].

When the ETT is in place, it is important to confirm the presence of gas exchange. An end-tidal CO_2 detector is attached to the proximal end of the ETT, and breaths are delivered by a BV device. It is important to confirm bilateral breath sounds and the absence of sound over the stomach. The ETT is secured once confirmation of correct placement is obtained. A CXR should then be obtained to confirm the depth of the ETT.

Bougie Stylet

A bougie may be needed with either DL or VL. If the clinician is only able to get a CL view of Grade 3 or 4, a bougie may need to be employed. When the best CL has been obtained, a bougie is placed into the clinician's right hand. The clinician advances the angled end of the bougie into the larynx and watches as the bougie is advanced just under the epiglottis. With further advancement, the clinician should be able to "feel" the bougie bouncing on the tracheal rings through the vibrations of the stylet. If the clinician is

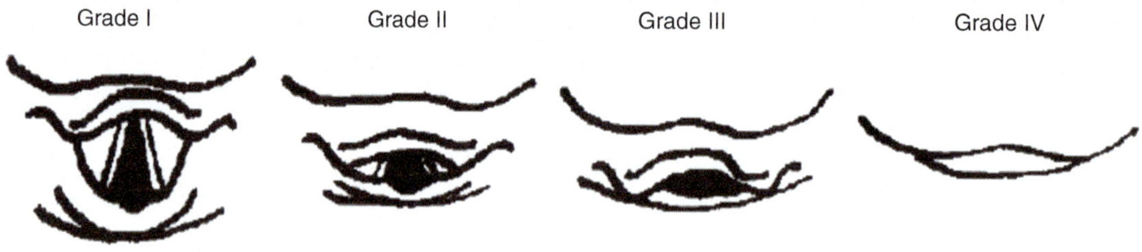

Fig. 2.11 Cormack–Lehane views of laryngoscopy. (Adapted from Samsoon and Young [19])

unable to sense this bouncing, then the bougie is most likely in the esophagus, which has no cartilaginous rings. The bougie is advanced until resistance is met.

At this point, when using DL, some clinicians elect to remove the laryngoscope, but maintaining the laryngoscope in place aids in easing the ETT placement by keeping the oral, pharyngeal, and laryngeal axes aligned. When using VL, most clinicians elect to keep the laryngoscope in place.

Regardless of whether or not the laryngoscope is used, the next step is to load a properly sized, leak-tested, and lubricated ETT onto the bougie. The ETT is advanced over the bougie using a Seldinger technique. When the ETT is unable to be advanced further, the bougie and laryngoscope (if being used) are withdrawn, while maintaining the ETT in place. Attach a BV device and confirm the presence of gas exchange by using the $ETCO_2$ and other clinical means. Assess the adequacy of bilateral breath sounds and oxygenation. If there are no left-sided breath sounds, then the ETT is likely too deep and will probably need to be withdrawn a few centimeters. When appropriate position of the ETT is confirmed, secure it in place.

Video Laryngoscopy

Dr. John Pacey introduced the Glidescope in 2001. The first academic paper was published in 2003 [44]. Since then, the use of VL for AM has skyrocketed, and its use is growing faster than other medical technologies [45]. From the ASA Practice Guidelines, over half of the clinicians surveyed strongly favor using VL on the first intubation attempt [5]. It is potential that DL will become a lost art form, similar to how automatics have largely replaced manual transmissions in cars. More than half (59%) of critical care fellowships in the United States offer specific training with VL and little training in DL [46].

VL was initially developed for difficult airways, but many clinicians are using VL for all intubations. In the OR, VL has a high frequency of success and a higher success on first pass attempts compared to DL [47]. When comparing successful intubation in emergent AM, VL was shown to be no better than DL [48].

VL does not decrease the amount of cervical spine movement compared to DL [49, 50]. In the 10th edition of the Advanced Trauma Life Support student manual, VL is an option for use by experienced providers in specific circumstances [51]. Despite a lack of evidence for improved outcome [52], many providers consider VL to be the primary AM tool for patients in a cervical collar.

Glidescope

The Glidescope (GS) is a video laryngoscope in which the hyperangulated blade design is an anatomically shaped curved blade with a 60° angle on the distal portion of the blade. There is a small camera at the tip that has an antifog feature. The blade is connected via a cable to a video screen. The GS does not use direct line of sight. The GVL is the original model, but there are several versions currently available (Fig. 2.12). There are several sizes of blades available for adult use. Size 3 is recommended to be used in a 10-kg patient to an average-sized adult. Size 4 is recommended for an average adult to morbidly obese patient. Size 5 is recommended for a large adult to morbidly obese patient, specifically "designed to accommodate anatomic anomalies sometimes associated with bariatric patients" [53].

To use the GS, carefully insert the blade into the mouth, either on the right side or more commonly in the midline. The mouth must open to at least 16 mm to accommodate the GVL. Advance the blade to the posterior oropharynx, taking care to avoid trauma to the oral structures. When the blade is in the posterior oropharynx, the operator then turns his or her attention to the video monitor. The blade is manipulated to obtain the best possible view of the glottis. Secretions, foreign bodies, or blood may obscure the view. Withdrawal of the GS and suctioning of the oropharynx may be necessary.

Once the best view of the vocal cords is obtained, the ETT is advanced into the mouth and through the vocal cords while watching the video monitor. Due to 60° angle of the distal tip of the hyperangulated blade, the stylet may need to be manipulated more than when using DL. For this

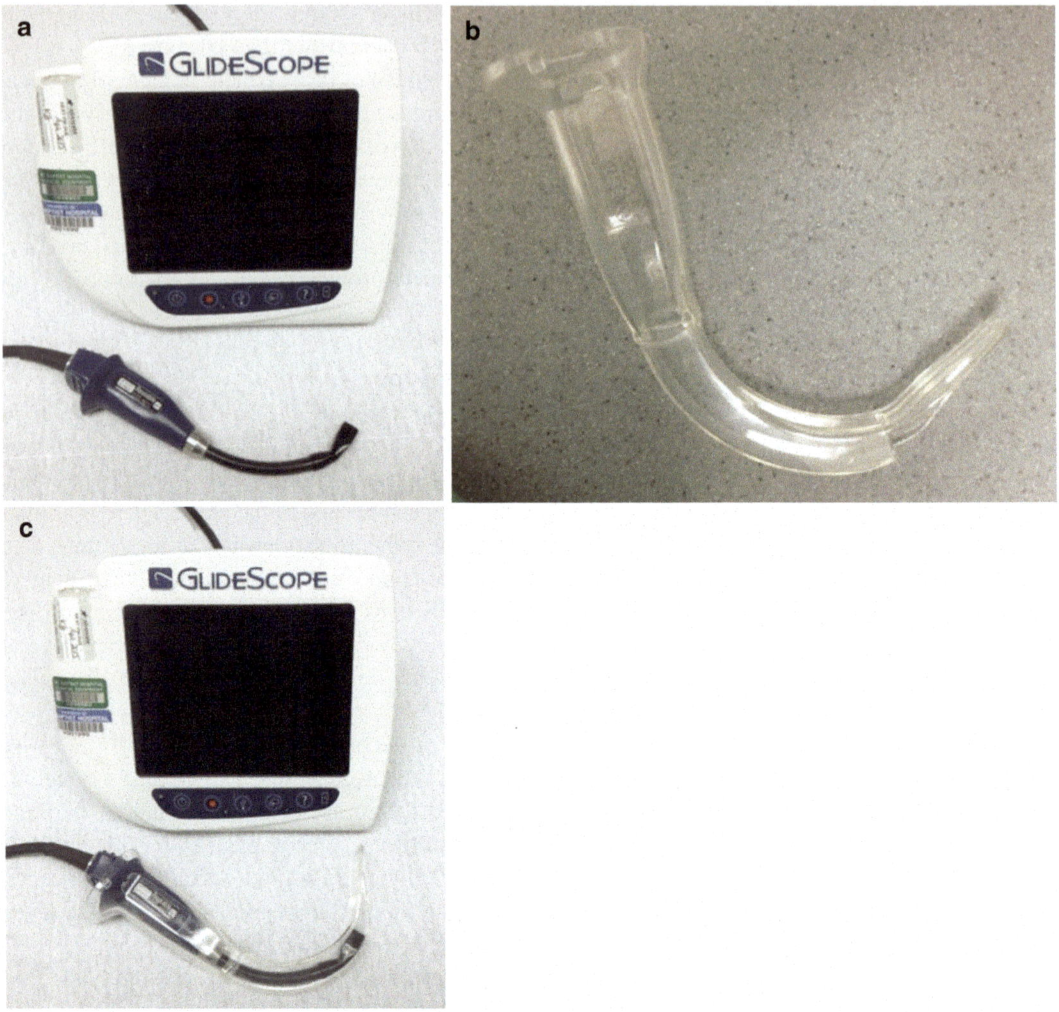

Fig. 2.12 Glidescope video laryngoscope. (**a**) AVL single-use model. (**b**) Disposable blade. (**c**) AVL with disposable blade

reason, Verathon recommends the use of their proprietary GlideRite rigid stylet (Fig. 2.13). There is some evidence that using the rigid stylet is more efficacious than using a malleable stylet in emergent AM settings [54]. Removing a rigid stylet may be difficult, so it may be necessary to have an assistant perform this part of the procedure.

After the ETT has been placed, withdraw the GS and confirm the presence of gas exchange by using the $ETCO_2$ and other clinical means. Secure the ETT once placement is confirmed.

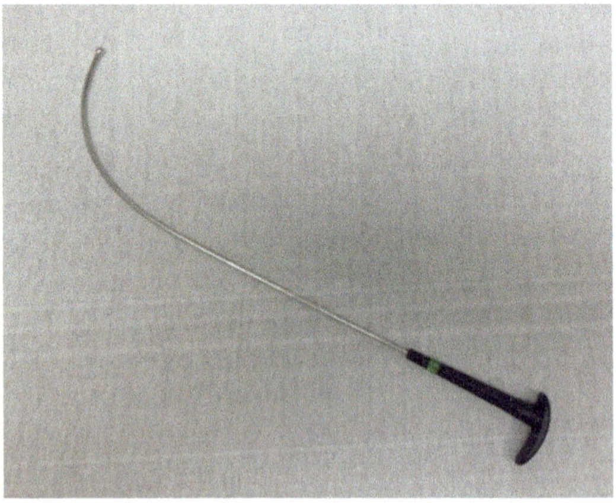

Fig. 2.13 Glidescope proprietary stylet

McGrath

The McGrath MAC enhanced direct laryngoscope (McGrath) merges the ability to perform DL or VL

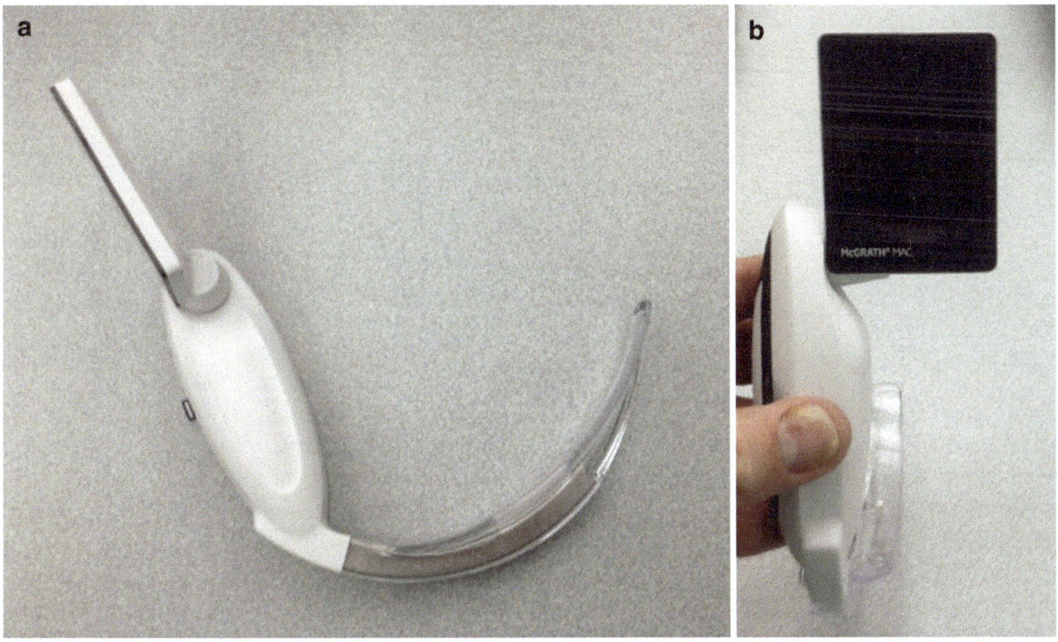

Fig. 2.14 (a, b) McGrath MAC enhanced direct laryngoscope

in one device. The device is handheld with a 2.5-inch video monitor on top of the handle (Fig. 2.14). A disposable curved blade (similar to a MacIntosh blade but more angulated) is connected such that the camera is inside the blade near the distal tip. There is only one size blade. An antifog material may need to be applied to the camera to enhance the graphics on the video monitor.

The technique for using the McGrath is the same as a curved blade for DL or as a GS for VL. After the ETT has been placed, withdraw the McGrath and confirm the presence of gas exchange by using an $ETCO_2$ and other clinical means. Secure the ETT once placement is confirmed.

C-MAC

The C MAC is a complete video laryngoscopy system, which has grown from the original device to include disposable, handheld, and fiberoptic devices. The original C-MAC is described further here. The C-MAC has the potential to be used for DL or VL. A curved blade (again, similar to a MacIntosh blade but more angulated) is attached to a handle that is connected by a cable to a video monitor. The antifog camera is inserted into the C-MAC handle. The C-MAC is available in multiple traditional blade sizes for adults. Currently, the C-MAC straight blades are only available in pediatric sizes.

The C-MAC is inserted and used just like a regular curved. After the ETT has been placed, withdraw the C-MAC and confirm the presence of gas exchange by using an $ETCO_2$ and other clinical means. Secure the ETT once placement is confirmed.

There is a potential training benefit of using the C-MAC. Due to the size of the video monitor, a trainee can use the C-MAC for DL and a supervisor is able to see what the trainee sees and offer guidance to improve technique. In a retrospective study of ED intubations, the C-MAC was shown to have better first-pass success compared to DL [55].

Fiberoptic Intubation

A flexible fiberoptic bronchoscope (FOB) is another method of VL that has a role in emergent AM. One of the biggest benefits of FOB for intubation is its use in an awake patient who poses an increased risk of a difficult airway if put to sleep

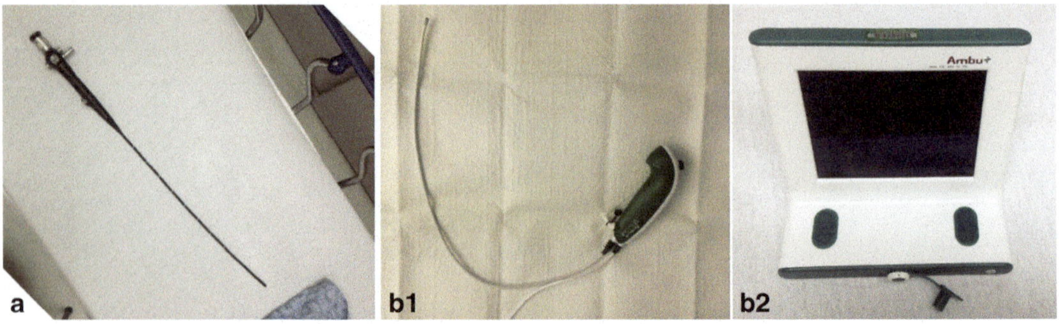

Fig. 2.15 (**a**) Fiberoptic scope with eyepiece. (**b**) 1–2. Fiberoptic scope with video monitor

for AM. FOB can also be used in patients who have unstable neck trauma. In patients with significant angioedema, nasal FOB is a good alternative to a surgical airway.

There are different FOB sizes and types (Fig. 2.15). Some have suction capabilities, while others do not. Some FOBs use an eyepiece, while others are attached to or only have a video monitor. It is important to use a FOB that will allow the use of an appropriately sized ETT. Depending on the manufacturer, a water-soluble lubricant may be placed on the FOB to help with passing the ETT off the FOB into the trachea.

The use of FOB in the ED is often restricted due to either a presumed emergent airway or familiarity with the equipment. Most AM situations in the ED or ICU are urgent, not emergent. Learning how to use a FOB is not complicated, but the process takes finesse and should not be rushed. FOB should be practiced on patients who are not predicted to have difficult airways. The skill requires experience and once mastered is an excellent resource for difficult AM.

To maximize the chances of success with FOB, it is important to prepare the patient properly. The patient may either be in a supine or an upright position. If supine, the FOB operator stands either at the head or to the side of the bed. If upright, the FOB operator stands to the side of the patient. An antisialogogue is recommended in an effort to minimize secretions. An ovassapian airway (Fig. 2.16) is a type of OPA that displaces the tongue and provides a channel through which the FOB and ETT may be passed. A Berman airway or a Williams airway are two other OPAs through which a fiberoptic scope can be passed. If none of these specialized airways are available, have an assistant grasp the tongue with gauze and pull it forward. A jaw thrust maneuver will also facilitate intubation.

To operate the scope, place one hand approximately 8–10 cm from the tip at the distal end of the FOB and the other hand on the control end. The control end will have a lever that flexes and retroflexes the distal end of the scope. The FOB will only move up and down. To move the FOB sideways, the clinician must rotate his or her wrist and shoulder as one unit. Perhaps the most important step to take to maximize success with FOB is to remember to always keep the scope taught. If the FOB is not mildly taught, whenever the operator twists his or her hand to twist the distal end, the distal end will not twist. Laxity in the FOB leads to the scope being twisted on itself like a snake or wet spaghetti.

For oral FOB, insert the scope into the mouth. Once the tip is beyond the back of the tongue, use the control end to bend the tip to follow the natural curvature of the airway. The tip will either be flexed if standing at the head of the bed or retroflexed if standing to the side of the patient. Continue advancing the scope in the midline until the operator's distal hand contacts the patient's mouth. At this point, the operator should focus attention on the eyepiece or video screen. The vocal cords should be in view. Avoid the temptation to "look around" to try to find the vocal cords unless the operator is confident that he or she is in the larynx. Too often, if the cords are not in view, the scope is in the esophagus. Withdraw the scope and try again. It may be necessary to place the distal hand closer to the tip of the FOB.

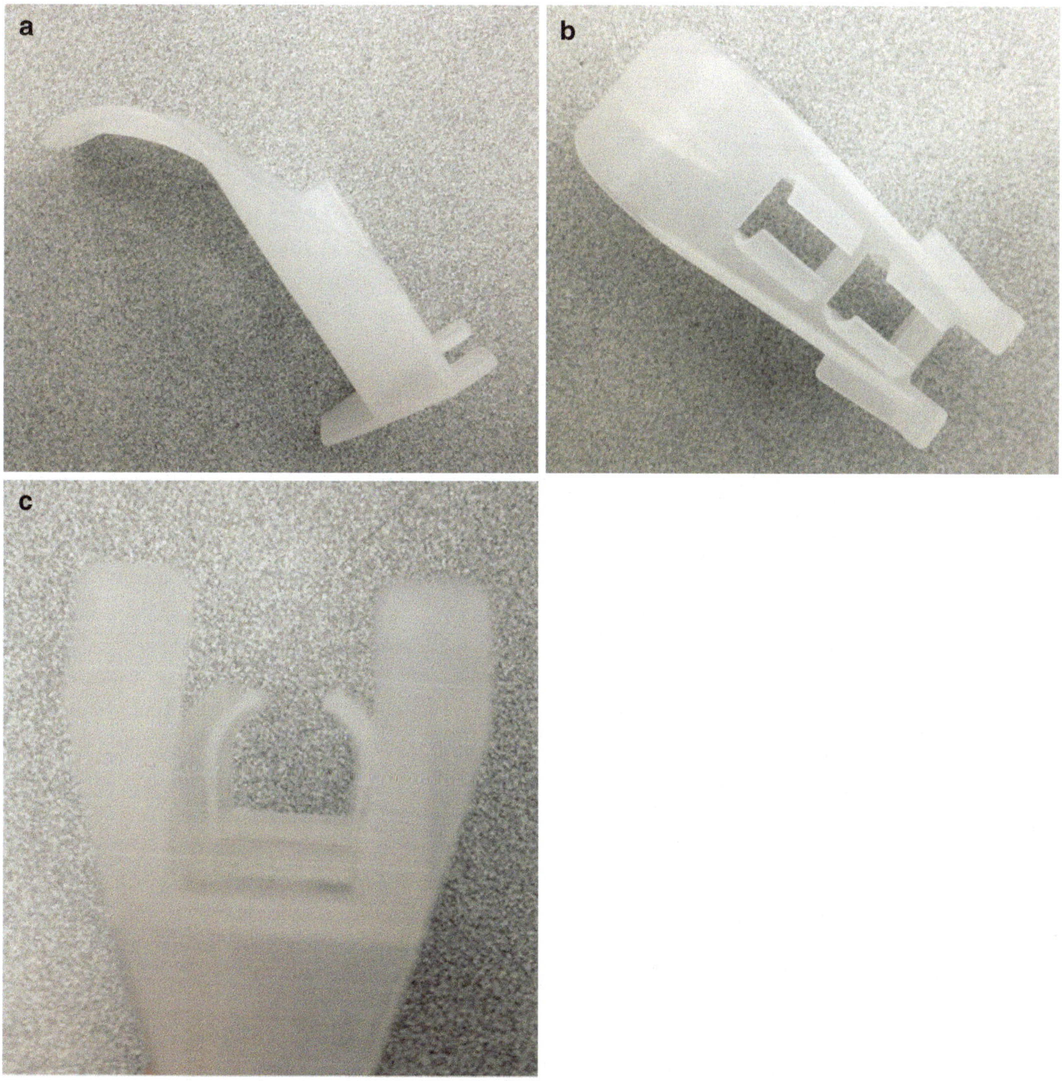

Fig. 2.16 (a–c) Ovassapian airway

For nasal FOB, insert the scope into the largest nare. Advance the FOB into the nasal passages. Once the operator's hand comes into contact with the patient's nose, look through the eyepiece or video screen. The tip should be in the posterior pharynx a few centimeters above the vocal cords. It may be necessary to flex (or retroflex depending on the operator's position relative to the patient) mildly to see the vocal cords.

With either technique, once the vocal cords are identified, advance the FOB by pulling the scope into the airway with the hand on the distal end, instead of pushing the FOB with the hand on the control end. Advancement of the scope should be done with deliberate action instead of slowly. If done slowly, there is a significant chance that the scope will contact the vocal cords and induce coughing, especially in a spontaneously breathing patient who is not fully anesthetized.

Once the FOB tip has been pulled into the trachea, advance the scope to the mid trachea or until the carina is visualized. At this point, hold the FOB in place and slide the ETT off the scope and slowly into position. Occasionally, the ETT will get caught up on redundant tissue in the larynx (especially if the patient is heavily sedated) or the vocal cords. If this occurs, gently rotate the ETT 90° and try to advance the ETT again. If this does not correct the situation, the ETT may be too big and a smaller size needs to be used.

When the ETT is in the trachea, use the FOB to confirm placement. Withdraw the FOB while an assistant holds the ETT in place. When the FOB has been removed, confirm the presence of gas exchange by using an $ETCO_2$ and other clinical means and then secure the ETT.

Supraglottic Airway Devices

In the ED and ICU, supraglottic airway devices are mainly used as a backup when the clinician is unable to place the ETT. SGAs are beneficial in situations in which the provider is not able to mask ventilate or oxygenate a patient [56]. Many prehospital emergency medical services place an SGA instead of an ETT. An SGA is not considered a definitive airway, so it is necessary to exchange an SGA for a tube in the trachea.

When performing an airway examination, it is important to identify conditions that may be associated with difficulty placing an SGA. The most prominent finding is a restricted mouth opening. If the SGA cannot fit into the oropharynx, then it cannot be placed appropriately. If there is an obstruction of the airway, then the obstruction must be removed before an SGA will function properly. Along those lines, SGA placement may be difficult in morbidly obese patients due to the amount of redundant tissue in the hypopharynx.

There are many different types of SGAs on the market. Some are disposable. Second generation SGAs allow an ETT to be passed through the SGA into the trachea. Some have two potential ventilation tubes. When inflated, SGAs form a seal around the hypopharynx. All SGAs function by forcing air into the trachea without actually having a tube in the trachea. Not all SGAs occlude the esophagus, so the clinician must always be aware of the potential for reflux and aspiration of gastric contents.

Laryngeal Mask Airway

The first version of the LMA marketed commercially is the LMA Classic. There are other versions now available. See Fig. 2.17, for example. These have slight modifications to the design. All LMAs are inserted in a similar fashion. An appropriate size LMA should be selected depending on the patient's weight. Adult sizes are #3 for patients 30–50 kg, #4 for patients 50–70 kg, and #5 for patients 70–100 kg. An LMA Classic is available for patients weighing >100 kg. If unsure about the patient's weight, it is advised to select the larger size.

Similar to an ETT, it is necessary to inflate the mask to ensure that there are no leaks. Next, remove all air from the mask and make sure that the tip is not folded over. Placing the LMA on a flat surface and applying a mild downward pressure as air is removed from the mask may help prevent the tip from folding over. This action will also help minimize wrinkles in the cuff.

Apply a water-soluble lubricant to both sides of the mask. Open the patient's airway and lift the

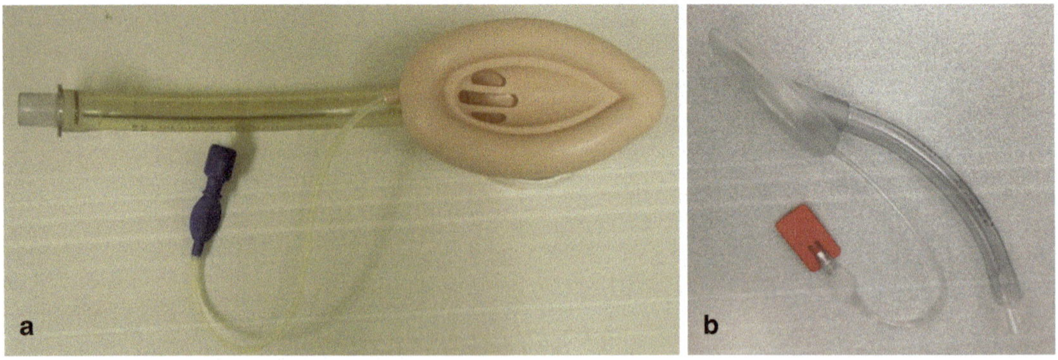

Fig. 2.17 Laryngeal mask airway (LMA): (**a**) Classic. (**b**) Unique

patient's jaw. With the tube side of the mask superiorly position, insert the LMA into the midline of the mouth and advance the mask along the hard palate and to the hypopharynx as far as possible. Cricoid pressure may make placement more difficult. When it is not possible to advance any more, inflate the LMA with air: 20 ml for a #3, 30 ml for a #4, and 40 ml for a #5. As the mask inflates, the LMA will seat itself into position over the larynx.

To minimize cuff leak, make sure that the tube portion of the LMA is in the midline of the mouth and that the head and neck are in a neutral position. If a cuff leak persists, it may be necessary to deflate the cuff, remove the LMA completely, and reinsert the LMA again. If the second insertion does not correct the problem, move to a different size, with the first choice being one size larger if possible.

Laryngospasm or the epiglottis occluding the trachea may cause obstruction of the LMA. In the case of suspected laryngospasm, the provider should attempt to bag the patient through the problem. Use paralytics with extreme caution, especially if the LMA is being placed as a backup airway device. In the case of an epiglottis obstructing the trachea, it may be necessary to remove the LMA and attempt reinsertion.

Once the LMA is properly positioned, attach a BV device and confirm the presence of gas exchange by using an $ETCO_2$ and other clinical means. Secure the LMA in place with tape once placement is confirmed.

It is possible to place an ETT through newer versions of the LMA. The different versions of LMAs have different maximum regular ETTs that can be used. It is recommended to use a FOB to accomplish ETT placement through a non-LMA-Fastrach.

Laryngeal Mask Airway-Fastrach

The LMA-Fastrach, also known as an intubating LMA (I-LMA) (Fig. 2.18), was also developed by Dr. Brain. The I-LMA has a different shape from the LMA Classic. The basis for the design came from MRI images of 50 normal subjects whose heads were in the neutral position [57]. The version with a metal handle may be reused 40 times. The version with the plastic handle is disposable. The Fastrach is available in sizes 3, 4, and 5, which correspond to the same sizes as a regular LMA.

The I-LMA is placed in a similar fashion to other LMAs. Because of the handle, it is often easier to place an I-LMA. Placement confirmation is also similar to other LMA products. Once the I-LMA has been appropriately positioned and oxygenation has been maximized, it is recommended to place an ETT to obtain a definitive airway. There are a few different options for placing an ETT through the I-LMA.

The first option of placing an ETT is done blindly with the wire reinforced ETT and stabilizing rod designed specifically for I-LMAs. The wire reinforced ETT has a distal cuff that conforms to the tube when deflated. This feature allows for the ETT to more easily pass

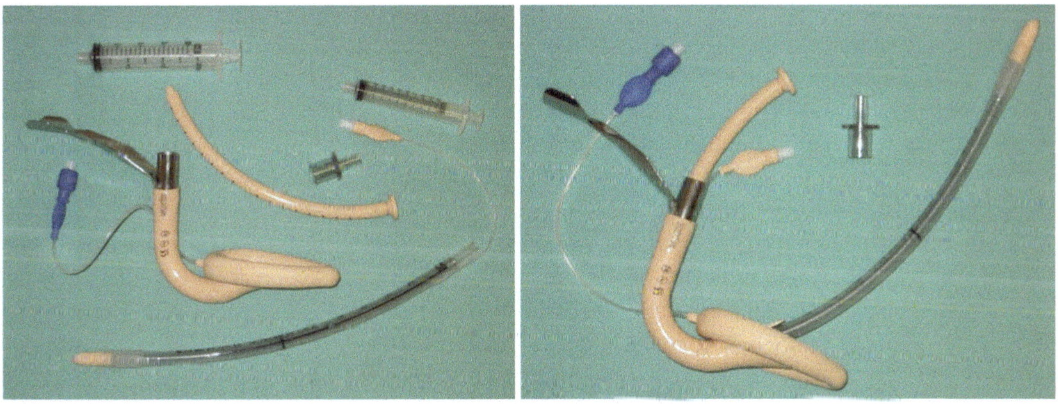

Fig. 2.18 LMA Fastrach. (**a**) LMA Fastrach and syringe, along with wire rimmed ETT, 15mm adapter, syringe, and stabilizing rod. (**b**) Wire rimmed ETT through LMA Fastrach with stabilizing rod in place simulating what the process of ETT placment looks like

through the I-LMA, especially compared to a regular ETT that has a balloon cuff that may get hung up on something as it passes through the I-LMA.

It is important to have the maximum airflow and least amount of resistance possible to ensure easy passage of the tube. There are many different named maneuvers that aim to achieve optimal airflow [58]. The Chandy maneuver, which is probably the most known, has two steps. First, maneuver the I-LMA ever so slightly in a coronal or sagittal plane. When the operator feels that the maximum airflow position has been achieved, the I-LMA is held in that plane and lifted up. This second step lifts the mask off of the posterior pharynx and allows for the ETT to be passed more easily. Use caution with disposable I-LMAs, as the plastic handle has the potential to break since it is not able to lift with as much force as a metal handle.

At this point, the clinician inserts the ETT. To place the wire reinforced ETT, apply a water-soluble lubricant to the ETT and test the cuff for leaks. There may be a bit of resistance as the tube must push through the epiglottic elevating bar, a piece of silicon in the midline of the mask aperture. It may be difficult to tell the depth of the ETT because the centimeter depth markings on the ETT are covered by the metal tube of the I-LMA. This problem does not occur if using the disposable Fastrach. When the tube has been inserted to an adequate depth, inflate the cuff and attach a BV device and confirm the presence of gas exchange by using an $ETCO_2$ and other clinical means.

After confirmation that the ETT is in the trachea and the patient is maximally oxygenated, it is necessary to remove the I-LMA. Optimally, the patient would be hemodynamically stable and maximally oxygenated before this step. Removing the I-LMA has inherent risk due to the possibility of dislodging the ETT and losing the patient's airway. It would be advantageous to have an assistant that is familiar with this process at bedside, as there is some level of dexterity required.

To remove the I-LMA, deflate the I-LMA cuff completely. Ensure that the cuff on the ETT is inflated. Remove the 15-mm adapter from the proximal end of the ETT. Place the stabilizing rod into the proximal end of the ETT. The pilot balloon for the ETT should be in the same hand (often the provider's nondominant hand) as that which is holding the stabilizing rod. The provider may choose to continue holding the rod/ETT or have an assistant take over. Slowly withdraw the I-LMA from the mouth over the ETT and stabilizing rod (often done with the provider's dominant hand). As the I-LMA is being withdrawn from the mouth, look for the ETT coming through the epiglottic elevating bar.

When the ETT is visualized, move the hand holding the stabilizing rod/ETT to the mouth and secure the ETT at that position in the mouth. Continue withdrawing the I-LMA until the ETT and stabilizing rod are completely clear of the mask. At this point, remove the stabilizing rod and place the 15-mm adapter back into the proximal end of the ETT. Attach a BV device with an $ETCO_2$ detector and use any other modality to confirm placement into the trachea. Once position is confirmed, the wire rimmed ETT can be either secured and used or exchanged for a regular ETT. If the wire rimmed ETT is used, there is a risk that the patient will bite down and clamp the ETT. If this occurs, the ETT will not go back to its normal shape because the wire will be bent and hold its shape and there is the risk of poor gas exchange.

Instead of blindly inserting the ETT, another option is to place a regular ETT by using a FOB. Lubricate the inside and outside of an appropriately sized ETT (up to 8.0 mm) and then place it onto a FOB. The ETT is placed the same as any other FOB intubation. Once tube position is confirmed, and the FOB has been withdrawn, it is necessary to remove the I-LMA.

When removing the I-LMA over a regular ETT, the stabilizing rod is not specifically designed for this type of ETT, so there is the potential for malposition of the rod. The cuff of a regular ETT will also be larger than the cuff on a wire reinforced ETT specifically designed for I-LMAs, so there is the potential that the ETT may be withdrawn from the airway.

In an effort to minimize the chances of dislodging the ETT from the airway, the FOB itself may be used to guide removal of the I-LMA via a Seldinger technique. Once the ETT position has been confirmed via the FOB and the ETT cuff is inflated, fully deflate the I-LMA cuff. Have an assistant hold the ETT in place. Remove the 15-mm adapter from the proximal end of the ETT and slide it to the proximal end of the FOB. Hold the FOB in place. Slowly withdraw the I-LMA from the mouth. As it is removed, the I-LMA will cover the proximal end of the ETT and slide toward the proximal end of the FOB. When the distal end of the ETT is visualized in the mouth as the mask is removed, the assistant secures the ETT at that position.

Once the I-LMA is completely out of the mouth, use the FOB to confirm that the ETT is still in the trachea. When ETT position has been confirmed, remove the FOB completely from the ETT. Remove the I-LMA and 15-mm adapter from the FOB and place the 15-mm adapter onto the proximal end of the ETT. Attach a BV device and confirm the presence of gas exchange by using an $ETCO_2$ and other clinical means. Secure the ETT once placement is confirmed.

i-gel

The i-gel is an SGA that does not use an inflatable cuff. Instead, the i-gel uses a noninflated cuff made of a gel-like material that rests on the laryngeal structures. Like any other component of AM, it is important to use the proper size. The i-gel comes in pediatric and adult sizes. Adult sizes are #3 for patients 30–60 kg, #4 for patients 50–90 kg, and #5 for patients >90 kg. If unsure about the patient's weight, it is advised to select the larger size.

The patient should be in a sniffing position or with the head tilted and chin lifted. Apply lubricant to all sides of the i-gel. The company recommends gentle pressure on the chin as the i-gel is inserted in the midline along the hard palate [59]. Continue advancing until continuous resistance is encountered. The patient's teeth should be at the black horizontal line, which is the bite block portion on the i-gel. At this point, the i-gel should be in its proper position and care must be taken to avoid dislodging it. Once the i-gel is properly positioned, attach a BV device and confirm the presence of gas exchange by using the $ETCO_2$ and other clinical means. Secure the i-gel in place with tape once placement is confirmed.

It is possible to place an ETT through an i-gel. A #3 i-gel will accommodate up to a 6.0-mm ETT, a #4 i-gel up to a 7.0-mm ETT, and a #5 i-gel up to an 8.0-mm ETT. To place an ETT through an i-gel, use a FOB and the same technique for placement of an ETT through an I-LMA.

Air-Q

The air-Q is another commercially available SGA that is available for AM. air-Q comes in a disposable or reusable (up to 60 times) version. There is a version with a self-pressurizing mask and a version that has an inflatable mask. It is possible to place an ETT through any air-Q. Adult and pediatric sizes are available. Adult sizes are #2.5 for patients 20–50 kg, #3.5 for patients 50–70 kg, and #4.5 for patients 70–100 kg. If unsure about the patient's weight, it is advised to select the larger size. There are minimum mouth apertures for the different sizes: 20 mm for #2.5, 23 mm for #3.5, and 25 mm for #4.5.

To place an air-Q, place the patient in a sniffing position or a head-tilt/chin-lift position. Lubricate the anterior and posterior portions of the mask. Perform a jaw lift or use a tongue blade to maximize ease of insertion. Insert the air-Q in the midline into the pharynx and advance it along the palate to the base of the tongue in an inward and downward motion. Continue advancing until resistance prohibits further advancement. At this point, the air-Q should be in position. Inflate the mask: 2–3 ml for a #2.5, 3–4 ml for a #3.5, and 4–5 ml for a #4.5 [60]. After mask inflation, attach a BV device and confirm the presence of gas exchange by using an $ETCO_2$ and other clinical means. Secure the air-Q in place with tape once placement is confirmed.

To place an ETT through an air-Q, either a FOB or a blind insertion with a bougie may be used. If using a FOB, the technique is similar to the placement of an ETT through other SGAs previously mentioned. For a blind technique, insert a bougie into the air-Q and advance it slowly. The provider places a hand on the patient's cricoid membrane and "feels" the bougie as it is advanced into the trachea, bouncing on the tracheal rings. With the other hand, the provider should attempt to feel the tracheal rings through the vibrations in the bougie as it is advanced. When the bougie meets resistance, deflate the air-Q and withdraw it from the pharynx and over the bougie, making sure to hold the bougie in place. Place an ETT on the bougie and advance it via Seldinger technique into the trachea. Once the ETT is inserted to an appropriate depth, remove the bougie and secure the ETT manually. Once the bougie has been removed, attach a BV device and confirm the presence of gas exchange by using an $ETCO_2$ and other clinical means. When appropriate position of the ETT is confirmed, secure it in place.

Combitube

The Combitube is a blind insertion SGA which consists of two tubes that are connected at the distal end and separate at the proximal end. There are two sizes available based on patient height: 37 Fr for patients 48–66″ and 41 Fr for patients >60″. A 15-mm adapter is attached to the proximal end of each tube. One tube is blue and is longer than the other tube which is clear. The blue tube is labeled "1," and the clear tube is labeled "2." Each tube has a balloon with a number that corresponds to the tube number. The balloon on tube 1 holds 85 ml for the 37-Fr size or 100 ml for the 41-Fr size. The balloon on tube 2 is smaller and holds 15 ml of air.

Before insertion, test both balloons to assess for a leak. Lubricate from the distal end of the tube to the base of the larger balloon. Place the patient so that the head is in a neutral position. While lifting the patient's jaw and tongue, grasp the Combitube like a pencil just distal to the two black circumferential lines and insert the Combitube in the midline into the pharynx. Continue advancing until the patient's upper incisors are between the two black circumferential lines. Advancement of the Combitube may take a moderate amount of force, since it usually goes into the esophagus and must traverse the upper esophageal sphincter.

Once the Combitube is in place, inflate the #1 cuff with either 85 or 100 ml of air (depending on the size of the Combitube). If the distal tube is in the esophagus, the large cuff (#1) should seat itself in the oral cavity and prevent air leakage during ventilation. Inflate the #2 cuff with 15 ml of air which will prevent air from leaking out of the trachea (if the tube is there) or from being pushed into the stomach (if the tube is in the esophagus).

After the two cuffs have been properly inflated, connect a BV device to the blue #1 tube and begin ventilation. If the distal tube is in the esophagus (the vast majority of cases), during ventilation, air passes down the #1 tube and out of the tube through several side ports and into the trachea. The distal tip of tube #1 is occluded. Use an $ETCO_2$ detector and any other modality to confirm gas exchange. If unable to confirm oxygenation through the blue #1 tube, attach the BV device to the clear #2 tube and assess for oxygenation through ventilation of that tube.

If adequate oxygenation still cannot be confirmed through either tube, the Combitube is likely too distal in the esophagus. Deflate the distal cuff fully and the proximal large cuff approximately 50% and withdraw the Combitube 1–2 cm. Inflate both cuffs fully. Attach the BV device to the blue #1 tube and begin ventilation and reattempt to confirm gas exchange.

If oxygenation is confirmed through tube #1, the Combitube is in the esophagus. A suction tube can be placed through tube #2 into the stomach to remove gastric contents. If oxygenation is confirmed through tube #2, the Combitube is in the trachea and is functioning like a regular ETT. Regardless of placement location, once the patient has been stabilized, it is recommended to exchange the Combitube for a regular ETT. If the Combitube is already in the trachea, it can be exchanged with a tube exchanger. If the Combitube is in the esophagus, there is no way to exchange it for a definitive airway. The Combitube must be completely removed in order to perform laryngoscopy to place a definitive airway.

King Laryngeal Tube

The King Laryngeal Tube (King) is a blindly inserted SGA with one tube and two balloons. Kings are available from newborn to adult, and each size corresponds to a different colored 15-mm adapter. An appropriately sized King should be selected depending on the patient's height. Adult sizes are #3 for patients 4–5 feet (122–155 cm), #4 for patients 5–6 feet (155–180 cm), and #5 for patients >6 feet (180 cm). If unsure about the patient's height, it is advised to select the larger size. There is a reusable version and a version that allows gastric access.

Prior to placement, inflate the balloons to assess for any leaks. Although there are two balloons, there is only one syringe port. After testing for leaks, lubricate the distal tip. With the patient supine and the head in a neutral position, lift the tongue and jaw and insert the King into the lateral aspect of the mouth. While advancing the King along the hard palate and toward the base of the tongue, move the distal portion of the King toward the midline of the oropharynx. Continue advancing the King until the distal portion of the 15-mm adapter is aligned with the patient's teeth (or gums if edentulous). Inflate the cuff depending on the size of the King: 50 ml for a #3, 70 ml for a #4, and 80 ml for a #5.

Once the balloons are inflated, attach a BV device and confirm the presence of gas exchange by using an $ETCO_2$ and other clinical means. Assess the adequacy of bilateral breath sounds and oxygenation. The King will likely need to be withdrawn 1–3 cm to achieve a position in which ventilation is easy and without much resistance. It may also be necessary to adjust the volume in the cuff to ensure a proper seal in the hypopharynx. Once the King is in its proper position, secure it in place with tape.

After the patient has been stabilized, it is recommended to place an ETT. It is possible to exchange a King directly to an ETT. This may be done with a bougie or a pediatric exchange catheter. Lubricate the catheter and advance it into the King. The catheter should go through the ventilation channel and into the trachea. Once this happens, deflate the King and withdraw it over the catheter. At this point, the process is just like any other ETT exchange. See section "Endotracheal Tube Exchange."

Surgical Airway

A surgical airway is the final option in any AM algorithm. The need for a surgical airway is a rarity, but a surgical airway is associated with high morbidity and mortality. A surgical airway is essentially always an emergency and a high anxiety situation. A cricothyrotomy (crich) is the procedure of choice for an emergent surgical airway. A crich can be performed in less than 30 seconds [61]. A tracheotomy takes too long to perform in an emergency, and there is a higher risk of bleeding, injuries, and long-term complications compared to a crich [62]. Commercial kits are available for either a scalpel incision or a needle crich. Some kits have the necessary equipment to perform either procedure.

The most difficult part of placing a surgical airway is to make the decision to do it. It is possible to limit the amount of anxiety by always being prepared for a surgical airway. It is important to integrate examining the CTM as part of the airway examination. In doing so, the clinician increases his or her familiarity with the CTM location and will know exactly where on the neck to perform the procedure.

There are some findings that may be associated with difficulty performing a crich. If these findings are present, it may be useful to have assistants who are trained in AM available. If the patient has a history of a mass, tumor, or prior radiation or surgery to the neck, the normal anatomy may be distorted and it may be difficult to perform a crich. Similarly, if the patient is obese or there is a significant amount of edema, hematoma, or subcutaneous air in the neck or submental area, a crich may be difficult. It is important to recognize these findings and incorporate them into the AM plan individualized for the patient.

Needle Cricothyrotomy

A needle cricothyrotomy is a temporizing procedure utilized to oxygenate a patient until an alternative method is available. A needle crich can be performed on any aged patient. Multiple companies manufacture needle crich kits that have all of the components necessary to perform the procedure. Some of the more common kits are the QuickTrach kit, the Portex kit, and the Pertrach kit.

To perform a needle crich, locate the CTM with the nondominant hand. Clean the area appropriately. Attach a 14- or 16-gauge intravenous catheter to a syringe. An 18-gauge intravenous cannula is recommended if the patient is less than 12 years old. Insert the needle through the CTM. Once the "pop" of the membrane is felt, aspirate air. If air is aspirated, advance the catheter through the membrane and aiming caudad toward the carina. Remove the needle and syringe, while keeping the catheter in place. If air is not aspirated, it is possible that the needle is either too deep, too shallow or off of the midline. Reposition the needle as necessary or withdraw completely and reinsert.

Firmly hold the catheter flange and attach a jet ventilation system. If a jet system is not available, attach a 3-ml syringe to the catheter and remove the plunger. Insert a 15-mm adapter from a 7.0 ETT into the cavity of the syringe. When either a jet or a syringe setup is in place, give the patient short positive-pressure breaths with 100% FiO_2 oxygen. It is important to watch for subcutaneous air or any other sign of barotrauma. It is highly likely that the patient will become hypercarbic due to the limited ability to exhale.

An alternative AM plan should be implemented quickly, as this method of oxygenation is only a temporary solution at best. It is relatively easy for the catheter to become dislodged or obstructed. Once the patient has been appropriately oxygenated and adequate resources are available, it is recommended that a definitive airway be placed.

Surgical Cricothyrotomy

A surgical cricothyrotomy differs from a needle crich in that an incision is made into the neck. The clinician does not have to be a surgeon to perform a surgical crich. Clinicians that perform AM should be proficient in this procedure. Surgical crichs should not be performed on patients less than 12 years old.

To perform a surgical crich, clean the area appropriately. Make a 1- to 2-cm scalpel incision in the skin. Conventionally, a vertical incision is used, but there is no evidence to recommend using a horizontal or vertical cut for the skin incision. Palpate the CTM, which may be obscured by blood or tissue. It may be necessary to use manual skin retractor(s). Once the CTM is identified, make a 1-cm horizontal scalpel incision in the CTM. The CTM incision may then be dilated by the back of the scalpel blade or a Trousseau dilator (Fig. 2.19). A tracheal hook (Fig. 2.20) may be needed to lift the distal portion of the airway.

A 4.0–6.0 Shiley is then placed into the trachea. A trach tube is easier to insert in a surgical

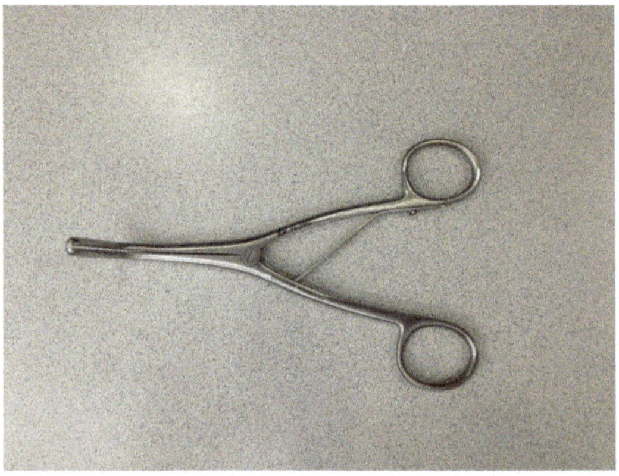

Fig. 2.19 Trousseau dilator

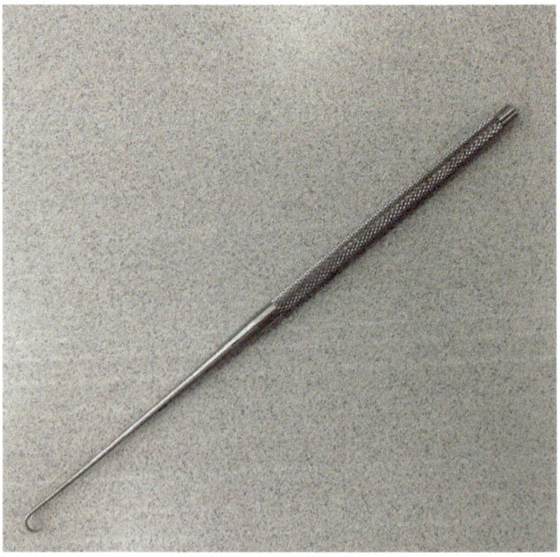

Fig. 2.20 Tracheal hook

airway than an ETT for several reasons. Trach tubes have smaller outer diameters and are more rigid than ETTs. An obturator may be used to facilitate trach tube insertion. Trach tubes are shorter and easier to suction. If a trach tube is not available, a 4.0–6.0 ETT may be used instead. Once a tube is in the trachea, manually hold it in place and inflate the balloon. Attach a BV device and confirm the presence of gas exchange by using an $ETCO_2$ and other clinical means. Secure the trach tube once placement is confirmed.

Regardless of what type of crich is performed, when the patient's oxygenation has been stabilized, the patient will need to have the crich changed to a tracheostomy. The tracheostomy should be performed within 72 hours, yet most clinicians elect to have this done as soon as the patient is stable enough to undergo the procedure.

Melker makes a crich kit (Fig. 2.21), which includes all of the equipment necessary for either a needle or surgical crich. For those clinicians who are more comfortable performing a surgical crich, the kit comes with a scalpel, a Trousseau dilator, and a tracheal hook. For clinicians who are more comfortable with a needle crich, there is the option of using a Seldinger technique to place a 5-mm trach tube instead of an 18-gauge catheter in the airway.

For the needle crich, a skin incision can be made but is not a necessity. If a skin incision is made, then the 18-gauge needle connected to the 12-ml syringe is placed directly into the CTM. If there is no skin incision, the needle is placed percutaneously into the CTM. Once in the airway, the syringe is removed from the needle. The Amplatz 0.38″ wire is placed through the 18-gauge needle advanced into the trachea. Using a Seldinger technique, the needle is removed and the blunt dilator is introduced into the trachea. The blunt dilator is then removed and inserted into the 5-mm trach tube. The dilator/trach tube is then inserted via Seldinger technique into the trachea. The wire and blunt dilator are then removed. At this point, attach a BV device and confirm the presence of gas exchange by using an $ETCO_2$ and other clinical means. Secure the trach tube once placement is confirmed.

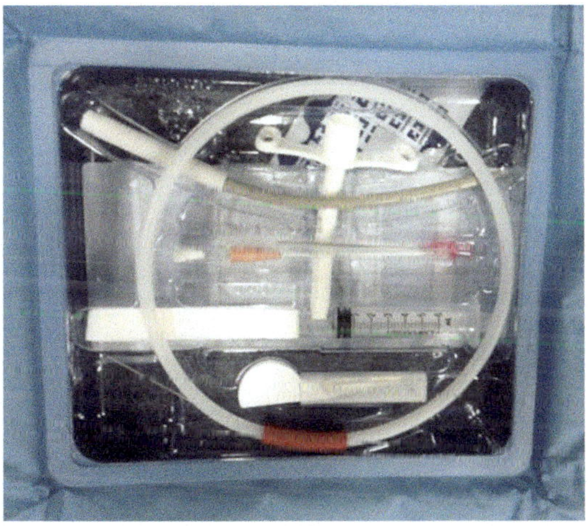

Fig. 2.21 Melker cricothyrotomy kit

Endotracheal Tube Exchange

Endotracheal tube exchange is a high-risk procedure and should be performed with all necessary resources because there is the potential to lose the patient's airway. There are several reasons for which an ETT may need to be exchanged. If the cuff or pilot balloon has a leak, the patient may not receive adequate tidal volumes. If the ETT is too small, the peak inspiratory pressures may be too high. It may not be possible to perform bronchoscopy through a small ETT.

Prior to ETT exchange, make sure that the patient is hemodynamically stable. If the patient has a functioning airway, there is rarely a need to exchange it emergently. Gather resources and personnel necessary to complete the exchange. While there is no evidence to support this practice, it is recommended to sedate and paralyze the patient prior to ETT exchange. With the patient sedated and paralyzed, there is less of a chance of the patient accidently coughing or moving and having the ETT become dislodged.

With the patient adequately sedated, paralyzed, and oxygenated, remove the securing mechanism for the ETT. A laryngoscope may be utilized to facilitate the procedure. Place an airway exchange catheter (AEC) into the ETT. A bougie or Aintree catheter may be used, but a Cook exchange catheter is specifically designed for ETT exchange and comes in several different sizes, from pediatric to adult. Advance the AEC until continuous resistance is met, which is usually a few centimeters longer than the length of the ETT to the teeth. Withdraw the old ETT from the patient's trachea while holding the AEC in place at the distal end. When the ETT has cleared the mouth, secure the AEC at that location and withdraw the old ETT completely from the AEC. Now, place the new ETT on to the AEC and advance the ETT to the patient's mouth. At this point, grab the distal end of the AEC and advance the ETT completely into the trachea.

When the ETT is in place, attach a BV device and confirm the presence of gas exchange by using an $ETCO_2$ and other clinical means. Assess the adequacy of bilateral breath sounds and oxygenation. The new ETT is likely too deep and will probably need to be withdrawn a few centimeters. When appropriate position of the new ETT is confirmed, secure it in place.

Conclusions

Airway management is more than putting a tube into the trachea. The process of airway management begins with evaluating a patient's clinical status and need for mechanical ventilation. The process continues with a physical examination and more importantly, an airway examination. The next step is to develop an initial and at least one backup plan for airway manipulation. Before beginning the actual procedure, it is important to prepare for all possible scenarios. The most crucial step is the actual placement of a tube into the trachea, but management does not stop there. It ends with conformation of tube placement and a return to pre-management hemodynamics.

This chapter does not cover every potential tool for AM, and a clinician will not become an expert or even proficient in AM just by reading the chapter. AM is a skill that is learned and developed over a significant period of time dealing with multiple different clinical scenarios. The best place to learn the basics of AM is the OR in a controlled atmosphere where there is ample time and the patient is usually not acutely decompensating, not the ED or the ICU where AM is usually urgent or emergent due to the patient's illness severity. Once the basics have been mastered, the clinician can build upon that knowledge in other clinical arenas, such as the ED or ICU. But, the clinician should not stop there. AM is a lifelong learning process that must be practiced and updated continuously.

References

1. Martin LD, Mhyre JM, Shanks AM, Tremper KK, Kheterpal S. 3,423 emergency tracheal intubations at a university hospital: airway outcomes and complications. Anesthesiology. 2011;114:42–8.
2. Benedetto WJ, et al. Urgent tracheal intubation in general hospital units: an observational study. J Clin Anesth. 2007;19:20–4.
3. Bair AE, Filbin MR, Kulkarni RG, Walls RM. The failed intubation attempt in the emergency department: analysis of prevalence, rescue techniques, and personnel. J Emerg Med. 2002;23:131–40.
4. Langvad S, Hyldmo PK, Nakstad AR, Vist GE, Sandberg M. Emergency cricothyrotomy – a systematic review. Scand J Trauma Resusc Emerg Med. 2013;21:43.
5. Apfelbaum JL, et al. Practice guidelines for management of the difficult airway: an updated report by the American Society of Anesthesiologists task force on management of the difficult airway. Anesthesiology. 2013;118:251–70.
6. Henderson JJ, Popat MT, Latto IP, Pearce AC. Difficult Airway Society guidelines for management of the unanticipated difficult intubation. Anaesthesia. 2004;59:675–94.
7. Shiga T, Wajima ZI, Inoue T, Sakamoto A. Predicting difficult intubation in apparently normal patients: a meta-analysis of bedside screening test performance. Anesthesiology. 2005;103:429–37.
8. Peterson GN, et al. Management of the difficult airway: a closed claims analysis. Anesthesiology. 2005;103:33–9.
9. Marshall S. The use of cognitive aids during emergencies in anesthesia: a review of the literature. Anesth Analg. 2013;117:1162–71.
10. Baillard C, et al. Noninvasive ventilation improves preoxygenation before intubation of hypoxic patients. Am J Respir Crit Care Med. 2006;174:171–7.
11. Wilcox SR, et al. Neuromuscular blocking agent administration for emergent tracheal intubation is associated with decreased prevalence of procedure-related complications. Crit Care Med. 2012;40:1808–13.
12. Mace SE. Challenges and advances in intubation: rapid sequence intubation. Emerg Med Clin North Am. 2008;26:1043–1068, x.
13. Bozeman WP, Kleiner DM, Huggett V. A comparison of rapid-sequence intubation and etomidate-only intubation in the prehospital air medical setting. Prehosp Emerg Care. 2006;10:8–13.

14. Weingart SD. Preoxygenation, reoxygenation, and delayed sequence intubation in the emergency department. J Emerg Med. 2011;40:661–7.
15. Walker IA, Reshamwalla S, Wilson IH. Surgical safety checklists: do they improve outcomes? Br J Anaesth. 2012;109:aes175. https://doi.org/10.1093/bja/aes175.
16. Kheterpal S, et al. Incidence and predictors of difficult and impossible mask ventilation. Anesthesiology. 2006;105:885–91.
17. Khan ZH, Kashfi A, Ebrahimkhani E. A comparison of the upper lip bite test (a simple new technique) with modified Mallampati classification in predicting difficulty in endotracheal intubation: a prospective blinded study. Anesth Analg. 2003;96:595–9.
18. Mallampati SR, et al. A clinical sign to predict difficult tracheal intubation; a prospective study. Can Anaesth Soc J. 1985;32:429–34.
19. Samsoon GL, Young JR. Difficult tracheal intubation: a retrospective study. Anaesthesia. 1987;42:487–90.
20. Mallampati SR. Clinical sign to predict difficult tracheal intubation (hypothesis). Can Anaesth Soc J. 1983;30:316–7.
21. Baraka AS, Taha SK, Aouad MT, El-Khatib MF, Kawkabani NI. Preoxygenation: comparison of maximal breathing and tidal volume breathing techniques. Anesthesiology. 1999;91:612–6.
22. Miguel-Montanes R, et al. Use of high-flow nasal cannula oxygen therapy to prevent desaturation during tracheal intubation of intensive care patients with mild to-moderate hypoxemia. Crit Care Med. 2014;43:574. https://doi.org/10.1097/CCM.0000000000000743.
23. van Zundert TCRV, Brimacombe JR, Ferson DZ, Bacon DR, Wilkinson DJ. Archie Brain: celebrating 30 years of development in laryngeal mask airways. Anaesthesia. 2012;67:1375–85.
24. Tran DTT, et al. Rocuronium versus succinylcholine for rapid sequence induction intubation. Cochrane Database Syst Rev. 2015;(10):CD002788.
25. Kim WY, et al. Factors associated with the occurrence of cardiac arrest after emergency tracheal intubation in the emergency department. PLoS One. 2014;9:e112779.
26. Walls RM, Brown CA, Bair AE, Pallin DJ, NEAR II Investigators. Emergency airway management: a multi-center report of 8937 emergency department intubations. J Emerg Med. 2011;41:347–54.
27. Doyle J. Topical and regional anesthesia for tracheal intubation. Anesthesiol News. 2014;40:8.
28. Reasoner DK, Warner DS, Todd MM, Hunt SW, Kirchner J. A comparison of anesthetic techniques for awake intubation in neurosurgical patients. J Neurosurg Anesthesiol. 1995;7:94–9.
29. Kohli S, et al. Topical airway anesthesia for awake fiberoptic intubation: comparison between airway nerve blocks and nebulized lignocaine by ultrasonic nebulizer. Saudi J Anaesth. 2014;8:15.
30. Kundra P, Kutralam S, Ravishankar M. Local anaesthesia for awake fibreoptic nasotracheal intubation. Acta Anaesthesiol Scand. 2000;44:511–6.
31. Shimizu T, Mizutani T, Yamashita S, Hagiya K, Tanaka M. Endotracheal tube extubation force: adhesive tape versus endotracheal tube holder. Respir Care. 2011;56:1825–9.
32. Miller KJ, Cornman L, Fenstermarker C et al. Utilization of Anchor Fast oral endotracheal tube fastener to reduce the incidence of lip ulcers. Respiratory Care Journal 2009 OPEN FORUM Abstracts 2009.
33. Fisher DF, Chenelle CT, Marchese AD, Kratohvil JP, Kacmarek RM. Comparison of commercial and noncommercial endotracheal tube-securing devices. Respir Care. 2014;59:1315–23.
34. Joffe AM, Hetzel S, Liew EC. A two-handed jaw-thrust technique is superior to the one-handed 'EC-clamp' technique for mask ventilation in the apneic unconscious person. Anesthesiology. 2010;113:873–9.
35. Sellick BA. Cricoid pressure to control regurgitation of stomach contents during induction of anaesthesia. Lancet. 1961;2:404–6.
36. Wraight WJ, Chamney AR, Howells TH. The determination of an effective cricoid pressure. Anaesthesia. 1983;38:461–6.
37. Hirsch NP, Smith GB, Hirsch PO. Alfred Kirstein: pioneer of direct laryngoscopy. Anaesthesia. 1986;41:42–5.
38. Miller RA. A new laryngoscope. Anesthesiology. 1941;2:317–20.
39. Macintosh RR. A new laryngoscope. Lancet. 1943;241:205.
40. Phillips L, Orford N, Ragg M. Prospective observational study of emergent endotracheal intubation practice in the intensive care unit and emergency department of an Australian regional tertiary hospital. Emerg Med Australas: EMA. 2014;26:368–75.
41. Cormack RS, Lehane J. Difficult tracheal intubation in obstetrics. Anaesthesia. 1984;39:1105–11.
42. Cherng C-H, Wong C-S, Hsu C-H, Ho S-T. Airway length in adults: estimation of the optimal endotracheal tube length for orotracheal intubation. J Clin Anesth. 2002;14:271–4.
43. Faris C, et al. Estimation of tracheostomy tube cuff pressure by pilot balloon palpation. J Laryngol Otol. 2007;121:869–71.
44. Cooper RM. Use of a new videolaryngoscope (GlideScope) in the management of a difficult airway. Can J Anaesth. 2003;50:611–3.
45. Raja AS, Sullivan AF, Pallin DJ, Bohan JS, Camargo CA. Adoption of video laryngoscopy in Massachusetts emergency departments. J Emerg Med. 2012;42:233–7.
46. Silverberg MJ, Kory P. Survey of video laryngoscopy use by U.S. critical care fellowship training programs. Ann Am Thorac Soc. 2014;11:1225–9.
47. Ibinson JW, Ezaru CS, Cormican DS, Mangione MP. GlideScope use improves intubation success rates: an observational study using propensity score matching. BMC Anesthesiol. 2014;14:101.
48. Lee Y-K, Chen C-C, Wang T-L, Lin KJ, Su Y-C. Comparison of video and direct laryngoscope for tracheal intubation in emergency settings: a meta-analysis. J Acute Med. 2012;2:43–9.
49. De Jesus CR, García Peña BM, Lozano JM, Maniaci V. Cervical spine motion during airway manage-

ment using two manual in-line immobilization techniques: a human simulator model study. Pediatr Emerg Care. 2014;31:627. https://doi.org/10.1097/PEC.0000000000000245.
50. Robitaille A, et al. Cervical spine motion during tracheal intubation with manual in-line stabilization: direct laryngoscopy versus GlideScope videolaryngoscopy. Anesth Analg. 2008;106:935–41, table of contents.
51. Henry, S. ATLS®: Advanced Trauma Life Support Student Course Manual. Chicago, IL: American College of Surgeons, 2018.
52. Aziz M. Use of video-assisted intubation devices in the management of patients with trauma. Anesthesiol Clin. 2013;31:157–66.
53. GlideScope GVL and Cobalt user's manual & quick reference guide [PDF file]. Retrieved from https://biomedicalmanuals.com/wp-content/uploads/2019/03/Glide-Scope-VLManual.pdf
54. Sakles JC, Kalin L. The effect of stylet choice on the success rate of intubation using the GlideScope video laryngoscope in the emergency department. Acad Emerg Med Off J Soc Acad Emerg Med. 2012;19:235–8.
55. Sakles JC, Mosier J, Chiu S, Cosentino M, Kalin L. A comparison of the C-MAC video laryngoscope to the Macintosh direct laryngoscope for intubation in the emergency department. Ann Emerg Med. 2012;60:739–48.
56. Ferson DZ, Rosenblatt WH, Johansen MJ, Osborn I, Ovassapian A. Use of the intubating LMA-Fastrach in 254 patients with difficult-to-manage airways. Anesthesiology. 2001;95:1175–81.
57. Kapila A, Addy EV, Verghese C, Brain AI. The intubating laryngeal mask airway: an initial assessment of performance. Br J Anaesth. 1997;79:710–3.
58. Verghese C. Laryngeal mask airway devices: three maneuvers for any clinical situation. Anesthesiol News. 2010;36:8.
59. i-gel User Guide (issue 4) [PDF file]. Retrieved from https://www.intersurgical.com/info/igel
60. air-Q® INTUBATING LARYNGEAL AIRWAY INDICATIONS [PDF file]. Retrieved from https://cookgas.com/ifu/
61. Buonopane CE, et al. Cricothyrotomy performed with the Melker™ set or the QuickTrach™ kit: procedure times, learning curves and operators' preference. Il G Chir. 2014;35:165–70.
62. Sise MJ, Shackford SR, Cruickshank JC, Murphy G, Fridlund PH. Cricothyroidotomy for long-term tracheal access. A prospective analysis of morbidity and mortality in 76 patients. Ann Surg. 1984;200:13–7.

Acute Respiratory Failure

3

Jarrod M. Mosier

Critical Points

1. A working knowledge of the pathophysiology of acute respiratory failure is necessary to tailor therapeutic maneuvers.
2. The respiratory system has two goals: ventilation and oxygenation. Both goals require work, which is due to both resistance and elastance.
3. The most common causes of hypoxemic respiratory failure are ventilation–perfusion mismatch and shunt.
4. Ventilatory failure is caused by any CO_2 load that is unable to be managed, either through decreased efficiency or drive or through increased production.
5. Ventilatory and oxygenation failure have varying invasive and noninvasive mechanical ventilation requirements, which should be optimized early by the emergency physician to improve outcomes and limit ventilator-induced lung injury.

Introduction

The respiratory system is a highly coordinated set of organs designed to accomplish two important goals: provide oxygen for aerobic metabolism and eliminate cellular waste in the form of carbon dioxide (CO_2). The respiratory system comprises the following:

- *Neurologic system*: The respiratory center in the medulla, phrenic nerve, and neuromuscular membrane coordinate muscular activity and adjustments to metabolic demand.
- *Upper airway*: It provides the conduit from the external environment to the lungs that regulates the temperature and humidity of the air entering the respiratory system and provides the first line of immunologic defense.
- *Lower airway*: The increased cross-sectional area at the lower airways allows flow to become diffusion rather than convection, allowing gas exchange to occur.
- *Cardiovascular system*: It fuels the respiratory pump and delivers CO_2 for exhalation, while supplying the respiratory pump with oxygen to perform work.
- *Lungs*: They provide the surface area for gas exchange.
- *Chest wall/diaphragm*: Because ambient air pressure cannot be altered to provide flow of air into the lungs, the chest wall and diaphragm are

J. M. Mosier (✉)
Department of Emergency Medicine, Department of Medicine, Division of Pulmonary, Allergy, Critical Care, and Sleep, University of Arizona, Tucson, AZ, USA
e-mail: jmosier@aemrc.arizona.edu

© Springer Nature Switzerland AG 2020

J. R. Shiber, S. D. Weingart (eds.), *Emergency Department Critical Care*,
https://doi.org/10.1007/978-3-030-28794-8_3

designed to lower intrathoracic pressure allowing air to flow down the pressure gradient from the external environment. This process makes breathing a metabolically active process. Exhalation, normally achieved by passive recoil of the chest wall and diaphragm, becomes an active process in pathologic conditions such as obstructive lung disease. This active exhalation greatly increases the work of breathing.

The two goals of respiration (eliminating CO_2 and providing adequate oxygen) require work. Work of breathing is the combination of resistive and elastic forces that inhibit airflow over a respiratory cycle. Resistive work of breathing is the work required to overcome resistance to airflow. The larynx provides a point of fixed resistance that must be overcome with normal respiration and can greatly increase the work of breathing due to increased resistance in laryngeal or subglottic disorders, such as laryngospasm, vocal cord dysfunction, and croup. Bronchospasm and mucosal inflammation are common etiologies of dramatically increased work of breathing in asthma exacerbations. Elastic work of breathing is that which overcomes the lung's desire to be at residual volume. Fibrotic lung disease and breathing at higher lung volumes such as the case with obstructive lung diseases increases the elastic work of breathing. The total work of breathing is the work per breath (both resistive and elastic) multiplied by the respiratory rate. Acute respiratory failure (ARF) occurs when any process prevents the respiratory system from adequately maintaining acid–base balance with CO_2 elimination or providing an adequate oxygen supply to maintain aerobic metabolism.

Pathophysiology

With any process that either increases work of breathing beyond the respiratory system's compensatory capacity or limits the respiratory system's ability to eliminate CO_2 or supply adequate oxygen, acute respiratory failure (ARF) occurs. There are four types of respiratory failure (Fig. 3.1):

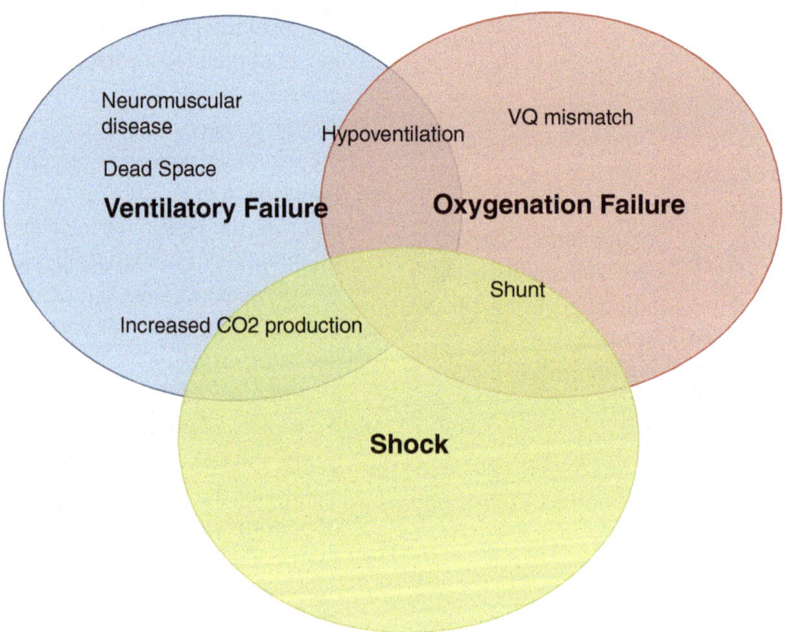

Fig. 3.1 Pathophysiology of acute respiratory failure. Acute respiratory failure can be due to ventilatory failure from hypercapnia (Type II), which is induced by hypoventilation, neuromuscular disease or chest wall abnormalities, increased dead space, or increased work of breathing. Ventilatory failure can also be secondary to increased CO_2 production seen in shock or toxic ingestions. Oxygenation failure (Type I) is most commonly due to VQ mismatch and shunt. Some precipitants of respiratory failure can cause both ventilation and oxygenation defects.

- *Type I* (hypoxemic respiratory failure): Most commonly due to shunt or ventilation/perfusion (*V*/*Q*) mismatch due to airspace disease or anatomic shunt.
- *Type II* (hypercapnic respiratory failure): Most commonly due to a decrease in alveolar ventilation.
- *Type III* (perioperative or mixed respiratory failure): Mixed hypoxemia and hypercapnia, most commonly due to atelectasis.
- *Type IV* (respiratory failure secondary to shock): Most commonly due to increased work of breathing or hypoperfusion to the respiratory muscles, endotoxemia, pulmonary hypertension, and hemorrhage.

Hypoxemic Respiratory Failure

Hypoxemic (Type I) respiratory failure occurs from any etiology that prevents the respiratory system from providing adequate oxygen for delivery to the cells. Hypoventilation can lead to hypoxemia due to the increased partial pressure of CO_2 in the alveolar space displacing oxygen [1]. Similarly, decreased barometric pressure at high elevations leads to a lower oxygen tension in the alveoli at any level of CO_2, given fixed fraction of inspired oxygen, nitrogen, and water vapor [2]. Diffusion abnormalities increase the distance for oxygen diffusion across the alveolar–capillary membrane and can cause hypoxemia in times of increased demand such as high cardiac output states [3]. Additionally, a low mixed venous oxygen saturation can result in systemic hypoxemia in patients with high cardiac output requirements and/or shunt physiology [4]. However, the most common clinically significant precipitants of hypoxemic respiratory failure are *V*/*Q* mismatch and shunt physiology [3].

Any deviation from the optimal ratio of alveolar ventilation to perfusion leads to *V*/*Q* mismatch. A disruption in this ratio leads to alveoli that are either relatively underperfused or underventilated. When alveoli have a relative lack of blood supply for the level of ventilation it receives, those alveoli have a high *V*/*Q* ratio or relative dead space. The respiratory system compensates by increasing blood supply to these areas through hypoxic vasoconstriction of other areas of the lung, optimizing *VQ* mismatch [5]. Disrupting this relationship can lead to hypoxemic respiratory failure. The opposite *V*/*Q* abnormality, perfusion that does not participate in gas exchange, leads to shunt physiology. Due to no ventilation, these alveoli are unable to provide oxygen to this portion of the blood supply, leading to hypoxemia. Shunt physiology is due to either anatomic shunt (e.g., pulmonary embolism or arteriovenous malformation) or physiologic shunt due to alveolar filling (i.e., cardiogenic or noncardiogenic pulmonary edema) or increased flow in the alveolar–capillary beds (i.e., hepatopulmonary syndrome). A commonly encountered shunt physiology is seen with acute respiratory distress syndrome (ARDS), where the degree of shunt increases as alveolar filling worsens, causing progressively worsened hypoxemia (Table 3.1) [6].

Any of these abnormalities lead to a decrease in dissolved oxygen available in the blood or pO_2. Although dissolved oxygen plays a small role in the amount of oxygen delivered to the cell compared to hemoglobin bound oxygen, dissolved

Table 3.1 Berlin definition of ARDS

Acute respiratory distress syndrome	
Timing	Within 1 week of a known clinical insult or new or worsening respiratory symptoms
Chest imaging	Bilateral opacities – not fully explained by effusions, lobar/lung collapse, or nodules
Origin of edema	Respiratory failure not fully explained by cardiac failure or fluid overload. Need objective assessment (i.e., echocardiography) to exclude hydrostatic edema if no risk factor present
Oxygenation	
Mild	200 mgHg $<PaO_2/FiO_2 \leq 300$ mmHg with PEEP or CPAP >5 cmH_2O
Moderate	100 mgHg $<PaO_2/FiO_2 <200$ mmHg with PEEP >5 cmH_2O
Severe	$PaO_2/FiO_2 <100$ mmHg with PEEP >5 cmH_2O

oxygen is required to allow oxygen to bind hemoglobin. The clinically important etiologies of hypoxemic respiratory failure commonly encountered are as follows:

- Pneumonia
- Cardiogenic pulmonary edema
- Noncardiogenic pulmonary edema (ARDS)

Hypercapnic Respiratory Failure

Hypercapnic (Type II) respiratory failure occurs when the patient is unable to maintain blood pH by increasing minute ventilation (V_E), or the amount of CO_2 exhaled per minute determined by tidal volume multiplied by the respiratory rate [3]. CO_2 is produced in the peripheral tissues by cellular metabolism and freely dissolves across the membrane into the blood stream, unlike oxygen, which requires being bound by hemoglobin. Thus, a linear increase in CO_2 production in the periphery requires a linear increase in minute ventilation to compensate and maintain normal blood pH. Unfortunately, not all of the surface area of the respiratory system participates in gas exchange, and thus, a portion of the minute ventilation is wasted or "dead space" ventilation [7]. Dead space (V_D) occurs from an increase in conducting airways such as is seen after parenchymal loss in emphysema or in any process that leads to a relative decrease in blood supply to the alveoli such as seen in pulmonary embolism. Consequently, alveolar ventilation (V_A) is the ventilation that participates in CO_2 removal and is determined by the minute ventilation minus dead space, meaning that any increase in dead space or decrease in minute ventilation will lead to decreased alveolar ventilation causing a drop in pH [3, 7, 8]. Additionally, a relative increase in CO_2 production compared to exhaled CO_2, such as seen with metabolic acidosis, will lead to a drop in pH. Thus, pCO_2 can be expressed as follows:

$$pCO_2 = [VCO_2 / RR \times V_E - V_D] \times 0.863 \text{ or } [VCO_2 / V_A] \times 0.863$$

where VCO_2 is the production of CO_2, RR is the respiratory rate, V_E is minute ventilation, V_A is alveolar ventilation, and V_D is dead space.

Unfortunately, while pCO_2 and CO_2 production are linear, the pCO_2 response to alveolar ventilation increases in supranormal alveolar ventilation [3, 7]. The result is that while respiratory acidosis is easily compensated for by increasing alveolar ventilation, metabolic acidosis due to increased CO_2 production will often exceed the ability to compensate by increased alveolar ventilation as is often seen in lactic acidosis, diabetic ketoacidosis, and toxic ingestions.

In summary, any condition that leads to decreased respiratory drive, decreased respiratory efficiency, or increased ventilatory demand beyond the respiratory system's capacity will lead to ventilatory failure. Common conditions include the following:

- Obstructive lung diseases such as asthma or chronic obstructive pulmonary disease (COPD)
- Increased ventilatory demand from shock
- Overdoses (opiates and sedatives)

Patient Presentation

Patients with acute respiratory failure present with many different syndromes, depending on the offending gas exchange disturbance. Following are typical presentations of common causes of acute respiratory failure:

- *COPD*: Patients are typically middle age or older with a history of smoking and present with cough, dyspnea, and often chest pain. Physical exam often demonstrates barrel chest, tripoding, pursed-lip breathing, and accessory muscle use with a severely prolonged expiratory phase and wheezing.
- *Asthma*: Patients are typically younger to middle age with acute onset of wheezing, chest pain, and dyspnea. Physical examination typically demonstrates tripoding, diminished breath sounds or wheezing, and accessory

muscle use. Depending on the amount of mucous plugging, patients may have crackles and hypoxemia as well.

- *Shock*: Patients typically present with severely increased minute ventilation with tachypnea and large tidal volumes. Patients may be anxious and hypotensive. Breath sounds are typically clear.
- *Cardiogenic pulmonary edema*: Patients are typically middle age or older. If the primary cause is systolic heart failure, patients typically have ischemic cardiomyopathy either acutely or chronically. If the primary cause is diastolic heart failure, patients typically have a longstanding history of hypertension. Patients typically present with dyspnea and orthopnea. Physical examination demonstrates crackles diffusely, jugular venous distension, accessory muscle use, and a displaced point of maximal impulse.
- *Pneumonia/ARDS*: Patients often present with productive cough, chest pain, and dyspnea. They may have diminished breath sounds or crackles either locally or diffusely. As the degree of shunt increases, the oxygen saturation will become less responsive to supplemental oxygen.

Diagnostics

All patients with acute respiratory failure should have a thorough investigation into the etiology of the respiratory failure. Evaluation should include the following:

- *Evaluation for mental status changes*: If altered, mental status, medication history, and drug use should be investigated.
- *Evaluation for airspace disease*: Patients should get a chest X-ray and/or bedside ultrasound to evaluate for pulmonary edema, atelectasis, or alveolar filling processes.
- *Evaluation of gas exchange and acid–base status*: Ventilatory status can be evaluated with a venous blood gas and a metabolic panel. Oxygenation evaluation requires an arterial blood gas. With an *arterial* blood gas, the alveolar–arterial (A–a) gradient can be evaluated. With primary hypoxemic conditions (VQ mismatch, shunt, fibrosis, etc.), the A–a gradient will increase as the inspired oxygen will not diffuse into the arterial blood. With hypoxemia due to hypoventilation, the A–a gradient will be normal. When the ventilatory and acid–base status is of interest, a venous blood gas will give an accurate pH and pCO_2. However, while in healthy adults, there is a predictable correlation in pO_2 between an ABG and VBG, increased oxygen consumption, regional blood flow variation, and inconsistent pulmonary oxygenation all make a VBG unreliable in critically ill patients.
- *Evaluation of cardiovascular status*: Bedside sonographic evaluation of cardiac performance and volume status can be both diagnostic and guide therapy for cardiogenic pulmonary edema or respiratory failure due to shock.

Initial Stabilization and Treatment

Stabilization and treatment for acute respiratory failure depend on etiology (Table 3.2). Reversible causes should be sought after and treated immediately. For example, depressed respiratory drive from narcotic overdose can be easily reversed with naloxone. In general, goals with management of acute respiratory failure include the following:

- Minimize work of breathing
- Limit risk with NIPPV and risk of ventilator-induced lung injury with invasive mechanical ventilation
- Improve patient–ventilator synchrony

Ventilatory Failure from COPD or Asthma

Noninvasive positive-pressure ventilation (NIPPV) improves work of breathing and reduces symptoms, mortality, and need for intubation and mechanical ventilation compared to oxygen sup-

Table 3.2 Treatment of acute respiratory failure by diagnosis

Diagnosis	ARF type	Mechanism of ARF	NIPPV use	Indication for intubation	Ventilator mode	Monitoring	Other treatment
COPD	Hypercapnic	Increased work of breathing due to hyperinflation, decreased respiratory muscle efficiency, and dynamic hyperinflation	Decreases work of breathing, need for intubation, and mortality compared to standard therapy	pCO_2 >100 mmHg, pH <7.05, persistently high work of breathing, impending respiratory arrest, persistent hypoxemia	Volume control, low respiratory rate	Monitor expiratory flow waveform on ventilator for air trapping, follow peak pressures, and monitor blood gasses	Bronchodilators and corticosteroids
Asthma	Mixed	Bronchospasm induces hyperinflation and hypercapnia, increased work of breathing. Mucous plugging induces VQ mismatch and hypoxemia.	May reduce work of breathing, lacking outcomes data				
Cardiogenic pulmonary edema	Hypoxemia	Pulmonary edema leads to VQ mismatch, increased work of breathing	Decreases work of breathing, reduces mortality and need for intubation compared to standard therapy; improves pulmonary edema by improving hemodynamics	Persistent hypoxemia, impending respiratory or cardiac arrest, inability to tolerate mask	Volume- or pressure-targeted mode, increase PEEP, lung protective tidal volumes	Monitor blood gas for improved hypoxemia, bedside ultrasound or chest x-ray for pulmonary edema resolution, monitor tidal volumes if pressure-targeted mode, monitor pressures if volume-targeted mode	Afterload reduction and inotropic agents if necessary, intervention if active ischemia
Pneumonia ARDS	Hypoxemia	Shunt due to alveolar filling	Controversial. High failure rate, increased mortality with failure. Improved outcomes with hematologic malignancy patients	If NIPPV trial attempted, PEEP >10 and/or FiO_2 >60% and PaO_2 <100 or PF ratio <200 2 hours after initiation	Volume-targeted mode preferred, pressure-targeted mode (APRV) can improve oxygenation in refractory hypoxemia, lung protective tidal volumes necessary	Monitor blood gas for improvement in hypoxemia, monitor tidal volumes and plateau pressures (<30 cmH_2O)	Early appropriate antibiotics if infectious, steroids if inflammatory ARDS. Refractory ARDS-neuromuscular blockers, proning, inhaled NO, ECMO
Shock	Mixed	Increased work of breathing, decreased blood supply to respiratory muscles, increased CO_2 production	Unsupported	Same as above	Volume or pressure-targeted mode with lung protective tidal volumes, may need higher respiratory rate	Monitor for improvement in shock	Appropriate therapy for etiology of shock

plementation alone in patients with COPD [9–14]. NIPPV for asthma is more controversial than in COPD as there is more regional hyperinflation due to mucous plugging and flow restriction due to bronchospasm, which make the use of PEEP a risk of pneumothorax. However, NIPPV may improve work of breathing and reduce symptoms [15]. In general, keep PEEP low in asthma exacerbation requiring mechanical ventilation.

Contraindications to NIPPV in all patients include the following:

- pCO_2 >100 or pH <7.05, inability to protect airway, vomiting, hemodynamic instability, GI bleed, hemoptysis, epistaxis, excessive secretions, inability to tolerate accidental removal of NIPPV mask.
- Indications for intubation are persistently high work of breathing with evidence of fatigue, respiratory or cardiac arrest, or persistent hypoxemia.

Monitoring while on NIPPV includes blood gas with initiation of NIPPV and frequently (q1–2 hours) until stable. For COPD patients with O_2Sat >92%, a VBG can be used instead of ABG (see section "Diagnostics"). If pCO_2 is not improving or work of breathing remains high (increased RR >20, accessory muscle use), increase IPAP by 5 until 20/5. If no improvement, consider intubation and invasive mechanical ventilation.

Invasive mechanical ventilation for COPD and asthma should be performed with a volume-targeted mode (assist control (AC), synchronized intermittent mandatory ventilation (SIMV), pressure-regulated volume control (PRVC)) with a low respiratory rate (10–12 per minute). Pressure control modes must be used cautiously due to the risk of regional hyperinflation and pneumothorax.

- Decrease the respiratory rate until expiratory flow returns to baseline prior to next mandatory breath. As COPD patients have outflow obstruction, peak pressures are often high. If the peak pressure alarms, evaluate the expiratory flow waveform on the ventilator monitor for air trapping and decrease ventilator rate as needed. Allow permissive hypercapnia if necessary.
- If no air trapping is present, perform inspiratory pause to evaluate plateau pressure. If plateau pressure >30 cmH_2O, a portable X-ray or bedside ultrasound should be performed to evaluate for pneumothorax.
- If no pneumothorax is present, perform expiratory pause to evaluate autopeep. If autopeep is elevated, then increase set PEEP and decrease respiratory rate. If hypotensive, disconnect ventilator from ETT and decompress chest with external compression to allow air to empty from the lungs. Needle decompression will not allow trapped air to escape in autopeep scenarios.
- Treat bronchospasm with bronchodilators.

Hypoxemic Respiratory Failure

NIPPV improves work of breathing and reduces symptoms, mortality, and need for intubation and mechanical ventilation in patients with cardiogenic pulmonary edema [16–19]. PEEP provides the benefit in cardiogenic pulmonary edema by improving cardiac performance. However, inspiratory pressure support may be desired if high work of breathing with inspiration. Initial NIPPV settings should be EPAP (PEEP) 8–10 cmH_2O or may use IPAP of 12–15. Monitoring while on NIPPV includes blood gas prior to initiation of NIPPV and following oxygen saturation and symptoms after initiation of NIPPV. If work of breathing remains high (increased RR >20, accessory muscle use, persistent hypoxemia), titrate PEEP up to 15. If still no improvement, consider intubation and invasive mechanical ventilation.

NIPPV is in general contraindicated for hypoxemic respiratory failure due to pneumonia or ARDS given high risk of failure (50+%) [14, 20–29]. However, if NIPPV is chosen for oxygenation support, very close observation is required to monitor response to therapy. If requiring PEEP >10 and/or FiO_2 >60% and PaO_2 <100 or PF ratio <200 (i.e., moderate or severe ARDS

Table 3.3 ARDSnet PEEP/FiO_2 table for mechanical ventilation

FiO_2	.30	.40	.40	.50	.50	.60	.70	.70	.70	.80	.90	.90	.90	1.0	1.0
PEEP	5	5	8	8	10	10	10	12	14	14	14	16	18	18	20–24

based on Berlin definition) by 2 hours after initiation, recommend intubation and mechanical ventilation [23].

Invasive mechanical ventilation for hypoxemic respiratory failure should be performed with a volume-targeted mode (assist control (AC), synchronized intermittent mandatory ventilation (SIMV), pressure-regulated volume control (PRVC)) with the following settings:

- Rate of 12–15 breaths per minute. May increase based on ventilatory requirement.
- Tidal volume of 6–8 ml/kg PBW (predicted body weight), must keep plateau pressure< 30 cmH_2O.
- Positive end-expiratory pressure (PEEP) of 5–8 cmH_2O.
- FiO_2 of 100% upon initiation and titration to SpO_2 >90.

Monitoring while undergoing mechanical ventilation should include the following:

- *Arterial* blood gas prior to intubation and q1 hour until hemodynamically stable and no active ventilator changes are needed.
- Continuous quantitative $EtCO_2$ and pulse oximetry.
- If requiring FiO_2 >60%, increase PEEP ×5 every 30 minutes until a PEEP of 15 is reached as outlined in the ARDSnet PEEP/FiO_2 table (Table 3.3) [30].
- If still persistently hypoxemic at a PEEP of 15, the patient has refractory hypoxemia.

Refractory hypoxemia (PaO_2 <60, PF <200 requiring FiO_2 >60% or PEEP ≥15 cmH_2O) is a critical problem encountered in many patients with ARDS and carries a high mortality [6, 31–33]. Many methods have been used to treat refractory hypoxemia with mixed results. At our hospital at the University of Arizona, we recommend the following therapies in ARDS patients with refractory hypoxemia.

- Consider airway pressure release ventilation (APRV mode) and adjust the high and low pressures and ensure tidal volumes are lung protective (6–8 ml/kg) as lung compliance improves [34, 35].
- Ensure adequate sedation and analgesia to minimize patient–ventilator dyssynchrony. If patient–ventilator dyssynchrony persists, consider continuous paralytic infusion [36]. Cisatracurium (Nimbex) is the preferred neuromuscular blocking agent, as it is long acting and not altered by hepatic or renal dysfunction.
- If sedation adequate and no patient–ventilator dyssynchrony, early prone positioning should be performed [37–41].
- If still persistently hypoxemic, consider inhaled nitric oxide at 10 ppm or inhaled epoprostenol (Flolan) [32].
- Discuss with intensivist colleagues if the patient is a candidate for extracorporeal membrane oxygenation (ECMO) [42].

Respiratory Failure Secondary to Shock

NIPPV is not recommended for shock-induced respiratory failure. Invasive mechanical ventilation reduces respiratory muscle oxygen consumption and diaphragm fatigue, and it reduces lung injury due to circulating cytokines and high ventilatory demand-induced volutrauma [8, 43, 44].

References

1. Roussos C, Macklem PT. The respiratory muscles. N Engl J Med. 1982;307(13):786–97.
2. Grocott MP, Martin DS, Levett DZ, McMorrow R, Windsor J, Montgomery HE, et al. Arterial blood gases and oxygen content in climbers on Mount Everest. N Engl J Med. 2009;360(2):140–9.
3. Mason RJ, Broaddus VC, Martin TR, King TE, Schraufnagel DE, Murray JF, et al. Murray and

Nadel's textbook of respiratory medicine. 5th ed. Philadelphia: Elsevier; 2010.
4. Rossaint R, Hahn SM, Pappert D, Falke KJ, Radermacher P. Influence of mixed venous PO2 and inspired O2 fraction on intrapulmonary shunt in patients with severe ARDS. J Appl Physiol. 1995;78(4):1531–6.
5. Swenson ER. Hypoxic pulmonary vasoconstriction. High Alt Med Biol. 2013;14(2):101–10.
6. Force ADT, Ranieri VM, Rubenfeld GD, Thompson BT, Ferguson ND, Caldwell E, et al. Acute respiratory distress syndrome: the Berlin definition. JAMA. 2012;307(23):2526–33.
7. Vincent JL, Abraham E, Moore FA, Kochanek P, Fink MP. Textbook of critical care. 6th ed. Philadelphia: Elsevier; 2011.
8. Roussos C, Koutsoukou A. Respiratory failure. Eur Respir J Suppl. 2003;47:3s–14s.
9. Bott J, Carroll MP, Conway JH, Keilty SE, Ward EM, Brown AM, et al. Randomised controlled trial of nasal ventilation in acute ventilatory failure due to chronic obstructive airways disease. Lancet. 1993;341(8860):1555–7.
10. Brochard L, Mancebo J, Wysocki M, Lofaso F, Conti G, Rauss A, et al. Noninvasive ventilation for acute exacerbations of chronic obstructive pulmonary disease. N Engl J Med. 1995;333(13):817–22.
11. Chandra D, Stamm JA, Taylor B, Ramos RM, Satterwhite L, Krishnan JA, et al. Outcomes of noninvasive ventilation for acute exacerbations of chronic obstructive pulmonary disease in the United States, 1998–2008. Am J Respir Crit Care Med. 2012;185(2):152–9.
12. Lightowler JV, Wedzicha JA, Elliott MW, Ram FS. Non-invasive positive pressure ventilation to treat respiratory failure resulting from exacerbations of chronic obstructive pulmonary disease: Cochrane systematic review and meta-analysis. BMJ. 2003;326(7382):185.
13. Plant PK, Owen JL, Elliott MW. Early use of non-invasive ventilation for acute exacerbations of chronic obstructive pulmonary disease on general respiratory wards: a multicentre randomised controlled trial. Lancet. 2000;355(9219):1931–5.
14. Schnell D, Timsit JF, Darmon M, Vesin A, Goldgran-Toledano D, Dumenil AS, et al. Noninvasive mechanical ventilation in acute respiratory failure: trends in use and outcomes. Intensive Care Med. 2014;40(4):582–91.
15. Soroksky A, Klinowski E, Ilgyev E, Mizrachi A, Miller A, Ben Yehuda TM, et al. Noninvasive positive pressure ventilation in acute asthmatic attack. Eur Respir Rev. 2010;19(115):39–45.
16. Girou E, Brun-Buisson C, Taille S, Lemaire F, Brochard L. Secular trends in nosocomial infections and mortality associated with noninvasive ventilation in patients with exacerbation of COPD and pulmonary edema. JAMA. 2003;290(22):2985–91.
17. Liesching T, Kwok H, Hill NS. Acute applications of noninvasive positive pressure ventilation. Chest. 2003;124(2):699–713.
18. Masip J, Betbese AJ, Paez J, Vecilla F, Canizares R, Padro J, et al. Non-invasive pressure support ventilation versus conventional oxygen therapy in acute cardiogenic pulmonary oedema: a randomised trial. Lancet. 2000;356(9248):2126–32.
19. Nava S, Carbone G, DiBattista N, Bellone A, Baiardi P, Cosentini R, et al. Noninvasive ventilation in cardiogenic pulmonary edema: a multicenter randomized trial. Am J Respir Crit Care Med. 2003;168(12):1432–7.
20. Carrillo A, Gonzalez-Diaz G, Ferrer M, Martinez-Quintana ME, Lopez-Martinez A, Llamas N, et al. Non-invasive ventilation in community-acquired pneumonia and severe acute respiratory failure. Intensive Care Med. 2012;38(3):458–66.
21. Delclaux C, L'Her E, Alberti C, Mancebo J, Abroug F, Conti G, et al. Treatment of acute hypoxemic nonhypercapnic respiratory insufficiency with continuous positive airway pressure delivered by a face mask: a randomized controlled trial. JAMA. 2000;284(18):2352–60.
22. Demoule A, Girou E, Richard JC, Taille S, Brochard L. Benefits and risks of success or failure of noninvasive ventilation. Intensive Care Med. 2006;32(11):1756–65.
23. Esteban A, Frutos-Vivar F, Ferguson ND, Arabi Y, Apezteguia C, Gonzalez M, et al. Noninvasive positive-pressure ventilation for respiratory failure after extubation. N Engl J Med. 2004;350(24):2452–60.
24. Ferrer M, Esquinas A, Leon M, Gonzalez G, Alarcon A, Torres A. Noninvasive ventilation in severe hypoxemic respiratory failure: a randomized clinical trial. Am J Respir Crit Care Med. 2003;168(12):1438–44.
25. Hilbert G, Gruson D, Vargas F, Valentino R, Gbikpi-Benissan G, Dupon M, et al. Noninvasive ventilation in immunosuppressed patients with pulmonary infiltrates, fever, and acute respiratory failure. N Engl J Med. 2001;344(7):481–7.
26. Keenan SP, Kernerman PD, Cook DJ, Martin CM, McCormack D, Sibbald WJ. Effect of noninvasive positive pressure ventilation on mortality in patients admitted with acute respiratory failure: a meta-analysis. Crit Care Med. 1997;25(10):1685–92.
27. Thille AW, Contou D, Fragnoli C, Cordoba-Izquierdo A, Boissier F, Brun-Buisson C. Non-invasive ventilation for acute hypoxemic respiratory failure: intubation rate and risk factors. Crit Care. 2013;17(6):R269.
28. Thille AW, Frat JP, Brun-Buisson C. Trends in use and benefits of non-invasive ventilation as first-line therapy in acute respiratory failure. Intensive Care Med. 2014;40(8):1179–80.
29. Williams JW, Cox CE, Hargett CW, Gilstrap DL, Castillo CE, Govert JA, et al. Noninvasive positive-pressure ventilation (NPPV) for acute respiratory failure. Rockville: Agency for Healthcare Research and Quality. Comparative Effectiveness Reviews; 2012.
30. Brower RG, Lanken PN, MacIntyre N, Matthay MA, Morris A, Ancukiewicz M, et al. Higher versus lower positive end-expiratory pressures in patients with the

acute respiratory distress syndrome. N Engl J Med. 2004;351(4):327–36.
31. Esan A, Hess DR, Raoof S, George L, Sessler CN. Severe hypoxemic respiratory failure: part 1--ventilatory strategies. Chest. 2010;137(5):1203–16.
32. Raoof S, Goulet K, Esan A, Hess DR, Sessler CN. Severe hypoxemic respiratory failure: part 2--nonventilatory strategies. Chest. 2010;137(6):1437–48.
33. Walkey AJ, Summer R, Ho V, Alkana P. Acute respiratory distress syndrome: epidemiology and management approaches. Clin Epidemiol. 2012;4:159–69.
34. Kawashima H, Go S, Nara S, Miura T, Ushio M, Miyahara A, et al. Extreme efficiency of airway pressure release ventilation (APRV) in a patient suffering from acute lung injury with pandemic influenza A (H1N1) 2009 and high cytokines. Indian J Pediatr. 2011;78(3):348–50.
35. Sundar KM, Thaut P, Nielsen DB, Alward WT, Pearce MJ. Clinical course of ICU patients with severe pandemic 2009 influenza A (H1N1) pneumonia: single center experience with proning and pressure release ventilation. J Intensive Care Med. 2012;27(3):184–90.
36. Papazian L, Forel JM, Gacouin A, Penot-Ragon C, Perrin G, Loundou A, et al. Neuromuscular blockers in early acute respiratory distress syndrome. N Engl J Med. 2010;363(12):1107–16.
37. Beitler JR, Shaefi S, Montesi SB, Devlin A, Loring SH, Talmor D, et al. Prone positioning reduces mortality from acute respiratory distress syndrome in the low tidal volume era: a meta-analysis. Intensive Care Med. 2014;40(3):332–41.
38. Guerin C, Reignier J, Richard JC, Beuret P, Gacouin A, Boulain T, et al. Prone positioning in severe acute respiratory distress syndrome. N Engl J Med. 2013;368(23):2159–68.
39. Hu SL, He HL, Pan C, Liu AR, Liu SQ, Liu L, et al. The effect of prone positioning on mortality in patients with acute respiratory distress syndrome: a meta-analysis of randomized controlled trials. Crit Care. 2014;18(3):R109.
40. Sud S, Friedrich JO, Adhikari NK, Taccone P, Mancebo J, Polli F, et al. Effect of prone positioning during mechanical ventilation on mortality among patients with acute respiratory distress syndrome: a systematic review and meta-analysis. CMAJ: Can Med Assoc J (journal de l'Association medicale canadienne). 2014;186:E381.
41. Sud S, Friedrich JO, Taccone P, Polli F, Adhikari NK, Latini R, et al. Prone ventilation reduces mortality in patients with acute respiratory failure and severe hypoxemia: systematic review and meta-analysis. Intensive Care Med. 2010;36(4):585–99.
42. Peek GJ, Elbourne D, Mugford M, Tiruvoipati R, Wilson A, Allen E, et al. Randomised controlled trial and parallel economic evaluation of conventional ventilatory support versus extracorporeal membrane oxygenation for severe adult respiratory failure (CESAR). Health Technol Assess. 2010;14(35):1–46.
43. Mascheroni D, Kolobow T, Fumagalli R, Moretti MP, Chen V, Buckhold D. Acute respiratory failure following pharmacologically induced hyperventilation: an experimental animal study. Intensive Care Med. 1988;15(1):8–14.
44. Ward ME, Magder SA, Hussain SN. Oxygen delivery-independent effect of blood flow on diaphragm fatigue. Am Rev Respir Dis. 1992;145(5):1058–63.

Noninvasive and Mechanical Ventilation

4

John P. Gaillard and Michael Schinlever

Critical Points

- NIPPV may be helpful in an easily reversible respiratory disease.
- Invasive PPV is the gold standard treatment for respiratory failure.
- Ventilators can be described in terms of parameters: control, trigger, cycle, and limit.
- The mode refers to the manner in which the ventilator provides inspiratory support to the patient.
- A/C and SIMV with PSV are the two modes most commonly used.
- To increase oxygenation, increase the FiO_2 or PEEP.
- To decrease pCO_2, increase the minute ventilation.
- 6 cc/kg should be the default tidal volume.
- Autopeep may occur if the patient is not given enough time to exhale.

J. P. Gaillard (✉)
Anesthesiology-Critical Care, Emergency Medicine, Internal Medicine-Pulmonary/Critical Care, Wake Forest Baptist Health, Winston-Salem, NC, USA
e-mail: jgaillar@wakehealth.edu

M. Schinlever
Surgery – Critical Care, Rochester Regional Health, Rochester, NY, USA

Introduction

Respiratory failure is a common complaint in emergency medicine (EM). The goal of treatment is to ensure that there is adequate gas exchange for the metabolic demands on the body. There are many techniques and tools with which to manage respiratory failure, and the list of options continues to expand. Noninvasive positive-pressure ventilation (NIPPV) and mechanical ventilation (MV) are tools commonly used for the management of acute respiratory failure. EM providers undergo a great deal of training in airway management, but there is often little training in the use of NIPPV and MV. It is important for EM providers to become more comfortable with initial and ongoing ventilation management because intubated critically ill patients are spending more time in the ED. This chapter discusses NIPPV and MV in an effort to provide the EM provider with the tools necessary to provide ICU-level respiratory care in the ED.

Physiologic Changes Due to Positive-Pressure Ventilation (PPV)

The process of induction, paralysis, and initiation of PPV has dramatic effects on a patient's physiology. Most patients who are emergently intubated in the ED are critically ill and have

© Springer Nature Switzerland AG 2020

J. R. Shiber, S. D. Weingart (eds.), *Emergency Department Critical Care*,
https://doi.org/10.1007/978-3-030-28794-8_4

poor physiologic reserve. Failure to account for and anticipate the physiologic changes that occur postintubation may lead to poor patient outcomes. Most commonly used induction medications cause vasodilation leading to hypotension. Some medicines, such as propofol, may also contribute directly to hypotension by inducing myocardial depression.

Once PPV is initiated, thoracic physiology is changed. Each breath is delivered by positive pressure from the ventilator rather than the negative pressure derived from diaphragm contraction and thoracic expansion. In addition, there is the contribution of PEEP that creates a baseline positive-pressure environment even at times of exhalation. The increase in intrathoracic pressure during and between each breath may cause a significant change in cardiovascular function.

Under normal circumstances, when a person inhales, venous return to the right atrium (RA) is assisted by the negative intrathoracic pressure. The negative-pressure gradient minimizes impedance on venous return and will provide an added gradient that helps draw venous blood into the RA. When on PPV, the positive intrathoracic pressure may dramatically decrease venous return and cardiac preload by negating the normal physiologic advantages. There will be loss of this favorable pressure gradient from abdomen to thorax which will also impede venous return to the RA.

PEEP reduces left ventricular (LV) afterload. This effect may be related to the decrease in venous return to the heart that causes a reduced preload that is translated into a decreased mean arterial pressure. The PEEP-induced decrease in LV afterload may also be due to the reduction in the LV end-systolic transmural pressure. This occurs when intrathoracic pressure is elevated and arterial pressure is constant. The LV needs less force to eject blood into the aorta. There is a pressure gradient between the left ventricle and the systemic circulation, which effectively lowers left ventricular afterload and increases cardiac output (CO) [1, 2]. See Fig. 4.1.

Using PEEP to increase MAP (mean airway pressure) is one of the primary methods for treating hypoxia, but there are also negative effects associated with elevated PEEP that must be considered. The effects of PEEP are dose dependent. In cases of poor pulmonary compliance, high levels of PEEP may dramatically decrease venous return to the RA and also significantly increase pulmonary vascular resistance. High PEEP will

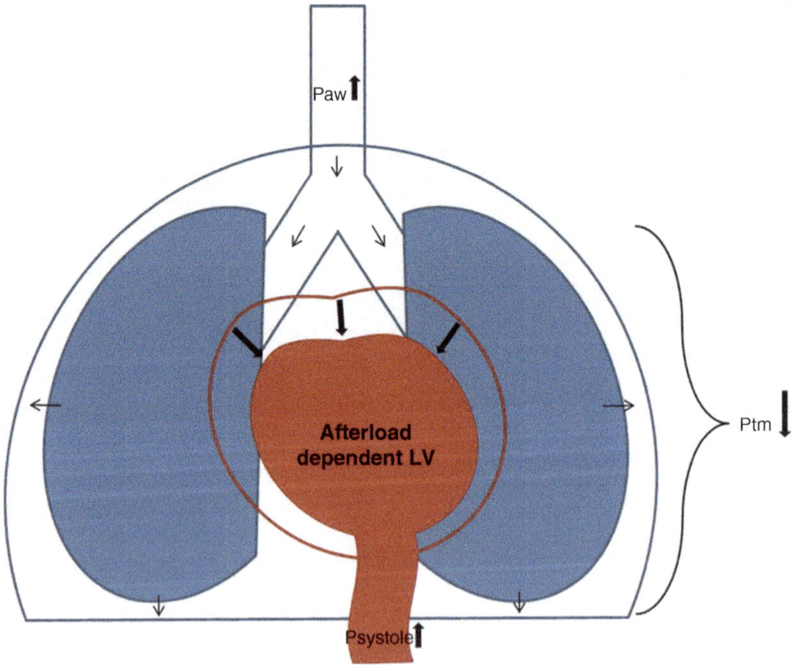

Fig. 4.1 The PEEP-induced decrease in LV afterload may also be due to the reduction in the LV end-systolic transmural pressure. This occurs when intrathoracic pressure is elevated, and arterial pressure is constant. The LV needs less force to eject blood into the aorta. There is a pressure gradient between the left ventricle and the systemic circulation, which effectively lowers left ventricular afterload and increases cardiac output (CO)

also cause an increase in right ventricular afterload.

It is clear that the initiation of PPV dramatically affects cardiovascular physiology. Many common processes requiring intubation (e.g., trauma, sepsis, or other shock states) are associated with hypovolemia and inadequate preload. Initiating PPV may be enough to lead to cardiovascular collapse. Hence, EM providers must take care to evaluate fluid and preload status prior to intubation. More importantly, it is necessary to reevaluate the patient's hemodynamics in the first 10–15 minutes following intubation.

Indications for NIPPV

Noninvasive PPV is a treatment strategy for patients with respiratory failure that is probably underutilized. In the correct patient population, NIPPV can decrease the need for intubation and MV. The most common modes of NIPPV are continuous positive airway pressure (CPAP) and bi-level positive airway pressure (BIPAP, not to be confused with BiPAP®, a proprietary trade name for Philips Respironics noninvasive ventilators). There are many other types of NIPPV that use different parameters to assist patients, but the modes are essentially the same.

NIPPV helps decrease a patient's work of breathing and relieve dyspnea. The most prudent indication for NIPPV is a case of respiratory failure that is easily reversible. NIPPV has been shown to decrease the need for intubation in patients with hypercapnic respiratory failure, although risk factors for NIPPV failure include pH <7.25, GCS <11, and RR >30 [3]. Other indications for NIPPV include "Do Not Intubate" patients or as a way to improve preoxygenation for patients to be intubated [5]. In patients with ARDS and acute cardiac pulmonary edema, NIPPV may decrease the number of intubations but does not change mortality [2, 4].

Patient selection is important when considering NIPPV. Patients who ultimately fail NIPPV and require invasive mechanical ventilation have a higher mortality [5]. An arterial blood gas should be obtained prior to beginning therapy, and patients should be reassessed often (every 30 minutes) until their respiratory failure has stabilized. NIPPV requires patient compliance. Patients must be able to protect their airway. See Fig. 4.2 for a flow diagram for the initial management of a patient on NIPPV. See Table 4.1 for contraindications to NIPPV.

Indications for Invasive PPV

There are four key indications for intubation: (1) inability to oxygenate, (2) inability to ventilate, (3) airway protection, and (4) anticipated clinical course [5]. It is important to understand how invasive PPV and MV benefit patients.

Oxygenation

Oxygenation includes all processes that lead to the delivery of O_2 from the upper airway to the tissues. Hypoxemia may be due to one or more of the following: *V*/*Q* mismatch, poor diffusion, low inspired FiO_2, or hypoventilation. Gas delivery to the alveolus is known as ventilation (*V*). Transport of gas across the alveolar–capillary membrane into the circulatory system is flow (*Q*). The ratio of alveolar ventilation (V_A technically but by convention, it is shortened to *V*) and capillary flow (*Q*) is an important consideration when treating a patient with hypoxic respiratory failure. In normal lungs, there is an inherent *V*/*Q* inequality that is related to gravity. More blood flows to the dependent areas of lung (i.e., there is more *Q*). This leads to different physiologic zones within the lung related to the gravity-dependent areas. In the most dependent areas, the *V*/*Q* ratio is lower. In higher areas, there is relatively more *V* and less *Q*, and thus, the *V*/*Q* ratio is higher. This is a normal physiologic situation, but there are certain disease processes that exaggerate this ratio and contribute to respiratory failure.

Two classic examples of *V*/*Q* mismatch are (1) the lung that is completely obstructed (e.g., main bronchus mucous plug) and (2) the lung that receives no blood flow (e.g., main pulmonary artery embolism). In the first example, the

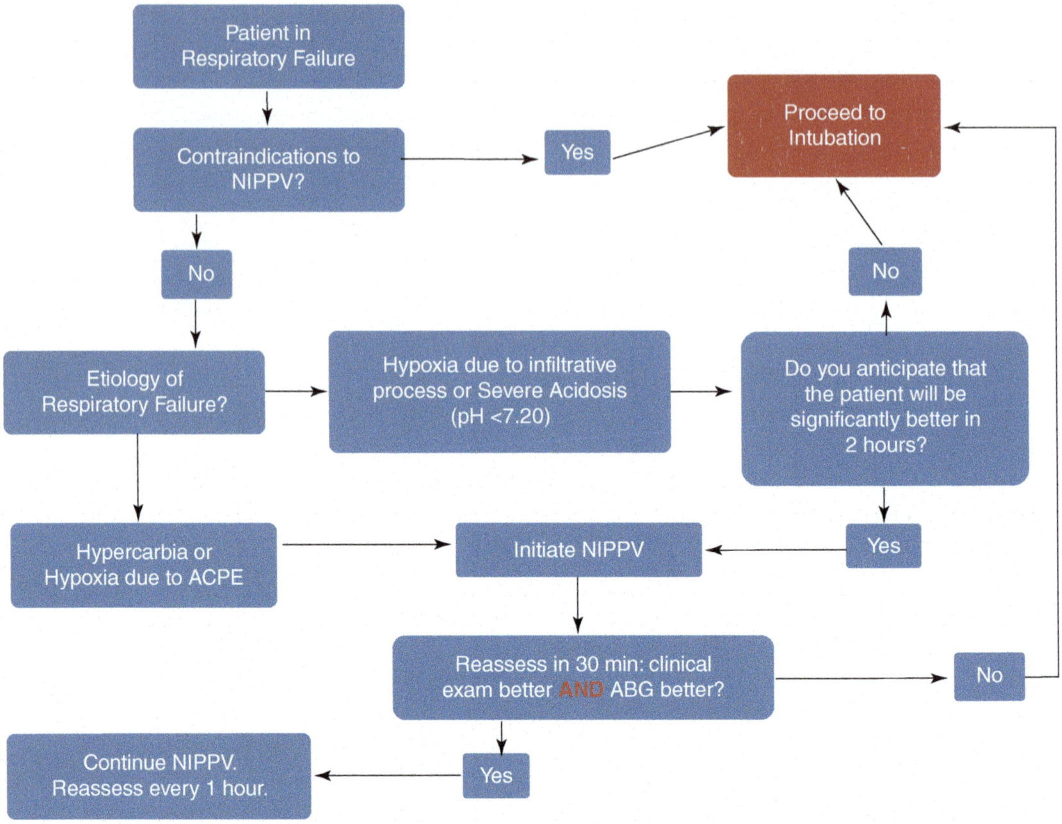

Fig. 4.2 Flow diagram for the initiation of NIPPV on a patient with respiratory failure

Table 4.1 Contraindications to NIPPV

Contraindications for NIPPV	
Uncooperative patient	Patient unable to protect airway
Apnea	Severe hypoxemia
Severe acidemia	Multiorgan failure
Inability to control secretions	Vomiting
Upper gastrointestinal bleeding	Airway obstruction
Severe hemodynamic instability	Anticipated prolonged respiratory failure

lung segment or alveolus has been completely obstructed so that no air gets to the alveoli. In this case, the $V = 0$ and Q remains the same. The $V/Q = 0$, which is known as a pulmonary shunt. In the second example, the lung segment has adequate ventilation but has no blood flow to the alveolar–capillary interface (i.e., during pulmonary embolism). This situation will have $V/Q = \infty$, which is known as dead space. In clinical terms, oxygenation will be poor in the setting of significant V/Q mismatch, regardless of the extreme end of the spectrum on which it lies [6].

Gas delivery to smaller airways may be disrupted by several mechanisms. It is possible to have ineffective delivery due to bronchial collapse. These conditions may be seen in external mass effect on airways, foreign bodies, or an ET placed into a main stem bronchus. There are also conditions that inhibit the ability of the alveoli to accommodate gasses. Alveolar collapse (atelectasis) will often cause hypoxia. Atelectasis is related to pressure compression of alveoli, insufficient thoracic negative pressure, surfactant deficiency/dysfunction, or mechanical obstruction of the smaller airways due to mucus. There are also a number of infiltrative processes in which alveolar gas exchange is limited because the alveolar space is occupied by simple fluid, blood, inflammatory cells, or debris.

Oxygen diffusion across the alveolar–capillary membrane is far less efficient than CO_2 diffusion. Therefore, even when gas delivery to alveoli has occurred, there may still be barriers to O_2 diffusion across the alveolar–capillary membrane. Acute processes that alter the interface between alveolus and capillary, like pulmonary edema and pneumonitis, are commonly seen in clinical practice. In each of these conditions, it is critical to identify the underlying cause and target treatment with appropriate anti-inflammatories, diuretics, or antibiotics. Supplemental O_2 will increase alveolar oxygen concentration and help improve most forms of hypoxemia.

Failure to oxygenate is easy to identify with clinical examination, pulse oximetry, or an arterial blood gas. When supplemental O_2 is unable to provide adequate oxygenation, NIPPV may be indicated. If the patient is not a candidate for NIPPV, then invasive PPV is indicated. PPV allows for the best optimization and control of oxygen delivery (DO_2) and MAP. There are numerous methods for supplementing O_2 concentration beyond the 21% fraction of inspired oxygen (FiO_2) of room air. Simple noninvasive tools primarily include nasal cannulas, face shields, and face masks. By increasing the O_2 concentration in the alveolar gas, a favorable O_2 gradient is created and O_2 diffuses from the alveolus to the alveolar–capillary beds. The FiO_2 delivered with supplemental O_2 can reach levels near 100%. There will be situations where hypoxia prevails despite maximizing FiO_2. These are cases where $V/Q = 0$, and PPV is required to improve the shunt physiology before the hypoxia will be corrected.

There are several factors that contribute to the MAP, including inspiratory time and inspiratory pressure, but the most clinically significant factor is positive end-expiratory pressure (PEEP). MAP augmentation is a critical tool in the treatment of hypoxia related to intrapulmonary shunting. PEEP is a continuous pressure that remains after completion of the exhaled phase. By keeping some positive airway pressure during exhalation, there is less alveolar collapse. This is the concept of open lung ventilation. The underlying pulmonary pathology, level of PEEP, and pulmonary compliance all factor into how well alveoli respond to PEEP. With time and increasing levels of PEEP, collapsed alveoli may open up. This is alveolar recruitment. Using PEEP is a way to try to expose more alveoli to an elevated MAP with each respiratory phase. Alveolar recruitment improves pulmonary compliance and improves shunt physiology by increasing the functional reserve capacity (FRC). As more alveoli open and are able to accommodate airflow, there is an increase in V_A that will help correct V/Q mismatching.

There is evidence that higher plateau pressures (>27 cm H_2O) are associated with right ventricular (RV) failure [7]. As MAP increases, the RV must work harder which causes the RV to fail [8, 9]. For patients with severe hypoxemia, there is a balance of making sure that the patient receives enough oxygen without causing RV failure. Prone positioning reduces airway pressure and pCO_2, which reduces RV overload. This may be the reason for which there were less cardiac arrests in the PROSEVA trial [8, 10].

Once a patient is connected to invasive PPV and V_A is optimized, it is important to account for the extrapulmonary components of oxygen delivery.

$$DO_2 = CO \times \left[\left(1.34 \times Hgb \times SaO_2\right) + \left(0.003 \times PaO_2\right)\right],$$

where CO = cardiac output, Hgb = hemoglobin

This equation highlights the efficiency of hemoglobin's oxygen transport and the importance of attaining adequate O_2 saturations. From the oxygen dissociation curve, at a pO_2 of 60, hemoglobin is 90% saturated. There is really no clinical difference for any further increase in the percentage saturation of hemoglobin. There are only a few situations (e.g., severe anemia or carbon monoxide poisoning) where focusing on the small contribution of dissolved oxygen (pO_2) will yield significant clinical effects. The techniques for optimizing CO and appropriate hemoglobin levels fall outside this discussion on MV, but their consideration is paramount in critically ill patients who show evidence of inadequate DO_2. Similarly, hyperbaric oxygen is a method to increase the oxygen content of the blood, but its use is also outside the realm of this discussion.

Ventilation

Ventilation is the removal of carbon dioxide (CO_2) from the body. This process is much less complex than oxygenation. Minute ventilation (V_E) is the volume of air entering or exiting the respiratory system per minute.

$$V_E = RR \times V_T,$$

where RR = respiratory rate and V_T = tidal volume

Ventilation is a dynamic process that relies on matching respiratory drive to metabolic demands. Hypoventilation is the result of a respiratory drive that is unable to match intrinsic metabolic demands, which results in an elevated pCO_2 level and acidosis (in an acute situation). This may be seen in times of normal or accelerated metabolism and cellular waste production. Inadequate ventilation is due to a relatively low RR, low V_T, or increased dead space ventilation. The alveolar–capillary CO_2 exchange is quite efficient. CO_2 exchanges across the alveolar–capillary interface are about 20 times more efficient than oxygen (O_2) [6]. As a result, dysfunctional gas exchange at the level of the alveoli is rarely a primary driver for hypoventilation.

It is critical to determine the acuity of pCO_2 elevation. Patients with chronic respiratory diseases like COPD or obesity hypoventilation syndrome may have pCO_2 levels that are elevated at baseline. This pCO_2 elevation has occurred over time, and compensatory mechanisms have been able to buffer the acidic CO_2, so that there should be no acidemia. The most prominent compensatory mechanism is the kidney's excretion of carbonic acid and increased bicarbonate absorption. This process, while powerful, takes 1–5 days to provide significant compensation. This is the key to differentiating the timing of an elevated pCO_2. An elevated pCO_2 with associated acidosis (pH <7.35) suggests an acute uncompensated hypoventilation. An elevated pCO_2 without acidosis warrants further clinical investigation because the patient may be at his or her baseline state.

While thinking of ventilation in the simple terms of RR and V_T is clinically helpful, it is important to account for the components of V_T.

$$V_T = V_A + V_D,$$

where V_A is alveolar ventilation and V_D is dead space ventilation

Dead space is any area in which there is no gas exchange taking place. This includes the endotracheal (ET) tube, trachea, and large airways. These are all fixed volumes and are the first volumes of gas exhaled. Since gas exchange does not occur in these areas, there is no ventilatory contribution. On a ventilator, the typical V_D in an adult is about 150 mL [6]. With this in mind, consider a typical adult patient with shallow breaths (V_T about 250 mL). The patient will only be exchanging about 100 mL of alveolar volume per breath. Even if the RR is 50, the V_E will be 5 L, which may be too little depending on the clinical situation.

The two parameters used to modify ventilation will be RR and V_T. If low RR is the only variable driving the acute hypercapnic respiratory failure, this should be evident when examining and monitoring the patient. Hypoventilation secondary to low RR typically stems from the central nervous system (CNS). The CNS may be affected by injury, disease, toxins, or medications (especially inappropriate narcotic and sedative ingestions). Reversing the underlying CNS cause of hypopnea will lead to adequate ventilation. If this is not possible or ineffective, the patient will require NIPPV (if there are no contraindications) or PPV to increase the patient's V_E.

There are also a number of conditions that lead to hypoventilation by way of inadequate V_T. One group of conditions is defined by poor respiratory muscle contraction, as seen in neuromuscular disorders like Guillain–Barre syndrome, Amyotrophic Lateral Sclerosis, or Myasthenia Gravis. Poor chest wall mechanics as seen in significant trauma or restrictive thoracic anatomy is another cause of low V_T. Lastly, low volumes of gas reaching alveoli (e.g., obesity, pulmonary edema, or pneumothorax) may contribute to inadequate ventilation.

When combined with treatment of the underlying problem, NIPPV or PPV may improve gas exchange by augmenting the patient's V_T.

Failure to ventilate adequately is identified with clinical examination (although not always reliable) and a blood gas (arterial or venous). Interpreting this information and determining the need for intubation is often more complicated. Patients may have a normal oxygen level but still be hypoventilating, which occurs when the pCO_2 is elevated to a point to disturb the patient's A–a gradient. It is important to take into account the patient's history (including baseline pCO_2 level), symptoms of hypercapnia, and response to therapy. Medications targeted at the underlying cause (e.g., naloxone) or NIPPV may be appropriate treatment options for patients with hypoventilation. If the patient fails to respond to these interventions or has hypercapnia with severe metabolic or mental status derangements, invasive PPV is most appropriate.

Airway Protection

This indication for MV is the most subjective. There are many different etiologies to consider when dealing with upper airway compromise. For patients with upper airway obstruction, intubation or other airway bypass means are often necessary. Many etiologies, like angioedema and neck hematoma, tend to worsen over time without definitive treatment. Early intubation while treating the underlying reason for needing airway protection is the best treatment plan. It is easier to identify obstructive airway tissues than it is to assess a patient's ability to protect his or her airway. There is a wide range of diseases that could compromise a patient's ability to protect his or her airway from occlusion or aspiration. Differentiating patients based on the etiology is helpful, especially if the underlying problem is immediately reversible.

However, many patients have metabolic or neurologic dysfunction that cannot be easily reversed. The provider must rely on subjective features, including alertness, swallow/speech function, and secretion quality, to make a determination regarding airway protection. There have been attempts to assign airway protection prognostication to more objective measures like the Glasgow Coma Scale (GCS) and the presence of a gag or cough. A depressed GCS of 8 or less has value in determining which patients require intubation, but it alone is not an adequate decision tool [11, 12]. In controlled experiments, 37% of healthy subjects did not have a gag reflex [13]. In every case, the provider must carefully consider the GCS and individual clinical situation when determining if intubation is needed for airway protection.

Anticipated Clinical Course

There are situations where the healthcare provider has to evaluate and treat the patient while trying to predict downstream events. Many times, careful foresight and a controlled intubation can prevent a crash airway emergency. Going back to the idea of improving gas exchange and maximizing DO_2, there are many instances where a patient may not have a problem with their respiratory system per se, but the patient would clearly benefit from being on MV.

Consider a patient with blunt trauma who arrives in the ED with a borderline hemodynamic status and waning mental status. One could argue that immediate intubation is unnecessary because the patient is protecting his or her airway, is oxygenating well, and has a GCS greater than 8. However, there is the high likelihood of serious injury and a clinical trajectory of decreasing mental and hemodynamic status. This patient will need prompt clinical and radiographic evaluation and possibly emergent operative intervention. Transporting the patient away from the ED for imaging, the operating room, or to another facility may put he or she at risk of aspiration or other airway failure. Preemptively securing a patient's airway in the ED is far safer than having to emergently manage an airway while in the halls of the hospital or in the back of an ambulance.

In addition to patients with multisystem trauma, there are medical patients who will benefit from early intubation. For example, in an elderly patient with pneumonia, mild hypoxia on supplemental O_2, tachypnea, and using some accessory muscles, fatigue is highly likely. Even with antibiotics and oxygen, the clinical picture is not likely to improve over the next several hours. Intubating the patient early in the clinical course is preferred instead of letting the patient become exhausted and use up his or her physiologic reserve. There are also patients with severe nonpulmonary illness who benefit from early intubation. Consider a patient with bacteremia and associated septic shock. This patient has increased metabolic demands and physiologic strain. The pulmonary function may be normal, but in states of critical illness, the respiratory system may account for up to 24% of metabolic demands [14]. Intubating these patients will offload physiologic strain and allow for increased DO_2 to the brain, heart, kidneys, and liver.

Ventilator Parameters and Modes

Current ventilators have a variety of modes. Many clinicians tout benefits of one mode over another, but most of this is based on anecdotes and personal preference. There is not one mode of ventilation that is best for all patients, but there are some modes that may be more appropriate than others in certain clinical situations [15]. The modes typically seen in the ED include assist control (AC), synchronized intermittent mandatory ventilation (SIMV), pressure support ventilation (PSV), and airway pressure release ventilation (APRV). There are many additional modes, but those are used less frequently. The variety of modes, numerous acronyms, and different terminology often lead to confusion, but breaking MV down to its basic parameters may aid in the understanding of each mode.

Parameters

Parameters are features and settings on the ventilator that determine how a breath is initiated, how large a breath will be, and how long a breath will last. Parameters are independent of the mode of ventilation. One mode may have several possible combinations of the same parameters. Regardless of the mode, there will always be the four parameters below. The selection and combination of the parameters help define the mode and determine how the patient and ventilator will interact.

As ventilators become more sophisticated, manufacturers develop proprietary nomenclature for these new advances. These new terms become confusing to practitioners because they may only be familiar with one manufacturer for all of their ventilators. When confusion occurs about a ventilator mode, remember to focus on the parameters of the ventilator and what you are trying to accomplish with the ventilator.

Control

The term control has two meanings when talking about MV. A ventilator breath can be referred to as controlled or assisted. Breaths that are initiated by the ventilator are termed controlled, and those that are initiated by the patient are termed assisted. Control, as a parameter of the ventilator, is what the ventilator delivers to the patient. Volume control or pressure control is most frequently used. For volume control, a specific V_T is set. The ventilator then modulates pressure delivery in order to attain the set volume. As pulmonary compliance worsens, the ventilator will use a higher pressure to achieve the set volume. Volume control is most commonly used when patients are initiated on MV because it allows for close control of V_E.

In pressure control (sometimes called PCV), a maximum pressure is set. Volume is delivered until the desired pressure is reached. With pressure control, V_T will vary with each breath. As pulmonary compliance worsens, the resultant V_T will be smaller. Since there may be dramatic breath-by-breath variation in the V_T during pressure control, it may be more difficult to ensure a consistent V_E.

Trigger

Trigger is the parameter that determines what initiates inhalation. In most cases, this will be time, pressure, or flow. There are some applications where esophageal pressure or neurologic impulses may be used as a trigger, but these are rarely seen in the ED. When time is used as the trigger, the RR is selected and each minute is divided into equal blocks based on that rate. The ventilator will then ensure that a time-triggered breath is given at least once in every time period. In some modes, the ventilator will not deliver a controlled breath if the patient initiates his or her own breath in that specified time block. For example, if the RR is set for 10 breaths per minute, there will be a time-triggered breath every 6 seconds. If the patient does not initiate a breath, then the ventilator will ensure that a controlled breath occurs every 6 seconds.

In addition to time, pressure or flow may be a trigger to initiate a breath. Pressure or flow triggering relies on the patient taking a breath. When the patient inhales, there will be a decrease in the pressure within the ventilator tubing. This attempted breath will also create negative flow. If the pressure decrease or negative flow meets the set threshold, then an assisted breath will be delivered. Pressure and flow triggering allows the ventilator to support or augment breaths in those patients with an intrinsic drive but insufficient strength. Some breaths within a set mode may be time triggered and others may be pressure or flow triggered.

Cycle

Cycle is what ends the inspiratory phase of the ventilator. This is different from starting exhalation. Exhalation is a passive process on a ventilator, unless using a high-frequency mode like high-frequency oscillatory ventilation. The cycle may be volume, pressure, flow, or time. Once the inspiratory phase has reached the set end point, the ventilator will stop delivering a positive-pressure breath. The patient may continue inhaling beyond this point, but the ventilator will no longer be assisting the patient's inspiratory effort. As soon as the inhalation stops, it gives way to the exhalation phase of breathing.

Limit

Limits are the safety mechanisms on the ventilator. A limit may be set to a specific pressure, volume, flow, or time. Limits are determined for the control, the trigger, and the cycle. If a limit is reached, then an alarm goes off. This alarm is a warning to the provider that there is a problem with the control, the trigger, or the cycle. The purpose of having a limit is that if the ventilator goes beyond the limit, then there is a higher likelihood of injury to the respiratory system.

Modes

The mode of ventilation refers to the manner in which the ventilator provides inspiratory support to the patient. Each mode uses some combination of the above parameters to ensure that gas is delivered to the patient. The mode will determine how the patient and ventilator interact. Some modes disregard a patient's intrinsic respiratory drive completely and focus only on delivering controlled breaths. Other modes may not deliver controlled breaths and only assist when the patient attempts a breath. Mode names may vary depending on the ventilator brand. Focusing on the underlying parameters and the nature of the patient–ventilator interaction will guide the appropriate mode choice for each clinical situation. Figure 4.3 shows ventilator waveforms for airway pressure, flow, and volume as each relates to the mode.

Continuous Mandatory Ventilation (CMV) and Assist Control (AC)

The oldest and simplest mode of mechanical ventilation is CMV. It may be volume or pressure controlled but will always be time triggered. The provider sets the desired volume or pressure and then sets the desired rate. A controlled breath will be delivered at the specified rate. It is an appropriate mode for patients who have no intrinsic respiratory drive or are paralyzed. The downside of CMV is when the patient has a RR greater than

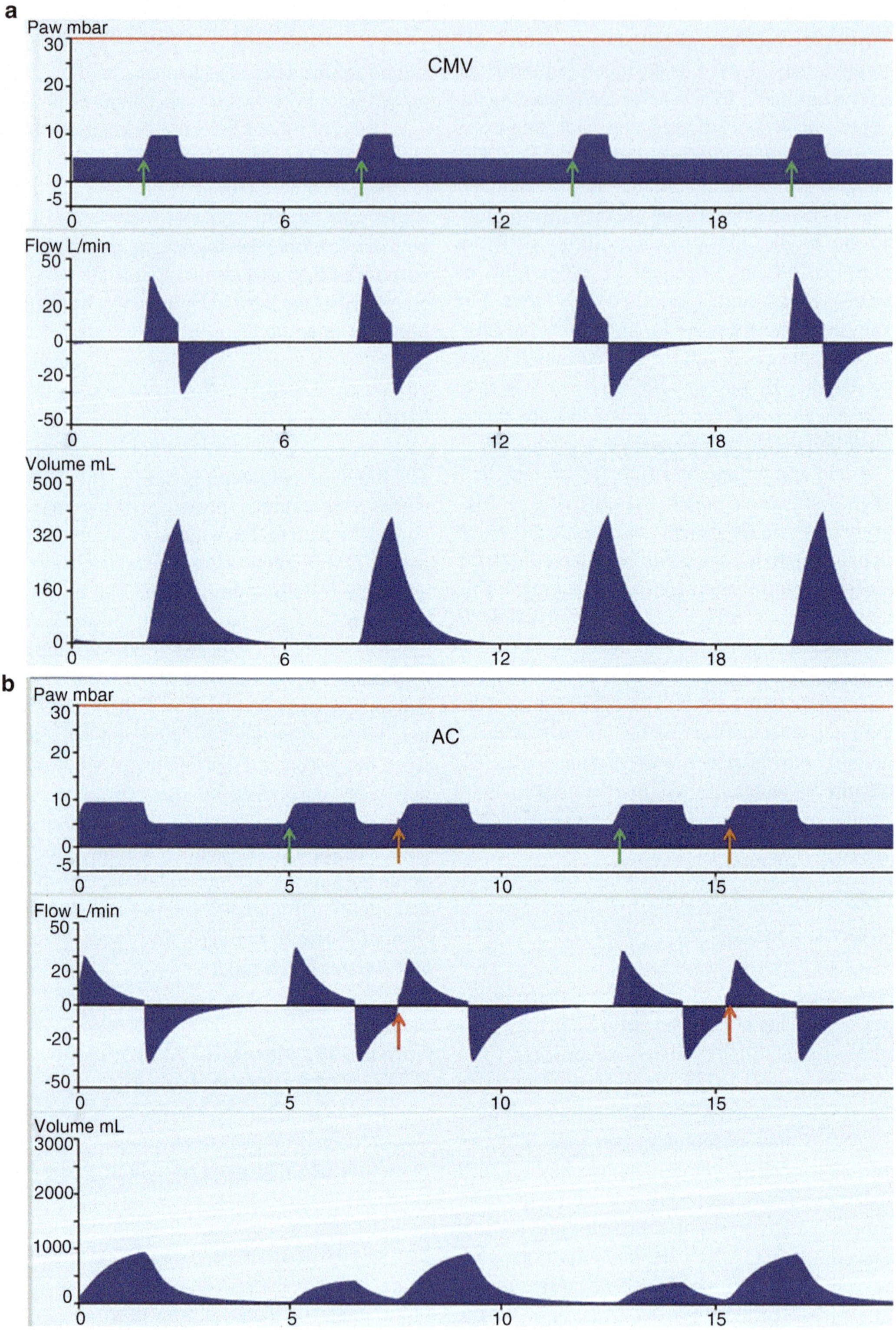

Fig. 4.3 Waveforms of different ventilator modes. (**a**) CMV, (**b**) AC, (**c**) IMV, (**d**) SIMV, (**e**) SIMV/PSV, (**f**) APRV. Green arrows are controlled breaths. Orange arrows are assisted breaths. Red arrows are patient attempts to breathe. (Images adapted from Dräger Evita V500 Product Demonstrator manual simulation available at www.Draeger.com)

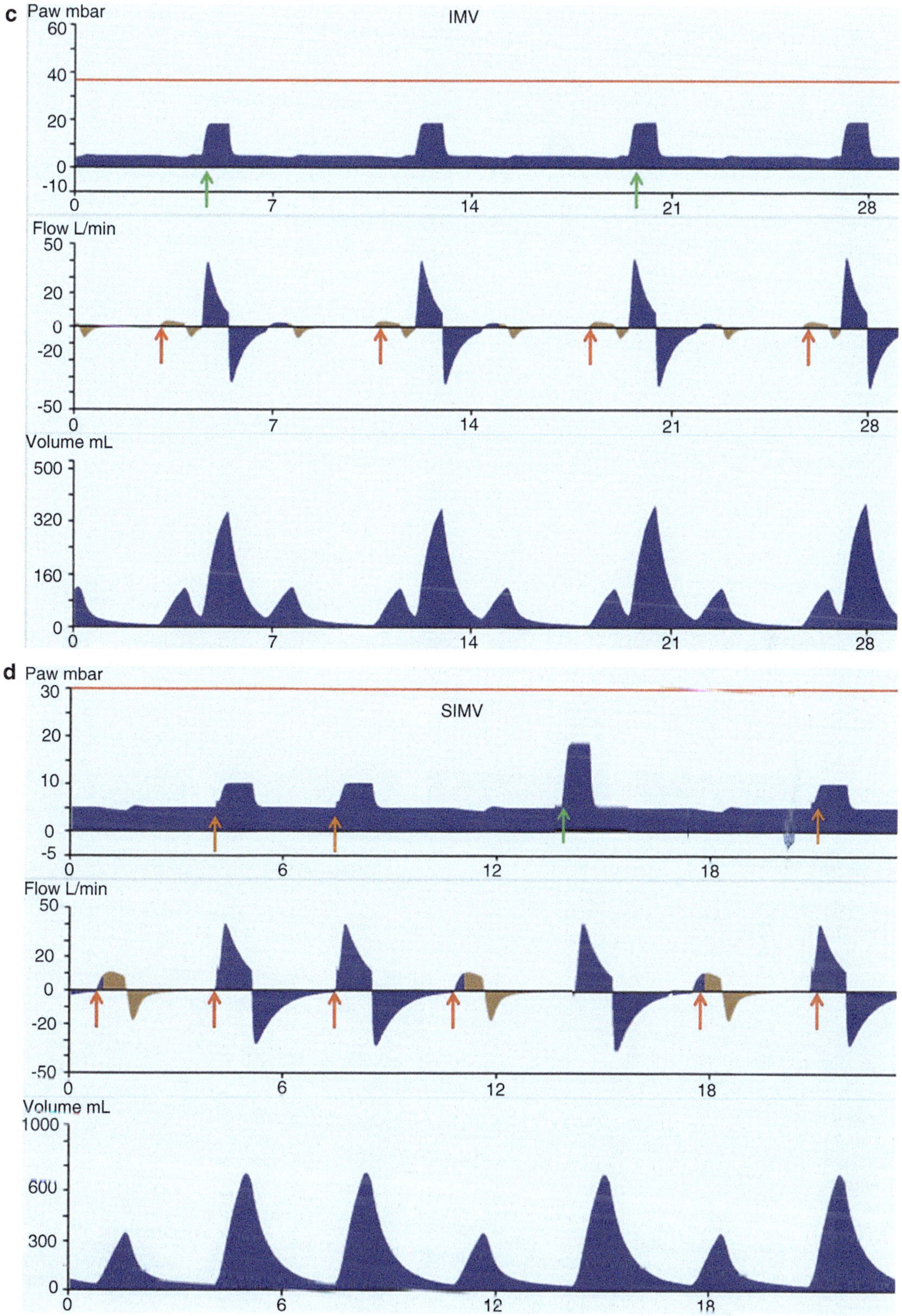

Fig. 4.3 (continued)

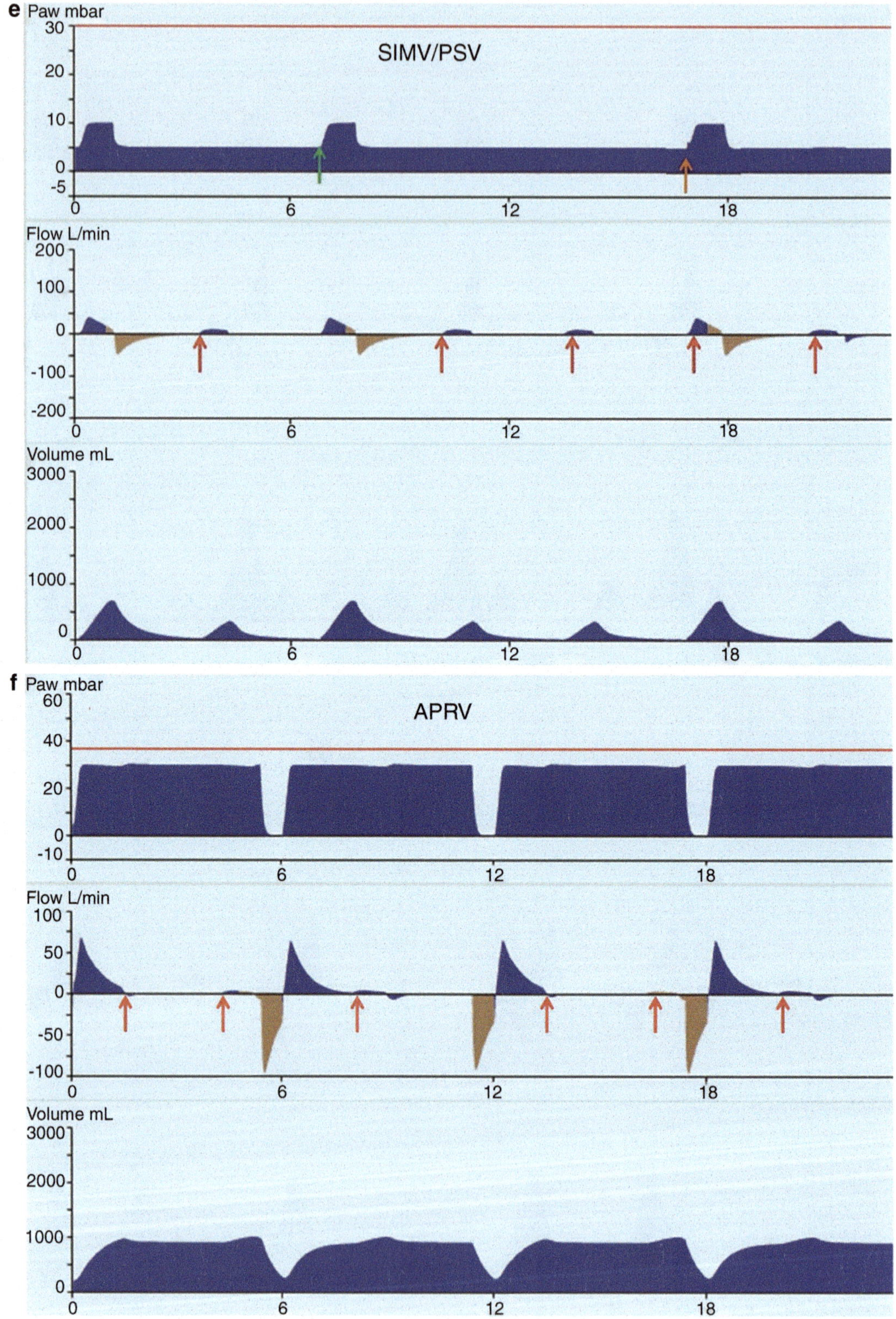

Fig. 4.3 (continued)

the set rate and attempts a spontaneous breath between controlled breaths. These spontaneous patient breaths occur against a closed circuit. For the patient, this is analogous to inhaling through a tube with a cork on the end. This creates discomfort and anxiety and may make weaning from MV difficult.

Because of the poor patient–ventilator interaction in CMV, it has largely been replaced by AC. If a patient is paralyzed or has an intrinsic RR less than that set on the ventilator, then CMV and AC are the same. The ventilator will deliver a volume- or pressure-controlled breath at the set time. The major difference between CMV and AC is how the ventilator responds when a patient initiates a spontaneous breath. Rather than the spontaneous breath being against a closed circuit as in CMV, in AC, this spontaneous patient breath will be assisted. The ventilator will still ensure that a breath occurs during each time cycle, using controlled breaths if the patient does not initiate a breath. In AC, the ventilator will also give an assisted breath whenever the patient attempts a spontaneous breath. AC is a well-tolerated and comfortable mode of ventilation that is able to dramatically decrease a patient's work of breathing. This feature makes AC a valuable mode in the treatment of respiratory failure related to shock or sepsis. However, since the patient receives the set V_T with each spontaneous effort, the V_E may be excessive. Patients with an inappropriately high RR will be at risk for hyperventilation [16, 17].

Intermittent Mandatory Ventilation (IMV) and Synchronized Intermittent Mandatory Ventilation (SIMV)

IMV is a volume or pressure-controlled mode of ventilation that uses a time trigger. There is a set rate of volume- or pressure-controlled breaths. At first glance, it appears to be the same as CMV. In patients with no respiratory drive or one with an intrinsic rate under that set on the ventilator, IMV is essentially the same as CMV. However, there is a major difference between CMV and IMV when a patient has a spontaneous breath. In IMV, those spontaneous breaths are against an open circuit. It is as if the patient is breathing through an open-ended tube rather than a tube that is occluded. The patient is able to breathe whenever he or she wants, but there are still time-triggered controlled breaths. This may lead to breath stacking when controlled breaths are delivered on top of a patient's spontaneous breaths. The resultant V_T may be quite large and put the patient at risk for barotrauma or volutrauma.

SIMV was developed in order to avoid these air stacking situations and create a better patient–ventilator interaction. SIMV is a modification of IMV that is time and patient (pressure or flow) triggered. For a set RR, the ventilator will divide a minute into equal blocks or segments. The ventilator will ensure that one controlled breath is delivered during each of those blocks. If the patient initiates a spontaneous breath during the block, the ventilator will deliver an assisted breath. That breath will satisfy the requirement for the specific block of time, and the ventilator will wait to give a full breath until the next time segment. If the patient does not take a spontaneous breath during the time segment, a time-triggered controlled breath will be delivered. The ventilator will wait until the end of the time segment before delivering a controlled breath, thereby giving the patient an opportunity to trigger a breath on his or her own. For example, if the ventilator's rate is set at 10, each minute will be divided into ten 6-second blocks. The patient may take spontaneous breaths in all or none of those blocks but will still get at least 10 full breaths per minute. If the patient initiates a breath 2 seconds into the block, then the ventilator will deliver an assisted breath, which will satisfy the breath requirement for that block. Like IMV, the patient is also able to take extra breaths. If the patient initiates two or more breaths during a block, only the first breath will be a fully assisted breath. The subsequent breaths in the same time block will not be assisted by the ventilator.

Since the additional breaths in a time period are unsupported, it is common to combine SIMV with pressure support ventilation (PSV). This new "mode" is called SIMV/PSV (although many practitioners commonly say SIMV when, in fact, they mean SIMV/PSV), but it is actually two ventilator modes working together. SIMV/PSV only differs from SIMV when taking into account the patient's extra spontaneous breaths in a time segment. In SIMV, the patient's extra breaths are unsupported, but in SIMV/PSV, these extra breaths are given a set amount of pressure support. The addition of PSV allows the patient's subsequent spontaneous breaths in a time period to contribute more to the minute ventilation. One of the main benefits of SIMV/PSV is thought to be its ease in weaning, though there is little evidence to support this [15]. Theoretically, there is also a more consistent V_E compared to AC. SIMV/PSV is especially advantageous in patients who have inappropriate tachypnea. Patients are less likely to hyperventilate compared to if they were on AC.

Pressure Support Ventilation (PSV)

PSV is a pressure-controlled mode of ventilation that is flow or pressure triggered. An oversimplified way to think of PSV is to think of PSV as invasive NIPPV. With PSV, there are two pressures that may be adjusted. The first is the inspiratory pressure, which is delivered when the patient generates enough pressure or flow to trigger the ventilator. The second pressure is PEEP. As the expiratory phase ends, the ventilator will keep a set level of PEEP, thereby preventing alveolar pressures from returning to 0 cm H_2O. Each breath the patient takes will get the same inspiratory pressure and PEEP. The rate is up to the patient. The resultant V_T will vary depending on the patient's pulmonary compliance, chest wall compliance, and respiratory effort.

A key difference between PSV and controlled modes, such as AC or SIMV, is that PSV is only pressure or flow triggered. There are no breaths unless the patient has respiratory effort; thus, there is no way to guarantee a minimum V_E. An apneic or very weak patient who is unable to mount a satisfactory inspiratory force will not trigger a breath. It is for this reason that PSV is not an acceptable mode for patients who are paralyzed, have profound diaphragm weakness, or are prone to apnea. (Note: all modern ventilators have backup safety mechanisms in place such that if the minimum V_E alarm is triggered, the ventilator will begin giving patients volume-controlled breaths.) PSV is, however, a comfortable and well-tolerated mode for patients with a good respiratory drive, for example, patients who have been intubated for airway protection only. There is less patient–ventilator dyssynchrony than with other modes of ventilation, and the patient is able to control his or her V_E. PSV is most commonly used in patients intubated for upper airway protection and those who are weaning toward extubation.

Airway Pressure Release Ventilation (APRV)

APRV (sometimes referred to as Bi-Level) is a mode that focuses on elevating the MAP for the purpose alveolar recruitment. It is typically used in patients with poor oxygenation and poor pulmonary compliance. It is a pressure-controlled and time-triggered mode of ventilation. Since it is pressure controlled, there is no specific V_T to set. Instead, the pressures (P_{high} and P_{low}) and times (T_{high} and T_{low}) are set and modified to attain adequate oxygenation and ventilation. The majority of oxygenation occurs at P_{high}, when the alveoli are subject to a sustained pressure. This pressure may force open alveoli and the continuous nature of it tends to keep the alveoli open, thereby leading to alveolar recruitment. The recruited alveoli increase V_A. With increased V_A, gas exchange should improve. This concept is most helpful with oxygenation. CO_2 removal primarily occurs during the patient's unassisted spontaneous respirations at P_{high} and during pressure drops (called "releases") from P_{high} to P_{low}. The pressure gradient from P_{high} to P_{low} is a major factor for determining the amount of CO_2 removed.

APRV is excellent for oxygenation, but adequate ventilation may be difficult. Since a good deal of CO_2 removal depends on the patient's

Table 4.2 Recommendations for initial ventilator settings based on different clinical pictures

	Airway protection	Hypoxia	COPD or asthma	Increased metabolic demands
Key concerns or considerations	Apnea	Lung protection	Auto-PEEP	Matching respiratory alkalosis
Mode	PSV, AC, SIMV+P	AC, SIMV+P	AC, SIMV+P	AC, SIMV+P
V_T (mL/kg of IBW)	6	6	6	6
RR	10–14	12–20	6–8	18–24
PEEP (cm H_2O)	5	8	0–5	5
FiO_2	0.4	0.8–1.0	0.4–1.0	0.4
I:E	1:2	1:2	1:3–1:5	1:2
Inspiratory flow (L/min)	60	60	100	60

Each setting should take into account the underlying pathology and key physiologic consideration

spontaneous breaths, this mode should be avoided in heavily sedated or paralyzed patients.

Dual-Mode Ventilation

Dual-mode ventilation is not really a ventilator mode, but rather an attempt to target a certain V_T by using a pressure limit. Going back to the idea of manufacturers trying to make their product marketable, they coin new terms and market these terms as "modes" when, in fact, they are not. PRVC (pressure-regulated volume control), Autoflow, and VC+ are examples of this marketing strategy that can easily confuse the practitioner, especially if he or she does not use ventilators every day. Despite the confusing nomenclature of ventilators, no one mode has a better mortality benefit over another.

PRVC is essentially VC+, which is found on Puritan Bennett ventilators, or Autoflow, which is found on Dräger ventilators. These three terms, PRVC, VC+, and Autoflow, can be used to describe a ventilator mode that is pressure limited and volume and time cycled. The ventilator is set up in a volume-cycled mode. The ventilator uses a constant pressure throughout inspiration, which causes a decelerating flow pattern. The ventilator compares the resistance and compliance and delivered V_T for each breath to determine the amount of pressure needed to deliver the set V_T. If the delivered V_T is too high, then the ventilator decreases the inspiratory pressure on the next breath. If the delivered V_T is too low, then the ventilator increases the inspiratory pressure on the next breath.

Initial Ventilator Settings

Whenever a patient is placed on MV, it is important to have an idea of why the patient needs the ventilator. This knowledge will help determine what the initial ventilator settings should be (Table 4.2). It is recommended to obtain an ABG soon after starting MV to ascertain the type of respiratory failure: hypoxic, hypercapnic, or both.

First, choose the mode. A volume-controlled mode with a time trigger, such as AC or SIMV/PSV, is usually the first choice for most clinicians since it will ensure a minimum V_E and is appropriate for apneic patients. PSV is a potential option but only in spontaneously breathing patients without risk of apnea.

Second, set (in the case of a volume-controlled mode) or target (in the case of a pressure-controlled mode) a V_T of 6 mL/kg ideal body weight (IBW). Low tidal volumes of 6 mL/kg of IBW have been shown to decrease mortality and ICU length of stay in patients with acute respiratory distress syndrome (ARDS) [18]. Even when the clinical scenario may not meet all criteria for ARDS, there is emerging evidence that patients without ARDS have better outcomes when using low V_T [19]. It is also important to use IBW to calculate V_T, which is based on a patient's height.

Approximately 10–15 minutes after initiating a V_T of 6 ml/kg IBW, it is important to assess the plateau pressure (P_{plat}). This is done by performing an inspiratory hold on the ventilator. Most modern ventilators have a button/knob for this feature. ARDSnet guidelines recommend a P_{plat} less than 30 cm H_2O. There is evidence that mortality is proportional to the P_{plat} [20], so it would be prudent to minimize the P_{plat}.

The third step in setting up the ventilator is to select the RR. The goal is to match or exceed the preintubation V_E. For clinical conditions where the patient has a high metabolic demand and V_E, such as septic shock, salicylate toxicity, or diabetic ketoacidosis (DKA), it is important to ensure that the postintubation V_E is high. For example, a patient with DKA may have a pH of 6.9 while generating his or her own V_E of 30 L/min. In this case, the patient is barely compensating for the severe metabolic acidosis despite an extremely high V_E. Choosing a V_T and RR that yields a lower V_E than the preintubation value of 30 L/min may lead to cardiac arrest since the lower V_E will allow CO_2 to rise which will cause the pH will fall below 6.9.

After setting the RR, it is important to frequently reassess the patient's pH and ventilator parameters. In a case such as this, end-tidal CO_2 measurement before, during, and after intubation may be particularly useful. Monitoring of real-time trends in ventilation may allow for quicker intervention than conventional titration by blood gases [21]. With regard to the severity of lung injury, if P_{plat} is elevated >30 cm H_20, a V_T of 4–5 mL/kg may be needed. In this situation, it is often necessary to increase the RR in order to maintain an appropriate V_E.

The next setting to consider is the breakdown of each breath into an inspiratory and expiratory phase. The most common inspiratory to expiratory ratio (I:E) is 1:2. This means that twice as much time is allotted to the expiratory phase of the breath. It is necessary to consider the patient's underlying lung pathology and monitor the ventilator outputs for evidence of auto-PEEP. Patients with a prolonged expiratory phase due to bronchospasm (e.g., COPD) who are prone to air trapping will often need a longer I:E, occasionally as high as 1:8.

The last major settings are FiO_2 and PEEP. As mentioned, each of these relates to oxygenation, and the choice of settings will rely heavily on the clinical situation. An FiO_2 up to 100% may be used initially, but this amount of FiO_2 is usually not needed when PEEP and FiO_2 are titrated to maintain an O_2 saturation of >89%. If a patient is intubated for airway protection and preintubation oxygenation was not an issue, then an FiO_2 of 40–60% with PEEP of 5 should be adequate. For those patients with significant hypoxia, an initial FiO_2 of 80–100% may be more appropriate. A higher PEEP of 8–12 cm H_2O would also be reasonable in an effort to raise the MAP and improve oxygenation.

Titrating PEEP can be a difficult process due to the fact that there is a balance between achieving adequate oxygenation and trying to avoid RV failure. The ARDS network has developed a set of tables (Fig. 4.4) in order to assist providers with initial choice and titration of PEEP and FiO_2. These tables help guide settings that optimize recruitment while minimizing the harmful effects of excessive PEEP [22]. It is important to know that there is no outcome difference between the different tables [23].

Bedside recruitment is another way to titrate PEEP. The ventilator must be in a square wave flow (not PRVC, Autoflow, or VC+). Observe the P_{plat} and PEEP values. Raise the PEEP by some determined amount, usually 2–5 cm H_2O. After approximately 10–15 minutes, if the new P_{plat} rises by less than the amount of PEEP increase, then recruitment has occurred. The reason for this is that compliance is higher. PEEP is opening lung units that are closed, so there is a minimal effect on P_{plat}. However, if the new P_{plat} rises by more than the increase in PEEP, then recruitment has NOT occurred. Instead, the PEEP increase is causing overdistension of already open lung units (volutrauma), which causes the P_{plat} to increase more than the increase in PEEP. Regardless of what strategy is used for PEEP titration, it is best to pick one and continue it throughout the clinical course.

When initiating APRV, P_{high} is set at approximately 5 cm H_2O above the plateau pressure with the usual maximum P_{high} of 35 cm H_2O. P_{low} is set

Lower PEEP/higher Fio2

Fio_2	0.3	0.4	0.4	0.5	0.5	0.6	0.7	0.7
PEEP	5	5	8	8	10	10	10	1.2

Fio_2	0.7	0.8	0.9	0.9	0.9	1.0
PEEP	14	14	14	16	18	18-24

Higher PEEP/Lower Fio2

Fio_2	0.3	0.3	0.3	0.3	0.3	0.4	0.4	0.5
PEEP	5	5	10	12	14	14	16	16

Fio_2	0.5	0.5-0.8	0.8	0.9	1.0	1.0
PEEP	18	20	22	22	22	24

Fig. 4.4 Tables from ARDSnet protocol summary showing different combinations of PEEP and FiO_2. The goal oxygenation is PaO_2 55–80 mmHg or SpO_2 88–95%. (Adapted from www.ARDSNET.org)

to 0 cm H_2O to provide the largest pressure gradient and optimize ventilation. There may be certain cases in which P_{high} is elevated to overcome chest wall or abdominal compliances issues, just as using ARDSnet the P_{plat} can be allowed >30 for same reasons. To optimize oxygenation, it is important to maximize the time with high airway pressure (T_{high}) and minimize time with low airway pressure (T_{low}). The net effect of this strategy will raise the MAP and improve oxygenation. The more time spent at T_{low} may lead to alveolar collapse or derecruitment. Derecruitment may be further minimized by setting a T_{low} that is short enough so that P_{high} restarts before the expiratory/release flow rate has gone below 50%. A common starting point is to set T_{high} for 5.4 seconds and T_{low} for 0.6 seconds. On these settings, there will be one release every 6 seconds or 10 releases per minute.

Specific Clinical Situations and Ventilator Considerations

Airway Protection

Patients who require intubation for airway protection are usually suffering from a neurologic insult. Whether the insult is related to a drug-induced encephalopathy or a direct damage to the brain, the patient, who is unable to protect his or her airway, will need a definitive airway. The ET tube is placed in an effort to protect the patient from aspiration and upper airway occlusion. Assuming that the patient has metabolized the induction medications and paralytics and still has an adequate respiratory drive, PSV may be an appropriate mode of ventilation. PSV would allow the patient to breathe comfortably with a protected airway, while controlling his or her own V_E.

Severe Hypoxemia and ARD (See Chap. 6 for Additional Discussion on ARDS)

ARDS is a condition of hypoxia that may stem from a variety of illnesses and is characterized by alveolar edema, endothelial damage, and neutrophil deposition [24]. Based on the Berlin Criteria [25], ARDS is characterized as acute (less than 1 week onset), noncardiogenic respiratory failure with bilateral opacities on chest radiograph, and PaO_2/FiO_2 ratio <300 mmHg. There are separate classifications for mild (PaO_2/FiO_2 ratio <300 mmHg), moderate (PaO_2/FiO_2

ratio <200 mmHg), and severe (PaO_2/FiO_2 ratio <100 mmHg) ARDS. Though the definition has changed, the clinical implication is the same.

Patients may not initially present to the ED with florid ARDS, but it does not take long for ARDS to develop. As critically ill patients spend more time in the ED, EM providers must become familiar with ventilation management in ARDS [26]. While many ARDS management options may have little utility in the ED, there is an ARDS management strategy that is easily applied upon initial presentation. The use of low V_T is the cornerstone of ARDS management. In the original ARMA trial, V_T of 12 mL/kg IBW was compared to V_T of 6 mL/kg IBW. The low V_T group was associated with a decrease in mortality (31% vs. 40% at 28 days) [18]. With this initial result as well as several follow-up studies and analyses, the estimate for number needed to treat is only about 10 to attain a mortality benefit [27]. The benefits of lower V_T ventilation in ARDS extend beyond mortality and include decreased time on ventilator and decreased ICU length of stay.

The evidence for using low V_T is quite strong, but there are a number of real-world implications that must be taken into consideration. First, low V_T is based on IBW. Providers tend to do a poor job of estimating a patient's height while he or she lies on the stretcher [28]. For this reason, providers should take a brief moment to measure a patient's height before calculating the goal V_T.

Another issue to consider is ventilation. When using a low V_T, V_E becomes more reliant on a higher RR. There are times when the RR is limited by obstructive issues or auto-PEEP. Other times, the metabolic demands are so high that even with a high RR, the patient's V_E may still be inadequate. Despite this, there should still be an emphasis of maintaining a low V_T. In fact, if this clinical situation occurs, it is tolerable to allow the pCO_2 to rise greater than 45 mmHg or allow the pH to drift below 7.35. This is termed permissive hypercapnia [29]. Even in patients with a significant respiratory acidosis (pH <7.2), it is recommended to continue low V_T ventilation. Treatment of the associated respiratory acidosis is controversial, but it is reasonable to add a buffer infusion like sodium bicarbonate or THAM to keep pH between 7.15 and 7.20 [30]. There is even some suggestion that permissive hypercapnia may itself carry some mortality benefit outside the strict adherence to low V_T [31–33].

Despite the benefits seen with ventilator strategies that rely on permissive hypercapnia, it is important to keep in mind the select patient populations that may be hurt by elevated pCO_2 levels. This includes patients with increased intracranial pressures or other significant neurologic issues, since the elevated pCO_2 will cause marked dilation of the cerebral arteries and an increase cerebral blood flow. Patients with significant arrhythmias, heart failure (especially right ventricle), or pulmonary hypertension may not tolerate hypercapnia well either.

As mentioned above, ARDS may not be apparent in the ED, and it is difficult to determine which patients with acute respiratory failure will progress to that severity of illness. Despite that, the dramatic benefits seen with low V_T make it reasonable to use this ventilation strategy even if ARDS criteria are not met. In summary, patients intubated for respiratory failure in the ED are likely to benefit from a V_T of 6 mL/kg IBW.

Obstructive Lung Disease and Auto-PEEP (See Chap. 6 for Additional Discussion on COPD)

The decision to intubate a patient with a COPD or asthma exacerbation is often difficult because it often depends more on subjective factors, such as work of breathing, anticipated respiratory fatigue, or mental status changes. Once the patient is intubated, the clinical management may become even more difficult. In the case of a COPD exacerbation, there is most likely going to be acute respiratory acidosis. Because of this and the need for close monitoring of V_E, a volume-controlled AC or SIMV is usually most appropriate. The provider can then set a minimum V_E in an effort to improve ventilation.

The obstructive nature of COPD and asthma makes these patients difficult to ventilate and also makes these patients prone to auto-PEEP [34] (also known as air stacking, breath stacking, or air trapping). When the end-expiratory volume exceeds the relaxed lung volume (at the end of lung elastic recoil), there will be dynamic pulmonary hyperinflation. This represents the volume component of auto-PEEP. There is also a pressure component related to the buildup of air volume in airways [35].

For most patients, an I:E of 1:2 is sufficient. However, in patients with obstructive lung disease who have expiratory flow limitation, an I:E of 1:2 may not allow for complete exhalation. For example, assume the patient is on a time-triggered volume-controlled mode that delivers a V_T of 500 mL every 5 seconds. The ventilator may deliver the 500 mL volume over 1 second, but with obstructive airway disease, it may take 5 seconds to fully exhale that volume. Monitoring of ventilator measurements may show inhaled V_T of 500 mL but measured expiratory V_T of only 400 mL. With each breath cycle, the problem is compounded and 100 mL of volume is added to the dead space. As this continues, there is increase alveolar distention and pressure. Eventually, the increasing airway pressures will inflict barotrauma, seen as pneumomediastinum or pneumothorax. The excess alveolar volume will overdistend and stretch the alveoli, causing volutrauma. Auto-PEEP also leads to a significant increase in intrathoracic pressure, which will cause cardiovascular compromise by impaired venous return to the RA and increased pulmonary vascular resistance. It is common to see hypotension or hypoxia as a result of these physiologic changes.

There are clinical clues and ventilator measurements that may help providers identify auto-PEEP early. From a clinical standpoint, it is helpful to auscultate the lungs during several respiratory cycles. If the next inspiration occurs while still auscultating the previous exhalation, then the patient has auto-PEEP. It is also important to monitor the patient's respiratory effort and synchrony with the ventilator. There are different ventilator values that may aid in diagnosis of auto-PEEP, but it is important to realize that the PEEP measured by the ventilator is greater than the PEEP set. Assuming no circuit or airway leak, the measured exhaled V_T should be approximately equal the inhaled V_T. If there is a significant difference between those two values, auto-PEEP is likely present. There are also ventilator graphics that show flow over time. If the negative flow (representing exhalation) deflection does not return to the baseline ($V = 0$) axis before another inspiration is initiated, then there will be air trapping [35]. See Fig. 4.5.

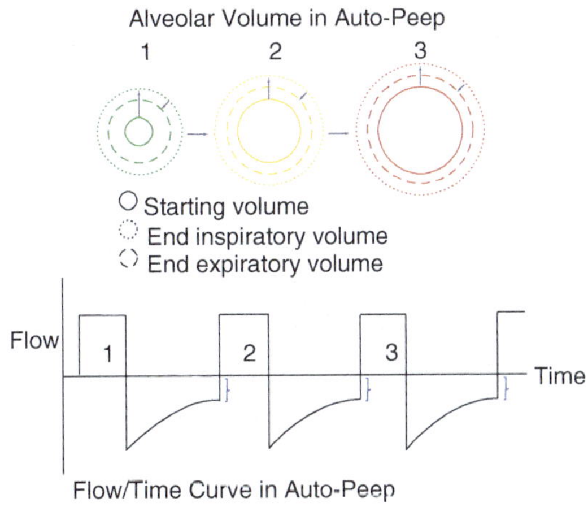

Fig. 4.5 Flow vs. time curve of Auto-PEEP. In the first two cycles, the expiratory flow does not reach 0 L/min before the next inspiratory phase starts. The outlined volume (red) represents auto-PEEP. The images below are a single alveolus acting as a model representing alveolar volume. With each inspiratory volume that has inadequate expiration, the alveolar volume is increasing. This volume stacking represents auto-PEEP. The third image shows alveolar volume after adequate expiration

Troubleshooting the Ventilator

As with any piece of equipment, it is crucial to understand what to do when problems develop. Since the overwhelming majority of ventilated patients in the ED are critically ill, it is important to be able to quickly recognize and rectify problems with the ventilator. Table 4.3 lists several common complications associated with MV.

Auto-PEEP

There are a number of interventions that may be used in patients with auto-PEEP. The first step is to lower the RR. If this does not work, lower the V_T. With less delivered volume, there is less volume to exhale. The next step is to shorten the inspiratory phase of each breath because it leaves more time for a longer expiratory phase. Rather

Table 4.3 Complications associated with mechanical ventilation

Common complications associated with MV	
Volutrauma	Barotrauma
Alveolar injury	Pneumothorax
Tracheal stenosis	Pneumomediastinum
Loss of muscle mass	Stress ulcer
RV failure due	Infections

than the typical I:E of 1:2, it may be necessary to set an I:E of 1:3–1:8. Lowering PEEP may also improve exhalation. Other interventions, such as increased sedation and suctioning, may improve patient–ventilator interaction and maintain a lower RR and V_T. Since the RR and V_T are lowered in response to auto-PEEP, hypoventilation is possible. Depending on the severity of the auto-PEEP, permissive hypercapnia, in an effort to protect from barotrauma and volutrauma, is reasonable.

Whenever a ventilated patient has a dramatic respiratory and cardiovascular decline, always consider auto-PEEP. Assess the pressures measured by the ventilator and look for clinical signs of auto-PEEP. If the patient has findings suggestive of auto-PEEP and has hypotension, immediately disconnect him from the ventilator and allow a prolonged exhalation. Keep the circuit disconnected until the full exhalation is complete. If this does not immediately resolve the cardiovascular decline, then the provider should rapidly evaluate for (and treat) a tension pneumothorax.

Air trapping may have dramatic effects on both respiratory and cardiovascular physiology. It is, therefore, imperative for providers to have a high index of suspicion and to frequently reassess their mechanically ventilated patients, especially those with obstructive lung disease or asthma. It is also important to keep in mind that MV does not treat the underlying disease. Parallel aggressive medical management aimed at bronchodilation is imperative.

Hypoxia

Hypoxia in the setting of MV is common and may be difficult to treat. When an intubated patient has an abrupt change in clinical status or more specifically oxygenation, first evaluate the machinery and circuit. A pneumonic (DOPE) is commonly used to guide this assessment. Look for a dislodged or displaced (D) ET tube. The patient may cough or tongue out the ET tube without warning. There are also times where position change may lead to the ET tube migrating either out of the trachea or down into the right mainstem bronchus. There may be an acute obstruction (O) in the ET tube or airway. Tube kinks, foreign bodies, or mucous plugging of airways are all potential obstructions that will cause hypoxia. With any PPV, there should always be a heightened suspicion for pneumothorax (P), especially in patients with trauma, high peak airway pressures, or asymmetric lung sounds. In addition to a physical examination, it is often necessary to evaluate the patient with some form of imaging: bedside ultrasound, chest X-ray, or chest CT. There is always the chance that some component of the ventilator or other equipment (E) has malfunctioned. In this case, simplify the respiratory circuit by removing the patient from the ventilator and manually using a bag valve mask (BVM). This will allow time to address specific machine issues. Table 4.4 addresses causes of sudden hypoxia in a patient on MV.

As discussed earlier, the two main ventilator settings that affect oxygenation are FiO_2 and PEEP. FiO_2 may be increased to 100%, but that may not be adequate for patients who are difficult to oxygenate. The concept of PEEP and alveolar recruitment highlights the importance of intervening on the underlying V/Q mismatch. Incrementally increasing PEEP will often improve oxygenation. When titrating PEEP, the aforementioned ARDS tables may be a valuable resource. There are times when patients with especially poor lung compliance require a PEEP of 20–24 cm H_2O. It is difficult to determine how quickly patients will respond to adjustments in PEEP. The oxygenation will typically improve within 10 minutes of increasing PEEP, but the full recruitment advantage at a given PEEP may not be seen for over 60 minutes [36]. There will also be diminishing returns on PEEP as the level is raised. At higher levels, the compliant alveoli may stretch to the point that flow of the alveolar–capillary bed is impaired. This will actu-

Table 4.4 Causes of sudden hypoxia in a patient on a ventilator

Causes of sudden hypoxia on a ventilator	
Tube dislodged	Pneumothorax
Tube disconnected from the ventilator	Self-extubation
Tube obstruction	Equipment malfunction
Pulmonary embolism	Autopeep
Bronchospasm	

ally worsen oxygenation as the perfusion of oxygen-rich alveoli decreases by creating more intrapulmonary shunt.

Aside from PEEP, there are other techniques that may be used to minimize the effect of *V*/*Q* mismatch. In patients with a focal consolidation or lateralization of the disease process, place the affected or bad lung up. This leaves the lung with better air exchange in a dependent or lower gravity position. Since pulmonary perfusion favors dependent areas, the lung with better ventilation will receive more perfusion.

There has been recent evidence that this concept can also be applied to some patients with diffuse lung involvement. For patients with ARDS, especially those with posterior lung field involvement, outcomes improved when placing them in a prone position [10]. This technique has shown promise in the ICU setting, but it requires training, staffing, and equipment. These factors may hinder its application in the ED.

There are other situations when a patient's poor interaction with the ventilator contributes to hypoxia. If a patient is agitated, he or she may be attempting to take breaths over controlled breaths or be trying to exhale against delivered breaths. This dyssynchrony with the ventilator inhibits air exchange and may contribute to hypoxia. The goal is to adapt the ventilator to the patient's need, rather than make the patient tolerate the ventilator. Sedation may often alleviate this dyssynchrony and allow adequate breath delivery. The choice of sedation depends heavily on the overall clinical scenario. For most cases, treat pain with intravenous narcotic boluses and agitation with a nonbenzodiazepine sedative, such as propofol. This regiment is typically effective and minimizes the delirium that has been seen with benzodiazepines [37]. In patients with ARDS and refractory hypoxia, heavy sedation may not be enough. Paralysis with neuromuscular blocking agents (for up to 48 hours) may eliminate patient–ventilator dyssynchrony, thereby improving survival and increasing ventilator-free days [38–40].

Alarms

As mentioned before, the limits on the ventilator are in place as a safety net. They can be adjusted to accommodate specific clinical situations, but once a limit is crossed, the alarm sounds. The alarming ventilator warns providers that either targets are not being met or the patient is at risk for injury. The most common alarms will be related to high or low pressures. Figure 4.6 is a flow diagram that shows how to systematically assess pressure alarms and the differentiation of possible etiologies. When faced with pressure alarms without a clear etiology, remove the ventilator circuit and use a BVM. This minimizes variables by isolating the patient from the ventilator and allows for better clinical assessment of compliance.

There may also be alarms related to V_E. A patient with hypopnea or apnea may trigger an alarm for low V_E. This is a warning to providers that the patient is at risk for hypoventilation. Depending on the situation, the patient may need sedation decreased, an increase in the set RR on the ventilator, or conversion from PSV to a mode with a time trigger (for guaranteed breaths). A patient who has high V_E alarms may be agitated with tachypnea or may be compensating for a severe metabolic acidosis. Regardless of the alarm type, the provider should immediately assess the patient at the bedside.

Conclusion

NIPPV and MV aid in stabilizing issues related to airway compromise, ventilation, oxygenation, and clinical course. The positive-pressure circuit enables providers to optimize gas delivery while recruiting collapsed alveoli and controlling V_E. When choos-

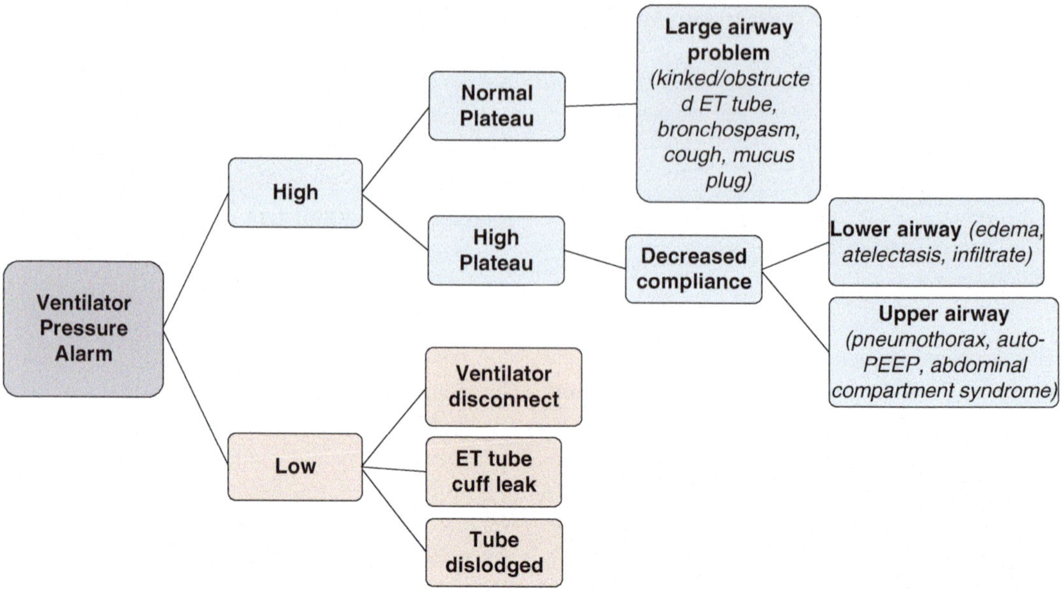

Fig. 4.6 A flow diagram that shows how to systematically assess pressure alarms and the differentiation of possible etiologies

ing between the variety of modes and parameters, it is important to account for the patient's specific needs. Focus on identifying the underlying etiology and complicating features of the patient's respiratory failure. Keep in mind the physiology of ventilation and how titration of RR and V_T control V_E. From an oxygenation stand point, consider the physiology of DO_2 and apply therapies that address the underlying problems. Use FiO_2 to maximize alveolar oxygen content while correcting *V*/*Q* mismatch with PEEP and MAP modulation. Frequently reassess the patient's tolerance of the ventilator, as well as the effects of different settings and interventions. Alarms warn of possible patient danger and should be promptly evaluated. Remember that ventilators can stabilize but do not treat respiratory failure. The goal of ventilator management is to provide time for aggressive treatment of the underlying problem while minimizing physiologic disruption and airway damage.

References

1. Luecke T, Pelosi P. Clinical review: positive end-expiratory pressure and cardiac output. Crit Care Lond Engl. 2005;9:607–21.
2. Gray A, et al. Noninvasive ventilation in acute cardiogenic pulmonary edema. N Engl J Med. 2008;359:142–51.
3. Confalonieri M, et al. A chart of failure risk for non-invasive ventilation in patients with COPD exacerbation. Eur Respir J. 2005;25:348–55.
4. Luo J, et al. Can non-invasive positive pressure ventilation prevent endotracheal intubation in acute lung injury/acute respiratory distress syndrome? A meta-analysis. Respirology Carlton VIC. 2014;19:1149–57.
5. Corrêa TD, et al. Performance of noninvasive ventilation in acute respiratory failure in critically ill patients: a prospective, observational, cohort study. BMC Pulm Med. 2015;15:144.
6. Walls RM, Murphy MF. Manual of emergency airway management. Philadelphia: Wolters Kluwer Health/Lippincott Williams & Wilkins; 2008.
7. West JB. Chapter 50: Acid–base management. In: Respiratory physiology. Baltimore: Lippincott Williams & Wilkins; 2012.
8. Jardin F, Vieillard-Baron A. Is there a safe plateau pressure in ARDS? The right heart only knows. Intensive Care Med. 2007;33:444–7.
9. Vieillard-Baron A, et al. Prone positioning unloads the right ventricle in severe ARDS. Chest. 2007;132:1440–6.
10. Guervilly C, et al. Right ventricular function during high-frequency oscillatory ventilation in adults with acute respiratory distress syndrome. Crit Care Med. 2012;40:1539–45.
11. Guérin C, et al. Prone positioning in severe acute respiratory distress syndrome. N Engl J Med. 2013;368:2159–68.

12. Chan B, Gaudry P, Grattan-Smith TM, McNeil R. The use of Glasgow Coma Scale in poisoning. J Emerg Med. 1993;11:579–82.
13. Donald C, Duncan R, Thakore S. Predictors of the need for rapid sequence intubation in the poisoned patient with reduced Glasgow coma score. Emerg Med J: EMJ. 2009;26:510–2.
14. Davies AE, Kidd D, Stone SP, MacMahon J. Pharyngeal sensation and gag reflex in healthy subjects. Lancet. 1995;345:487–8.
15. Magder S. Bench-to-bedside review: ventilatory abnormalities in sepsis. Crit Care Lond Engl. 2009;13:202.
16. Hess DR. Ventilator modes: where have we come from and where are we going? Chest. 2010;137:1256–8.
17. Bersten AD, Soni N. Oh's intensive care manual: expert consult: online. London: Elsevier Health Sciences; 2013.
18. Agasti TK. Textbook of anaesthesia for postgraduates. New Delhi St. Louis: JP Brothers Medical Publishers Ltd; 2011.
19. The Acute Respiratory Distress Syndrome Network. Ventilation with lower tidal volumes as compared with traditional tidal volumes for acute lung injury and the acute respiratory distress syndrome. N Engl J Med. 2000;342:1301–8.
20. Futier E, et al. A trial of intraoperative low-tidal-volume ventilation in abdominal surgery. N Engl J Med. 2013;369:428–37.
21. Hager DN, Krishnan JA, Hayden DL, Brower RG, ARDS Clinical Trials Network. Tidal volume reduction in patients with acute lung injury when plateau pressures are not high. Am J Respir Crit Care Med. 2005;172:1241–5.
22. Weingart S. Podcast 3 – Laryngoscope as a Murder Weapon (LAMW) Series – Ventilatory Kills – Intubating the patient with Severe Metabolic Acidosis. EMCrit Blog. Published on May 22, 2009; Accessed on November 22nd 2019. Available at https://emcrit.org/emcrit/tube-severe-acidosis/.
23. Kallet RH, Branson RD. Respiratory controversies in the critical care setting. Do the NIH ARDS Clinical Trials Network PEEP/FIO2 tables provide the best evidence-based guide to balancing PEEP and FIO2 settings in adults? Respir Care. 2007;52:461–75; discussion 475–477.
24. Brower RG, et al. Higher versus lower positive end-expiratory pressures in patients with the acute respiratory distress syndrome. N Engl J Med. 2004;351:327–36.
25. Fanelli V, et al. Acute respiratory distress syndrome: new definition, current and future therapeutic options. J Thorac Dis. 2013;5:326–34.
26. Ferguson ND, et al. The Berlin definition of ARDS: an expanded rationale, justification, and supplementary material. Intensive Care Med. 2012;38:1573–82.
27. Mikkelsen ME, et al. The epidemiology of acute respiratory distress syndrome in patients presenting to the emergency department with severe sepsis. Shock Augusta Ga. 2013;40:375–81.
28. Petrucci N, Iacovelli W. Ventilation with lower tidal volumes versus traditional tidal volumes in adults for acute lung injury and acute respiratory distress syndrome. Cochrane Database Syst Rev. 2004:CD003844. https://doi.org/10.1002/14651858.CD003844.pub2.
29. Stehman CR, et al. Bedside estimation of patient height for calculating ideal body weight in the emergency department. J Emerg Med. 2011;41:97 101.
30. Hickling KG. Permissive hypercapnia. Respir Care Clin N Am. 2002;8:155–169, v.
31. Bidani A, Tzouanakis AE, Cardenas VJ, Zwischenberger JB. Permissive hypercapnia in acute respiratory failure. JAMA. 1994;272:957–62.
32. Kregenow DA, Rubenfeld GD, Hudson LD, Swenson ER. Hypercapnic acidosis and mortality in acute lung injury. Crit Care Med. 2006;34:1–7.
33. Ni Chonghaile M, Higgins B, Laffey JG. Permissive hypercapnia: role in protective lung ventilatory strategies. Curr Opin Crit Care. 2005;11:56–62.
34. Curley G, Hayes M, Laffey JG. Can 'permissive' hypercapnia modulate the severity of sepsis-induced ALI/ARDS? Crit Care Lond Engl. 2011;15:212.
35. Reddy VG. Auto-PEEP: how to detect and how to prevent--a review. Middle East J Anaesthesiol. 2005;18:293–312.
36. Laghi F, Goyal A. Auto-PEEP in respiratory failure. Minerva Anestesiol. 2012;78:201–21.
37. Chiumello D, et al. Time to reach a new steady state after changes of positive end expiratory pressure. Intensive Care Med. 2013;39:1377–85.
38. Barr J, Pandharipande PP. The pain, agitation, and delirium care bundle: synergistic benefits of implementing the 2013 pain, agitation, and delirium guidelines in an integrated and interdisciplinary fashion. Crit Care Med. 2013;41:S99–115.
39. Needham CJ, Brindley PG. Best evidence in critical care medicine: the role of neuromuscular blocking drugs in early severe acute respiratory distress syndrome. Can J Anaesth. 2012;59:105–8.
40. Papazian L, et al. Neuromuscular blockers in early acute respiratory distress syndrome. N Engl J Med. 2010;363:1107–16.

Asthma and COPD

5

Jonathan Auerbach and Lillian Emlet

Asthma Background

"Asthma," a Greek word that means *short of breath* [1], dates back to some of the earliest writings. Asthma pathophysiology, however, was first described in detail in 1892 by Sir William Osler [1], the father of modern-day medicine.

Epidemiology

Asthma afflicts over 330 million people worldwide and has been increasing in prevalence among poorer countries [2]. In the United States, asthma afflicted over 25 million people of all age groups in 2017 [3]. Asthma is slightly more common in women than in men, affecting African Americans and Puerto Ricans at higher rates [3]. Asthma is also more common among lower-income individuals, accounted for 1.8 million ED visits in 2016, and led to over 3500 deaths in 2016 [3]. The annual economic cost of asthma in the United States has been estimated to be approximately 56 billion dollars in 2011 [43].

J. Auerbach
Critical Care Medicine, University of Miami Hospital, Miami, FL, USA

L. Emlet (✉)
Critical Care Medicine and Emergency Medicine, University of Pittsburgh Medical Center, Pittsburgh, PA, USA
e-mail: emlell@ccm.upmc.edu

Pathophysiology

Asthma, a condition that results in recurrent episodes of reversible bronchial obstruction, is in reality a heterogeneous group of conditions [4]. Asthma presentation can be quite variable including symptoms of shortness of breath, wheezing, cough, and/or chest tightness and by reduction in expiratory airflow [17]. Typically, asthma presents in childhood, although it has been described as presenting in all age groups [4]. Of note, symptomology of asthma including airflow limitation and intensity of symptoms varies over time, with variability due to triggers, including allergens, irritant exposure, exercise, respiratory infections, and weather changes [17].

Asthma sufferers are defined into what has been described in the literature as "asthma phenotypes." These phenotypes describe various severities of asthmatic patients [19–21]. Some of the most common phenotypes of asthma are as follows:

- *Allergic asthma*: This form often starts in childhood and is associated with a family history of or a personal history of allergic disease. These patients sputum often reveal eosinophilia. These patients often respond well to inhaled corticosteroids [17].
- *Nonallergic asthma*: In these patients, asthma is not related to allergy. The sputum of these patients may be predominantly eosinophilic and neutrophilic or only contain few

© Springer Nature Switzerland AG 2020

J. R. Shiber, S. D. Weingart (eds.), *Emergency Department Critical Care*,
https://doi.org/10.1007/978-3-030-28794-8_5

inflammatory cells. These patients also typically respond well to inhaled corticosteroids [17].

- *Late-onset asthma:* This subgroup of adults, particularly women, present later in life with asthma. These patients tend to be nonallergenic and can be refractory to corticosteroid therapy [21].
- *Asthma with fixed airflow limitation:* Some asthmatics develop fixed airflow limitation. This is likely due to airway remodeling [17].

Special Populations

Pregnancy [10]

The most common respiratory disorder of pregnancy is asthma, affecting up to one-eighth of pregnant patients [10]. Prevalence rates of asthma during pregnancy appear to be increasing [11], with approximately 20% of asthmatic pregnant patients requiring medical interventions and 6% requiring hospital admission [13]. It has been thought that approximately one-third of asthmatic pregnant patients have worsening of symptoms, one-third stay the same, and one-third improve [15]; however, more recent evidence calls this into question [11]. Of note, the pathophysiology of asthma exacerbations during pregnancy has not been fully described. Likely, medication nonadherence, obesity, upper respiratory tract infection, smoking [12], and physiological changes contribute to this condition [14].

Asthma during pregnancy has been associated with multiple medical comorbidities, including pre-eclampsia, pregnancy-induced hypertension, premature rupture of membranes, gestational diabetes, Cesarean section, hyperemesis, chorioamnionitis, and antepartum and postpartum hemorrhage. Additionally, numerous fetal complications have been described, including increased neonatal intensive care use, hyperbilirubinemia, asphyxia, respiratory distress syndrome, anemia, intracerebral hemorrhage, transient tachypnea of the newborn low birth rate, preterm birth, congenital malformations, intrauterine growth restriction, and small for gestational age babies. In addition to all the above complications, such babies are likely at increased risk for long-term health complications associated with prematurity [10].

Adequate control of asthma during pregnancy is crucial as asthma is associated with poor maternal and fetal outcomes, and appropriate control leads to improved health outcomes of mothers and babies. Appropriate asthma control has been defined by the National Heart, Lung and Blood Institute as: "minimal or no chronic symptoms day or night; minimal or no exacerbations; no limitations of activities; maintenance of (near) normal pulmonary function; minimal use of short-acting inhaled β2-agonists; minimal or no adverse effects from medications" [16].

In general, asthma therapy during pregnancy is considered "safer" than nontreatment. Literature in the past has called into question the notion that short-acting beta-agonists are safe during pregnancy, suggesting a possible increase in congenital abnormalities with their use [11]. Anti-inflammatory agents have been associated with slightly increased risk of birth defects, including cleft palate and/or cleft lip, although this data is controversial [11]. Newer literature calls into question these associations [10]. Avoiding environmental exposures, in particular smoking, is an important safe way to help prevent asthma exacerbations in pregnancy. In light of morbidity and mortality of asthma by itself, medications should be used in the emergency department as needed, in order to stabilize the asthmatic pregnant patient.

Work-Related Asthma

Work-related asthma has been described to account for 5–25% of adult asthma cases [6, 7] and is among the most common occupational diseases [5]. This leads to significant social economic burdens. Multiple agents have been described to cause this condition. Some overlap has been described between work-related chronic obstructive pulmonary disease and work-related asthma. Thus, prevention of work-related asthma will likely decrease work-related chronic obstructive pulmonary disease. Work-related asthma has both direct and indirect costs that have been shown in the literature to be quite high, costing the United States an estimated 1.6 billion dollars in 1996 [9] or approximately 0.13% of total US healthcare costs [5].

Early diagnosis is important to prevent progression, enable appropriate treatment, and prevent future exposure to such allergens. Hundreds of agents in the workplace have been reported to cause work-related asthma [8]. Most commonly reported agents include isocyanates, flower and grain dust, latex, soldering fluxes, animals, wood dust, aldehydes, and colophony [5]. Occupations that are highest associated with such exposures include bakers and pastry makers, paint sprayers, chemical workers, nurses, welders, animal handlers, food processing workers, timber workers, and hairdressers [5]. Work-related asthma is directly related to the causative agent and exposure level [5]. There is no single test that can diagnose work-related asthma [5]. Diagnosis and treatment start with primary prevention of exposure to presumed causative agent [5]. If this is not possible, reduction of exposure should be tried and personal protection equipment should be used [5].

Diagnosis

There are multiple features that increase the probability that a patient has asthma. These include two or more of the following: wheezing, cough, shortness of breath, and chest tightness, especially in the adult patient. Specific triggers of symptoms are as follows: exercise, changes in weather, viral infections, allergens, and irritants. Symptoms are usually worse at night and early morning and vary over time and intensity. Ultimately, asthma is diagnosed based on the history of symptoms and confirmed variable expiratory airflow limitations. Spirometry is the cornerstone to diagnosis of asthma versus COPD, with asthmatics usually exhibiting normal or reversible FEV_1/FVC with an increase in $FEV_1 > 12\%$ or 200 ml from baseline after albuterol administration. Spirometry in COPD usually exhibits postbronchodilator $FEV_1/FVC < 0.7$ [17, 18].

There also features that have been shown in the literature to decrease the probability that a patient has asthma. These include chronic production of sputum, chest pain, isolated cough, exercise-induced dyspnea, and shortness of breath associated with dizziness, lightheadedness, or paresthesias [17].

It is important to be aware that asthma severity is defined by number of clinical characteristics, including heart rate >120, RR > 30, oxygen saturation <90% on room air, peak expiratory flow rate ≤50%, and accessory muscle use and/or agitation. An ABG, although unnecessary, if obtained, would show a $PaO_2 < 60$ mm Hg and a $PaCO_2 > 45$ mm Hg. Ultimately, a late-stage clinical presentation is respiratory doom and would present with exhaustion, respiratory fatigue, altered mental status, bradypnea via, and/or cardiac arrhythmias [17]. Also, one should be aware that degree of tachycardia has been shown to correlate with asthma severity [44]. It is also important to realize the studies show that heart rate falls in response to bronchodilator therapy [45]. Therefore, tachycardia should not be ascribed to the bronchodilator therapy; but rather to worsening asthma [45].

Treatment

Is important to note there are various factors that increase the risk of asthma-related death. Among these factors are hospitalization or emergency care visit for asthma within the past year, not using inhaled corticosteroids, a history of asthmatic attack requiring intubation and mechanical ventilation, active use or recent use of oral corticosteroids, overuse of short-acting beta-agonist, poor adherence to asthma treatment, history of psychiatric illness or psychosocial problems, and/or food allergies [17].

Treatment of the asthmatic patient begins with bronchodilation via a short-acting beta-agonist. Summary of medication options is listed in Table 5.1. Immediate rescue medication for asthma exacerbation usually is albuterol or levalbuterol. Although the appropriate frequency of administration is controversial [25, 26], based

Table 5.1 Medications for asthma and COPD (GOLD and GINA and NEJM 2010 Niewoehner et al.)

Medications class	Subtype	Dosage	SE
Short-acting beta-2 adrenergic agonists (SABA)			Headache, dizziness, tremor, tachycardia, hypersensitivity reaction ->1.4 canister/month use associated with increased risk of asthma-related death
	Albuterol	2.5 mg q1–q4 hrs	
	Levalbuterol	1.25 mg q6–q8 hrs	
Long-acting beta-2 adrenergic agonists (LABA)			Headache, dizziness, tremor, hypersensitivity reaction
	Salmoterol	Inhaled only 50 mcg per inhalation BID	
	Formoterol	1. Inhaled: 12 mcg per puff, 1 puff BID 2. Nebulized: 20 mcg BID	
	Arformoterol	Nebulized: 15 mcg BID	
Anticholinergic agents	Tiotropium (LAMA)	18 mcg per inhalation, 1 inhalation QAM	Dry mouth, urinary retention, narrow angle glaucoma, hypersensitivity reaction
Corticosteroids			
	Prednisone	50 mg daily for 5 days	
	Dexamethasone	16 mg oral or IV daily for 2 days	
Inhaled corticosteroids (ICS)			Sore throat, dysphonia, headache, nasopharyngitis, thrush, hypersensitivity reaction
	Fluticasone	1. Dry powder 250 mcg inhalation 1–2 × daily 2. Aerosolized form: 220 mcg inhaled 1–2 × daily	
	Budesonide	Inhaled 160 mcg per inhalation, 2 inhalations BID	
	Beclomethasone	Inhalation 80 mcg per inhalation, 2 inhalations BID	
	Mometasone	220 mcg per inhalation, 1–2 inhalations BID	
SABA/SAMA	Salbutamol/ipratropium	100mcg/20mcg 2 puffs QID	
LABA/LAMA	Olodaterol/tiotropium	2.5mcg/2.5mcg 2 puffs daily	
Combination LABA + ICS			
	Fluticasone (250 mcg) + Salmetolol (50 mcg)	Dry powder, 1 inhalation BID	
	Budesonide (150 mcg) + Formetorol (4.5 mcg)	2 inhalations BID	
Short-term anticholinergic agents (SAMA)	Ipratropium bromide	0.5 mg q20 min nebulized	
Aminophylline	Theophylline	Call pulmonologist to start, no indication in emergent stabilization	Dry mouth, bitter taste, urinary retention, narrow angle glaucoma, hypersensitivity reaction, nausea, vomiting, tremors, seizures, insomnia
PDE-4 inhibitors	Roflumilast	Call pulmonologist to start, no indication in emergent stabilization	N/V, diarrhea

Table 5.1 (continued)

Medications class	Subtype	Dosage	SE
Epinephrine		0.3 ml 1:1000 IM	GI symptoms, arrhythmias, seizures, death
Magnesium		2 g over 20 minutes	No benefit in acute asthma
antibiotics: Typical organisms to cover: *H. influenzae*, *S. pneumonia*, and *M. catarrhalis*			
First-line uncomplicated			
	Amoxillin +/– clavulanic acid	875/125 mg p.o. BID × 7 days or 875 mg p.o. BID × 7 days	
	Macrolide (i.e., azithromycin)	Azithromycin 500 mg p.o. daily × 5 days	
	Doxycycline	100 mg BID × 10 days	
First-line complicated: concern for pseudomonas and other resistant pathogens			
	Ciprofloxacin		
	Levofloxacin		
	Gemifloxacin		
	Moxifloxacin		
Second line			
	Ceftriaxone	1 gram IM qd × 7 days	
	Clarithromycin	500 mg bid × 14 days	
	Cefuroxime–axetil	250 mg BID × 7 days	
	Trimethoprim–sulfamethoxazole	160/800 mg BID × 10 days	
Future directions			
	Inhaled antibiotics		

on current data, continuous therapy should initially be used followed by intermittent on-demand therapy [17]. Appropriate oxygenation should be maintained, and supplemental oxygen should be administered to a goal saturation of 93–95% [22, 23]. There is some data to suggest that aiming for higher oxygen saturations may be harmful [22–24]. Epinephrine (SQ) is indicated for acute asthma exacerbation only when associated with anaphylaxis and/or angioedema [17].

Systemic steroids should be administered to patients who present with moderate-to-severe asthma exacerbation [27, 28]. Of note, oral and intravenous administrations are equally efficacious [28]. Since the oral route is cheaper and one can administer it more rapidly, it is, in general, the preferred route [17]. In certain cases, for instance, if a patient is too short of breath, has persistent vomiting, does not have enteral access, and/or is having anaphylaxis or angioedema, then intravenous route is preferred [17]. Dosing of systemic steroids should be equivalent to 50 mg of prednisolone or 200 mg of hydrocortisone [17]. Duration of therapy is typically 5–7 days [29, 30]. Inhaled corticosteroids appear to show decreased risk of admission [27]. This does not seem to be the case when oral steroids are also given [17]. Utility of inhaled corticosteroids in acute ED management is, therefore, controversial [17].

Addition of a short-acting anticholinergic such as ipratropium bromide has been shown when added to short-acting beta-agonist to decrease the amount of hospitalizations and improve PEF and FEV_1 in these patients [17, 31]. Aminophylline and theophylline should not be used in the management of asthma exacerbation based on poor efficacy and potential severe and life-threatening side effects [32]. Magnesium is controversial: Some literature shows a reduction in hospital admissions in certain patient groups [33], while other literature shows no differences [34]. It would appear based on current literature that magnesium may improve severe asthma outcomes [33, 34]. The dosage is typically 2 grams intravenously over 20 minutes [34].

Heliox is controversial [17]; There is data to suggest decreased admission rate to hospitals with moderate-to-severe asthma exacerbation [35]. However, costs and necessary equipment may preclude its use [35].

Care must be taken not to give sedatives to patients with asthma exacerbations. This can lead to respiratory depression and has been associated in the literature with avoidable asthma deaths [36].

Noninvasive ventilation can potentially be used for respiratory support in the asthmatic patient; however, there is scant literature to suggest that it improves outcomes [37]. If used judiciously, one must monitor the patient extremely closely and still retain a low threshold for endotracheal intubation and mechanical ventilation to unload work of breathing [17]. Sedatives have been shown in the literature to increase mortality; one should not use sedatives for the purpose of being able to apply noninvasive positive pressure ventilation to the asthmatic patient [36].

Intubation of the asthmatic patient must be approached with care. Indications for intubation include impending respiratory failure including alterations in the mental status and exhaustion, respiratory distress including silent chest and weak breathing effort, hypercapnia and respiratory acidosis, hypoxemia and cyanosis, and cardiovascular compromise including arrhythmias and hypotension [17, 73]. Ketamine is an excellent induction agent due to its bronchodilator effects and ability to decrease airway resistance. At usual induction dose of 2 mg/kg ketamine maintains both laryngeal and pharyngeal protective reflexes. This medication is considered by many the "go to medication" for asthmatics who need intubation. Additionally, ketamine is very well tolerated hemodynamically due to its sympathomimetic activity [74, 75].

Ketamine does have some disadvantages. For instance, ketamine can cause bronchorrhea, and although this may be advantageous by decreasing mucus plugging, this can make visualization of the airway difficult. One can treat and/or prevent this by administering 0.1 mg of glycopyrrolate every 2 minutes as needed. Additionally, ketamine can cause an emergence reaction, while not deadly, this can be quite traumatizing to patients family members and staff. Co-administration of benzodiazepines may decrease the incidence of this, and it is also the treatment for this condition. Ketamine is contraindicated in pregnancy. Additionally, although controversial, one must use caution when using ketamine in patients with increased intracranial pressure and in patients with cardiogenic shock [74, 75].

Another induction agent is propofol (2 mg/kg) also favored due to its bronchodilator properties. Propofol can also provide continuous infusion to maintain sedation. Continuous infusion rates usually are in the range of 25–50 micrograms per kilogram per minute. Propofol does have some side effects, including hypotension, bradycardia, and cardiovascular collapse [74].

A technique that is commonly used in the management of mechanical ventilation of severe asthmatics is permissive hypercapnia. By allowing hypercarbia and respiratory acidosis of values up to 80 mmHg of $PaCO_2$ and pH down to 7.15, this well-tolerated technique by patients allows us to minimize subsequent barotrauma and volutrauma [76]. Additionally, just as low oxygen is harmful for patients, elevated oxygen is also harmful. One wants to minimize lung injury and atelectasis by keeping the lowest FiO_2 tolerated by the patient. Ideally, FiO_2 less than 40% should be used. The goal oxygen saturation for the asthmatic is 90–93%.

Disposition

Ultimate disposition of the patient is based on PEF [17] after 1 hour of therapy, as this has been shown to correlate better when compared to hospital arrival evaluation [38, 39]. Please be aware that there are factors that are associated with increased need for admission, including older age [40], nonwhite race [41], female sex [40], history of severe exacerbations [41], severity of exacerbation [41], use of more than eight beta-2-agonists puffs in the 24 hours [40], and/or prior need for oral corticosteroids [40]. There are numerous indications for hospital admission. These include pretreatment PEF or $FEV_1 < 25\%$ predicted or posttreatment PEF or $FEV_1 < 40\%$ predicted [17]. Posttreatment PEF or FEV_1 of 40–60% predicted can be considered for discharge pending risk factors and follow-up [17]. PEF or $FEV_1 > 60\%$ predicted are, in general, discharged unless there are extenuating circumstances, including risk factors and poor follow-up [17]. For patients who are discharged from the emergency department to their home, a follow-up appointment should be made within 1 week [42]. Additionally, appropriate medication management, in particular, inhaler skill set, should be demonstrated [42]. Prescribing spacer for MDI administration allows potential for adequate medication adherence.

COPD Background

The earliest known description of COPD was in 1679 by Bonet who described "voluminous lungs" [46]. It was not, however, until 1814 when Badham started the quest toward clinical understanding of COPD [46]. COPD is now known as a condition that is characterized by persistent airflow limitation [49]. This condition is associated with chronic inflammatory changes of the lungs due to noxious substances [49]. Additionally, this condition is usually progressive [49]. COPD is caused by parenchymal destruction, that is, emphysema and small airway disease and obstructive bronchiolitis [49]. Chronic inflammatory changes lead to structural changes and narrowing of the small airways [49]. This leads to decreased lung elasticity and diminishes ability of airways to remain open during expiration phase [49].

COPD Epidemiology

According to the World Health Organization, moderate-to-severe COPD affects approximately 65 million people worldwide [47]. Additionally, more than 3 million people died in 2005 due to COPD [47]. This corresponds to 5% of world deaths [47]. Furthermore, in 2002, COPD was the fifth-leading cause of death and is expected to become the third-leading cause of death by 2030 [47].

In the United States, COPD mortality rates were 48 per 100,000 people as of 2010 [48]. Mortality rates among men have declined from 1999 to 2010; however, they are essentially unchanged among women [48]. As of 2011, prevalence rates range from approximately 3–9% depending on state, with highest rates in the Ohio and lower Mississippi river area [48].

COPD Pathophysiology

Noxious substances, including cigarette smoke in particular, cause lung inflammation [50]. Chronic inflammation may disrupt the body's repair defense mechanisms, leading to small airway fibrosis, and induce parenchymal tissue destruction, leading to emphysema [50]. These changes lead to air-trapping and progressive airflow limitation [50]. These changes increase with disease severity and persist with removal of offending agents [50].

Ultimately, inflammation and narrowing of small airways lead to decreased FEV_1 [49]. Additionally, destruction of parenchyma further contributes to limitations of airflow and ultimately leads to decreased gas diffusion [49]. Reduction in FEV_1 correlates with the extent of inflammation, small airway exudates, and fibrosis [49]. This leads to progressive air-trapping during the expiratory phase causing hyperinflation [49], which ultimately leads to decreases in inspiratory capacity in every cycle of increasing dyspnea, and limited exercise capacity [49].

Furthermore, oxygen and carbon dioxide diffusion worsens as COPD progresses [52]. This ultimately leads to worsening ventilation perfusion mismatch. There is a particular subset of COPD patients who have mucus hyper secretion [52]. These patients have increased number of goblet cells and enlarged submucosal glands that are due to the noxious substances [49].

Pulmonary hypertension, a potential complication of COPD, is due to hypoxic vasoconstriction of pulmonary arterioles, leading to intimal and smooth-muscle hyperplasia [53]. This ultimately leads to progressive worsening pulmonary hypertension, RV strain, and hypertrophy, and eventually cor pulmonale [49, 53]. Systemic complications associated with COPD include skeletal muscle wasting and cachexia, heart failure, heart disease, anemia, osteoporosis, metabolic syndrome, diabetes, and depression [54].

COPD Diagnosis

Patients with chronic cough or sputum production, dyspnea, and any history of exposure to risk factors for COPD should be considered for the diagnosis of COPD [49]. Exposure risk factors include tobacco smoke, occupational dust and chemicals, and smoke from cooking and heating fuels [49]. Spirometry is required to make the diagnosis [55], and postbronchodilator FEV_1/FVC < 0.70 confirms persistent airflow limitation for the clinical diagnosis of COPD [49].

COPD Acute Exacerbation Treatment

A COPD acute exacerbation is defined as any event associated with worsening patient respiratory status that changes from the normal day-to-day variations, often associated with medication changes [56–58]. COPD exacerbations lead to decreased quality of life, accelerated lung function decline, increased socioeconomic costs, and increased mortality and morbidity [49, 59, 60]. In particular, in hospital, mortality of patients with hypercapnic respiratory acidosis is above 10% [61]. Patients who required mechanical support showed over 40% mortality [62]. It, therefore, behooves us to prevent exacerbations as best as possible using current medical therapies. Table 5.4 classifies the different types of COPD exacerbations with associated admission and mortality.

Arterial blood gases can be used to assess the degree of acute ventilatory failure [49], and when unavailable, central venous gases can be used. Chest X-ray should be obtained to rule out other pathology [49]. Numerous indications for admission are discussed in the disposition section. Severe COPD is complicated by frequent exacerbations, significant worsening of symptom intensity, associated serious comorbidities, and failure of exacerbation to respond to medical management is associated with older age and poor home environment [49].

Oxygen

Oxygen therapy should be administered when needed to maintain an oxygen saturation of only 88–92%, as higher oxygen saturations have been associated with increased mortality and morbidity [49, 63]. According to the international consortium, one needs to check an ABG within 30–60 minutes of initiating oxygen on a patient to ensure that carbon dioxide is not rising [49]. There are, however, data to suggest that venous blood gas sample can be used to rule out hypercarbia when the level of PCO_2 is ≤45 mm Hg [81].

Ventilatory Support

Noninvasive mechanical ventilation has been shown to decrease respiratory rate, decrease work of breathing, improve acute respiratory acidosis [49], and decrease length of hospital stay [64]. Additionally, both mortality and intubation rates are decreased with this intervention [64].

Indications for noninvasive mechanical ventilation include severe dyspnea with clinical signs of respiratory fatigue and/or increased work of breathing [49]. Additionally, pH ≤ 7.36 and/or $PaCO_2 \geq 45$ mm Hg are further indications [49]. In general, noninvasive ventilation should be used for 1 hour before reassessment is made; if not improved in 1 hour, the patient is unlikely to improve and will need intubation. Additionally, noninvasive ventilation should only be used in cooperative patients who are able to protect their airways.

Table 5.3 Ventilator troubleshooting

Hypoxia
Confirm proper endotracheal tube placement
Ensure endotracheal tube not obstructed
Rule out shunt:
Pus
Blood
Water
Atelectasis
Hypotension
Detach from ventilator (Auto-PEEP)
Volume resuscitate
Rule out pneumothorax
Check for myocardial infarction and sepsis

Invasive Mechanical Ventilation

There are multiple indications for invasive mechanical ventilation (Table 5.2). In general, invasive mechanical ventilation is considered when one is unable to tolerate or fails noninvasive ventilation [49]. Table 5.3 discusses ventilator troubleshooting techniques. Careful observation of ventilator waveforms for this patient population is critical in order to prevent ventilator dyssynchrony, inadequate mechanical support, all potentially resulting in air-trapping and auto-PEEP, and eventually pneumothorax. Similar to asthmatics, permissive hypercapnia is tolerated well, and watching to ensure adequate time for exhalation, adequate PEEP, and low tidal volumes (Table 5.4).

Table 5.2 Indication for intubation (GOLD 2015)

Airway
Respiratory arrest
Inability to protect airway: that is, AMS, massive aspiration
Breathing
Refractory hypoxemia
Irreversible respiratory acidosis
Silent chest
Progressive exhaustion
Inability to tolerate or contraindication to NIV
pH < 7.2
CO_2 increasing by 5 mm Hg/hr
CO_2 > 55–70 mm Hg
PaO_2 < 60
Circulation
Cardiac arrest
HR < 50 with mental status changes
Refractory hemodynamic instability
Severe ventricular arrhythmias

Short-Acting Bronchodilators

Inhaled short-acting anticholinergics and/or short-acting beta-agonist are the preferred modality for treatment of acute exacerbation [65]. Appropriate MDI use appears to be as efficacious as nebulization therapy [66]. Intravenous methylxanthines, for example, aminophylline and theophylline are considered third-line agents in select patients who do not respond to the short-acting bronchodilators and long-acting anticholinergies or long-acting beta-agonists [49] (Table 5.1). The reason for them being third-line agents is due to their significant toxicity (narrow therapeutic index), including mortality risk and limited beneficial effects [49, 77, 78].

Corticosteroids

Corticosteroids are a primary therapy for COPD exacerbation. The reason for this is that they have been shown to improve lung function, in particular, FEV_1 [67], shorten recovery time, and improve arterial hypoxemia [67, 69, 70]. They also have been shown to reduce treatment failure risk, decreased duration of length of stay to the hospital, and reduce early relapse [67, 69, 70]. Recommended doses are

Table 5.4 Gold criteria classification of airflow limitation in COPD patients based on postbronchodilator FEV_1

			Yearly exacerbations	Yearly hospitalizations	3 year mortality
Gold 1	Mild	$FEV_1 \geq$ 80% predicted			
Gold 2	Moderate	FEV_1 <80% and ≥ 50% predicted	0.7-0.9	0.11-0.2	11%
Gold 3	Severe	FEV_1 <50% and ≥ 30% predicted	1.1-1.3	0.25-0.3	15%
Gold 4	Very Severe	FEV_1<30% predicted	1.2-2	0.4-0.54	24%

40 mg daily of prednisone for 5 days [49], although this is somewhat controversial [68, 69]. Tapering doses of prednisone are not typically necessary, although there is a subset of patients who will require longer-term steroid therapy.

Antibiotics

Use of antibiotics, outside of ICU patients, are quite controversial [71]. Antibiotics are recommended for patients who have increased purulence of sputum with either increased sputum volume and/or increased dyspnea or who require mechanical ventilation: both invasive and noninvasive [49]. Duration of antibiotic use is generally recommended for 5–10 days [49]. Initial antibiotics are typically a macrolide, aminopenicillin with or without clavulanic acid, or tetracycline [49] (Table 5.1). Patients requiring mechanical ventilation, or who are at increased risk for resistant organisms such as ones with frequent exacerbations, should be covered for resistant organisms such as pseudomonas [49, 79, 80] (Table 5.1).

Disposition

Indications for Hospital/ ICU Admission

Indications for hospital admission are numerous. These include worsening symptoms (i.e., resting dyspnea), new physical symptoms (i.e., cyanosis), severe underlying COPD, frequent exacerbations, serious comorbidities, older age, and poor home support [49]. There are numerous indications for ICU admission. These include altered mental status, severe dyspnea refractory to initial therapy, hemodynamic instability requiring pressers, persistent or worsening hypoxia (PaO_2 < 40 mm Hg) and/or worsening respiratory acidosis despite therapy (pH < 7.25), and need for mechanical ventilation [49].

Indications for Discharge

Indications for discharge from the hospital are as follows: understanding the correct use of medications and demonstrating proper use of long-acting bronchodilators, therapy need no more often than every 4 hours, ambulatory (if at baseline), ABG and patient stable for 12–24 hours, has appropriate follow-up, and able to eat and sleep without dyspnea [49]. In general, these patients should be followed up in 4–6 weeks from discharge [49]. Additionally, it is crucial to discuss with these patients about smoking cessation, appropriate inhaler technique used, and need for influenza and pneumococcal vaccines [49].

COPD/Asthma Overlap Syndrome

Please be aware that COPD and asthma, although associated with chronic inflammation of the respiratory tract, have different pathophysiology [51]. This leads to different symptoms, physiological effects, and response to therapies [51].

With this in mind, there is a condition called asthma–COPD overlap syndrome or ACOS [17]. This condition is characterized by persistent airflow limitation that has equal asthmatic and COPD features [17]. This overlap syndrome is a heterogeneous disease, as it is not resented by a single disease process [17]. Diagnoses of ACOS are made when a patient has a differential diagnosis that is equally split between asthma and COPD [17]. In general, treatment is with inhaled corticosteroids (ICS) and either a long-acting beta-agonist (LABA) or long-acting antimuscarinic agonist (LAMA) [17]. Modifiable risk factors should be treated [17]. Ultimately, much research needs to be done on this condition to further elucidate the etiology [17]. Of interest, there is some literature to support the notion that there are asthmatics who are on a continuum with COPD [72, 82].

Conclusion

Asthma, COPD, and ACOS are different diseases that are treated similarly. In particular, the emergency medicine physician needs to be aware of treatment algorithms most notably what medications to use and indications for NPPV, intubation, hospital admission, and discharge.

References

1. Holgate ST. A brief history of asthma and its mechanisms to modern concepts of disease pathogenesis. Allergy Asthma Immunol Res. 2010;2:165–71.
2. The Global Initiative for Asthma. https://ginasthma.org/gina-reports/ last accessed December 11, 2019.
3. CDC Asthma Stats. https://www.cdc.gov/asthma/asthma_stats/documents/AsthmStat_Mortality_2001-2016-H.pdf last accessed December 11, 2019.
4. Martinez FD, Vercelli D. Asthma. Lancet. 2013;382(9901):1360–72.
5. Baur X, Aasen TB, Sherwood Burge P, et al. The management of work-related asthma guidelines: a broader perspective. Eur Respir Rev. 2012;21(124):125–39.
6. Toren K, Blanc PD. Asthma caused by occupational exposures is common – a systematic analysis of estimates of the population-attributable fraction. BMC Pulm Med. 2009;9:7.
7. Mannino DM. How much asthma is occupationally related? Occup Med. 2000;15:359–68.
8. Balmes J, Becklake M, Blanc P, et al. American Thoracic Society statement: occupational contribution to the burden of airway disease. Am J Respir Crit Care Med. 2003;167:787–97.
9. Leigh JP, Romano PS, Schenker MB, et al. Costs of occupational COPD and asthma. Chest. 2002;121:264–72.
10. Bain E, Pierides KL, Clifton VL, Hodyl NA, Stark MJ, Crowther CA, Middleton P. Interventions for managing asthma in pregnancy. Cochrane Database Syst Rev. 2014;(10):Art. No.: CD010660. https://doi.org/10.1002/14651858.CD010660.pub2.
11. Katz O, Sheiner E. Asthma and pregnancy: a review of two decades. Expert Rev Respir Med. 2008;2(1):97–107.
12. McCallister JW. Asthma in pregnancy management strategies. Curr Opin Pulm Med. 2013;19(1):13–7.
13. Murphy VE, Clifton VL, Gibson PG. Asthma exacerbations during pregnancy: incidence and association with adverse pregnancy outcomes. Thorax. 2006;61(2):169–76.
14. Gluck J. The change of asthma course during pregnancy. Clin Rev Allergy Immunol. 2004;26(3):171–80.
15. Juniper E, Newhouse M. Effect of pregnancy on asthma: a systematic review and meta-analysis. In: Schatz M, Zaiger RS, Claman HC, editors. Asthma and immunological diseases in pregnancy and early infancy. New York: Marcel Dekker; 1993. p. 401–27.
16. National Asthma Education and Prevention Program Working Group (NAEPP). Report on managing asthma during pregnancy: recommendations for pharmacologic treatment. Update 2004. National Institutes of Health, National Heart, Lung, and Blood Institute, 2005.
17. From the Global Strategy for Asthma Management and Prevention, Global Initiative for Asthma (GINA) 2015. Available from: http://www.ginasthma.org/

18. Lougheed MD, Lemiere C, Ducahrme FM, Licskai C, et al. Canadian Thoracic Society 2012 guideline update: diagnosis and management of asthma in preschoolers, children and adults: executive summary. Can Respir J. 2012;19:6 e81–8.
19. Bel EH. Clinical phenotypes of asthma. Curr Opin Pulm Med. 2004;10:44–50.
20. Moore WC, Meyers DA, Wenzel SE, et al. Identification of asthma phenotypes using cluster analysis in the Severe Asthma Research Program. Am J Respir Crit Care Med. 2010;181:315–23.
21. Wenzel SE. Asthma phenotypes: the evolution from clinical to molecular approaches. Nat Med. 2012;18:716–25.
22. Perrin K, Wijesinghe M, Healy B, et al. Randomised controlled trial of high concentration versus titrated oxygen therapy in severe exacerbations of asthma. Thorax. 2011;66:937–41.
23. Rodrigo GJ, Rodriquez Verde M, Peregalli V, Rodrigo C. Effects of short-term 28% and 100% oxygen on PaCO2 and peak expiratory flow rate in acute asthma: a randomized trial. Chest. 2003;124:1312–7.
24. Chien JW, Ciufo R, Novak R, et al. Uncontrolled oxygen administration and respiratory failure in acute asthma. Chest. 2000;117:728–33.
25. Rodrigo GJ, Rodrigo C. Continuous vs intermittent beta-agonists in the treatment of acute adult asthma: a systematic review with meta-analysis. Chest. 2002;122:160–5.
26. Camargo CA Jr, Spooner CH, Rowe BH. Continuous versus intermittent beta-agonists in the treatment of acute asthma. Cochrane Database Syst Rev. 2003:CD001115.
27. Edmonds ML, Milan SJ, Camargo CA Jr, Pollack CV, Rowe BH. Early use of inhaled corticosteroids in the emergency department treatment of acute asthma. Cochrane Database Syst Rev. 2012;12:CD002308.
28. Rowe BH, Spooner CH, Ducharme FM, Bretzlaff JA, Bota GW. Corticosteroids for preventing relapse following acute exacerbations of asthma. Cochrane Database Syst Rev. 2007:CD000195.
29. Hasegawa T, Ishihara K, Takakura S, et al. Duration of systemic corticosteroids in the treatment of asthma exacerbation; a randomized study. Intern Med. 2000;39:794–7.
30. Jones AM, Munavvar M, Vail A, et al. Prospective, placebo-controlled trial of 5 vs 10 days of oral prednisolone in acute adult asthma. Respir Med. 2002;96:950–4.
31. Rodrigo GJ, Castro-Rodriguez JA. Anticholinergics in the treatment of children and adults with acute asthma: a systematic review with meta-analysis. Thorax. 2005;60:740–6.
32. Nair P, Milan SJ, Rowe BH. Addition of intravenous aminophylline to inhaled beta(2)-agonists in adults with acute asthma. Cochrane Database Syst Rev. 2012;12:CD002742.
33. Rowe BH, Bretzlaff JA, Bourdon C, Bota GW, Camargo CA Jr. Magnesium sulfate for treating exacerbations of acute asthma in the emergency department. Cochrane Database Syst Rev. 2000;2:CD001490.
34. Goodacre S, Cohen J, Bradburn M, Gray A, Benger J, Coats T. Intravenous or nebulised magnesium sulphate versus standard therapy for severe acute asthma (3Mg trial): a double-blind, randomised controlled trial. Lancet Respir Med. 2013;1:293–300.
35. Rodrigo GJ, Castro-Rodriguez JA. Heliox-driven beta2-agonists nebulization for children and adults with acute asthma: a systematic review with meta-analysis. Ann Allergy Asthma Immunol. 2014;112:29–34.
36. Joseph KS, Blais L, Ernst P, Suissa S. Increased morbidity and mortality related to asthma among asthmatic patients who use major tranquillizers. BMJ. 1996;312:79–82.
37. Lim WJ, Mohammed Akram R, Carson KV, et al. Non-invasive positive pressure ventilation for treatment of respiratory failure due to severe acute exacerbations of asthma. Cochrane Database Syst Rev. 2012;12:CD004360.
38. Kelly A-M, Kerr D, Powell C. Is severity assessment after one hour of treatment better for predicting the need for admission in acute asthma? Respir Med. 2004;98:777–81.
39. Wilson MM, Irwin RS, Connolly AE, Linden C, Manno MM. A prospective evaluation of the 1-hour decision point for admission versus discharge in acute asthma. J Intensive Care Med. 2003;18:275–85.
40. Rowe BH, Villa-Roel C, Abu-Laban RB, et al. Admissions to Canadian hospitals for acute asthma: a prospective, multicentre study. Can Respir J. 2010;17:25–30.
41. Weber EJ, Silverman RA, Callaham ML, et al. A prospective multicenter study of factors associated with hospital admission among adults with acute asthma. Am J Med. 2002;113:371–8.
42. Schatz M, Rachelefsky G, Krishnan JA. Follow-up after acute asthma episodes: what improves future outcomes? Proc Am Thorac Soc. 2009;6:386–93.
43. Centers for Disease Control and Prevention, (May 2011) Asthma in the U.S. Vital Signs, http://www.cdc.gov/vitalsigns/asthma/.
44. Hodder R, Lougheed MD, Rowe BH, FitzGerald JM, Kaplan AG, McIvor RA. Management of acute asthma in adults in the emergency department: Nonventilatory management. CMAJ. 2010;182:E55–67.
45. Aldington S, Beasley R. Asthma exacerbations 5: assessment and management of severe asthma in adults in hospital. Thorax. 2007;62:447–58.
46. Petty TL. The history of COPD. Int J Chron Obstruct Pulmon Dis. 2006;1:3–14.
47. Chronic respiratory diseases: Burden of COPD. Geneva: World Health Organization. Available from URL: http://www.who.int/respiratory/copd/burden/en/.
48. Chronic Obstructive Pulmonary Disease (COPD): Data and statistics. United States: Centers for Disease Control and Prevention. Available from URL: http://www.cdc.gov/copd/data.htm.

49. From the Global Strategy for the Diagnosis, Management and Prevention of COPD, Global Initiative for Chronic Obstructive Lung Disease (GOLD) 2015. Available from: http://www.goldcopd.org/.
50. Barnes PJ, Shapiro SD, Pauwels RA. Chronic obstructive pulmonary disease: molecular and cellular mechanisms. Eur Respir J. 2003;22:672–88.
51. Fabbri LM, Romagnoli M, Corbetta L, et al. Differences 84. In airway inflammation in patients with fixed airflow obstruction due to asthma or chronic obstructive pulmonary disease. Am J Respir Crit Care Med. 2003;167:418–24.
52. Rodriguez-Roisin R, Drakulovic M, Rodriguez DA, Roca J, Barbera JA, Wagner PD. Ventilation-perfusion imbalance and chronic obstructive pulmonary disease staging severity. J Appl Physiol. 2009;106:1902–8.
53. Peinado VI, Pizarro S, Barbera JA. Pulmonary vascular involvement in COPD. Chest. 2008;134:808–14.
54. Barnes PJ, Celli BR. Systemic manifestations and comorbidities of COPD. Eur Respir J. 2009;33:1165–85.
55. Zwar NA, Marks GB, Hermiz O, Middleton S, Comino EJ, Hasan I, et al. Predictors of accuracy of diagnosis of chronic obstructive pulmonary disease in general practice. Med J Aust. 2011;195(4):168–71.
56. Rodriguez-Roisin R. Toward a consensus definition for COPD exacerbations. Chest. 2000;117:398S–401S.
57. Burge S, Wedzicha JA. COPD exacerbations: definitions and classifications. Eur Respir J. 2003;41(Suppl):46s–53s.
58. Celli BR, Barnes PJ. Exacerbations of chronic obstructive pulmonary disease. Eur Respir J. 2007;29:1224–38.
59. Spencer S, Calverley PM, Burge PS, Jones PW. Impact of preventing exacerbations on deterioration of health status in COPD. Eur Respir J. 2004;23:698–702.
60. Donaldson GC, Seemungal TA, Bhowmik A, Wedzicha JA. Relationship between exacerbation frequency and lung function decline in chronic obstructive pulmonary disease. Thorax. 2002;57:847–52.
61. Connors AF Jr, Dawson NV, Thomas C, et al. Outcomes following acute exacerbation of severe chronic obstructive lung disease. The SUPPORT investigators (Study to Understand Prognoses and Preferences for Outcomes and Risks of Treatments). Am J Respir Crit Care Med. 1996;154:959–67.
62. Seneff MG, Wagner DP, Wagner RP, Zimmerman JE, Knaus WA. Hospital and 1-year survival of patients admitted to intensive care units with acute exacerbation of chronic obstructive pulmonary disease. JAMA. 1995;274:1852–7.
63. Austin MA, Wills KE, Blizzard L, Walters EH, Wood-Baker R. Effect of high flow oxygen on mortality in chronic obstructive pulmonary disease patients in prehospital setting: randomised controlled trial. BMJ. 2010;341:c5462.
64. Brochard L, Mancebo J, Wysocki M, et al. Noninvasive ventilation for acute exacerbations of chronic obstructive pulmonary disease. N Engl J Med. 1995;333:817–22.
65. National Institute for Clinical Excellence (NICE). Chronic obstructive pulmonary disease. Management of chronic obstructive pulmonary disease in adults in primary and secondary care. https://pathways.nice.org.uk/pathways/chronic-obstructive-pulmonary-disease.
66. Turner MO, Patel A, Ginsburg S, FitzGerald JM. Bronchodilator delivery in acute airflow obstruction. A meta-analysis. Arch Intern Med. 1997;157:1736–44.
67. Davies L, Angus RM, Calverley PM. Oral corticosteroids in patients admitted to hospital with exacerbations of chronic obstructive pulmonary disease: a prospective randomised controlled trial. Lancet. 1999;354:456–60.
68. Maltais F, Ostinelli J, Bourbeau J, et al. Comparison of nebulized budesonide and oral prednisolone with placebo in the treatment of acute exacerbations of chronic obstructive pulmonary disease: a randomized controlled trial. Am J Respir Crit Care Med. 2002;165:698–703.
69. Niewoehner DE, Erbland ML, Deupree RH, et al. Effect of systemic glucocorticoids on exacerbations of chronic obstructive pulmonary disease. Department of Veterans Affairs Cooperative Study Group. N Engl J Med. 1999;340:1941–7.
70. Thompson WH, Nielson CP, Carvalho P, Charan NB, Crowley JJ. Controlled trial of oral prednisone in outpatients with acute COPD exacerbation. Am J Respir Crit Care Med. 1996;154:407–12.
71. Vollenweider DJ, Jarrett H, Steurer-Stey CA, Garcia-Aymerich J, Puhan MA. Antibiotics for exacerbations of chronic obstructive pulmonary disease. Cochrane Database Syst Rev. 2012;12:CD010257.
72. Tai A, Tran H, Roberts M, Clarke N, Wilson J, Robertson CF. The association between childhood asthma and adult chronic obstructive pulmonary disease. Thorax. 2014;69(9):805–10.
73. Hodder R, Lougheed MD, Fitzgerald JM, et al. Management of acute asthma in adults in the emergency department: assisted ventilation. CMAJ. 2010;182:265–72.
74. Burburan SM, Xisto DG, Rocco PRM. Anaesthetic management in asthma. Minerva Anesthesiol. 2007;73:357–65.
75. Denmark TK, Crane HA, Brown L. Ketamine to avoid mechanical ventilation in severe pediatric asthma. J Emerg Med. 2006;30:163–6.
76. Brenner B, Corbridge T, Kazzi A. Intubation and mechanical ventilation of the asthmatic patient in respiratory failure. J Emerg Med. 2009;37:S23–34.
77. Donohue JF, Hanania NA, Ciubotaru RL, et al. Comparison of levalbuterol and racemic albuterol in hospitalized patients with acute asthma or COPD: A 2-week, multicenter, randomized, open-label study. Clin Ther. 2008;30(6):989–1002.
78. Lin RY, Pesola GR, Bakalchuk L, et al. Superiority of ipratropium plus albuterol over albuterol alone in the emergency department management of adult

asthma: a randomized clinical trial. Ann Emerg Med. 1998;31(2):208–13.

79. Daniels JM, Snijders D, de Graaff CS, Vlaspolder F, Jansen HM, Boersma WG. Antibiotics in addition to systemic corticosteroids for acute exacerbations of chronic obstructive pulmonary disease. Am J Respir Crit Care Med. 2010;181:150–7.
80. Castaldo RS, Celli BR, Gomez F, LaVallee N, Souhrada J, Hanrahan JP. A comparison of 5-day courses of dirithromycin and azithromycin in the treatment of acute exacerbations of chronic obstructive pulmonary disease. Clin Ther. 2003;25(2):542–57.
81. McCanny P, Bennett K, Staunton P, McMahon G. Venous vs arterial blood gases in the assessment of patients presenting with an exacerbation of chronic obstructive pulmonary disease. Am J Emerg Med. 2012;30:896–900.
82. Postma DS and Rabe KF. The Asthma-COPD Overlap Syndrome. NEJM 2015;373:1241–9.

Acute Respiratory Distress Syndrome

6

Zachary D. Levy, Todd L. Slesinger, and Brian J. Wright

Introduction

> Be thou assured, if words be made of breath
> And breath of life, I have no life to breathe
> What thou hast said to me.
>
> – Hamlet, Act III, Scene IV

Defining ARDS

Throughout the 1970s and 1980s, ARDS remained a nebulous entity. Without clinicians and researchers speaking the same language, it proved difficult to have meaningful and externally valid discussions on epidemiology, pathophysiology, treatment, and prognosis. This changed in 1994, when the American–European Consensus Conference (AECC) on ARDS gathered in an international effort to standardize the definition of ARDS and promote future clinical research. This represented the first major collaborative and objective step forward in our efforts to understand ARDS and to develop effective treatment algorithms. A standardized definition of ARDS was developed and has undergone continuous scrutiny and revision over the past 20 years. The most recent update to that consensus conference, known as the Berlin definition [2], was drafted in 2011. Per the Berlin criteria, ARDS is characterized as follows:

> ...a type of acute diffuse, inflammatory lung injury, leading to increased pulmonary vascular permeability, increased lung weight, and loss of aerated lung tissue. The clinical hallmarks are hypoxemia and bilateral radiographic opacities, associated with increased venous admixture, increased physiological dead space, and decreased lung compliance [2].

Note the similarities between the narrative description here and Ashbaugh, et al. prior observations. Indeed, the real nuts and bolts of the Berlin definition are the objective diagnostic criteria.

There are a few notable departures from the 1994 AECC definition. First, in the older AECC definition, hydrostatic pulmonary edema had to be excluded before a diagnosis of ARDS could be established. This was previously accomplished by measuring the pulmonary artery wedge pressure (PAWP) using a cutoff of <18 mm Hg [3]. In the Berlin definition, hydrostatic edema (CHF) must not be the *primary* cause of respiratory failure (Table 6.1). It is recognized that hydrostatic edema and ARDS can coexist. Second, the Berlin criteria require that a minimum of 5 cm H_2O of PEEP be applied when analyzing the oxygenation criteria by the fraction of arterial oxygen to inspired oxygen (PaO_2/FiO_2) ratio. Finally, the

Z. D. Levy
Emergency Medicine and Neurosurgery, Zucker School of Medicine at Hofstra/Northwell, Hempstead, NY, USA

T. L. Slesinger
Herbert Wertheim College of Medicine, Florida International University, Miami, FL, USA

B. J. Wright (✉)
Emergency Medicine and Neurosurgery, Stony Brook University School of Medicine, Stony Brook, NY, USA

© Springer Nature Switzerland AG 2020

J. R. Shiber, S. D. Weingart (eds.), *Emergency Department Critical Care*,
https://doi.org/10.1007/978-3-030-28794-8_6

Table 6.1 The Berlin definition

ARDS: the Berlin definition
1. Onset <7 days from a defined illness or traumatic event
2. Bilateral opacities on chest X-ray or CT scan consistent with pulmonary edema
3. The degree of respiratory failure cannot entirely be attributed to congestive heart failure (CHF) and/or fluid overload

Table 6.2 ARDS severity categories

ARDS Berlin severity categories
Mild ARDS: PaO_2/FiO_2 ratio 200–300 (~27% mortality)
Moderate ARDS: PaO_2/FiO_2 ratio 100–200 (~32% mortality)
Severe ARDS: PaO_2/FiO_2 < 100 (~45% mortality)

Berlin criteria removed the diagnosis of acute lung injury (ALI), which was effectively "mild" ARDS, and replaced it with three ARDS disease severity categories based on the PaO_2/FiO_2 ratio (Table 6.2).

The Berlin diagnostic criteria and risk stratification scores are part of the continuing effort to objectively define ARDS, to improve the external validity of ARDS research, and to develop meaningful treatment considerations. In addition to addressing limitations of the prior AECC definition, the Berlin criteria have better predictive validity for mortality [2], may better risk stratify patients for different treatment strategies, and also help researchers define patient populations for experimental treatments. There is also evidence that the Berlin criteria have a better sensitivity and specificity (82% and 52%, respectively) for predicting the presence of diffuse alveolar damage (DAD) at autopsy, compared to the AECC definition (76% and 47%), though both performed marginally [4].

Epidemiology

The quoted incidence of ARDS has varied widely. This is likely a reflection of several variables, including an ever-changing understanding of the disease, geographic, cultural factors, and a heterogeneously ill patient population. Estimates have historically been higher in North America compared to Europe, recently ranging from 7.2 per 100,000 [5] (Spain) to 78.9 per 100,000 [6] (the United States). Some of these discrepancies may normalize as we approach greater uniformity in diagnosing ARDS.

For similar reasons, mortality estimates are also variable. Aside from the mortality rates conferred by the mild/moderate/severe Berlin categories, a recent meta-analysis [7] reported an overall mortality of 43%, with wide variations reported among included studies (ranging from 15% to 72%). Interestingly, the overall mortality in ARDS declined about 1% per year over the 12-year study period 1994–2006.

Pathophysiology

ARDS can develop through two separate mechanisms. Precipitating factors may be primary pulmonary events, such as smoke inhalation, aspiration, and pneumonia. However, nearly half of all cases are caused by extrapulmonary triggers, including sepsis, multitrauma (but especially chest injury and pulmonary contusions), pancreatitis, and blood product administration [4, 8]. These two distinct pathways have contributed to the delay in standardizing the definition of ARDS and are consistent with Ashbaugh, et al. initial observation nearly 50 years ago of a disorder that can truly be precipitated by "a variety of stimuli" [1].

The Three-Phase Model

ARDS is characterized by a number of abnormal processes on the cellular level. First, a triggering event occurs, acting either via direct cellular insult or via indirect systemic inflammatory response [9, 10]. Regardless of whether the initial trigger is pulmonary or extrapulmonary, ARDS then proceeds down a common pathway. An initial *exudative phase*, lasting several days to a week, is defined by multiple inflammatory processes [10]. These include neutrophil influx, cytokine release, loss of surfactant, and endothelial dysfunction. Consequently, the exudative phase is characterized by significant pulmonary edema.

The *proliferative phase* follows, where type II pneumocytes multiply and attempt to replace damaged type I pneumocytes on the epithelial surface [11]. The proliferative phase is also characterized by thickening of the alveolar capillaries, organization of exudate, and early fibroblast activity [12]. These processes result in progressive airspace narrowing, and pulmonary hypertension may result from destruction of the pulmonary vasculature. Hypoxemia may worsen secondary to restricted diffusion.

Finally, a variable *fibrotic phase* sets in, with collagen deposition resulting in decreased lung compliance and progressive VQ mismatch. A decline in neutrophils is seen on bronchoalveolar lavage (BAL), with a relative increase in both lymphocytes and macrophages. Not all patients will progress through the fibrotic phase of ARDS, and there is some evidence that the degree of fibrotic change is correlated with increased overall mortality [13].

Ventilator-Induced Lung Injury

It is worth noting that many of the pathologic processes associated with ARDS may be iatrogenic, related to overzealous use of invasive ventilation. There are four distinct mechanisms in which the ventilator can be a primary source of lung injury in ARDS (or any condition requiring mechanical ventilation, for that matter):

- Excessive tidal volumes that result in alveolar strain (*volutrauma*)
- High airway pressures (*barotrauma*)
- Cyclic collapse of alveoli during the respiratory cycle (*atelectotrauma*)
- Inflammatory cytokine release in response to these mechanical lung stressors (*biotrauma*)

Collectively, these four mechanisms are referred to as ventilator-induced lung injury (VILI) [14], and much of the supportive care in ARDS revolves around avoiding these iatrogenic insults.

Diagnosis

The diagnosis of ARDS is now relatively straightforward and involves a clinical suspicion coupled with an imaging study, in accordance with the previously mentioned Berlin criteria. Imaging studies in ARDS typically include standard chest X-ray and lung computerized tomography (CT). Bilateral interstitial infiltrates are typically present in a "patchy" or "fluffy" distribution and are often readily apparent on plain films (see Fig. 6.1). These infiltrates are the result of protein-rich fluid leaking into the alveolar space secondary to alveolar epithelial insult and diffuse alveolar damage. CT will demonstrate bilateral ground-glass opacities with dense consolidations that appear worse in the dependent sections of the lungs (see Fig. 6.2). Lung ultrasound may also be beneficial and may demonstrate B lines in the presence of pleural abnormalities (Fig. 6.3). Finally, capillary permeability may be directly measured with positron emission tomography (PET) scanning of the chest, though this modality is rarely (if ever) utilized.

A number of serum biomarkers have been studied to aid in the diagnosis of ARDS. These include, but are not limited to, C-reactive protein (CRP), laminin, desmosine, protein C, serum surfactant, soluble receptor of advanced glyca-

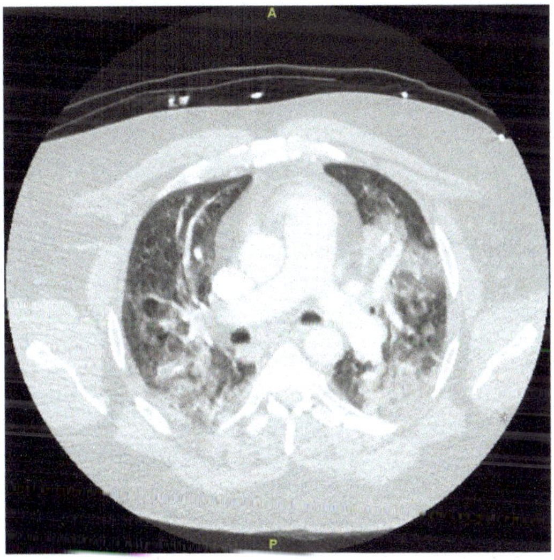

Fig. 6.1 Typical ARDS plain film

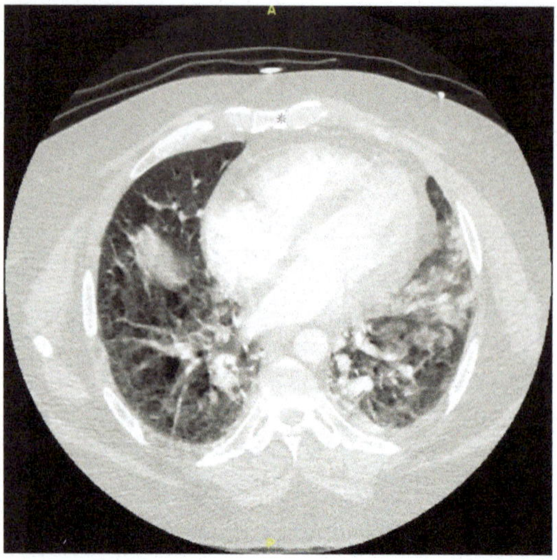

Fig. 6.2 Typical ARDS chest CT, axial image

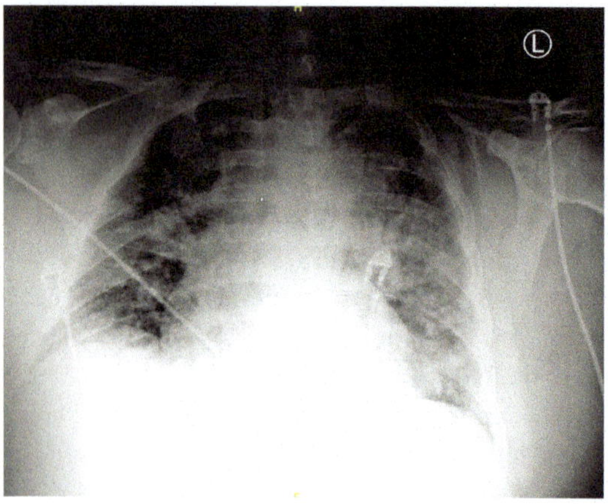

Fig. 6.3 Typical ARDS lung u/s

tion end products (RAGE), various interleukins, and various growth factors. To date, none of these have demonstrated significant diagnostic or prognostic value and are not used in clinical practice [15].

Is It ARDS or Is It Pneumonia?

The X-ray appearance of ARDS can mimic that of multifocal pneumonia, and both processes may emerge in critically ill, ventilated patients. Unfortunately, there is no consistently reliable way to differentiate the two, and misdiagnosis of ARDS as ventilator-associated pneumonia (and vice versa) may be inevitable to some extent. The diffuse nature of the infiltrates may serve to differentiate ARDS from pneumonia, along with a lack of clear stigmata of infection (such as fever, copious thick secretions, or leukocytosis). However, these features are sometimes present in ARDS as well. Additionally, the lack or presence of other precipitating causes (pancreatitis, trauma, blood transfusion, or nonpulmonary sepsis) in the patient's history and physical examination, along with the use of appropriate laboratory and imaging studies, can sometimes help clue the clinician to the correct diagnosis. When in doubt, treat the pneumonia – in sepsis, a delay in antibiotic use is associated with increased mortality [16].

Treatment

Invasive Ventilation

Except for the most mild cases, invasive ventilation is needed to appropriately manage ARDS. However, the specter of VILI invokes Virgil – *aegrescit medendo*, the remedy is worse than the disease. With this in mind, the National Institute of Health established the ARDS Network (ARDSNet) in 1994 in order to facilitate large, multicenter trials involving treatment of ARDS patients [17], including a determination of the ideal ventilator approach. The most widely cited and groundbreaking ARDSNet study to date demonstrated that a "lung-protective" ventilation strategy (LPVS) (see Table 6.3), which utilized volume-assist-control ventilation to deliver tidal

Table 6.3 Lung-protective ventilation strategy

ARDSnet lung-protective ventilation strategy
1. Volume-assist-control ventilation set at 6 cc/kg predicted body weight (PBW) Male patients: PBW (kg) = 50 + 2.3 ∗ (height in inches – 60) Female patients: PBW (kg) = 45.5 + 2.3 ∗ (height in inches – 60)
2. Maintain plateau pressure <30 cm of water
3. If plateau pressures >30 cm of water, decrease tidal volume by 1 cc/kg to a minimum of 4 cc/kg
4. If plateau pressures <30 cm with severe dyspnea, increase tidal volume by 1 cc/kg to a maximum of 8 cc/kg

volumes of 4–8 cc per kg of Ideal Body Weight and maintained plateau pressures <30 cm of water, significantly improved mortality and time off the ventilator in the first 28 days of illness [18]. This has effectively become the standard of care for invasive ventilation in ARDS. These tidal volumes often approximate resting tidal volumes – "physiologic" or "normal" ventilation may be a more accurate description than "lung-protective" ventilation. In a similar vein, a recent meta-analysis by Neto et al. [19] suggested that LPVS may improve clinical outcomes across a spectrum of non-ARDS disease processes.

When providing LPVS, it is important to keep in mind that decreased tidal volumes will result in decreased alveolar ventilation. PCO_2 and pH need to be monitored closely. While patients with intact respiratory drives will often compensate on their own, sedated and/or paralyzed patients will require the ventilator rate to be increased in order to prevent significant hypercarbia. Increased respiratory rates, in turn, will decrease expiratory times and expose patients to a greater risk of air-trapping and auto-PEEP, which itself may lead to decreased venous return and hypotension. This is particularly true among patients with underlying obstructive pulmonary disease.

Recruitment Maneuvers

Persistent hypoxemia in ventilated patients with ARDS and/or severe pneumonia – assuming that the ventilator circuit is intact, the endotracheal tube is proper position, and the patient has not developed a pulmonary embolism or pneumothorax – is often due to shunting of deoxygenated blood back to the heart. With significant pulmonary edema and atelectasis, venous blood may not encounter functional oxygenated alveoli as it courses through the lungs, resulting in deoxygenated blood being pumped into the systemic circulation. In this case, increasing the FiO_2 may have little impact. PEEP is intended to ameliorate this effect, but in severe cases, recruitment maneuvers may be beneficial.

There are various iterations (including "sighs," "extended sighs," and "sustained inflation") that all involve transient increases in mean airway pressure in order to open collapsed lung segments. A common example of sustained inflation would be to apply continuous positive airway pressure (CPAP) at 10 cm of water higher than the current plateau pressure (Pplat) for 30–45 seconds. Other variations exist as well. The use of recruitment maneuvers has not been demonstrated to be beneficial in the routine management of ARDS, and given the risks of significantly elevated airway pressures, it should be considered only for significant and refractory hypoxemia [20].

Advanced Ventilatory Modes

More advanced ventilation strategies, such as airway pressure release ventilation (APRV) and high-frequency oscillation, have also been studied. APRV is an example of inverse ratio ventilation except that it allows for spontaneous breathing so that the I:E ratio is irrelevant; if no spontaneous breathing occurs, then minute ventilation is only from the release volume. The majority of the respiratory cycle is spent in sustained pressure hold (known as P High for a time period know as T High), followed by brief pressure release (P Low) that is short enough (T Low) to prevent alveolar collapse. Spontaneous breathing during the inspiratory phase promotes natural diaphragmatic excursion and increases recruitment in the dependent portions of the lung. Some degree of CO_2 retention may be tolerated, given the brief expiratory phase ("permissive hypercapnia"). It is worth noting that use of APRV has not been shown to decrease mortality in ARDS compared to volume- or pressure-controlled ventilation, but is associated with lower rates of ARDS and mortality in high-risk patient populations [21], and APRV should be viewed simply as an alternative approach for patients who remain hypoxemic on more traditional volume-assist-control ventilator settings.

High-frequency oscillation ventilation (HFOV) is a form of rapid cycle ventilation that delivers miniscule tidal volumes up to several hundred times per minute at elevated airway pressures. It can be conceptualized as rapid, shallow tidal breaths that are "oscillating" around a markedly elevated level of continuous positive end-expiratory pressure (CPAP) (see Fig. 6.3). HFOV has traditionally been used as a last ditch ventilation strategy for severe refractory hypoxemia and should not generally be used as a substitute for traditional LPVS. In one large randomized multicenter study, Ferguson, et al. demonstrated a significant increase in mortality (RR 1.33) when HFOV was used in placed of LPVS – a trial that was actually stopped by the data monitoring committee due to harm after enrolling fewer than half of the intended sample size [22].

Intravenous Fluids

The judicious use of resuscitative and maintenance fluids is worth mentioning. The ARDSnet FACTT trial compared liberal versus conservative fluid management strategies, and it also compared central venous catheter (CVC) versus pulmonary artery catheter (PAC) placement to guide fluid therapy. The protocol resulted in a net even fluid balance in the conservative group over the first week of treatment, while patients in the liberal group were positive 7 L, on average. A 60-day mortality was equal between the groups, though patients in the conservative group enjoyed fewer days on the ventilator and fewer days in the ICU [23]. There was no significant difference between groups regarding the need for renal replacement therapy (RRT).

Regarding the use of invasive monitoring in ARDS, PAC-guided therapy was associated with a significant increase in complications as compared to CVC-guided therapy [24] while providing no overall mortality benefit in the first 60 days after randomization. Complications of PAC therapy were primarily catheter-induced arrhythmias. In the intervening years since FACTT was published, PAC-guided therapy has fallen largely out of favor.

Pharmacotherapy

Of the various pharmacotherapies for ARDS, corticosteroids have historically been among the most commonly used and the most controversial. In one ARDSnet trial examining the potential benefit of methylprednisolone in ARDS, patients in the treatment group appeared to have improved oxygenation, better hemodynamics, and more time off the ventilator, but these changes were not associated with any short- or long-term mortality benefits [25]. More importantly, corticosteroid use was associated with increased mortality when initiated more than 2 weeks after the onset of symptoms. The lack of overall benefit for corticosteroids more or less confirmed the findings of two prior studies that failed to show a mortality benefit for high-dose methylprednisolone in early ARDS [26, 27].

Neuromuscular blocking agents (NMBAs) have also been heavily studied. The ACURASYS trial indicated that a short course of the neuromuscular blocking agent cisatracurium may improve mortality and decrease the incidence of barotrauma, likely by optimizing patient–ventilator synchrony [28, 29]. There is also some evidence that the use of NMBAs is associated with a decrease in serum inflammatory markers [30], which is either secondary to a decrease in mechanical stressors or results from some other independent mechanism. The potential benefit of NMBAs was again demonstrated in a recent systematic review that found a decrease in both in-hospital mortality and rates of barotrauma without significant adverse events [31]. Using both steroids and neuromuscular blocking agents simultaneously should be avoided, as it is believed to increase the incidence of ICU-acquired muscle weakness [32]. If NMBAs are going to be utilized, it is important to administer analgesics and sedatives as well, to prevent a fully conscious (and likely uncomfortable) patient from enduring several days of total paralysis.

On the whole, effective pharmacologic treatments remain elusive. In fact, we know a great deal more about what *does not work* in ARDS rather than what does. ARDSnet has carried out several negative studies regarding experimental pharmacotherapies, including the use of both ketoconazole [33] and lisofylline [34]. Other medications that have failed to show conclusive benefit include inhaled nitric oxide, inhaled prostacyclins, systemic prostaglandins, neutrophil elastase inhibitors, albumin, endobronchial surfactant, and N-acetylcysteine [35].

Inhaled vasodilators (nitric oxide and prostacyclins) deserve special mention, as these medications have been used extensively in ARDS patients with refractory hypoxemia. Inhaled vasodilators selectively increase blood flow to alveolar units that are participating in gas exchange. This increase in pulmonary blood flow should (theoretically) decrease the amount of shunted blood that reaches the systemic circulation and improve arterial oxygenation. Numerous studies have examined the efficacy of these agents (particularly inhaled nitric oxide) in ARDS; while there is evidence for a transient improvement in PaO_2 to FiO_2 ratios, there is no evidence for any reduction in morbidity or mortality [36].

Nutritional Support

To call ARDS an inflammatory state is an understatement – it is inflammation gone haywire. Patients will be hypercatabolic, and as a result, will have significant dietary needs. Early nutritional support has been demonstrated to temper the systemic inflammatory response by staving off gut atrophy. This prevents the translocation of gut bacteria through leaky, permeable epithelial junctions that otherwise results from a prolonged fasting state [37]. A diminished bacterial burden results in diminished systemic inflammation.

However, overfeeding is not without its own risks. These include hypercapnia, hyperglycemia, hepatic steatosis, azotemia, and electrolyte imbalances, to name a few [38]. Hyperglycemia itself is linked to an increased infectious risk and poor wound healing, and so clinicians have to walk a fine line between too little nutritional support and too much. The current American Society for Parenteral and Enteral Nutrition (ASPEN) guidelines recommend that patients with ARDS receive early enteric feeding when feasible using tube feeds with an anti-inflammatory lipid profile (including borage seed oils and omega-3 fish oils) [37]. A subset of the ARDSNet EDEN study attempted to determine if adding omega-3 supplements to tube feeds would positively impact ventilator-free days, but was stopped early for futility [39]. That same study also found no difference in outcomes with the use of full enteric feeds versus lower volume "trophic" feeds in the first 6 days of illness [39].

Prone Positioning

Simpler interventions have been studied as well. Prone positioning, which had fallen out of favor for a time, is regaining interest after the prone positioning in severe ARDS (PROSEVA) trial demonstrated significant improvements in 28- and 90-day mortality when patients with severe ARDS were proned for a minimum of 16 hours per day [40]. The beneficial effects of proning are thought to include reduced VQ mismatch, redistribution of secretions and extravascular lung water, and more effective diaphragmatic excursion. These effects are partially accomplished by relieving atelectasis that tends to form in dependent portions of the lung when patients are placed in the supine position for extended periods of time.

Prone positioning can be accomplished either via specialized pronating beds or by traditional log-rolling techniques using standard hospital beds. It may be technically difficult to perform, and the greatest risks involve dislodging or obstructing the endotracheal tube, as well as the development of pressure ulcers [41]. Proning in ARDS is a perfect example of the adage "everything old is new again," as the theoretical benefits of proning have been described in infants since the 1970s [42, 43].

Extracorporeal Membrane Oxygenation (ECMO)

ECMO is emerging as a viable treatment option in severe ARDS, particularly with the advent of more portable ECMO devices and dual-lumen catheters that allow for single-puncture venovenous (VV) access [44]. In the VV ECMO model, the pulmonary support provided by the ECMO device relieves the burden placed on the ventilator, which can be set to minimal LPVS parameters. The potential benefits of ECMO were demonstrated in the CESAR study [45], where patients with severe ARDS (defined by a Murray Score > 3 or a pH <7.2 on optimum conventional management) who received ECMO experienced a reduction in 6-month mortality compared to conventional management (63% vs. 47%, RR 0.69; CI 0.05–0.97). Enthusiasm for these findings is tempered by a lack of uniformity in the control group, where nearly a third of patients did not receive lung-protective ventilation. Other studies [46] examining the efficacy of ECMO in severe ARDS are ongoing.

Recent advances notwithstanding, ECMO is resource-intense, and is generally not available outside of large academic centers. Additionally, the use of anticoagulants in the ECMO circuit, coupled with the large bore catheters required for the exchange process, present significant bleeding risks. Other risks include hemolysis and the development of DIC, and these factors, for the time being preclude the use of ECMO in all but the sickest patients.

Interest is emerging in a subtype of ECMO therapy that focuses primarily on extracorporeal CO_2 removal (ECCO2R). By "uncoupling" ventilation from oxygenation, LPVS can be performed without fear of hypercarbia or the need to adjust the respiratory rate. A benefit of ECCO2R versus traditional ECMO is that the low flow requirements of these newer systems require smaller, single catheter venous access. A recent meta-analysis by Fitzgerald, et al. could not find a mortality benefit for ECCO2R in ARDS, but it was limited by a lack of high-quality studies [47].

Life after ARDS

ARDS survivors have been noted to have persistent functional limitations, even years after their illness [48]. Somewhat paradoxically, symptoms are predominantly extrapulmonary in nature, including muscle weakness and generalized depression. Chronic muscle weakness may account for the fact that diminished exercise capacity up to 5 years after suffering from ARDS has been demonstrated despite normal to near-normal pulmonary function testing, particularly in younger patients [48, 49].

The lingering effects of ARDS may be a function of prolonged ICU stays and multiorgan system failure in general, the use of corticosteroids and neuromuscular blocking agents, something inherent to ARDS itself, or most likely some contribution from all of the above. This unfortunately means that the societal costs of ARDS continue long after these patients are discharged from the hospital and include a decreased quality of life and an increased utilization of health-care resources. By some estimates, ARDS survivors cost the health-care system $1100 to $3200 per person per year more than healthy controls [48].

Summary

ARDS is a debilitating illness brought on by a variety of pulmonary and extrapulmonary insults. The improved Berlin criteria allow practitioners to diagnose ARDS objectively, risk-stratify patients based on disease severity, and engage in meaningful research collaboratives. Several landmark studies in ARDS have been published in the last two decades (see Table 6.4) to guide therapy. Clinical recommendations include the following:

Table 6.4 Landmark trials in ARDS

Summary of landmark trials in ARDS
ARDSNet – Lower vs. Traditional Tidal Volumes (*NEJM* 2000)
ARDSNet – Fluid and Catheter Treatment Trial (FACTT) (*NEJM* 2006)
Conventional Ventilatory Support Versus ECMO for Severe Adult Respiratory Failure (CESAR) (*Lancet* 2009)
Neuromuscular Blocking Agents in ARDS (ACURASYS) (*NEJM* 2010)
Prone Positioning in Severe ARDS (PROSEVA) (*NEJM* 2013)

- Lung-protective ventilation in ARDS has become the standard of care, and it should be considered in non-ARDS patients as well.
- Once ARDS sets in, physicians should aim for neutral fluid balance.
- There is insufficient evidence to support routine use of any specific medication in ARDS, though a brief course of NMBAs may be beneficial in reducing VILI and systemic inflammation.
- Inhaled nitric oxide may transiently improve oxygenation without affecting mortality.
- Corticosteroids remain controversial and are largely contraindicated.
- Early enteric feeding, unless contraindicated, should be instituted with anti-inflammatory tube feed preparations; trophic feeds may be equivalent to full enteric feeding.
- Prone positioning and ECMO may be advantageous in severe ARDS, particularly if the patient is not responding to standard therapies.

Finally, one should keep in mind that ARDS is not simply an acute process. After recovery and hospital discharge, patients continue struggle with muscle weakness, mood disorders, increased health-care expenditures, and an overall decreased quality of life.

References

1. Ashbaugh DG, Bigelow DB, Petty TL, Levine BE. Acute respiratory distress in adults. Lancet. 1967;2(7511):319–23.
2. Ranieri VM, Rubenfeld GD, Thompson BT, et al. Acute respiratory distress syndrome: the Berlin definition. JAMA. 2012;307(23):2526–33.
3. Bernard GR, Artigas A, Brigham KL, et al. The American-European consensus conference on ARDS. Definitions, mechanisms, relevant outcomes, and clinical trial coordination. Am J Respir Crit Care Med. 1994;149(3 Pt 1):818–24.
4. Frohlich S, Doolan A, Murphy N, Crotty T, Boylan J. Comparison of the accuracy of the AECC and Berlin definitions in diagnosing ARDS. Am J Respir Crit Care Med. 2013;187:A2211.
5. Villar, et al. Intensive Care Med 2011;37(12): 1932–41.
6. Rubenfield, et al. N Engl J Med. 2005;353(16): 1685–93.
7. Zambon M, Vincent JL. Mortality rates for patients with acute lung injury/ARDS have decreased over time. Chest. 2008;133(5):1120–7.
8. Gajic O, Dabbagh O, Park PK, et al. Early identification of patients at risk of acute lung injury: evaluation of lung injury prediction score in a multicenter cohort study. Am J Respir Crit Care Med. 2011;183(4):462–70.
9. Tomashefski JF. Pulmonary pathology of the adult respiratory distress syndrome. Clin Chest Med. 1990;11(4):593–619.
10. Walkey AJ, Summer R, Ho V, Alkana P. Acute respiratory distress syndrome: epidemiology and management approaches. Clin Epidemiol. 2012;4:159–69.
11. Bellingan GJ. The pulmonary physician in critical care * 6: the pathogenesis of ALI/ARDS. Thorax. 2002;57(6):540–6.
12. Mendez JL, Hubmayr RD. New insights into the pathology of acute respiratory failure. Curr Opin Crit Care. 2005;11(1):29–36.
13. Martin C, Papazian L, Payan MJ, Saux P, Gouin F. Pulmonary fibrosis correlates with outcome in adult respiratory distress syndrome. A study in mechanically ventilated patients. Chest. 1995;107(1):196–200.
14. Slutsky AS, Ranieri VM. Ventilator-induced lung injury. N Engl J Med. 2013;369(22):2126–36.
15. Bhargava M, Wendt CH. Biomarkers in acute lung injury. Transl Res. 2012;159(4):205–17.
16. Kumar A, Roberts D, Wood KE, et al. Duration of hypotension before initiation of effective antimicrobial therapy is the critical determinant of survival in human septic shock. Crit Care Med. 2006;34(6):1589–96.
17. http://www.ardsnet.org.
18. Ventilation with lower tidal volumes as compared with traditional tidal volumes for acute lung injury and the acute respiratory distress syndrome. The acute respiratory distress syndrome network. N Engl J Med. 2000;342(18):1301–8.
19. Serpa Neto A, Cardoso SO, Manetta JA, et al. Association between use of lung-protective ventilation with lower tidal volumes and clinical outcomes among patients without acute respiratory distress syndrome: a meta-analysis. JAMA. 2012;308(16):1651–9.
20. Guerin C, Debord S, Leray V, et al. Efficacy and safety of recruitment maneuvers in acute respiratory distress syndrome. Ann Intensive Care. 2011;1(1):9.
21. Daoud EG, Farag HL, Chatburn RL. Airway pressure release ventilation: what do we know? Respir Care. 2012;57(2):282–92.
22. Ferguson ND, Cook DJ, Guyatt GH, et al. High-frequency oscillation in early acute respiratory distress syndrome. N Engl J Med. 2013;368(9):795–805.
23. Wiedemann HP, Wheeler AP, Bernard GR, et al. Comparison of two fluid-management

strategies in acute lung injury. N Engl J Med. 2006;354(24):2564–75.
24. Wheeler AP, Bernard GR, Thompson BT, et al. Pulmonary-artery versus central venous catheter to guide treatment of acute lung injury. N Engl J Med. 2006;354(21):2213–24.
25. Steinberg KP, Hudson LD, Goodman RB, et al. Efficacy and safety of corticosteroids for persistent acute respiratory distress syndrome. N Engl J Med. 2006;354(16):1671–84.
26. Luce JM, Montgomery AB, Marks JD, Turner J, Metz CA, Murray JF. Ineffectiveness of high-dose methylprednisolone in preventing parenchymal lung injury and improving mortality in patients with septic shock. Am Rev Respir Dis. 1988;138(1):62–8.
27. Bernard GR, Luce JM, Sprung CL, et al. High-dose corticosteroids in patients with the adult respiratory distress syndrome. N Engl J Med. 1987;317(25):1565–70.
28. Papazian L, Forel JM, Gacouin A, et al. Neuromuscular blockers in early acute respiratory distress syndrome. N Engl J Med. 2010;363(12):1107–16.
29. Shafeeq H, Lat I. Pharmacotherapy for acute respiratory distress syndrome. Pharmacotherapy. 2012;32(10):943–57.
30. Forel JM, Roch A, Marin V, et al. Neuromuscular blocking agents decrease inflammatory response in patients presenting with acute respiratory distress syndrome. Crit Care Med. 2006;34(11):2749–57.
31. Alhazzani W, Alshahrani M, Jaeschke R, et al. Neuromuscular blocking agents in acute respiratory distress syndrome: a systematic review and meta-analysis of randomized controlled trials. Crit Care. 2013;17(2):R43.
32. De jonghe B, Lacherade JC, Sharshar T, Outin H. Intensive care unit-acquired weakness: risk factors and prevention. Crit Care Med. 2009;37(10 Suppl):S309–15.
33. Ketoconazole for early treatment of acute lung injury and acute respiratory distress syndrome: a randomized controlled trial. The ARDS network. JAMA. 2000;283(15):1995–2002.
34. Randomized, placebo-controlled trial of lisofylline for early treatment of acute lung injury and acute respiratory distress syndrome. Crit Care Med. 2002;30(1):1–6.
35. Boyle AJ, MacSweeney R, Mcauley DF. Pharmacological treatments in ARDS; a state-of-the-art update. BMC Med. 2013;11:166.
36. Afshari A, Brok J, Møller AM, Wetterslev J. Inhaled nitric oxide for acute respiratory distress syndrome (ARDS) and acute lung injury in children and adults. Cochrane Database Syst Rev. 2010;(7):CD002787.
37. Mcclave SA, Martindale RG, Vanek VW, et al. Guidelines for the provision and assessment of nutrition support therapy in the adult critically ill patient: Society of Critical Care Medicine (SCCM) and American Society for Parenteral and Enteral Nutrition (A.S.P.E.N.). JPEN J Parenter Enteral Nutr. 2009;33(3):277–316.
38. Krzak A, Pleva M, Napolitano LM. Nutrition therapy for ALI and ARDS. Crit Care Clin. 2011;27(3):647–59.
39. Rice TW, Wheeler AP, Thompson BT, et al. Enteral omega-3 fatty acid, gamma-linolenic acid, and antioxidant supplementation in acute lung injury. JAMA. 2011;306(14):1574–81.
40. Guérin C, Reignier J, Richard JC, et al. Prone positioning in severe acute respiratory distress syndrome. N Engl J Med. 2013;368(23):2159–68.
41. Lee JM, Bae W, Lee YJ, Cho YJ. The efficacy and safety of prone positional ventilation in acute respiratory distress syndrome: updated study-level meta-analysis of 11 randomized controlled trials. Crit Care Med. 2014;42(5):1252–62.
42. Bryan AC. Conference on the scientific basis of respiratory therapy. Pulmonary physiotherapy in the pediatric age group. Comments of a devil's advocate. Am Rev Respir Dis. 1974;110(6 Pt 2):143–4.
43. Wagaman MJ, Shutack JG, Moomjian AS, Schwartz JG, ShaVer TH, Fox WW. Improved oxygenation and lung compliance with prone positioning of neonates. J Pediatr. 1979;94:787–91.
44. Brodie D, Bacchetta M. Extracorporeal membrane oxygenation for ARDS in adults. N Engl J Med. 2011;365(20):1905–14.
45. Peek GJ, Mugford M, Tiruvoipati R, et al. Efficacy and economic assessment of conventional ventilatory support versus extracorporeal membrane oxygenation for severe adult respiratory failure (CESAR): a multicentre randomised controlled trial. Lancet. 2009;374(9698):1351–63.
46. Clinicaltrials.gov ID: NCT01470703.
47. Fitzgerald M, Millar J, Blackwood B, et al. Extracorporeal carbon dioxide removal for patients with acute respiratory failure secondary to the acute respiratory distress syndrome: a systematic review. Crit Care. 2014;18(3):222.
48. Herridge MS, Tansey CM, Matté A, et al. Functional disability 5 years after acute respiratory distress syndrome. N Engl J Med. 2011;364(14):1293–304.
49. Davidson TA, Caldwell ES, Curtis JR, Hudson LD, Steinberg KP. Reduced quality of life in survivors of acute respiratory distress syndrome compared with critically ill control patients. JAMA. 1999;281(4):354–60.

Pulmonary Embolism and Massive DVT for Emergency Critical Care

7

Timothy J. Ellender, David Hackenson, and Emily Gundert

Introduction

Venous thromboembolism (VTE) as a first event occurs in 100 per 100,000 persons each year in the United States with an incidence that rises exponentially with age [1]. More than 60% of symptomatic VTE cases manifest as deep vein thrombosis (DVT) alone, whereas one-third of patients present with pulmonary embolism (PE) [1]. Recurrence occurs in approximately 7% of patients and happens more frequently with PE than DVT [1, 2]. The incidence of death within 30 days of diagnosis occurs in 6% of patients with DVT and 12% with PE [1]. Less common manifestations of venous thrombosis include phlegmasia alba dolens, phlegmasia cerulea dolens (PCD), and venous gangrene, which form a clinical spectrum that carries significant morbidity [3, 4]. It is important for the emergency practitioner (EP) to appropriately recognize and treat VTE, as delays in diagnosis and treatment may result in a significant increase in morbidity and mortality.

T. J. Ellender (✉)
Department of Emergency Medicine, IU School of Medicine, IU Health-Methodist Hospital, Indianapolis, IN, USA
e-mail: tellende@iupui.edu

D. Hackenson
Emergency Medicine, University of Michigan, Ann Arbor, MI, USA

E. Gundert
Emergency Medicine, UT Southwestern Medical Center, Dallas, TX, USA

Phlegmasia Alba Dolens, Phlegmasia Cerulea Dolens, and Venous Gangrene

Phlegmasia has been described in the medical literature as far back as the sixteenth century, though much of the formative work describing the pathophysiology was completed over the last 200 years [5–8]. All three manifestations result from acute massive venous thrombosis and obstruction of the venous drainage of an extremity. Phlegmasia alba dolens, PCD, and venous gangrene are more common during the fifth and sixth decades of life, but can occur at any age [3, 8–10]. The incidence of all three entities is higher in females than in males. Malignancy is the most commonly associated trigger and is present in approximately 20–40% of patients with PCD [3, 11].

Other associated risk factors include thrombophilia, trauma, surgery, heparin-induced thrombocytopenia, inflammatory bowel diseases, heart failure, vena cava filter insertion, and pregnancy [9, 11, 12]. Finally, 10% of patients with phlegmasia have no apparent risk factors identifiable [10]. PCD of the upper extremities is rare (<5% of patients), while PCD of the lower extremities is more common with the left-sided occurrence being three to four times more common than the right-sided occurrence [4, 12].

© Springer Nature Switzerland AG 2020
J. R. Shiber, S. D. Weingart (eds.), *Emergency Department Critical Care*,
https://doi.org/10.1007/978-3-030-28794-8_7

Pathophysiology

Phlegmasia is caused by massive thrombosis and occlusion of the major venous channels (commonly iliofemoral veins), causing significant compromise to venous outflow and venous hypertension [12]. In phlegmasia alba dolens, the thrombosis involves only major deep venous channels of the extremity and spares the collateral veins. The venous drainage, though decreased, is still present, which reduces venous congestion and the resultant tissue ischemia which differentiates this entity from PCD. In PCD, the thrombosis extends to collateral veins causing near complete occlusion of outflow, resulting in venous congestion with massive fluid sequestration, significant edema, and tissue ischemia with bluish discoloration [3, 12, 13]. Early phases of phlegmasia are reversible if proper measures are taken to prevent venous gangrene. Capillary involvement occurs in 40–60% of PCD cases which results in irreversible venous gangrene that extends to the skin, subcutaneous tissue, or muscle [12–15]. Under this extreme, the hydrostatic pressure in arterial and venous capillaries exceeds oncotic pressure, causing fluid sequestration in the interstitium and increased compartment pressures [16, 17]. Venous pressure may increase rapidly, and fluid sequestration may reach 6–10 L [11, 18]. Circulatory shock and arterial insufficiency may ensue. Though the exact mechanism for the arterial compromise is not completely clear, it is believed to be associated with the dysregulation of coagulation and fibrinolysis and circulatory collapse from the loss of venous return [9, 12].

Key Points

- Phlegmasia occurs more commonly with advancing age (greatest in the fifth and sixth decades of life) and is more common in females.
- All three clinical entities more commonly occur in the lower extremity.
- Of the causative factors associated with VTE, cancer is most commonly associated with phlegmasia.
- The pathophysiology of phlegmasia is caused by massive thrombosis and occlusion of the major venous channels (commonly iliofemoral veins) causing significant compromise to venous outflow and venous hypertension which can eventually encroach on tissue perfusion causing tissue gangrene.

Patient Presentation

Manifestations of phlegmasia may be insidious or fulminant. Of PCD cases, 50–60% are preceded by phlegmasia alba dolens, with symptoms of edema, pain, and blanching (alba) without cyanosis [12]. The blanching, which previously was thought to be caused by arterial vasospasm, is caused by subcutaneous edema, without overwhelming venous congestion and ischemia, leaving the leg swollen and white appearing giving rise to the term "milk leg" [12].

Patients with PCD present with the clinical triad of severe edema, agonizing pain, and cyanosis [12]. Massive fluid sequestration may lead to bleb and bullae formation. Though the pathognomonic cyanosis (cerulea) in PCD usually starts distally and extends proximally, the constant pain usually starts at the femoral triangle and progresses to the entire extremity [12]. When venous gangrene occurs, it usually follows a similar distribution to the cyanosis [4, 19]. Arterial pulses may be present if venous compromise is superficial; however, when gangrene involves the muscular compartment, the resultant increased compartment pressures may produce a pulse deficit [9]. Arterial signals may be intact though difficult to appreciate because of the significant edema [12]. Patients with fulminant disease usually present with sudden severe pain, swelling, cyanosis, venous gangrene, and compartment syndrome that together impair venous outflow and arterial supply, such that circulatory collapse and shock frequently ensue [9].

Diagnostics

The diagnoses of phlegmasia alba dolens, phlegmasia cerulea dolens (PCD), and venous gangrene can be made mainly by clinical presentation with the assistance of additional imaging for confirmation. Although contrast venography was once considered the standard for diagnosis, technical difficulties can be common (in as many as 20–25% of patients) [9, 15]. Venography, an invasive test, relies on timely support from our radiology or vascular surgery colleagues. Ascending venography can be challenging as the presence of extensive deep system thrombosis can result in nonvisualization of the deep system and a nondiagnostic study result [12, 15]. Continued improvements in ultrasonography have made this modality a faster, less expensive, and noninvasive way to assess the venous system. It has in many ways become a more reliable and accurate way to assess for proximal deep venous thrombosis (DVT) with less morbidity and can be repeated as needed to monitor for thrombus propagation or vessel recanalization (Fig. 7.1). Computer tomographic angiography (CTA) and venography may be used to evaluate clot burden, and if time allows, magnetic resonance venography can provide additional diagnostic data about vessel integrity and tissue compromise.

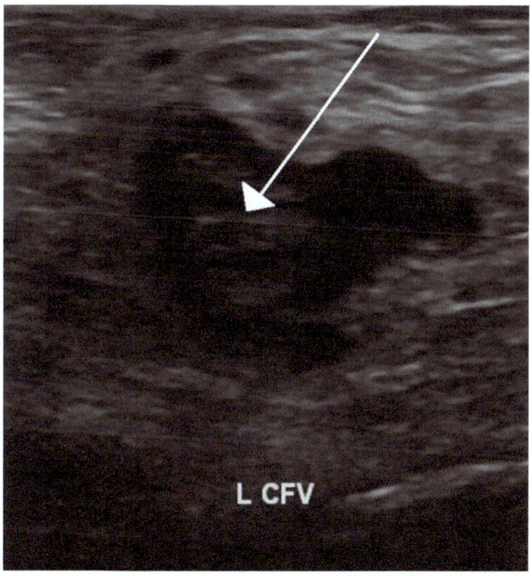

Fig. 7.1 Duplex ultrasound showing clot propagation into the common femoral vein (CMV)

Medical Therapy

The standard treatment of phlegmasia and venous gangrene is still evolving as the disease presentation is rare. The optimal therapeutic modality remains under debate and most data on therapeutic trends have been generated by case series and expert consensus [20]. So far, the results of treatment for early forms of phlegmasia have been moderately successful. Therapeutic intervention is typically multimodal, and successful intervention relies on expert consultation from interventional radiology, vascular surgery, surgery, and/or medicine depending on expert availability and institutional procedures. Therapy is aimed at preventing progression to venous gangrene by reducing venous hypertension and high interstitial pressures through restoring venous outflow to the affected extremity [12]. Conservative medical treatments, such as steep limb elevation, anticoagulation with intravenous administration of heparin, and fluid resuscitation, should be the initial course of therapy for phlegmasia alba dolens and mild nongangrenous forms of PCD [12, 20]. More invasive treatment options for severe disease include systemic or local thrombolysis, percutaneous suction or other mechanical thrombus removal techniques, percutaneous transluminal angioplasty with or without stenting, surgical thrombectomy with or without fasciotomy, or a combination of these techniques [20].

Steep leg elevation remains the best method to reduce significant leg edema and should be deployed in conjunction with anticoagulants. The purpose of rapid heparin anticoagulation is to decrease the risk of proximal clot propagation or thromboembolism. Heparin should be initiated with an intravenous bolus of 80–100 U/kg, followed by a continuous infusion of 15–18 U/kg/h and titrated to an activated partial thromboplastin time (aPTT) goal range of 2–2.5 times the laboratory reference range [21]. With heparin infusion, it is recommended that platelet counts be monitored to allow for early detection of heparin-induced thrombocytopenia. Low-molecular-weight heparins are safe and effective in the treatment of proximal deep venous thrombosis (DVT) and pulmonary embolism (PE); however, there is lesser evidence available to support the use of these agents in phlegmasia and venous gangrene, especially where the potential need for surgical intervention is high [15].

In PCD without gangrene, (1) if no clinical improvement is seen within 6–12 hours, (2) if thrombus burden is significant, or (3) if there is severe symptomatic swelling and tissue ischemia, catheter-directed thrombolysis is employed [15]. Some experts propose catheter-directed thrombolysis directly into the vein with high doses of urokinase or tissue plasminogen activator (t-PA) [12, 22], while others support intra-arterial low-dose thrombolysis via the common femoral artery, reasoning that the arterial route delivers the thrombolytic agent to the arterial capillaries and, subsequently, to the venules, which is seemingly more effective in cases with venous gangrene [20, 23]. There is some debate regarding thrombolysis given that the risk of relevant hemorrhage can be as high as 10–12% [20]; thus, recent reports of therapeutic techniques often involve a combination of direct catheter-based thrombolysis and mechanical thrombectomy [15, 20, 22, 24–26]. Percutaneous transluminal angioplasty with or without stenting has also been used [15, 20] with success though decision for modality and patient selection have not been well illustrated.

Surgical thrombectomy alone is the classically described approach to PCD with massive clot burden and ischemic compromise [19, 27]. However, isolated surgical or catheter-based thrombectomy in combination with heparin anticoagulation in patients with PCD is associated with a high rate of rethrombosis and valvular incompetence or postphlebitic syndrome [12, 23, 28]. Thrombectomy cannot open the small venules that are affected in venous gangrene; thus, a combination of therapies along with thrombolysis is often used for the successful resolution of symptoms [12, 15]. Surgical fasciotomy is indicated in patients with progressive compartment syndrome and venous gangrene. Fasciotomy alone or in conjunction with thrombectomy or thrombolysis reduces compartmental pressures; however, it can significantly increase morbidity because of prolonged wound healing and infection risk [12]. Finally, if all efforts fail, amputation might be required in up to 20% of cases [12].

Key Points

- Phlegmasia may be insidious or fulminant. Most patients presenting with an early form of the disease spectrum (phlegmasia alba dolens) present with symptoms of edema, pain, and blanching (alba) without cyanosis.
- As the disease progresses to phlegmasia cerulea dolens, the blanching caused by subcutaneous edema, venous congestion, and ischemia gives way to progressive arterial compromise leaving the extremity swollen and cyanotic (blue).
- Patients with PCD present with the clinical triad of severe edema, agonizing pain, and cyanosis. Patients with fulminant disease usually present with sudden severe pain, swelling, cyanosis, venous gangrene, and compartment syndrome.
- Ultrasonography, a faster, less expensive, and noninvasive way to assess the venous system, has become a more reliable and accurate way to assess for proximal deep venous thrombosis (DVT) with less morbidity and can be repeated as needed to monitor for thrombus propagation or vessel recanalization.
- The therapeutic intervention for phlegmasia is often multimodal and optimally involves several disciplines. Therapy is aimed at preventing progression to

venous gangrene by reducing venous hypertension and high interstitial pressures through restoring venous outflow to the affected extremity.

- Steep leg elevation remains the best method to reduce significant leg edema and should be deployed in conjunction with anticoagulants. Heparin should be initiated to decrease the risk of proximal clot propagation or thromboembolism with an intravenous bolus of 80–100 U/kg, followed by a continuous infusion of 15–18 U/kg/h and titrated to an activated partial thromboplastin time (aPTT) goal range of 2–2.5 times the laboratory reference range.
- More invasive treatment options for severe disease include systemic or local thrombolysis, percutaneous suction or other mechanical thrombus removal techniques, percutaneous transluminal angioplasty with or without stenting, surgical thrombectomy with or without fasciotomy, or a combination of these techniques.

Pulmonary Embolism

Acute pulmonary embolism is a common diagnosis in the emergency department, and it may present with a wide range of signs and symptoms, from mild dyspnea to sudden and refractory cardiovascular collapse. The diagnosis and treatment of PE cause considerable consternation among EM physicians. Physicians order a substantial number of computed tomography pulmonary angiogram (CT-PA) studies, despite the fact that gestalt, bedside screening metrics, and readily available laboratory tests like d-dimer could obviate some cross-sectional imaging and the concomitant risks [29]. Fortunately, for the majority of patients with a PE, this excess worry is unwarranted. For the patient with a large obstructive burden and marked cardiovascular compromise, minimizing the time to diagnosis and treatment is imperative, as the majority of those patients who die as a result of their PE will do so in the first few hours after the inciting event [30, 31].

Incidence of PE is 69 per 100,000, favoring women in the cohort under 55 years of age, and men in the cohort over 55 years of age [32], and is thought to result in 200,000–300,000 deaths per year. Mortality for untreated PE is up to 30%. With more timely diagnosis and treatment, the mortality can be reduced significantly. The pulmonary embolism severity index (PESI) can be used to predict 30-day mortality, but in patients requiring urgent or emergent evaluation for lysis, it may not be readily available or useful in the decision process (Table 7.1) [33]. Morbidity, in particular, related to the effects of clot burden on RV function and progression to pulmonary hypertension, is a subject of current research interest driving the pursuit of fibrinolysis in patients with signs of right ventricular (RV) compromise but without hemodynamic instability [34–36]. For patients at the far opposite ends of the PE spectrum, for example, those with hemodynamically insignificant PE or cardiovascular collapse, the decision to treat and mode of therapy is based on in the former preventing progression of clot and symptom management, and unloading the RV by relieving clot burden and restoring adequate cardiopulmonary function in the latter.

There are several patient subsets in the emergency department which warrant special regard with respect to PE. In the pediatric population, PE is less common overall than in adults and more common in association with a provoking event or condition, such as a central line, recent cardiac surgery, malignancy, or history of thromboembolic disease [37, 38]. Obstetric populations have an increased incidence of VTE beginning in the first trimester, with a plateau in the second and third trimesters, and a sharp peak immediately postpartum [39–41]. The overall rate of PE is in the postpartum phase is 15 times that of pregnancy, with PE risk concentrated in the first week postpartum, and in mothers over 35 years of age [39, 42]; 96.9% of postpartum PE occurred in the first 6.5 weeks after delivery,

Table 7.1 Pulmonary Embolism Severity Index (PESI) [33]

Criteria	*Score*	*Range*
Age	1 point per year of life	1–100
Gender	Male = 10 points	0 or 10
Heart failure	Active = 10 points	0 or 10
Chronic lung disease	Active or past = 10 points	0 or 10
Heart rate	Heart rate > 110 bpm = 20 points	0 or 20
Respiratory rate	Respiratory rate > 30 bpm = 20 points	0 or 20
Temperature	Temperature < 36 C = 20 points	0 or 20
Oxygenation	Oxygen saturation < 90% = 20 points	0 or 20
Cancer	Active or past = 30 points	0 or 30
Systolic blood pressure	Systolic pressure < 100 mmHg = 30 points	0 or 30
Mental status	Altered mentation = 60 points	0 or 60
Interpretation	*Score*	*Mortality risk*
Class 1	Score < 66	Very low mortality risk (0–1.6%)
Class 2	Score 66–85	Low mortality risk (1.7–3.5%)
Class 3	Score 86–105	Moderate mortality risk (3.2–7.1%)
Class 4	Score 106–126	High mortality risk (4.0–11.4%)
Class 5	Score > 126	Very high mortality risk (10.0–24.5%)

*Predicts 30-day mortality from pulmonary embolism
*Risk stratified management
Thrombolytic treatment of massive pulmonary embolism (Class 4–5)
Consider outpatient management for low-risk pulmonary embolism (Class 1)

indicating a rapid return to baseline risk after delivery [39]. Among patients with genetic thrombophilias, factor V Leiden is the most common, and homozygous patients are at significantly increased risk for thromboembolic events [43]. While a PE may be the event that leads to diagnosis, the workup and therapy is the same as for patients with normal factor V activity. This holds true for patients with other genetic thrombophilias except ATIII deficiency, which will be resistant to Heparin. The literature recommends using Heparin for cancer-induced hypercoagulable state (Trousseau's syndrome). Other disease processes associated with PE, such as antiphospholipid syndrome (often associated with Lupus), heparin-induced thrombocytopenia (HIT), paroxysmal nocturnal hemoglobinuria, and sickle cell anemia, can be evaluated and initially treated as any other patient presenting with similar symptoms, with the exception of anticoagulant choice in those patients suspected to have HIT. A history of multiple miscarriages may offer a diagnostic clue in patients with primary or secondary antiphospholipid syndrome. Patients with hepatic dysfunction, specifically cirrhosis, are known to have increased risk of thromboembolic disease, despite relative coagulopathy as indicated by testing such as the international normalized ratio (INR) [44].

Pathophysiology

Thromboembolic disease is characterized by Virchow's triad: hypercoagulable state, alterations in blood flow including stasis and turbulence, and endothelial dysfunction. These three broad categories help explain why the normal equilibrium between clot formation and breakdown may be skewed to favor the formation, propagation, and/or embolization of clots. Small emboli may present with minimal to no symptoms, or they may present with pleuritic chest pain, due to the irritation of the visceral pleura cause by hypoperfusion. Large emboli may cause acutely increased right ventricular and right pulmonary artery pressures. Since the right heart poorly accommodates acute increases in afterload, this may result in relative ischemia, acute right heart failure, cardiovascular collapse, and PEA arrest. It is important to note that while PE is typically thought of as a thromboembolic phenomenon, any substance that is introduced intravenously and is relatively immiscible in blood can produce similar symptoms. Other embolic phenomenon include fat, amniotic fluid, air, talc (intravenous drug abuse), and iatrogenic emboli, including devices, adhesives, and cements [45–47].

Patient Presentation

There is a reason why physician gestalt ("presence of an alternative diagnosis that was as likely as or more likely than pulmonary embolism") is included in the Wells' criteria for PE [48]; there are no signs or symptoms that are both specific and sensitive to the diagnosis of PE. Despite the absence of a common presentation, experienced clinicians can make reasonable estimations about the presence of this disease state. Perhaps, the most obvious presentation would be the patient with a known acute DVT and no other medical history, who is noncompliant with therapy, and who presents with new-onset dyspnea and pleu ritic chest pain. While few patients will present in this way, over three quarters of patients with a PE have evidence of lower extremity deep vein thrombosis (DVT) on clinical examination or imaging [49]. Thus, similar historical risk factors heralding DVT (Table 7.2) are expected in PE. Additional risk factors and historical elements, captured in screening tools like the Wells criteria [48, 50–52], PE Rule Out Criteria (PERC) [53], and Geneva scores [54–56], include oral contraceptive or exogenous estrogen use, hemoptysis, recent intubation, history of DVT/PE, recent fracture, recent surgery, and known hypercoagulable, hemoconcentrated, or hyperviscous states (including polycythemias/leukemias) (Table 7.3) [57, 58]. Common presenting symptoms of PE are nonspecific and can include dyspnea, chest pain, and cough (Table 7.4). Vital signs may be of some assistance and are part of multiple clinical decision rules. Tachycardia, tachypnea, and hypoxia commonly present either singly or in combination with PE;

Table 7.2 Top five most common historical risk factors in patients with confirmed DVT [98]

Risk factors present in patients with DVT	%
>48 h limited mobility in the prior month	45
Recent (<3 months) prior hospitalization	39
Recent surgery	34
Recent malignancy	34
Recent infection	34

Table 7.3 Common clinical scoring systems used in the evaluation of pulmonary embolus

Clinical scoring system	Components
Wells PE risk: 0–1 low, 1–6 moderate, >6 high	Clinical signs and symptoms of DVT = 3 points PE is most or equally likely as a diagnosis = 3 points Heart rate > 100 = 1.5 points Immobilization >3 days, surgery in the prior 4 weeks = 1.5 points Previous, objectively diagnosed PE/DVT = 1.5 points Hemoptysis = 1 point Malignancy with treatment in the prior 6 mo, or palliative = 1 point
Geneva PE risk: 0–3 < 10% incidence of PE, 4–10 intermediate risk, ≥11 high risk >60% incidence of PE	Age > 65 = 1 point Previous PE/DVT = 3 points Surgery required general anesthesia or lower extremity fracture in the prior month = 2 points Active malignancy in prior year = 2 points Unilateral lower extremity pain = 3 points Hemoptysis = 2 points Pain on deep palpation of lower extremity = 4 points Heart rate < 75 = 0 point, 75–94 = 3 points, ≥95 = 5 points
PERC PE risk: if pretest probability is low (<15%), then no further testing is required if none of the criteria are met	Age ≥ 50 HR ≥ 99 O_2 saturation on room air <95% History of venous thromboembolism Trauma or surgery in prior 4 weeks Hemoptysis Exogenous estrogen Unilateral leg swelling

Table 7.4 Common symptoms at presentation in one cohort of patients with confirmed PE [61]

Common presenting complaints in patients with pulmonary embolism	%
Dyspnea	73
Pleuritic pain	66
Cough	37
Leg swelling	28
Leg pain	26
Hemoptysis	13

however, they are hardly specific to PE. On cardiac examination, PE patients may have a split S2 with a prominent P2 due to the effect of elevated pulmonary artery pressure on the pulmonic valve [49]. An extremity, if affected by a DVT, may be tender, swollen, erythematous, or warm to the touch. Fever, if greater than 38° Celsius, or wheezes on pulmonary auscultation are typically indicative of etiology other than PE [59].

Key Points

- The mortality rate for pulmonary embolus exceeds 15% in the first 3 months of treatment, and the majority of deaths due to pulmonary embolism occur in the first 1–2 hours of care.
- Common presenting symptoms of PE are nonspecific and can include dyspnea, chest pain, and cough. Tachycardia, tachypnea, and hypoxia commonly present either singly or in combination with PE.
- The most common arrhythmia seen in PE is sinus tachycardia.

Diagnostics

Once PE enters the differential diagnosis, there are several means to elucidate the diagnosis. There are, as demonstrated by the Wells', PERC, and Geneva scores, a number of historical and exam elements that can be used to generate a pretest probability of PE as a diagnosis. The Wells' score uses physician gestalt in addition to physical findings and historical context, whereas PERC and the Geneva score remove reliance on physician gestalt in an attempt to make application of the criteria more uniform, despite variations in clinician experience [48, 53, 54].

For almost all patients presenting with chest pain or dyspnea, initial evaluation should include a chest radiograph. Plain chest radiography, while frequently abnormal in PE [60], is rarely diagnostic of PE [61]. A normal or mildly abnormal radiograph does help to eliminate other potential diagnoses and will identify patients in whom V/Q scans are likely to be of assistance. Commonly, plain radiographs show nonspecific findings such as atelectasis and small pleural effusions. Uncommon plain radiographic findings more strongly associated with PE (but not diagnostic) are as follows: The Westermark sign, which is the absence of pulmonary vasculature consistent with pulmonary artery hypoperfusion or vasoconstriction; Hampton's hump, which is a dome-shaped peripheral density consistent with infarction and subsequent localized hemorrhage; and the Fleischner sign, which is the dilation of the central pulmonary artery seen in some patients with elevated pulmonary artery pressures [61]. In patients at risk for underlying cardiac etiology of their symptoms, an EKG will be of some assistance. EKG findings concerning for and consistent with PE include sinus tachycardia, the famed but uncommon S1Q3T3, a new right bundle branch block, a new rightward axis, or pulseless electrical activity (PEA) arrest [62].

Laboratory studies (Table 7.5), though nonspecific for PE, can help identify other etiologies and establish whether or not renal function is sufficient to tolerate contrasted CT for PE. While

Table 7.5 Common laboratory abnormalities associated with pulmonary embolus

Laboratory study	Abnormality
CBC	Normal, leukocytosis
BMP	Normal
ABG	Normal, respiratory alkalosis, hypoxemia, increased A-a gradient
d-dimer	Elevated
BNP	Normal, elevated (right heart strain)
Troponin	Normal, elevated (right heart strain)

contrasted angiography might be avoided in at risk patients, it might be worth considering in those patients with high-risk features that might benefit from early aggressive care. Additionally, laboratory studies in suspected PE may be used to support the diagnosis and further classify PE. Laboratory studies ordered in evaluation of a potential PE patient may reasonably include a complete blood count, basic metabolic panel, troponin, brain natriuretic peptide, arterial blood gas, and a d-dimer. D-dimer has a significant role in PE with the exception of rare false negatives; it is highly unlikely that a patient with a negative, or normal, d-dimer has a PE [63]. The converse, however, is not true, and many patients with an abnormal d-dimer do not have a PE as many common conditions presenting similarly to PE can elevate d-dimer levels (e.g., aortic dissection). Age and pregnancy can also alter d-dimer values in a predictable sequence [64]. Hence, a d-dimer should not be ordered casually, as a positive test, might necessitate further explanation and three-dimensional imaging.

Direct visualization of a PE is ideal and is the only way to definitely diagnose a PE. Computed tomography with a timed contrast bolus corresponding to opacification of the pulmonary arteries (CT-PE) provides optimal visualization [65]. CT-PE, however, bears significant radiation and contrast burdens, both of which have potential long-term consequences. Patients who receive a CT-PE have a nearly 40% chance of having a subsequent CT within 2 years [66], and the oncogenic and nephrotoxic risks of repeated exposures are significant [67, 68]. Pulmonary angiography, ventilation/perfusion (V/Q) scanning, and lower extremity venous Doppler are alternative testing modalities, but do not offer definitive confirmation. Pulmonary angiography carries similar risks as CT-PE, and the number of practitioners and facilities equipped to perform and evaluate these studies is decreasing. V/Q scanning is a reasonable alternative in the patient with a previously normal chest radiograph [69], and it may be the preferred chest imaging modality in pregnant patients, if imaging is indicated. Additionally, for pregnant patients or in patients with contrast contraindications, d-dimer and lower extremity duplex might serve as first-step strategies. Some argue that if both the d-dimer and the Dopplers are positive, then there is no need for confirmatory chest imaging, and the patient can be started on therapeutic anticoagulation [64]. If, however, the Dopplers do not reveal an extremity deep vein thrombosis, then chest imaging is indicated, and V/Q, as mentioned, might be the preferred imaging modality [64]. Magnetic resonance angiography is an alternate diagnostic modality if the facility is equipped to perform and evaluate such a test [70], but image quality limits use in a significant number of patients.

Echocardiography, while not always providing direct visualization of the clot within the right ventricle or pulmonary artery, can help identify patients with significant clot burden, right ventricular dilation, and contractile dysfunction. Transthoracic echocardiography can be obtained formally, though a finalized read of that study may not be available in a timeframe necessary to support diagnosis or therapy decisions. For those practitioners comfortable with limited bedside echocardiography, a parasternal short-axis view demonstrating paradoxical septal bowing (toward the left ventricle), septal flattening, and/or evidence of right ventricular volume overload (RV diameter ≥ LV) are indicative of significant clot burden and impending hemodynamic compromise. Echocardiography can also identify a potential alternative diagnosis like pericardial effusion. Coupling the cardiac evaluation with pulmonary and DVT ultrasonography dramatically improves the sensitivity and specificity of bedside diagnosis for PE [71].

Key Points

- Because the symptoms of PE can be vague and can mimic other diseases, several clinical scoring systems (e.g., Wells', PERC, and Geneva scores) have been developed to generate a pretest probability of PE as a diagnosis and to help guide further intervention.

- ECGs can be normal in 10–15% of PE patients but are useful to determine other underlying cardiac etiologies of patient symptoms.
- Chest radiographs are rarely diagnostic though are abnormal in 76–90% of PE patients. A normal or mildly abnormal radiograph does help to eliminate other potential diagnoses and will identify patients in whom V/Q scans are likely to be of assistance.
- Bedside ultrasound can provide information regarding cardiac performance and delineate possible differential diagnoses. A parasternal short-axis view demonstrating paradoxical septal bowing (toward the left ventricle), septal flattening, and/or evidence of right ventricular volume overload (RV diameter ≥ LV) are indicative of significant clot burden and impending hemodynamic compromise.
- Right ventricular (RV) dilation can easily be determined by left ventricular (LV) comparison in the subcostal or apical view.
  - RV size = LV size: moderate RV dilation
  - RV size > LV size: marked RV dilation

Medical Therapy

The medical and interventional strategies in PE can best be stratified by subgroups that are based on the severity of the PE and by acute and subacute strategies of therapy [72]. Traditionally, PE has been classified based on the character of the hemodynamic stability and clot burden. Treatment approaches for PE subtypes vary based on the severity of patient illness making practitioners more likely to deploy high-risk therapies in those patients with significant cardiopulmonary compromise and more likely to die from their PE. In the medical literature, PE has traditionally been classified as either "massive" (with hemodynamic instability), "submassive" (now termed intermediate-risk PE), or "nonmassive" though the definitions vary and can be ambiguous [72]. For the EP, it is important to know how to manage the acutely ill PE patient, understand the goals of treatment, and command the varied options for management. The overall goal of therapy is not only to stabilize the acutely ill patient and reduce mortality but also to also prevent downstream sequella of PE, such as right ventricular (RV) dysfunction, right heart strain, and chronic thromboembolic pulmonary hypertension (CTEPH) [72–74].

Goldhaber and Lualdi first described acute pulmonary embolism as a spectrum of six syndromes: the first two syndromes, "massive PE" and "moderate-to-large PE," apply to patients with substantial pulmonary perfusion defects and right ventricular dyskinesis [75]. These two can be distinguished from one another by a transition from relatively normal blood pressures (moderate-to-large PE; 30% perfusion obstruction) to persistent arterial hypotension (massive PE; >50% obstruction) [75]. Thus, "massive" from "submassive" pulmonary emboli can be distinguished on the basis of hemodynamic stability, and the use of this distinction is often used as part of an overall strategy for risk stratification and treatment [76].

Massive PE (MPE) is best defined by consensus as an "acute PE with sustained hypotension (systolic blood pressure <90 mm Hg for at least 15 minutes or requiring inotropic support, not due to a cause other than PE, such as arrhythmia, hypovolemia, sepsis, or left ventricular [LV] dysfunction), pulselessness, or persistent profound bradycardia (heart rate <40 bpm with signs or symptoms of shock)" [72]. MPE with shock is one of the more anxiety-provoking conditions seen in the ED and is a condition that carries a high mortality despite optimal care [43, 72]. Diagnosis alone can be challenging, thus familiarity with the optimal management of these unstable patients should optimize delivery of time-dependent therapy.

Resuscitation and Initial Cardiopulmonary Stabilization

Patients with MPE often present with moderately marginal to persistently unstable hemodynamics. Initial efforts should be aimed at stabilizing the patient by utilizing a combination of fluids, vasopressors, and inotropic agents. The initial reaction of the EP to hypotension in most cases is to begin with a fluid bolus, regardless of an assessment of the patient's fluid status. However, the use of fluid loading in acute massive pulmonary embolism remains controversial. Though fluids might initially improve blood pressure response, the added strain on the right heart in the form of increased end-diastolic volume may actually serve to worsen RV failure. Therefore, current literature supports a 250- to 500-ml bolus and the avoidance of excessive fluid resuscitation in the absence of a clear understanding of the patient's right heart physiology [77].

Hypotension in MPE is the result of RV outflow obstruction leading to poor pulmonary perfusion and circulatory collapse secondary to RV strain and right-sided heart failure. Though vaso constriction may seem counterintuitive; it is important to realize that the RV is perfused in both diastole and systole [78, 79]. Therefore, in the setting of shock with increased myocardial oxygen demand, maintaining the mean arterial pressure head can improve myocardial perfusion and hibernating RV function. In MPE, the ideal agent would increase systemic vasoconstriction without increasing pulmonary vascular resistance, though no currently available agent achieves this goal. Data extrapolated from animal models and case studies suggest that norepinephrine (NE) is the vasopressor of choice for shock secondary to MPE [77, 80–85]. Epinephrine as a second-line agent has been advocated in case-based literature for treatment of refractory shock complicating PE [86], and vasopressin has also been used in low doses to treat hypotension without detriment to cardiac output or pulmonary artery pressures [87]. Often, a single vasopressor is insufficient to overcome the hemodynamic instability seen in massive PE; thus, a combination of vasoactive agents (Table 7.6) is often needed. Of the available inotropes, dobutamine is considered the inotropic agent of choice for the treatment of PE-related cardiac failure. Dobutamine beta-adrenergic positive inotropic and pulmonary vasodilating properties lead to increased right ventricular contractility and decreased pulmonary vascular resistance [77].

Table 7.6 Common vasoactive agents used in pulmonary embolism management

Vasoactive agent	Dosing
Norepinephrine	2–30 mcg/min
Epinephrine	2–10 mcg/min
Vasopressin	0.01–0.04 u/min
Dobutamine	2–20 mcg/kg/min

Key Points

- Hypotension can be managed with a small fluid bolus (250–500 ml) to avoid complicating RV failure and followed with the addition of vasopressors (norepinephrine) in those patients with ongoing hemodynamic instability.
- Epinephrine and vasopressin as well as dobutamine can be considered in refractory hypotension.

While supplementary oxygen is practical in all patients with pulmonary compromise, the oxygen debt and respiratory distress in MPE often necessitate more advanced pulmonary support. The EP must approach the respiratory support of the patient with MPE with some degree of caution as negative interactions between the heart and lungs can further destabilize an already unstable situation. Positive-pressure ventilation alters thoracic physiology and may decrease venous return to the heart and further increase right heart pressure and systolic dysfunction.

Intubation in MPE can be complicated by cardiovascular collapse for several reasons. Sedatives can blunt catecholamine-directed peripheral vasoconstriction and central pulmonary vasodilation. Lung overinflation can increase pulmonary vascular resistance and decrease venous return. Thus, EPs considering rapid sequence intubation in MPE should consider sedative agents that preserve hemodynamic function (i.e., etomidate and ketamine), select ventilator settings that limit overinflation, and have vasopressors immediately available or already infusing in preparation for worsened hypotension.

Mechanical ventilation, often a necessary adjunct in the management of patients with MPE, can lead to elevated airway pressures, increased transpulmonary pressures, decreased venous return, limited RV diastolic filling, and increased RV afterload that impedes RV systolic function [88, 89]. Limiting positive end-expiratory pressure (PEEP; 5 cm H_2O) and tidal volumes (6–8 ml/kg) might decrease airway pressures and minimize RV dysfunction. Ventilation management strategies must be tailored to limit hypercarbia and hypoxemia, which can exacerbate pulmonary vasoconstriction and hypertension if adequate ventilation or oxygenation is not maintained. Close monitoring and fine-tuning of tidal volume and respiratory rate can help maintain normocarbia, while the maintenance of recruitment (PEEP) and modulation of gas trapping (expiratory time) can improve oxygenation [81, 88, 90].

Key Points

- Supplemental O_2 should be used to treat hypoxia/hypoxemia secondary to shunting.
- NIPPV/ventilation may be necessary in patients suffering from acute PE with a goal of using low tidal volume and low peep ventilation to avoid further altering hemodynamics.
- Prepare for worsened hypotension with intubation and ventilation; it is often necessary to have vasopressors immediately available or already infusing when preparing for induction.
- Avoid lung hyperventilation as this can worsen hemodynamic instability.

Clot Management

Beyond the acute management of the hemodynamic stability and potential respiratory failure seen in PE, the treatment of the pulmonary embolism itself is controversial. Fibrinolytics, the mainstay of acute PE treatment, act directly on the clot itself promoting hydrolysis of fibrin and leading to clot break down [72, 74]. There is a general consensus that the use of fibrinolytics in the critically ill, hemodynamically unstable patient with pulmonary embolism, in the absence of major contraindications, is recommended (Class IIa, Level of Evidence B) [72]. A meta-analysis and formal Cochrane Review strongly endorse the use of rapid fibrinolytic therapy versus the use of heparin alone as a means to potentially reduce recurrence (OR 0.63; 95% CI 0.33–1.20) and death (OR 0.89; 95% CI 0.45–1.78) in MPE [91]. For the EP, administration of rapid fibrinolytic therapy is less invasive and is the primary method of treatment for the hemodynamically unstable PE patient who lacks contraindications to systemic therapy. Three thrombolytic agents are currently approved for use in patients with acute PE: streptokinase, urokinase, and rt-PA (Table 7.7). A 2005 meta-analysis aimed at identifying differences among thrombolytic regimens failed to demonstrate any statistically significant differences in efficacy [92]. Despite the lack of data proving superiority, the American College of Chest Physicians (ACCP) guidelines suggest using the thrombolytic regimen with the shortest infusion time (currently Alteplase) [21, 93].

The EP is more likely through the course of his or her career to encounter the patient with submassive (intermediate risk) PE in whom the treatment

Table 7.7 Thrombolytic regimens for acute pulmonary embolism

Drug	Dosing regimens
Alteplase (rt-PA)	Initial dose: 10 mg bolus, then infusion: 90 mg over 2 h
Streptokinase	Initial dose: 250,000 units over 30 min, then infusion: 100,000 units/h over 24 h
Urokinase	Initial dose: 4400 units/kg over 10 min, then infusion: 4400 units/kg/h over 12 h

options can be varied and sometimes controversial. This patient, unlike the hemodynamically compromised patient, often presents normotensive with minimal to no respiratory distress and often appears less sick. The optimal treatment strategy is less clear in submassive PE. The EP treatment choices include the use of supportive measures and therapeutic anticoagulation, alternative anticoagulants such as Xa inhibitors, in some cases systemic fibrinolytics (in full or altered doses), and in some institutions referral for catheter-directed fibrinolysis or direct clot extraction.

The most widely accepted initial management for submassive PE is anticoagulation with either unfractionated heparin or low-molecular-weight heparin (LMWH) [72] aimed at reducing further clot propagation and preventing additional VTE. Early anticoagulation is suggested in PE regardless of downstream management style, as it remains a relatively low risk and is an easily titratable and reversible treatment (Table 7.8). The decision to pursue fibrinolysis should not delay the onset of anticoagulation as it can be held for fibrinolysis delivery and restarted after the completion of lytic therapy. For many community EPs, basic anticoagulation will be the mainstay of treatment as it easily initiated and followed by the initiation of oral anticoagulants (OACs), though anticoagulation often requires hospital admission. Heparin therapy can be initiated with a bolus or without. In patients without contraindications, a bolus of heparin (80 u/kg) should be given followed by a titratable infusion (18 u/kg/h initially and then adjusted to a goal aPTT of two times the normal reference range).

One of the more controversial treatment options includes the use of systemic fibrinolysis for submassive PE. Fibrinolysis in submassive PE in recent research has been focused on evaluating the efficacy of early fibrinolysis at mitigating unwanted debilitation and chronic complications resultant from chronic RV remodeling and pulmonary artery hypertension in VTE [35]. Specifically, the MOPETT trial found that a lower dose (50 mg) of TPA was as efficacious in reducing PA pressures as the traditional 100-mg dose (better than the use of LMWH alone) and did not show an increased risk of major bleeding (including intracranial hemorrhage) in their treatment group [36]. What remains controversial is whether or not the risk of major bleeding outweighs the potential benefits seen in reducing downstream debilitation that can accompany PE. EPs should be aware that fibrinolysis is a reasonable option (including lower doses) and that this option might best apply in the "borderline" patient without hemodynamic compromise but who demonstrates signs of acute right heart dysfunction. Additionally, patients above the age of 75 are at higher risk of bleeding and might benefit from reduced dose fibrinolysis [72, 94]. Ultimately, the submassive patient who is stratified as high risk for chronic VTE-related cardiopulmonary compromise should be involved in the decision-making process and the bleeding risks reviewed prior to using fibrinolysis.

In the extremely low-risk group, recent PE research suggests that patients with segmental and nonobstructing submassive PE might easily be managed with outpatient regimens [95–97]. For those patients who present with minimal symptoms, and without evidence of right heart strain, the relatively new Xa inhibitors are a reasonable option. They may be used in conjunction with a

Table 7.8 Anticoagulants used in the treatment of venous thromboembolic disease

Anticoagulant	Initial dose	Restriction	Time to peak
Unfractionated heparin	17 U/kg then 70 U/kg/hr, IV	Heparin-induced thrombocytopenia	1 hour
Enoxaparin	1 mg/kg subcutaneously[a]	Creatinine clearance <30 ml/min	3 hours
Dalteparin	200 U/kg subcutaneously[a]	Creatinine clearance <30 ml/min	4 hours
Fondaparinux	5–10 mg subcutaneously[a]	Creatinine clearance <30 ml/min	3 hours
Rivaroxaban	15 mg orally with food	Creatinine clearance <30 ml/min	2–4 hours
Apixaban	10 mg orally with or without food	Creatinine clearance <30 ml/min	3–4 hours

[a]Although low-molecular-weight heparin compounds are usually injected subcutaneously, no trials have been conducted to justify this route over intravenous injection. Intravenous injection achieves more rapid anticoagulation and does not produce more bleeding.

single therapeutic dose of LMWH, such as enoxaparin and confer immediate anticoagulation.

Several of the Xa inhibitors, also known as the novel oral anticoagulants (NOACs), are now FDA approved for the management of acute PE and are easy to use without the need for titration or outpatient monitoring. Thus, these agents are ideally suited for the low-risk PE patient who could potentially be discharged from the ED.

The remaining available therapies, such as catheter-directed fibrinolysis or thrombectomy and clot extraction, are becoming increasingly available in larger institutions. These therapies may be the best option in moderately ill PE patients for whom bleeding risks are too great. Thus, these novel interventional approaches in a complex patient subtype might require patient transfer to another institution. The focus of optimization and advanced technique availability has fueled recent discussion as to whether "PE Centers" are needed to impart best available practices.

Key Points

- UFH/LMWH should be initiated as soon as the dx of PE is suspected. It can be stopped to administer fibrinolytics and resumed following.
- Submassive PE treatment options are varied, including the potential outpatient management with NOACs, patient transfer to specialty centers for advanced therapies, and the use of altered doses of fibrinolytics in the borderline patient.

Summary

Complex venous thromboembolic disease requires rapid evaluation, diagnosis, and management. It is clear that the clinician with an understanding of the pathophysiology of complex VTE can better guide therapy according to clinical acumen. Beginning resuscitation and escalating support while initiating definitive therapy are the mainstays of ED care. Finally, heparinization and thrombolytic therapy play an essential role in the successful treatment of the patient with complex VTE. The EP armed with a standardized approach to therapy in VTE will likely play a key role in limiting patient morbidity and mortality.

References

1. White RH. The epidemiology of venous thromboembolism. Circulation. 2003;107:I4–8.
2. Cushman M, Tsai AW, White RH, et al. Deep vein thrombosis and pulmonary embolism in two cohorts: the longitudinal investigation of thromboembolism etiology. Am J Med. 2004;117:19–25.
3. Sarwar S, Narra S, Munir A. Phlegmasia cerulea dolens. Tex Heart Inst J. 2009;36:76–7.
4. Haimovici H. The ischemic forms of venous thrombosis. 1. Phlegmasia cerulea dolens. 2. Venous gangrene. J Cardiovasc Surg. 1965;5(Suppl):164–73.
5. Lee R. A contribution to the pathology of Phlegmasia Dolens. Med chir Trans. 1829;15:132–45.
6. Lee R. Further researches on the pathology of Phlegmasia Dolens. Med Chir Trans. 1853;36:281–314.
7. Mackenzie FW. Researches on the pathology of obstructive phlebitis, and the nature and proximate cause of Phlegmasia Dolens. Med Chir Trans. 1853;36:169–244.
8. De BM, Ochsner A. Phlegmasia cerulea dolens and gangrene associated with thrombophlebitis; case reports and review of the literature. Surgery. 1949;26:16–29.
9. Perkins JM, Magee TR, Galland RB. Phlegmasia caerulea dolens and venous gangrene. Br J Surg. 1996;83:19–23.
10. Mumoli N, Invernizzi C, Luschi R, Carmignani G, Camaiti A, Cei M. Phlegmasia cerulea dolens. Circulation. 2012;125:1056–7.
11. Brockman SK, Vasko JS. Phlegmasia cerulea dolens. Surg Gynecol Obstet. 1965;121:1347–56.
12. Suwanabol PA, Tefera G, Schwarze ML. Syndromes associated with the deep veins: phlegmasia cerulea dolens, May-Thurner syndrome, and nutcracker syndrome. Perspect Vasc Surg Endovasc Ther. 2010;22:223–30.
13. Mahomed A, Williams D. Phlegmasia caerulea dolens and venous gangrene. Br J Surg. 1996;83:1160–1.
14. Warkentin TE, Elavathil LJ, Hayward CP, Johnston MA, Russett JI, Kelton JG. The pathogenesis of venous limb gangrene associated with heparin-induced thrombocytopenia. Ann Intern Med. 1997;127:804–12.
15. Chinsakchai K, Ten Duis K, Moll FL, de Borst GJ. Trends in management of phlegmasia cerulea dolens. Vasc Endovasc Surg. 2011;45:5–14.
16. Brockman SK, Vasko JS. The pathologic physiology of phlegmasia cerulea dolens. Surgery. 1966;59:997–1007.

17. Qvarfordt P, Eklof B, Ohlin P. Intramuscular pressure in the lower leg in deep vein thrombosis and phlegmasia cerulae dolens. Ann Surg. 1983;197:450–3.
18. Haller JA Jr, Mays T. Experimental studies on Iliofemoral venous thrombosis. Am Surg. 1963;29:567–71.
19. Laohapensang K, Hanpipat S, Aworn S, Orrapin S. Surgical venous thrombectomy for phlegmasia cerulea dolens and venous gangrene of the lower extremities. J Med Assoc Thai Chotmaihet thangphaet. 2013;96:1463–9.
20. Klok FA, Huisman MV. Seeking optimal treatment for phlegmasia cerulea dolens. Thromb Res. 2013;131:372–3.
21. Kearon C, Akl EA, Comerota AJ, et al. Antithrombotic therapy for VTE disease: antithrombotic therapy and prevention of thrombosis, 9th ed: American College of Chest Physicians Evidence-Based Clinical Practice Guidelines. Chest. 2012;141:e419S–94S.
22. Vedantham S. Interventional approaches to acute venous thromboembolism. Semin Respir Crit Care Med. 2008;29:56–65.
23. Kalagher SD, Kane DD. Phlegmasia cerulea dolens: before and after lysis. Intern Emerg Med. 2015;10:103–4.
24. Oo TH. Thrombolytic therapy and thrombectomy in phlegmasia cerulea dolens. J R Coll Physicians Edinb. 2010;40:92.
25. Erdoes LS, Ezell JB, Myers SI, Hogan MB, LeSar CJ, Sprouse LR 2nd. Pharmacomechanical thrombolysis for phlegmasia cerulea dolens. Am Surg. 2011;77:1606–12.
26. Kuo I, Smith J, Abou-Zamzam AM Jr. A multimodal therapeutic approach to phlegmasia cerulea dolens in a pediatric patient. J Vasc Surg. 2011;53:212–5.
27. Brockman SK, Vasko JS. Observations on the pathophysiology and treatment of Phlegmasia Cerulea Dolens with special reference to Thrombectomy. Am J Surg. 1965;109:485–92.
28. Meissner MH. Rationale and indications for aggressive early thrombus removal. Phlebology/Venous Forum of the Royal Society of Medicine. 2012;27(Suppl 1):78–84.
29. Venkatesh AK, Kline JA, Courtney DM, et al. Evaluation of pulmonary embolism in the emergency department and consistency with a National Quality Measure. Arch Intern Med. 2012;172:1028–32.
30. Alpert JS, Smith R, Carlson J, et al. Mortality in patients treated for pulmonary embolism. JAMA. 1976;236:1477–80.
31. Coon WW, Willis PW. Deep venous thrombosis and pulmonary embolism. Am J Cardiol. 1959;4:611–21.
32. Silverstein MD, Heit JA, Mohr DN, et al. Trends in the incidence of deep vein thrombosis and pulmonary embolism. Arch Intern Med. 1998;158:585–93.
33. Aujesky D, Obrowsky DS, Stone RA, et al. Derivation and validation of a prognositic model for pulmonary embolism. Am J Respir Crit Care Med. 2005;172:1041–6.
34. Kline JA, Nordenholz KE, Courtney DM, et al. Treatment of submassive pulmonary embolism with tenecteplase or placebo: cardiopulmonary outcomes at 3 months: multicenter double-blind, placebo-controlled randomized trial. J Thromb Haemost. 2014;12:459–68.
35. Meyer G, Vicaut E, Danays T, et al. Fibrinolysis for patients with intermediate-risk pulmonary embolism. N Engl J Med. 2014;370:1402–11.
36. Sharifi M, Bay C, Skrocki L, Rahimi F, Mehdipour M, Investigators M. Moderate pulmonary embolism treated with thrombolysis (from the "MOPETT" Trial). Am J Cardiol. 2013;111:273–7.
37. Monagle P, Adams M, Mahoney M, et al. Outcomes of pediatric thromboembolic disease: a report from the Canadian Childhood Thrombophilia Registry. Pediatr Res. 2000;47:763–6.
38. Patocka C, Nemeth J. Pulmonary embolism in pediatrics. J Emerg Med. 2012;42:105–16.
39. Heit JA, Kobbervig CE, James AH, et al. Trends in the incidence of venous thromboembolism during pregnancy or postpartum: a 30-year population-based study. Ann Intern Med. 2005;143:697–706.
40. Ghaji N, Boulet SL, Tepper N, Hooper WC. Trends in venous thromboembolism among pregnancy-related hospitalizations, United States, 1994-2009. Am J Obstet Gynecol. 2013;209:433 e1-8.
41. Kline JA, Kabrhel C. Emergency evaluation for pulmonary embolism, part 1: clinical factors that increase risk. J Emerg Med. 2015;48:771–80.
42. James AH, Jamison MG, Brancazio LR, Myers ER. Venous thromboembolism during pregnancy and the postpartum period: incidence, risk factors, and mortality. Am J Obstet Gynecol. 2006;194:1311–5.
43. Goldhaber SZ, Elliott CG. Acute pulmonary embolism: part I: epidemiology, pathophysiology, and diagnosis. Circulation. 2003;108:2726–9.
44. Tripodi A, Anstee QM, Sogaard KK, Primignani M, Valla DC. Hypercoagulability in cirrhosis: causes and consequences. J Thromb Haemost. 2011;9:1713–23.
45. Gorospe L, Blanchard-Rodriguez MJ, Chinea-Rodriguez A. Cement pulmonary embolism after percutaneous vertebroplasty in multiple myeloma. Asian Cardiovasc Thorac Ann. 2016;24(4):400–1.
46. Nagai H, Maeda H, Kuroda R, et al. Lethal pulmonary air embolism caused by the removal of a double-lumen hemodialysis catheter. Am J Forensic Med Pathol. 2014;35:237–8.
47. Haider I, Gupta R, Song S. Mobile vegetation leading to septic pulmonary embolism. Lung India. 2014;31:429–30.
48. Wells PS, Ginsberg JS, Anderson DR, et al. Use of a clinical model for safe management of patients with suspected pulmonary embolism. Ann Intern Med. 1998;129:997–1005.
49. Tapson VF. Acute pulmonary embolism. N Engl J Med. 2008;358:1037–52.
50. Wells PS, Anderson DR, Rodger M. Derivation of a simple clinical model to categorize patients' probability of pulmonary embolism: increasing the model's

utility with the SimliRED D-dimer. Thromb Haemost. 2000;83:416–20.
51. Wells PS, Anderson DR, Rodger M. Excluding pulmonary embolism at the bedside without diagnostic imaging: management of patients with suspected pulmonary embolism presenting to the emergency department by using a simple clinical model and d-dimer. Ann Intern Med. 2001;135:98–107.
52. Wells PS, Hirsh J, Anderson DR, et al. Accuracy of clinical assessment of deep-vein thrombosis. Lancet. 1995;345:1326–30.
53. Kline JA, Courtney DM, Kabrhel C, et al. Prospective multicenter evaluation of the pulmonary embolism rule-out criteria. J Thromb Haemost. 2008;6:772–80.
54. Klok FA, Mos ICM, Nijkeuter M, et al. Simplification of the revised Geneva score for assessing clinical probability of pulmonary embolism. Arch Intern Med. 2008;168:2131–6.
55. Le Gal G, Righini M, Roy P, et al. Prediction of pulmonary embolism in the emergency department: the revised Geneva score. Ann Intern Med. 2006;144:165–71.
56. Wicki J, Perneger TV, Junod AF, et al. Assessing clinical probability of pulmonary embolism in the emergency ward. Arch Intern Med. 2001;161:92–7.
57. Khouzam R, Gallahan MJ. Polycythemia rubra vera: an unlikely cause of severe pulmonary embolism. JAAPA. 2011;25:51–3.
58. Vu K, Luong NV, Hubbard J, et al. A retrospective study of venous thromboembolism in acute leukemia patients treated at the University of Texas MD Anderson Cancer Center. Cancer Med. 2015;4:27–35.
59. Miniati M, Bottai M, Monti S, Salvadori M, Serasini L, Passera M. Simple and accurate prediction of the clinical probability of pulmonary embolism. Am J Respir Crit Care Med. 2008;178:290–4.
60. Elliott CG, Goldhaber SZ, Visani L, DeRosa M. Chest radiographs in acute pulmonary embolism. Results from the international cooperative pulmonary embolism registry. Chest. 2000;118:33–8.
61. Stein PD, Terrin ML, Hales CA, et al. Clinical, laboratory, roentgenographic and electrocardiographic findings in patients with acute pulmonary embolism and no pre-existing cardiac or pulmonary disease. Chest. 1991;100:598–603.
62. Kukla P, McIntyre WF, Fijorek K, et al. Electrocardiographic abnormalities in patients with acute pulmonary embolism complicated by cardiogenic shock. Am J Emerg Med. 2014;32:507–10.
63. Kabrhel C, Mark Courtney D, Camargo CA Jr, et al. Potential impact of adjusting the threshold of the quantitative D-dimer based on pretest probability of acute pulmonary embolism. Acad Emerg Med. 2009;16:325–32.
64. Kline JA, Kabrhel C. Emergency evaluation for pulmonary embolism, part 2: diagnostic approach. J Emerg Med. 2015;49:104–17.
65. Stein PD, Fowler SE, Goodman LR, et al. Multidetector computed tomography for acute pulmonary embolism. NEJM. 2006;354:2317–27.
66. Kline JA, Courtney DM, Beam DM, King MC, Steuerwald M. Incidence and predictors of repeated computed tomographic pulmonary angiography in emergency department patients. Ann Emerg Med. 2009;54:41–8.
67. Einstein AJ, Henzlova MJ, Rajagopalan S. Estimating risk of cancer associated with radiation exposure from 64-slice computed coronary angiography. JAMA. 2007;298:317–23.
68. Mitchell AM, Kline JA, Jones AE, Tumlin JA. Major adverse events one year after acute kidney injury after contrast-enhanced computed tomography. Clin J Am Soc Nephrol. 2010;5:4–9.
69. Worsley DF, Alavi A. Comprehensive analysis of the results of the PIOPED study. J Nucl Med. 1995;36:2380–7.
70. Stein PD, Chenevert TL, Fowler SE, et al. Gadolinium-enhanced magnetic resonance angiography for pulmonary embolism. Ann Intern Med. 2010;152:434.
71. Nazerian P, Vanni S, Volpicelli G, et al. Accuracy of point-of-care multiorgan ultrasonography for the diagnosis of pulmonary embolism. Chest. 2014;145:950–7.
72. Jaff MR, McMurtry MS, Archer SL, et al. Management of massive and submassive pulmonary embolism, iliofemoral deep vein thrombosis, and chronic thromboembolic pulmonary hypertension: a scientific statement from the American Heart Association. Circulation. 2011;123:1788–830.
73. Jeffrey A, Kline MTS, Marchick MR, Hernandez-Nino J, Rose GA. Prospective evaluation of right heart function and functional status at 6 months after acute submassive pulmonary embolism. Chest. 2009;136:1202–10.
74. Kline JANK, Courtney DM, et al. Treatment of submassive pulmonary embolism with tenecteplase or placebo: cardiopulmonary outcomes at 3 months: multicenter double-blind, placebo-controlled randomized trial. J Thromb Haemost. 2014;12:459–68.
75. Lualdi JC, Goldhaber SZ. Right ventricular dysfunction after acute pulmonary embolism: pathophysiologic factors, detection, and therapeutic implications. Am Heart J. 1995;130:1276–82.
76. Fengler BT, Brady WJ. Fibrinolytic therapy in pulmonary embolism: an evidence-based treatment algorithm. Am J Emerg Med. 2009;27:84–95.
77. Layish DT, Tapson VF. Pharmacologic hemodynamic support in massive pulmonary embolism. Chest. 1997;111:218–24.
78. Mebazaa A, Karpati P, Renaud E, Algotsson L. Acute right ventricular failure--from pathophysiology to new treatments. Intensive Care Med. 2004;30:185–96.
79. Lee FA. Hemodynamics of the right ventricle in normal and disease states. Cardiol Clin. 1992;10:59–67.
80. Angle MR, Molloy DW, Penner B, Jones D, Prewitt RM. The cardiopulmonary and renal hemodynamic effects of norepinephrine in canine pulmonary embolism. Chest. 1989;95:1333–7.
81. Torbicki A, Perrier A, Konstantinides S, et al. Guidelines on the diagnosis and management of acute pulmonary embolism. Eur Heart J. 2008;29:2276–315.

82. Hirsch LJ, Rooney MW, Wat SS, Kleinmann B, Mathru M. Norepinephrine and phenylephrine effects on right ventricular function in experimental canine pulmonary embolism. Chest. 1991;100:796–801.
83. Layish DTMD, Tapson VFMD. Pharmacologic hemodynamic support in massive pulmonary embolism*. [review]. Chest. 1997;111:218–24.
84. deBoisblanc BP. Treatment of massive pulmonary embolism. Clin Pulm Med. 1995;2:353–8.
85. Molloy WD, Lee KY, Girling L, Schick U, Prewitt RM. Treatment of shock in a canine model of pulmonary embolism. Am Rev Respir Dis. 1984; 130:870–4.
86. Boulain T, Lanotte R, Legras A, Perrotin D. Efficacy of epinephrine therapy in shock complicating pulmonary embolism. Chest. 1993;104:300–2.
87. Gold J, Cullinane S, Chen J, et al. Vasopressin in the treatment of milrinone-induced hypotension in severe heart failure. Am J Cardiol. 2000;85:506–8, A11.
88. Jardin F, Vieillard-Baron A. Right ventricular function and positive pressure ventilation in clinical practice: from hemodynamic subsets to respirator settings. Intensive Care Med. 2003;29:1426–34.
89. Haddad F, Couture P, Tousignant C, Denault AY. The right ventricle in cardiac surgery, a perioperative perspective: I. anatomy, physiology, and assessment. Anesth Analg. 2009;108:407–21.
90. Smulders YM. Pathophysiology and treatment of haemodynamic instability in acute pulmonary embolism: the pivotal role of pulmonary vasoconstriction. Cardiovasc Res. 2000;48:23–33.
91. Wan S, Quinlan DJ, Agnelli G, Eikelboom JW. Thrombolysis compared with heparin for the initial treatment of pulmonary embolism: a meta-analysis of the randomized controlled trials. Circulation. 2004;110:744–9.
92. Capstick T, Henry MT. Efficacy of thrombolytic agents in the treatment of pulmonary embolism. Eur Respir J. 2005;26:864–74.
93. Kearon C, Kahn SR, Agnelli G, Goldhaber S, Raskob GE, Comerota AJ. Antithrombotic therapy for venous thromboembolic disease: American College of Chest Physicians Evidence-Based Clinical Practice Guidelines (8th edition). Chest. 2008;133:454S–545S.
94. Sharifi MBC, Skrocki L, et al. Moderate pulmonary embolism treated with thrombolysis (from the "MOPETT" trial). J Cardiol. 2013;111:273–7.
95. Aujesky D, Roy P-M, Verschuren F, et al. Outpatient versus inpatient treatment for patients with acute pulmonary embolism: an international, open-label, randomised, non-inferiority trial. Lancet. 2011;378:41–8.
96. Zondag W, Mos IC, Creemers-Schild D, et al. Outpatient treatment in patients with acute pulmonary embolism: the Hestia study. J Thromb Haemost. 2011;9:1500–7.
97. Yoo HHB, Queluz T, El Dib R. Outpatient versus inpatient treatment for acute pulmonary embolism (review). Cochrane Collab. 2014:CD010019.
98. Spencer FA, Emery C, Lessard D, et al. The Worcester venous Thromboembolism study: a population-based study of the clinical epidemiology of venous thromboembolism. J Gen Intern Med. 2006;21:722–7.

Acute Coronary Syndrome and Myocardial Infarction

8

Zachary D. Levy and Qiuping Zhou

Introduction

The human heart begins beating approximately 4–5 weeks after conception. During a typical lifespan, it will send more than 2 billion gallons of blood through a network of blood vessels that, if placed end-on-end, would stretch out over 60,000 miles, enough to circle the Earth twice and still have enough room leftover to connect New York City to Antarctica. Not bad for a muscular pump that beats for more than seven decades, on average, without fatiguing.

Although the heart is amazingly resilient, it is also prone to disease, particularly the intricate network of coronary vessels that can narrow after years of cumulative inflammation and fatty deposits. Here, we will examine the patterns, pathology, and treatment of acute coronary syndrome (ACS) and myocardial infarction (MI), with a particular focus on emergency department (ED) management and stabilization. We will discuss evidence-based treatment options and also explore future avenues of research. The authors promise to put their heart into it.

Z. D. Levy (✉)
Emergency Medicine and Neurosurgery, Zucker School of Medicine at Hofstra/Northwell, Hempstead, NY, USA

Q. Zhou
Emergency Medicine and Cardiothoracic Surgery, Zucker School of Medicine at Hofstra/Northwell, Hempstead, NY, USA

Epidemiology

In the United States, approximately 620,000 people are either hospitalized due to acute MI or die from the disease annually, with about one heart attack occurring every 34 seconds and one death secondary to MI occurring every 83 seconds [1]. These figures are intimately related to the health of the average American. About 32 million adults >20 years of age have hyperlipidemia (13.8% of the adult population), and 78 million have hypertension (33% of the adult population). More than two-thirds of the adult population is overweight, a third of whom are obese (BMI >30 kg/m^2) [1]. We have (quite literally) a big problem on our hands.

However, despite our expanding waistlines, mortality trends in ACS give room for optimism. Although more Americans still die of heart disease every year than any other cause, according to figures from the National Registry of Myocardial Infarction, mortality rates for STEMI and NSTEMI in 1994 were 11.5% and 7.1%, respectively; by 2006, these figures had declined to 8% and 5.2%, with a pooled mortality reduction of 23.6% during the 12-year study period [2]. Both inpatient and outpatient factors have contributed, including an emphasis on early percutaneous coronary intervention (PCI) [3–5] and public awareness campaigns aimed at reducing cardiovascular risk factors (i.e., smoking cessation and blood pressure control) [6, 7]. As clinicians on the front line in the war against

© Springer Nature Switzerland AG 2020

J. R. Shiber, S. D. Weingart (eds.), *Emergency Department Critical Care*,
https://doi.org/10.1007/978-3-030-28794-8_8

ACS, the vigilance, judgment, and actions of emergency physicians will continue to play a central role [8, 9].

Pathophysiology

ACS is a spectrum of disease that collectively refers to unstable angina (UA), non-ST-segment elevation MI (NSTEMI), and ST-segment elevation MI (STEMI). All three conditions have a first step in common – namely, the narrowing of one of the coronary vessels. Although chronic, progressive occlusions do occur, ACS most commonly is the result of frank plaque rupture [10]. This occurs when a thick, inflamed deposit of lipids and macrophages lining the coronary vessel wall breaks through its fibrous cap. When circulating platelets encounter the exposed collagen and plaque contents, they begin to adhere and aggregate, occluding the vessel and resulting in cardiac ischemia.

The degree of obstruction will determine the pathology. Mild, intermittent ischemia will result in UA. As ischemia progresses and myocytes die off, there is a detectable leakage of cardiac enzymes into the bloodstream, and the patient progresses to an NSTEMI. The end stage of ACS involves significant vessel occlusion with both the release of cardiac enzymes and electrographic evidence of myocyte conduction abnormalities – the patient now has a full-blown STEMI.

Diagnosis

Electrocardiography

In March 1912, Wilhelm Einthoven described "the human electrocardiogram" before the Chelsea Clinical Society, expounding on the value of the test in determining "the time relations between the action of the ventricles and auricles" [11]. Although modern medicine has seen more than a century of progress since Einthoven's address, the humble ECG is still the most important diagnostic tool in the initial evaluation of potential ACS and will quickly identify STEMI patients so that they can be evaluated for reperfusion therapy. ECGs can be performed rapidly, can be repeated, are noninvasive, and provide a wealth of clinical information, which likely explains their longevity in the clinical arsenal.

An ECG should be rapidly obtained for almost every patient presenting to the emergency department with chest pain. In ACS (and STEMI in particular), deviations from the "normal" 12-lead ECG occur in typical distributions that allow one to estimate the vessel(s) involved, and ST-segment elevations in one distribution may be accompanied by reciprocal ST-segment depressions in another. In general:

- Inferior infarcts are seen in leads II, III, and aVF.
- Anterior infarcts are seen in V2–V4.
- Lateral infarcts are seen in V5 and V6.
- High lateral infarcts are seen in leads I and aVL.
- Septal infarcts are seen in V1 and V2.

ECG interpretation in the presence of a left bundle branch block (LBBB) deserves special mention. The presence of a new LBBB is classically thought of as a STEMI equivalent, though the evidence suggests that it may not be quite as ominous. Recent studies from Kontos et al. [12] and Jain et al. [13] indicated an ACS prevalence of 29% and 33%, respectively, in patients with new LBBB (or presumed new LBBB due to lack of prior ECG) presenting to the emergency department with chest pain or symptoms concerning for ACS.

In the setting of chronic LBBB, it may be difficult to identify a STEMI given the normally elevated appearance of the ST segment in the anterior precordial leads. The Sgarbossa criteria may be useful in diagnosing STEMI in chronic LBBB. A meta-analysis by Tabas et al. indicated that a score of >/= 3 was 98% specific but only 20% sensitive for ACS, while a score of 0 was not useful for excluding the diagnosis [14]. For a description of the Sgarbossa scoring system, see Table 8.1.

Table 8.1 Sgarbossa criteria

ST-segment elevation >/= 1 mm in a lead concordant with QRS complex	5 points
ST-segment depression >/= 1 mm in V1–V3	3 points
ST-segment elevation >/= 5 mm in a lead discordant with QRS complex	2 points

Adapted from Sgarbossa EB, Pinski SL, Barbagelata A, et al. Electrocardiographic diagnosis of evolving acute myocardial infarction in the presence of left bundle-branch block. GUSTO-1 (Global Utilization of Streptokinase and Tissue Plasminogen Activator for Occluded Coronary Arteries) Investigators. *N Engl J Med.* 1996;334(8):481–7

Table 8.2 2013 ESC/ACC definition of acute MI

Rise and/or fall of cardiac biomarker values (preferably cardiac troponin, cTn) with at least one value above the 99th percentile upper reference limit, with at least one of the following:
Symptoms of ischemia
New ST-segment changes or new LBBB
Development of pathological Q waves
Imaging evidence of new loss of viable myocardium or regional wall motion abnormality
Identification of an intracoronary thrombus by angiography (or autopsy)

Serum Biomarkers

Serum biomarkers are less important when a massive STEMI is staring you down on the initial ECG, but take a more central role in the diagnosis of NSTEMI and UA. The most commonly used are the cardiac troponins (I and T), and to a lesser extent, the creatine kinase–MB fraction and serum myoglobin. (Incidentally, "cardiac enzyme" as a catchall term is a misnomer, as cardiac troponins are structural proteins released from dead and dying myocytes, and have no enzymatic function. The term is a holdover from the days of diagnosing ACS using aspartate transaminase (AST) and lactate dehydrogenase (LDH) levels, although technically, CK-MB *is* an enzyme.) The integral nature of serum troponins in the diagnosis of ACS was cemented in 2000, when a consensus definition of myocardial infarction by The Joint European Society of Cardiology (ESC) and the American College of Cardiology (ACC) included troponin elevation as a key component [15]. The 2013 ESC/ACC update to the consensus definition of acute myocardial infarction is outlined in Table 8.2.

Cardiac biomarkers rise and fall in predictable patterns after acute injury [16]. cTn rises after 4–9 hours, peaks within the first 24 hours, and returns to normal in 1–2 weeks. CK/CK-MB also appears within 4–9 hours and peaks within the first 24 hours, but normalizes rapidly compared to cTn (within 48–72 hours). Finally, myoglobin may be elevated within 1 hour, peaks within 12 hours, and then returns to normal in 24 hours. Both CK-MB and myoglobin are limited by poor specificity for ACS compared to cTn [16].

High-sensitivity troponin (hST) has garnered widespread attention over the last several years, and their use has particularly exploded in the United States following FDA approval in January 2017. As the name implies, these assays have the potential to detect evidence of ischemia within 1 hour of ED arrival [43], though the ideal way to incorporate them into clinical practice and treatment algorithms is still murky [44]. Criticisms include the fact that the enhanced sensitivity of hs-cTn comes at the cause of a significantly reduced specificity for acute MI [45].

Cardiac Imaging

The advent of high-resolution, multislice computed tomography (CT) has opened the door for noninvasive imaging of the coronary vessels themselves. In the realm of emergency medicine, cardiac CT is generally reserved for patients in whom STEMI and NSTEMI have been ruled out, and for whom the diagnosis of UA still lingers. The idea of a rapid, noninvasive imaging test that could provide information on par with coronary angiography is a game changer – unfortunately, that promise has yet to fully materialize. In the "Rule Out Myocardial Infarction using Computer Assisted Tomography" (ROMICAT) II trial, performance of cardiac CT decreased overall length of stay and increased rates of direct ED discharge among low- and intermediate-risk patients with suspected ACS, but was not associated with any improvement in outcomes and did not appear to be superior to traditional care [17]. Similarly, Litt et al. reported a decrease in ED length of stay without any improvement in the rates of AMI or cardiac death at 30 days compared to the traditional care group [18]. Cardiac CT remains an option in cases of suspected ACS among a lower risk patient population as an alternative to conventional stress testing following a normal ECG and negative cardiac enzymes. One definitive benefit of cardiac CT is that it obviates the need for repeat cardiac workup in a patient with radiographically normal coronary arteries who returns to the ED with recurrent chest pain in the subsequent weeks and months after their initial presentation.

Treatment

Primary Percutaneous Coronary Intervention (PCI)

STEMI PCI, when available, is the standard of care and single best intervention for STEMI, definitively surpassing lytic therapy toward the end of the twentieth century [19]. Accordingly, the number of PCI-capable centers is growing rapidly. In 2001, 1176 of 4609 US hospitals (~25%) had PCI programs, a number that grew to 1695 of 4673 US hospitals (~36%) by 2006 [20]. Interestingly, the proportion of the population with access to PCI centers remained virtually unchanged between the two periods (79% vs. 79.9%), suggesting that the bulk of newly established PCI centers are simply competing with other local hospitals for the same patient population. This unfortunately means that one-in-five Americans continue to lack access to the single best intervention for a prevalent and morbid disease.

There has been an emphasis on reducing "door-to-balloon time" (i.e., time from presentation to angioplasty and stenting) to 90 minutes or less, based on several studies indicating an increased in-hospital mortality for door-to-balloon time in excess of 90 minutes [21, 22]. Although more recent evidence from the CathPCI registry suggests that widespread implementation of the 90-minute goal may not have the impact on mortality that was once imagined [23], almighty JCAHO has adopted it as a Quality Core Measure (AMI-8a), which means it is here to stay. Faster door-to-balloon times may be facilitated by "heart alert" or "code STEMI" teams that are activated by the ED physician (or in some cases, prehospital personnel) in order to alert cardiologists to the presence of STEMI patients in the ED while simultaneously preparing catheterization lab personnel for patient arrival.

NSTEMI/UA In NSTEMI, the role of PCI is less straightforward, though it is clear that a subset of the population may benefit from a more aggressive approach. The Global Registry of Acute Coronary Events (GRACE) score has been used to risk stratify ACS patients into low-, medium-, and high-risk categories, and this scoring system may help identify NSTEMI patients who would benefit from PCI. The AHA currently endorses invasive therapy for NSTEMI patients who have been deemed high risk, as defined by a GRACE score > 140 [24]. For the individual elements of the GRACE score, see Table 8.3.

Fibrinolytic Therapy

STEMI Fibrinolytics are a viable alternative in STEMI when PCI is unavailable. The 2013 STEMI management guidelines from the AHA recommend fibrinolytic therapy for any patient at a non-PCI center where the first medical contact (FMC)-to-device time is expected to exceed 120 minutes [25]. FMC-to-device time is marked by either (a) arrival of EMS personnel in the prehospital setting or (b) ED arrival for patients transported by private vehicle. The AHA gives a Ia recommendation for fibrinolytic therapy as outlined above within 12 hours of ischemic symptoms, and a IIa recommendation for up to 24 hours if there is evidence of ongoing ischemia and a large area of myocardium "at risk," or in the presence of hemodynamic instability [25]. Streptokinase, the original "wonder drug" first used in 1958 by Sol Sherry and colleagues to treat myocardial infarction [26], has

Table 8.3 The GRACE score

Clinical variable	Value	Points
Age (years)	<30	0
	30–39	8
	40–49	25
	50–59	41
	60–69	58
	70–79	75
	80–89	91
	>90	100
Heart rate (beats per minute)	<50	0
	50–69	3
	70–89	9
	90–109	15
	110–149	24
	150–199	38
	>200	46
Systolic blood pressure (mm Hg)	<80	58
	80–99	53
	100–119	43
	120–139	34
	140–159	24
	160–199	10
	>200	0
Creatinine (mg/dL)	0–0.39	1
	0.40–0.79	4
	0.80–1.19	7
	1.20–1.59	10
	1.60–1.99	13
	2.00–3.99	21
	>4	28
Cardiac arrest on admission?	Y/N	39
STEMI?	Y/N	28
Elevated cardiac markers?	Y/N	14

Adapted from Fox KA, Dabbous OH, Goldberg RJ, et al. Prediction of risk of death and myocardial infarction in the six months after presentation with acute coronary syndrome: prospective multinational observational study (GRACE). *BMJ*. 2006;333(7578):1091

now been joined by alteplase, reteplase, tenecteplase, and anistreplase.

NSTEMI/UA Fibrinolytics are generally contraindicated in NSTEMI/UA, for several reasons. First and foremost, compared to STEMI, there is unlikely to be a complete vessel occlusion amenable to thrombolysis. Additionally, NSTEMI/UA is by nature a less emergent diagnosis, which alters the risk–benefit ratio of lytic administration. This was borne out in the TIMI IIIB trial, which indicated no benefit (and possible harm) for lytics in NSTEMI compared to conservative treatment [27].

Antiplatelet Agents

Aspirin (ASA), first isolated from the bark of the willow tree, is a permanent inhibitor of platelet activation and aggregation that acts by inhibiting COX-1 and preventing the formation of thromboxane A2. In suspected ACS, chewed aspirin is recommended in doses of either 162 or 325 mg, with evidence from the GUSTO I and GUSTO III trials, suggesting that the lower dose may be safer and equally effective in STEMI patients being treated with lytic therapy [28]. Aspirin should be administered in the prehospital setting immediately after symptom onset, or at the latest, on arrival to the hospital.

Clopidogrel, prasugrel, and ticagrelor are thienopyridines that also permanently inhibit platelet activation, acting by interfering with platelet ADP receptors (P2Y12 inhibitors). Compared to clopidogrel, use of prasugrel results in a greater inhibition of platelet aggregation but carries a higher bleeding risk. Prasugrel has been shown to reduce ischemic complications related to PCI, but this comes at a cost, including significantly increased rate of fatal bleeding events [29]. Clopidogrel is usually administered as a 600-mg loading dose in PCI patients, followed by 75-mg daily maintenance dosing. Prasugrel is given as a 60-mg loading dose, followed by 10-mg daily dosing. Ticagrelor is given as a 180-mg loading dose, followed by 90 mg twice daily dosing.

The ACC currently recommends 600 mg of clopidogrel (in addition to either 162 or 325 mg of aspirin) for STEMI patients prior to undergoing PCI [25]. In STEMI patients receiving fibrinolytic therapy, dual aspirin and clopidogrel therapy has been shown to increase vessel patency and reduce ischemic complications [30]. Accordingly, patients receiving fibrinolytics should also receive either 300 mg (<75 years old) or 75 mg (>75 years old) of clopidogrel in addition to 162 or 325 mg of aspirin [25].

Intravenous glycoprotein IIb/IIIa receptor antagonists are antiplatelet agents that may be considered in addition to dual antiplatelet therapy (DAPT) in STEMI patients undergoing PCI. Examples include abciximab, tirofiban, and eptifibatide. Evidence for the use of these agents for improving outcomes in STEMI is equivocal [31, 32].

For patients with NSTEMI and UA, aspirin at either 162 or 325 mg is the primary antiplatelet therapy. For patients with aspirin sensitivity, clopidogrel should be administered instead [33]. DAPT can be given to UA/NSTEMI patients who are higher risk and will undergo invasive therapy.

Anticoagulation

Anticoagulant therapy in ACS involves one of the three medications in the heparin family, including unfractionated heparin (UFH), low-molecular-weight heparin (LMWH), or the synthetic low-molecular-weight alternative fondaparinux. A fourth agent, bivalirudin, is a synthetic congener of leech saliva. The heparin agents activate antithrombin III, inhibiting both factor Xa and thrombin itself. Bivalirudin, by contrast, is a direct thrombin inhibitor.

In STEMI patients undergoing PCI, administering unfractionated heparin to an activated partial thromboplastin time (aPTT) target is recommended in addition to DAPT. There is evidence from the ATOLL trial that the LMWH enoxaparin may be superior to UFH in this setting [34], though its routine use is not yet recommended in the current ACC guidelines [25]. Fondaparinux, by contrast, is contraindicated as the only anticoagulative agent in PCI therapy due to the risk of guiding catheter thrombosis [35].

For STEMI patients undergoing fibrinolytic therapy, UFH, LMWH, and fondaparinux are all viable anticoagulant therapies. UFH titrated to an aPTT target has been used extensively in this setting. Enoxaperin is an alternative that may provide net clinical benefit despite an increased bleeding risk [36], and it should be dosed in consideration with patient weight, age, and renal function. Fondaparinux is also an alternative to UFH with lytic therapy, and there is evidence that compared to UFH, fondaparinux may reduce reinfarction without any increased risk of bleeding [35].

For NSTEMI and UA patients, the use of any one particular anticoagulant (UFH, LMWH, or fondaparinux) and the duration of therapy are complicated and dependent on many factors. These include whether or not the patient undergoes stress testing and/or angiography, whether or not those studies indicate the presence of significant coronary artery disease, and which subsequent therapies (PCI, coronary artery bypass grafting [CABG], or medical management) are selected [33].

Anti-Ischemic Therapy

Traditional anti-ischemic therapy in ACS consists of supplemental oxygen, morphine, nitrates, and β-blockers. These will be considered individually.

Oxygen The use of supplemental oxygen in suspected ACS is longstanding, but there is remarkably little literature to support the habit. While it is still prudent to provide supplemental oxygen for hypoxic patients, the routine use of supplemental oxygen in all cases of ACS is not evidence based. In fact, some studies have indicated that routine oxygen use may increase infarct size and mortality, owing to a hyperoxia-related decrease in coronary blood flow [37]. A prospective, randomized trial is badly needed but not forthcoming.

Morphine Morphine is the prototypical mu-opioid agonist. Much like oxygen, the use of morphine to relieve ischemia-related chest pain and anxiety is widespread but not evidence based. The AHA still recommends morphine as the analgesic of choice in ACS [25], despite evidence from the large CRUSADE database indicating an increased mortality associated with morphine use in NSTEMI [38]. This is believed to be the result of morphine masking the symptoms of ongoing ischemia and may be analogous to giving a paralytic agent to a seizing patient (in that the "symptom" will resolve, but the underlying pathology may continue unabated).

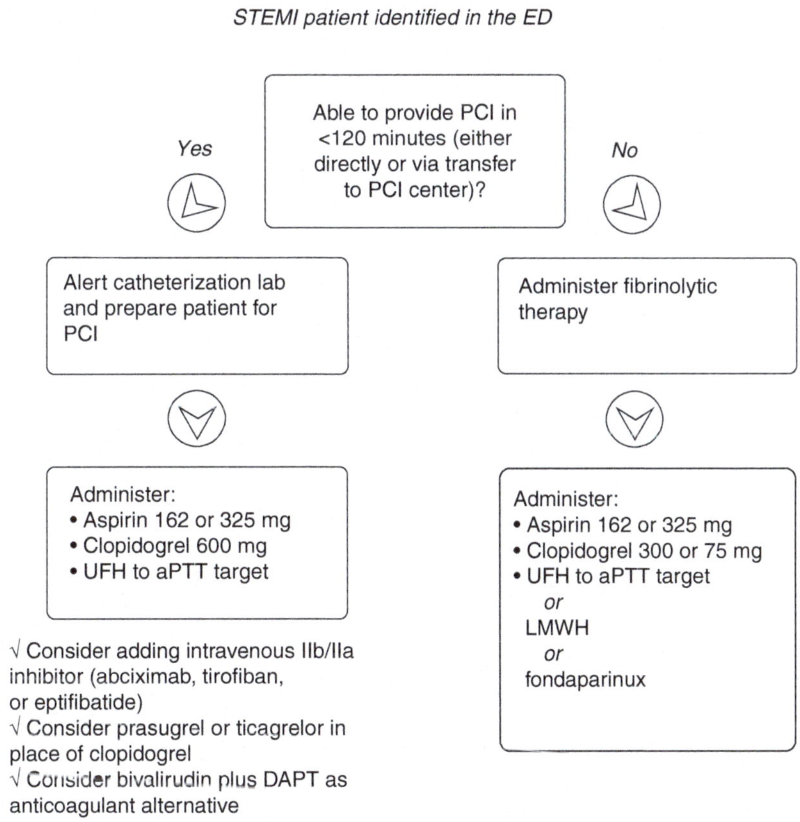

Fig. 8.1 STEMI treatment algorithm. (Adapted from O'Gara et al. [25]). Note: <120 minutes refers to FMC-to-device time

Nitrates Nitrates induce venous and arterial dilation, reducing both cardiac preload and afterload. Nitrates may be beneficial in heart failure related to ACS and ACS, in general, but the evidence is modest [39, 40]. Nitrates are contraindicated in the presence of hypotension or recent phosphodiesterase inhibitor use, and they should be used with great caution in patients with inferior wall or right ventricular infarcts.

β-blockers β-blockers decrease the heart rate and reduce cardiac contractility, curtailing myocardial oxygen demand. Evidence from the COMMIT trial indicated that the use of β-blockers may reduce the rate of reinfarction and ventricular fibrillation in ACS, but it may also increase the risk of developing cardiogenic shock [41], particularly in the first 24 hours after admission. Tachycardia may be a mechanism of compensated shock, which can progress to decompensated shock when the heart rate is actively reduced and cardiac output falls. The risks and benefits should be weighed accordingly. The AHA recommends oral β-blocker therapy in the first 24 hours for patients without any evidence of heart failure and gives a IIa recommendation for intravenous β-blocker use in the ED for patients without contraindications who are hypertensive or have ongoing signs of ischemia (Fig. 8.1) [25].

Disposition

STEMI patients and higher risk NSTEMI patients, particularly those undergoing invasive therapy, do not pose much of a dilemma concerning their disposition: Virtually all will be admitted to the hospital, preferably to the cardiac intensive care unit. There is, however, abundant controversy regarding whether UA or lower risk NSTEMI patients being admitted to the hospital should be placed on cardiac telemetry. There is evidence that the practice is grossly overused and was recently targeted by the Society for Hospital

Table 8.4 Example of a guideline-based model for determining duration of telemetry monitoring

24-hour monitoring:	*48-hour monitoring:*	*Indefinite monitoring:*
Chest pain/rule out MI	Acute MI	Cardiac surgery during this admission
Elective PCI	CHF exacerbation	Use of wearable automatic defibrillator
Defibrillator/pacemaker placement	Syncope, suspected arrhythmia	Complex cardiac disorders (i.e., incessant ventricular tachycardia)
Uncomplicated ablation	Thoracic surgery	
Syncope, unknown origin	Acute stroke	
Major surgery	Complex major surgery	

Adapted from Dressler et al. [44]

Medicine (SHM) as a behavior that should be curtailed for the "Choosing Wisely" campaign [42]. It has been shown that adhering to the 2004 AHA guidelines on cardiac telemetry [43] (see Table 8.4) can drastically reduce the use of telemetry without having a deleterious impact on patient outcomes [44].

More difficult still are the decisions which arise when deciding on the disposition for low-risk chest pain patients being evaluated for UA. Practice varies and may include traditional hospital admission; admission to "short stay" or clinical decision units (CDUs); discharge from the emergency department after one, two, or three sets of cardiac enzymes; or discharge home with no further workup following the history and physical examination. Patients admitted to the hospital or the CDU will usually receive further diagnostic testing, including exercise or nuclear stress testing, cardiac CT, or, in some cases, conventional angiography. For patients whom are deemed low enough risk for discharge but whom still require further diagnostic testing, 72-hour stress testing appears to be a safe approach [45].

What's Next?

Cardiac CT is an area in which rapid technological advances are inevitable and already underway. Despite the limitations noted above, the attractiveness of noninvasive cardiac angiography means that the use of the technology will continue. Recent breakthroughs include the development of 128-slice dual-source scanners, which have been shown to reduce radiation exposure by more than 60% compared to conventional 64-slice scanners, with no apparent decay in image quality [46].

Summary

ACS includes a spectrum of disease processes that range from unstable angina to the increasingly morbid non-ST elevation MI and ST elevation MI. Higher-risk patients with evidence of profound or ongoing ischemia will be treated with a combination of antiplatelet, anticoagulant, and anti-ischemic therapies, and some may be candidates for PCI, fibrinolysis, or CABG. Lower-risk patients pose a greater diagnostic dilemma, with some requiring inpatient evaluations while others will be suitable for discharge and outpatient follow-up. Emergency physicians will be the point of first contact for large numbers of these patients as they enter the health-care system, and coordinated efforts between the ED and our cardiology colleagues will continue to prove necessary to risk stratify patients appropriately and improve patient outcomes.

References

1. Go AS, Mozaffarian D, Roger VL, et al. Executive summary: heart disease and stroke statistics--2014 update: a report from the American Heart Association. Circulation. 2014;129(3):399–410.
2. Rogers WJ, Frederick PD, Stoehr E, et al. Trends in presenting characteristics and hospital mortality among patients with ST elevation and non-ST elevation myocardial infarction in the National Registry of Myocardial Infarction from 1990 to 2006. Am Heart J. 2008;156(6):1026–34.
3. Yan AT, Yan RT, Tan M, et al. In-hospital revascularization and one-year outcome of acute coronary syndrome patients stratified by the GRACE risk score. Am J Cardiol. 2005;96(7):913–6.
4. Terkelsen CJ, Christiansen EH, Sørensen JT, et al. Primary PCI as the preferred reperfusion therapy in STEMI: it is a matter of time. Heart. 2009;95(5):362–9.

5. Navarese EP, De servi S, Politi A, et al. Impact of primary PCI volume on hospital mortality in STEMI patients: does time-to-presentation matter? J Thromb Thrombolysis. 2011;32(2):223–31.
6. Ritchey MD, Wall HK, Gillespie C, George MG, Jamal A. Million hearts: prevalence of leading cardiovascular disease risk factors--United States, 2005-2012. MMWR Morb Mortal Wkly Rep. 2014;63(21):462–7.
7. Lloyd-jones DM, Hong Y, Labarthe D, et al. Defining and setting national goals for cardiovascular health promotion and disease reduction: the American Heart Association's strategic impact goal through 2020 and beyond. Circulation. 2010;121(4):586–613.
8. Body R, Cook G, Burrows G, Carley S, Lewis PS. Can emergency physicians 'rule in' and 'rule out' acute myocardial infarction with clinical judgement? Emerg Med J. 2014;31(11):872–6.
9. Lee CP, Hoffmann U, Bamberg F, et al. Emergency physician estimates of the probability of acute coronary syndrome in a cohort of patients enrolled in a study of coronary computed tomographic angiography. CJEM. 2012;14(3):147–56.
10. Arroyo LH, Lee RT. Mechanisms of plaque rupture: mechanical and biologic interactions. Cardiovasc Res. 1999;41(2):369–75.
11. Einthoven W. The different forms of the human electrocardiogram and their signification. Lancet. 1912;179(4622):853–61.
12. Kontos MC, Aziz HA, Chau VQ, Roberts CS, Ornato JP, Vetrovec GW. Outcomes in patients with chronicity of left bundle-branch block with possible acute myocardial infarction. Am Heart J. 2011;161(4):698–704.
13. Jain S, Ting HT, Bell M, et al. Utility of left bundle branch block as a diagnostic criterion for acute myocardial infarction. Am J Cardiol. 2011;107(8):1111–6.
14. Tabas JA, Rodriguez RM, Seligman HK, Goldschlager NF. Electrocardiographic criteria for detecting acute myocardial infarction in patients with left bundle branch block: a meta-analysis. Ann Emerg Med. 2008;52(4):329–336.e1.
15. Alpert JS, Thygesen K, Antman E, Bassand JP. Myocardial infarction redefined--a consensus document of The Joint European Society of Cardiology/American College of Cardiology Committee for the redefinition of myocardial infarction. J Am Coll Cardiol. 2000;36(3):959–69.
16. Lewandrowski K, Chen A, Januzzi J. Cardiac markers for myocardial infarction. A brief review. Am J Clin Pathol. 2002;118(Suppl):S93–9.
17. Hoffmann U, Truong QA, Schoenfeld DA, et al. Coronary CT angiography versus standard evaluation in acute chest pain. N Engl J Med. 2012;367(4):299–308.
18. Litt HI, Gatsonis C, Snyder B, et al. CT angiography for safe discharge of patients with possible acute coronary syndromes. N Engl J Med. 2012;366(15):1393–403.
19. Keeley EC, Boura JA, Grines CL. Primary angioplasty versus intravenous thrombolytic therapy for acute myocardial infarction: a quantitative review of 23 randomised trials. Lancet. 2003;361(9351):13–20.
20. Concannon TW, Nelson J, Goetz J, Griffith JL. A percutaneous coronary intervention lab in every hospital? Circ Cardiovasc Qual Outcomes. 2012;5(1):14–20.
21. Mcnamara RL, Wang Y, Herrin J, et al. Effect of door-to-balloon time on mortality in patients with ST-segment elevation myocardial infarction. J Am Coll Cardiol. 2006;47(11):2180–6.
22. Antman EM, Hand M, Armstrong PW, et al. 2007 Focused update of the ACC/AHA 2004 guidelines for the management of patients with ST-elevation myocardial infarction: a report of the American College of Cardiology/American Heart Association Task Force on Practice Guidelines: developed in collaboration with the Canadian Cardiovascular Society endorsed by the American Academy of family physicians: 2007 Writing Group to review new evidence and update the ACC/AHA 2004 guidelines for the management of patients with ST-elevation myocardial infarction, writing on behalf of the 2004 Writing Committee. Circulation. 2008;117(2):296–329.
23. Menees DS, Peterson ED, Wang Y, et al. Door-to-balloon time and mortality among patients undergoing primary PCI. N Engl J Med. 2013;369(10):901–9.
24. Jneid H, Anderson JL, Wright RS, et al. 2012 ACCF/AHA focused update of the guideline for the management of patients with unstable angina/non-ST-elevation myocardial infarction (updating the 2007 guideline and replacing the 2011 focused update): a report of the American College of Cardiology Foundation/American Heart Association Task Force on Practice Guidelines. J Am Coll Cardiol. 2012;60(7):645–81.
25. O'Gara PT, Kushner FG, Ascheim DD, et al. 2013 ACCF/AHA guideline for the management of ST-elevation myocardial infarction: a report of the American College of Cardiology Foundation/American Heart Association Task Force on Practice Guidelines. Circulation. 2013;127:e362–452.
26. Sikri N, Bardia A. A history of streptokinase use in acute myocardial infarction. Tex Heart Inst J. 2007;34(3):318–27.
27. Effects of tissue plasminogen activator and a comparison of early invasive and conservative strategies in unstable angina and non-Q-wave myocardial infarction. Results of the TIMI IIIB Trial. Thrombolysis in Myocardial Ischemia. Circulation. 1994;89(4):1545–56.
28. Berger JS, Stebbins A, Granger CB, et al. Initial aspirin dose and outcome among ST-elevation myocardial infarction patients treated with fibrinolytic therapy. Circulation. 2008;117(2):192–9.
29. Wiviott SD, Braunwald E, Mccabe CH, et al. Prasugrel versus clopidogrel in patients with acute coronary syndromes. N Engl J Med. 2007;357(20):2001–15.
30. Sabatine MS, Cannon CP, Gibson CM, et al. Addition of clopidogrel to aspirin and fibrinolytic therapy for

myocardial infarction with ST-segment elevation. N Engl J Med. 2005;352(12):1179–89.
31. Stone GW, Grines CL, Cox DA, et al. Comparison of angioplasty with stenting, with or without abciximab, in acute myocardial infarction. N Engl J Med. 2002;346(13):957–66.
32. Brener SJ, Barr LA, Burchenal JE, et al. Randomized, placebo-controlled trial of platelet glycoprotein IIb/IIIa blockade with primary angioplasty for acute myocardial infarction. ReoPro and Primary PTCA Organization and Randomized Trial (RAPPORT) Investigators. Circulation. 1998;98(8):734–41.
33. Jneid H, Anderson JL, Wright RS, et al. 2012 ACCF/AHA focused update of the guideline for the management of patients with unstable angina/non-ST-elevation myocardial infarction (updating the 2007 guideline and replacing the 2011 focused update): a report of the American College of Cardiology Foundation/American Heart Association Task Force on practice guidelines. Circulation. 2012;126(7):875–910.
34. Montalescot G, Zeymer U, Silvain J, et al. Intravenous enoxaparin or unfractionated heparin in primary percutaneous coronary intervention for ST-elevation myocardial infarction: the international randomised open-label ATOLL trial. Lancet. 2011;378(9792):693–703.
35. Yusuf S, Mehta SR, Chrolavicius S, et al. Effects of fondaparinux on mortality and reinfarction in patients with acute ST-segment elevation myocardial infarction: the OASIS-6 randomized trial. JAMA. 2006;295(13):1519–30.
36. Assessment of the Safety and Efficacy of a New Thrombolytic Regimen (ASSENT)-3 Investigators. Efficacy and safety of tenecteplase in combination with enoxaparin, abciximab, or unfractionated heparin: the ASSENT-3 randomised trial in acute myocardial infarction. Lancet. 2001;358(9282):605–13.
37. Wijesinghe M, Perrin K, Ranchord A, Simmonds M, Weatherall M, Beasley R. Routine use of oxygen in the treatment of myocardial infarction: systematic review. Heart. 2009;95(3):198–202.
38. Meine TJ, Roe MT, Chen AY, et al. Association of intravenous morphine use and outcomes in acute coronary syndromes: results from the CRUSADE quality improvement initiative. Am Heart J. 2005;149(6):1043–9.
39. Wakai A, Mccabe A, Kidney R, et al. Nitrates for acute heart failure syndromes. Cochrane Database Syst Rev. 2013;8:CD005151.
40. ISIS-4: a randomised factorial trial assessing early oral captopril, oral mononitrate, and intravenous magnesium sulphate in 58,050 patients with suspected acute myocardial infarction. ISIS-4 (fourth international study of infarct survival) Collaborative Group. Lancet. 1995;345(8951):669–85.
41. Chen ZM, Pan HC, Chen YP, et al. Early intravenous then oral metoprolol in 45,852 patients with acute myocardial infarction: randomised placebo-controlled trial. Lancet. 2005;366(9497):1622–32.
42. Bulger J, Nickel W, Messler J, et al. Choosing wisely in adult hospital medicine: five opportunities for improved healthcare value. J Hosp Med. 2013;8(9):486–92.
43. Drew BJ, Califf RM, Funk M, et al. Practice standards for electrocardiographic monitoring in hospital settings: an American Heart Association scientific statement from the councils on cardiovascular nursing, clinical cardiology, and cardiovascular disease in the young: endorsed by the International Society of Computerized Electrocardiology and the American Association of Critical-Care Nurses. Circulation. 2004;110(17):2721–46.
44. Dressler R, Dryer MM, Coletti C, Mahoney D, Doorey AJ. Altering overuse of cardiac telemetry in non-intensive care unit settings by hardwiring the use of American Heart Association Guidelines. JAMA Intern Med. 2014;174(11):1852–4.
45. Meyer MC, Mooney RP, Sekera AK. A critical pathway for patients with acute chest pain and low risk for short-term adverse cardiac events: role of outpatient stress testing. Ann Emerg Med. 2006;47(5):427–35.
46. Chinnaiyan KM, Bilolikar AN, Walsh E, et al. CT dose reduction using prospectively triggered or fast-pitch spiral technique employed in cardiothoracic imaging (the CT dose study). J Cardiovasc Comput Tomogr. 2014;8(3):205–14.

Cardiac Dysrhythmias

9

Neil Christopher and Wan-Tsu W. Chang

Introduction

Cardiac dysrhythmias encountered in the emergency and critical care setting are often life-threatening situations, requiring emergent diagnosis as well as therapeutic intervention. In some cases, intervention may be required to stabilize the patient even prior to establishing a firm diagnosis. Thus, a structured approach to dysrhythmias is essential to ensure that key diagnostics and appropriate treatment modalities are not overlooked. In this chapter, we review the most common dysrhythmias encountered in the emergency department and their management.

Bradydysrhythmias

Bradydysrhythmias can result from a wide range of underlying pathologies. While cardiovascular etiologies are common, thorough evaluation should not overlook respiratory (hypoxia), traumatic, intracranial, and intra-abdominal causes. Hemodynamic instability is rare, but the clinician must be prepared with emergent interventions as needed to stabilize the patient. These include medications as well as procedures such as transcutaneous and transvenous pacing.

Pathophysiology

The etiologies of bradydysrhythmias are diverse and include ischemia, infarction, hypothermia, toxin-mediated causes, electrolyte abnormalities, age-related degeneration among many others. Patients may present with a range of symptoms from fatigue to altered mental status and syncope. Bradydysrhythmias can be categorized into sinus node dysfunction and atrioventricular block (Table 9.1). Sinus node dysfunctions are due to failure to generate appropriate cardiac potentials from the sinus node. Atrioventricular blocks occur when conduction from the atria to the atrioventricular node and into the bundle of His is disrupted.

Emergency Evaluation

Initial Assessment

Patients with significant bradydysrhythmias must be promptly identified in the emergency department. A quick assessment of airway, breathing, and circulation can help in the initial determination of stability. Additionally, assessment of the

The authors have nothing to disclose.

N. Christopher
Department of Emergency Medicine, Icahn School of Medicine at Mount Sinai, New York, NY, USA

W.-T. W. Chang (✉)
Department of Emergency Medicine, University of Maryland School of Medicine, Baltimore, MD, USA
e-mail: wchang1@som.umaryland.edu

© Springer Nature Switzerland AG 2020
J. R. Shiber, S. D. Weingart (eds.), *Emergency Department Critical Care*,
https://doi.org/10.1007/978-3-030-28794-8_9

Table 9.1 Definitions of bradydysrhythmias

Sinus node dysfunctions	Sinus bradycardia	Rate <60, regular P waves with normal PR interval, preceding each QRS
	Sinus arrest	Absent atrial depolarization $\geq$2 seconds.
	Tachycardia–bradycardia (Tachy–Brady) syndrome	Episodes of sinus bradycardia or sinus arrest interspersed with episodes of supraventricular tachycardia. Atrial fibrillation is the most common underlying rhythm
	Chronotropic incompetence	Sinus node fails to regulate heart rate in response to changes in metabolic demand
Atrioventricular blocks	First-degree AV block	PR interval >20 msec, 1:1 P:QRS conduction
	Second-degree AV block Mobitz type I (Wenckebach)	Progressive prolongation of PR interval prior to a nonconducted QRS
	Second-degree AV block Mobitz type II	Fixed PR intervals prior to a nonconducted QRS. More likely to degrade to third-degree AV block
	Third-degree AV block (complete heart block)	No relation between atrial and ventricular depolarization that occur at regular but independent rates

character and regularity of the pulse can help to identify dysrhythmias even prior obtaining the ECG. Finally, initial vital signs are an essential part of assessing hemodynamic stability.

Focused history and physical examination can aid in characterizing the etiology of the dysrhythmia. History of an implantable defibrillator or pacemaker may suggest a known underlying unstable dysrhythmia. Severe abdominal tenderness on examination can suggest an intra-abdominal insult causing reflex bradycardia.

Diagnostic Studies

An EKG and continuous cardiac monitoring are essential for the diagnosis of bradydysrhythmias. Laboratory studies should be directed at the possible etiologies suggested by the history and physical. Electrolyte levels, especially potassium, calcium, and magnesium, should be obtained. Drug levels for digoxin are essential if consistent with medication history. Cardiac biomarkers (e.g., troponin, creatine kinase, CK-MB, B-type natriuretic peptide) may be helpful in the diagnosis of myocardial infarction or heart failure. Thyroid function testing as well as testing for Lyme and Syphilis may also be indicated if other etiologies have been ruled out. Lactate levels may also be useful if there is concern for alteration in perfusion. Imaging studies should be limited and based on the clinical history. Suspicion of an intracranial cause of bradydysrhythmia requires CT imaging of the head. Abdominal imaging may be useful to support a diagnosis of reflex or relative bradycardia. Finally, a chest X-ray may help in the diagnosis of heart failure by revealing an enlarged cardiac silhouette or pulmonary edema.

Treatment

The treatment strategy for patients with bradydysrhythmias is guided by the patient's clinical stability. Signs of instability include hypotension, altered mental status, acute heart failure, and evidence of poor perfusion. Unstable patients require transcutaneous pacing emergently, which can be utilized while medications are being prepared.

Pacing

The standard of care for the unstable patient with bradycardia is utilization of a pacemaker. The transcutaneous approach is most accessible, thus should be the first-line therapy. A consideration prior to initiation of pacing is sedation. Transcutaneous pacing can be very painful for the awake patient as electrical discharges pass through skin and muscle. Choice of sedation in this clinical scenario may be difficult as many commonly used agents also cause hypotension, but some options with minimal deleterious cardiovascular effects include ketamine (begin with 1 mg/kg IV) and etomidate (begin with 0.15 mg/kg IV).

Once preparations are complete, pacing should be started with an initial rate that is at least as high as the patient's intrinsic rate. Usually, a rate of 60–80 beats/minute is chosen to assess effectiveness of capture. Current can be started at 10–20 mA and increased progressively until a clear QRS and T wave is found following each pacer spike (electrical capture). The patient's pulse should also correspond to pacing spikes demonstrating mechanical capture. Some adjuncts to aid in determining capture include looking at the heart rate on the pulse oximetry waveform as well as looking for an increase in CO_2 levels on capnometry. Once capture is achieved, the current level should be set to 5–10 mA above the threshold for capture. Generally, the threshold required for pacing should be 40–80 mA but can vary.

There will be patients in whom transcutaneous pacing is either not capturing or not improving the hemodynamic status (i.e., perfusion). In these patients, utilization of pharmacotherapy while transvenous pacing is prepared would be the next step. A more in-depth discussion of the procedure is beyond the scope of this chapter, but can be found in various texts.

Medical Management

As for all unstable patients, support of their airway and breathing may be necessary. When a bradydysrhythmia is the source of the patient's circulatory instability, the first-line medication for this patient is atropine, which has been shown to improve heart rate and conduction blocks [1]. The recommended dose is 0.5 mg intravenously every 3–5 minutes to a maximum of 3 mg. However, it is important to note that atropine may be ineffective in cardiac transplant patients due to lack of vagal innervation [2]. Additionally, it will have no effect in the case of second-degree type II or third-degree atrioventricular block.

If atropine is ineffective, the next agent of choice should be a beta-adrenergic agent. These include dopamine, epinephrine, or isoproterenol. Recall that varying doses of dopamine can have different effects; thus, we recommend a dose of 5–10 mcg/kg/min. Epinephrine is another option with an infusion rate of 2–10 mcg/min [3]. Isoproterenol specifically targets beta-adrenergic activity, and in our experience, is useful in the setting of post heart transplant bradycardia and sinus arrest. However, this has not been extensively studied [4] and one must consider the potential hypotension mediated by beta 2 activity when using this agent.

Bradydysrhythmias induced by drug toxicity may require specific management tailored to the drug ingested. Beta-blockers and calcium channel blockers are the most likely medications to cause bradydysrhythmias and are often unintentional overdoses of prescribed medications [5]. In cases of beta-blocker or calcium channel blocker overdose, glucagon has potential for clinical effect [6]. Digoxin is another common cause of bradydysrhythmias often with concomitant atrioventricular block in up to 35% of patients owing to its narrow therapeutic window [7]. Treatment of specific drug toxicities should be initiated with consultation of local poison control centers and with consideration of decontamination and additional supportive care.

For the stable patient, the initial management focus shifts from correcting a malignant dysrhythmia to diagnosing and treating the underlying cause. Constant reassessment of clinical stability is important in these patients as they may quickly deteriorate. With certain etiologies such as electrolyte abnormalities or toxic ingestions leading to bradydysrhythmias, definitive treatment should start expeditiously in the ED to reduce the chance for clinical instability. However, other etiologies (e.g., CHF, MI, infection) may require hospital admission and specialty consultation for definitive management (Table 9.2).

Tachydysrhythmias

Tachydysrhythmias can originate from the sinus node, atria, AV node, or ventricular myocardium. An approach to tachydysrhythmias starts with determining whether the QRS complex is narrow or wide and whether the rhythm is regular or irregular (Fig. 9.1).

Table 9.2 Differential diagnosis and management of bradydysrhythmias

Etiology		History	Diagnostics	Management
Ischemia – inferior MI, right coronary artery occlusion		Preceding angina	ST elevations/depressions, troponinemia	Aspirin, statin, GP IIb/IIIa inhibitor, PCI / stents, tPA
Elevated ICP		Headache, AMS, head trauma, falls	Papilledema, CT scan	Hyperventilation, hypertonic saline/mannitol, neurosurgical intervention
Hyperkalemia		History of ESRD on HD	EKG – peaked T waves, sine wave, electrolytes	Calcium infusion, albuterol, insulin + glucose, binders, hemodialysis
Hypothyroidism		Cold intolerance, weight gain, fatigue	TSH, free T4	Levothyroxine
Hypothermia		Prolonged exposure to cold	EKG – Osborn waves	Warming
Infectious – Chagas, Lyme, Parvovirus, Coxsackie, Syphilis		Fever, tick bite, travel to endemic areas	Specific antigen testing	Antibiotics
Vasovagal		Severe pain, anxiety, strong emotion	None	None
Toxidromes	Beta-blockers	History of overdose, medication change, polypharmacy	Bradycardia with AV block	Glucagon (5 mg IV Q10 minutes up to 3 doses)
	Calcium channel blockers		Bradycardia with AV block	Calcium gluconate, insulin (1 u/kg bolus then 0.5 u/kg/hr) + glucose
	Digitalis	Nausea, vomiting, yellow/green vision discoloration, palpitations, confusion	Slow AF, AV block (first, second, or third), regularized AF, VT, scooped ST segment	Digoxin immune Fab, 10–20 vials or dose based on levels
	Opioids	Miosis, bradypnea	Response to naloxone	Naloxone 0.4 mg IV then 2 mg IV if no response
	Organophosphates	Salivation, lacrimation, urination, defecation, gastrointestinal motility, emesis, miosis	None	Atropine 2 mg IV every 3–5 minutes (PRN bradycardia or bronchorrhea) + pralidoxime (2-PAM) 2 g IV over 10–15 minutes

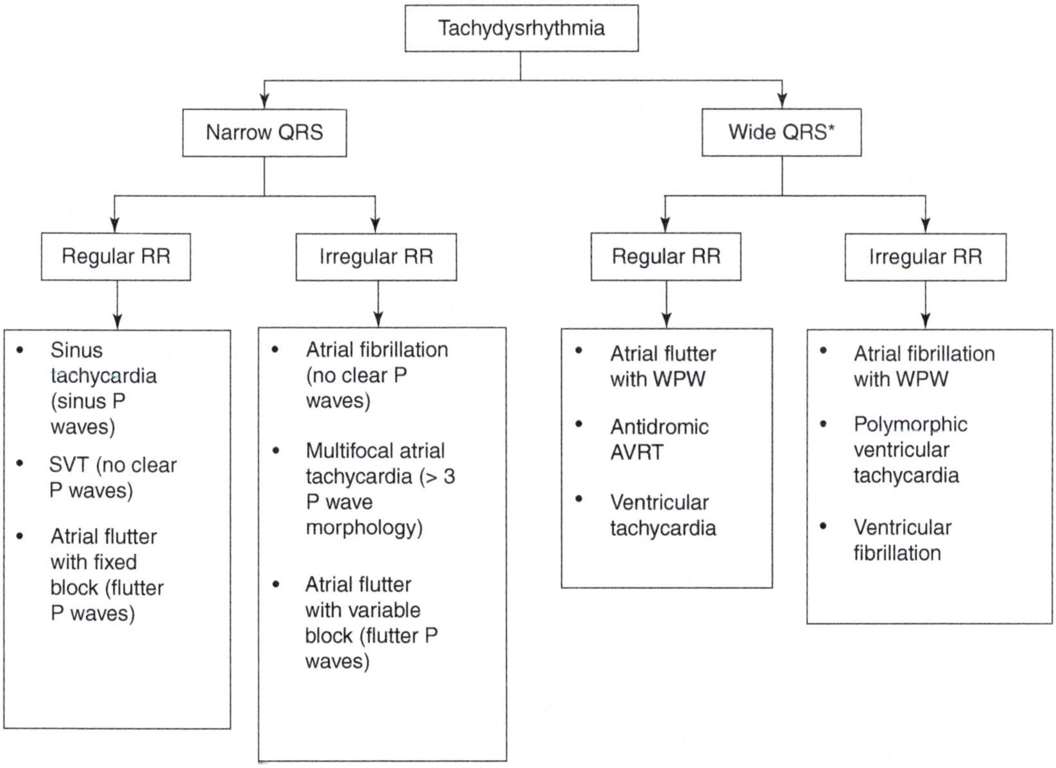

Fig. 9.1 Approach to tachydysrhythmias. An approach to tachydysrhythmias includes determining whether the QRS complex is narrow or wide and whether the rhythm is regular or irregular. *Wide QRS tachydysrhythmias include any tachydysrhythmias with bundle branch block or aberrancy

Pathophysiology

Sinus Tachycardia (ST)

A sinus rate greater than 100 beats/min defines sinus tachycardia and is often caused by enhanced automaticity of the SA node. The P-wave configuration is the same as in sinus rhythm with upright morphology in leads II, III, and aVF, negative in AVR, biphasic in V1–V2, and positive in leads V3–V6. Generally, the maximum predicted atrial rate can be estimated by the simple formula of 220 - age, although this can underestimate true maximum [8]. Sinus tachycardia results from increased adrenergic drive, found in exercise, hyperthyroidism, acute sepsis, decompensated heart failure, anemia, fever, pulmonary embolism, myocardial ischemia, hypovolemia, and many other conditions. This situation is termed physiologic sinus tachycardia, and management historically involves treatment of the underlying cause, although more recently there has been evidence to suggest that controlling rate in the setting of septic shock may impact outcome [9].

A persistently elevated resting heart rate in the absence of obvious triggers is known as inappropriate sinus tachycardia. The underlying cause is either enhanced automaticity or abnormal autonomic regulation of the sinus node. This is a diagnosis of exclusion, as all other causes of sinus tachycardia must be addressed. Postural orthostatic tachycardia syndrome is a constellation of signs and symptoms that include marked orthostatic sinus tachycardia (rate >120 or increase >30 beats/min within 10 minutes of positional change) without orthostatic hypotension in a patient without autonomic neuropathy.

Supraventricular Tachycardia (SVT)

Supraventricular tachycardia refers to a wide range of tachydysrhythmias that originate from the sinus node, atria, and/or atrioventricular node. This includes sinus node reentry tachycardia (SNRT), AV nodal reentry tachycardia (AVNRT), AV reentry tachycardia (AVRT), unifocal atrial tachycardia (UAT), multifocal atrial tachycardia (MAT), and junctional tachycardia (JT). Atrial fibrillation and atrial flutter may degenerate into SVT and may require a slightly different approach. SVT originates from a combination of enhanced automaticity and the presence of reentrant paths for conduction. Enhanced automaticity allows cells to depolarize earlier than normal in diastole, with the resulting impulses overriding the sinus node as the predominant pacemaker of the heart. There are many areas of the heart that can exhibit enhanced automaticity, including tissues of the atria, AV node, His bundle, pulmonary veins, or vena cava [10, 11]. Reentry occurs as repetitive excitation of a region of the heart that begins from a specific focus and moves through a defined circuit. Often, the location of the reentrant circuit will characterize the type of SVT with the majority of reentrant tachycardias originating from the AV node or from an AV circuit [12].

Sinus Node Reentry Tachycardia (SNRT)

Sinus node reentry is a rare tachycardia that presents as paroxysmal tachycardia with abrupt onset and termination. The P-wave morphology is similar to sinus rhythm, resulting from a reentrant circuit located near the sinus node. One clue to the diagnosis is a RP interval that is longer than the PR interval [13]. This rhythm is often triggered by a PAC. Vagal maneuvers are useful in terminating sinus node reentry.

AV Nodal Reentry Tachycardia (AVNRT)

AVNRT is the most common SVT and is more prevalent in women [14]. AVNRT is not usually associated with underlying heart disease, and typical heart rates range from low 100 s to over 250 beats/min [15]. In AVNRT, the reentrant circuit is localized to the AV node itself and is composed of fast pathways and slow pathways. Normal conduction through a fast pathway usually leads to normal P & QRS morphology. However, if rate is too high, conduction may switch to the slow pathway and create a reentrant loop. Following conduction through the AV node, impulses are carried by the His–Purkinje system, which leads to a narrow QRS (<120 ms) without any bundle branch block (BBB).

AV Reentry Tachycardia (AVRT)

AVRT is the second most common SVT with typically a heart rate between 120 and 250 beats/min [14–17]. In AVRT, a normal AV node with a single conduction pathway is paired with an accessory pathway between the atria and ventricles. An example of this type of conduction occurs in Wolff–Parkinson–White (WPW) syndrome in which the accessory pathway is termed bundle of Kent.

Normal conduction in WPW occurs through both the AV node and bundle of Kent, leading to a short PR interval from rapid conduction through the accessory pathway and a slurred QRS (delta wave) from the early ventricular depolarization through the accessory pathway. As conduction through the AV node catches up, the remainder of the QRS takes on a narrow morphology. Orthodromic AVRT occurs when conduction travels anterograde through the AV node and retrograde through the accessory pathway. This results in a narrow complex without aberrancy or BBB and no delta wave. Antidromic AVRT occurs with anterograde conduction through the accessory pathway and retrograde conduction through the AV node. Since the accessory pathway depolarized the ventricular myocardium, this arrhythmia is a wide-complex regular tachycardia indistinguishable from VT.

In patients with atrial fibrillation, impulses may be conducted through the accessory pathway, AV node, or both, which results in a rapid, irregular tachycardia with variable QRS morphology. This preexcited AF can degenerate to ventricular fibrillation. It is important to distinguish this irregular wide-complex tachycardia from others, such as atrial fibrillation with RVR and a BBB. Some clues that suggest the presence of an accessory pathway include a ventricular rate greater than 250 beats/min, beat-to-beat variability of QRS-complex morphology, and atypical bundle branch morphology [18, 19].

Unifocal Atrial Tachycardia (UAT)

Unifocal atrial tachycardia is a paroxysmal narrow-complex regular tachycardia generated from a pacemaker not in the SA node, which has a rate between 100 and 250 beats/min and a monomorphic P wave. This P wave is often obscured by the T wave due to an underlying first-degree AV block, which helps differentiate this SVT from AVRT and AVNRT. UAT can be caused by abnormal automaticity or micro-reentry, which is differentiated by a gradual versus sudden heart rate increase, respectively. Nonsustained UAT is often asymptomatic, while sustained UAT can account for 10–15% of SVTs that require ablation [20]. UAT is frequently seen in children (10–23%) and at much higher rates in patients with congenital heart disease, even after repair [21–24]. UAT usually occurs in patients before the age of 40 and is associated with cardiovascular disease [17, 25].

Multifocal Atrial Tachycardia (MAT)

Multifocal atrial tachycardia manifests as an irregularly irregular tachycardia with three or more distinct P-wave morphologies and an atrial rate greater than 100 beats/min. It is responsible for 1–2% of all SVT, and most cases are associated with underlying severe pulmonary disease. It can also occur in the setting of pneumonia, sepsis, heart failure, digoxin toxicity, and theophylline toxicity and in the postoperative period [26]. Each distinct P wave originates from a separate atrial focus and results in a variable PP, PR, and RR interval. Calcium channel blockers may be indicated for rate control, but antiarrhythmic drugs or DC cardioversion are ineffective. Correction of the underlying electrolyte disorder or treatment of pulmonary disease is most successful at controlling this arrhythmia.

Junctional Tachycardia (JT)

Junctional tachycardia arises from either the AV node or common His bundle. It can be broken down into paroxysmal or nonparoxysmal. Paroxysmal junctional tachycardia is seen in children with congenital heart abnormalities or young adults in the setting of stress or exercise [27]. Nonparoxysmal junctional tachycardia (NPJT) results from enhanced automaticity from cells in the AV node or common His bundle [28] or as a response to a trigger. NPJT is associated with acute myocardial infarction, hypokalemia, chronic obstructive lung disease with hypoxia, post-valvular cardiac surgery, CABG, myocarditis, and digitalis toxicity [25].

Junctional tachycardia is a narrow-complex regular tachycardia. Rates can be as high as 250 beats/min if paroxysmal, while nonparoxysmal JT rarely exceeds 120 beats/min. The P wave may precede, follow, or be buried in the QRS complex. The QRS complex can be wide if a BBB or aberrancy is present. The relationship between the atrial and ventricular rates is variable. If retrograde AV block is present, there will be AV dissociation and the atria may be in sinus rhythm. Otherwise, there will be a constant relationship between the QRS and the P wave with the P wave inverted in II, III, and aVF. If a junctional tachycardia is associated with atrial fibrillation, digitalis toxicity should be suspected [29].

Atrial Flutter with Fixed Conduction

Atrial flutter is a macro-reentrant atrial tachyarrhythmia with atrial rates ranging from 250 to 350 beats/min and a fixed or variable ventricular conduction. When there is a fixed atrioventricular block (usually 2:1), the resulting rhythm is narrow complex with a rate of approximately 150 beats/min. This characteristic rate should raise the suspicion for atrial flutter with a 2:1 block if it is steady. ECGs typically show a sawtooth appearance of the P wave with negative deflections in leads II, III, and aVF and no return to an isoelectric baseline. Ventricular rate varies based on AV nodal conduction and ranges from 1:1 to 4:1. In 1:1 conduction, ventricular depolarizations may appear as wide complex and can be associated with significant hemodynamic instability. When atrioventricular conduction is variable, the EKG will show an irregular narrow-complex tachycardia, which can be differentiated from atrial fibrillation or MAT by the presence of uniform flutter waves inferiorly or in V1.

Emergency Evaluation

Initial Assessment

In the initial evaluation of patients with SVT, assessment of clinical stability is paramount and will guide initial management decisions. In stable patients, a focused history and physical can aid in the diagnosis. Typical symptoms include palpitations, chest discomfort, dyspnea, fatigue, presyncope, and syncope. The regularity and character of onset of palpitations also provides useful information, as abrupt onset and termination with vagal stimulus (e.g., cough, Valsalva) are more likely to be related to an SVT while gradual onset is more likely sinus tachycardia. Syncope related to SVT can occur at the initiation and termination of SVT episodes due to low cardiac output or prolonged sinus pause, respectively. However, these are not typical and syncope with SVT may suggest an accessory pathway or structural heart disease. Finally, the diagnosis of hyperthyroidism should always be considered in patients with a first episode of SVT.

Physical examination is often noncontributory to the diagnosis of SVT. However, careful assessment of volume status can aid in evaluation of sinus tachycardia. Furthermore, evaluation for signs of hyperthyroidism, anemia, underlying cardiac disease (MVP, CHF), and chronic lung disease can help to delineate further essential workup. Directed diagnostic workup for SVT can include toxicologic screens for sympathomimetics or anticholinergics, thyroid function evaluation, chest X-ray to evaluate for signs of CHF or pulmonary disease, and cardiac troponin levels in patients with symptoms consistent with ischemia. However, mild troponinemia can be seen as a consequence of SVT and may lead to inappropriate anti-anginal therapy and coronary angiography.

Diagnostic Studies

ECG evaluation is the diagnostic test of choice and should focus on details previously discussed but should also include evaluation for signs of ischemia and underlying conduction abnormalities (e.g., Brugada). Additionally, one study shows that using an increased paper speed of 50 mm/sec can improve the diagnostic accuracy of physicians and prevent inappropriate dosing of adenosine [30]. Further studies include echocardiography to evaluate for structural heart disease and Holter monitor or event monitor to characterize transient arrhythmias, but these modalities are not usually emergently applicable.

Treatment

Patients with mild symptoms but without cardiovascular compromise may be managed on the outpatient basis with avoidance of precipitating factors (i.e., caffeine, alcohol, and illicit drugs) and further workup in primary care and cardiology clinic evaluations. However, patients with significant symptoms or sustained tachydysrhythmias must be managed expeditiously (Table 9.3). Initial evaluation and support of the patients' ABCs should be followed by appropriate placement of cardiopulmonary monitors and intravenous access. Patients who are unstable *due to their tachydysrhythmia* should be prepared for immediate synchronized cardioversion. Note that there are patients with atrial fibrillation with rapid ventricular response from septic shock who would benefit from aggressive volume repletion rather than focusing on the dysrhythmia, so management decisions clearly need to be in the context of the clinical evaluation. While preparing for cardioversion, vagal maneuvers and/or adenosine administration may be attempted if immediately available.

AV Nodal Blockade

Vagal maneuvers such as carotid sinus massage, Valsalva, and cold water facial immersion have been shown to terminate SVT in 30% of patients [31]. Valsalva was shown to be the most effective, accounting for 54% of successful terminations [32]. These maneuvers are most successful if the SVT is recent in onset as sympathetic tone increases with the duration of SVT [33].

Adenosine is an AV nodal blocking agent that has a short half-life (<10 s) and rapid onset of action. It can be used to determine the underlying rhythm or terminate certain SVTs (preferred for reentrant SVT). The initial dose of 6 mg should be given as a rapid push through a large bore proximal IV followed by a rapid saline

Table 9.3 Specific treatment considerations for supraventricular tachycardias

Diagnosis	Recommendations
Sinus tachycardia	Address underlying cause; beta-blockers for post-MI/CHF, thyrotoxicosis and anxiety-related symptoms.
Sinoatrial nodal reentrant tachycardia	Catheter ablation reserved for patients with significant symptomatic episodes not responsive to AV nodal blockade.
AVNRT	"Pill in the Pocket" approach may be recommended for patients with infrequent, well-tolerated AVNRT. Single-dose diltiazem + propranolol superior to flecainide and placebo. Chronic therapy with AV blockade or digoxin; second-line agents are flecainide/propafenone. Catheter ablation recommended if symptomatic and sustained AVNRT.
AVRT	Narrow complex (orthodromic): Treat with vagal maneuvers, AV blockade (can degenerate to VFib if WPW present). Wide complex (antidromic): Treat as VT, consider procainamide/amiodarone if stable and DC cardioversion if not. AFib/flutter with paroxysmal wide complex: Treat with cardioversion but procainamide or ibutilide can be used if stable. Catheter ablation is an option.
UAT	Secondary to micro-reentry. Sensitive to AV blockade and cardioversion but may require antiarrhythmics (Ia, Ic, III). UAT with AV block - > dig toxicity. Catheter ablation 86% success rate; 8% generate new focus.
MAT	Correct underlying pulmonary disease (hypoxia) and electrolyte abnormalities. Beta-blockade useful but controversial if caused by pulmonary disease.
Junctional tachycardia	AV blockade effective, antiarrhythmics (Ia, Ic, III) if refractory. Catheter ablation is definitive but 5–10% risk AV block. Consider dig toxicity, hypokalemia, COPD, MI, and myocarditis as causes.

flush, which is often facilitated with a three-way stopcock. If no change is noted, a second dose of 12 mg can be given. A randomized, double-blinded, placebo-controlled study has shown successful conversion of up to 60% of SVT with a 6-mg dose and 90% with a 12-mg dose [34, 35]. When given centrally, dosing should be halved (3 mg and 6 mg for initial and subsequent doses).

When not successful at conversion to sinus rhythm, adenosine can still provide information about the underlying rhythm, often with demonstration of atrial tachycardia with a high-grade AV block or the presence of an accessory pathway. Alternatively, the patients' rate may gradually slow and then resume the prior arrhythmia. Typically, AVRT, AVNRT, and SNRT will terminate with adenosine, while ST and JT will slow and then resume their prior rate. Atrial tachycardia, flutter, and fibrillation will reveal their underlying atrial rhythm with an AV block. Adenosine administration may be associated with significant side effects, including flushing, chest pain, headache, nausea, and a "sense of doom," all of which are usually self-limited [35], but it is prudent to advise the patient of these effects prior to administration. Some significant bradydysrhythmias and ventricular tachydysrhythmias have been reported with its use [36]. Adenosine should be used in lower doses (1–3 mg) in heart transplant patients, as they are particularly sensitive. Theophylline and caffeine may blunt the response to adenosine, while dipyridamole and carbamazepine may lead to heart block [25]. If WPW is suspected, nodal blocking agents should be avoided.

Nondihydropyridine calcium channel blockers slow conduction and increase refractoriness of the AV node, which can terminate reentrant arrhythmias and control ventricular rate. While they may decrease blood pressure, these effects can be mitigated with a continuous infusion [37] and/or pretreatment with calcium [38]. Studies have shown equivalence in efficacy and relapse with both diltiazem and verapamil [37]. Diltiazem can be given at an initial dose of 0.25 mg/kg and subsequent dose of 0.35 mg/kg if no response, while verapamil can be dosed at

2.5–5 mg initially with subsequent doses of 5–10 mg. However, these agents are not recommended in the setting of heart failure [25].

Beta-adrenergic blockade can decrease heart rate as well as blood pressure, with side effects including bradycardias and AV conduction delays. Metoprolol can be given as a 5 mg infusion over 2 minutes with repeat doses every 15 minutes. Propranolol infusion of 0.15 mg/kg can be given over 2 minutes, and esmolol can be bolused at 250–500 mcg/kg over 1 minute followed by 50 mcg/kg/min with titration to control heart rate (maximum dose 200 mcg/kg/min). These agents are contraindicated in second- and third-degree heart block, severe heart failure, lung disease with bronchospasm, and WPW.

Antidysrhythmic Therapy

Procainamide, ibutilide, flecainide, propafenone, and amiodarone can all be used for rhythm control in both SVT and atrial fibrillation/flutter with WPW. Procainamide (class IA) slows conduction by prolonging the refractory period of cardiac tissue and accessory pathways. It is given at a rate of 20 mg/min until the arrhythmia is suppressed, QRS duration prolongs more than 50%, hypotension occurs, or maximum dose is reached (17–20 mg/kg). If successful, continuous infusion of 1–4 mg/min can be initiated. Amiodarone is preferred in patients with severely depressed LVEF and is given as a bolus of 150 mg over 10 minutes followed by 1 mg/min for 6 hours and 0.5 mg/min over 18 hours. Initial treatment can include repeated boluses prior to starting an infusion if the clinical effects are not complete. Hypotension and bradycardia can occur as side effects which are mitigated by slowing the infusion.

DC Cardioversion

Synchronized cardioversion is the recommended treatment when the patient is unstable and is the preferred treatment for the patient with atrial fibrillation/flutter with WPW [19, 25, 39]. Shock delivery should be synchronized to prevent R on T phenomenon, which can degenerate into ventricular fibrillation. The initial dose for cardioversion is 50–100 J monophasic (30–50 J biphasic). However, some clinicians and studies report higher success rates by starting at higher energy levels. When possible, patients should be sedated prior to cardioversion. Cardioversion is not likely to be successful for junctional tachycardia or MAT.

Atrial Fibrillation

Atrial fibrillation (AF) is the most common atrial dysrhythmia encountered in the hospital setting, and the presentations range from asymptomatic to life threatening [40–42]. It is associated with increased strokes and thromboembolic events and accounts for significant healthcare expense with over 350,000 hospitalizations and 276,000 emergency department visits [43–45]. Risk factors include valvular heart disease, conduction system disorders, and pericardial disease [46]. Atrial fibrillation is often associated with electrolyte abnormalities, infection, hypoxia, thyrotoxicosis, pulmonary embolism, and digoxin toxicity [47–49]. AF is also common in the post-MI patient with up to 15% of ED patients with new-onset AF as a presenting sign of an MI [50–53].

Pathophysiology

AF originates from disorganized atrial depolarization, which is frequently associated with areas of fibrosis and loss of myocardium. These areas are prone to reentry circuits, which have a shortened refractory period and action potential [54]. AF can be triggered by many mechanisms, including autonomic stimulation, premature atrial beats, tachycardia, accessory pathways, atrial stretch, or abnormal foci in the pulmonary veins or vena cava [55]. Disorganized atrial activity results loss of contractile force, which when coupled with a rapid ventricular rate can lead to hemodynamic compromise [56, 57]. Prolonged AF with rapid ventricular rates can lead to dilated cardiomyopathy, which can make restoration and maintenance of sinus rhythm difficult [54, 58, 59].

Emergency Evaluation

Initial Assessment

The management of AF begins with an assessment of stability based on the patient's airway, breathing, and circulation. If signs of significant instability are present, early cardioversion is indicated. However, in the stable patient, additional information from the history, physical, and diagnostic tests may be useful in directing management. For example, cases of AF secondary to sepsis or hypovolemia may require an alternate resuscitation route than cardioversion.

A focused history should assess for clinical symptoms, including anxiety, palpitations, chest pain, dizziness, shortness of breath, or generalized weakness. In addition to vitals, the examination should focus on etiologies by evaluating for hyperthyroidism, DVT or pulmonary embolus, and signs of valvular disease or heart failure.

Diagnostic Studies

AF is distinguished on ECG with the presence of low-amplitude fibrillation with lack of discernable P waves and an irregularly irregular ventricular rhythm with a ventricular rate of up to 160 beats/minute. When coupled with WPW, the rhythm can look like VT, but is distinguished by its irregularity, variable QRS morphology, and rates above 250 beats/min.

Initial labs should focus on presumed etiologies and may include electrolyte panel, CBC, liver function tests, and coagulation profile. Thyroid function should be evaluated in patients older than 55, those which clinical symptoms consistent with hyperthyroidism, or those with difficult to control AF [60]. If risk factors or ECG findings of an acute coronary syndrome are present, cardiac markers should be drawn. Additional studies including drug screening, digoxin levels, theophylline levels, and pregnancy testing should be done when appropriate.

A chest X-ray may aid in the diagnosis of heart failure with the presence of pulmonary edema, valvular disease evidenced by an enlarged left atrium, or pulmonary embolism suggested by a Westermark sign. Focused cardiac ultrasound can help identify signs of right heart strain indicative of pulmonary embolism or dilated cardiomyopathy associated with valvular disease [61–63]. Additionally, ultrasound can help rule out other causes of hypotension, including tamponade and abdominal aortic aneurysm, as well as evaluate for signs of intravascular volume depletion [64, 65]. Formal transthoracic ultrasound may be obtained as part of the inpatient workup of AF, and can indicate causative factors as well as predict successful conversion to sinus rhythm based on left atrial size [66]. Transesophageal echocardiography may be necessary to evaluate for atrial thrombus if the duration of arrhythmia is unknown [67–73].

Treatment

The initial management of AF should focus on ensuring hemodynamic stability while treating symptoms and preventing thromboembolism [70]. As with all arrhythmias, initial stability does not preclude the potential for decompensation, so the provider should be prepared with cardiac monitoring, IV access, and supplemental oxygen.

Unstable Patient

ACLS guidelines state that cardioversion should be performed in patients with signs of shock or hemodynamic instability, which may include altered mental status, chest pain, or acute heart failure [74]. Additionally, patients with a wide-complex QRS which may suggest an accessory pathway should be treated with cardioversion. However, cardioversion may be unsuccessful if the AF is secondary to another disease process (sepsis, pulmonary embolism, tamponade, hypovolemia) or if it is longstanding. In these cases, treatment of hypovolemia with crystalloid resuscitation (30 ml/kg) [61] should be started early. Additionally, appropriate antibiotics, thrombolytics, pericardiocentesis, transfusion, and revascularization should be considered based on the etiology of AF.

Electrical cardioversion is a first-line treatment of AF, which can convert the patient to sinus rhythm. If indicated by hemodynamic instability, this therapy should not be withheld based on the concern for thromboembolism.

Synchronized cardioversion may be attempted starting with 50 J (biphasic) or 100 J (monophasic). However, studies have shown higher success rates with higher power (100 J – 60% conversion, 200 J – 90%) [75]. In addition, the application of manual pressure to the pads during cardioversion may enhance electrical conduction and increase success rates [76]. In an unstable patient who fails cardioversion, an alternative strategy is to pretreat with push dose phenylephrine (50–200 mcg Q1-2 minutes) to a goal diastolic pressure >60 mmHg prior to a slow infusion of amiodarone (150 mg bolus) or diltiazem (2.5 mg/min drip) [77]. Additionally, calcium pretreatment (5–10 ml of calcium gluconate or 1–3 ml of calcium chloride) may reduce the hypotensive effects of some calcium channel blockers [78–81].

Stable Patient

In the stable patient, the major management consideration is rate versus rhythm control. Multiple studies have shown no difference in mortality and stroke rate in patients treated with rate or rhythm control [82–88]. However, rhythm control may have the added benefit of decreasing hospital admissions for low-risk patients with new-onset AF of <48 hours [89–94]. Caveats to this practice include the fact that many patients cannot identify the onset of AF reliably [55, 95, 96]. Additionally, it is unclear whether rate control prior to cardioversion affects success rates [97, 98]. Alternatively, since nearly 50% of patients spontaneously convert, selected patients may be started on rate control and managed as an outpatient with next day follow-up.

Rate Control

Most rate control agents work by slowing conduction through the atrioventricular node. These agents should be avoided if there is any concern for preexcitation (accessory pathway). Typical agents include beta-blockers (e.g., esmolol, metoprolol, and propranolol) and nondihydropyridine calcium channel blockers (e.g., diltiazem, verapamil). Digoxin is a weak AV nodal blocker that works by increasing vagal tone.

Beta-blockers are the drug of choice in patients with heart failure, hypertension, or acute coronary syndrome. Propranolol is especially useful in the setting of hyperthyroidism. Beta-blockers should be used with caution in acute decompensated heart failure as well as in patients with obstructive pulmonary disease.

Nondihydropyridine calcium channel blockers are also first-line agents especially useful when there is a contraindication to beta blockade. Verapamil tends to have more potent negative inotropy and vasodilation [99]. Diltiazem has a faster onset than both propranolol and metoprolol [100, 101] and is more effective at rate control than digoxin or amiodarone [102].

Digoxin has both negative chronotropy and positive inotropy, which makes it particularly useful in heart failure with AF. It does not cause significant hypotension, but its action may take up to 3 hours [103]. Thus, digoxin is particularly useful as an adjunct to beta-blockers or calcium channel blockers and exerts a synergistic effect [104]. It should be noted though that the combination of atenolol with digoxin may precipitate severe bradycardia [118], while verapamil can increase digoxin levels [105].

Amiodarone is a second-line agent due to its slower onset and significant side effect profile [106]. It has less negative inotropy and, thus, may be useful in patients with significant hypotension or heart failure [107]. It can also promote cardioversion, so it should be used with caution in patients with high risk of thromboembolism.

Magnesium supplementation is an adjunctive therapy, which slows AV nodal conduction [108–113] without significant negative inotropy or other side effects. Rapid infusion, however, can be associated with respiratory muscle weakness, hypotension, and sinus pauses [108]. Magnesium can also promote conversion to sinus rhythm [109].

Rhythm Control

Rhythm control can be achieved through electrical or pharmacologic cardioversion. Studies have shown shorter ED length of stay as well as reduced recurrence of AF with cardioversion

[89, 90]. If electrical cardioversion is selected, the patient should be sedated prior to the procedure. Additionally, pretreatment with an antidysrhythmic (amiodarone, flecainide, ibutilide, propafenone) can increase the success of electrical cardioversion and should be considered if the initial electrical cardioversion attempt is unsuccessful.

Prior to pharmacologic cardioversion, a patient's electrolyte abnormalities should be corrected and QTc should be checked as many antidysrhythmics can prolong the QT. Procainamide (1 g over 60 minutes) is the most common choice with a success rate of up to 58% and low rate of adverse events. The most common complication is temporary hypotension [114]. Ibutilide (1 mg over 10 minutes) is another option, which side effects including QT prolongation and torsades. Amiodarone (5–7 mg/kg over 30–60 min followed by 1.2–1.8 g/day) is another alternative. Other agents include flecainide, propafenone, dofetilide, and quinidine.

Thromboembolic Risk

AF is strongly associated with increased risk of thromboembolic disease, especially in the postconversion period [115]. Stagnant blood flow due to poor contractility can predispose to clot formation. Cardioversion may also lead to atrial "stunning" in which atrial contraction may be impaired for weeks [116]. The rate of thromboembolic events after cardioversion ranges from 5% to 7% but drops to <2% if patients are anticoagulated for 2–4 weeks and have a negative transesophageal echocardiogram. If cardioversion is carried out within the first 48 hours of AF onset, the incidence of embolism is similar to that of anticoagulated patients [117]. However, studies have reported the presence of a clot in 13% of patients with AF for less than 72 hours.

Current recommendations from the ACC/AHA suggest that if patients require immediate cardioversion, they should be concurrently started on a heparin drip with a bolus and goal PTT of 1.5-2x normal. If cardioversion is not emergently required, the patient should be anticoagulated (INR 2–3) for 3 weeks prior and 4 weeks after cardioversion. Alternatively, a transesophageal echo can reliably rule out an atrial thrombus prior to cardioversion. However, these patients should also be concurrently anticoagulated with heparin. If a thrombus is identified, patients should be anticoagulated for at least 3 weeks prior and 4 weeks after cardioversion.

In patients who are not undergoing cardioversion, the risk of stroke should be evaluated in order to determine the need for anticoagulation. Multiple studies have validated the CHADS2-VASc scoring system for classifying risk of stroke in patients with AF. This method stratifies patients into low, moderate, and high risk. High-risk patients (>2 points) should be started on anticoagulation, while low-risk patients can be safely managed without anticoagulation. Moderate-risk patients require further risk stratification. However, even in the high-risk group, the yearly risk of stroke ranges from 2.2% to 11.2%, which extrapolates to a maximum daily risk of 0.03%. These numbers suggest that anticoagulation may be delayed without any significant increase in stroke risk, which may be appropriate for patients the potential for significant bleeding.

If a patient is considered low risk (<2% stroke risk per 100 patient years if on aspirin), the risk of bleeding with vitamin K antagonists is significantly higher than the benefits of stroke reduction [118]. For patients considered high risk (>4% stroke risk per 100 patient-years), the usage of vitamin K antagonists has been shown to improve survival [119]. Vitamin K antagonists reduce stroke risk by 66%, while aspirin alone reduces risk by 22% [120]. Adding clopidogrel to aspirin reduces stroke risk at the expense of increased major bleeding [120]. However, vitamin K antagonists carry a 0.4% increased risk of intracranial hemorrhage [121]. Other potential agents include rivaroxaban, dabigatran, and apixaban, which have been shown to be noninferior to warfarin for thromboembolism prevention. However, these agents carry additional risk due to the lack of available reversal agents.

Wide-Complex Tachycardias

Wide-complex tachycardias (WCT) are arrhythmias that occur with frequent concomitant clinical instability. Common etiologies of WCT include SVT with aberrant ventricular conduction, ventricular tachycardia (VT), preexcitation tachycardias, as well as toxic and metabolically mediated WCT. While a safe and effective treatment for most WCT includes DC cardioversion, a systematic approach to the diagnosis of WCT can suggest additional interventions likely to prevent recurrent episodes.

WCT is defined by a ventricular rate greater than 100 beats/min with a QRS duration of 120 ms or longer in adults. This significant dysrhythmia is one that is seen frequently in the emergency setting, with numbers ranging from 2 to 7 cases seen per month [122, 123]. The breakdown for causes of WCT is variable, with some studies showing 80% of WCT diagnosed as VT, while other studies suggest that the actual number is much lower (16%) when accounting for SVT with aberrancy and atrial fibrillation [124, 125].

Pathophysiology

In the most basic terms, WCT occurs when the conduction of electrical impulses through the ventricular myocardium is delayed. This delay can be secondary to a dysfunctional or damaged conduction system or the lack of utilization of the intact conduction system.

Ventricular Tachycardia

Ventricular tachycardia most often originates from a scar in the myocardium usually secondary to coronary artery disease and myocardial infarction [126, 127]. EPS studies in patients with prior MI often show significant inducible monomorphic ventricular tachycardia. Nonischemic cardiomyopathy also tends to generate scars which can promote VT.

Preexcitation Tachycardia

Preexcitation tachycardia can also manifest as a wide-complex tachycardia. This typically occurs in WPW as the impulse from the atria travels down the accessory pathway to the ventricular myocyte and propagates through the myocardium, resulting in a wide QRS. In this situation, the underlying rhythm may be atrial fibrillation, SVT, or antidromic reciprocating tachycardia.

Toxic and Metabolic Causes of Wide-Complex Tachycardia

Metabolic derangements and toxidromes can also generate WCT, with the most classic cases secondary to TCA overdose, hyperkalemia, and antiarrhythmic toxicity. The underlying pathophysiology of these derangements is a poisoning of the conduction system by an alteration of the function of ion channels. This effect can lead to both atrial and ventricular arrhythmias. Often, arrhythmias generated from toxic and metabolic causes can be refractory to standard management strategies. One common antidysrhythmics that can lead to malignant ventricular arrhythmias is sodium channel blockers (Class IC – propafenone, flecainide, with flecainide associated with high mortality in overdose [128]). Many other drugs, including class Ia and III antidysrhythmics, can lead to arrhythmias due to QT prolongation, which leads to torsades de pointes [129]. TCA toxicity is also associated with WCT that is worsened with acidosis and hyperthermia [130, 131]. This is typically manifested with an anticholinergic toxidrome and ECG findings of a deep S wave in lead I and a terminal R in aVR [132]. Hyperkalemia is another common source of conduction abnormalities. Elevated extracellular potassium causes persistent membrane depolarization, which slows conduction and leads to widened QRS rarely with a rate greater than 140. Slowing of conduction is evidenced on ECG by the lack of any rapid deflections in the QRS complex [133–136].

Pacemaker-Related Wide-Complex Tachycardia

In rare cases, a malfunctioning pacemaker can lead to VT. This runaway pacemaker can induce ventricular fibrillation and needs to be addressed emergently. In most modern pacemakers, the placement of a magnet over the device will default the device into asynchronous mode. If this does not terminate the rhythm, more drastic measures such as cutting the leads or removal of the pacemaker may be necessary. Other pacemaker-mediated WCT includes sensor-mediated tachycardia, where the activity sensor, which is meant to adjust heart rate to patient demands during exercise, inappropriately senses and elevates the ventricular rate. This can also occur if a pacemaker is sensing the atrial rate and responding during an SVT. Finally, if a retrograde pathway is present, impulses from pacemaker activation of the ventricle can travel to the atria and be sensed by the pacemaker as an atrial depolarization, inducing a response. These WCTs are usually limited by maximum rates, which are programmed into the device [137–140].

Emergency Evaluation

One of the fundamentals of management of VT is the recognition that typical interventions for VT will not have deleterious effects if the actual arrhythmia is SVT, but the converse is not true. Accordingly, if there is any uncertainty, the default diagnosis of VT should be assumed and treatment should proceed along this algorithm. Another common misconception is that hemodynamic stability in the setting of WCT favors SVT [141]. However, hemodynamic instability should trigger an immediate intervention including telemetry monitoring and frequent BP checks [142–144], deferring the history and physical until stability is achieved.

Initial Assessment

Certain specific history elements can significantly increase the likelihood of a ventricular arrhythmia. These include history of MI, CHF, or unstable angina. In one retrospective univariate analysis, these features were associated with high positive likelihood ratios (>6) and low negative likelihood ratios (<0.5). Additional useful historical elements include ESRD, presence of pacemaker or ICD, history of ingestion of suicide attempt, and home medications that are dysrhythmogenic (TCA, digoxin, antidysrhythmics). These elements have been shown to differentiate VT from SVT with statistical significance [125] and can hint at the cause of the WCT, leading to specific steps in management (i.e., empiric treatment of hyperkalemia). History of CABG, PCI, or valvular disease does not carry the same weight in differentiating VT from SVT as these diagnoses are not necessarily associated with myocardial scarring, which is the prime etiology of VT. Age less than 35 also should not favor SVT over VT as approximately 10% of cases of WCT in this age group are VT.

Physical exam findings are rarely useful, but specific findings of AV dissociation include irregular cannon "a" waves and variations in the intensity of the first heart sound (S1) [145]. Additionally, the physical presence of a dialysis catheter, AV graft, or pacemaker can identify a patient's risk for VT.

Diagnostic Studies

The single most important laboratory test for the management of WCT is electrolytes, as derangements in potassium and magnesium can trigger arrhythmias as well as reduce the success of electrical conversion. Troponin and BNP may be helpful in determining etiology but rarely change initial management. Laboratory studies which can generate results within minutes (i.e., blood gas with electrolytes) are most useful as pH and electrolyte measurements can significantly change the initial management.

Detailed analysis of the ECG to differentiate supraventricular and ventricular WCT should be forgone in patients with hemodynamic instability. These patients should receive immediate electrical cardioversion. However, it should be kept in mind that WCT resulting from metabolic or drug toxicities may be resistant to cardioversion.

The first step toward the diagnosis of WCT is to obtain a 12-lead ECG. This will help to differentiate artifacts and pacemaker-related WCT (revealed by pacer spikes) from other etiologies.

If possible, a prior ECG can significantly aid in the diagnosis of WCT. If the wide QRS beats during sinus rhythm have a significantly different morphology or axis from the QRS complexes during WCT, a diagnosis of VT is strongly suggested. The converse can be cautiously suggested but significant exceptions exist [146–148]. A baseline ECG with a narrow complex is less helpful in the diagnosis of WCT.

Given the patient is still hemodynamically stable, the WCT can be classified into irregular or regular rhythm. Irregular WCT is usually polymorphic VT, AF with AVC, or AF with antegrade conduction down an accessory pathway (AF with WPW). Polymorphic VT is characterized by a rate >200 beats/min and significant variability in QRS amplitude [149]. AF with AVC usually has a rate <200 beats/min with a relatively stable QRS amplitude. AF with preexcitation usually has rates >200 beats/min with beat-to-beat variability of QRS morphology and amplitude. Regular WCT can be broken down into monomorphic VT, regular SVT with AVC, SVT with preexcitation, or pacemaker-related WCT.

There are numerous criteria to distinguish different etiologies of WCT. These include the Brugada criteria as well as the Griffith criteria. In order to be clinically useful, these criteria must be sensitive, simple, and easy to recall. The Griffith criteria come close to these standards and provide a way to characterize both regular and irregular WCT. These criteria use the QRS morphology, axis, and presence of AV dissociation to identify VT. The presence of AV dissociation (fusion or capture beats) in any case is pathognomonic for VT, but this occurs rarely. The remainder of the Griffith criteria deal with the QRS morphology and axis. Using this framework, a regular WCT with a classic RBBB without a northwest axis (180–270°) is suggestive of SVT with AVC. Alternatively, a regular WCT with classic LBBB without a right (90–180) or northwest (180–270) axis is suggestive of SVT with AVC. All other WCT should be considered VT. While these criteria can lead to misdiagnosis of SVT with AVC or preexcitation as VT, it leads to safer ED management the use of VT appropriate drugs. In diagnosing irregular WCT, polymorphic VT must first be excluded (rate >200 beats/min with variable amplitude QRS complexes). If a classic LBBB or RBBB is present, the suggested diagnosis is AF with AVC. Otherwise, all other irregular WCTs should be labeled AF with preexcitation. Again, this methodology can misclassify AF with AVC as AF with preexcitation, but this leads to a safer management algorithm rather than the opposite.

Treatment

The treatment of WCT is primarily dependent on the clinical presentation and degree of hemodynamic stability of the patient (Table 9.4.). As

Table 9.4 Differential diagnosis for wide-complex tachycardia

Diagnosis	Considerations
Supraventricular tachycardia with aberrancy	Abnormal intraventricular conduction delay in His–Purkinje system during SVT (transient or preexisting)
Ventricular tachycardia	Originates from the ventricular myocardium Monomorphic – secondary to scar tissue (structural HD, prior MI, NICM) – more inducible in patients with prior MI than in those with CAD Polymorphic
Preexcitation tachycardia	WPW – impulse flows down accessory pathway external to AV node and His–Purkinje Subtypes – antidromic reciprocating tachycardia, atrial fib with preexcitation, SVT with preexcitation
Toxic and metabolic causes	Poisoning of the conduction system – requires specific interventions Antiarrhythmic overdose – sodium channel blockade – leads to arrhythmia, electromechanical dissociation, asystole Flecainide overdose – high mortality (8%) – mechanism QRS prolongation and torsades TCA toxicity – hypotension and WCT – sinus with BBB, VT, VF
Pacemaker-related WCT	Runaway pacemaker, sensor-mediated WCT, endless loop tachycardia

discussed earlier, an analysis of the rhythm is useful to direct therapy, but it is not essential for appropriate and safe medical management. Clinical instability is evidenced by hypoperfusion, coronary ischemia, altered mental status, pulmonary edema, or a rapid rate. Any WCT can rapidly deteriorate into VF and the presence of signs of instability should prompt immediate interventions (i.e., defibrillation).

For the unstable patient, synchronized cardioversion is the treatment of choice and should be performed as many times as necessary. Patients with recurrent unstable VT should also receive an IV antiarrhythmic. First-line agent is amiodarone (bolus 300 mg, 150 mg, then 1 mg/min × 6 hours and 0.5 mg/min × 18 hours), and lidocaine is another option (1–1.5 mg/kg IV with repeat doses 0.5–0.75 mg/kg up to max 3 mg/kg and infusion of 1–4 mg/min).

For stable patients, synchronized cardioversion should be immediately available but attempts at medical management can be made. Procainamide is the drug of choice for termination of stable VT (77% termination rate) versus amiodarone (30%) and lidocaine (27%) [150–153]. Additionally, procainamide blocks accessory pathways which can terminate preexcitation tachycardias. Procainamide can be given until the arrhythmia terminates or one of the following: hypotension, QRS prolongation >50% of baseline, worsening tachycardia, or total 17 mg/kg administered. Rapid loading can be achieved with rates of 100 mg/min to a max dose of 10 mg/kg [151]. Maintenance dosing is 1–4 mg/min with lower doses for renal insufficiency.

Amiodarone and lidocaine are also viable options for the treatment of stable VT or preexcitation tachycardia. Amiodarone is given as a bolus dose of 150 mg over 10 minutes with maintenance of 1 mg/min over 6 hours and 0.5 mg/min over 18 hours. Additional bolus doses can be given as needed. Lidocaine is less effective than amiodarone and procainamide [153–155] for both VT and preexcitation tachycardia. For stable VT, the dose is 0.5–1.5 mg/kg over 2 minutes with repeat doses of 0.5–0.75 mg/kg every 5–10 minutes and an infusion of 1–4 mg/min (max dose 3 mg/kg) [150, 156, 157].

If there is a strong suggestion based on the Griffith criteria that a WCT is actually SVT with AVC (if regular) or AF with AVC (if irregular), then the treatment algorithm can proceed in a slightly different path for the stable patient. Take note that if there is any doubt to the diagnosis, the default treatment path should be that of VT/preexcitation, as the consequences of using AV nodal blockade in the setting of preexcitation can lead to cardiovascular collapse.

In patients with SVT with AVC, AV nodal blocking agents are the drugs of choice after attempts at vagal maneuvers. Adenosine is the first line, with the initial dose of 6 mg rapid IV push through a large IV followed by 12 mg if unsuccessful. Typically this will result in conversion to sinus rhythm or slowing of the ventricular response. Alternative agents are beta-blockers and calcium channel blockers. Diltiazem can be given as multiple bolus doses (0.25 mg–0.35 mg/kg per dose) followed by a maintenance dose (5–15 mg/hr) or oral loading dose if successful. Metoprolol can be given as 5 mg IV doses every 5 minutes for up to 3 doses. Alternatively, esmolol can be started as a loading dose of 0.5 mg/kg over 1 minute followed by an infusion of 0.05 mg/kg/min over 4 minutes. This can be repeated with an increase in the infusion to 0.1 mg/kg/min if unsuccessful. Significant side effects for these agents include bradycardias, hypotension, and pulmonary edema.

Polymorphic VT is another WCT characterized by a high rate (>200 beats/min) and significant QRS amplitude variability. This rhythm can quickly degenerate into VF. Sustained polymorphic VT is typically an unstable rhythm, but some patients can demonstrate recurrent episodes that are self-limited. If unstable, the treatment of choice is cardioversion. Otherwise, the first step to management is determination of the QT interval as polymorphic VT with a prolonged QT is torsades de pointes, while a normal QT interval suggests myocardial ischemia. In the case of suspected myocardial ischemia, the treatment of choice is beta blockade, amiodarone, and early cardiac catheterization. Beta blockade can be with propranolol (0.15 mg/kg over 10 minutes and 3–5 mg Q6 hours), esmolol (300–500 mg/kg over 1 minute and 25–50 mg/kg/min maintenance), or metoprolol (5 mg IV every 5 minutes for 3 doses with an oral dose of 50 mg every 6 hours). Amiodarone is typically dosed as 150-mg bolus followed by an infusion. Lidocaine can also be used as an alternative at previously mentioned doses. If torsades de pointes is suspected, rapid correction of electrolytes, especially magnesium and potassium, is essential. Patients should be given 2-gm bolus dose of IV magnesium sulfate, which can be repeated if VT persists. Since tachycardia shortens QT intervals, other treatment modalities may also be useful. Transvenous or transcutaneous pacing can be initiated, especially if the underlying rhythm is bradycardic. Alternatively, isoproterenol (1–4 mcg/min) can be used as long as the patient does not have significant hypertension, myocardial ischemia, or history of congenital long QT syndrome, which can predispose the patient to malignant arrhythmias. Finally, while lidocaine can also be used for polymorphic VT with a prolonged QT, amiodarone should be avoided as it causes QT prolongation.

Pacemaker-mediated WCT is a rare cause of wide-complex tachycardia whose management is significantly different than other etiologies. If this diagnosis is suspected, an ECG should be obtained before and after placement of a magnet on the pacemaker. Pacer spikes should be clearly seen before each QRS complex. The application of a magnet to the pacemaker will terminate most pacemaker-mediated WCT. Specific changes to pacemaker settings can then be made in consultation with a cardiologist.

WCT mediated by drug toxicity or metabolic derangements can often be resistant to cardioversion. These patients can present with significant hemodynamic instability, requiring inotropes, pressors, and even mechanical support (ECMO, balloon pump) [158]. Toxicity secondary to class 1 antiarrhythmic toxicity (propafenone, flecainide) can be treated with sodium bicarbonate. The increased concentration of sodium overcomes the channel blockade and can terminate the dysrhythmia. Often times, the amount of sodium bicarbonate required is high (ranging from 200 to 450 meq, 3 meq/kg) [159–161]. Sodium bicarbonate is also essential to treatment of TCA toxicity, with the initial dose of 1–2 meg/kg given as an IV bolus with continuous monitoring of the ECG. Treatment is titrated to narrowing of the QRS complex and goal pH of 7.5–7.55. Lidocaine and amiodarone are also options for treatment of flecainide toxicity [162, 163]. The treatment of hyperkalemia involves the use of membrane-stabilizing agents (calcium), transient shifting agents (sodium bicarbonate, albuterol, insulin, dextrose, magnesium sulfate), and removal agents (polystyrene binding resins and hemodialysis).

Conclusion

Cardiac dysrhythmias are often life-threatening problems requiring immediate and appropriately directed interventions to stabilize the patient. However, a systematic approach can lead to the correct diagnostic and treatment steps whether dealing with bradydysrhythmias or tachydysrhythmias. In many cases, treatment of the dysrhythmia and stabilization of the patient may precede the determination of the etiology. Regardless, a reasoned approach as is laid out in this chapter should lead to the safe and effective management of cardiac dysrhythmias in the emergency and critical care setting.

References

1. Brady WJ, et al. The efficacy of atropine in the treatment of hemodynamically unstable bradycardia and atrioventricular block: prehospital and emergency department considerations. Resuscitation. 1999;41(1):47–55.
2. Bernheim A, et al. Atropine often results in complete atrioventricular block or sinus arrest after cardiac transplantation: an unpredictable and dose-independent phenomenon. Transplantation. 2004;77(8):1181–5.
3. The American Heart Association in collaboration with the International Liaison Committee on Resuscitation. American Heart Association Guidelines for Cardiopulmonary Resuscitation and Emergency Cardiovascular Care. Part 7.3: Management of symptomatic bradycardia and tachycardia. Circulation. 2005;112(24_supplement):IV-67-IV-77.
4. Momeni M, et al. Anaphylactic shock in a beta-blocked child: usefulness of isoproterenol. Paediatr Anaesth. 2007;17(9):897–9.

5. Truitt CA, et al. Outcomes of unintentional beta-blocker or calcium channel blocker overdoses: a retrospective review of poison center data. J Med Toxicol. 2012;8(2):135–9.
6. Love JN, et al. A potential role for glucagon in the treatment of drug-induced symptomatic bradycardia. Chest. 1998;114(1):323–6.
7. Ma G, et al. Electrocardiographic manifestations: digitalis toxicity. J Emerg Med. 2001;20(2):145–52.
8. Tanaka H, Monahan KD, Seals DR. Age-predicted maximal heart rate revisited. J Am Coll Cardiol. 2001;37(1):153–6.
9. Morelli A, et al. Effect of heart rate control with esmolol on hemodynamic and clinical outcomes in patients with septic shock: a randomized clinical trial. JAMA. 2013;310(16):1683–91.
10. Cheung DW. Electrical activity of the pulmonary vein and its interaction with the right atrium in the guinea-pig. J Physiol. 1980;314:445–56.
11. Cheung DW. Pulmonary vein as an ectopic focus in digitalis-induced arrhythmia. Nature. 1981;294(5841):582–4.
12. Wellens HJ. 25 years of insights into the mechanisms of supraventricular arrhythmias. Heart Rhythm. 2004;1(5 Suppl):19C–25C.
13. Gomes JA, Mehta D, Langan MN. Sinus node reentrant tachycardia. Pacing Clin Electrophysiol. 1995;18(5 Pt 1):1045–57.
14. Goyal R, et al. Comparison of the ages of tachycardia onset in patients with atrioventricular nodal reentrant tachycardia and accessory pathway-mediated tachycardia. Am Heart J. 1996;132(4):765–7.
15. Kumar UN, Rao RK, Scheinman MM. The 12-lead electrocardiogram in supraventricular tachycardia. Cardiol Clin. 2006;24(3):427–37, ix.
16. Delacretaz E. Supraventricular tachycardia. N Engl J Med. 2006;354(10):1039–51.
17. Rodriguez LM, et al. Age at onset and gender of patients with different types of supraventricular tachycardias. Am J Cardiol. 1992;70(13):1213–5.
18. Lau EW, et al. Electrocardiographic criteria for diagnosis of irregular broad complex tachycardia with a high sensitivity for preexcited atrial fibrillation. Pacing Clin Electrophysiol. 2000;23(12):2040–5.
19. Fengler BT, et al. Atrial fibrillation in the Wolff-Parkinson-white syndrome: ECG recognition and treatment in the ED. Am J Emerg Med. 2007;25:576–83.
20. Steinbeck G, Hoffmann E. 'True' atrial tachycardia. Eur Heart J. 1998;19(Suppl E):E10-2, E48.
21. Ko JK, et al. Supraventricular tachycardia mechanisms and their age distribution in pediatric patients. Am J Cardiol. 1992;69(12):1028–32.
22. Gillette PC. The mechanisms of supraventricular tachycardia in children. Circulation. 1976;54(1):133–9.
23. Wu MH, et al. Radiofrequency catheter ablation of tachycardia in children with and without congenital heart disease: indications and limitations. Int J Cardiol. 2000;72(3):221–7.
24. Garson A, Gillette PC. Electrophysiologic studies of supraventricular tachycardia in children. I. Clinical-electrophysiologic correlations. Am Heart J. 1981;102(2):233–50.
25. Blomstrom-Lundqvist C, et al. ACC/AHA/ESC guidelines for the management of patients with supraventricular arrhythmias--executive summary: a report of the American College of Cardiology/American Heart Association Task Force on Practice Guidelines and the European Society of Cardiology Committee for Practice Guidelines (Writing Committee to develop guidelines for the management of patients with Supraventricular Arrhythmias). Circulation. 2003;108(15):1871–909.
26. McCord J, Borzak S. Multifocal atrial tachycardia. Chest. 1998;113(1):203–9.
27. Ruder MA, et al. Clinical and electrophysiologic characterization of automatic junctional tachycardia in adults. Circulation. 1986;73(5):930–7.
28. Lee KL, et al. Effect of adenosine and verapamil in catecholamine-induced accelerated atrioventricular junctional rhythm: insights into the underlying mechanism. Pacing Clin Electrophysiol. 1999;22(6 Pt 1):866–70.
29. Castellanos A, Sung RJ, Myerburg RJ. His bundle electrocardiography in digitalis-induced "atrioventricular junctional" Wenckebach periods with irregular H-H intervals. Am J Cardiol. 1979;43(3):653–6.
30. Accardi AJ, Miller R, Holmes JF. Enhanced diagnosis of narrow complex tachycardias with increased electrocardiograph speed. J Emerg Med. 2002;22(2):123–6.
31. Lim SH, et al. Comparison of treatment of supraventricular tachycardia by Valsalva maneuver and carotid sinus massage. Ann Emerg Med. 1998;31(1):30–5.
32. Mehta D, et al. Relative efficacy of various physical manoeuvres in the termination of junctional tachycardia. Lancet. 1988;1(8596):1181–5.
33. Ferguson JD, DiMarco JP. Contemporary management of paroxysmal supraventricular tachycardia. Circulation. 2003;107(8):1096–9.
34. Dimarco JP, Miles W, Akhtar M. Adenosine for paroxysmal supraventricular tachycardia: dose ranging and comparison with verapamil. Assessment in placebo-controlled, multicenter trials. The Adenosine for PSVT Study Group. Ann Intern Med. 1990;113(2):104–10.
35. Holdgate A, Ching N, Angonese L. Variability in agreement between physicians and nurses when measuring the Glasgow Coma Scale in the emergency department limits its clinical usefulness. Emerg Med Australas. 2006;18(4):379–84.
36. Mallet ML. Proarrhythmic effects of adenosine: a review of the literature. Emerg Med J. 2004;21(4):408–10.
37. Lim SH, Anantharaman V, Teo WS. Slow-infusion of calcium channel blockers in the emergency management of supraventricular tachycardia. Resuscitation. 2002;52(2):167–74.

38. Moser LR, Smythe MA, Tisdale JE. The use of calcium salts in the prevention and management of verapamil-induced hypotension. Ann Pharmacother. 2000;34(5):622–9.
39. Tijunelis MA, Herbert ME. Myth: intravenous amiodarone is safe in patients with atrial fibrillation and Wolff-Parkinson-white syndrome in the emergency department. CJEM. 2005;7(4):262–5.
40. Fuster V, et al. ACC/AHA/ESC guidelines for the Management of Patients with Atrial Fibrillation: executive summary a report of the American College of Cardiology/American Heart Association Task Force on practice guidelines and the European Society of Cardiology Committee for practice guidelines and policy conferences (Committee to develop guidelines for the management of patients with Atrial Fibrillation) developed in collaboration with the North American Society of Pacing and Electrophysiology. Circulation. 2001;104(17):2118–50.
41. European Heart Rhythm Association, E.A.f.C.-T.S, Camm AJ, et al. Guidelines for the management of atrial fibrillation: the Task Force for the management of atrial fibrillation of the European Society of Cardiology (ESC). Eur Heart J. 2010;31(19):2369–429.
42. Naccarelli GV, et al. Increasing prevalence of atrial fibrillation and flutter in the United States. Am J Cardiol. 2009;104(11):1534–9.
43. Lanzarotti CJ, Olshansky B. Thromboembolism in chronic atrial flutter: is the risk underestimated? J Am Coll Cardiol. 1997;30(6):1506–11.
44. Ghali WA, et al. Atrial flutter and the risk of thromboembolism: a systematic review and meta-analysis. Am J Med. 2005;118(2):101–7.
45. Coyne KS, et al. Assessing the direct costs of treating nonvalvular atrial fibrillation in the United States. Value Health. 2006;9(5):348–56.
46. Kannel WB, et al. Epidemiologic features of chronic atrial fibrillation: the Framingham study. N Engl J Med. 1982;306(17):1018–22.
47. Benjamin EJ, et al. Independent risk factors for atrial fibrillation in a population-based cohort. The Framingham Heart Study. JAMA. 1994;271(11):840–4.
48. Pollock GF. Atrial fibrillation in the ED: cardioversion, rate control, anticoagulation, and more. Emergency Medicine Practice. 2002;4(8):1–28.
49. Badheka AO, et al. Influence of obesity on outcomes in atrial fibrillation: yet another obesity paradox. Am J Med. 2010;123(7):646–51.
50. Friedman HZ, et al. Acute complications associated with new-onset atrial fibrillation. Am J Cardiol. 1991;67(5):437–9.
51. Zimetbaum PJ, et al. Incidence and predictors of myocardial infarction among patients with atrial fibrillation. J Am Coll Cardiol. 2000;36(4):1223–7.
52. Laurent G, et al. Atrial fibrillation during myocardial infarction with and without ST segment elevation. Arch Mal Coeur Vaiss. 2005;98(6):608–14.
53. Meshkat N, et al. Troponin utilization in patients presenting with atrial fibrillation/flutter to the emergency department: retrospective chart review. Int J Emerg Med. 2011;4(1):25.
54. Fuster V, et al. ACC/AHA/ESC 2006 guidelines for the management of patients with atrial fibrillation-executive summary: a report of the American College of Cardiology/American Heart Association Task Force on practice guidelines and the European Society of Cardiology Committee for practice guidelines (Writing Committee to revise the 2001 guidelines for the management of patients with atrial fibrillation). Eur Heart J. 2006;27(16):1979–2030.
55. Allessie MA, et al. Pathophysiology and prevention of atrial fibrillation. Circulation. 2001;103(5):769–77.
56. Ruskin J, et al. Pressure-flow studies in man: effect of atrial systole on left ventricular function. J Clin Invest. 1970;49(3):472–8.
57. Rahimtoola SH, et al. Left atrial transport function in myocardial infarction. Importance of its booster pump function. Am J Med. 1975;59(5):686–94.
58. Grogan M, et al. Left ventricular dysfunction due to atrial fibrillation in patients initially believed to have idiopathic dilated cardiomyopathy. Am J Cardiol. 1992;69(19):1570–3.
59. Iga K, et al. Reversible left ventricular dysfunction secondary to rapid atrial fibrillation. Int J Cardiol. 1993;41(1):59–64.
60. Frost L, Vestergaard P, Mosekilde L. Hyperthyroidism and risk of atrial fibrillation or flutter: a population-based study. Arch Intern Med. 2004;164(15):1675–8.
61. Weekes AJ, Zapata RJ, Napolitano A. Symptomatic hypotension: ED stabilization and the emerging role of sonography. EM Pract. 2007;9:1–28.
62. Perera P, et al. The RUSH exam: rapid ultrasound in SHock in the evaluation of the critically ill. Emerg Med Clin North Am. 2010;28(1):29–56, vii.
63. Atkinson PR, et al. Abdominal and Cardiac Evaluation with Sonography in Shock (ACES): an approach by emergency physicians for the use of ultrasound in patients with undifferentiated hypotension. Emerg Med J. 2009;26(2):87–91.
64. Dipti A, et al. Role of inferior vena cava diameter in assessment of volume status: a meta-analysis. Am J Emerg Med. 2012;30(8):1414–1419.e1.
65. Barbier C, et al. Respiratory changes in inferior vena cava diameter are helpful in predicting fluid responsiveness in ventilated septic patients. Intensive Care Med. 2004;30(9):1740–6.
66. Brodsky MA, et al. Factors determining maintenance of sinus rhythm after chronic atrial fibrillation with left atrial dilatation. Am J Cardiol. 1989;63(15):1065–8.
67. Silverman DI, Manning WJ. Role of echocardiography in patients undergoing elective cardioversion of atrial fibrillation. Circulation. 1998;98(5):479–86.
68. Moreyra E, Finkelhor RS, Cebul RD. Limitations of transesophageal echocardiography in the risk assessment of patients before nonanticoagulated cardio-

version from atrial fibrillation and flutter: an analysis of pooled trials. Am Heart J. 1995;129(1):71–5.
69. Manning WJ, et al. Cardioversion from atrial fibrillation without prolonged anticoagulation with use of transesophageal echocardiography to exclude the presence of atrial thrombi. N Engl J Med. 1993;328(11):750–5.
70. Black IW, et al. Evaluation of transesophageal echocardiography before cardioversion of atrial fibrillation and flutter in nonanticoagulated patients. Am Heart J. 1993;126(2):375–81.
71. Corrado G, et al. Atrial thrombi resolution after prolonged anticoagulation in patients with atrial fibrillation. Chest. 1999;115(1):140–3.
72. Klein AL, et al. Use of transesophageal echocardiography to guide cardioversion in patients with atrial fibrillation. N Engl J Med. 2001;344(19):1411–20.
73. Klein AL, et al. Cardioversion guided by transesophageal echocardiography: the ACUTE Pilot Study. A randomized, controlled trial. Assessment of cardioversion using transesophageal echocardiography. Ann Intern Med. 1997;126(3):200–9.
74. Neumar RW, et al. Part 8: adult advanced cardiovascular life support: 2010 American Heart Association guidelines for cardiopulmonary resuscitation and emergency cardiovascular care. Circulation. 2010;122(18 Suppl 3):S729–67.
75. Page RL, et al. Biphasic versus monophasic shock waveform for conversion of atrial fibrillation: the results of an international randomized, double-blind multicenter trial. J Am Coll Cardiol. 2002;39(12):1956–63.
76. Cohen TJ, et al. Active compression cardioversion for refractory atrial fibrillation. Am J Cardiol. 1997;80(3):354–5.
77. Weingart S. The crashing atrial fibrillation patient. In: Weingart S, editor. The EMCrit blog; 2012. http://emcrit.org/podcasts/crashing-a-fib/.
78. Allen R. Preventing hypotension effect of calcium channel blockers. Am Fam Physician. 2003;67(5):940; author reply 940–1.
79. Lipman J, et al. Intravenous calcium chloride as an antidote to verapamil-induced hypotension. Intensive Care Med. 1982;8(1):55–7.
80. Midtbo K, Hals O. Can blood pressure reduction induced by slow calcium channel blockade (verapamil) be reversed by calcium infusion? Pharmacol Toxicol. 1987;60(5):330–2.
81. Weiss AT, et al. The use of calcium with verapamil in the management of supraventricular tachyarrhythmias. Int J Cardiol. 1983;4(3):275–84.
82. Hohnloser SH, Kuck KH, Lilienthal J. Rhythm or rate control in atrial fibrillation--Pharmacological Intervention in Atrial Fibrillation (PIAF): a randomised trial. Lancet. 2000;356(9244):1789–94.
83. Wyse DG, et al. A comparison of rate control and rhythm control in patients with atrial fibrillation. N Engl J Med. 2002;347(23):1825–33.
84. Van Gelder IC, et al. A comparison of rate control and rhythm control in patients with recurrent persistent atrial fibrillation. N Engl J Med. 2002;347(23):1834–40.
85. Carlsson J, et al. Randomized trial of rate-control versus rhythm-control in persistent atrial fibrillation: the Strategies of Treatment of Atrial Fibrillation (STAF) study. J Am Coll Cardiol. 2003;41(10):1690–6.
86. Opolski G, et al. Rate control vs rhythm control in patients with nonvalvular persistent atrial fibrillation: the results of the polish how to treat chronic atrial fibrillation (HOT CAFE) study. Chest. 2004;126(2):476–86.
87. Roy D, et al. Rhythm control versus rate control for atrial fibrillation and heart failure. N Engl J Med. 2008;358(25):2667–77.
88. Ogawa S, et al. Optimal treatment strategy for patients with paroxysmal atrial fibrillation: J-RHYTHM Study. Circ J. 2009;73(2):242–8.
89. Stiell IG, et al. Association of the Ottawa Aggressive Protocol with rapid discharge of emergency department patients with recent-onset atrial fibrillation or flutter. CJEM. 2010;12(3):181–91.
90. Scheuermeyer FX, Grafstein E, Stenstrom R. Thirty-day outcomes of emergency department patients undergoing electrical cardioversion for atrial fibrillation or flutter. Acad Emerg Med. 2010;17(4):408–15.
91. Cristoni L, et al. Cardioversion of acute atrial fibrillation in the short observation unit: comparison of a protocol focused on electrical cardioversion with simple antiarrhythmic treatment. Emerg Med J. 2011;28(11):932–7.
92. Doyle B, Reeves M. "Wait and see" approach to the emergency department cardioversion of acute atrial fibrillation. Emerg Med Int. 2011;2011:545023.
93. Stiell IG, Macle L, C.C.S.A.F.G. Committee. Canadian Cardiovascular Society atrial fibrillation guidelines 2010: management of recent-onset atrial fibrillation and flutter in the emergency department. Can J Cardiol. 2011;27(1):38–46.
94. Bellone A, et al. Cardioversion of acute atrial fibrillation in the emergency department: a prospective randomised trial. Emerg Med J. 2012;29(3):188–91.
95. Abarbanell NR, et al. Prehospital management of rapid atrial fibrillation: recommendations for treatment protocols. Am J Emerg Med. 2001;19(1):6–9.
96. Camm AJ, Camm CF, Savelieva I. Medical treatment of atrial fibrillation. J Cardiovasc Med (Hagerstown). 2012;13(2):97–107.
97. Blecher GE, et al. Use of rate control medication before cardioversion of recent-onset atrial fibrillation or flutter in the emergency department is associated with reduced success rates. CJEM. 2012;14(3):169–77.
98. Scheuermeyer FX, et al. Thirty-day and 1-year outcomes of emergency department patients with atrial fibrillation and no acute underlying medical cause. Ann Emerg Med. 2012;60(6):755–765.e2.
99. Phillips BG, et al. Comparison of intravenous diltiazem and verapamil for the acute treatment of atrial fibrillation and atrial flutter. Pharmacotherapy. 1997;17(6):1238–45.

100. Demircan C, et al. Comparison of the effectiveness of intravenous diltiazem and metoprolol in the management of rapid ventricular rate in atrial fibrillation. Emerg Med J. 2005;22(6):411–4.
101. Lip GYH, Tse H-F. Management of atrial fibrillation. Lancet. 2007;370(9587):604–18.
102. Siu C-W, et al. Intravenous diltiazem is superior to intravenous amiodarone or digoxin for achieving ventricular rate control in patients with acute uncomplicated atrial fibrillation. Crit Care Med. 2009;37(7):2174–9; quiz 2180.
103. Jacob S, et al. Pharmacotherapy of atrial fibrillation: a pathophysiological perspective and review. Am J Ther. 2011;18(3):241–60.
104. Cheng JWM, Rybak I. Use of digoxin for heart failure and atrial fibrillation in elderly patients. Am J Geriatr Pharmacother. 2010;8(5):419–27.
105. Lee G. A review of the literature on atrial fibrillation: rate reversion or control? J Clin Nurs. 2007;16(1):77–83.
106. Hou ZY, et al. Acute treatment of recent-onset atrial fibrillation and flutter with a tailored dosing regimen of intravenous amiodarone. A randomized, digoxin-controlled study. Eur Heart J. 1995;16(4):521–8.
107. Lie KI, van Gelder IC. Therapy of recent onset atrial fibrillation and flutter in haemodynamically compromised patients: chemical conversion or control of the ventricular rate? Eur Heart J. 1995;16(4):433–4.
108. Brodsky MA, et al. Magnesium therapy in new-onset atrial fibrillation. Am J Cardiol. 1994;73(16):1227–9.
109. Chiladakis JA, et al. Intravenous magnesium sulfate versus diltiazem in paroxysmal atrial fibrillation. Int J Cardiol. 2001;79(2–3):287–91.
110. Chu K, et al. Magnesium sulfate versus placebo for paroxysmal atrial fibrillation: a randomized clinical trial. Acad Emerg Med. 2009;16(4):295–300.
111. Gullestad L, et al. The effect of magnesium versus verapamil on supraventricular arrhythmias. Clin Cardiol. 1993;16(5):429–34.
112. Hays JV, Gilman JK, Rubal BJ. Effect of magnesium sulfate on ventricular rate control in atrial fibrillation. Ann Emerg Med. 1994;24(1):61–4.
113. Moran JL, et al. Parenteral magnesium sulfate versus amiodarone in the therapy of atrial tachyarrhythmias: a prospective, randomized study. Crit Care Med. 1995;23(11):1816–24.
114. Stiell IG, et al. Emergency department use of intravenous procainamide for patients with acute atrial fibrillation or flutter. Acad Emerg Med. 2007;14(12):1158–64.
115. Berger M, Schweitzer P. Timing of thromboembolic events after electrical cardioversion of atrial fibrillation or flutter: a retrospective analysis. Am J Cardiol. 1998;82(12):1545–7, A8.
116. Falcone RA, Morady F, Armstrong WF. Transesophageal echocardiographic evaluation of left atrial appendage function and spontaneous contrast formation after chemical or electrical cardioversion of atrial fibrillation. Am J Cardiol. 1996;78(4):435–9.
117. Weigner MJ, et al. Risk for clinical thromboembolism associated with conversion to sinus rhythm in patients with atrial fibrillation lasting less than 48 hours. Ann Intern Med. 1997;126(8):615–20.
118. Gage BF, Cardinalli AB, Owens DK. Cost-effectiveness of preference-based antithrombotic therapy for patients with nonvalvular atrial fibrillation. Stroke. 1998;29(6):1083–91.
119. Hart RG, et al. Antithrombotic therapy to prevent stroke in patients with atrial fibrillation: a meta-analysis. Ann Intern Med. 1999;131(7):492–501.
120. Investigators A, et al. Effect of clopidogrel added to aspirin in patients with atrial fibrillation. N Engl J Med. 2009;360(20):2066–78.
121. Aguilar MI, Hart R, Pearce LA. Oral anticoagulants versus antiplatelet therapy for preventing stroke in patients with non-valvular atrial fibrillation and no history of stroke or transient ischemic attacks. Cochrane Database Syst Rev. 2007;3:CD006186.
122. Domanovits H, et al. Sustained ventricular tachycardia in the emergency department. Resuscitation. 1999;42(1):19–25.
123. Herbert ME, et al. Failure to agree on the electrocardiographic diagnosis of ventricular tachycardia. Ann Emerg Med. 1996;27(1):35–8.
124. Akhtar M, et al. Wide QRS complex tachycardia. Reappraisal of a common clinical problem. Ann Intern Med. 1988;109(11):905–12.
125. Baerman JM, et al. Differentiation of ventricular tachycardia from supraventricular tachycardia with aberration: value of the clinical history. Ann Emerg Med. 1987;16(1):40–3.
126. Josephson ME. Electrophysiology of ventricular tachycardia: an historical perspective. J Cardiovasc Electrophysiol. 2003;14(10):1134–48.
127. Stevenson WG. Catheter ablation of monomorphic ventricular tachycardia. Curr Opin Cardiol. 2005;20(1):42–7.
128. Koppel C, et al. Clinical course and outcome in class IC antiarrhythmic overdose. Clin Toxicol. 1990;28(4):433–44.
129. Al-Khatib SM, et al. What clinicians should know about the QT interval. JAMA. 2003;289(16):2120–7.
130. Thanacoody HKR, Thomas SHL. Tricyclic antidepressant poisoning : cardiovascular toxicity. Toxicol Rev. 2005;24(3):205–14.
131. Bradberry SM, et al. Management of the cardiovascular complications of tricyclic antidepressant poisoning: role of sodium bicarbonate. Toxicol Rev. 2005;24(3):195–204.
132. Liebelt EL, Francis PD, Woolf AD. ECG lead aVR versus QRS interval in predicting seizures and arrhythmias in acute tricyclic antidepressant toxicity. Ann Emerg Med. 1995;26(2):195–201.
133. Dittrich KL, Walls RM. Hyperkalemia: ECG manifestations and clinical considerations. J Emerg Med. 1986;4(6):449–55.
134. Mattu A, Brady WJ, Robinson DA. Electrocardiographic manifestations of hyperkalemia. Am J Emerg Med. 2000;18(6):721–9.

135. Fisch C. Relation of electrolyte disturbances to cardiac arrhythmias. Circulation. 1973;47(2):408–19.
136. Danaberg J. Electrolyte abnormalities affecting the heart. In: Schwartz GR, editor. Principles and practice of emergency medicine. Baltimore: Williams & Wilkins; 1999. p. 425–7.
137. Sobel RM, et al. Pacemaker-mediated tachycardia: management by pacemaker interrogation/reprogramming in the ED. Am J Emerg Med. 2002;20:336–9.
138. Love CJ. Pacemaker troubleshooting and follow-up. In: KA KGE, Lau C, et al., editors. Clinical cardiac pacing, defibrillation, and resynchronization therapy. Philadelphia: Saunders; 2007. p. 1047–53.
139. Griffin J, Smithline H, Cook J. Runaway pacemaker: a case report and review. J Emerg Med. 2000;19(2):177–81.
140. Makaryus AN, Patrick C, Maccaro P. A rare case of "runaway" pacemaker in a modern CPU-controlled pacemaker. Pacing Clin Electrophysiol. 2005;28(9):993–6.
141. Stewart RB, Bardy GH, Greene HL. Wide complex tachycardia: misdiagnosis and outcome after emergent therapy. Ann Intern Med. 1986;104(6):766–71.
142. Steinman RT, et al. Wide QRS tachycardia in the conscious adult. Ventricular tachycardia is the most frequent cause. JAMA. 1989;261(7):1013–6.
143. Delbridge TR, Yealy DM. Wide complex tachycardia. Emerg Med Clin North Am. 1996;13:902–24.
144. Wrenn K. Management strategies in wide QRS complex tachycardia. Am J Emerg Med. 1991;9(6):592–7.
145. Gupta AK, Thakur RK. Wide QRS complex tachycardias. Med Clin North Am. 2001;85(2):245–66, ix.
146. Dongas J, et al. Value of preexisting bundle branch block in the electrocardiographic differentiation of supraventricular from ventricular origin of wide QRS tachycardia. Am J Cardiol. 1985;55(6):717–21.
147. Guo H, et al. Ventricular tachycardia with QRS configuration similar to that in sinus rhythm and a myocardial origin: differential diagnosis with bundle branch reentry. Europace. 2001;3(2):115–23.
148. Oreto G, et al. Wide complex tachycardia with atrioventricular dissociation and QRS morphology identical to that of sinus rhythm: a manifestation of bundle branch reentry. Heart. 1996;76(6):541–7.
149. Chou TC. Electrocardiography in clinical practice: adult and pediatric. 4th ed. Philadelphia: WB Saunders Company, 1996.
150. Zipes DP, et al. ACC/AHA/ESC 2006 guidelines for management of patients with Ventricular Arrhythmias and the prevention of sudden cardiac death: a report of the American College of Cardiology/American Heart Association Task Force and the European Society of Cardiology Committee for practice guidelines (writing committee to develop guidelines for management of patients with Ventricular Arrhythmias and the prevention of sudden cardiac death): developed in collaboration with the European Heart Rhythm Association and the Heart Rhythm Society. Circulation. 2006;114(10):e385–484.
151. Gorgels AP, et al. Comparison of procainamide and lidocaine in terminating sustained monomorphic ventricular tachycardia. Am J Cardiol. 1996;78(1):43–6.
152. Marill KA, et al. Amiodarone is poorly effective for the acute termination of ventricular tachycardia. Ann Emerg Med. 2006;47(3):217–24.
153. Ho DS, et al. Double-blind trial of lignocaine versus sotalol for acute termination of spontaneous sustained ventricular tachycardia. Lancet. 1994;344(8914):18–23.
154. Dorian P, et al. Amiodarone as compared with lidocaine for shock-resistant ventricular fibrillation. N Engl J Med. 2002;346(12):884–90.
155. Somberg JC, et al. Intravenous lidocaine versus intravenous amiodarone (in a new aqueous formulation) for incessant ventricular tachycardia. Am J Cardiol. 2002;90(8):853–9.
156. Association, A.H. AHA guidelines for cardiopulmonary resuscitation and emergency cardiovascular care management of symptomatic Bradycardia and Tachycardia. Circulation. 2005;112(Suppl I):IV–67-IV-77.
157. Tomlinson DR, Cherian P, Betts TR. Should intravenous amiodorone be utilized for haemodynamically tolerated sustained monomorphic ventricular tachycardia? J Am Coll Cardiol. 2007;49(9):19A. Suppl A.
158. Timperley J, et al. Flecainide overdose--support using an intra-aortic balloon pump. BMC Emerg Med. 2005;5:10.
159. Goldman MJ, Mowry JB, Kirk MA. Sodium bicarbonate to correct widened QRS in a case of flecainide overdose. J Emerg Med. 1997;15(2):183–6.
160. Brubacher J. Bicarbonate therapy for unstable propafenone-induced wide complex tachycardia. CJEM. 2004;6(5):349–56.
161. Salerno DM, et al. Reversal of flecainide-induced ventricular arrhythmia by hypertonic sodium bicarbonate in dogs. Am J Emerg Med. 1995;13(3):285–93.
162. Bauman JL, et al. Flecainide-induced sustained ventricular tachycardia successfully treated with lidocaine. Chest. 1987;92(3):573–5.
163. Siegers A, Board PN. Amiodarone used in successful resuscitation after near-fatal flecainide overdose. Resuscitation. 2002;53(1):105–8.

Left Ventricular Assist Devices and Pacemakers

10

Ayan Sen

Section I: Ventricular Assist Devices

Left Ventricular Assist Devices

Mechanical circulatory devices have become common to support a failing heart, often as a temporizing measure prior to cardiac transplantation, and occasionally as destination therapy [1]. It restores tissue circulation by optimizing blood supply thereby enabling organ function. However, these devices could be associated with several challenges and complications and with increasing number of devices being implanted both as a bridge to transplant and destination therapy, it is necessary for the critical care and emergency physicians unfamiliar with them to understand the physiology, clinical presentations, and management of complications.

Mechanical circulatory assist devices [2, 3] or left ventricular assist devices (LVAD) can be inserted in these following situations:

- Bridge to transplant (BT): Supporting the cardiac function prior to patient being able to receive a heart transplant.
- Bridge to recovery: Supporting cardiac function before the native heart shows signs of recovery.
- Bridge to decision: Decision about whether patient is a candidate for transplant/may have cardiac recovery.
- Destination therapy (DT): Supporting the cardiac function until the end of life.

Some of the device-related terminologies are as follows:

- *Paracorporeal devices*: The pumping chamber can be placed outside the patient's body (extra- or paracorporeal devices).
- *Intracorporeal devices*: The pumping chamber is placed within the abdomen in a preperitoneal position immediately under the diaphragm or above the diaphragm in the pericardial space (intracorporeal devices).
- *Blood flow in LVADs can be pulsatile or continuous.*
- *Pulsatile flow LVAD:* Pulsatile or displacement pumps were the first generation of left ventricular support devices. These pumps consist of inflow and outflow conduits, unidirectional valves, a pumping chamber, a battery pack, and a system controller and may be driven pneumatically or electrically. Due to size and frequent complication rate of pulsatile devices, continuous-flow VADs have become more common.
- *Continuous-flow VAD*: CF rotary pumps generally consist of blood inlet and outlet ports and a single rotating element that imparts

A. Sen (✉)
Critical Care Medicine, Emergency Medicine, Mayo Clinic College of Medicine, Mayo Clinic Arizona, Phoenix, AZ, USA

© Springer Nature Switzerland AG 2020
J. R. Shiber, S. D. Weingart (eds.), *Emergency Department Critical Care*, https://doi.org/10.1007/978-3-030-28794-8_10

energy to the blood to increase arterial blood flow and pressure [4]. Blood is pulled into the impeller of the pump via an inlet cannula connected to the left ventricular apex and delivered to the systemic circulation via an outflow cannula connected to either the ascending or the descending aorta. The rigid stationary housing(s) that surrounds and/or lies in the center of the rotating element incorporates some combination of motor windings, permanent magnets, electromagnets, or mechanical bearing surfaces that act to drive and support the rotating element. Newer generation continuous-flow LVADs are designed for less mechanical wear and doubled 2-year survival compared with pulsatile LVADs and improved quality of life for BTT and DT patients [5–7]. Continuous-flow VADs have two types of blood flow: centrifugal or axial [8].

- *Centrifugal pump:* Rotating elements act as a spinning disk with blades that work as a "thrower" where the fluid is captured and thrown tangentially out of the blade tips.
- *Axial pump*: Axial CF pump rotating elements operate like a propeller in a pipe and can be viewed as a "pusher." This mechanism can also be viewed as an "auger" trying to screw itself into the inlet fluid, against the "resistance force" at the outlet, to overcome the difference between preload and afterload.

A classification of different kinds of devices and type of cardiac support provided are shown in Table 10.1:

Another classification that is used as follows:

- First generation (pulsatile blood flow), for example, Novacor
- Second generation (continuous axial blood flow), for example, HeartMate II
- Third generation (continuous centrifugal blood flow), for example, HeartWare

Table 10.1 Mechanical Circulatory Devices

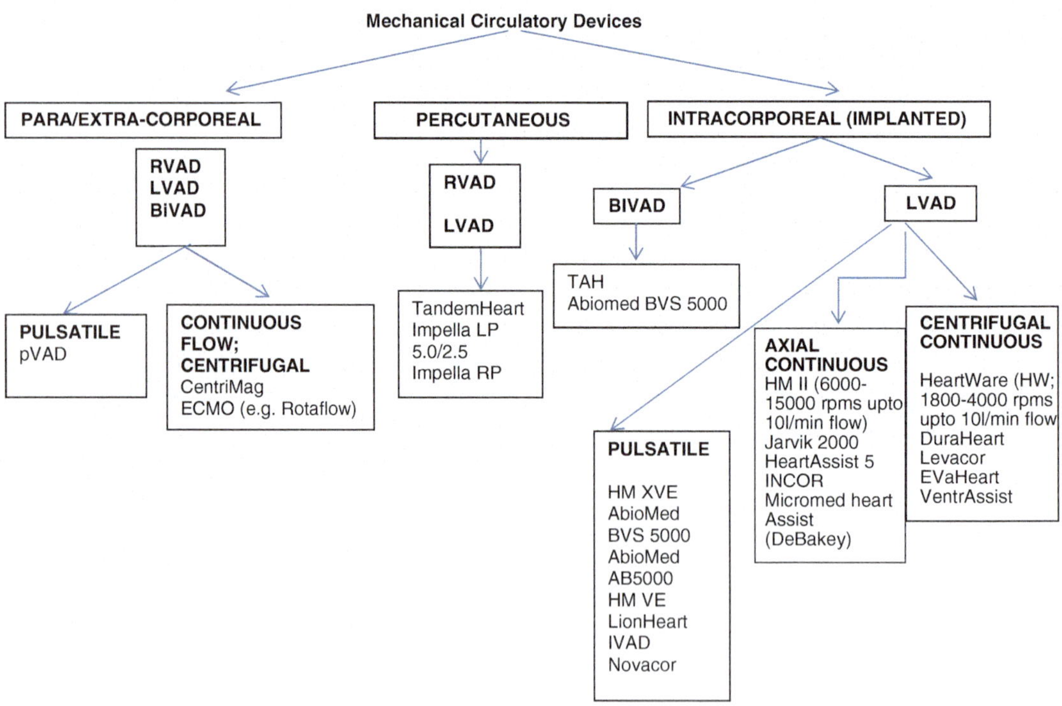

Radiographic Images of (A) Novacor, (B) HeartMate II, and (C) HeartWare [9]

Terms and Numbers

Revolutions per Minute (RPM) This value is entered by the provider and it is the pump RPMs that create VAD flows. It is directly measured through the motor. RPMs are modified based on flows needed. Usual range is 6000–15,000 for HM II and 1500–4000 for HW device.

Flows The continuous flow of the LVAD is created from a circulating impeller device in the bloodstream which generates forward flows [10]. A change in pump function or patient condition leads to changes in flow. The device flow is directly proportional to the rotor speed and inversely related to the difference of pressure in the inflow and outflow cannulas.

$$\text{Device Flow} = \text{Rotor Speed} / \text{Pinflow} - \text{Poutflow}.$$

Therefore, low device flows are caused by:

1. Low intravascular volume/low preload to the device
2. RV failure/tamponade/thrombus/kinking in the inflow cannula/low preload to the device
3. Hypertensive emergency/outflow cannula obstruction/high afterload to device

Pump Power LVAD pump power is a measure of the current and voltage applied to the motor. It varies directly with pump speed and flow [10]. Flow obstruction without contact with LVAD rotor results in reduced power, while thrombus in contact with the rotor will lead to increased power with low flows.

Pulsatility Index This corresponds to magnitude of flow pulse through the pump. The magnitude of flow pulse is measured and averaged over a 15-second interval to produce pulsatility index on the HM II but not the HW [11]. PI fluctuates with change in volume status and heart's contractility.

Increased PI

1. Increased preload
2. Increased contractility

Decreased PI

1. Decrease volume status
2. Reduced afterload
3. Inflow/outflow obstruction with low flows and abnormal power

Suction Events A suction event occurs when there is reduced filling of the pump/reduced preload, which increases negative pressure within the left ventricle. A part of the ventricle wall is sucked over and covers the pump inlet cannula. The pump alarms and leads to decrease in speed to release suction. The causes are:

1. Low volume
2. RV failure/tamponade causing low LV filling
3. Inflow cannula obstruction

Suction events can lead to low VAD flows and trigger ventricular arrhythmia. The management includes turning down RPMs and administering fluid [10].

Clinical Presentations

Picture of a Typical HeartMate II Device on a Patient

Always look at the patient first, and then, look at the device

- A = Assess ability to protect airway
- B = Assess breathing (RR, pulse oximetry [may not reliable]), use of accessory muscles, work of breathing
- C = Check Doppler MAP and HR/EKG/listen to hear sounds – continuous whirling sound
- Check device – Which device/pump speed/flows/power/PIs/suction events
- *Call the VAD coordinator/CT surgeon/heart failure cardiologist*

- Backup bag = two extra fully charged batteries, second controller
- D = Neuro assessment
- E = Exposure under environmental control
- DEFG = Do not ever forget glucose

Blood Pressure Measurement [12] (Fig. 10.1)

Steps

1. Use Doppler ultrasound monitor, 8–9 MHz, pencil style
2. Appropriate BP cuff with sphygmomanometer
3. Ultrasound gel
4. Artery location with probe at 15 degree angle to skin; do not press too hard
5. Inflate to 30 mm above where sound disappears
6. Release bulb slowly and note pressure at which sound reappears

Device Failure

Providers taking care of a patient with an LVAD should be aware of the following emergency drill if there is concern for LVAD failure with alarms:

- Call VAD coordinator/center.
- Check instruction booklet/color of the tag (on the controller around the waist).
- Check batteries (do not remove both batteries at the same time).

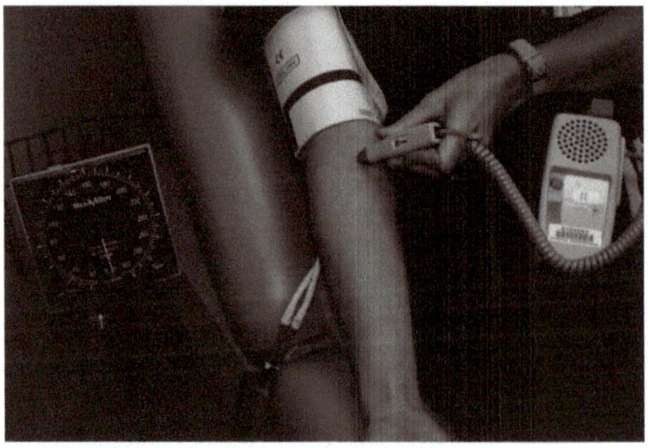

Fig. 10.1 Using a Doppler probe to determine BP in a patient with a continuous flow LVAD

- Batteries drain simultaneously, replace as a pair when drained (exchange one battery at a time).
- One battery will briefly run the LVAD while changing power sources.
- Check controller (green light).
- Check for loose connections.
- Assess for alarms (usually if flows <2.5 lpm) (Fig. 10.2a, b).

Some Common Alarms in a Patient with an LVAD

Emergency Pump Drill

Pump is *running*…

A. Controller is *not* alarming
   - Patient issue, not a pump issue
B. Controller *is* alarming:
   - Continuous tone = Urgent
   - Beeping = Warning
   - Check all cable connections
   - Check power source
   - Change controller if needed (follow product manual)

Pump is *stopped*…

A. Controller alarm lights/sounds should be alarming continuously
   - Check all cable connections
   - Check power source
   - Change controller if needed
B. Patient:
   - Connect EKG
   - Check Doppler pressure
   - Support blood pressure
   - Advanced cardiac life support (ACLS, except CPR unless unable to restart pump)
   - Start CPR if unable to restart pump
   - Heparin bolus recommended if ACLS and CPR needed

Other abnormal LVAD-related alarms and differential diagnosis is described below [6, 13] (Figs. 10.3 and 10.4):

a

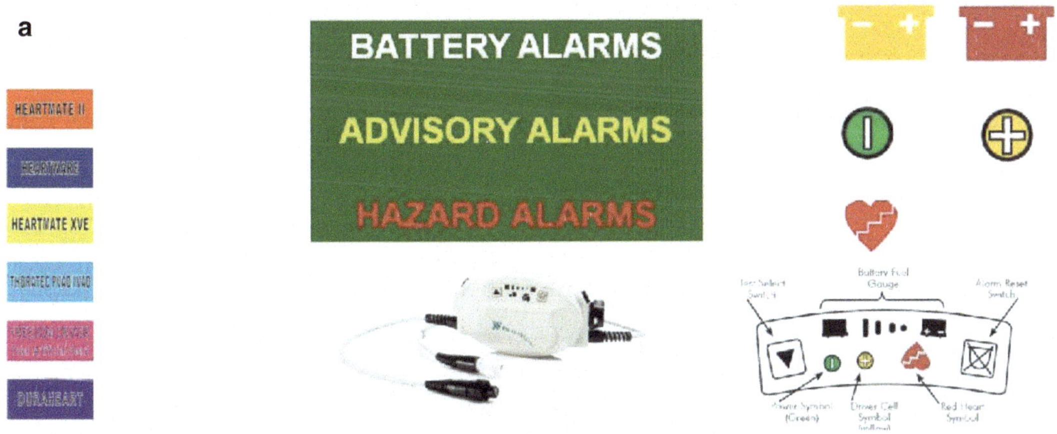

b

System Controller Warning Lights & Sounds

Warning Lights	Audio Tone	Alarm Message	Meaning	Action
Red Heart	Steady Audio Tone	LOW FLOW HAZARD (on Display Module) LOW FLOW, PUMP OFF and/or PUMP DISCONNECTED (on System Monitor)	Pump flow < 2.5 lpm, pump has stopped, perc lead is disconnected, or pump is not working properly	1. Make sure System Controller is connected to the pump 2. Make sure System Controller is connected to a power source (batteries, PBU/Power Module, or Emergency Power Pack [EPP]) 3. If alarm continues, immediately seek additional help
NONE: No Warning Lights and No Green Power Symbol	Steady Audio Tone	NONE	System Controller is not receiving power	1. Make sure System Controller is connected to a power source (batteries, PBU/Power Module, or EPP) 2. If connected and alarm continues, switch to alternate power source 3. If alarm continues after switching power source, replace Controller (see otherside for instructions.)
Red Battery	Steady Audio Tone	LOW VOLTAGE	Less than 5 minutes of battery power remain, voltage is too low, or the System Controller is not getting enough power from the PBU/Power Module	Immediately replace depleted batteries with new, fully-charged set. Change batteries **one at a time**. If fully-charged batteries are not available, switch to PBU/PowerModule or EPP. **WARNING! Do NOT remove power from both power leads at the same time, or the pump will stop.** **Note**: Pump speed will gradually decrease to save power (i.e., "Power Saver Mode") until the condition is resolved and the alarm clears
Yellow Battery	1 Beep Every 4 Seconds	Low Voltage Advisory	Less than 15 minutes of battery power remain, voltage is too low, or the System Controller is not getting enough power from the PBU/Power Module	Immediately replace depleted batteries with new, fully-charged set. Change batteries **one at a time**. If fully-charged batteries are not available, switch to PBU/PowerModule or EPP. **WARNING! Do NOT remove power from both power leads at the same time, or the pump will stop.**
NONE: No Warning Light	Broken Audio Tone (repeating cycle: 1 beep per second for 2 seconds, followed by 2 seconds of silence)	REPLACE SYSTEM CONTROLLER (on System Monitor) REPLACE SYSTEM DRIVER (on Display Module)	System Controller is operating in back-up mode	1. Replace the System Controller (see other side for instructions) 2. Notify the patient's physician 3. Obtain a new backup System Controller 4. Program the new backup Controller with settings prescribed for this patient
Yellow Controller Cell	1 Beep Every 4 Seconds	SC CELL MODULE LOW (on System Monitor) Driver Cell Low (on Display Module)	The battery module that powers the System Controller audible alarm is depleted.	Replace the System Controller Battery Module
Rapidly Flashing Green Power Symbol and 4 Green Battery Fuel Gauge Lights Flashing Once Per Second	1 Beep Every Second	POWER CABLE DISCONNECTED	One of the power leads is damaged or disconnected	1. Reconnect or tighten disconnected/loose power lead 2. If alarm continues, check System Controller power lead and PBU/Power Module patient cable for damage 3. If System Controller power lead is damaged, replace the Controller (see other side for instructions) If PBU/Power Module patient cable is damaged, replace PBU/Power Module patient cable 4. Obtain a new, backup System Controller for this patient, if necessary
NONE: No Warning Light	NONE on PBU w/ System Monitor 1 Beep Every 4 Seconds when on Batteries or PBU (w/Display Module)	WARNING: Low Speed Operation	Pump is operating below low speed limit	Connect System Controller to System Monitor (audio alarm will stop) and increase fixed speed setting or reduce low speed limit

Fig. 10.2 LVAD System Controller Warning Lights and Sounds

The Short of Breath "VAD" Patient

These can be noted in a patient who presents to the emergency department or a fresh postoperative LVAD patient in a cardiothoracic ICU. VAD-specific diagnoses include:

1. LV failure (new MI, worsening LV failure)
2. Device failure (pump thrombus, cannula obstruction, mechanical failure)
3. RV failure
4. Valvular regurgitation
5. Tamponade

Abnormalities	Causes	Interventions
High Flows	Vasodilation causes; SALAD- Sepsis/ Anaphylaxis/Liver Dysfunction/Adrenal Insufficiency/Drugs-Device	Identify and treat causes of sepsis; vasopressors if low MAP
Low Flows	Hypovolemia/Bleeding	Give IV fluids/blood
	RV failure/Tamponade/ Hypertensive	Assess and treat
	Arrhythmias	Assess and treat
Suction events	All causes of Low flow	Give volume
	Excessive LV unloading	Lower pump speed

Fig. 10.3 LVAD Trouble- Shooting 1

Abnormalities	Cause	Interventions
High Power	Pump thrombus	Anticogulation, pump exchange
Low power	Device problem	Check batteries, power
High PI	Recovery of LV function	
	Lead damage	Check LVAD/driveline
Low PI	Worse native ventricular function	Increase pump speed, intropes
	Hypovolemia	Give fluids
	Excess pump speed	Lower pump speed

Fig. 10.4 LVAD Trouble- Shooting 2

6. Arrhythmias
7. Hypovolemia

Other primary pulmonary, CNS, and metabolic problems should be considered in the differential diagnosis. Measure ABG, lactate, continuous pulse oximetry, chest X-ray, and if necessary, CT scan should be considered. Worsening hypoxia, hypercarbia, or acidosis and inability to protect airway may warrant intubation and mechanical ventilation. Mechanical ventilation should adopt lung protective ventilation strategies. Low tidal volume/adequate PEEP strategies are helpful. Care must be taken not to increase PEEP too much for risk of causes worsening RV dysfunction. Therapeutic management may include drainage of pleural effusion, chest tube for pneumothorax, bronchoscopy, and optimizing hemodynamics.

The Hypotensive VAD Patient

Hypotension is usually defined as mean arterial pressure <60 as measured by Doppler. Patients may have cold, mottled extremities or warm peripheries based on the etiology as described in the figure below. LVAD flows should be assessed. Bedside echocardiography can help provide valuable clinical data. Assess inferior vena cava collapsibility/tamponade signs. Check RV and LV functions. On echocardiographic examination, the ventricular septum should be flat and lie in a neutral position, the LV should be adequately filled but not distended and the drainage cannula (if placed in the LV apex) should be well aligned with the mitral valve. The aortic valve should be competent and open only intermittently, every second or third beat. Central access and arterial line access should be instituted. Hematocrit should be measured to assess for bleeding (Table 10.2).

The VAD-specific causes of *shortness of breath* and *cardiogenic shock* are described as follows:

(a) *New LV dysfunction:* This may manifest as fluid overload and other signs of cardiogenic shock as listed above. The etiology may be due to worsening LV function, new MI, arrhythmias, and aortic valve degeneration causing aortic regurgitation. The management includes adjusting pump speed, use of

Table 10.2 Algorithm for evaluation and management of hypotension/shock in a patient witha LVAD

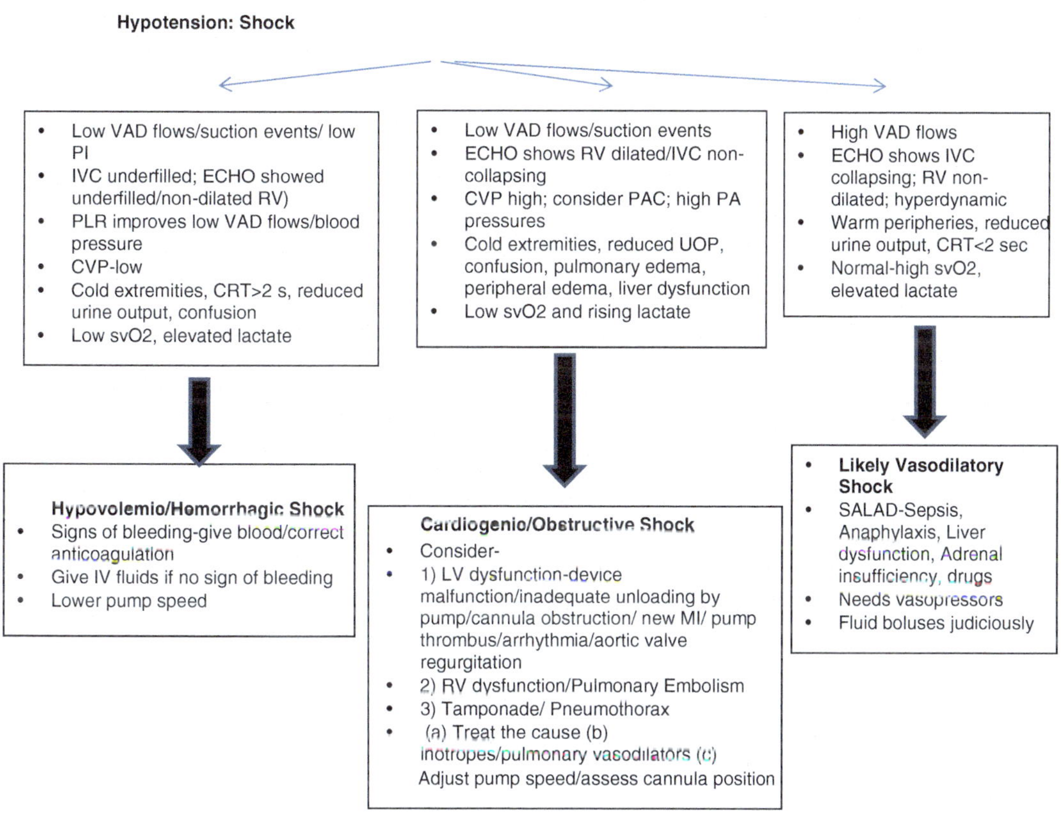

inotropes/diuretics, antiarrhythmics, relieving tamponade, if present.

(b) *New MI:* Acute myocardial infarction (AMI) can occur in LVAD patients and may be due to coronary plaque rupture or thromboembolism from a deep vein thrombus if there is a right–left shunt [14]. Left heart catheterization should be performed for symptom relief, prevention of arrhythmias, supporting the right ventricle function if AMI is causing right ventricle failure.

(c) *RV failure:* Right heart failure can occur in 5–10% of patients after LVAD implantation [15]. This can be diagnosed through bedside echocardiography. If a central venous catheter is inserted, a high CVP will be noted. Pulmonary artery catheter (PAC) may be needed to assess pulmonary artery pressures. Inodilator support for the right heart may be needed (e.g., milrinone, dobutamine, or low-dose epinephrine). LVAD settings may be titrated to keep the ventricular septum in a neutral position. Avoidance of hypoxia, hypercarbia, and limiting positive end-expiratory pressure (PEEP) is beneficial. If pulmonary vascular resistance is increased (as measured through a PAC), inhaled nitric oxide or sildenafil may be required [16]. Continued worsening right heart failure may necessitate insertion of right ventricular device support in the form of an RVAD/Impella/TandemHeart [17].

(d) *Tamponade/pneumothorax–cardiac tamponade:* Hypotension and low VAD flows with/without suction events may indicate developing cardiac tamponade. Late tamponade is possible. Bleeding is a risk factor. Stat bedside echo may reveal the cause. TEE may be necessary for regional tamponade.

(e) *Arrhythmias:* Atrial fibrillation/flutter has been reported to be present in patients with LVADs and associated with worse clinical outcomes despite the absence of an increased risk of bleeding and thromboembolism. Loss of AV synchrony results in reduced ventricular filling and decompensated right heart failure [18]. Antiarrhythmic therapy is standard including beta-blockers, amiodarone, sotalol, digoxin, if tolerated, but may not be very successful for maintenance. Ventricular arrhythmias have been reported to occur in 22–59% of LVAD recipients [7, 19]. Some patients can experience right heart failure, hemodynamic deterioration, ICD shocks, and cardiac arrest with ventricular arrhythmias. Beta-blockers and intravenous amiodarone and lidocaine can be used acutely. Close attention to potassium and magnesium levels and avoidance of QT prolonging medications should be considered. Patients with an LVAD should have an automatic implanted cardioverted defibrillator (AICD). AICD interrogation and optimization may be needed to treat ventricular rhythms. Uncontrollable ventricular arrhythmias can be an indication for temporary ECMO, bi-VAD, total artificial heart, or heart transplantation.

(f) *Aortic valve degeneration:* Continuous-flow LVADs can lead to aortic valve degeneration and aortic regurgitation with long-term use. Changes in the blood flow mechanics causing increased mechanical stress on the valve causes the above changes [20, 21]. This has been reported in more than 90% of patients with long-term VAD support, although the time course is variable [22, 23]. Echocardiography can help diagnose the problem. Aortic valve degeneration increases the risk of thromboembolism, infection, congestive heart failure, and cardiogenic shock. Antihypertensives should be used to improve forward flow. Surgical patch closure or valve replacement should be considered early, prior to the development of heart failure. VAD pump RPM may be adjusted so that the aortic valve opens once every three cardiac cycles to improve hemodynamics. Serial echocardiography may be needed [24].

(g) *Cannula obstruction:* Cannula obstruction is one potential cause for low pump flow despite adequate volume and can occur because of malpositioning or blockage of the cannula with thrombus. Reduced power consumption is noted on the VAD. Auscultation over the device may elicit an intermittent chattering sound, as the device is unable to obtain fill because of the obstruction. Echocardiography can determine whether the inflow orifice points toward the mitral valve (desirable) or is malpositioned toward the septum or LV free wall and becoming intermittently occluded. Cannula obstruction must be surgically repaired.

(h) *Pump thrombosis:* One of the common causes of low cardiac output state is pump thrombosis which occurs in around 8% of continuous-flow LVADs [25]. Predisposing factors include blood–VAD surface interactions, low flow states, cannula malposition, hypercoagulable states including development of heparin-induced thrombocytopenia, and protein C and S deficiency. There is low occurrence of pump thrombosis with INR range above 1.5. Apart from signs of cardiogenic shock, including shortness of breath, hypotension, and tachycardia, they may have "scratchy, grating, rough sounds" on auscultation, power spikes, and low flow alarms, and increased native pulsatility (new aortic valve opening or significantly increased pulse pressure). Laboratory evidence of hemolysis (lactate dehydrogenase [LDH] levels greater than three times the upper limit of normal and/or plasma free hemoglobin [pfHb] greater than 40 mg/dL should raise concern for possible thrombus). Serial recording of LV end-diastolic diameter with increasing VAD speeds (so-called ramp study) may diagnose pump thrombus or other obstructions to blood flow within the rotary pump and cannula system [14, 26]. Pump exchange is the definitive treatment. Intracavitary thrombolysis to resolve LVAD thrombosis has been used in select patients deemed inoperable candidates for pump exchange or urgent transplantation [27]. If heparin-induced thrombocytopenia is diagnosed, alternative anticoagulants should be used (e.g., antifactor Xa fondaparinux, direct thrombin inhibitors – bivalirudin, argatroban) [28, 29].

LVAD Patient with GI Bleed

The incidence of GI bleeding in LVAD patients has been reported to be around 22–40% in various studies [30]. The etiology of the bleeding is considered due to altered blood flow patterns (Heyde's syndrome) in continuous-flow LVAD patients and also due to acquired von Willebrand factor deficiency [31]. Gastric and colonic AVMs have been reported. Octreotide is a long-acting somatostatin analog used in GI bleeding because it reduces splanchnic arterial and portal blood flow, most probably by decreasing smooth muscle tone. Case reports using octreotide have shown a significant reduction in hospital admissions and number of administered blood units and increase in mean hemoglobin values in patients with chronically bleeding AVMs [32, 33]. Management steps include stopping anticoagulation, correcting coagulopathy, blood transfusion, octreotide, proton pump inhibitors, and endoscopy. Injection/clipping and cauterization may be needed. If source of bleeding is not identifiable, capsule study or push enteroscopy may be required. If all else fails, mesenteric angiography and embolization should be considered. Resumption of anticoagulation is controversial. Some authors propose resuming warfarin with INR goal of 1.5, while others have used aspirin only or a combination of the two.

Acute Kidney Injury in an LVAD Patient

Patients with an LVAD may present with new onset of acute kidney injury (AKI) as manifested by oliguria, abdominal pain, fatigue, nausea, vomiting, dysuria, hematuria, and lower extremity edema. The incidence of AKI after LVAD implantation has been reported to range from 7% to 56% [34]. Some patients may have abnormal renal function prior to LVAD due to low flow states. Postdevice implantation they show improvement of their renal perfusion and function. Mortality is high among patients who have postimplantation AKI. VAD-specific causes of AKI include shock states (cardiogenic/hypovolemic/vasodilatory) leading to poor renal perfusion and prerenal azotemia and acute tubular necrosis from hemolysis. Patients who do not improve by optimization of hemodynamics and volume status may need CRRT or hemodialysis.

Criteria for renal replacement therapy remain the same as for non-VAD patients (AEIOU; A = acidosis, E = electrolyte imbalance [HyperkK, hyperphosphatemia, etc.], I = intoxicants, O = overload [fluid], U = uremic encephalopathy/pericarditis). Emergent dialysis will require temporary catheter placement. Hemodialysis can be done and is preferred through an AV graft placement to avoid tunneled catheters introducing infections and causing bacteremia.

LVAD Patient with Stroke

As with any patient, the initial assessment of an LVAD patient with altered mental status or new onset of focal or global neurologic deficit should be seen in the emergency department and subsequently admitted to the ICU. Examination should be focused on ABCDEs (airway, breathing, circulation, disability, exposure assessment). LVAD device should be checked along with the patient examination. Full neurologic examination should be done/CT scan and MRI will be needed; full blood count, hemolysis panel (LDH/haptoglobin, bilirubin, plasma-free Hb), and coagulation panel should be sent. A study comparing the use of a pulsatile-flow LVAD versus a continuous-flow LVAD showed the rate of hemorrhagic stroke to be 11% in the continuous-flow group and 8% in the pulsatile-flow group [35]. Risk factors of stroke in LVAD patients include diabetes, preimplant strokes, aortic cross-clamping with cardioplegic arrest during their LVAD implant [36] and systemic infection [37]. Supratherapeutic INR due to anticoagulation is a risk factor for hemorrhagic stroke. Acquired von Willebrand syndrome (aVWS) is also a risk factor leading to impaired hemostasis of the vascular endothelium. Of all strokes that occurred, 58% were found to occur in the right hemisphere compared to a left hemisphere rate of 28%, bilateral hemispheres 6.5%, and vertebrobasilar 6.5%. The authors suggested a significant correlation between infection and the development of stroke. The predilection of right hemispheric stroke was explained by the anatomic alignment of the outflow cannula directing material toward the brachiocephalic trunk [38]. Management of hemorrhagic stroke includes reversal of coagulopathy (FFP, vitamin K, and/or prothrombin complex concentrate [PCC] if patient is on warfarin). Desmopressin has been used if patient has been on antiplatelet agents along with platelet transfusion. The risk of pump thrombosis is high, but risks–benefits must be ascertained by a multidisciplinary team. Ischemic stroke in a patient with LVAD may warrant endovascular stroke therapies based on new literature (especially as systemic thrombolytics may be contraindicated).

VAD-Related Infections

Second-generation continuous-flow LVADs have lower overall infection rates compared with first-generation devices, ranging from 30% to 50% [9, 39]. Destination therapy patients were more likely to develop infections compared with those who received LVADs as a bridge to transplant because destination therapy patients tend to be more ill and have a longer duration of LVAD support. A classification of VADs and associated infections are as follows [9, 40].

Driveline Infections They occur in 17–30% of patients. Cutaneous migration of bacteria and local trauma is a causative factor. Exit site cellulitis may be noted. Ultrasound/CT may be helpful in diagnosis. Common organisms include *Staphylococcus*, *Enterococcus*, *Pseudomonas*, *Enterobacter*, *Candida*, etc. Oral/IV antibiotics are needed based on severity. Two-week therapy may suffice.

Pump Pocket Infection With a prevalence rate of 1.8–10%, they may present as abscess beneath skin, purulent drainage, and systemic signs of infection (sepsis). Ultrasound/CT scan can help in diagnosis. *Staphylococcus* is a common cause; gram-negative bacteria and *Candida* have been reported. Management includes drainage and debridement of pump pocket with empiric broad-spectrum antibiotics. Chronic antimicrobial suppressive therapy is indicated and omental wrapping of pump pocket has been described.

Cannula/Pump Infection/Endocarditis Although rare at around 0.6%, this is associated with high mortality. Diagnosis is usually presumptive when other sources of infection cannot be found, and usually patients are in septic shock. Device removal is necessary and urgent transplantation is the norm in bridge-to-transplant patients.

Bloodstream Infection Bloodstream infections are high with a reported rate of 20–27%. Fever, leukocytosis, septic shock, and septic embolization have been described. This may be as a result of central catheter or LVAD related. If blood cultures grow same organism from peripheral and catheter culture less than 2 hours from each other, then this is usually LVAD-related bacteremia. More than 2 hours between the two cultures could indicate catheter-related infections. Empiric antibiotics should be commenced with removal of central catheter source. If continued bacteremia is noted, device replacement and transplantation are indicated, although associated with low survival.

Other contiguous sources of infection should be investigated: pneumonia, urinary tract infections, sinusitis, cholecystitis, wound infections, cellulitis, etc. should be assessed in patients presenting with signs of infection or sepsis.

Pregnancy

Although favorable outcomes have been reported with one case report indicating successful cesarean section and childbirth [41], the lack of data on placental blood flow and pregnancy risks during support with a left ventricular assist device continues to make pregnancy a contraindication after its placement. Pregnancy counseling is therefore necessary prior to device placement.

Involved in Trauma

Management of trauma in a patient with an LVAD should be as per Advanced Trauma Life Support (ATLS) protocols. Device malfunction must be ruled out. Early involvement of the VAD coordinator and heart failure/cardiac surgery team is necessary. Trauma-related failure of a continuous-flow left ventricular assist device (LVAD) has been reported [42]. Damage to the cables and displacement of the pump from its original position have been described. The mechanism has been due to fall or blow to the chest. Pump exchange has been undertaken.

Cardiac Arrest

Cardiac arrests may occur in patients with indwelling left ventricular assist devices. A stepwise approach is helpful. VAD coordinator/perfusionist should be contacted. Stat VAD equipment should be assessed to check if critical connections are intact. Driveline and power should be checked and reconnected if disconnected. Alarms should be assessed. Presence of VAD hum should be auscultated. Doppler should be used to check blood pressure. If pump stays off, backup controller should be switched on or alternately power sources should be switched. ACLS should be continued with *no chest compressions* unless the pump cannot be restarted.

Section II: Pacemakers

Pacemakers

Temporary cardiac pacing consists of an artificial electrical stimulus to the heart to produce cardiac cell depolarization [43]. This is necessary when the patient's own intrinsic pacemaker fails or is aberrant leading to ineffective depolarization. Cardiac pacemaker problems can arise from degeneration of the conduction system, atherosclerosis, ischemia, drug induced, electrolyte problems, and postcardiac surgery. Urgent temporary pacing may be necessary. Electrophysiological abnormalities that may benefit from temporary cardiac pacing [44, 45] are as follows.

Conduction Abnormality

- Prolonged AV delay (common after cardiac surgery)
- AV block, third degree or type II second degree
- Bifascicular block with first degree block
- New onset bifascicular block (indicative of active ischemia)
- Prolonged QT syndrome in the presence of significant bradycardia (to prevent torsades de pointes)

Tachycardia

- AV junctional tachycardia (common after cardiopulmonary bypass) may be terminated by a brief period of pacing, which can then be discontinued
- To terminate reentrant SVT or VT
- Type I atrial flutter (rate <320–340 beats/min)
- Prophylaxis of atrial fibrillation

Other

- Sick sinus syndrome
- Neurocardiogenic syncope
- To restore AV mechanical synchrony in underlying third degree block, AV junctional or ventricular rhythms
- Hypertrophic obstructive cardiomyopathy (in particular if effective in reducing systolic anterior motion of the anterior mitral leaflet)
- Following heart transplantation

The types of pacing are as follows.

Temporary Transvenous Pacing
- Transcutaneous pacing
- Epicardial pacing

Permanent Pacing
- Single chamber
- Dual chamber
- Biventricular

Transcutaneous pacing is quick to apply, noninvasive, but should only be used for a short time.

Transvenous pacing should be provided when available: Easiest route is right internal jugular or left subclavian; fluoroscopy should be used, but it can be attempted without it in an emergency.

If the patient has epicardial wires postcardiac surgery, then this is the primary method of pacing.

Some common terminologies are as follows:
- *Pacing* – Deliver an electrical impulse.
- *Pacing spike* – Stimulus from the pacemaker recorded on the EKG, a short narrow deflection.
- *Capture* – Depolarization of the heart by an artificial stimulus; myocardial cells capture the impulse delivered by the pacemaker; pacer spike followed by a QRS complex (Fig. 10.5).

Pacing Threshold It is the amount of energy required to initiate depolarization for the cells to capture the impulse and depolarize. It is measured in mA. This should be checked regularly in order to see how much "leeway" you have to go up in milliamps. Turn the mA down until there is no capture, that is, the stimulation threshold. The mA should be set at double or triple that number (Fig. 10.6).

Different hearts may require different amounts of energy to elicit a depolarization and contrac-

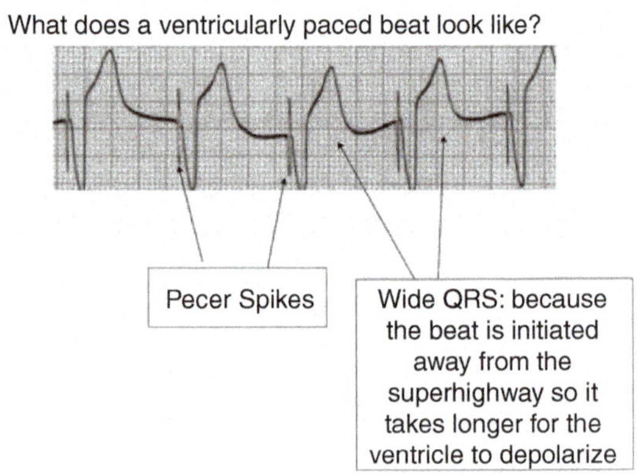

Fig. 10.5 Pacemaker spike with QRS showing capture

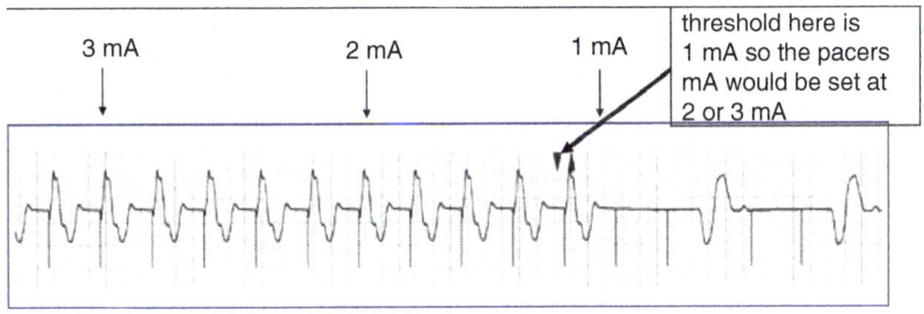

Fig. 10.6 As mA is reduced below the threshold required ventricular capture is lost

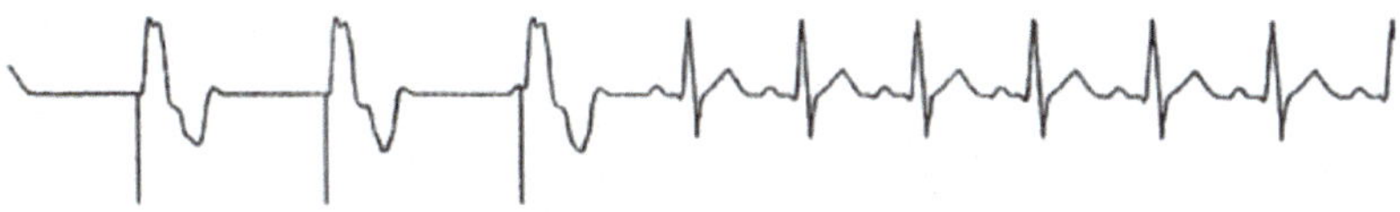

Fig. 10.7 Appropriate sensing inhibits the pacemaker when the intrinisic rate is above the pacing minimum rate

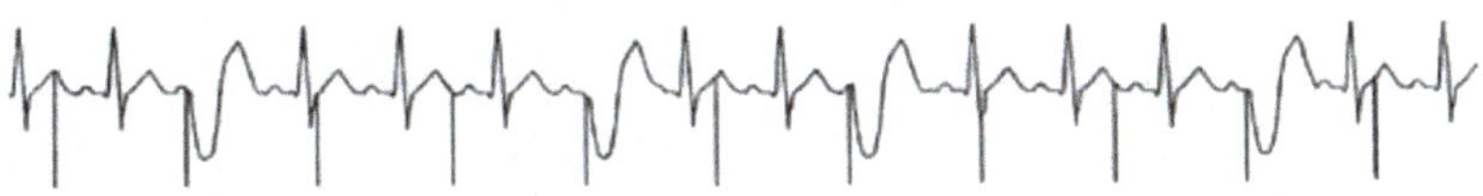

Fig. 10.8 Pacing in the asynchronous mode without any sensing risks R on T phenomena since pacing spikes occur despite intrinsic depolariazations

tion; the variables that could affect the amount of energy required include the following:

- Position of electrode
- Contact with viable myocardial tissue
- Level of energy delivered through wire; presence of hypoxia, acidosis, or electrolyte imbalances
- Other medications being used
- Degree of inflammation/fibrosis at the needle site

Demand (Synchronous) Mode

- In demand mode, the stimulus is provided when the patient's heart rate drops below at predetermined rate.
- Pacemaker detects or senses the patient's intrinsic electrical activity and inhibits the pacemaker from firing an electrical stimulus.
- If the pacer is set at 60, it will not pace until the heart rate falls below 60.
- This avoids competition between the native heart rate and that of the pacer box.
- Adequate sensing must be present (Fig. 10.7).

Fixed (Asynchronous) Mode

- In fixed mode, the stimulus is provided at a preset rate and the pacer fires at that rate regardless of what the patient's heart is doing.
- If fixed rate is used and the patient has an underlying rhythm, the rate must be set greater than the patient's inherent rate to avoid competition.
- There is a great risk for "R on T" phenomena with asynchronous pacing (Fig. 10.8).

Sensing and Sensitivity

Sensing involves the ability of the pacemaker to detect intrinsic cardiac electric activity in the patient. This is the minimum native current that the pacemaker is able to sense. A lower number corresponds to greater sensitivity. This is beneficial when synchronous or demand pacing is applied. Sensitivity is measured in millivolts (mV). The sensitivity is set low enough so that the smallest electric activity of the heart is detected and inappropriate pacing is not activated. The sensitivity is set to detect the mini-

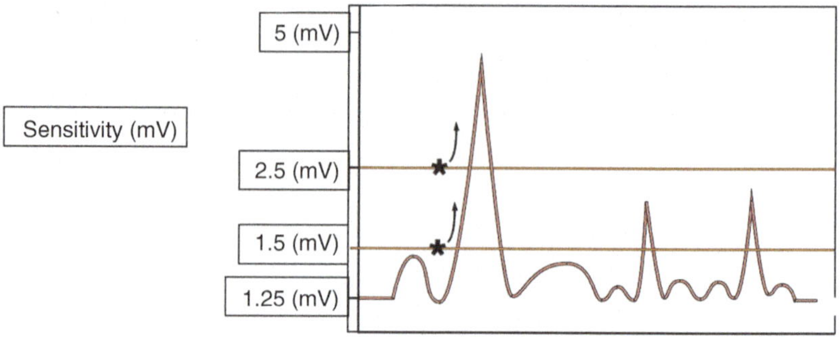

Fig. 10.9 Setting the pacemaker sensitivity at 2 mA when there is no intrinisic heart rate

mum R wave amplitude and subsequently set two to three times lower. It is usually assessed in demand modes (VVI, AAI, DDD) and allowed to pace asynchronously before being dialed down until the "sense" indicator flashes. If sensitivity *value* is set too low (too sensitive), it may have interference. Sensitivity depends on the device being used. If there is no endogenous rhythm, it is impossible to determine the pacemaker sensitivity, in which case the sensitivity is typically set to 2 mV (Fig. 10.9).

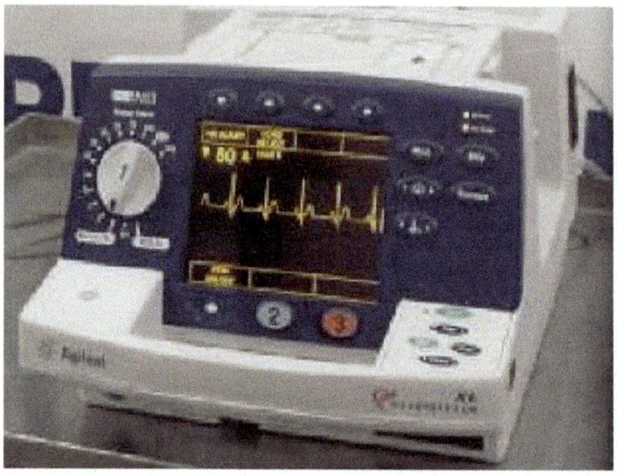

Fig. 10.10 An external defibrillator with trascutaneous pacing

Rate

The rate set on pacemakers is the rate at which we want the heart to beat to achieve adequate cardiac output. Usually it is set at 80–90 beats/min. Occasionally, a backup rate can be set which allows patients to have their native rhythm until the pacemaker sets in when the rate falls too low leading to hemodynamic collapse.

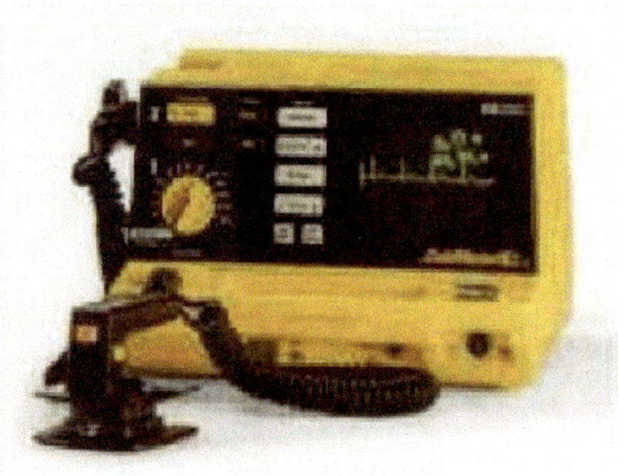

Fig. 10.11 Another model

Other Pacing Variables

The less commonly adjusted variables, such as the maximum tracking rate, AV interval, and postventricular (pacing spike) atrial refractory period (PVARP) should be noted.

Transcutaneous Pacing

External transcutaneous pacing is done in emergency situation. Most defibrillators have the ability to deliver this pacing.(Figs. 10.10 and 10.11).

- The Philips defibrillator machines are capable of delivering either demand or nondemand fixed (asynchronous) pacing.
- Both the rate and current level (mA), called "output" on this machine, can be controlled.
- Although it is sensing when you are in demand mode, you are not able to control the sensitivity.

- Pacing is done through two disposable electrodes which are self-adhering.
- ECG leads should be plugged into defibrillator machine.
- Like defibrillation, anterolateral and anteroposterior placement of patches with electrodes can be done.
- High outputs (~200 mA) may be necessary for capture due to tissue impedance.

Femoral pulse should be checked to assess if the electrical capture is leading to cardiac output (Fig. 10.12)

Pulse Generators

Pulse generators are small, battery-powered medical devices designed to electrically stimulate the heart muscle. They are used with either transvenous or epicardial pacing wires in situ. With these pacer boxes you can choose and adjust:

- Asynchronous or demand pacing.
- The rate at which you pace the patient's heart.
- The amount of energy in milliamps (mA) required for to cause a depolarization in the myocyte, referred to as "capture."
- How sensitive you want the pacer box to be to the intrinsic activity of the heart (Figs. 10.13 and 10.14).

Medtronic Temporary Pacemaker [46] (Fig. 10.15)

Green LED is for pacing stimulus. Orange LED for sensing indication. Set-up indicators identify chambers set up to pace/sense (Figs. 10.16 and 10.17).

Pacing range 30–200 PPM
Atrial output range 0.1–20 mA
Ventricular output range 0.1–25 mA

The menu key activates the lower screen and the four menus

- Sensitivity/AV interval/tracking
- Upper rate/PVARP
- Rapid atrial pacing
- Dial-a-mode (Fig. 10.18)

Atrial and ventricular sensitivity have been described in previous section.

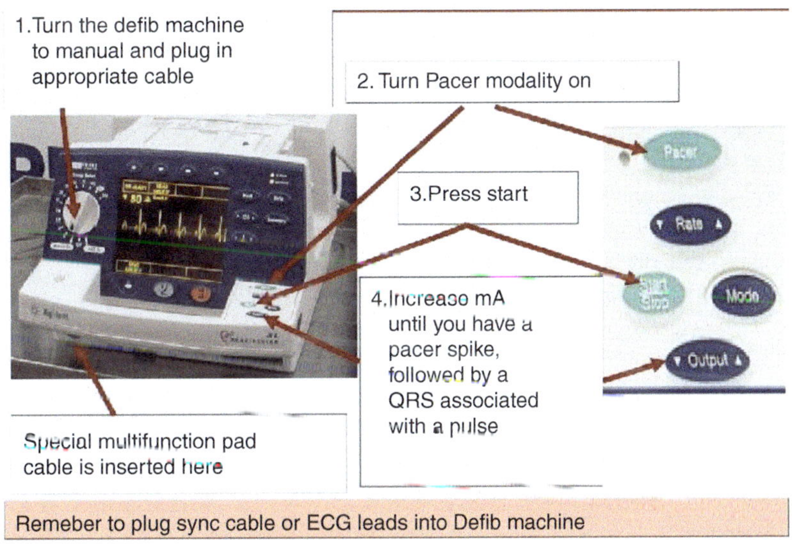

Fig. 10.12 An upclose image showing controls and settings

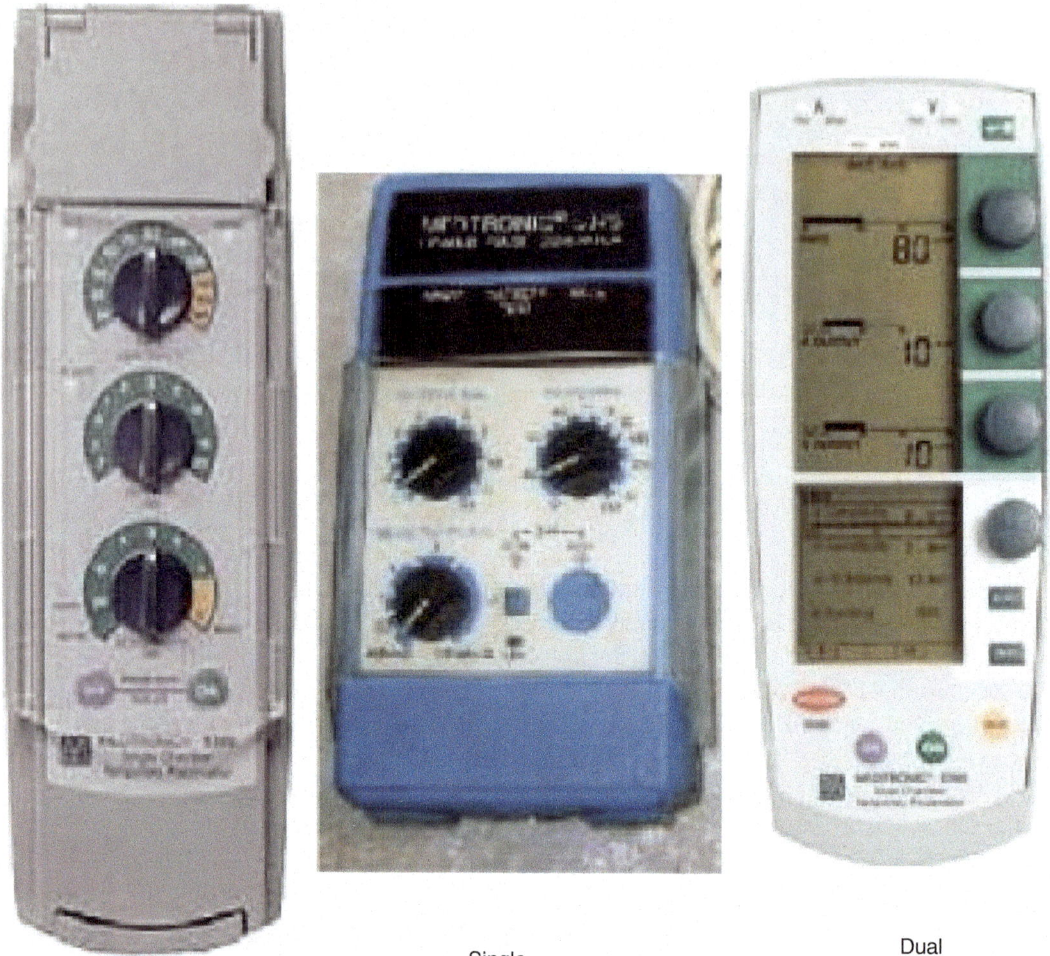

Single

Single

Dual

Fig. 10.13 Varoius models of pulse generators for transvenous or epicardial pacing

AV Interval

This represents the interval following atrial depolarization before a ventricular spike is delivered. The default is usually set at 170 millisec. The pacemaker takes on the function of the AV node. No change is usually necessary from default settings.

PVARP

This time interval is needed to prevent retrograde conduction between the ventricle and atrium through the AV node or accessory pathway. Retrograde pulses may trigger a loop and trigger ventricular contraction leading to a reentry tachycardia. PVARP ensures that the atrium is refractory during the ventricular depolarization, but this may limit atrial tracking. Typical settings are 300 msec.

Upper Rate Limit

This rate indicates the fastest the pacemaker will pace the ventricle in response to a sensed atrial event and protects against overpacing of ventricle in atrial tachycardia. It lengthens the AV interval until it is long enough for the next atrial depolar-

1. Pace/Sense LEDs
2. Lock/Unlock Key
3. Lock Indications
4. Rate Dial
5. Atrial Output Dial
6. Ventricular Output Dial
7. Menu Parameter Dial
8. Parameter Selection Key
9. Menu Selection Key
10. Pause Key
11. Power On Key
12. Power Off Key
13. Emergency/Asynchronous Pacing Key
14. Lower Screen
15. Ventricular Output Graphics
16. Artial Output Graphics
17. Upper Screen
18. Rate Graphics
19. Setup Indicators
20. DDI Indicator
21. Low Battery Indicator
22. Setup Labels

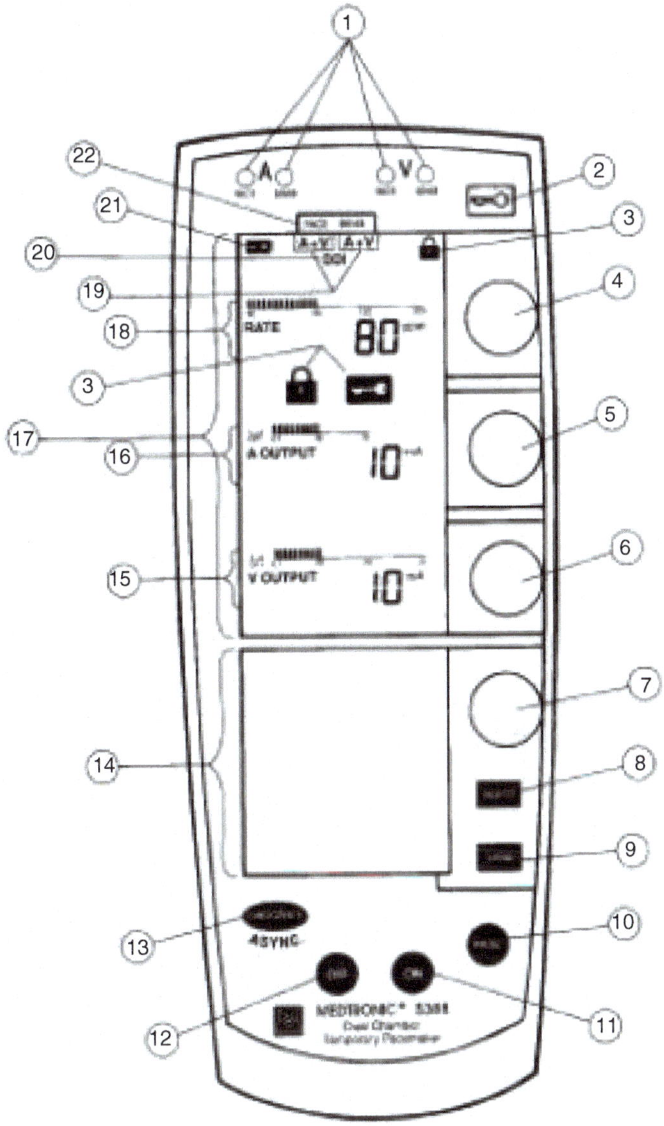

Fig. 10.14 An up close image of a pulse generator showing the controls and setting

ization to fall within the PVARP Most generators set this automatically.

Blanking Period

Atrial or ventricular blanking periods are time periods that begin after an impulse is delivered into the other cardiac chamber, thereby preventing cross-talk between leads. This is preset.

Atrial Tracking

Atrial tracking enables ventricle depolarizing at the same rate as the atria. If the patient's intrinsic rate is 80 and the pacemaker set rate is 70, it will *sense* the higher atrial rate and will not *pace* the atria. It will wait for preset AV interval and if the ventricle does not depolarize, the pacer will *trigger* and *pace* the ventricle at the intrinsic rate of atria.

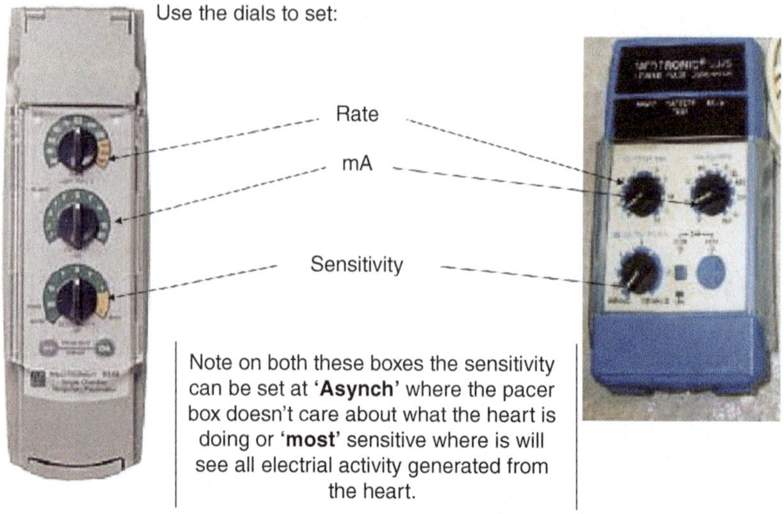

Fig. 10.15 Pulse Generators settings of Rate, Output (mA) and Sensitivity

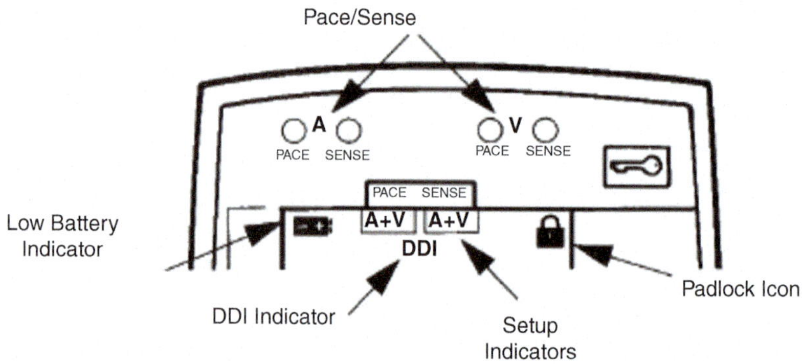

Fig. 10.16 Pulse Generator indicators

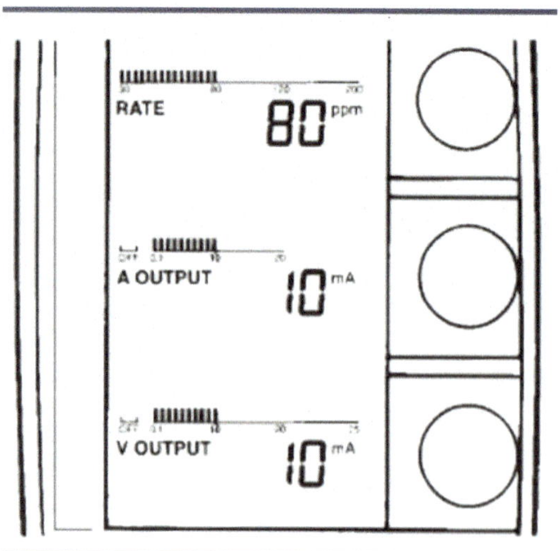

Fig. 10.17 Pulse Generator screen showing possible setttings

Antitachycardia Pacing

Overdrive pacing can be used to terminate tachyarrhythmias. When attempting *overdrive pacing, ventricular tachycardia or fibrillation may result and so DC cardioversion must be immediately available.*

Rhythms that *cannot* be controlled by pacing:

1. Atrial fibrillation
2. Sinus tachycardia
3. Ventricular fibrillation

Transvenous Pacing Wire Insertion

Transvenous wires are inserted through an introducer placed in a large central vessel like

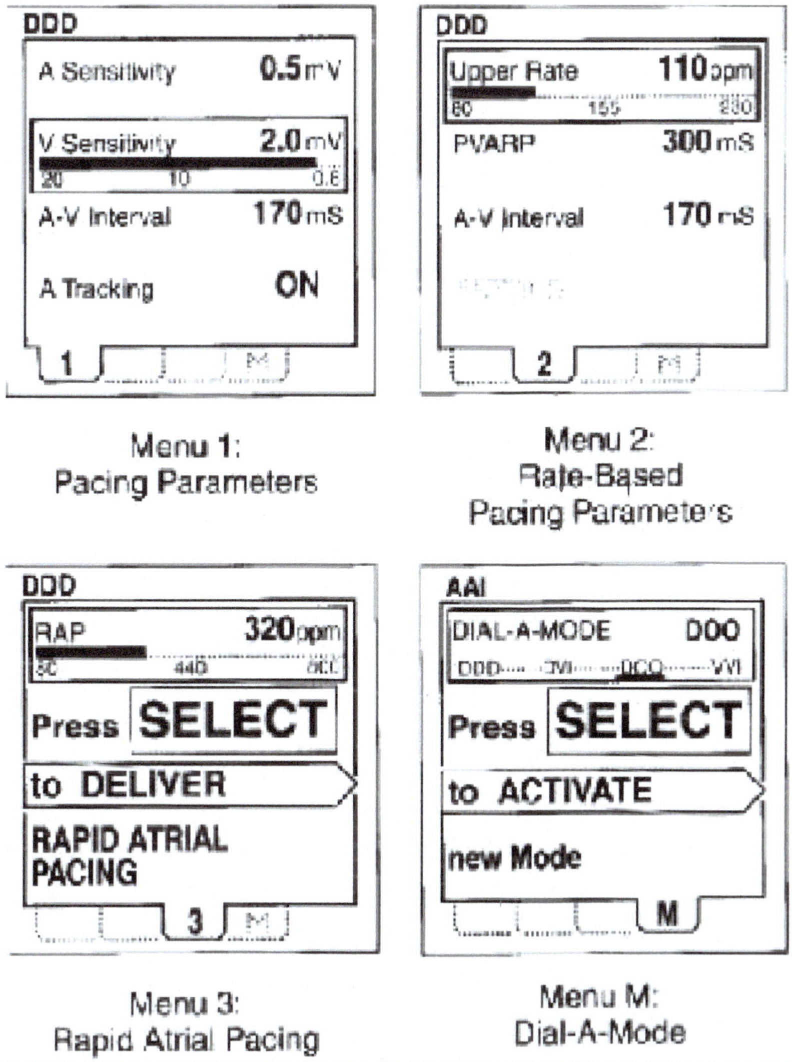

Fig. 10.18 Pulse Generator menu options

the internal jugular vein or subclavian vein. The introducer is one size bigger than the size of the wire (e.g., 6Fr introducer for 5Fr wire; 7Fr for a 6Fr wire, etc.). The pacer wire should not be put in through an existing PA catheter introducer, as the size is larger and will lead to leakage around the wire. The best way to ensure proper placement is to do the procedure under fluoroscopy, but if transvenous pacing requires stat, it can be inserted without fluoroscopy.

Epicardial Pacing Wires (Figs. 10.19 **and** 10.20)

The risk of epicardial wires is small, but it does exist. They include myocardial damage, infection, perforation, tamponade, or disruption of coronary anastomoses [47, 48]. Epicardial wires are manufactured with a small needle on one end. This is used to embed the wire in the myocardium. The lead should be sufficiently well anchored in the myocardium to avoid premature dislodgement,

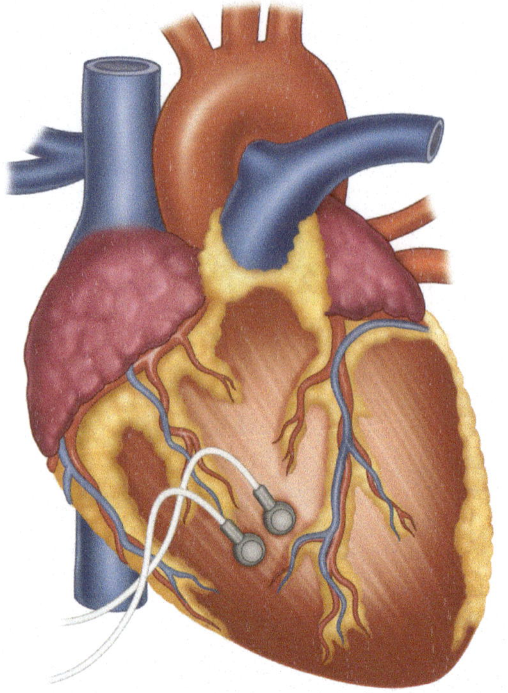

Fig. 10.19 Epicardial pacing wires

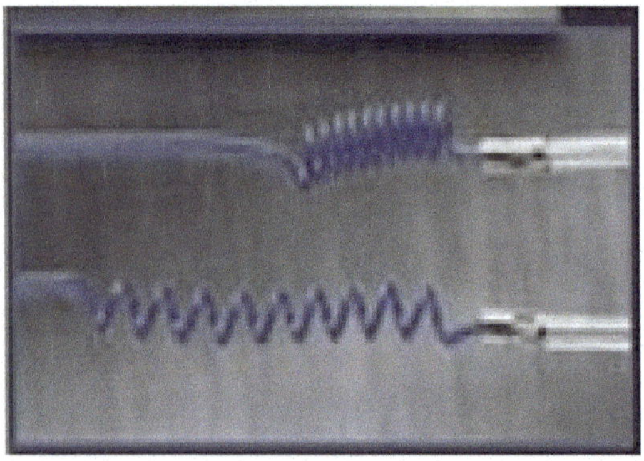

Fig. 10.20 Up close image

while still allowing eventual removal by gentle traction. Epicardial pacing wires can be unipolar and bipolar [43, 49] (Figs. 10.21 and 10.22).

Unipolar Single wire (anode) attached to epicardium and positive electrode at a distance in the subcutaneous tissue.

Bipolar Single wire with two conductors insulated from one another run to the epicardial surface. The ends of the conductor are 8 mm apart. Better in dual-chamber applications as current needed for sensing and pacing is much less due to less susceptibility to interference. Unipolar has a larger spike.

Wires attached to the right atrium are brought out through skin on the right of the sternum. They are usually blue in color. Wire attached to right ventricle emerges on the left of the sternum. They are usually brown in color.

One of the problems with epicardial wires is development of an inflammatory reaction around wire/myocardial surface [47, 50, 51]. Inflammation is increased with higher energy. Increased resistance with inflammation may lead to increased need for current or voltage to pace perpetuating a vicious cycle. Bipolar electrodes require less energy. Epicardial wires fail to sense and capture after a few days. Variations in placement site and use of steroids have been tried to extend wire longevity with variable results. Steroid-eluting endovascular wires have been used in permanent systems.

NASPE/BPEG codes for temporary pacemakers are as follows [52] (Fig. 10.23).

Temporary Pacemaker Modes [52]

1. *VVI*
   V – Ventricular pacing: The pacing device is located in the *ventricle. V* – Ventricular sensing: The device is sensing for *ventricular* activity. *I* – Inhibit mode: The pacing device will *inhibit* itself from pacing when it senses intrinsic ventricular activity. It should be used for bradycardia with AV block, sick sinus syndrome, atrial fibrillation, atrial flutter, or overdrive suppression of ectopic beats.
2. *AAI*
   A – Atrial pacing: The pacing device is located in the *atria. A* – Atrial sensing: The device is sensing for *atrial* activity. *I* – Inhibit mode: The pacing device will *inhibit* itself from pacing when it senses any intrinsic atrial activity. Bradycardia, with an endogenous atrial rhythm (or frequent ectopics), sufficiently quick to compete with the pacemaker rate is an indication. It should not be used in atrial tachycardias, fibrillation, flutter, or AV nodal block.

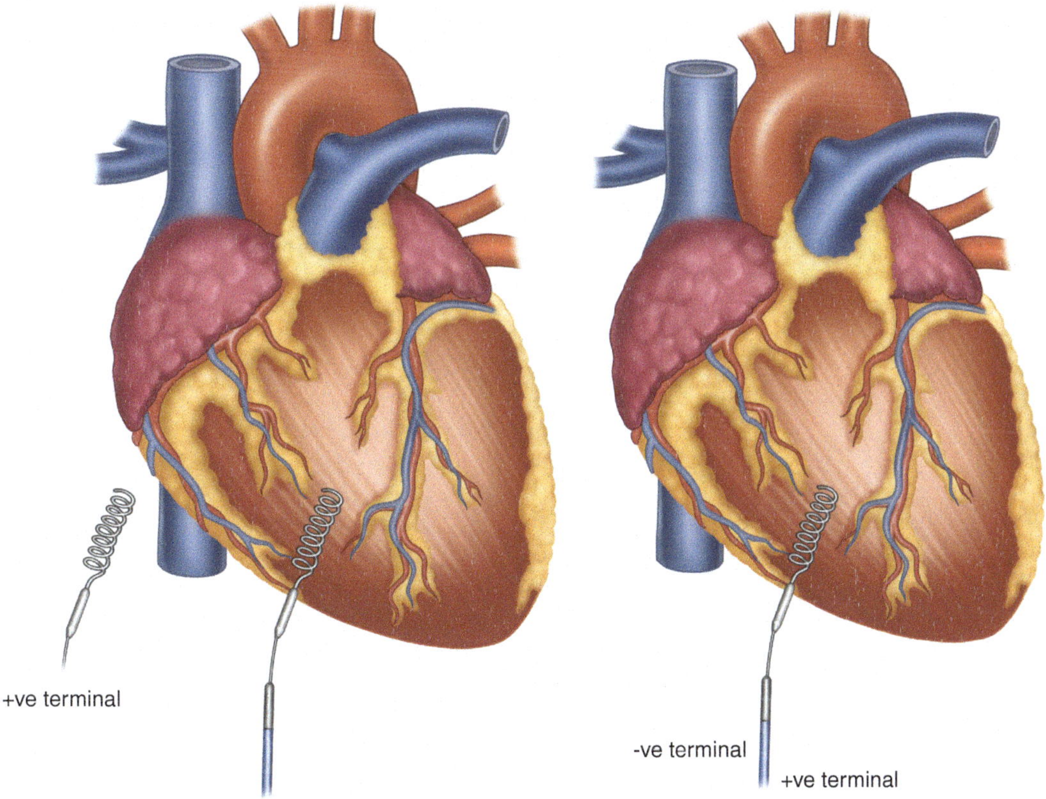

Fig. 10.21 Unipolar and Bipolar pacing wires

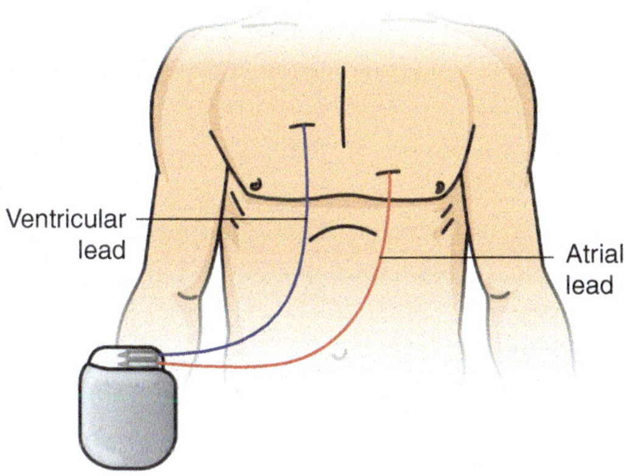

Fig. 10.22 Bipolar pacing schematic

3. *VOO*

   VOO is fixed asynchronous pacing of the ventricle. The pacer does not care what the patient's heart is doing, it is just going to pace at the set rate. This may cause an R-on-T phenomenon and should only be used in bradycardia without reliable AV node conduction where sensing may be a problem (e.g., electrocautery interference).

4. *AOO*

   This is atrial asynchronous mode. Pacing spikes are delivered to the atrium at a set rate, regardless of electrical activity in either chamber of the heart. The conduction must be intact through the AV node. It is contraindicated in atrial tachycardia, fibrillation, flutter, AV nodal block, and can be used only in bradycardia with intact AV conduction, especially when sensing may not be possible (e.g., electrocautery).

5. *DDD*

   This indicates dual function, with pacing and sensing of both atria and ventricle with inhibition when there is intrinsic activity in either of the chambers. This is also described as AV synchronous/universal pacing. This is indi-

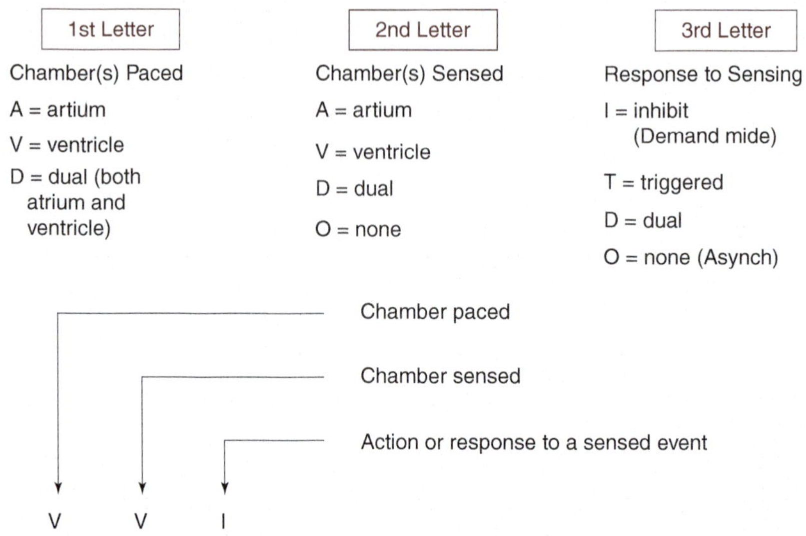

Fig. 10.23 Codes for temporary pacemakers

cated for pacing for all indications except atrial tachyarrhythmias.

6. *DOO*
   Dual-chamber pacing, but no sensing function. This can be used like VOO with additional atrial contribution. R-on-T phenomenon can occur.
7. *DVI*
   This is also described as AV sequential pacing. There is no atrial sensing. When ventricular depolarization is sensed (due to intrinsic or paced atrial beat), the ventricular spike is inhibited. This is preferred mode if there is retrograde conduction of a ventricular paced beat up the AV node. Atrial sensing in DDD and DDI modes may misinterpret this as intrinsic activity and lead to pacemaker-induced tachycardia. DVI mode, which resets the AV interval, avoids this complication. This mode is contraindicated in atrial tachycardias and fibrillation.
8. *DDI*
   This is a form of AV sequential dual-chamber sensing pacing. It adds atrial sensing to DVI, avoiding atrial pacing spike to compete with intrinsic atrial rhythm. DDI is better than DDD in rapid atrial tachyarrhythmias.
9. *VDD*
   Only the ventricle is paced here. Sensed intrinsic atrial beat will lead to ventricular depolarization if there is none; if there is no atrial beat, the ventricular will still be paced.

   This mode is unusual among the dual-chamber modes in that only the ventricle is paced.

   The pulse generator inhibits its ventricular spike in response to a sensed ventricular depolarization. A sensed atrial depolarization, however, triggers a ventricular spike if an endogenous ventricular depolarization is not sensed. If there is no endogenous atrial depolarization, a ventricular pacing spike is delivered. This is helpful in patients with an AV node block and intact sinus node.
10. *Triggered modes*
    Triggered modes (VAT, AAT, and DAT) are more commonly employed in permanent pacemakers. Triggered modes prevent inappropriate inhibition from oversensing (such as with electrocautery) [5], but in practice, asynchronous modes are more commonly used for this indication (Fig. 10.24).

A tabular form of set-up indications is described in Fig. 10.24.

Table 5-3. *Model 5388 Pacing Setup Table.*

	AOO*	VOO	AAI	VVI	DOO	DVI	DDD	DDI
Setup Indicators	**A**	**V**	**A A**	**V V**	**A+V**	**A+V V**	**A+V A+V**	**A+V A+V DDI**
Instructions								
1. Set Output								
A Output	On	Off	On	Off	On	On	On	On
V Output	Off	On	Off	On	On	On	On	On
2. Set Sensitivity								
A Sensitivity	ASYNC	NA	On	NA	ASYNC	ASYNC	On	On
V Sensitivity	NA	ASYNC	NA	On	ASYNC	On	On	On
3. Set A Tracking	NA	NA	NA	NA	NA	NA	On	Off

* **Caution:** DAD and OOO are accessible modes, but are not recommended. Refer to "Controls, Indicators, and Other Features" in the technical manual.

Fig. 10.24 Temporary Pacemaker Set Up

Appropriate modes for different arrhythmias postcardiac surgery

1. *AV junctional tachycardia* – AOO, VOO, AV sequential overdrive pacing; pacing rate increased to 120% of intrinsic rate; after 1:1 capture is achieved, pacemaker rate is reduced and a sinus rhythm should be established.
2. *Paroxysmal reentrant SVT* – AOO, AV sequential overdrive pacing.
3. *Atrial flutter* – Overdrive pacing in type 1 atrial flutter (<320–340 beats/min), but not in type II flutter with higher rates. Typically 10–20 bpm higher than flutter rate.
4. *Supraventricular tachycardias with rapid ventricular response: failure to revert to sinus rhythm* – If overdrive pacing fails, rapid atrial pacing up to 800 beats/min may terminate SVT.
5. *Ventricular tachycardia* – Although overdrive pacing may be beneficial, the risk of precipitating VF makes DC cardioversion the acceptable preferred standard of care.

Pacemaker Problems

In a study of 1675 patients undergoing cardiac surgery over 18 months, the incidence of temporary epicardial pacemakers requiring troubleshooting was 0.4%. The following steps should be adopted if any pacemaker problem is suspected:

1. Are the wires secure if patient has epicardial wires postop? Confirm the wire connection with pacer.
2. The pacer box needs to be checked for settings, mode, battery lights, and cable.
3. Check the ECG strip rate of rhythm, pacer capturing every stimulus, sensing all intrinsic activity?
4. Check underlying rhythm.
5. Check underlying rate (ideal to walk the rate down to give intrinsic rate to evolve).
6. Check stimulus threshold – pacer rate is turned to 10 above intrinsic rate and then mA is turned down until capture is lost. This is the threshold and the set threshold should be double or triple the number.

Failure to Pace

With failure to pace, the pacer does not produce a stimulus when it is required. Check for:

1. Failure of pacemaker battery or pulse generator so both may need to be changed.
2. Loose cable connections in the pacing system.
3. Fracture or dislodgement of the pacing lead wire.
4. With epicardial pacing, check ground is in place/strip everything down to wires can be seen.
5. Eliminate sources of external interference.
6. If cross-talk is suspected, sensitivities may be adjusted (Fig. 10.25).

Failure to Capture

Failure to capture is when the cardiac cells are unable to depolarize in response to the stimulus being generated by the pacemaker. It happens because of one of the following:

- Lack of enough milliamps (mA) being generated by the pacer for the cells to depolarize.
- The cells are unable to depolarize because of issues such as ischemia, fibrosis, electrolyte imbalance; the lead has perforated the myocardium.
- There is an issue with the pacing system.
- This is the most common problem encountered with temporary pacemakers (Fig. 10.26).

The following steps should be followed:

1. View rhythm in different leads; verify with a-line or pulse oximeter.
2. Check to make sure the battery light on the pacer is not on. Change battery if required.
3. Increase the mA.
4. Check and change the lead cables, connections, and the pacer itself; if dealing with epicardial wires, ensure the ground is intact.
5. If you have a transvenous wire, it may need to be repositioned.
6. Try changing polarity (change which wire is in the positive and negative port).

Undersensing

Undersensing involves the pacemaker firing without regard to patient's own rhythm. It does not sense the intrinsic activity of patient's heart. This may lead to ventricular tachycardia or fibrillation. *Undersensing* indicates *overpacing*. Undersensing can occur because of inadequate QRS signal, myocardial ischemia, fibrosis, myocardial edema, electrolyte imbalances, bundle branch block, or a poorly positioned lead (Fig. 10.27).

1. Sensitivity of pacemaker needs to be checked. Lower number indicates more ability to sense and not fire indiscriminately (decrease mV).
2. Check that the battery light is not on.
3. Check all lead connections and ground connection.
4. Check electrolytes/pH/ABG.
5. Switch polarity on epicardial wires.
6. If the patient has an adequate underlying rhythm, you may have to turn the pacer off.

Oversensing

When oversensing occurs, the pacemaker thinks it detects a QRS complex so it inhibits itself from producing a pacing stimulus. What the pacer could be seeing is the following:

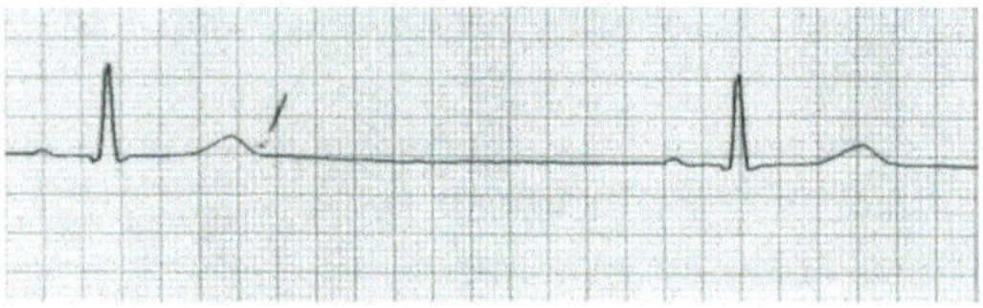

Fig. 10.25 Failure to pace

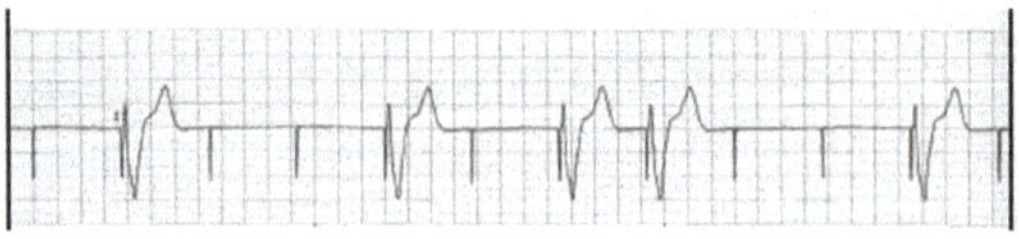

Fig. 10.26 Failure to capture

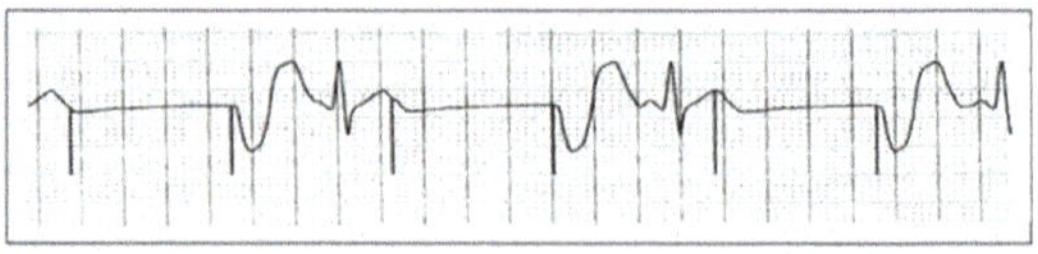

Fig. 10.27 Undersensing

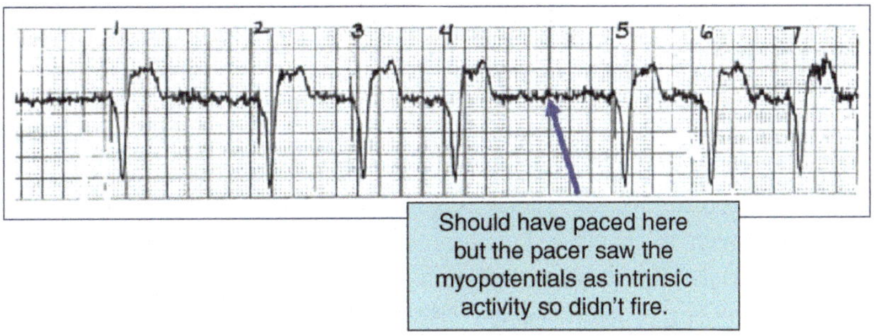

Fig. 10.28 Oversensing

- Tall or peaked P waves or T waves
- Myopotentials (electrical signals produced by skeletal muscle contraction as with shivering or seizures) (Fig. 10.28)

1. Pacemaker needs to be made less sensitive (increase mV).
2. Check all connections, change cables, switch pacer.
3. Reverse polarity on epicardial wires.

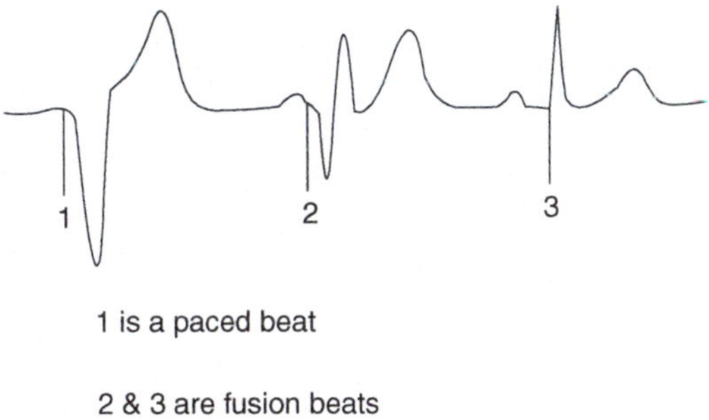

Fig. 10.29 Fusion beats

Competition and Fusion Beats

There will be times, especially if the heart is recovering when both the intrinsic rate and the paced rate are very close. This can lead to competition between the two. This can lead to fusion beats. Competition can also occur when there is asynchronous pacing, failure to sense, mechanical failure, or loose connections (Fig. 10.29).

Cross-Talk

This occurs in a dual-chamber system with AV pacing and ventricular sensing (DVI, DDD, and DDI). Sensing of one lead depolarization by another causes an inappropriate response. In atrial sensing systems, this is less serious because ventricular pacing persists. Of more concern is the system that allows such atrial sensing "cross-talk" to trigger a ventricular pacemaker spike. This will cause a form of pacemaker-mediated tachycardia. The steps to eliminating cross-talk are:

- Reduce the sensitivity (increase the lowest power that is sensed) in the atrial or ventricular channel.
- Reduce the power delivered to the ventricular or atrial pacing wire.

Pacemaker-Mediated Tachycardia

This usually occurs in VDD or DDD mode. Atrial sensing of a ventricular depolarization interpreted as intrinsic atrial spike and leads to new ventricular depolarization. This can occur also when reentrant pathways are present. Atrial blanking period can prevent this. Prolonging the PVARP period may be helpful, especially if a reentrant pathway is present. Alternative is to change mode to DVI or VVI. However, this may lead to loss of AV synchrony.

Atrial Electrogram: Temporary Wires for Diagnostic Use

Atrial pacemaker wires can be used to create an atrial electrogram (AEG). The advantage of atrial electrograms over routine ECGs recorded from skin electrodes is that the P waves are much larger on atrial electrograms, a characteristic that aids in diagnosis of arrhythmias. This helps in differentiating atrial and junctional arrhythmias [53]. They can be valuable in the following circumstances [43, 53]:

- Atrial depolarization is not visible with surface ECG leads (bedside monitor or standard 12-lead ECG).
- The relationship between atrial and ventricular electrical activity is unclear.
- Wide QRS complex rhythms need to be defined (e.g., distinguishing ventricular tachycardia from supraventricular tachycardia with a bundle branch block or aberrant conduction).
- Clarification of tachycardias with a narrow QRS complex is needed when the arrhythmia mechanism is unclear.

Some new ECG recorders have three leads used specifically for this purpose: two for bipolar atrial wires and a third for skin electrode. AEG channel set to lead I reveals large deflection with atrial depolarization, but no signal with ventricular depolarization. Lead II or III will lead to larger ventricular waveform. If the machine does not have AEG leads, the right and left arm leads can be attached to bipolar atrial wires. Lead I will reveal an AEG. Some recommend connecting the wires to chest leads as the AEG using limb leads will not record simultaneously from chest leads [43] (Fig. 10.30).

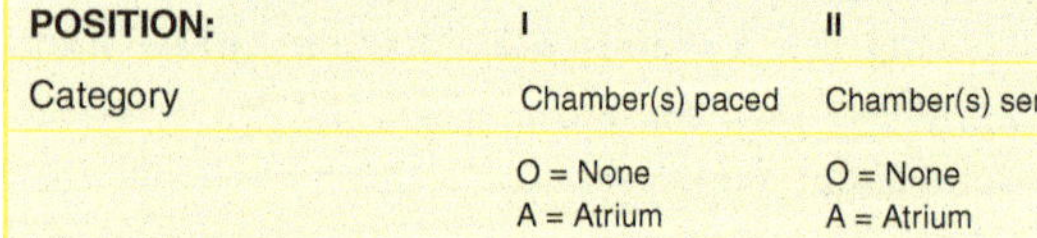

Fig. 10.30 Rhythm strip showing paced beats and PVCs in 2 leads simultaneously

Removal of the Epicardial Wires

Pacing wires are usually removed after 4–5 days when they may stop capturing or need higher current. If pacing is still needed, permanent pacemaker should be placed. Gentle traction should be applied. Excessive traction may lead to risk of tamponade, ventricular arrhythmia, or damage to coronary anastomosis [54].

Permanent pacemakers have the following codes [52] (Fig. 10.31).

Special Circumstances

MRI is not possible in a patient dependent on temporary epicardial pacing as it may precipitate arrhythmia or cause heating [55]. When a patient has an IABP in situ, high-frequency filter should be applied. If filter is disabled, spikes may be misinterpreted by balloon pump as QRS complex. IABP should be timed to the arterial pulse. If atrial spike is also being misinterpreted, timing cannot be adjusted and filter needs to be applied.

POSITION:	I	II	III	IV	V
Category	Chamber(s) paced	Chamber(s) sensed	Response(s) to sensing	Rate modulation	Multi-site pacing
	O = None A = Atrium V = Ventricle D = Dual (A+V)	O = None A = Atrium V = Ventricle D = Dual (A+V)	O = None T = Triggered I = Inhibited D = Dual (T+I)	O = None R = Rate modulation	O = None A = Atrium V = Ventricle D = Dual (A+V)
Manufacturers' designation only	S = Single (A or V)	S = Single (A or V)	*Note:* Position I through III are used exclusively for antibradyarrhythmia function.		

From Bernstein AD, Doubert JC, Fletcher RD, et al: The revised NASPE/BPEG generic code for antibradycardia, adaptive-rate and multisite pacing. North American Society of Pacing and Electrophysiology/British Pacing and Electrophysiology Group, Pacing Clin Electrophysiol 25-260–264, 2002.

Fig. 10.31 Permanent pacemaker coding

References

1. Slaughter MS, et al. Clinical management of continuous-flow left ventricular assist devices in advanced heart failure. J Heart Lung Transplant. 2010;29(4 Suppl):S1–39.
2. Kormos RL, Miller LW. Mechanical circulatory support: a companion to Braunwald's heart disease: expert consult. Philadelphia, PA: Elsevier; 2011.
3. Joyce D, Joyce L, Locke M. Mechanical circulatory support: principles and applications 2011. New York: McGraw-Hill Professional.
4. Agarwal S, High KM. Newer-generation ventricular assist devices. Best Pract Res Clin Anaesthesiol. 2012;26(2):117–30.
5. Rogers JG, et al. Continuous flow left ventricular assist device improves functional capacity and quality of life of advanced heart failure patients. J Am Coll Cardiol. 2010;55(17):1826–34.
6. Pratt AK, Shah NS, Boyce SW. Left ventricular assist device management in the ICU. Crit Care Med. 2014;42(1):158–68.
7. Miller LW, et al. Use of a continuous-flow device in patients awaiting heart transplantation. N Engl J Med. 2007;357(9):885–96.
8. Moazami N, et al. Axial and centrifugal continuous-flow rotary pumps: a translation from pump mechanics to clinical practice. J Heart Lung Transplant. 2013;32(1):1–11.
9. Nienaber J, Wilhelm MP, Sohail MR. Current concepts in the diagnosis and management of left ventricular assist device infections. Expert Rev Anti-Infect Ther. 2013;11(2):201–10.
10. Slaughter MS. Long-term continuous flow left ventricular assist device support and end-organ function: prospects for destination therapy. J Card Surg. 2010;25(4):490–4.
11. Uriel N, et al. Development of a novel echocardiography ramp test for speed optimization and diagnosis of device thrombosis in continuous-flow left ventricular assist devices: the Columbia ramp study. J Am Coll Cardiol. 2012;60(18):1764–75.
12. O'Shea G. Ventricular assist devices: what intensive care unit nurses need to know about postoperative management. AACN Adv Crit Care. 2012;23(1):69–83; quiz 84–5
13. Feldman D, et al. The 2013 International Society for Heart and Lung Transplantation Guidelines for mechanical circulatory support: executive summary. J Heart Lung Transplant. 2013;32(2):157–87.
14. Kapur NK, Jumean MF Management of continuous flow left ventricular assist device patients in the Cardiac Catheterization Laboratory. www.cathlabdigest.com 2014. 22.
15. Morgan JA, et al. Impact of continuous-flow left ventricular assist device support on right ventricular function. J Heart Lung Transplant. 2013;32(4):398–403.
16. Imamura T, et al. Bosentan improved persistent pulmonary hypertension in a case after implantation of a left ventricular assist device. J Artif Organs. 2013;16(1):101–4.
17. Goldstein JA, Kern MJ. Percutaneous mechanical support for the failing right heart. Cardiol Clin. 2012;30(2):303–10.
18. Hottigoudar RU, et al. Catheter ablation of atrial flutter in patients with left ventricular assist device improves symptoms of right heart failure. Congest Heart Fail. 2013;19(4):165–71.
19. Nakahara S, et al. Ventricular arrhythmias after left ventricular assist device. Circ Arrhythm Electrophysiol. 2013;6(3):648–54.
20. Rajagopal K, et al. Natural history and clinical effect of aortic valve regurgitation after left ventricular assist device implantation. J Thorac Cardiovasc Surg. 2013;145(5):1373–9.
21. Patil NP, et al. De novo aortic regurgitation after continuous-flow left ventricular assist device implantation. Ann Thorac Surg. 2014;98(3):850–7.
22. John R, et al. Aortic valve pathophysiology during left ventricular assist device support. J Heart Lung Transplant. 2010;29(12):1321–9.
23. Allen SJ, Sidebotham D. Postoperative care and complications after ventricular assist device implantation. Best Pract Res Clin Anaesthesiol. 2012;26(2):231–46.
24. Morgan JA, et al. Management of aortic valve insufficiency in patients supported by long-term continuous flow left ventricular assist devices. Ann Thorac Surg. 2012;94(5):1710–2.
25. Mehra MR, Stewart GC, Uber PA. The vexing problem of thrombosis in long-term mechanical circulatory support. J Heart Lung Transplant. 2014;33(1):1–11.
26. Adatya S, et al. Loading conditions influence reliability of the echocardiographic ramp test in continuous-flow left ventricular assist devices. J Heart Lung Transplant. 2013;32(11):1142–4.
27. Kapur NK, et al. Left ventricular assist device thrombosis presenting as an acute coronary syndrome. J Thorac Cardiovasc Surg. 2014;147(6):e72–3.
28. Velagic V, et al. Management of heparin-induced thrombocytopenia with fondaparinux in a patient with left ventricular assist device. Int J Organ Transplant Med. 2014;5(2):83–6.
29. Schroder JN, et al. Heparin-induced thrombocytopenia in left ventricular assist device bridge-to-transplant patients. Ann Thorac Surg. 2007;84(3):841–5; discussion 845–6.
30. Morgan JA, et al. Gastrointestinal bleeding with the HeartMate II left ventricular assist device. J Heart Lung Transplant. 2012;31(7):715–8.
31. Meyer AL, et al. Acquired von Willebrand syndrome in patients with an axial flow left ventricular assist device. Circ Heart Fail. 2010;3(6):675–81.
32. Coutance G, et al. Octreotide for recurrent intestinal bleeding due to ventricular assist device. Asian Cardiovasc Thorac Ann. 2014;22(3):350–2.
33. Rennyson SL, et al. Octreotide for left ventricular assist device-related gastrointestinal hemorrhage: can we stop the bleeding? ASAIO J. 2013;59(4):450–1.

34. Patel AM, et al. Renal failure in patients with left ventricular assist devices. Clin J Am Soc Nephrol. 2013;8(3):484–96.
35. Wilson TJ, et al. Management of intracranial hemorrhage in patients with left ventricular assist devices. J Neurosurg. 2013;118(5):1063–8.
36. Morgan JA, et al. Stroke while on long-term left ventricular assist device support: incidence, outcome, and predictors. ASAIO J. 2014;60(3):284–9.
37. Kato TS, et al. Pre-operative and post-operative risk factors associated with neurologic complications in patients with advanced heart failure supported by a left ventricular assist device. J Heart Lung Transplant. 2012;31(1):1–8.
38. Kato TS, et al. Asymmetric pattern of cerebrovascular lesions in patients after left ventricular assist device implantation. Stroke. 2012;43(3):872–4.
39. Gordon RJ, et al. Prospective, multicenter study of ventricular assist device infections. Circulation. 2013;127(6):691–702.
40. Nienaber JJ, et al. Clinical manifestations and management of left ventricular assist device-associated infections. Clin Infect Dis. 2013;57(10):1438–48.
41. LaRue S, et al. Left ventricular assist device in pregnancy. Obstet Gynecol. 2011;118(2 Pt 2):426–8.
42. Sarsam SH, et al. Trauma in patients with continuous-flow left ventricular assist devices. Am J Cardiol. 2013;112(9):1520–2.
43. Reade MC. Temporary epicardial pacing after cardiac surgery: a practical review: part 1: general considerations in the management of epicardial pacing. Anaesthesia. 2007;62(3):264–71.
44. Rozner MA, Trankina M. Cardiac pacing and defibrillation. In: Kaplan JA, Reich DL, Lake CL, Konstadt SN, editors. Kaplan's cardiac anesthesia. Philadelphia: W. B. Saunders; 2006. p. 827–43.
45. Atlee JL, Bernstein AD. Cardiac rhythm management devices (part II): perioperative management. Anesthesiology. 2001;95(6):1492–506.
46. Scales G Medtronic model 5388 dual chamber temporary pacemaker technical manual. 2006.
47. Timothy PR, Rodeman BJ. Temporary pacemakers in critically ill patients: assessment and management strategies. AACN Clin Issues. 2004;15(3):305–25.
48. Bojar RM, editor. Manual of perioperative care in adult cardiac surgery. 4th ed. Malden: Blackwell Publishing; 2004.
49. Spotnitz HM. Optimizing temporary perioperative cardiac pacing. J Thorac Cardiovasc Surg. 2005;129(1):5–8.
50. Elmi F, Tullo NG, Khalighi K. Natural history and predictors of temporary epicardial pacemaker wire function in patients after open heart surgery. Cardiology. 2002;98(4):175–80.
51. Daoud EG, et al. Randomized, double-blind trial of simultaneous right and left atrial epicardial pacing for prevention of post-open heart surgery atrial fibrillation. Circulation. 2000;102(7):761–5.
52. Bernstein AD, et al. The revised NASPE/BPEG generic code for antibradycardia, adaptive-rate, and multisite pacing. North American Society of Pacing and Electrophysiology/British Pacing and Electrophysiology Group. Pacing Clin Electrophysiol. 2002;25(2):260–4.
53. Miller JN, Drew BJ. Atrial electrograms after cardiac surgery: survey of clinical practice. Am J Crit Care. 2007;16(4):350–6; quiz 357; discussion 358–9.
54. Carroll KC, et al. Risks associated with removal of ventricular epicardial pacing wires after cardiac surgery. Am J Crit Care. 1998;7(6):444–9.
55. Luechinger R, et al. In vivo heating of pacemaker leads during magnetic resonance imaging. Eur Heart J. 2005;26(4):376–83; discussion 325–7.

11 Cardiac Arrest and the Post-arrest Syndrome

Torben K. Becker and Jonathan Elmer

Abbreviations

CNS	Central nervous system
$PaCO_2$	Partial pressure of carbon dioxide
COPD	Chronic obstructive pulmonary disease
CT	Computed tomography
CXR	Chest X-ray
DKA	Diabetic ketoacidosis
ECG	Electrocardiogram
ED	Emergency department
EEG	Electroencephalogram
EMS	Emergency medical services
FOUR	Full outline of unresponsiveness
GI	Gastrointestinal
ICU	Intensive care unit
MAP	Mean arterial pressure
MRI	Magnetic resonance imaging
OHCA	Out-of-hospital cardiac arrest
PaO_2	Partial pressure of oxygen
ROSC	Return of spontaneous circulation
RV	Right ventricle
SAH	Subarachnoid hemorrhage
TTM	Targeted temperature management
UA	Urinalysis

T. K. Becker
Department of Emergency Medicine, University of Florida, Gainesville, FL, USA

J. Elmer (✉)
Departments of Emergency Medicine, Critical Care Medicine and Neurology, University of Pittsburgh School of Medicine, Pittsburgh, PA, USA
e-mail: elmerjp@upmc.edu

Critical Points

- More than 300,000 Americans suffer out-of-hospital cardiac arrest annually; about 40,000 achieve return of spontaneous circulation (ROSC) and are treated in the emergency department.
- Initial management of the pulseless patient should follow American Heart Association cardiac arrest guidelines based on the presenting rhythm:
  - High-quality chest compressions and early defibrillation of shockable rhythms are treatment priorities. Both improve patient outcomes.
  - Secondary priorities that are not shown to improve outcomes are intravenous access, code medications, and placement of an advanced airway.
- Patients with ROSC who remain comatose are at significant risk for poor outcome without early and advanced critical care interventions including:
  - Active temperature management.
  - Identification and treatment of the underlying etiology of arrest, with emergent cardiac catheterization if indicated.
  - Avoidance of hyperoxia, hyperventilation, and cerebral hypoperfusion.
  - Delayed neurological prognostication by experts.

© Springer Nature Switzerland AG 2020
J. R. Shiber, S. D. Weingart (eds.), *Emergency Department Critical Care*,
https://doi.org/10.1007/978-3-030-28794-8_11

- Anoxic brain injury is the most common cause of death after cardiac arrest, but accurate neurological prognostication is impossible for at least 72 h after ROSC.
  - Before this time, no clinical sign or combination of signs precludes favorable outcome.
  - The diagnosis of brain death cannot be made for at least 24 h following cardiac arrest.
- Comatose cardiac arrest survivors should be transferred to a hospital capable of providing advanced cardiac and neurological care, including cardiac catheterization, specialized neurocritical care, and neurological prognostication.

Introduction

Sudden cardiac arrest is the most common cause of death in America, with over 500,000 Americans suffering cardiac arrest annually. About two-thirds of these occur outside of the hospital and are assessed by emergency medical service (EMS) providers. Half of these are treated by EMS and a quarter of EMS-treated out-of-hospital cardiac arrest (OHCA) patients have return of spontaneous circulation (ROSC) and survive at least 1 hour after emergency department (ED) arrival. With increasing use of implantable defibrillators and other cardiac care, the proportion of patients with shockable rhythms on presentation is decreasing over time, and now represents a minority of patients. In recent years, rates of ROSC and survival from OHCA have improved in some patient populations, such as bystander-witnessed cardiac arrest, however, overall survival and favorable neurological recovery after OHCA remain low at about 10.6% and 8.3%, respectively [1].

Pathophysiology

Cardiac arrest can result from many different underlying disease processes, such as acute coronary syndrome, pulmonary embolism, sepsis, or stroke, among many other causes. Rapid identification and treatment of the underlying etiology of an individual patient's cardiac arrest is mandatory, as is supportive critical care treatment of the postcardiac arrest syndrome. During pulselessness, total body ischemia develops, which is then compounded by reperfusion injury in the minutes after ROSC. This ischemia–reperfusion injury results in significant derangements of normal physiology and a systemic inflammatory response, often leading to multisystem organ failure. Common pathophysiological manifestations of the postcardiac arrest syndrome include anoxic brain injury, respiratory failure, post-arrest myocardial dysfunction, and vasodilatory shock [2].

Patient Presentation

A patient in cardiac arrest will typically be obvious to recognize. However, it is important to note that in the absence of a definitive pulse in an otherwise unresponsive patient, cardiac arrest is to be assumed and resuscitative measures should not be delayed by attempting to verify whether other signs of circulatory collapse can be ruled in or out. After ROSC, the severity of multisystem organ failure will be variable and must be assessed systematically. For example, patients may rapidly regain consciousness or remain comatose; myocardial dysfunction and shock may range from mild to profound. Cardiac arrest is not an uncommon presentation resulting from ST-elevation myocardial infarction or other acute coronary syndrome. This and other possible underlying etiologies of arrest (see below) must not be obscured by the more dramatic presentation of full cardiac arrest, and ruled in or out based on clinical suspicion or directed diagnostic testing.

Initial Diagnostics

During cardiac arrest, clinicians should search for reversible causes of cardiovascular collapse: hypovolemia, hypoxia, hypothermia, acidosis, abnormal serum potassium levels, tension pneumothorax, cardiac tamponade, toxins, acute coronary syndrome, and pulmonary embolism [3]. A focused history may be helpful to rule in or out many of these possible causes of cardiac arrest. Therefore, it is important to gather as much information as possible from EMS personnel or family. In addition, in our practice, a standardized approach to evaluate for reversible causes includes a physical examination, a fingerstick glucometer test, a blood gas with electrolytes, and a focused ultrasound of the heart and lungs for signs of pericardial effusion, right ventricular failure, pneumothorax, or pulmonary edema. However, a definitive cause is often difficult to determine before ROSC and thus clinicians must often continue to investigate the etiology of arrest after ROSC. Without identifying and reversing the primary disease process, cardiac arrest will likely recur.

Intra-arrest Management

The fundamentals of cardiac arrest treatment include high-quality chest compressions and early defibrillation of ventricular fibrillation or pulseless ventricular tachycardia. The American Heart Association 2010 cardiac arrest algorithm provides an easy-to-follow and systematic approach to the management of a patient in cardiac arrest (Fig. 11.1). For a few select patients with cardiac arrest refractory to standard treatment, invasive extracorporeal support may be considered [4].

Post-arrest Diagnostics

After ROSC, several rapid diagnostic and therapeutic options must be considered. It is important to perform and document an initial neurologic examination, including a brainstem and motor examination, as it has prognostic value [5]. The full outline of unresponsiveness (FOUR) score (Table 11.1) has been validated in both the emergency department (ED) and the intensive care unit (ICU) with good interrater reliability [6]. We recommend its use over the Glasgow Coma Scale, since the FOUR score includes a brainstem examination and allows for a more differentiated assessment of intubated patients. In addition, the following minimum diagnostic work-up should be performed on virtually every postcardiac arrest patient:

- ECG to evaluate for underlying cardiac etiology, since patients with underlying, and often undiagnosed, coronary artery disease are at particularly elevated risk to suffer from cardiac arrest [1].
- Laboratory tests to include complete blood count, comprehensive chemistry, coagulation studies, arterial blood gas, lactic acid, and troponin.
- Noncontrast CT of the head to evaluate for underlying etiology, such as subarachnoid hemorrhage, and for prognostic purposes [7, 8].
- Additional workup guided by clinical context and results of the above-mentioned studies (Table 11.2).

Post-arrest Management

Neurological Early studies demonstrated that therapeutic hypothermia after OHCA improved neurological outcomes compared to no temperature management for selected comatose patients. The more recent and larger targeted temperature management (TTM) trial found that active temperature management to a goal of 33 °C was equivalent to active temperature management to a goal of 36 °C [9–11]. Unlike earlier studies, the TTM study included subjects with nonshockable initial rhythms. Regardless of the goal temperature, active temperature management should be strongly considered in all comatose post-arrest patients unless an absolute contraindication (such as significant intracranial hemorrhage or uncontrolled bleeding) exists

Cardiovascular Consideration must be given to emergent cardiac catheterization after OHCA, particularly for patients with signs or symptoms of acute coronary syndrome as the cause of cardiac arrest. Such signs may include a shockable initial arrest rhythm. The post-arrest ECG is neither specific nor sensitive for coronary occlusion,

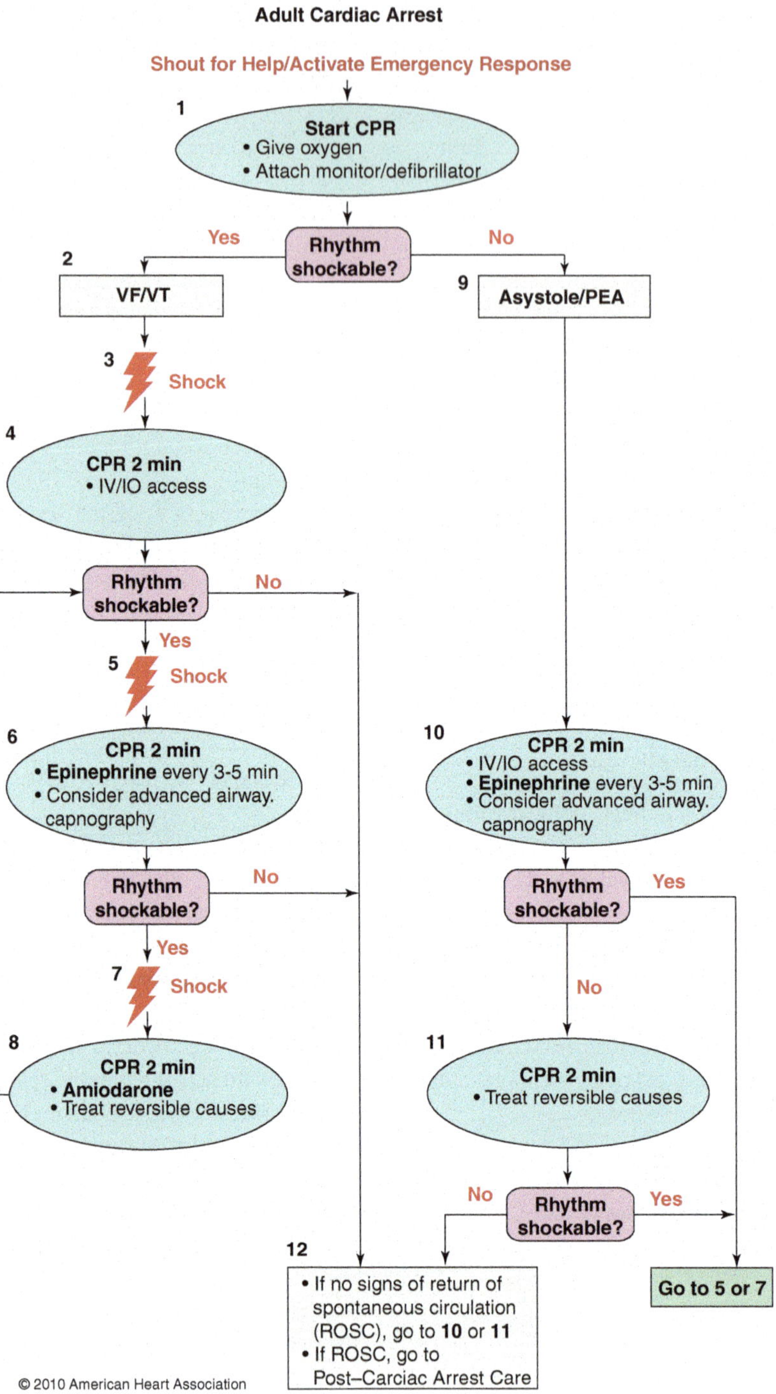

Fig. 11.1 Cardiac arrest algorithm by the American Heart Association (Source: American Heart Association. Available at: http://circ.ahajournals.org/content/122/18_suppl_3/S729/F1.large.jpg)

Table 11.1 Full outline of unresponsiveness (FOUR) score

	Response	Score
Eyes	Open spontaneously, track, blinks to command	4
	Open but do not track or blink to command	3
	Open to loud voice	2
	Open to painful stimuli	1
	Remain closed with painful stimuli	0
Motor	Follows commands	4
	Localizes pain	3
	Flexes to pain	2
	Extends to pain	1
	No response to pain or myoclonic status	0
Brainstem	Pupil and corneal reflexes present	4
	One pupil wide and fixed	3
	Pupil or corneal reflexes absent	2
	Pupil and corneal absent	1
	Absent pupil, corneal, and cough	0
Respiration	Not intubated, regular breathing pattern	4
	Not intubated, Cheyne–Stokes breathing	3
	Not intubated, irregular breathing pattern	2
	Intubated, overbreathing ventilator	1
	Intubated, breathing at set rate or apnea	0

Table 11.2 Symptom-guided diagnostic evaluation of the postcardiac arrest patient

Underlying etiology	Work-up to consider
Cardiac Acute coronary syndrome Structural heart disease Cardiomyopathies RV failure (e.g., pulmonary hypertension, pulmonary embolus) Arrhythmia	ECG for ischemic changes, rhythm, and intervals Troponin BNP Echocardiogram CT angiography of chest Cardiac catheterization
Pulmonary Primary respiratory failure (e.g., COPD, asthma) Large airway obstruction	CXR Blood gas Peak pressures Bronchoscopy
Trauma Exsanguination Nontrauma exsanguination (e.g., GI bleed) Pneumothorax Cardiac tamponade	Detailed history Complete blood count CT chest/abdomen/pelvis
Catastrophic neurological event Stroke Subarachnoid hemorrhage	CT head MRI head
Septic shock	Cultures (blood, urine, +/− sputum) CXR Inflammatory markers
Metabolic derangements Diabetic ketoacidosis Hypoglycemia Hyperkalemia	Comprehensive chemistry
Exposures Toxicological Environmental (e.g., electrocution, hypothermia)	Detailed history Toxicology studies ECG for intervals

and catheterization should not be withheld based on a relatively normal ECG only, as risk-adjusted analyses have shown catheterization to be associated with improved neurological outcomes in patients surviving OHCA [12–14]. Cerebral autoregulation is commonly impaired after ROSC, and the already injured brain may be vulnerable to secondary brain injury for several days. Observational data suggest that targeting a mean arterial pressure (MAP) of 80 mmHg or higher in the early postcardiac arrest phase, regardless of the need for vasopressor support, improves neurological outcomes [15]. If there is no contraindication, a higher than typical MAP goal may be considered to ensure adequate cerebral blood flow. Conversely, hypotension must be avoided.

Respiratory Most post-arrest patients are comatose and will require endotracheal intubation for airway protection and to ensure adequate oxygenation and ventilation. Multiple observational studies have associated early arterial hyperoxia with worse patient outcomes, presumably due to increased oxidative injury during ischemia–reperfusion [16]. This observation has not been consistently replicated in all studies; regardless, no studies have associated hyperoxia with improved outcomes. We believe that hyperoxia should therefore be avoided. From a practical perspective, clinicians should target a pulse oximetry of not above 99%, or a PaO2 of less than 300 mmHg. Additionally, mild hypercapnia ($PaCO_2$ 40 to 45 mmHg) has been associated with improved neurological outcome, presumably by increasing cerebral blood flow [17]. Blood gas results must be temperature corrected in patients who are hypothermic or undergoing TTM.

Prognosis Neurological prognostication in the ED must be avoided. Evidence-based guidelines recommend delaying withdrawal of life-sustaining therapy based on neurological prognosis for at least 72 hours after ROSC. Prior to this time, no clinical sign or test precludes a favorable neurological outcome [18], and patients who remain comatose days after ROSC may still awaken and have favorable recoveries [19]. Formal brain death testing should not be conducted for at least 24 hours after ROSC.

Disposition Patients who have achieved ROSC but remain comatose should be transferred to a hospital capable of providing advanced critical care interventions, including cardiac catheterization, expert neurological evaluation, and electroencephalogram (EEG) monitoring [20].

References

1. Mozaffarian D, Benjamin EJ, Go AS, Arnett DK, Blaha MJ, Cushman M, et al. Heart disease and stroke statistics--2015 update: a report from the American Heart Association. Circulation. 2015;131(4):e29–322. Epub 2014/12/19.
2. Stub D, Bernard S, Duffy SJ, Kaye DM. Post cardiac arrest syndrome: a review of therapeutic strategies. Circulation. 2011;123(13):1428–35. Epub 2011/04/06
3. Field JM, Hazinski MF, Sayre MR, Chameides L, Schexnayder SM, Hemphill R, et al. Part 1: executive summary 2010 American Heart Association guidelines for cardiopulmonary resuscitation and emergency cardiovascular care. Circulation. 2010;122(18 suppl 3):S640–S56.
4. Wang C-H, Chou N-K, Becker LB, Lin J-W, Yu H-Y, Chi N-H, et al. Improved outcome of extracorporeal cardiopulmonary resuscitation for out-of-hospital cardiac arrest–a comparison with that for extracorporeal rescue for in-hospital cardiac arrest. Resuscitation. 2014;85(9):1219–24.
5. Coppler PJ, Elmer J, Calderon L, Sabedra A, Doshi AA, Callaway CW, et al. Validation of the Pittsburgh Cardiac Arrest Category illness severity score. Resuscitation. 2015;89:86–92.
6. Rittenberger JC, Doshi AA, Reynolds JC, Service PCA. Postcardiac arrest management. Emerg Med Clin North Am. 2015;33:691.
7. Cocchi MN, Lucas JM, Salciccioli J, Carney E, Herman S, Zimetbaum P, et al. The role of cranial computed tomography in the immediate post-cardiac arrest period. Intern Emerg Med. 2010;5(6):533–8.
8. Metter RB, Rittenberger JC, Guyette FX, Callaway CW. Association between a quantitative CT scan measure of brain edema and outcome after cardiac arrest. Resuscitation. 2011;82(9):1180–5.
9. Bernard SA, Gray TW, Buist MD, Jones BM, Silvester W, Gutteridge G, et al. Treatment of comatose survivors of out-of-hospital cardiac arrest with induced hypothermia. N Engl J Med. 2002;346(8):557–63.
10. Nikolov NM, Cunningham AJ. Mild therapeutic hypothermia to improve the neurologic outcome after cardiac arrest. Survey Anesthesiol. 2003;47(4):219–20.
11. Nielsen N, Wetterslev J, Cronberg T, Erlinge D, Gasche Y, Hassager C, et al. Targeted temperature management at 33 C versus 36 C after cardiac arrest. N Engl J Med. 2013;369(23):2197–206.
12. Camuglia AC, Randhawa VK, Lavi S, Walters DL. Cardiac catheterization is associated with superior outcomes for survivors of out of hospital cardiac arrest: review and meta-analysis. Resuscitation. 2014;85(11):1533–40.
13. Reynolds JC, Rittenberger JC, Toma C, Callaway CW, Service TPCA. Risk-adjusted outcome prediction with initial post-cardiac arrest illness severity: implications for cardiac arrest survivors being considered for early invasive strategy. Resuscitation. 2014;85(9):1232–9.
14. Redfors B, Råmunddal T, Angerås O, Dworeck C, Haraldsson I, Ioanes D, et al. Angiographic findings and survival in patients undergoing coronary angiography due to sudden cardiac arrest in Western Sweden. Resuscitation. 2015;90:13–20.
15. Beylin ME, Perman SM, Abella BS, Leary M, Shofer FS, Grossestreuer AV, et al. Higher mean arterial pressure with or without vasoactive agents is associated with increased survival and better neurological outcomes in comatose survivors of cardiac arrest. Intensive Care Med. 2013;39(11):1981–8.
16. Elmer J, Scutella M, Pullalarevu R, Wang B, Vaghasia N, Trzeciak S, et al. The association between hyperoxia and patient outcomes after cardiac arrest: analysis of a high-resolution database. Intensive Care Med. 2015;41(1):49–57.
17. Vaahersalo J, Bendel S, Reinikainen M, Kurola J, Tiainen M, Raj R, et al. Arterial blood gas tensions after resuscitation from out-of-hospital cardiac arrest: associations with long-term neurologic outcome∗. Crit Care Med. 2014;42(6):1463–70.
18. Sandroni C, Cavallaro F, Callaway CW, D'Arrigo S, Sanna T, Kuiper MA, et al. Predictors of poor neurological outcome in adult comatose survivors of cardiac arrest: a systematic review and meta-analysis.

Part 2: patients treated with therapeutic hypothermia. Resuscitation. 2013;84(10):1324–38.
19. Gold B, Puertas L, Davis SP, Metzger A, Yannopoulos D, Oakes DA, et al. Awakening after cardiac arrest and post resuscitation hypothermia: are we pulling the plug too early? Resuscitation. 2014;85(2):211–4.
20. Institute of Medicine. Strategies to Improve Cardiac Arrest Survival: A Time to Act. 2015; Available from: http://iom.nationalacademies.org/~/media/Files/Report%20Files/CardiacArrestReportBrief.pdf.

12 Heart Failure

Christopher J. Hogan

Acute Heart Failure

Critical Points

- Assess if preserved versus reduced ejection fraction heart failure: old records, echocardiography.
- Evaluate early for myocardial infarction or acute ischemia: ECG, serial cardiac enzymes.
- Use noninvasive pressure support ventilation often and early.
- Hypotension (do not overlook *relative* hypotension) is ominous and should be corrected early and aggressively (fluids, dobutamine).
- N-terminal brain natriuretic peptide (NT-proBNP) or B-type natriuretic peptide (BNP) measurements are of limited use in renal failure patients.
- If using nitrates, higher doses may be more beneficial, but may be of less value in patients who are on chronic nitrate therapy.
- If the initial dose of loop diuretics fails to be effective, consider adding a low-dose second agent such as thiazides or spironolactone.

Introduction

Acute heart failure (AHF) affects approximately 5.7 million Americans, with 87,000 new AHF cases annually [1]. For every large myocardial infarction saved by an intervention, another heart failure patient is created. Projections suggest that the prevalence of AHF will increase 46% from 2012 to 2030, resulting in over 8 million people with the disease [2, 3]. A disease of the elderly [4], up to 75% of AHF patients also have preceding hypertension, another reason why emphasizing follow-up for uncontrolled hypertension in emergency department (ED) patients presenting with other complaints is important. Because AHF disproportionally affects minorities, urban medical centers evaluate and treat AHF-related problems more frequently.

AHF is particularly germane to emergency physicians because 80% of patients hospitalized with the disease are admitted through the ED [5], accounting

C. J. Hogan (✉)
Department of Emergency Medicine, Department of Surgery, Division of Trauma/Critical Care, VCU Medical Center, Medical College of Virginia Campus, Richmond, VA, USA
e-mail: chogan@mcvh-vcu.edu

© Springer Nature Switzerland AG 2020
J. R. Shiber, S. D. Weingart (eds.), *Emergency Department Critical Care*,
https://doi.org/10.1007/978-3-030-28794-8_12

for almost a million ED visits annually in the United States. Once admitted, patients stay for a median of 3.4 days, a duration that has not changed in a decade [4]. While most of the cost of AHF is from post-discharge care [6–8], the cost of ED evaluation and subsequent admission are expensive as well [4]. The treatment rendered by ED physicians impacts patient outcome and cost [9], not only in those patients discharged from the ED [10], but those who are admitted as outpatients as well [11, 12].

Pathophysiology

The nomenclature of AHF has undergone several iterations. The classic concept of "heart failure" has a reduced ejection fraction in which the left ventricle is dilated with reduced systolic function (defined as an ejection fraction less than 40%). This occurs in ~50% of AHF patients. While in the United States the leading cause is uncontrolled hypertension and post-myocardial infarction loss of myocardium, the worldwide cause is Chagas disease. To offset falling cardiac output and perfusion, vasoconstriction is enhanced by upgrading the renin–angiotensin axis. Unfortunately, this further taxes a failing heart, exacerbating the diminished forward flow.

The other half of HF patients has a normal ejection fraction, defined as an EF equal to or greater than 50% [13]. Previously, this was referred to as diastolic AHF because it was thought that most patients with the symptoms of AHF and a normal EF had diastolic dysfunction, but this has been found to not be the case. The current prevailing theory is that prolonged hypertension causes left ventricular hypertrophy, decreased renal function, and vascular changes, all of which impair microvascular perfusion and cause local ischemia. This disrupts the balance of autoregulation and vasodilation, causing organ remodeling, myocardial fibrosis, hypertrophy, and necrosis. Additionally, pulmonary hypertension occurs in about 80% [14] of patients with preserved EF AHF. One potential clue of the presence of preserved EF AHF is decreased exercise tolerance – as stroke volume fails to rise, patients develop dyspnea and fatigue.

Although the initial evaluation and treatment of preserved EF AHF is not drastically different from classic AHF, the overall behavior of the disease differs. Secondary analyses of the Irbesartan in Heart Failure with Preserved Ejection Fraction (I-PRESERVE) trial reported an annual death rate of 5.2%, 26% of which was due to sudden death, 14% AHF, 5% myocardial infarction, and 9% from stroke death [5]. Most of these presentations will be to the ED.

Classic teaching has centered around two main components of heart failure: The degree of fluid overload (wet vs. dry) and the perfusion from diminished cardiac output (warm vs. cold) [15, 16]. While most presentations are warm and wet, patients can be hypovolemic from over-diuresis and can demonstrate a low perfusion state (cold) that will initially require resuscitation. Cardiogenic shock is caused by fluid overload and diminished perfusion (cold and wet) and is difficult to treat because it requires resuscitation despite fluid overloaded patients.

Patient Presentation

The traditional evaluation for acute AHF relies on qualitative measures and clinical gestalt based on physical examination findings, patient symptoms, and chest radiograph findings [17]. ED physicians in particular are not good at estimating the perfusion and fluid status, as one study found that one in five patients thought to have AHF in the ED did not have that as a final diagnosis [18]. This is echoed by an older study suggesting AHF patients admitted with an AHF diagnosis were misdiagnosed in approximately 10% of hospital admissions [19].

In patients presenting with what appears to be AHF, but who do not carry the diagnosis, a further evaluation in necessary. In patients from South or Central America, the presence of a systolic murmur may be an indication of valvular damage from Chagas disease. In patients with a drug abuse history, valvular disease should also be considered, necessitating a formal echocardiogram. All patients need an ECG to evaluate for acute or recent infarct as well as left ventricular hypertrophy or pulmonary hypertension.

Although the Forrester AHF classification was developed in AMI patients, it lends itself well to the acutely decompensated reduced EF AHF population [16]. Patients are classified clinically on the basis of peripheral perfusion (cool/clammy skin, cyanosis, altered mental status, or oliguria) and pulmonary congestion (rales, abnormal chest X-ray). If the hemodynamic component of the classification is not readily available in the ED (cardiac index $\leq$2.2 L/min/m^2 or pulmonary capillary pressure >18 mmHg), they may be found in old records. Treatment strategy is based according to the clinical and hemodynamic status and its approach is still valuable when assessing AHF patients. For instance, even though a patient may be grossly fluid overloaded, she may still need intravascular volume if hypoperfusion is present [16]. Mortality was 2.2% in group I, 10.1% in group II, 22.4% in group III, and 55.5% in group IV – not too different from the current cardiogenic shock population [20].

The one universal finding in compensated AHF, regardless of its etiology, is hypertension. This is from a combination of the worsening renin–angiotensin feedback loop and anxiety. It also enables the use of afterload reduction and diuresis, giving a buffer to the treating physician.

Physical examination findings, review of systems, and the elements of the history are by themselves limited in attempting to determine the presence of AHF, but the lack of these findings does not mean it is not present. While the specificity of physical examination findings such as a cardiac third heart sound (S3) (99%), rales (78%), or JVD (92%) are reasonable, the respective sensitivities are poor (13%, 60%, and 39%) for evaluating for AHF [21, 22] as are the likelihood ratios. In one study, rales on lung examination were absent in 80% of patients who were found by pulmonary artery catheter pressure monitoring to have elevated filling pressures [23]. Wang et al published a thorough analysis of physical examination and chest radiographs findings in acutely decompensated AHF, concluding that the most useful piece of history is preexisting AHF and the presence of paroxysmal nocturnal dyspnea, orthopnea, and peripheral edema on physical examination have an acceptable positive likelihood ratios for the presence of acute decompensated systolic AHF [22].

In patients with preserved EF AHF, decreased ventricular compliance predisposes them to pulmonary edema because small changes in volume can lead to large changes in left ventricular diastolic pressure. The ventricle is unable to tolerate venous return without elevated diastolic pressures, so small changes in fluid balance will manifest clinically, such as hypertension and dyspnea. This makes patients very sensitive to vasodilation and vasoconstriction, and they can also develop hypotension with aggressive diuresis or vasodilation [14].

Cardiogenic shock is usually obvious and ominous, as patients have hypotension and other indicators of poor perfusion, coupled with dyspnea and lung rales usually associated with classic AHF. Although there is usually a component of dyspnea with cardiogenic shock, poor perfusion can also manifest itself in other ways, such as altered mental status or worsening renal failure. These presentations can be more subtle than straightforward acute AHF decompensation.

Diagnostics

Traditionally, chest radiographs (CXR) are the mainstay of AHF evaluation, looking for pulmonary edema or other causes of dyspnea (Table 12.1). But pulmonary edema or increased vascular markings [24, 25] found on CXR are poor indicators of the degree of AHF present [22, 25], and chronic heart failure can also account for findings that can be confused with acute disease [24, 25]. While pulmonary venous congestion, cardiomegaly, and interstitial edema are the most specific test findings for AHF, their absence will not rule it out [22]. Twenty percent of AHF ED patients can demonstrate no evidence of congestion on CXR [26].

Surrogate markers have had limited success in guiding treatment for AHF [27], and risk stratification models have yet to prove long-term accu-

Table 12.1 Summary of diagnostic accuracy of findings on chest radiography and electrocardiography for acute heart failure in emergency department patients presenting with dyspnea

	Pooled		Summary LR (95% CI)	
Finding	Sensitivity	Specificity	Positive	Negative
Chest radiography				
Pulmonary venous congestion	0.54	0.96	12.0 (6.8–21.0)	0.48 (0.28–0.83)
Interstitial edema	0.34	0.97	12.0 (5.2–27.0)	0.68 (0.54–0.85)
Alveolar edema	0.06	0.99	6.0 (2.2–16.0)	0.95 (0.93–0.97)
Cardiomegaly	0.74	0.78	3.3 (2.4–4.7)	0.33 (0.23–0.48)
Pleural effusion	0.26	0.92	3.2 (2.4–4.3)	0.81 (0.77–0.85)
Any edema	0.70	0.77	3.1 (0.60–16.0)	0.38 (0.11–1.3)
Pneumonia	0.04	0.92	0.50 (0.29–0.87)	1.0 (1.0–1.1)
Hyperinflation	0.03	0.92	0.38 (0.20–0.69)	1.1 (1.0–1.1)
Electrocardiography				
Atrial fibrillation	0.26	0.93	3.8 (1.7–8.8)	0.79 (0.65–0.96)
New T-wave changes	0.24	0.92	3.0 (1.7–5.3)	0.83 (0.74–0.92)
Any abnormal finding	0.50	0.78	2.2 (1.6–3.1)	0.64 (0.47–0.88)
ST-segment elevation	0.05	0.97	1.8 (0.80–4.0)	0.96 (0.95–1.0)
ST-segment depression	0.11	0.94	1.7 (0.97–2.9)	0.95 (0.90–1.0)

LR likelihood ratio, *CI* confidence interval
Used with permission from Collins et al. [35]

racy in long-term outpatients. However, they are of good value in the ED setting. The mainstay of the suspected AHF diagnostic armamentarium are N-terminal brain natriuretic peptide (NT-proBNP) and B-type natriuretic peptide (BNP). Serum natriuretic testing is supported as a Level B guideline in the ACEP Clinical Guidelines for heart failure [17] and is highly recommended by the American College of Cardiology Foundation (ACCF)/American Heart Association [28]. The ACEP Guidelines for AHF specifically stating that a single BNP or NT-proBNP level can improve the diagnostic accuracy for the presence of AHF when compared to standard clinical judgment alone. When ruling out AHF in the acutely dyspneic patient, a BNP < 100 pg/dL or NT-proBNP < 300 pg/dL makes AHF less likely (negative LR = 0.1). When trying to rule in ADHF, a BNP > 500 pg/dL or NT-proBNP > 1000 pg/dL is present (positive LR = 6) [17].

Natriuretic peptide measurement is most useful when trying to rule out the presence of AHF in patients presenting with dyspnea [29, 30]. Specifically, a value <100 pg/mL yields a negative LR = 0.11 (95% CI, 0.07–0.16) [22, 31]. In one study, BNP had greater utility than CXR for diagnosing AHF [29]. There are limitations to the usefulness of BNP, namely that it increases with age and are affected by weight and ethnicity [31]. Since BNP is released from atrial stretching, conditions that cause distention can also cause false elevated levels, such as pulmonary embolism, pulmonary hypertension, and hemodialysis. Since it is cleared renally, chronic or acute kidney disease will also cause elevated levels. Finally, genetic variation can alter BNP levels and obesity can cause falsely low BNP values [32].

BNP levels can also help guide initial treatment. If a prior BNP level is known, a level greater than 50% suggests volume overload, as does a dyspneic patient with a history of AHF found with a BNP level >600 pg/ml for BNP or >6000 pg/ml for proBNP. If being discharged from the ED, remember a decrease in BNP in response to treatment is important, as the final BNP level seems to be the most accurate predictor of death or readmission. A BNP in the 350–400 pg/ml or NT-proBNP in the 4000 pg/ml range at the time of discharge predicts a stable posthospital course [33].

Bedside cardiac ultrasonography is a more recent addition to diagnostics that holds promise for determining the etiology of dyspnea. It provides a real-time assessment of left ventricular function and volume status, and can be repeated as treatment is rendered. ED physicians can estimate ejection fraction with good interrater reliability [34], and volume status can be estimated by inferior vena cava (IVC) diameter and its degree of change with respiratory variation, specifically looking for dilation without any respiratory variation, consistent with fluid overload [35]. Pulmonary edema may be evident on pulmonary ultrasound (US) by looking for sonographic B lines, which occur most commonly in patients with AHF and correlate with elevated PCWP and pulmonary edema [36]. When used in conjunction with serum markers, US accuracy improves [37]. For further discussion on US, see Chap. 35.

More recently, bedside ultrasound has been used to augment the diagnosis of AHF, particularly when there are other potential causes of dyspnea, such as COPD or end-stage renal disease. One study ($n = 130$) prospectively examined patients presenting with dyspnea and for the diagnosis of reduced EF AHF and found cardiopulmonary ultrasound had an accuracy of 90% (95% CI: 84–95) versus 81% (95% CI: 72–88) for the com bination clinical examination, NT-proBNP and CXR. In addition to evaluating AHF in the setting of dyspnea, cardiopulmonary ultrasound can also shed light into the presence of pneumonia or pleural effusion with an accuracy of 86% (95% CI, 80–92) and decompensated chronic obstructive pulmonary disease or asthma with an accuracy of 95% (95% CI, 92–99) [38].

Previously stable AHF often is exacerbated by other comorbidities. Considerations include:

- Unstable angina/myocardial infarction (particularly involving right ventricle)
- Myocarditis
- Poor dietary or medication compliance (NSAID use)
- Arrhythmias +/− electrolyte abnormalities
- Hypertensive crisis
- Chordae tendineae rupture or other valvular regurgitation
- Acute kidney injury/failure
- Aortic valve stenosis
- Sympathomimetic (cocaine) abuse
- High-output syndromes (wet beriberi)
- Sepsis/SIRS
- Cardiac tamponade
- Aortic dissection
- Postpartum cardiomyopathy
- Pulmonary hypertension/asthma/COPD
- Pheochromocytoma or thyrotoxicosis crisis
- Critical anemia

Initial Stabilization

Acute HF patients typically present with dyspnea, ranging from wheezing to complete respiratory failure. Often, comorbidities such as COPD or asthma may accompany AHF, and preserved EF AHF patients often have a component of pulmonary hypertension that can complicate presentation and management. The majority of AHF patients are hypertensive upon presentation, as this is part of the AHF pathophysiology. Hypotension in the AHF population is ominous and makes the usual management (diuresis, afterload reduction) more challenging. Resuscitation with small volume of intravenous fluids or initiation of an inotropic agent is reasonable first moves.

An ECG early in the presentation is important to evaluate for an acute myocardial infarction or cardiac ischemia (particularly in hypotensive patients), which may alter the trajectory of the patient's care (Table 12.2). A CXR will also allow a more thorough differential diagnosis, including pneumonia, pleural effusion, or the presence of chronic pulmonary disease, in addition to serum lab work.

Patients with underlying AHF are at risk for a variety of cardiac arrhythmias, sometimes from ischemic myocardium or hypokalemia. For ventricular fibrillation or tachycardia, the usual ACLS guidelines apply. Low doses of beta blockade (metoprolol or esmolol) can be used to treat sinus or supraventricular tachycardias. Atrial fibrillation or flutters are occasional arrhythmias that require cardioversion (if unstable), β blockade, or amiodarone to slow AV conduction without compromising left ventricular function. Rarely, theophylline is required in AMI patients with atropine-resistant bradycardia [15]. If the bradycardia is nonresponsive to medications,

Table 12.2 Suggested workup in patients with acute heart failure

Complete blood count	Always
Electrocardiogram	Always
PT/PTT/INR	If patient anticoagulated or may need anticoagulation
Basic metabolic panel	Always
Cardiac enzymes (troponin)	Always
BNP or NT-proBNP	Always except in renal failure patients
Echocardiography	If no recent one available or if new issue suspected
Arterial blood gas	If acidosis or hypoxia suspected
Serum lactate	Always
Liver function tests	If hepatic dysfunction suspected or AMS
Urinalysis	If infection suspected
Chest radiograph	Always
Chest radiograph	Always

consider temporary transcutaneous or transvenous pacing.

Noninvasive Pressure Support Ventilation

The urgency to treat AHF and cardiogenic shock is dictated primarily by the pulmonary status of the patient. Dyspnea and impending respiratory failure from fluid overload are often the presenting complaint and main issue to address. Patients with chronic AHF, regardless of whether it is preserved versus reduced EF, know their disease, and often before ED presentation, will increase their diuretic dose as previously instructed by their cardiologist based on their daily weight in an attempt to mobilize excess fluid.

Noninvasive pressure support ventilation (NIPSV), either bilevel positive airway pressure support or continuous positive pressure airway support, is the greatest innovation available for AHF. It improves respiratory distress from cardiogenic pulmonary edema by preventing alveolar collapse and, to a small extent, helps to redistribute intra-alveolar fluid that improves pulmonary compliance. These reduce the work of breathing that has translated into clinical studies, as a recently updated Cochrane Review concluded that when compared to standard care without NIPSV, its use significantly reduced hospital mortality (relative risk reduction of 0.66) and endotracheal intubation (relative risk reduction of 0.52). While this did not translate into decreases in hospital length of stay, intensive care unit stay was reduced by 1 day. NPPV is an effective and safe intervention for the treatment of adult patients with acute cardiogenic pulmonary edema based on several small trials [39].

Although only a temporary measure, NIPSV can buy time while diuresis and afterload reduction therapy offload excess fluid [17]. It also frequently avoids endotracheal intubation in a subset of patients who are at a high likelihood of prolonged intubation because of their comorbidities. Altered mental status can sometimes cause NIPSV to fail because of an uncooperative patient, and it should also be avoided in patients at risk for vomiting or aspiration. NPPV, particularly the EPAP (or CPAP), reduces preload as well as afterload and acts as a mild LV assist device.

Definitive Treatment

Before initiating treatment, get a sense of the cardiac function, specifically the degree of preload, afterload, and contractility. This can be done with a chart review for the patient's most recent echocardiography or catheterization report. Not only is systolic function important, but particular consideration should be given to the patient's diastolic function.

If a recent cardiac assessment is unavailable, a bedside-limited transthoracic echocardiography (LTTE) examination can be done to get a rough idea of fluid status and contractility, as well as determine the presence of a pleural or cardiac effusion. Collins et al. [35] suggest an approach based on presenting blood pressure that is helpful (Table 12.3). Therapy can be guided based on patient blood pressure: hypertensive (SBP > 140 mm Hg), normotensive (SBP 100–140 mm Hg), or hypotensive (SBP < 100 mm Hg) [40, 41]. Hypertension is an important target

Table 12.3 Associated clinical characteristics and treatment approaches based on emergency department presentation phenotype

ED presentation phenotype	Clinical characteristics	Treatment
Low BP (SBP < 100 mm Hg)	Known/suspected low LVEF Likely CAD and CRI	Diuretics (+++) Inotropes/vasopressors (++) Mechanical support (+)
Normal BP (SBP 100–140 mm Hg)	Subacute symptoms Preserved or reduced LVEF Dietary/medical indiscretion	Diuretics (++) IV vasodilators (+) Topical nitrates (++)
High BP (SBP > 140 mm Hg)	History of HTN Abrupt symptom onset Flash pulmonary edema Multiple non-CV comorbidities	Topical/SL nitrates (++) Diuretics (+) IV vasodilators (+++) NIV

Adapted from and used with permission from Collins et al. [35]
+ relative intensity of use, *BP* blood pressure, *SBP* systolic blood pressure, *LVEF* left ventricular ejection fraction, *CAD* coronary artery disease, *CRI* chronic renal insufficiency, *IV* intravenous, *HTN* hypertension, *SL* sublingual, *NIV* noninvasive ventilation

because AHF patients may present with volume redistribution rather than volume overload, in which congestion is due to increased afterload rather than excess fluid. This is also important in diastolic AHF patients, who are known to present with a rapid onset of dyspnea and flash pulmonary edema. While for volume overloaded patients, intravenous loop diuretics remain the primary ED pharmacologic therapy, patients with volume redistribution may respond better to vasodilation therapy [42].

There are specific instances when emergent surgery is required in patients presenting with new or suddenly worsening AHF (of note, a bedside echocardiogram will help diagnose a majority of the following):

- Cardiogenic shock after AMI
- Postinfarction ventricular septal defect or free wall rupture
- Prosthetic valve failure or thrombosis
- Aortic aneurysm or aortic dissection rupture into the pericardial sac
- Acute mitral regurgitation from infection, ischemia or trauma
- Acute aortic regurgitation from infection, ischemia, dissection
- Mechanical assist device failure

The classic medication class used as an initial intervention for AHF for both EMS [43] and ED physicians [35] is loop diuretics, most commonly furosemide (Table 12.4). Despite its widespread usage (88% of the patients in on large database received IV diuretics during their admission) [44], there have been limited studies evaluating this drug class. Diuretics cause a decrease in plasma and extracellular fluid volume, leading to reduced ventricular filling pressures, peripheral congestion, and pulmonary edema. They also cause an early but temporary vasodilation effect with the first dose, as well as a reduction in neurohormonal activation [45]. Failure to respond to diuretics may be caused by intravascular volume depletion, rebound sodium uptake after volume loss, decreased tubular secretion from renal failure or nonsteroidal drug use (NSAIDs), and decreased renal or gut perfusion (not absorbing oral diuretics) from low cardiac output.

If the patient fails to respond to the initial dose of loop diuretics, consider adding a thiazide, as low-dose combinations can be more effective with fewer secondary effects than the use of higher doses of a single drug. Similarly, using diuretics in conjunction with dobutamine, dopamine, or nitrates can be effective and produce fewer secondary effects than increasing the dose of the diuretic [15]. The use of diuretics alone is further discouraged by the ACEP guidelines that caution against "aggressive" diuretic monotherapy, as it is unlikely to prevent the need for endotracheal intubation compared with aggressive nitrate monotherapy. These guidelines further recommend if diuretics are used,

Table 12.4 Medications commonly used in acute decompensated heart failure

Medication	Indication	Dosing	Side effect	Miscellaneous
Vasodilators				
Nitroglycerin	Afterload reduction, blood pressure control	Start 10 μg/min, increase by 10, Max 200 μg/min	Hypotension, headache	Decreased efficacy with chronic use
Isosorbide dinitrate	Afterload reduction, blood pressure control	Start 1 mg/h, Max 10 mg/h	" "	Decreased efficacy with chronic use
Nitroprusside	Hypertensive urgency or emergency	0.3–5 μg/kg/min	Hypotension, CN toxicity	Watch for cyanide toxicity in renal failure
Natriuretic peptides				
Nesiritide[a]	Acute HF, failed other measures	2 μg/kg IV bolus, then 0.01–0.03 μg/kg/min	Hypotension, atrial fibrillation	Infusion only if hypotension a concern
Loop diuretics				
Furosemide	Afterload reduction, diuresis	Mild to moderate: 40 mg PO/IV Severe: 80 mg IV	Dehydration, ototoxicity renal injury	If first dose fails, consider adding another agent below
Bumetanide	Prior patient use, diuresis	0.5–4 mg PO or IV	" "	Monitor Na, K, and creatinine closely
Torasemide	Prior patient use, diuresis	10–20 mg PO or IV	" "	Monitor Na, K, and creatinine closely
Thiazide diuretics				
Metalozone	Augment loop diuresis	2.5–5.0 mg PO	Worsening renal failure	Use in renal insufficiency
Hydrochlorothiazide	↓ sodium reabsorption in distal tubule	25–50 mg PO	" "	" "
Inotropes				
Dobutamine	Enhances cardiac contractility and diuresis if used with diuretics	2–20 μg/kg/min IV infusion, no bolus	Tachycardia (try fluid bolus), hypotension	Insert arterial and central catheters
Milrinone	Enhances cardiac contractility	50 μg/kg bolus, then 0.3–0.7 μg/kg/min	Arrhythmias, hypotension tachycardia	Insert arterial and central catheters

" "Same as Above

they should be administered judiciously, given the potential for worsening renal and long-term mortality [17].

Nitrates are another classic drug class that has been a mainstay for treatment of acute AHF with a paucity of convincing evidence. The mechanism of action addresses the arterial endothelial dysfunction and impaired endothelium-dependent dilation [46] known to occur in AHF, relieving pulmonary congestion without compromising stroke volume or increasing myocardial oxygen demand in AHF. While at low doses, nitrates should only induce venous dilation, and as the dose is gradually increased, arterial dilatation occurs as well. When titrated properly, nitrates can reduce left ventricular pre- and afterload without impairing tissue perfusion.

A recent Cochrane review [47] looked at four studies (634 participants) that met their inclusion criteria, with no significant difference in the rapidity of symptom relief between intravenous nitroglycerin and intravenous furosemide/morphine after 0.5, 3, or 24 hours, suggesting little evidence to support the use of intravenous nitrate vasodilator therapy in the AHF population. Other measures, such as the need for mechanical ventilation, change in blood pressure, and progression to myocardial infarction, suggest there was a significantly higher incidence of adverse events after 3 hours with nitroglycerin compared with placebo (odds ratio 2.29, 95% CI 1.26–4.16), but this was based on a single study. A more recent meta-analysis suggests intravenous vasodilators, when used in acute AHF in the ED, are safe and improve short-term symptoms but have no impact on mortality [48].

The studies evaluating nitrates used relatively lower doses that may have a limited effect in improving clinical status, so consider higher doses with the understanding that it is also best to avoid nitrates in hypotensive and *relatively* hypotensive patients, meaning patients who on any given day are profoundly hypertensive, but have what would be considered a normal blood pressure when you are considering treatment. In patients who are chronically on nitrates, even higher doses may not work because of the rapid development (12–24 h) of tolerance (especially when given intravenously) [15].

Sodium nitroprusside is another short-acting vasodilator that can be considered in patients with severe heart failure, particularly those with predominantly increased afterload (hypertension or mitral regurgitation). It must be titrated cautiously and requires an arterial line. Also, prolonged administration can accumulate thiocyanide and cyanide, so should be used with caution in renal or hepatic failure patients. To further argue against its use, it may cause "coronary steal syndrome" in ischemic patients by shifting blood toward healthy myocardium whose coronaries dilate and away from those areas where the vessels are diseased or obstructed and cannot dilate [15].

Inotropes

Typically, the use of inotropic support has been a last resort in the ED, as using these medication means an ICU bed will be needed for admission, and patients need arterial and central lines (except for dobutamine or milrinone, since no alpha effects) to safety titrate these medications. Of all of the sympathomimetics used in the management of acute heart failure, dopamine and dobutamine are the most common. Both target beta-adrenergic receptors and have positive inotropic effects at lower doses. Dopamine, at higher doses, can increase systemic vascular resistance which may impact cardiac output, making dobutamine a better choice for patients with normal MAPs who need an inotropic agent. Dobutamine is not without its drawbacks, as the peripheral vasodilatory effects that make it useful in acute AHF can also cause tachyarrhythmias. For further discussion on vasopressors, see Chap. 32.

Although initiating vasopressors in the ED is time-consuming, earlier initiation of vasoactive therapy may impact outcomes based on the large Using the Acute Decompensated Heart Failure (ADHERE) registry [9]. Although this study was not prospective or randomized, the investigators evaluated if vasoactive agents were used early (defined as <6 hours) versus later impacted inpatient mortality and found in-hospital mortality was significantly lower in the early group (OR = 0.87; 95% CI: 0.79–0.96; P = .006). Furthermore, the adjusted odds of death increased 6.8% for every 6 hours of treatment delay (95% CI, 4.2–9.6; $p < .0001$). Thus, the therapy initiated in the ED may impact overall mortality and should be considered earlier rather than later.

Milrinone in one prospective study showed that there was no difference when compared against placebo in days of hospitalization, but there were significant occurrences of hypotension, ventricular fibrillation, and tachycardia. These results suggest that routine use of milrinone in most patients admitted with AHF is not indicated, but those select patients with low cardiac output (cold) and hypervolemia (wet) might benefit if other modalities are contraindicated or have failed [49].

Even in hypotensive patients, an assessment of volume is important because they may still be fluid overloaded. For such patients, inotropes should be used as a last resort or if there is clear evidence of shock or organ hypoperfusion [35].

ACE-I

ACE inhibitors work by interrupting the renin–angiotensin system that results in decreased preload and decreased afterload. To date, no controlled, randomized clinical trials exist that evaluate the use of ACE inhibitors in AHF, but they are well accepted in chronic management [28].

Beta Blockers

While beta-blocker therapy is commonly used in chronic AHF because they reverse cardiac remodeling, improve the quality of life, and reduce mortality [28], it has come under greater scrutiny in those patients with preserved EF [50]. Overall, there is no role of beta-blockers in the acute management of AHF. That being said, in patients with preserved EF, tachycardia can decrease preload and cardiac output, and a small dose of beta blocker (for instance, metoprolol 5 mg IV, slow push) that lowers the heart rate may paradoxically improve output.

Hydralazine

As a vasodilator primarily targeting arteries and arterioles, hydralazine decreases peripheral resistance and decreasing afterload and should be an ideal agent for acute AHF. However, for treatment of AHF, it has been poorly studied and data is limited [48]. Should urgent blood pressure reduction be needed in an AHF patient, hydralazine would be a prudent choice, but be aware of rebound hypertension once its effects wear off.

Calcium Sensitizers

Levosimendan is a newer drug class for the treatment of AHF currently available in Europe, but not in the United States. Its mechanism of action is increasing calcium activity inside the cardiac cell (therefore increasing contractility); and relaxation of smooth muscle (causing vasodilation) [51]. Currently, it is under consideration at the FDA for clinical use.

Ultrafiltration

In patients with chronic renal failure, removal of excess fluids is a prudent indication for those with respiratory failure or in embarrassment. In patients without chronic renal failure, continuous renal replacement therapy, specifically ultrafiltration, may be considered in refractory cases in which fluid overload and pulmonary congestion from a specific source (renal failure, acute myocardial infarction) is identified. Those patients with persistent congestion despite diuretic therapy, with or without impaired renal function, may be candidates for continuous venovenous ultrafiltration after discussion with cardiology and renal consultants [15].

Disposition

With aggressive treatment in the ED, impending respiratory failure can be reversed effectively, sometimes making disposition (ICU vs. floor) a challenge. A trial of time off NIPSV or follow-up ABG can assist in disposition. Positive cardiac markers or new/worsened renal failure can also help an ICU disposition occur.

Both fields of cardiology and emergency medicine struggle with how to disposition those patients with mild heart failure, as these patients often have subclinical inadequate perfusion whose symptoms are reversed but have not had the underlying pathophysiology addressed [52]. This accounts for the high readmission rate encountered with AHF. If close follow-up can be arranged or the patient is well known by their primary physician, discharge home is possible. Otherwise, an observation stay may be in order.

References

1. Ambrosy AP, Fonarow GC, Butler J, et al. The global health and economic burden of hospitalizations for heart failure: lessons learned from hospitalized heart failure registries. J Am Coll Cardiol. 2014;63(12):1123–33.
2. Bobrow BJ, Clark LL, Ewy GA, et al. Minimally interrupted cardiac resuscitation by emergency medical services for out-of-hospital cardiac arrest. JAMA. 2008;299(10):1158–65.
3. Heidenreich PA, Trogdon JG, Khavjou OA, et al. Forecasting the future of cardiovascular disease in the United States: a policy statement from the American Heart Association. Circulation. 2011;123(8):933–44.
4. Storrow AB, Jenkins CA, Self WH, et al. The burden of acute heart failure on U.S. emergency departments. JACC Heart Fail. 2014;2(3):269–77.

5. Zile MR, Gaasch WH, Anand IS, et al. Mode of death in patients with heart failure and a preserved ejection fraction: results from the Irbesartan in Heart Failure with Preserved Ejection Fraction study (I-PRESERVE) trial. Circulation. 2010;121(12):1393–405.
6. McDermott MM, Feinglass J, Lee P, et al. Heart failure between 1986 and 1994: temporal trends in drug-prescribing practices, hospital readmissions, and survival at an academic medical center. Am Heart J. 1997;134(5 Pt 1):901–9.
7. McCullough PA, Philbin EF, Spertus JA, Kaatz S, Sandberg KR, Weaver WD. Confirmation of a heart failure epidemic: findings from the resource utilization among congestive heart failure (REACH) study. J Am Coll Cardiol. 2002;39(1):60–9.
8. Haldeman GA, Croft JB, Giles WH, Rashidee A. Hospitalization of patients with heart failure: National hospital discharge survey, 1985 to 1995. Am Heart J. 1999;137(2):352–60.
9. Peacock WF, Emerman C, Costanzo MR, Diercks DB, Lopatin M, Fonarow GC. Early vasoactive drugs improve heart failure outcomes. Congest Heart Fail. 2009;15(6):256–64.
10. Rame JE, Sheffield MA, Dries DL, et al. Outcomes after emergency department discharge with a primary diagnosis of heart failure. Am Heart J. 2001;142(4):714–9.
11. Brar S, McAlister FA, Youngson E, Rowe BH. Do outcomes for patients with heart failure vary by emergency department volume? Circ Heart Fail. 2013;6(6):1147–54.
12. Singer AJ, Birkhahn RH, Guss D, et al. Rapid emergency department heart failure outpatients trial (REDHOT II): a randomized controlled trial of the effect of serial B-type natriuretic peptide testing on patient management. Circ Heart Fail. 2009;2(4):287–93.
13. Angeja BG, Grossman W. Evaluation and management of diastolic heart failure. Circulation. 2003;107(5):659–63.
14. Volpe M, McKelvie R, Drexler H. Hypertension as an underlying factor in heart failure with preserved ejection fraction. J Clin Hypertens (Greenwich). 2010;12(4):277–83.
15. Nieminen MS, Böhm M, Cowie MR, et al. Executive summary of the guidelines on the diagnosis and treatment of acute heart failure. Eur Heart J. 2005;26(4):384–416. https://doi.org/10.1093/eurheartj/ehi044.
16. Forrester JS, Diamond G, Chatterjee K, Swan HJ. Medical therapy of acute myocardial infarction by application of hemodynamic subsets (second of two parts). N Engl J Med. 1976;295(25):1404–13.
17. Silvers SM, Howell JM, Kosowsky JM, Rokos IC, Jagoda AS. American College of Emergency Physicians. Clinical policy: critical issues in the evaluation and management of adult patients presenting to the emergency department with acute heart failure syndromes. Ann Emerg Med. 2007;49(5):627–69.
18. Chaudhry A, Singer AJ, Chohan J, Russo V, Lee C. Interrater reliability of hemodynamic profiling of patients with heart failure in the ED. Am J Emerg Med. 2008;26(2):196–201.
19. Fonarow GC. The acute decompensated heart failure national registry (ADHERE): opportunities to improve care of patients hospitalized with acute decompensated heart failure. Rev Cardiovasc Med. 2003;4(Suppl 7):S21–30.
20. Mozaffarian D, Benjamin EJ, Go AS, et al. Executive summary: heart disease and stroke statistics-2015 update: a report from the American Heart Association. Circulation. 2015;131(4):434–41.
21. Lok CE, Morgan CD, Ranganathan N. The accuracy and interobserver agreement in detecting the "gallop sounds" by cardiac auscultation. Chest. 1998;114(5):1283–8.
22. Wang CS, FitzGerald JM, Schulzer M, Mak E, Ayas NT. Does this dyspneic patient in the emergency department have congestive heart failure? JAMA. 2005;294(15):1944–56.
23. Cody RJ. Clinical trials of diuretic therapy in heart failure: research directions and clinical considerations. J Am Coll Cardiol. 1993;22(4 Suppl A):165A–71A.
24. Chakko S, Woska D, Martinez H, et al. Clinical, radiographic, and hemodynamic correlations in chronic congestive heart failure: conflicting results may lead to inappropriate care. Am J Med. 1991;90(3):353–9.
25. Mahdyoon H, Klein R, Eyler W, Lakier JB, Chakko SC, Gheorghiade M. Radiographic pulmonary congestion in end-stage congestive heart failure. Am J Cardiol. 1989;63(9):625–7.
26. Collins SP, Lindsell CJ, Storrow AB, Abraham WT, ADHERE Scientific Advisory Committee, Investigators and Study Group. Prevalence of negative chest radiography results in the emergency department patient with decompensated heart failure. Ann Emerg Med. 2006;47(1):13–8.
27. Gheorghiade MF, Adams KF Jr, Gattis WA, Teerlink JR, Orlandi C, O'Connor CM. Surrogate end points in heart failure trials. Am Heart J. 2003;145(2 Suppl):S67–70.
28. Yancy CW, Jessup M, Bozkurt B, et al. 2013 ACCF/AHA guideline for the management of heart failure: a report of the American College of Cardiology Foundation/American Heart Association task force on practice guidelines. J Am Coll Cardiol. 2013;62(16):e147–239.
29. Maisel AS, Krishnaswamy P, Nowak RM, et al. Rapid measurement of B-type natriuretic peptide in the emergency diagnosis of heart failure. N Engl J Med. 2002;347(3):161–7.
30. McCullough PA, Nowak RM, McCord J, et al. B-type natriuretic peptide and clinical judgment in emergency diagnosis of heart failure: analysis from breathing not properly (BNP) multinational study. Circulation. 2002;106(4):416–22.
31. Maisel AS, Clopton P, Krishnaswamy P, et al. Impact of age, race, and sex on the ability of B-type natriuretic peptide to aid in the emergency diagno-

sis of heart failure: results from the breathing not properly (BNP) multinational study. Am Heart J. 2004;147(6):1078–84.
32. Wang TJ, Larson MG, Levy D, et al. Heritability and genetic linkage of plasma natriuretic peptide levels. Circulation. 2003;108(1):13–6.
33. Maisel A, Mueller C, Adams K Jr, et al. State of the art: using natriuretic peptide levels in clinical practice. Eur J Heart Fail. 2008;10(9):824–39.
34. Pivetta E, Goffi A, Lupia E, et al. Lung ultrasound-implemented diagnosis of acute decompensated heart failure in the emergency department - a SIMEU multicenter study. Chest. 2015;148(1):202–10.
35. Collins S, Storrow AB, Albert NM, et al. Early management of patients with acute heart failure: state of the art and future directions. A consensus document from the Society for Academic Emergency Medicine/ Heart Failure Society of America Acute Heart Failure Working Group. J Card Fail. 2015;21(1):27–43.
36. Agricola E, Bove T, Oppizzi M, et al. "Ultrasound comet-tail images": a marker of pulmonary edema∗: a comparative study with wedge pressure and extravascular lung water. Chest. 2005;127(5):1690–5.
37. Liteplo AS, Marill KA, Villen T, et al. Emergency thoracic ultrasound in the differentiation of the etiology of shortness of breath (ETUDES): Sonographic B-lines and N-terminal pro-brain-type natriuretic peptide in diagnosing congestive heart failure. Acad Emerg Med. 2009;16(3):201–10.
38. Gallard E, Redonnet JP, Bourcier JE, et al. Diagnostic performance of cardiopulmonary ultrasound performed by the emergency physician in the management of acute dyspnea. Am J Emerg Med. 2014.
39. Vital FM, Ladeira MT, Atallah AN. Non-invasive positive pressure ventilation (CPAP or bilevel NPPV) for cardiogenic pulmonary oedema. Cochrane Database Syst Rev. 2013;5:CD005351.
40. Levy P, Compton S, Welch R, et al. Treatment of severe decompensated heart failure with high-dose intravenous nitroglycerin: a feasibility and outcome analysis. Ann Emerg Med. 2007;50(2):144–52.
41. Collins S, Storrow AB, Kirk JD, Pang PS, Diercks DB, Gheorghiade M. Beyond pulmonary edema: diagnostic, risk stratification, and treatment challenges of acute heart failure management in the emergency department. Ann Emerg Med. 2008;51(1):45–57.
42. Cotter G, Metra M, Milo-Cotter O, Dittrich HC, Gheorghiade M. Fluid overload in acute heart failure ? re-distribution and other mechanisms beyond fluid accumulation. Eur J Heart Fail. 2008;10(2):165–9.
43. Cotter G, Metzkor E, Kaluski E, et al. Randomised trial of high-dose isosorbide dinitrate plus low-dose furosemide versus high-dose furosemide plus low-dose isosorbide dinitrate in severe pulmonary oedema. Lancet. 1998;351(9100):389–93.
44. Adams KF Jr, Fonarow GC, Emerman CL, et al. Characteristics and outcomes of patients hospitalized for heart failure in the United States: rationale, design, and preliminary observations from the first 100,000 cases in the acute decompensated heart failure national registry (ADHERE). Am Heart J. 2005;149(2):209–16.
45. Johnson W, Omland T, Hall C, et al. Neurohormonal activation rapidly decreases after intravenous therapy with diuretics and vasodilators for class IV heart failure. J Am Coll Cardiol. 2002;39(10):1623–9.
46. den Uil CA, Brugts JJ. Impact of intravenous nitroglycerin in the management of acute decompensated heart failure. Curr Heart Fail Rep. 2015;12(1):87–93.
47. Wakai A, McCabe A, Kidney R, et al. Nitrates for acute heart failure syndromes. Cochrane Database Syst Rev. 2013;(8):CD005151.
48. Alexander P, Alkhawam L, Curry J, et al. Lack of evidence for intravenous vasodilators in ED patients with acute heart failure: a systematic review. Am J Emerg Med. 2015;33(2):133–41.
49. Cuffe MS, Califf RM, Adams KF Jr, et al. Short-term intravenous milrinone for acute exacerbation of chronic heart failure: a randomized controlled trial. JAMA. 2002;287(12):1541–7.
50. Lund LH, Benson L, Dahlstrom U, Edner M, Friberg L. Association between use of beta-blockers and outcomes in patients with heart failure and preserved ejection fraction. JAMA. 2014;312(19):2008–18.
51. Pathak A, Lebrin M, Vaccaro A, Senard JM, Despas F. Pharmacology of levosimendan: inotropic, vasodilatory and cardioprotective effects. J Clin Pharm Ther. 2013;38(5):341–9.
52. Hogan CJ, Dalawari J, Nassiry A, Ward KR. Sublingual microvascular perfusion defects in acutely decompensated heart failure. Acad Emerg Med. 2008;15(5):S61.

Hypertensive Emergencies

13

Aimee Wendelsdorf and Brian T. Wessman

Introduction

Systemic hypertension effects an estimated 1 billion persons worldwide and is responsible for 7.1 million deaths per year making it one of the most ubiquitous medical disorders seen and treated by the medical community [1]. Approximately 30% of the United States population, 65 million Americans, will suffer from high blood pressure by the age of 20 [2]. True hypertensive crisis, however, is less common, effecting only 1–2% of patients with chronic hypertension, yet still accounting for up to 25% of all medical emergencies and 3% of all emergency department (ED) visits [3, 4]. Hypertensive emergencies are the result of acute and rapid elevations in blood pressure. They may develop from a number of different etiologies (Table 13.1) and manifest across a variety of different organ systems making it both a diagnostic and a management challenge for the treating emergency medicine physician.

A. Wendelsdorf
Emergency Medicine and Critical Care Medicine, Presbyterian Hospital, Albuquerque, NM, USA

B. T. Wessman (✉)
Divisions of Critical Care Medicine and Emergency Medicine, Washington University in Saint Louis, School of Medicine, St. Louis, MO, USA
e-mail: brianwessman@wustl.edu

Table 13.1 Causes of hypertensive crisis [5, 6]

Essential hypertension
Medication noncompliance
Collagen vascular diseases (lupus)
Aortic dissection
Cardiac
Unstable angina
Myocardial ischemia/infarction
Acute left ventricular failure
Renal parenchymal disease
Acute renal failure
Acute glomerulonephritis
Vasculitis
Hemolytic uremic syndrome
Thrombotic thrombocytopenic purpura
Renal transplant rejection
Renovascular disease
Renal artery stenosis
Endocrine
Pheochromocytoma
Cushing's syndrome
Renin-secreting tumors
Mineralocorticoid hypertension
Thyroid storm
Illicit drugs/toxins
Cocaine, methamphetamines, PCP, lead poisoning
Rebound hypertension (s/p stopping BP agent such as clonidine)
Prescription drugs
Sympathomimetics, oral contraceptives, erythropoietin, cyclosporine, antihypertensive withdrawal (clonidine), monoamine-oxidase inhibitors (tyramine)
Alcohol withdrawal
Central nervous system disorders
Traumatic brain injury, cerebral infarction/hemorrhage, tumors

© Springer Nature Switzerland AG 2020
J. R. Shiber, S. D. Weingart (eds.), *Emergency Department Critical Care*,
https://doi.org/10.1007/978-3-030-28794-8_13

Pregnancy
Preeclampsia
Eclampsia
Autonomic hyperreactivity
Guillain–Barré syndrome, acute intermittent porphyria
Postoperative hypertension

Definition [1]

Systemic hypertension is defined as a systolic blood pressure (SBP) >140 mmHg or a diastolic blood pressure (DBP) >90 mmHg as classified by the Joint National Committee on Prevention, Detection, Evaluation, and Treatment of High Blood Pressure (Table 13.2) [7]. Although not recognized as a formal classification, hypertensive crisis is often defined as an acute elevation of blood pressure *greater than SBP ≥180 mmHg or a DBP ≥110 mmHg*. Of note, the below definitions are devoid of absolute blood pressure numbers due to the fact that end-organ damage can be patient specific and variable with the rapidity of blood pressure elevation.

- Hypertensive crisis: Nonspecific term for severe elevations in blood pressure that have the *potential* to cause end-organ damage (brain, heart, aorta, kidneys, eyes, vasculature).
- Hypertensive urgency: Blood pressure is severely elevated, but end organs have yet to be effected.
- Hypertensive emergency: Severe elevation of blood pressure with evidence of ongoing acute end-organ damage.
  - Hypertensive encephalopathy: Specific subset of hypertensive emergency characterized by headaches, irritability, and mental status changes (usually due to very rapid elevations of blood pressure).
  - Accelerated–malignant hypertension: Specific subset of hypertensive emergency characterized by fundoscopic findings of papilledema and/or acute retinal hemorrhages and exudates.

Table 13.2 Joint National Committee VII guidelines for defining hypertension

Blood pressure classification	Systolic blood pressure (mmHg)	Diastolic blood pressure (mmHg)
Normal	<120	and <80
Prehypertension	120–139	or 80–89
Stage 1 hypertension	140–159	or 90–99
Stage 2 hypertension	≥160	or ≥100

Pathophysiology

The pathophysiology related to hypertensive emergencies and the resulting end-organ damage is not well understood. Given evidence that the rapidity of blood pressure elevation contributes to the development of end-organ damage, one mechanism of action is believed to be a sudden increase in systemic vascular resistance due to circulating humoral vasoconstrictors that occur as a response to some acute insult. Whatever the underlying mechanism for the sudden increase in blood pressure, the end result is thought to be beyond that of which end-organ compensatory mechanisms can manage. This change in vascular resistance leads to fluid shifts, capillary leaks, edema, and fibrin deposits which can alter elasticity of the vessels responsible for augmenting blood flow to the organs [1, 5].

Presentation

Whether classified as hypertensive emergency or urgency, uncontrolled blood pressure can have numerous deleterious effects on varied organ systems as shown in Table 13.3. These multiple manifestations of disease may result in a variety of initial presenting signs and symp-

Table 13.3 Manifestations of hypertensive crisis [1, 4, 8]

Hypertensive urgencies
Shortness of breath
Severe anxiety
Epistaxis
Hypertensive emergencies
Hypertensive encephalopathy
Aortic dissection
Intracerebral hemorrhage
Acute coronary syndrome/myocardial infarction
Acute left ventricular failure
Pulmonary edema
Hypertensive retinopathy
Subarachnoid hemorrhage
Acute ischemic stroke
Sympathetic crisis
Acute postoperative hypertension

toms requiring a thorough history and physical examination to assess for both etiology and end-organ damage. A complete neurologic examination and fundoscopic examination assessing for findings concerning for stroke, papilledema, retinal hemorrhage, or exudates should be performed when focal neurologic symptoms, altered mental status, or visual disturbances exist. Appreciation of a third heart sound, gallop, peripheral edema of jugular venous distension may indicate acute decompensated heart failure or myocardial infarction, while a fourth heart sound may be present indicating a stiff LV due to elevated aortic afterload. Blood pressure should be measured in both arms as disparities may indicate aortic dissection (further discussed below) [1, 9].

Diagnostics

When blood pressure is severely elevated, laboratory and radiographic workup should be tailored based on found signs, symptoms, and suspicion for end-organ damage. In the presence of chest pain or signs of acute congestive heart failure, a CXR, EKG, serial troponins, and d-dimer are important to rule out other life-threatening causes of chest pain such as myocardial infarction or pulmonary embolus. When altered mental or focal neurologic signs are present, head computed tomography (CT) imaging is warranted to rule out any intracranial hemorrhage or acute stroke. A complete blood count with peripheral smear should be analyzed for low platelets and schistocytes indicating potential microvascular hemolysis (microangiopathic hemaolytic anemia). Urea, creatinine, and electrolytes should be monitored given the potential for renal dysfunction. Urinalysis may be analyzed for proteinuria, microscopic hematuria, or illicit substances [1, 2, 6, 9].

Initial Stabilization

The first priority in the management of hypertensive emergencies is the controlled yet rapid *reduction of mean arterial pressure (MAP) by 20–25% in the first hour of presentation with a target blood pressure of 160/110 in the first 3–6 hours* in most cases [4, 10–12]. This requires administration of appropriate intravenous antihypertensive medications and often invasive blood pressure monitoring in the form of an arterial line. The choice of antihypertensive medication should be tailored to the underlying etiology of hypertensive crisis and ideally should be short-acting (Figs. 13.1 and 13.2). Careful consideration of potential side effects should be considered as too great of a reduction in blood pressure may worsen outcomes in certain instances such as acute ischemic stroke, renal failure, or coronary ischemia. Any pain should be appropriately treated as it may contribute to uncontrolled hypertension. *Diuretics should be avoided in most cases* (except pulmonary edema or myocardial infarction), as patients are usually hypovolemic despite elevated blood pressure, as activation of the renin angiotensin system and pressure natriuresis leads to systemic free water loses. Some patients may actually require gentle crystalloid fluid resuscitation for precipitous drops in blood pressure on initiation of antihypertensive therapy [1].

Comorbidity	Acceptable Intravenous Agent(s)
Aortic dissection	Esmolol[a], labetalol[a], nicardipine, sodium nitroprusside
Acute congestive heart failure	Nitroglycerin, nitroprusside
Acute intracranial hemorrhage/ischemic stroke	Labetalol, nicardipine, nitroglycerin
Subarachnoid hemorrhage (SAH)	Esmolol, labetalol, nicardipine
Acute myocardial infarction	Clevidipine, esmolol, labetalol, nicardipine, nitroglycerin
Acute hypertensive pulmonary edema	Enalapril, nicardipine, nitroglycerin, nitroprusside
Acute renal failure	Clevidipine, fenoldompam, nicardipine
Encephalopathy/posterior reducible encephalopathy syndrome (PRES)	Nicardipine, clevidipine
Sympathetic crisis or catecholamine toxicity	Benzodiazipine, fenoldopam, nicardipine, nitroglycerin, phentolamine
Acute post-operative hypertension	Clevidipine, esmolol, narcotics (pain control) nicardipine, nitroglycerin, nitroprusside
Eclampsia or preeclamsia	Hydralazine, labetalol, nicardipine, nifedipine

Fig. 13.1 Hypertensive emergencies and recommended antihypertensive therapies. Medications are listed in alphabetical order, not order of preference. [a]Effective beta blockade should be achieved prior to institution of a vasodilator when treating aortic dissection

Drug	Drug Class	Initial dose	Titration	Max dose	Onset	Duration	Side-effects	Contra-indications
Clevidipine	Dihydropyridine calcium-channel blocker	1-2 mg/hr	May be doubled every 90 seconds till goal achieved	21 mg/hr	2-4 mins	5-15 mins	Reflex tachycardia hypertriglyceridemia with prolonged use at high doses	Severe aortic stenosis, allergies to soy or egg (emulsified), disordered lipid metabolism
Enalaprilat	ACE-inhibitor	1.25 mg IV push	Repeat dosing every 6 hrs	5 mg every 8 hours	15-30 mins	12-24 hrs	Delayed peak effect of 4 hrs	Renal artery stenosis, reduce dose in azotemia, pregnancy
Esmolol	Beta-1 selective blocker	500 mcg/kg IV bolus; 50 mcg/kg/min infusion	Bolus 500mcg/kg if no effect in 5 mins and increase infusior by 50 mcg/kg/min	300 mcg/kg/min	1-5 mins	15-30 mins	Local necrosis if extravasation occurs, bradycardia	LVH, COPD/asthma, high-grade heart block, bradycardia, cocaine-toxicity (controversial)
Fenoldopam	Dopamine-1 receptor agonist, vasodilator	0.1 to 0.3 mcg/kg/min	0.05 to 0.1 mcg/kg/min every 15 mins	1.6 mcg/kg/min	5-10 mins	1 hour	Flushing, headache, nausea, hypokalemia so potassium should be monitored	Glaucoma, sulfite sensitivity
Hydralazine	Arteriolar vasodilator	10 mg slow IV bolus/IM	10-20 mg IV bolus every 4 to 6 hours	20 mg/dose	10-30 mins	2-4 hours	Reflex tachycardia, less predictable response	Coronary disease, aortic dissection (administer beta-blocker prior)
Labetalol	Beta-blocker	20 mg IV push; 0.5 to 2 mg/min infusion	20-80 mg IV push every 10 mins	300 mg/day	5-10 mins	2-6 hrs	Bradycardia, orthostatic hypotension	Asthma, COPD, CHF, bradycardia, heart block
Nicardipine	Dihydropyridine calcium channel blocker	5 mg/hr	Increase by 2.5 mg/hr every 15 mins	15 mg/hr	15 mins	< 8 hours, 50% decrease in effect seen 30 mins after discontinuation	Long half-life, poor rapid titration	Heart block, recent AMI, renal failure
Nitroglycerin	Venous vasodilator	5 mcg/min IV infusion	Increase by 5 mcg/min every 3-5 mins	200mcg/min	2-5 mins	5-10 mins	Increases ICP, headache, decreased pre-load, nitrate tolerance	Right-sided AMI, HTN encephalopathy, stroke, ICH
Nitroprusside	Afteriolar and venous vasodilator	0.3-0.5 mcg/kg/min	Increase by 0.5 mcg/kg/min	10 mcg/kg/min	Within seconds	2-3 mins	Cyanide toxicity with prolonged use > 24-, 48 hrs	MI, renal failure, pregnancy

Fig. 13.2 Initial dosing and contraindications of commonly used intravenous antihypertensive agents ([10, 11], UpToDate. https://www.uptodate.com/contents/drugs-used-for-the-treatment-of-hypertensive-emergencies?source=see_link)

Definitive Treatment

The necessity for tight blood pressure control by continuous infusion and invasive monitoring warrants intensive care unit (ICU) admission [4, 7]. In cases of hypertensive urgency without end-organ damage, the goal should be symptom management such as analgesia for headache or nasal packing for epistaxis. If symptoms persist, then blood pressure control with cautious administration of oral medications or home antihypertensive regimens may be warranted followed by several hours of observation [7]. For *asymptomatic patients, intravenous antihypertensive should not routinely be initiated in the ED* as there is no proven benefit of blood pressure reduction in the first 24 hours in these patients, and uncontrolled reduction may lead to worsened outcomes and prolonged hospital stays [1, 2]. *Patients with hypertensive urgency may be discharged from the hospital as long as a reliable follow-up is available within 24–48 hours* [7]. For patients with limited resources and lack of reliable follow-up, ED physicians may want to initiate long-term antihypertensive therapy and admission to the hospital may be warranted [13]. Specific management of other hypertensive emergencies not listed below is discussed elsewhere in this book.

Critical Points

- The difference between hypertensive urgency and hypertensive emergency is the presence of end-organ damage.
- For hypertensive emergency, mean arterial pressure (MAP) should be rapidly reduced by 25% over the first hour of presentation.
- Elevated blood pressure in hypertensive urgency should be treated within 24 hours and if follow-up is arranged, patients can be discharged from the ED.
- Intravenous antihypertensive medications should not be administered to asymptomatic patients.
- Easily titratable, short-acting, intravenous antihypertensives are first-line therapy for initial stabilization and tight blood pressure control.

Aortic Dissection

Introduction

One of the most life-threatening hypertensive emergencies is acute aortic dissection. Occurring at a rate of 3 cases per 100,000 persons, it is a relatively rare disease, making it a diagnostic challenge that requires a high degree of suspicion on the part of the emergency medicine physician [14]. There are several underlying risk factors and etiologies for aortic dissection (Table 13.4), however, the most common causes seen in upward of 75% of cases is uncontrolled, severe hypertension (acute or chronic). Genetic disorders such as Marfan's syndrome account for approximately 20% of dissection cases [15].

Definition [14, 15]

Dissection may occur anywhere along the aorta. The location origin of the dissection is used to classify the disease process by either the Stanford or DeBakey system (Fig. 13.3). The DeBakey system further differentiates dissections of the ascending aorta.

- Stanford type A: Aortic dissection involving the ascending aorta, which begins proximal to the brachiocephalic artery and may or may not include the descending aorta.
- Stanford type B: Aortic dissection isolated to the descending aorta alone.
- DeBakey type I: Aortic dissection involving the ascending aorta, with extension to at least the aortic arch and often involving the descending aorta.
- DeBakey type II: Aortic dissection involving the ascending aorta alone.
- DeBakey type III: Aortic dissection isolated to the descending aorta.

Pathophysiology

Despite many different etiologies, the common pathophysiology leading to an aortic dissection is a defect in the intima of the aortic wall. This can

Table 13.4 Aortic dissection [14–17]

Risk factors
Hypertension (75%)
Dyslipidemia
Smoking
Genetic disorders
Marfan's syndrome (20%)
Loeys–Dietz syndrome
Ehlers–Danlos syndrome
Bicuspid aortic valve
Familial TAA/D (thoracic aortic aneurysm and dissection)
Congenial disorders
Coarctation of the aorta
Turner syndrome
Cocaine/amphetamine/stimulant use
Pheochromocytoma
Heavy weight lifting (with prolonged valsalva)
Pregnancy (during labor/early postpartum)
Autoimmune disorders
Infections
Syphilis
Tuberculosis
Blunt trauma/decelerating injuries
Iatrogenic injury
Intraaortic balloon pump
Catheter/stent placement
Presenting signs/symptoms
Sudden, sharp, severe chest, back and/or abdominal pain
Migratory/radiating pain (17%)
Painless aortic dissection (6%)
Hemodynamically unstable (50% of type A dissections)
Asymmetric/deficit pulses (19% type A, 9% type B)
Aortic regurgitation/new diastolic murmur (41–76% type A)
Syncope (9%)
Left-sided pleural effusion (20%)
Complications
Cardiac tamponade (9% type A)
Acute congestive heart failure (7%)
Acute myocardial infarction/right coronary artery dissection (1–2% type A)
Neurologic complications (more common in type A)
Stroke (6%)
Spinal cord ischemia
Ischemic neuropathy
Hypoxic encephalopathy
Mesenteric ischemia (5%)
Renal ischemia/infarction (5–10%)
Upper and lower limb ischemia
Diagnostics
CBC, renal and liver function studies, troponin, d-dimer, type and cross
CXR mediastinal widening (normal in 12–15%)
CT (most common)/MRI/TEE (dependent on availability and patient stability)

Nonspecific EKG changes (ST elevation in 1–2%)

be due to chronic weakening over time or an acute injury such as with trauma. A defect in the intima allows blood to dissect along the media creating both false and true aortic lumens. Chronic and poorly controlled hypertension is one of the most common underlying causes due to the chronic calcification, intimal thickening, and adventitial fibrosis that occur with repeated hypertensive insults. Once a tear in the intima develops, hematoma expansion and sheer forces (dP/dT) generated by the pulsatile blood flow within the aorta propagate the dissection allowing for extension along the aorta usually in an antegrade fashion. As the false lumen expands, it compresses the true lumen supplying blood to vital organs therefore leading to malperfusion syndromes. The ascending aorta is most susceptible to intimal tears as 65% of dissections occur here with only 30% and 10% evolving from the descending aorta and aortic arch, respectively [14, 15].

Presentation

Adding to the diagnostic challenge is the fact that aortic dissection can present in a variety of different ways. Depending on the location of the dissection along the aorta, blood flow may be compromised to the spinal cord, coronary arteries, intestines, kidneys, and limbs (Table 13.5). By far, the most common symptom on presentation is the sudden onset of severe chest pain (often described as ripping) that may radiate to the back, abdomen, or extremities. It is important to note that the resolution or absence of chest pain on evaluation *does not exclude dissection* and the diagnosis should still be considered in high-risk individuals especially in those without evidence of myocardial ischemia.

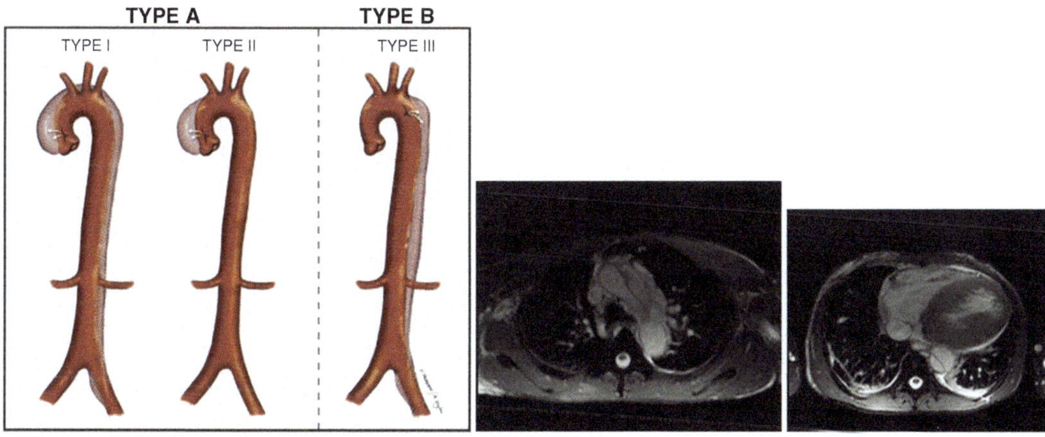

Fig. 13.3 Stanford (bold letter) and DeBakey (Roman numerical system) classification for aortic dissection [14] and MRI images of type A (arch and descending)

Table 13.5 Posterior reversible encephalopathy syndrome (PRES) [4, 18, 19]

Risk factors/causes
Hypertension/fluctuations in blood pressure
Chemotherapy and/or immunosuppressant therapy
Autoimmune disorder
Renal failure
Eclampsia
Signs and symptoms
Altered mental status/encephalopathy (50–80%)
Headache (50%)
Seizures (60–75%)
Visual disturbances/cortical blindness (33%)
Retinal arteriolar hemorrhage/exudates
Papilledema
Status epilepticus (5–15%)
Radiographic findings on MRI
Bilateral vasogenic cerebral edema
Cytotoxic cerebral edema
Frontal and temporal involvement (75%)
Intracranial hemorrhage (10–25%)
Microhemorrhage (58%)
Vasoconstriction (15–30%)
Normal
Management
Invasive blood pressure monitoring
Blood pressure reduction by 25% in first few hours
Antiepileptic therapy
Temporarily discontinue any inciting drugs
Standard treatment of any underlying autoimmune disorder or eclampsia

Although hypertension is a risk factor for dissection, patients *may be normotensive or even hypotensive* on presentation if active hemorrhage or cardiac tamponade is a factor. In fact, 50% of Type A dissections are hemodynamically unstable on presentation due to increased risk of tamponade, aortic valve dysfunction, and heart failure when compared to Type B dissections, which are more likely to present with hypertension [15].

Initial Stabilization

Mortality with acute aortic dissection is high especially if diagnosis and interventions are delayed; mortality increases by 1–2% every hour the first 24 hours of symptom onset. If untreated, 20% of patients will die within the first day, 30% within 48 hours, and 50% by 1 week [14]. This is unsettling given that only 39% of aortic dissections are diagnosed within the first 24 hours of symptom onset [17]. An early priority in the hemodynamically stable patient is blood pressure control to a goal systolic of 100–120 mmHg or the lowest pressure tolerated for organ perfusion. This should be achieved with intravenous medications that are easily titratable and "fast on and off" such as nicardipine or classically sodium nitroprusside (though this has fallen out of favor given risk for cyanide toxicity with prolonged use or high doses); see Figs. 13.1 and 13.2. *It is crucial, however, that effective beta blockade be achieved before reducing systemic blood pressure* in order to reduce sheer forces (dP/dt) that may worsen the dissection or lead to aortic rupture. This can be accomplished by reducing the heart rate to a goal rate of <60 bpm with a beta-blocker infusion such as esmolol [10, 11, 14].

Definitive Treatment

All aortic dissections require ICU admission for invasive blood pressure monitoring and titration of anti-hypertensive drips. Type B dissections isolated to the descending aorta can often be managed with medical therapy alone. However, for dissections involving the ascending aorta, the life-saving management is *prompt surgical intervention* [14–17]. Type B dissections resulting in complications involving the vasculature to the kidneys, bowel, or limbs may also require surgical intervention which is why *cardiothoracic and vascular surgery should be consulted for all aortic dissections no matter their location* to insure proper therapy is being instituted. After initial stabilization and blood pressure control, all patients requiring surgical intervention should be transferred to a tertiary care facility with an available interventional radiology service, cardiology consultation, and cardiothoracic–vascular surgeon [14].

Hypertensive Encephalopathy

It is defined as an acute encephalopathy or delirium in the setting of severe hypertension. Hypertensive encephalopathy results when an acute rise in systemic blood pressure overwhelms the brain's ability to autoregulate cerebral vascular resistance and therefore cerebral blood flow (Table 13.5) [6]. Normal autoregulation allows for controlled cerebral blood flow by adjusting vasoconstriction in the setting of blood pressure fluctuations. Inappropriate dilation of cerebral vessels in the setting of hypertension leads to disruption of the blood–brain barrier, extravasation of plasma into the surrounding tissues, and consequently cerebral edema [4]. The resulting consequences may vary widely from headache and confusion to seizures, intracranial hemorrhage, and ultimately coma. On the spectrum of hypertensive neurologic disorders is posterior reversible encephalopathy syndrome (PRES) where symptoms are resultant of characteristic edema isolated to the occipital and cerebellum of the brain that is detected on MRI during routine workup for altered mental status. As the name suggests, the rate of recovery from PRES is high (75–90%) with resolution of symptoms usually occurring within the first week of symptom onset in most cases [18, 19].

Critical Points

- Aortic dissection should be considered in any patient presenting with chest pain regardless of presenting blood pressure.
- A negative CXR and/or d-dimer do not rule out aortic dissection especially in high-risk patients.
- All dissections involving the ascending aorta require surgical intervention.
- Dissections of the descending aorta that compromise other vital organs or limbs may require surgical intervention along with standard medical therapy.

Critical Points

- A stat head CT should be obtained in all patients with altered mental status, seizure, or focal neurologic findings when hypertensive emergency is suspected.
- Targeted reduction of MAP by 25% is required to prevent any concurrent hypoperfusion to insulted brain tissue.
- Posterior reversible encephalopathy syndrome (PRES) often resolves with improved control of blood pressure fluctuations.

Flash Pulmonary Edema

More than half of patients in hypertensive crisis are euvolemic or hypovolemic. However, patients with underlying renal, hepatic, or congestive heart failure are often chronically hypervolemic. In this setting, dramatic increases in blood pressure may lead to development of sudden, "flash," pulmonary edema and hypoxic respiratory failure. If profoundly hypoxic or unable to tolerate increased work of breathing, patients may require mechanical ventilator support. Noninvasive ventilation strategies and careful use of diuretic therapy may avoid the need for invasive interventions, though most recent studies show no improvement in outcomes with diuretic therapy [9]. Preload reduction with nitroglycerin or nitroprusside is often recommended in the setting of pulmonary edema. Afterload reduction may be achieved with intravenous hydralazine or angiotensin-converting enzyme inhibitors (ACE inhibitors), however, renal function must be taken into consideration as administration of an ACE inhibitor may lead to further kidney injury [9–11].

Critical Points

- Noninvasive ventilation should be considered a first-line intervention for the management of hypoxemia secondary to flash pulmonary edema.
- Preload reduction through short-acting vasoactive infusions should be considered early in the management algorithm of pulmonary edema.

References

1. Marik PE, Rivera R. Hypertensive emergencies: an update. Curr Opin Crit Care. 2001;17:569–80.
2. Marik PE, Varon J. Hypertensive crises: challenges and management. Chest. 2007;131:1949–62.
3. Zampaglione B, Pascale C, Marchisio M, Cavallo-Perin P. Hypertensive urgencies and emergencies. Hypertension. 1996;27:144–7.
4. Price RS, Kasner SE. Hypertension and hypertensive emergency. In: Biller J, Ferro JM, editors. Handbook of clinical neurology, Vol. 119. Neurologic aspects of systemic disease part I. Edinburgh/London/New York: Elsevier; 2014. p. 161–7.
5. Rodriguez MA, Kumar SK, De Caro M. Hypertensive crisis. Cardiol Rev. 2010;18:102–7.
6. Vaughan CJ, Delanty N. Hypertensive emergencies. Lancet. 2000;356:411–7.
7. Chobanian AV, Bakris GL, Black HR, Cushman WC, Green LA, Izzo JL, et al. Seventh report of the Joint National Committee on Prevention, Detection, Evaluation and Treatment of High Blood Pressure. Hypertension. 2003;42:1206–52.
8. Cline DM, Machado AJ. Systemic and pulmonary hypertension. In: Tintinalli JE, Stapczynski JS, editors. Emergency medicine: a comprehensive study guide. 7th ed. New York: McGraw-Hill; 2011. p. 411–50.
9. Adebayo O, Rogers RL. Hypertensive emergencies in the emergency department. Emerg Med Clin North Am. 2015;33:539–51.
10. Rhoney D, Peacock WF. Intravenous therapy for hypertensive emergencies, part 1. Am J Health Syst Pharm. 2009;66:1343–52.
11. Rhoney D, Peacock WF. Intravenous therapy for hypertensive emergencies, part 2. Am J Health Syst Pharm. 2009;66:1448–57.
12. Salkic S, Brkic S, Batic-Mujanovic O. Emergency room treatment of hypertensive crises. Med Arch. 2015;69:302–6.
13. Wolf SJ, Lo B, Shih RD, Smith MD, Fesmire FM. Clincal policy: critical issues in the evaluation and management of adult patients in the emergency department with asymptomatic elevated blood pressure. Ann Emerg Med. 2013;62:59–68.
14. Nienaber CA, Clough RE. Management of acute aortic dissection. Lancet. 2015;385:800–11.
15. Braverman AC. Diseases of the aorta. In: Mann DL, Zipes DP, Libby P, Bonwo RO, editors. Braunwald's heart disease: a textbook of cardiovascular medicine. 10th ed. Philadelphia: Elsevier; 2015. p. 1277–311.
16. Braverman AC. Acute aortic dissection: clinical update. Circulation. 2010;122:184–8.
17. Klompas M. Does this patient have an acute thoracic aortic dissection? JAMA. 2002;287:2262–72.
18. Fugate JE, Rabinstein AA. Posterior reversible encephalopathy syndrome: clinical and radiological manifestations, pathophysiology and outstanding questions. Lancet Neurol. 2015;14:914–25.
19. Thompson RJ, Sharp B, Pothof J, Hamedani A. Posterior reversible encephalopathy syndrome in the emergency department: case series and literature review. West J Emerg Med. 2015;16:5–10.

14 Management of Emergency Department Patients with Gastrointestinal Hemorrhage

Adam B. Schlichting and Nicholas M. Mohr

Introduction

Emergency physicians care for a large number of patients with gastrointestinal (GI) bleeding; however, few of these patients develop life-threatening GI hemorrhage [1–3]. In these selected patients, prompt recognition, aggressive resuscitation, and definitive therapy saves lives. This chapter will discuss GI bleeding in general, but will focus on management of massive GI hemorrhage and the acute management of the critically ill patient.

Identifying a source of bleeding can be challenging. Although significant effort is often spent determining the location of bleeding, for the purposes of emergency department (ED) resuscitation, principles are similar regardless of the source.

Relevant Anatomy and Physiology

The upper and lower GI tract have traditionally been divided by the ligament of Treitz (*musculus suspensorius duodenii*), a suspensory muscle at the level of the duodenal–jejunal junction, where the retroperitoneal duodenum meets the intraperitoneal jejunum. This anatomic landmark was first described in 1853 by Vaclav Treitz, and bears his eponymous name. Proximal to this landmark is considered the upper GI tract and entails the esophagus, stomach, and first segment of the small intestine known as the duodenum. Distal to this division is considered the lower GI tract, and includes the distal portion of the duodenum, the remainder of the small bowel, the colon, and the anus.

Within the past decade, technologies including video capsule endoscopy and double-balloon push enteroscopy have potentially changed the definition of upper versus lower GI tract source by introducing the concept of the "mid-GI" tract. Lesions from the esophagus to ampulla of Vater are considered upper GI bleeding, and can generally be visualized and intervened upon via esophagogastroduodenoscopy (EGD). Mid-GI lesions are located between the ampulla of Vater and the terminal ileum within 6–7 m of small intestine, and can be visualized by double-balloon enteroscopy and capsule endoscopy. Bleeding distal to the terminal ileum is now considered to be of a lower GI source, and can best be visualized by colonoscopy [4–6]. This terminology is not yet widely adopted in the literature, and references in this chapter referring to upper versus lower GI bleeding largely predate the introduction of mid-GI bleeding, unless specifically noted.

A. B. Schlichting (✉)
Department of Emergency Medicine, Department of Internal Medicine, University of Iowa Healthcare, Iowa City, IA, USA
e-mail: adam-schlichting@uiowa.edu

N. M. Mohr
Department of Emergency Medicine, Department of Anesthesia, University of Iowa Carver College of Medicine, Iowa City, IA, USA

© Springer Nature Switzerland AG 2020
J. R. Shiber, S. D. Weingart (eds.), *Emergency Department Critical Care*,
https://doi.org/10.1007/978-3-030-28794-8_14

Understanding the origins of arterial and venous supply to the gastrointestinal tract is important in elucidating the causes and treatments of hemorrhage. Because of its important role in absorbing nutrients, the gastrointestinal tract has a robust blood supply, and this blood supply is well preserved, even in patients in shock. This is one factor that contributes to the severity of GI hemorrhage and the urgency of definitive hemorrhage control. Figure 14.1a and b details the respective arterial and venous supply to the GI tract.

Increased resistance to venous return leads to collateral connections between the portal and systemic circulation. For instance, patients with cirrhosis have chronically elevated portal venous pressures, so these portosystemic shunts develop in the form of esophageal varices, gastric varices, and even rectal varices. These connections are constructed of thin-walled veins that empty large volumes of portal blood into systemic circulation, and the high pressures that these venous structures can experience predispose them to bleeding. Hemorrhage from these sites may be particularly difficult to control, and large volumes of blood may drain into the lumen of the GI tract very quickly.

Special note must be made of patients with prior aortic surgery who present with GI bleeding. Because of postoperative scarring and remodeling, fistulae can develop between the aorta and the lumen of the GI tract. These aortoenteric fistulae are associated with high mortality and can be very difficult to repair. The astute clinician should maintain a low threshold to image these patients even in the absence of hemodynamic instability, and consulting a surgical specialist skilled in aortic surgery should be done early in patients for whom the diagnosis is suspected.

Epidemiology

Upper GI bleeding is responsible for 63–76% of bleeding for which gastroenterologists are consulted [1, 7]. Few studies have compared outcomes in patients with GI bleeding from upper versus lower sources, but overall, upper GI bleeding is associated with more recurrent GI bleeding, increased need for surgery, and higher mortality compared with lower GI bleeding or indeterminate source of GI bleeding (24.6% vs. 18.9% vs. 9.0%, respectively, $p = 0.008$) [8].

There is wide variety of etiologies causing upper GI bleeding, and epidemiologic investigations of etiology vary significantly between geographic regions, largely due to variation in prevalence of alcohol consumption, use of nonsteroidal anti-inflammatory medications, and hepatitis. In the United States, the most common cause of acute upper GI bleeding is peptic ulcer disease, which is responsible for approximately 50% of all acute upper GI bleeding episodes [3]. Other etiologies of acute upper GI bleeding include esophageal or gastric varices (10%), mucosal erosive diseases including esophagitis and gastritis (10%), Mallory–Weiss tears (5%), and malignancy (2%). Overall, mortality for acute upper GI bleeding is 5–10%. Of note, esophageal variceal bleeding is the cause of only 50–60% of acute upper GI bleeding in cirrhotic patients, suggesting that even patients at high risk develop nonvariceal bleeding [3, 9]. Gastric varices are also common in patients with portal hypertension, occurring in 5–33%. Risk of hemorrhage of known esophageal or gastric varices is 5–15% per year. Approximately 40% of bleeding esophageal varices stop bleeding spontaneously, but overall mortality for bleeding esophageal varices approaches 20% by 6 weeks [10].

Fewer studies describe the epidemiology of acute lower GI bleeding, and acute lower GI bleeds occur approximately 20% as frequently as upper GI bleeds [11]. The most common etiology is diverticulosis (20–40%) [2, 11, 12]. Other common causes of acute lower GI bleeding include ischemic colitis (5–25%), colitis (5–12%), hemorrhoids (5–28%), malignancy (6–14%), and postpolypectomy bleeding (1–8%). In-hospital mortality from an acute lower GI bleeding episode is 2–5% [11, 13]. Approximately 80% of lower GI bleeds resolve spontaneously [14]; however, there exists no reliable method for predicting which cases will resolve.

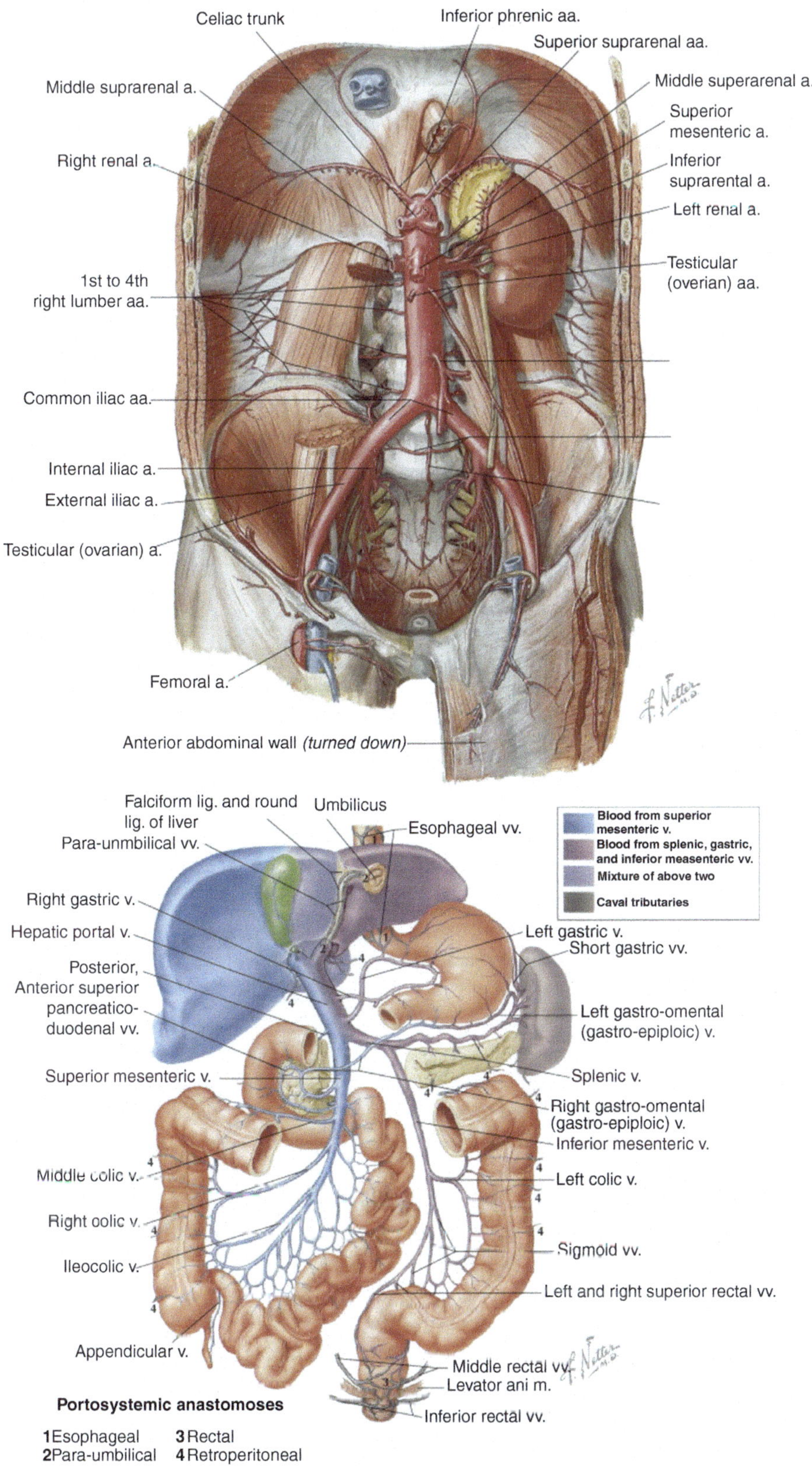

Fig. 14.1 Arterial and venous supply of upper and lower gastrointestinal tract

No source of bleeding (obscure bleeding) is found by EGD or colonoscopy in approximately 5% of patients who present with acute GI bleeding, and nearly 75% of these patients are found to have a small bowel lesion [15]. On further evaluation, nearly 80% of patients with an obscure source of bleeding will be found to have angiectasia, and nearly 50% of lesions may rebleed [5, 6].

Complicating the identification of a source of bleeding is the fact that nearly 10% of patients presenting with bright red blood per rectum or maroon-colored stool (typically associated with lower GI bleeding) actually have an upper GI source with rapid transit of the blood through the GI tract [16]. This reinforces the primary role of the emergency clinician to resuscitate the hemorrhaging patient, and not to be overly focused on identifying the exact source.

Diagnosis and Testing

Resuscitation and planning definitive therapy should be initiated prior to or in concert with significant investigation, especially in those who are hemodynamically unstable.

Physical Examination

Physical examination of the patient with an acute GI hemorrhage should follow a systematic approach. The airway should be assessed for both obstructing blood and the patient's level of consciousness (e.g., ability to protect the airway). In patients with advanced liver disease with GI bleeding, hepatic encephalopathy should be considered. Examination for stigmata of liver disease such as presence of ascites, spider angiomata, caput medusa, hemorrhoids, jaundice, or scleral icterus may help detect evidence for portal hypertension in a patient with undiagnosed cirrhosis.

Hematochezia, or bloody stools, are unreliable at predicting an upper versus lower source of GI bleeding [16]. Rectal examination for the presence of melena (digested blood) can be helpful to identify the source of bleeding (positive likelihood ratio 25, 95% CI 4–174), and is the single most important sign to help determine if a GI bleed is from an upper or lower GI source [1]. Not surprisingly, patients and physicians rarely agree when it comes to descriptive terms used for stool color [17].

Nasogastric Lavage

The use of nasogastric (NG) lavage for localizing the source of upper versus lower GI bleeding remains controversial. Patients presenting without hematemesis, but with either melena or hematochezia, may have either an upper GI source or a lower GI source. The potential for rupturing esophageal varices with the placement of an NG tube is an unfounded myth, and even known varices are not a contraindication for placement of an NG tube if necessary [18]. The process of NG lavage involves insertion of an NG tube, aspiration of gastric contents for gross appearance, and then instillation of a volume of saline or water followed by aspiration of that fluid for examination of the gross appearance of the fluid. An NG lavage is traditionally considered positive if it is blood red or coffee ground colored, whereas a negative NG lavage would be clear or green, bile colored [19]. There is a wide degree of heterogeneity with regard to reports on sensitivity and specificity of NG lavage, likely due to evolving gold standards and varying definitions of "positive" lavage, ranging from trace coffee ground colored to gross blood. Overall, nasogastric lavage is a poor test for localizing GI bleeding (sensitivity 42–90%; specificity 19–95%), and is infrequently used [1, 20]. The insensitivity of NG lavage is likely due to the inability of an NG lavage to detect postpyloric bleeding from the duodenum. More important than the very heterogeneous reports of test characteristics is that NG lavage has no effect on mortality (OR 0.84, 95% CI 0.37–1.92), hospital length of stay (7.3 vs. 8.1 days, $p = 0.57$), need for surgery (OR 1.51, 95% CI, 0.42–5.43), or the number of transfusions required (3.2 vs. 3.0 units, $p = 0.94$) [21]. Emergency department NG lavage was significantly associated with earlier time to endoscopy (HR 1.49, 95% CI, 1.09–2.04).

Laboratory and Ancillary Studies

Diagnostic laboratory studies for a patient with known or suspected GI hemorrhage should include a complete blood count, blood typing and screening for antibodies, and a chemistry profile. Additional routine studies to obtain include coagulation profile, liver function tests, troponin and electrocardiogram, and lactate.

Assessment of the ratio between blood urea nitrogen (BUN) and creatinine can suggest the location of the bleeding, and one study showed a significantly higher BUN/creatinine ratio in patients with an upper GI bleed as compared to those with a lower GI bleed (22.5 ± 11.5 vs. 15.9 ± 8.2; $p = 0.0001$). Using a BUN/creatinine ratio ≤ 33 resulted in sensitivity 96% and specificity 17% for a lower GI source, making the ratio suggestive but not diagnostic of upper versus lower GI source [22]. Another study found that a BUN/creatinine ratio ≥ 36 is predictive of upper GI bleeding, but a ratio <36 was not helpful in localizing the source [23].

We recommend assessment of ECG and troponin in patients with acute GI hemorrhage as there is a high incidence of acute coronary syndrome in patients with acute GI hemorrhage [24–26]. This is likely due to the supply–demand mismatch in acutely bleeding patients. Furthermore, the incidence of both coronary artery disease and GI bleeding increases with age.

The utility of serum lactate measurement as a clinical predictor for mortality has also been recently examined and found to be significant. Patients in this retrospective study presenting GI hemorrhage and a lactate >4 mmol/L had 6.44 times higher odds of death (OR 6.44, 95% CI 3.3–12.6), even when controlled for age, heart rate, and hematocrit [27]. Although this is preliminary, prospective validation of lactate as a predictor of mortality in GI hemorrhage may be on the horizon.

Nuclear Medicine

An obscure source of bleeding in a patient with GI hemorrhage can be difficult to manage. It is possible to help localize a source of bleeding noninvasively using a tagged red blood cell scan, typically utilizing technetium-99m-labeled red blood cells. Angiography (discussed below under section "Interventional Radiology") affords the benefit of being both diagnostic and, if a lesion is found, therapeutic, but requires 1–1.5 mL/min of blood extravasation to be detected. Using technetium-99m-labeled red blood cells, hemorrhage at rates as low as 0.05 mL/min can be detected in animal models of obscure GI bleeding [28]. In clinical practice, technetium-99 scans detect bleeding rates of 0.1–0.4 mL/min [29]. Since nuclear scans are not therapeutic, bleeding at this rate often stops by the time intervention is arranged. Additionally, localization errors ranging from 3% to 25% have been reported with this technique [30–32]. A tagged blood cell scan also requires that the patient be transferred from the ED to a radiology suite for imaging that often takes 1–2 h. For these reasons, we do not recommend routinely obtaining tagged red blood cell scans for GI hemorrhage, especially in hemodynamically unstable patients.

Capsule Endoscopy

Capsule endoscopy was introduced as a means to visualize the small bowel for evaluation and localization of an occult GI bleed. There have been several recent feasibility studies demonstrating that emergency physicians with minimal training can accurately interpret images obtained via capsule endoscopy, achieving sensitivity of 0.94 (95% CI 0.91–0.96) and specificity of 0.87 (95% CI 0.80–0.92) as compared to gold standard gastroenterologist interpretation of the images [33]. A pilot study also demonstrated emergency physician interpretation of capsule endoscopy is cost effective in managing patients at low and moderate risk (as determined by Glasgow–Blatchford score, see below) of GI hemorrhage [34]. In the next few years, the use of this diagnostic modality may become more common for low and moderate risk patients with GI bleeding, however, as capsule endoscopy is not a therapeutic option, it will likely not be employed in patients at high risk of GI hemorrhage nor in patients who require urgent endoscopic therapy.

Resuscitation

Airway

Patients with massive GI hemorrhage and hemorrhagic shock require aggressive resuscitation. Because massive hemorrhage can lead to both airway compromise and shock, endotracheal intubation is often required. Early endotracheal intubation should be performed for all patients with GI hemorrhage who are unable to protect their airways due to massive hematemesis, obtundation, or concurrent hepatic encephalopathy. Endotracheal intubation should be strongly considered for hemodynamically unstable patients who will be leaving the ED for procedures including EGD and for those patients requiring transfer to another hospital for definitive care. Recall that many medications used for rapid sequence induction can result in worsening of hypotension, so the choice of pharmacologic agents and the side effects of those agents should be considered; this must be balanced with the risk that many patients with GI hemorrhage will further decompensate, so early intubation in a hemodynamically unstable patient is preferred.

Endotracheal intubation is best achieved using rapid sequence induction with paralytics, as paralysis may reduce the risk of aspiration of hematemesis during the intubation procedure. Unfortunately, most muscles involved in vomiting are smooth muscles, which are unaffected by neuromuscular paralysis, so chemical paralysis does not completely eliminate the risks of intubating these high-risk patients. Patients who have been actively vomiting may benefit from placement of an NG tube prior to intubation to try to reduce gastric distention and emesis during intubation; however, there is no published literature to support this hypothesis. Indirect video laryngoscopy may be difficult because of large volumes of blood in the oropharynx, and fiberoptic intubation is generally contraindicated in a hemodynamically unstable patient with large volumes of blood obscuring visualization. During intubation, availability of two rigid suction catheters may help improve visualization of airway anatomy and enhance success. Supraglottic devices, in general, are not preferred in these patients because of the risk of large volume vomitus with an unprotected airway. Noninvasive ventilation is contraindicated in patients with massive hematemesis and marked hemodynamic instability, so should not be considered. Refer to Chap. 2 of this book for in-depth discussion of airway management.

Vascular Access

Another priority in the patient with life-threatening hemorrhage is vascular access. Patients exsanguinating from GI hemorrhage require intravenous volume and blood resuscitation, and the rapidity with which resuscitation fluids can be administered influence the speed with which shock can be reversed. Large-bore, short intravenous catheters have the least resistance to flow, making these catheters preferred for their use in resuscitation (Table 14.1). In vivo

Table 14.1 Approximate IV flow rate by catheter size [97–101]

	Published approximate infusion rate	
	Gravity (80 cm)	Pressure bag (300 mmHg)
Catheter		
22 Gauge PIV	10–30 mL/min	40 mL/min
20 Gauge PIV	30–40 mL/min	60 mL/min
18 Gauge PIV	50–60 mL/min	120–180 mL/min
16 Gauge PIV	90–125 mL/min	200–250 mL/min
14 Gauge PIV	125–160 mL/min	250–300 mL/min
Triple lumen catheter		
16 Gauge	50 mL/min	420 mL/min
18 Gauge	27 mL/min	300 mL/min
18 Gauge	25 mL/min	300 mL/min
8.5 French introducer	200 mL/min	400–600 mL/min
15 Gauge EZ-IO needle, tibial	4–70 mL/min	6–200 mL/min
15 Gauge EZ-IO needle, humeral	80 mL/min	140–220 mL/min

studies have failed to achieve flow rates similar to predicted values [35–38], but the advantages of large catheters are clear.

Large peripheral IVs are not always rapidly available due to body habitus, volume depletion, and poor peripheral vasculature. Multiple peripheral IVs can achieve more rapid volume administration than a single catheter [38]. Although no studies of intraosseous (IO) infusion for volume resuscitation of patients with GI bleeding exist, the rapid placement of an IO catheter seems prudent for patients in extremis for whom intravenous access has proven elusive. Central access is also an option in the patient for whom peripheral cannulation is impossible, but use of a large-bore trauma introducer will allow for more rapid resuscitation than a smaller gauge, longer triple-lumen catheter. Peripherally inserted central catheters have significant resistance to flow in rapid resuscitation scenarios and should not be used exclusively for volume resuscitating a hemorrhaging patient.

Volume Resuscitation and Transfusion

The initial fluid for resuscitation of an unstable patient with a GI bleeding should be a crystalloid, either 0.9% sodium chloride or lactated Ringer's solution. Crystalloid resuscitation may stabilize a hemorrhagic shock patient while blood products are prepared and while bleeding is managed. Transfusion of packed red blood cells should be initiated early in the presence of hemodynamic instability (e.g., hemorrhagic shock) or concomitant acute coronary or cerebral ischemia. The optimal goal of hemoglobin in a patient with acute blood loss anemia secondary to GI bleeding is unknown; however, evidence suggests that a more conservative threshold for transfusion has mortality benefits [39]. In a study of 921 patients with acute upper GI bleeding, survival at 6 weeks was significantly higher in patients who were transfused only for anemia with hemoglobin concentration less than 7 g/dL compared to transfusion for hemoglobin less than 9 g/dL (95% vs. 91%, $p = 0.02$). Patients in the latter group received fewer blood transfusions, had fewer rebleeding events, had fewer transfusion reactions, and less pulmonary edema. An important consideration is that patients with "massive exsanguinating bleeding," acute coronary syndrome, lower GI bleeding, stroke, or transient ischemic attack were excluded from this study, so restrictive transfusion practices may not apply in these populations. For patients with acute upper GI bleeding secondary to varices, one theory (based on a rat model) suggests that higher hemoglobin may increase portal pressure and result in higher incidence of rebleeding [40, 41]. A large trial of heterogeneous ICU patients has demonstrated more conservative transfusion thresholds result in improved mortality [42] and transfusion of packed red blood cells is independently associated with morbidity and mortality in critically ill adults [43, 44].

In addition to packed red blood cells, administration of platelets and plasma should be considered. Massive bleeding (usually defined as requiring 10 units of packed red blood cells over 24 h) leads to consumptive coagulopathy, so transfusing blood components to replete coagulation factors decreases the total amount of blood required. The ideal ratio of packed red blood cells, plasma, and platelets is debated [45], but this strategy has been effective at reducing mortality in exsanguinating trauma patients. An observational study of trauma patients receiving more than three units of blood products within 24 h of arrival has suggested "massive transfusion protocols" involving early administration of plasma with packed red blood cells may improve mortality at 24 h, but did not demonstrated a 30-day mortality benefit [46]. Similarly, another observational trial of trauma patients receiving plasma within the first 2.5 h or as part of the first 3–6 units of blood products demonstrated improved 24 h and 30-day mortality, whereas more gradual replacement of coagulation factors did not improve mortality [47]. Such protocols have not been studied in patients with acute GI bleeding, but we advocate for aggressive factor replacement early in massive hemorrhage patients.

Pharmacotherapy

Multiple classes of medications have been studied for pre-endoscopic management of undifferentiated GI bleeding, but few available in the United States have demonstrated a significant mortality benefit. Nonetheless, many of these agents continue to be used in hospitals nationwide for treatment of GI bleeding for significant reductions in need for endoscopic intervention, rebleeding, and need for transfusion (Table 14.2). A 2003 Cochrane meta-analysis of 15 randomized controlled clinical trials comparing emergent endoscopic sclerotherapy to pharmacotherapy (vasopressin ± nitroglycerine, terlipressin, somatostatin, or octreotide) for acute cirrhosis-associated variceal bleeding found equivalent efficacy. Acute bleeding was stopped by pharmacotherapy alone in 83% of patients [48].

Proton Pump Inhibitors

Gastric acidity impairs clot formation and stability, and coagulation and platelet aggregation show 50% reduction in activity with increased gastric acidity [49]. Randomized controlled trials and meta-analysis have demonstrated that histamine-2 (H2) blockers have no role in the management of acute gastric ulcer bleeding [50], however, proton pump inhibitors (PPIs) offer some benefits. Controversy remains as to whether PPIs prior to endoscopy provide clinical benefits.

Administration of IV omeprazole prior to endoscopy accelerated resolution of signs of bleeding on endoscopy (6.4% vs. 14.7%, $p = 0.01$), reduced the need for endoscopic intervention (19.1% vs. 28.4%, $p = 0.007$), and reduced the number of patients with a hospital length of stay more than 3 days (60.5% vs. 49.2%, $p = 0.005$) [51]. There were no significant effects on the number of units of blood transfused (1.5 vs. 1.9 units, $p = 0.12$), the percentage of patients with recurrent bleeding (5.9% vs. 4.2%, $p = 0.49$), the percentage of patients requiring emergent surgery (1.6% vs. 2.1%, $p = 1.0$), or the 30-day mortality rate (4.3% vs. 3.7%, $p = 0.78$). A 2010 Cochrane review also demonstrated that administration of proton pump inhibitors prior to endoscopy reduced the risk of finding stigmata of recent hemorrhage on endoscopy (OR 0.67, 95% CI 0.54–0.84) and reduced the risk of lesions requiring intervention on endoscopy (OR 0.68, 95% CI 0.5–0.93) [52]. There was no benefit of PPI administration prior to endoscopy on clinical outcomes of the need for emergent surgery (OR 0.90, 95% CI 0.65–1.25), rates of blood transfusion (OR 0.95, 95% CI 0.78–1.16), rates of rebleeding (OR 0.81, 95% CI 0.62–1.06), or 30-day mortality (OR 1.12, 95% CI 0.75–1.68). Because of the discordance between endoscopic and clinical outcomes, clinicians disagree on the utility of intravenous proton pump inhibitors in the undifferentiated bleeding patient. While there is not a mortality benefit, we recommend administration of PPIs to patients with acute upper GI bleeding for the benefits of reducing the necessity of future endoscopic intervention and reducing stigmata of recent hemorrhage.

Somatostatin Analogs

Patients with acute upper GI hemorrhage resulting from varices have increased splanchnic pres-

Table 14.2 Recommended pharmacotherapy of GI hemorrhage

Drug	Dose	Indication	Benefit
Pantoprazole or Esomeprazole	Bolus 80 mg IV; Consider infusion at 8 mg/h	Peptic ulcer, known or suspected Empiric upper GI bleed	Pre-endoscopy: reduces signs of recent bleeding on endoscopy, reduces need for endoscopic intervention, reduces hospital length of stay
Octreotide	Bolus: 50 μg IV; Consider infusion at 50 μg/h	Know ovr high suspicion of esophageal varices	Pre-endoscopy: significantly lower transfusion requirement; lower risk of initial hemostasis failure
Ceftriaxone or Ciprofloxacin	1 g IV daily 400 mg IV Q12 h	GI hemorrhage in patients with cirrhosis, with or without ascites	Reduced rates of rebleeding, bacterial infections, reduced mortality, reduced hospital length of stay

sure, so decreasing splanchnic circulation should decrease variceal bleeding. Administration of the synthetic somatostatin analog octreotide results in direct splanchnic vasoconstriction and reductions in splanchnic blood flow as well as inhibition of pepsin and acid secretion. In patients with acute bleeding from esophageal varices, treatment with octreotide improved initial hemostasis (RR 0.58, 95% CI 0.42–0.81) with fewer major complications (RR 0.31, 95% CI 0.11–0.87), compared with vasopressin [53]. In a 2008 Cochrane review of 21 trials involving 2588 patients with suspected bleeding esophageal varices, patients in blinded trials who were treated with somatostatin analogs octreotide or vapreotide were transfused 0.67 units less blood (95% CI, 95% CI 0.21–1.13) and had a lower risk of failure of initial hemostasis (RR 0.67, 95% CI 0.49–0.9) [54]. There was no improvement in patients treated with octreotide with regard to rebleeding episodes (RR 0.84, 95% CI 0.52–1.37) and no improvement in mortality (RR 0.97, 95% CI 0.75–1.25). Of note, 12 of the 21 trials required endoscopic confirmation of esophageal varices prior to randomization, which is rarely possible in the ED setting. Based on these findings, we recommend against empiric administration of octreotide for undifferentiated upper GI bleeding, however, in patients with known esophageal varices with active GI hemorrhage, particularly those with recent endoscopy or therapy of bleeding varices, octreotide should be considered.

Tranexamic Acid

Tranexamic acid (TXA) is an antifibrinolytic agent which reduces the degradation of the fibrin component of a blood clot. Trauma literature has promoted the use of tranexamic acid (TXA); however, several trials of TXA for patients with GI hemorrhage have failed to show significant benefit. A 2012 Cochrane review of seven clinical trials published between 1973 and 2001 found a significant decrease in mortality in patients with upper GI bleeding treated with TXA compared to placebo (5% vs. 8%, RR 0.61, 95% CI 0.42–0.89). This mortality effect, however, was not significant when the studies were controlled for potential bias or when a worst-case scenario analysis was performed (in which all cases lost to follow-up were assigned a treatment failure outcome, of which 21% of patients were assigned). Similarly, the Cochrane review showed no benefit with TXA with respect to rebleeding, number of units of blood transfused, nor need for operative intervention [55]. Based on these conclusions, we do not recommend using TXA in patients with acute GI hemorrhage.

Desmopressin (DDAVP)

Patients with end-stage renal disease have increased rates of both upper and lower GI bleeding, thought to be due to several factors including increased exposure to anticoagulants such as heparin with dialysis, uremic platelet dysfunction, increased propensity to develop arteriovenous malformations, and concomitant use of NSAIDS and antiplatelet medications such as clopidogrel. As uremic platelet dysfunction likely contributes to bleeding in patients with renal failure and concomitant gastrointestinal hemorrhage, some patients may benefit from administration of desmopressin (DDAVP) [56]. Therapy with DDAVP has not been studied specifically in the setting of GI hemorrhage, but bleeding time can be significantly reduced [57], so may be considered in uremic patients with GI hemorrhage. DDAVP in these patients should be administered intravenously in a single dose of 0.4 μg/kg.

Vasoactive Substances

Similar to the resuscitation of a trauma patient with hemorrhagic shock, resuscitation of a hemorrhaging patient with a GI bleed should focus on source control and controlling bleeding rather than administration of vasoactive medications or vasopressors. That said, prolonged hypoperfusion while awaiting definitive therapy is also likely undesirable.

Vasopressin

Vasopressin is a potent vasoconstrictor of splanchnic circulation, and causes decreased portal venous pressure, making it seemingly an ideal medication for upper GI bleeding, especially episodes resulting from increased portal pressure. Clinical trials, however, have not demonstrated a benefit to treatment of GI bleeding with vasopressin 40 units/h, and with no benefit to initial hemostasis, rebleeding, or mortality [58]. Vasopressin has been associated with significant side effects including ischemia and infarction of myocardium, bowel, and extremities. Addition of nitroglycerin therapy in an attempt to decrease the unintended ischemic complications of vasopressin has demonstrated a mild decrease in side effects, but no benefits with regard to rebleeding or mortality [59, 60]. Since the introduction of pharmacotherapy with octreotide, which has far fewer side effects than vasopressin, use of vasopressin with or without nitroglycerine has largely ceased as a therapy for GI bleeding, and we recommend against using vasopressin in patients with an acute GIB.

Terlipressin

Terlipressin is a synthetic analog of vasopressin that has significantly fewer side effects and has demonstrated a mortality benefit when compared with placebo in patients with acute GI bleeding due to varices. Within 1 min of administration of either octreotide or terlipressin, the hepatic venous pressure gradient and heart rate have been shown to decrease and the mean arterial pressure increases; these effects are short lived with octreotide, but terlipressin has sustained effects [61]. Furthermore, treatment of patient with acute upper GI bleeding due to varices with terlipressin, compared to placebo, has been shown in a 2003 Cochrane review to result in a significant reduction in all-cause mortality (RR 0.66, 95% CI 0.49–0.88) [62]. At the time of publication, however, terlipressin is not approved for use in the United States.

Antibiotics

Patients with cirrhosis-associated upper GI bleeding have high rates of developing spontaneous bacterial peritonitis (SBP) and other secondary infections. These infections are associated with increased rates of rebleeding and mortality [63, 64]. A short course of prophylactic antibiotics in patients with GI hemorrhage and cirrhosis, with or without ascites, has been shown to decrease rates of bacterial infection, decrease rates of rebleeding, and reduce mortality [65–67]. A 2011 meta-analysis supports these findings, with reduced rates of rebleeding (RR 0.53, 95% CI 0.38–0.74), reduced rates of bacterial infections (RR 0.35, 95% CI 0.26–0.47), reduced rates of mortality resulting from infection (RR 0.43, 95% CI 0.19–0.97), and reduced all-cause mortality (RR 0.79, 95% CI 0.63–0.98). In addition, hospital length of stay was reduced by administration of antibiotic prophylaxis, with a mean reduction in hospital length of stay by 1.9 days (95% CI −0.02 to −3.80 days) [68]. Intravenous ceftriaxone has demonstrated superiority over enteral antibiotics [69], so in the setting of an acute GI bleed in a patient with cirrhosis, we recommend administration of ceftriaxone 1 g IV daily for 7 days (or until hospital discharge). In patients with a cephalosporin allergy, IV ciprofloxacin is an acceptable alternative.

Definitive Therapy

Endoscopy

For upper GI bleeding, definitive therapy begins with EGD. The definition of "early" endoscopy varies by study, but often includes within 24 h after presentation. Patients who undergo EGD within 8 h of presentation have significantly higher rates of endoscopic findings of active bleeding, visible vessels, or adherent clots [70]. Despite no mortality benefit, endoscopy within 24 h of presentation is associated with decreased hospital length of stay, treatment cost, recurrent bleeding episodes, and need for surgery [71, 72].

The focus of this chapter is on the resuscitation of gastrointestinal hemorrhage and not on specific endoscopic techniques. The American College of Gastroenterology has published guidelines for the management of upper GI bleeding due to ulcer, varices, and lower GI bleeding [9, 32, 73]. Most patients presenting to the ED with GI hemorrhage have an undifferentiated etiology of bleeding, making these guidelines less applicable to the ED setting.

Following resuscitation, the majority of patients with GI bleeding that is not clearly from a lower GI source will undergo upper endoscopy first. Via endoscopy, esophageal varices can be banded or sclerosed, gastric varices can be injected with tissue adhesive, and nonvariceal lesions can be treated with thermal or chemical cautery, injection, or coagulation. It is recommended that patients presenting with hematochezia or bright red blood per rectum are evaluated with upper endoscopy first, as 10–15% of patients have an upper GI tract source with rapid transit through the GI tract [16, 74, 75]. Emergency lower GI endoscopy is not frequently performed for these patients as bowel prep is frequently necessary and therapeutic interventions via colonoscope are more limited than esophagogastroduodenoscopic interventions. A case series of 409 patients who underwent colonoscopic evaluation without purge bowel prep still had a 76% diagnostic yield of a lower GI source [76]; yet, in a randomized trial of urgent (<12 h) versus elective (36–60 h) colonoscopy, there were no differences in recurrent bleeding episodes, units of blood transfused, subsequent interventions, hospital length of stay, or costs [74].

Interventional Radiology

Both lower and upper GI bleeding can be managed definitively with interventional radiology (IR). For upper sources unable to be controlled endoscopically, embolization of vessels can be lifesaving. Transjugular intrahepatic portosystemic shunt (TIPS) can also be performed urgently, dramatically reducing portal pressure for treatment of varices and subsequently controlling hemorrhage. For lower GI sources, interventional radiology may be the initial attempt at definitive therapy, with the ability to perform diagnostic angiography and therapeutic intervention. As discussed above, angiography requires hemorrhage at a rate of at least 1–1.5 mL/min to be detected and localized. For less acute bleeding, some gastroenterologists may also perform a diagnostic endoscopy and, if an actively bleeding lesion is identified, place hemoclips to localize a source that can be identified by IR if rebleeding occurs.

Surgery

With effective endoscopic and IR interventions for GI bleeding, surgical options for definitive therapy are becoming infrequent. Complete or partial esophagectomy, gastrectomy, bowel resection, colectomy, or other procedures are, however, employed for the management of bleeding due to ischemic bowel and may occasionally be required for other causes of bleeding. Surgical portosystemic shunt creation and gastroesophageal disconnections are rarely performed, and few surgeons are experienced with these procedures even at tertiary referral centers.

Balloon Tamponade Devices

In cases of upper GI bleeding with hemorrhagic shock, patients are sometimes too unstable to undergo emergent EGD. Additionally, freestanding EDs or EDs in rural, remote hospitals may not have gastroenterology services immediately available. In both cases, placement of a gastroesophageal balloon tamponade device, commonly known as a Sengstaken–Blakemore or Minnesota tube, should be considered as a temporizing measure for an unstable hemorrhaging patient until more definitive therapy can be provided (Fig. 14.2). When utilized as a definitive therapy, balloon tamponade is inferior to endoscopy with sclerotherapy for mortality, hemostasis, and rebleeding [77]. Balloon tamponade can, however, prevent death from acute exsanguination when used temporarily while awaiting or transferring a patient for definitive care when such therapies are not immediately available [78].

Sengstaken and Blakemore first described use of this device in 1950, when they published their

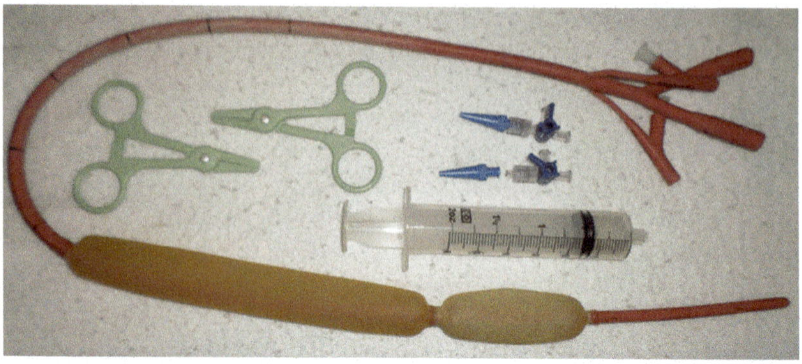

Fig. 14.2 Minnesota balloon tamponade tube (C.R. Bard, Covington, GA, USA) and specialized supplies suggested for insertion

experience in 30 patients with bleeding esophageal varices. They concluded, "There were no deaths from shock due to hemorrhage and, in our opinion, many pints of blood were saved" [79]. They further described how the device had been used for up to 7 weeks in patients with refractory bleeding. It must be understood that at the time, endoscopic interventions for acute bleeding were not available. Mortality in other series of esophageal bleeding treated with the device was significantly higher, with one case series reporting 90% mortality in 39 patients with 50 episodes of bleeding, and 8% of patients sustained esophageal rupture from the procedure that resulted in their death [80]. This case series did note that hemorrhage was controlled for more than 24 h in 40% of patients. Multiple case reports examining complications of Sengstaken–Blakemore tubes have reported esophageal rupture [81], jejunal rupture [82], airway obstruction [83], cardiac tamponade [84], tracheal rupture [85], and bilateral parotiditis [86].

Despite these potential complications, balloon tamponade devices may be the only chance at survival among a select cohort of patients for which EGD is not immediately available or is unsuccessful. In more recent literature, balloon tamponade used as a resuscitative, temporizing measure while awaiting more definitive interventional GI, radiological procedures, or surgical procedures, or as a rescue therapy for rebleeding after other interventions, and has demonstrated efficacy with relatively low mortality [78, 87].

In a 2006 series of 100 patients with variceal bleeding treated with balloon tamponade, the therapy was effective at stopping hemorrhage in 61% of patients with no cases of esophageal rupture reported, and balloon tamponade was employed after failed attempts at endoscopic therapy in 48% of patients [78].

In a multicenter study of 725 patients with variceal bleeding, initial balloon tamponade therapy was employed in 5.5% of patients; mortality for all variceal bleeds in this study was 12.9% and 83% of which were treated with EGD with banding and/or sclerotherapy as the initial therapy [88]. For the 92 patients who presented again within 2 weeks of their index variceal bleed, balloon tamponade was employed in 17.4% as the initial therapy for rebleeding.

A 2013 case series of 1308 episodes of gastric variceal bleeding also demonstrated potential efficacy of balloon tamponade, which was the index, nonpharmacologic therapy in 25 patients (1.9%), 76% of whom achieved hemostasis [87]. This case series also reported 28% mortality in patients who underwent balloon tamponade as the index therapy for gastric varices.

When used alone, somatostatin and balloon tamponade have similar success at achieving initial hemostasis by 4 h (74% vs. 60%) [89]. One study reported 80% success at initial hemostasis when balloon tamponade was used for control of acute variceal bleeding, but higher rates of rebleeding were observed compared to patients treated with octreotide or combined therapy with balloon tamponade and octreotide [90]. While this study compares the two therapies, for the ED resuscitation of a patient exsanguinating from variceal bleeding, we recommend initiation of octreotide and, if hemostasis is not rapidly achieved, careful consideration of placement of a balloon tamponade device.

Insertion Technique

Due to the multiple pieces of equipment necessary for expeditious and safe insertion of a balloon tamponade device, we strongly recommend assembling a kit with all necessary components so that the clinician directing the resuscitation can focus his time on insertion and ongoing resuscitation. Furthermore, we recommend ongoing training to refresh providers on the insertion technique, as this procedure is not often employed. Table 14.3 is a recommended list of items to assemble prior to inserting the device and Fig. 14.2 is an image of many of these individual specialized parts. Figures 14.3a and b are images of the parts combined to functionally inflate the balloon tamponade device and measure the pressure in the balloon. Unfortunately, the latex balloon devices can become cracked as they age, so the devices need to be replaced as they expire.

As with any procedure, insertion of a gastroesophageal tamponade balloon should follow a stepwise process. Our suggested general process is outlined in Table 14.4, and specific caveats are described subsequently.

As this device is being used as a temporizing method for hemorrhagic shock, all patients undergoing ED placement of a balloon tamponade catheter should be endotracheally intubated. This allows for adequate sedation and administration of a long-acting neuromuscular blocking agent.

In our experience, we strongly support using manometry and radiographic confirmation for insertion of balloon tamponade devices. To use manometry, the clinician must inflate the gastric balloon with serial volumes of air and record subsequent pressures prior to inserting the device into the patient. After insertion of

Table 14.3 Suggested list of supplies for insertion of a balloon tamponade device

Equipment		Equipment	
Insertion of device	Number	Securing of device	Number
Balloon tamponade catheter	1	Length of cord or oxygen tubing	1
Large wash basin (for ice bath)	1	1 L crystalloid for counter-traction	1
Manometer for manual blood pressure	1		
Three-way IV stopcock	2		
"Christmas tree" catheter adapter	2		
Plastic Kelly-type (dialysis) clamp	2		
Copy of Table 14.2 for recording pressure	1		
Laryngoscope or indirect videolaryngoscopy device	1		
Water-based lubricant	–		
McGill forceps	1		

Please refer to Fig. 14.1 for images of many of these specialized supplies

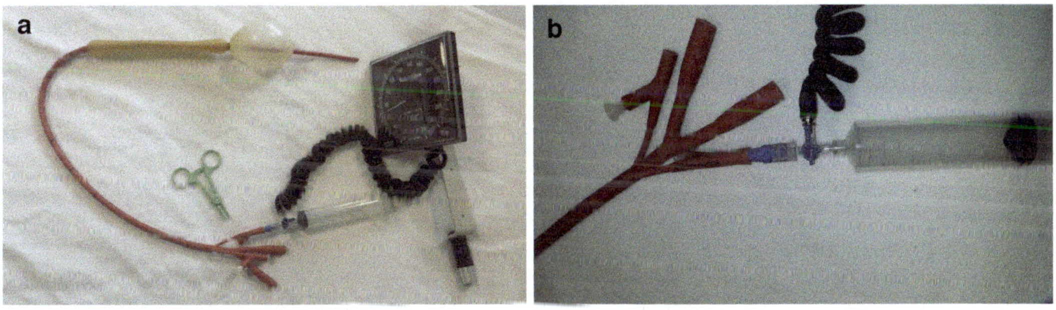

Fig. 14.3 (**a**) Assembled Minnesota tube and supplies for measuring pressure in balloon. (**b**) Detailed image of assembly of three-way stopcock, 60 mL syringe, manometer, fitting, and Minnesota tube

the device, a chest X-ray should be obtained prior to inflating the gastric balloon to ensure that the tube is in the stomach rather than the esophagus or airway. Recall that there is 10–15 cm of tube distal to the balloon, so having only the tip of the device in the stomach will not result in the balloon within the stomach, as illustrated in Figs. 14.4 and 14.5. Only after radiographic confirmation is obtained should the gastric balloon be inflated. If the device is inserted and the balloon is inflated with subsequent pressure more than 10 mmHg greater than the preinsertion pressure for the same volume of air, the balloon is likely positioned in either the esophagus or the duodenum, and should be repositioned prior to inflation. Table 14.5 is an example of a method for recording pressure–volume relationships within the gastric balloon. Following inflation of the balloon with air and confirmation via pressure readings, an additional chest radiograph should be obtained to further ensure proper positioning (Fig. 14.6).

Insertion of a balloon tamponade device is substantially more difficult than insertion of a standard orogastric tube due to the lack of rigidity of the latex balloon catheter. In our experience, we have found several techniques to improve placement success of balloon tamponade catheters.

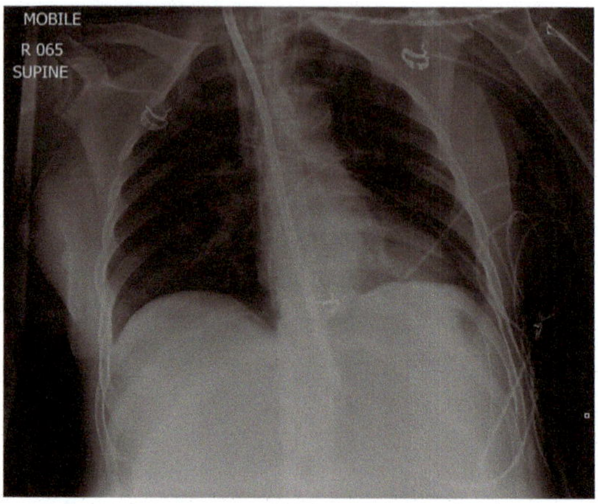

Fig. 14.4 Minnesota tube in proximal stomach

Table 14.4 Protocol for insertion of a balloon tamponade device

1.	Endotracheal intubation
2.	Notify X-ray technician they will be needed for multiple STAT images
3.	Gather necessary equipment (Table 14.3)
4.	Prepare balloon tamponade device by measuring and recording preinsertion balloon pressures for serial volumes of air (Fig. 14.2 and Table 14.5)
5.	Immerse balloon tamponade device in bedside ice bath
6.	Ensure adequate sedation and then administer pharmacologic paralysis to patient
7.	Using direct or indirect laryngoscopy, visualize proximal esophagus
8.	Have assistant rapidly remove device from ice bath, coat in water-based lubricant, and hand to operator
9.	Visualize tip of device entering proximal esophagus and advance to 50 cm depth; if necessary, use fingers or McGill forceps to advance down esophagus but do not force the device
10.	Obtain chest radiograph to ensure balloon is in the stomach and not airway, esophagus, or duodenum
11.	Inflate gastric balloon with 100 mL air and measure and record pressure; if this pressure is >10 mmHg greater than the pressure obtained prior to insertion of the device, deflate the balloon and reposition
12.	Inflate serial volumes of air into gastric balloon, recording pressure with each subsequent volume of air; if any pressure is >10 mmHg greater than the pressure for the corresponding volume of air obtained prior to insertion of the device, deflate the balloon and reposition
13.	Clamp the gastric inflation port with the plastic hemostat to prevent inadvertent leakage of air from the balloon or the three-way stopcock
14.	After inflation of the gastric balloon to a total volume of 300 mL of air, pull tension on the device coming out of the patients mouth and, using a hemostat and rope or oxygen tubing, secure the tube with traction applied by hanging a 1-L bag of fluid from the foot of the bed
15.	Obtain chest radiograph
16.	If tamponade of bleeding is not achieved, the esophageal balloon may be inflated with a volume of air titrated to stop bleeding; pressure should never exceed 50 mmHg to avoid esophageal rupture or pressure necrosis

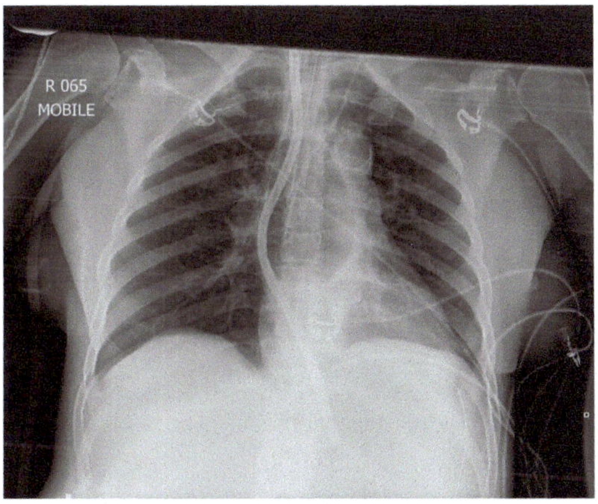

Fig. 14.5 Same patient after inflation of Minnesota tube gastric balloon in esophagus with resultant hemodynamic instability. This is the argument for manometry

Table 14.5 Recording pre- and postballoon inflation pressure–volume

Volume of air	Pressure (preinsertion)	Pressure (in situ)
50 mL	____ mmHg	____ mmHg
100 mL	____ mmHg	____ mmHg
200 mL	____ mmHg	____ mmHg
300 mL	____ mmHg	____ mmHg
400 mL	____ mmHg	____ mmHg
500 mL	____ mmHg	____ mmHg

If pressure in the balloon is >10 mmHg, different for the same volume of air preinsertion compared to in situ, the balloon is likely in the esophagus or duodenum and needs to be immediately deflated

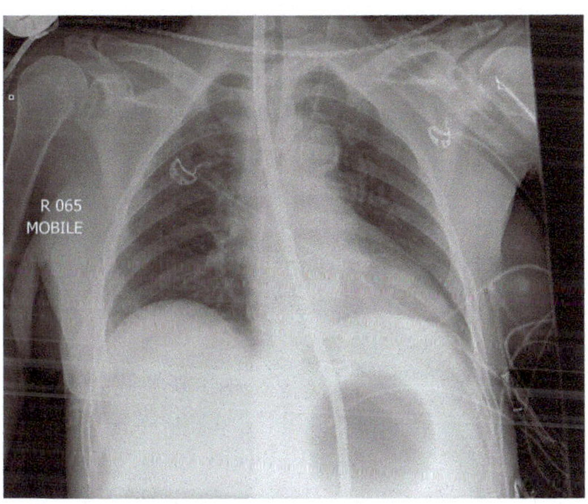

Fig. 14.6 Radiographic confirmation of correct position of Minnesota tube with balloon inflated in the stomach

Using a length of suture (0 silk), a standard nasogastric tube can be tied along the side of the balloon tamponade device to provide additional rigidity to the tube. If using a Sengstaken–Blakemore tube, this NG can serve as a suction of the esophagus proximal to the gastric balloon, whereas a Minnesota tube has both gastric and esophageal suction capabilities.

Cooling of a silicone Sengstaken–Blakemore tube does not improve rigidity of the device; however, cooling of a latex tube will provide mildly increased rigidity for approximately 30 s when exposed to body temperature after removal from the cold [91]. The majority of Minnesota and Sengstaken–Blakemore devices available in the United States are constructed of latex, and we feel that the very transient increase in rigidity of the latex device afforded by immersing it in a bedside ice water bath provides improved directability of the distal tip of the catheter down the esophagus. Once the device is removed from the ice bath, it is immediately coated in water-soluble lubricant and rapidly directed down the esophagus. Using direct or indirect laryngoscopy may help direct the tip of the catheter to the esophagus (Fig. 14.7). We recommend the operator visualize the esophagus with indirect laryngoscopy, then have an assistant remove the tube from the ice bath, coat it with lubricant, and hand quickly to the operator. Pharmacologic paralysis will facilitate advancing the device down the esophagus by inserting McGill forceps or the fingers of the operator into the mouth of the patient, as needed.

After insertion of the balloon tamponade catheter to a depth of 50 cm, the operator should examine the patient's oropharynx visually and by palpation to ensure that the tube is not coiled. A preinflation X-ray should then be obtained prior to inflating the gastric balloon as described above, checking and recording the pressure in the gastric balloon with each subsequent 100 mL of air. Care must be taken to ensure the three-way stopcock is closed at all times unless actively injecting air to avoid inadvertent deflation of the balloon. We recommend using a plastic hemostat or "dialysis clamp" to clamp the inflation port of the gastric

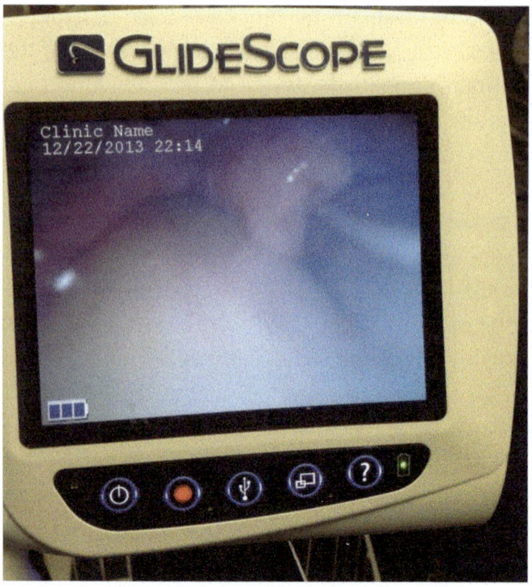

Fig. 14.7 Indirect laryngoscopic view of a Minnesota tube being advanced into the esophagus. Note the endotracheal tube at the 3 o'clock position and the Minnesota tube toward the bottom of the screen

balloon distal to the three-way stopcock to avoid leakage of air and resultant loss of pressure in the gastric balloon.

Securing the Balloon Tamponade Device

A variety of methods for securing the balloon tamponade device have been devised. As initially described by Sengstaken and Blakemore, the tube was inserted nasally and was secured with tape to the bridge of the nose [79]. More recently, with oral insertion of balloon tamponade devices, a technique involving placement of the patient in an American football helmet and securing the balloon tamponade device to the facemask of the helmet has been described. Unfortunately, this dramatically limits access to the patient's face, head, and neck and if the patient remained supine in the football helmet for several hours, pressure necrosis to the posterior head could develop. The alternate use of a baseball umpire mask slightly improves access, but continues to encumber the face and neck and can result in pressure necrosis to the anterior face. Use of an endotracheal tube-securing device has been proposed for securing a balloon tamponade tube, but does not allow for a

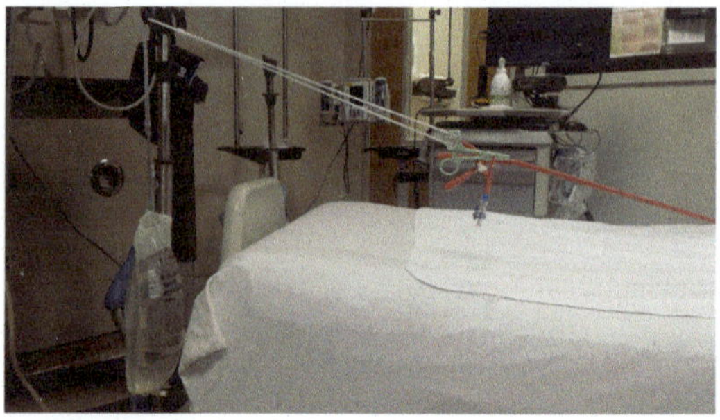

Fig. 14.8 Suggested application of traction to balloon tamponade device using nasal cannula and 1 L crystalloid solution

consistent amount of traction to be applied to the tube, thereby hindering the tamponade effect of the balloon. Finally, it has been suggested that simply tying the end of the balloon tamponade device to a length of traction rope and hanging a 500- to 1000-mL bag of crystalloid to the other end of the rope suspended from the head or foot of the bed will provide a consistent 0.5–1 Newton for traction on the balloon. As rope may not be readily accessible in the ED, a length of oxygen tubing or a nasal cannula could serve the same purpose (Fig. 14.8). For securing a balloon tamponade device in a patient in the ED, we recommend this final technique until more definitive therapy is available.

Transfer

Patients presenting to a hospital without the availability of gastroenterology or ICU services will often require transfer to a tertiary referral center. Refer to Chap. 34 of this book for an in-depth discussion of interhospital transfer of critically ill patients. When arranging the interhospital transfer of a patient with significant GI hemorrhage, particular attention should be focused on ensuring appropriate venous access and ensuring the patient's airway is protected. If there is doubt that the patient will maintain a protected airway, endotracheal intubation should be completed in the ED of the transferring facility prior to departure. Transfusion of blood products and administration of PPI and, if varices are suspected, octreotide, can be initiated prior to transfer.

Disposition and Risk Stratification

This chapter focuses on resuscitation of critically ill ED patients with GI bleeding, nearly all of whom should be admitted to a critical care unit. These patients are a minority of patients with a GI bleeding who present to the ED, but based on the potential for clinical decompensation, maintaining a low threshold for ICU admission is prudent until the patient has undergone endoscopic evaluation.

Several risk stratification tools for assessing the severity of upper GI bleeds have been developed, including the Rockall score [92] and the Glasgow–Blatchford score (GBS) [93] (Table 14.6). The Rockall score was originally devised to predict mortality for patients presenting with upper GI bleeding, and incorporates both clinical and endoscopic variables. An abbreviated version includes only pre-endoscopy variables and can be calculated in the ED prior to endoscopy [92].

The GBS was developed to identify a very low-risk cohort of patients who dare predicted not to require blood transfusion, surgery, or endo-

Table 14.6 Comparison of clinical scoring criteria for risk assessment in GI hemorrhage [92, 93, 96]

Pre-endoscopy Rockall score		Glasgow–Blatchford score		AIMS65 score	
Criteria	Points	Criteria	Points	Component	Points
Age		**BUN (mg/dL) (mmol/L)**		Albumin < 3 g/dL	1
<60 years	0	<18.2 (<6.5)	0	INR > 1.5	1
60–79 years	1	≥18.2 to <22.4 (≥6.5 to <8.0)	2	Mental status change (GCS < 14)	1
≥80 years	2	≥22.4 to <28 (≥8.0 to <10.0)	3	Systolic blood pressure < 90 mmHg	1
Shock		≥28 to <70 (≥10.0 to <25)	4	Age > 65 years	1
SBP ≥ 100 mmHg, HR < 100	0	≥70 (≥25.0)	6		
SBP ≥ 100 mmHg, HR ≥ 100	1	**Hemoglobin for men (g/dL)**			
SBP < 100 mmHg	2	>13.0	0		
Comorbidity		≥12.0 to <13.0	1		
No major comorbidity	0	≥10.0 to <12.0	3		
Cardiac failure, ischemic heart disease, any major comorbidity	2	<10.0	6		
Renal failure, liver failure, disseminated malignancy	3	**Hemoglobin for women (g/dL)**			
		>12.0	0		
		≥10.0 to 12.0	1		
		<10.0	6		
		Systolic blood pressure (mmHg)			
		≥110	0		
		100–109	1		
		90–99	2		
		<90	3		
		Other markers			
		HR ≥ 100/min	1		
		Presentation with melena	1		
		Presentation with syncope	2		
		Hepatic disease	2		
		Cardiac failure	2		

HR heart rate, *INR* international normalized ratio, *SBP* systolic blood pressure

scopic intervention to control bleeding [93]. Endoscopic findings are not included in the GBS, making it more applicable to use in the ED. Only those who have no risk factors on the GBS are considered low risk.

A study in the United Kingdom suggested that patients with a GBS of 0 could be safely discharged from the ED for outpatient follow-up [94]. In the derivation phase of the study, none of the 105 patients with a GBS of 0 required a transfusion, intervention to control bleeding, or died. Of the 184 patients with a Rockall score of 0, however, 17% had a complication: 23 required transfusion, 21 required endoscopy or surgery to control bleeding, and 1 died. In the validation phase of this study, 22% were found to have a GBS score of 0, of which 68% were discharged home and none of the 123 patients required transfusion, endoscopic or surgical intervention, or died during the subsequent 6 months.

Although use of the GBS demonstrated promise in the United Kingdom, a US study found that both the GBS and Rockall scores failed to identify several cases where endoscopy was felt to be necessary within the subsequent 24 h. Of 18% of patients with a Rockall score of 0, 7.4% required endoscopy within 24 h. Only 9% of patients had a GBS of 0 and 13% of patients who were admitted despite a GBS score of 0 required endoscopic therapy for bleeding within 24 h. The authors speculate that the poorer performance of both the Rockall and GBS scores are due to the retrospective design of their study and variation in patient and gastroenterologist practice between the United Kingdom and the United States [95].

The AIMS65 risk score was first described in 2011, and is intended to predict inpatient mortality, length of stay, and costs associated with an upper GI bleed (Tables 14.6 and 14.7). The score was derived by analysis of nearly 30,000 patients presenting to EDs in the United States with upper GI bleeding and was validated in 32,500 patients. The score identified five risk factors that accurately predicted in-hospital mortality, length of stay, and cost for the admission. Inpatient mortality was 0.3% for patients with no risk factors and 31.8% in patients with all five risk factors ($p < 0.001$) [96]. This score has not yet been validated in a prospective trial, but again demonstrates that even patients with no risk factors can die from acute GI hemorrhage.

Combining low risk factors from the Blatchford, GBS, and AIMS65 will still not eliminate the need for additional investigation, but these factors may help to guide decisions about the urgency of intervention (Table 14.8).

Table 14.7 Interpretation of AIMS65 scoring

Points	Mortality ($p < 0.001$)	Length of stay (days) ($p < 0.001$)	Inpatient cost ($p < 0.001$)
0	0.3%	3.44	$5,647
1	1.2%	4.37	$6,466
2	2.8%	5.35	$7,980
3	8.5%	6.23	$10,042
4	15.1%	7.21	$12,986
5	24.5%		$15,776

Table 14.8 Low-risk criteria for patients with GI hemorrhage

Low risk by pre-endoscopy Rockall score	Low risk by Glasgow–Blatchford score
Age <60 years SBP ≥ 100 mmHg and HR < 100/min Absence of: Cardiac failure Ischemic heart disease Renal failure Hepatic failure Disseminated malignancy Other major comorbidity	Urea < 18.2 mg/dL Hemoglobin ≥13 g/dL (male) or ≥12 g/dL (female) SBP ≥ 110 mmHg Pulse < 100/min Absence of: Melena Syncope Cardiac failure Liver disease
Low risk by AIMS65	
Albumin > 3 INR < 1.5 Normal mentation SBP > 90 Age <65 years	

SBP systolic blood pressure, *INR* international normalized ratio

Conclusions

Hemorrhage from the gastrointestinal tract is a common presenting complaint to EDs in the United States. Many of these bleeding events will resolve spontaneously, but for select cases, emergency physicians must rapidly assess and intervene. The determination of upper versus lower source of bleeding can be challenging and it should not preclude the necessary resuscitation of an acutely bleeding patient. Large-bore IV access and airway protection should be promptly obtained and volume resuscitation initiated. Blood transfusion may be required, but with a hemoglobin goal of 7 g/dL in a patient without hemorrhagic shock. Additionally, pharmacologic therapies may benefit patients with specific diagnoses. Definitive therapies may include endoscopy, interventional radiology, or surgery, but such therapies are often not available to all patients at all times, so temporizing measures including balloon tamponade tubes should be in the toolbox of emergency physicians. Additionally, if definitive therapy is not available locally, the patient should be resuscitated and transferred to a facility capable of providing this therapy.

References

1. Srygley FD, Gerardo CJ, Tran T, Fisher DA. Does this patient have a severe upper gastrointestinal bleed? JAMA. 2012;307:1072–9.
2. Ghassemi KA, Jensen DM. Lower GI bleeding: epidemiology and management. Curr Gastroenterol Rep. 2013;15:333.
3. van Leerdam ME. Epidemiology of acute upper gastrointestinal bleeding. Best Pract Res Clin Gastroenterol. 2008;22:209–24.
4. Ell C, May A. Mid-gastrointestinal bleeding: capsule endoscopy and push-and-pull enteroscopy give rise to a new medical term. Endoscopy. 2006;38:73–5.
5. Raju GS, Gerson L, Das A, Lewis B, American Gastroenterological Association. American Gastroenterological Association (AGA) Institute technical review on obscure gastrointestinal bleeding. Gastroenterology. 2007;133:1697–717.
6. Raju GS, Gerson L, Das A, Lewis B, American Gastroenterological Association. American Gastroenterological Association (AGA) Institute medical position statement on obscure gastrointestinal bleeding. Gastroenterology. 2007;133:1694–6.
7. Peura DA, Lanza FL, Gostout CJ, Foutch PG. The American College of Gastroenterology Bleeding Registry: preliminary findings. Am J Gastroenterol. 1997;92:924–8.
8. Afessa B. Triage of patients with acute gastrointestinal bleeding for intensive care unit admission based on risk factors for poor outcome. J Clin Gastroenterol. 2000;30:281–5.
9. Garcia-Tsao G, Sanyal AJ, Grace ND, Carey W, Practice Guidelines Committee of the American Association for the Study of Liver Diseases, Practice Parameters Committee of the American College of Gastroenterology. Prevention and management of gastroesophageal varices and variceal hemorrhage in cirrhosis. Hepatology. 2007;46:922–38.
10. Carbonell N, Pauwels A, Serfaty L, Fourdan O, Levy VG, Poupon R. Improved survival after variceal bleeding in patients with cirrhosis over the past two decades. Hepatology. 2004;40:652–9.
11. Longstreth GF. Epidemiology and outcome of patients hospitalized with acute lower gastrointestinal hemorrhage: a population-based study. Am J Gastroenterol. 1997;92:419–24.
12. Hreinsson JP, Gumundsson S, Kalaitzakis E, Bjornsson ES. Lower gastrointestinal bleeding: incidence, etiology, and outcomes in a population-based setting. Eur J Gastroenterol Hepatol. 2013;25:37–43.
13. Laine L, Yang H, Chang SC, Datto C. Trends for incidence of hospitalization and death due to GI complications in the United States from 2001 to 2009. Am J Gastroenterol. 2012;107:1190–5; quiz 6.
14. Zuccaro G. Epidemiology of lower gastrointestinal bleeding. Best Pract Res Clin Gastroenterol. 2008;22:225–32.
15. Szold A, Katz LB, Lewis BS. Surgical approach to occult gastrointestinal bleeding. Am J Surg. 1992;163:90–2; discussion 2–3.
16. Byers SE, Chudnofsky CR, Sorondo B, Dominici P, Parrillo SJ. Incidence of occult upper gastrointestinal bleeding in patients presenting to the ED with hematochezia. Am J Emerg Med. 2007;25:340–4.
17. Zuckerman GR, Trellis DR, Sherman TM, Clouse RE. An objective measure of stool color for differentiating upper from lower gastrointestinal bleeding. Dig Dis Sci. 1995;40:1614–21.
18. Ritter DM, Rettke SR, Hughes RW Jr, Burritt MF, Sterioff S, Ilstrup DM. Placement of nasogastric tubes and esophageal stethoscopes in patients with documented esophageal varices. Anesth Analg. 1988;67:283–5.
19. Witting MD, Magder L, Heins AE, Mattu A, Granja CA, Baumgarten M. Usefulness and validity of diagnostic nasogastric aspiration in patients without hematemesis. Ann Emerg Med. 2004;43:525–32.
20. Palamidessi N, Sinert R, Falzon L, Zehtabchi S. Nasogastric aspiration and lavage in emergency department patients with hematochezia or melena without hematemesis. Acad Emerg Med. 2010;17:126–32.
21. Huang ES, Karsan S, Kanwal F, Singh I, Makhani M, Spiegel BM. Impact of nasogastric lavage on outcomes in acute GI bleeding. Gastrointest Endosc. 2011;74:971–80.
22. Chalasani N, Clark WS, Wilcox CM. Blood urea nitrogen to creatinine concentration in gastrointestinal bleeding: a reappraisal. Am J Gastroenterol. 1997;92:1796–9.

23. Richards RJ, Donica MB, Grayer D. Can the blood urea nitrogen/creatinine ratio distinguish upper from lower gastrointestinal bleeding? J Clin Gastroenterol. 1990;12:500–4.
24. Bhatti N, Amoateng-Adjepong Y, Qamar A, Manthous CA. Myocardial infarction in critically ill patients presenting with gastrointestinal hemorrhage: retrospective analysis of risks and outcomes. Chest. 1998;114:1137–42.
25. Emenike E, Srivastava S, Amoateng-Adjepong Y, al-Kharrat T, Zarich S, Manthous CA. Myocardial infarction complicating gastrointestinal hemorrhage. Mayo Clin Proc. 1999;74:235–41.
26. Prendergast HM, Sloan EP, Cumpston K, Schlichting AB. Myocardial infarction and cardiac complications in emergency department patients admitted to the intensive care unit with gastrointestinal hemorrhage. J Emerg Med. 2005;28:19–25.
27. Shah A, Chisolm-Straker M, Alexander A, Rattu M, Dikdan S, Manini AF. Prognostic use of lactate to predict inpatient mortality in acute gastrointestinal hemorrhage. Am J Emerg Med. 2014;32:752–5.
28. Thorne DA, Datz FL, Remley K, Christian PE. Bleeding rates necessary for detecting acute gastrointestinal bleeding with technetium-99m-labeled red blood cells in an experimental model. J Nucl Med. 1987;28:514–20.
29. Zuckerman DA, Bocchini TP, Birnbaum EH. Massive hemorrhage in the lower gastrointestinal tract in adults: diagnostic imaging and intervention. AJR Am J Roentgenol. 1993;161:703–11.
30. Suzman MS, Talmor M, Jennis R, Binkert B, Barie PS. Accurate localization and surgical management of active lower gastrointestinal hemorrhage with technetium-labeled erythrocyte scintigraphy. Ann Surg. 1996;224:29–36.
31. Hunter JM, Pezim ME. Limited value of technetium 99m-labeled red cell scintigraphy in localization of lower gastrointestinal bleeding. Am J Surg. 1990;159:504–6.
32. Zuccaro G Jr. Management of the adult patient with acute lower gastrointestinal bleeding. American College of Gastroenterology. Practice Parameters Committee. Am J Gastroenterol. 1998;93:1202–8.
33. Meltzer AC, Pinchbeck C, Burnett S, et al. Emergency physicians accurately interpret video capsule endoscopy findings in suspected upper gastrointestinal hemorrhage: a video survey. Acad Emerg Med. 2013;20:711–5.
34. Meltzer AC, Ward MJ, Gralnek IM, Pines JM. The cost-effectiveness analysis of video capsule endoscopy compared to other strategies to manage acute upper gastrointestinal hemorrhage in the ED. Am J Emerg Med. 2014;32:823–32.
35. McPherson D, Adekanye O, Wilkes AR, Hall JE. Fluid flow through intravenous cannulae in a clinical model. Anesth Analg. 2009;108:1198–202.
36. Aeder MI, Crowe JP, Rhodes RS, Shuck JM, Wolf WM. Technical limitations in the rapid infusion of intravenous fluids. Ann Emerg Med. 1985;14:307–10.
37. Dutky PA, Stevens SL, Maull KI. Factors affecting rapid fluid resuscitation with large-bore introducer catheters. J Trauma. 1989;29:856–60.
38. Li SF, Cole M, Forest R, et al. Are 2 smaller intravenous catheters as good as 1 larger intravenous catheter? Am J Emerg Med. 2010;28:724–7.
39. Villanueva C, Colomo A, Bosch A, et al. Transfusion strategies for acute upper gastrointestinal bleeding. N Engl J Med. 2013;368:11–21.
40. Castaneda B, Morales J, Lionetti R, et al. Effects of blood volume restitution following a portal hypertensive-related bleeding in anesthetized cirrhotic rats. Hepatology. 2001;33:821–5.
41. Kravetz D, Sikuler E, Groszmann RJ. Splanchnic and systemic hemodynamics in portal hypertensive rats during hemorrhage and blood volume restitution. Gastroenterology. 1986;90:1232–40.
42. Hebert PC, Wells G, Blajchman MA, et al. A multicenter, randomized, controlled clinical trial of transfusion requirements in critical care. Transfusion Requirements in Critical Care Investigators, Canadian Critical Care Trials Group. N Engl J Med. 1999;340:409–17.
43. Marik PE, Corwin HL. Efficacy of red blood cell transfusion in the critically ill: a systematic review of the literature. Crit Care Med. 2008;36:2667–74.
44. Corwin HL, Gettinger A, Pearl RG, et al. The CRIT study: Anemia and blood transfusion in the critically ill--current clinical practice in the United States. Crit Care Med. 2004;32:39–52.
45. Baraniuk S, Tilley BC, Del Junco DJ, et al. Pragmatic Randomized Optimal Platelet and Plasma Ratios (PROPPR) Trial: design, rationale and implementation. Injury. 2014;45:1287–95.
46. Holcomb JB, del Junco DJ, Fox EE, et al. The prospective, observational, multicenter, major trauma transfusion (PROMMTT) study: comparative effectiveness of a time-varying treatment with competing risks. JAMA Surg. 2013;148:127–36.
47. del Junco DJ, Holcomb JB, Fox EE, et al. Resuscitate early with plasma and platelets or balance blood products gradually: findings from the PROMMTT study. J Trauma Acute Care Surg. 2013;75:S24–30.
48. D'Amico G, Pietrosi G, Tarantino I, Pagliaro L. Emergency sclerotherapy versus vasoactive drugs for variceal bleeding in cirrhosis: a Cochrane meta-analysis. Gastroenterology. 2003;124:1277–91.
49. Green FW Jr, Kaplan MM, Curtis LE, Levine PH. Effect of acid and pepsin on blood coagulation and platelet aggregation. A possible contributor prolonged gastroduodenal mucosal hemorrhage. Gastroenterology. 1978;74:38–43.
50. Gisbert JP, Gonzalez L, Calvet X, Roque M, Gabriel R, Pajares JM. Proton pump inhibitors versus H2-antagonists: a meta-analysis of their efficacy in treating bleeding peptic ulcer. Aliment Pharmacol Ther. 2001;15:917–26.

51. Lau JY, Leung WK, Wu JC, et al. Omeprazole before endoscopy in patients with gastrointestinal bleeding. N Engl J Med. 2007;356:1631–40.
52. Sreedharan A, Martin J, Leontiadis GI, et al. Proton pump inhibitor treatment initiated prior to endoscopic diagnosis in upper gastrointestinal bleeding. Cochrane Database Syst Rev. 2010;(7):CD005415.
53. Corley DA, Cello JP, Adkisson W, Ko WF, Kerlikowske K. Octreotide for acute esophageal variceal bleeding: a meta-analysis. Gastroenterology. 2001;120:946–54.
54. Gotzsche PC, Hrobjartsson A. Somatostatin analogues for acute bleeding oesophageal varices. Cochrane Database Syst Rev. 2008;(3):CD000193.
55. Gluud LL, Klingenberg SL, Langholz E. Tranexamic acid for upper gastrointestinal bleeding. Cochrane Database Syst Rev. 2012;(1):CD006640.
56. Kalman RS, Pedrosa MC. Evidence-based review of gastrointestinal bleeding in the chronic kidney disease patient. Semin Dial. 2015;28(1):68–74.
57. Hedges SJ, Dehoney SB, Hooper JS, Amanzadeh J, Busti AJ. Evidence-based treatment recommendations for uremic bleeding. Nat Clin Pract Nephrol. 2007;3:138–53.
58. Fogel MR, Knauer CM, Andres LL, et al. Continuous intravenous vasopressin in active upper gastrointestinal bleeding. Ann Intern Med. 1982;96:565–9.
59. Gimson AE, Westaby D, Hegarty J, Watson A, Williams R. A randomized trial of vasopressin and vasopressin plus nitroglycerin in the control of acute variceal hemorrhage. Hepatology. 1986;6:410–3.
60. Tsai YT, Lay CS, Lai KH, et al. Controlled trial of vasopressin plus nitroglycerin vs vasopressin alone in the treatment of bleeding esophageal varices. Hepatology. 1986;6:406–9.
61. Baik SK, Jeong PH, Ji SW, et al. Acute hemodynamic effects of octreotide and terlipressin in patients with cirrhosis: a randomized comparison. Am J Gastroenterol. 2005;100:631–5.
62. Ioannou G, Doust J, Rockey DC. Terlipressin for acute esophageal variceal hemorrhage. Cochrane Database Syst Rev. 2003;(1):CD002147.
63. Bernard B, Cadranel JF, Valla D, Escolano S, Jarlier V, Opolon P. Prognostic significance of bacterial infection in bleeding cirrhotic patients: a prospective study. Gastroenterology. 1995;108:1828–34.
64. Goulis J, Armonis A, Patch D, Sabin C, Greenslade L, Burroughs AK. Bacterial infection is independently associated with failure to control bleeding in cirrhotic patients with gastrointestinal hemorrhage. Hepatology. 1998;27:1207–12.
65. Bernard B, Grange JD, Khac EN, Amiot X, Opolon P, Poynard T. Antibiotic prophylaxis for the prevention of bacterial infections in cirrhotic patients with gastrointestinal bleeding: a meta-analysis. Hepatology. 1999;29:1655–61.
66. Hou MC, Lin HC, Liu TT, et al. Antibiotic prophylaxis after endoscopic therapy prevents rebleeding in acute variceal hemorrhage: a randomized trial. Hepatology. 2004;39:746–53.
67. Soares-Weiser K, Brezis M, Tur-Kaspa R, Leibovici L. Antibiotic prophylaxis for cirrhotic patients with gastrointestinal bleeding. Cochrane Database Syst Rev. 2002;(2):CD002907.
68. Chavez-Tapia NC, Barrientos-Gutierrez T, Tellez-Avila F, et al. Meta-analysis: antibiotic prophylaxis for cirrhotic patients with upper gastrointestinal bleeding – an updated Cochrane review. Aliment Pharmacol Ther. 2011;34:509–18.
69. Fernandez J, Ruiz del Arbol L, Gomez C, et al. Norfloxacin vs ceftriaxone in the prophylaxis of infections in patients with advanced cirrhosis and hemorrhage. Gastroenterology. 2006;131:1049–56; quiz 285.
70. Tsoi KK, Ma TK, Sung JJ. Endoscopy for upper gastrointestinal bleeding: how urgent is it? Nat Rev Gastroenterol Hepatol. 2009;6:463–9.
71. Cooper GS, Chak A, Way LE, Hammar PJ, Harper DL, Rosenthal GE. Early endoscopy in upper gastrointestinal hemorrhage: associations with recurrent bleeding, surgery, and length of hospital stay. Gastrointest Endosc. 1999;49:145–52.
72. Lee JG, Turnipseed S, Romano PS, et al. Endoscopy-based triage significantly reduces hospitalization rates and costs of treating upper GI bleeding: a randomized controlled trial. Gastrointest Endosc. 1999;50:755–61.
73. Laine L, Jensen DM. Management of patients with ulcer bleeding. Am J Gastroenterol. 2012;107:345–60; quiz 61.
74. Laine L, Shah A. Randomized trial of urgent vs elective colonoscopy in patients hospitalized with lower GI bleeding. Am J Gastroenterol. 2010;105:2636–41; quiz 42.
75. Jensen DM, Machicado GA. Diagnosis and treatment of severe hematochezia. The role of urgent colonoscopy after purge. Gastroenterology. 1988;95:1569–74.
76. Rossini FP, Ferrari A, Spandre M, et al. Emergency colonoscopy. World J Surg. 1989;13:190–2.
77. Paquet KJ, Feussner H. Endoscopic sclerosis and esophageal balloon tamponade in acute hemorrhage from esophagogastric varices: a prospective controlled randomized trial. Hepatology. 1985;5:580–3.
78. Pinto-Marques P, Romaozinho JM, Ferreira M, Amaro P, Freitas D. Esophageal perforation--associated risk with balloon tamponade after endoscopic therapy. Myth or reality? Hepato-Gastroenterology. 2006;53:536–9.
79. Sengstaken RW, Blakemore AH. Balloon tamponage for the control of hemorrhage from esophageal varices. Ann Surg. 1950;131:781–9.
80. Chojkier M, Conn HO. Esophageal tamponade in the treatment of bleeding varices. A decadel progress report. Dig Dis Sci. 1980;25:267–72.
81. Zeid SS, Young PC, Reeves JT. Rupture of the esophagus after introduction of the Sengstaken-Blakemore tube. Gastroenterology. 1959;36:128–31.
82. Schleinitz P. Jejunal rupture by Sengstaken-Blakemore tube. Gastroenterology. 1982;83:159.

83. Kelly DJ, Walsh F, Ahmed S, Synnott A. Airway obstruction due to a Sengstaken-Blakemore tube. Anesth Analg. 1997;85:219–21.
84. De Cock D, Monballyu P, Voigt JU, Wauters J. Extra-cardiac compression and left ventricular inflow obstruction as a complication of a Sengstaken-Blakemore tube. Eur J Echocardiogr. 2011;12:973.
85. Thomas P, Auge A, Lonjon T, et al. Rupture of the thoracic trachea with a Sengstaken-Blakemore tube. J Cardiovasc Surg. 1994;35:351–3.
86. Tekin F, Ozutemiz O, Bicak S, Oruc N, Ilter T. Bilateral acute parotitis following insertion of a Sengstaken-Blakemore tube. Endoscopy. 2009;41(Suppl 2):E206.
87. Kim MY, Um SH, Baik SK, et al. Clinical features and outcomes of gastric variceal bleeding: retrospective Korean multicenter data. Clin Mol Hepatol. 2013;19:36–44.
88. Sorbi D, Gostout CJ, Peura D, et al. An assessment of the management of acute bleeding varices: a multicenter prospective member-based study. Am J Gastroenterol. 2003;98:2424–34.
89. Jaramillo JL, de la Mata M, Mino G, Costan G, Gomez-Camacho F. Somatostatin versus Sengstaken balloon tamponade for primary haemostasia of bleeding esophageal varices. A randomized pilot study. J Hepatol. 1991;12:100–5.
90. Avgerinos A, Klonis C, Rekoumis G, Gouma P, Papadimitriou N, Raptis S. A prospective randomized trial comparing somatostatin, balloon tamponade and the combination of both methods in the management of acute variceal haemorrhage. J Hepatol. 1991;13:78–83.
91. Dearden JC, Hellawell GO, Pilling J, Besherdas K, Van Someren N. Does cooling Sengstaken-Blakemore tubes aid insertion? An evidence based approach. Eur J Gastroenterol Hepatol. 2004;16:1229–32.
92. Rockall TA, Logan RF, Devlin HB, Northfield TC. Risk assessment after acute upper gastrointestinal haemorrhage. Gut. 1996;38:316–21.
93. Blatchford O, Murray WR, Blatchford M. A risk score to predict need for treatment for upper-gastrointestinal haemorrhage. Lancet. 2000;356:1318–21.
94. Stanley AJ, Ashley D, Dalton HR, et al. Outpatient management of patients with low-risk upper-gastrointestinal haemorrhage: multicentre validation and prospective evaluation. Lancet. 2009;373:42–7.
95. Meltzer AC, Burnett S, Pinchbeck C, et al. Pre-endoscopic Rockall and Blatchford scores to identify which emergency department patients with suspected gastrointestinal bleed do not need endoscopic hemostasis. J Emerg Med. 2013;44:1083–7.
96. Saltzman JR, Tabak YP, Hyett BH, Sun X, Travis AC, Johannes RS. A simple risk score accurately predicts in-hospital mortality, length of stay, and cost in acute upper GI bleeding. Gastrointest Endosc. 2011;74:1215–24.
97. Cabañas JG, Manning JE, Cairns CB. Chapter 26. Fluid and blood resuscitation. In: Tintinalli JE, Stapczynski JS, Ma OJ, et al., editors. Tintinalli's emergency medicine: a comprehensive study guide. 7th ed. New York: The McGraw-Hill Companies; 2011.
98. de la Roche MR, Gauthier L. Rapid transfusion of packed red blood cells: effects of dilution, pressure, and catheter size. Ann Emerg Med. 1993;22:1551–5.
99. Lairet J, Bebarta V, Lairet K, et al. A comparison of proximal tibia, distal femur, and proximal humerus infusion rates using the EZ-IO intraosseous device on the adult swine (*Sus scrofa*) model. Prehosp Emerg Care. 2013;17:280–4.
100. Ngo AS, Oh JJ, Chen Y, Yong D, Ong ME. Intraosseous vascular access in adults using the EZ-IO in an emergency department. Int J Emerg Med. 2009;2:155–60.
101. Tan BK, Chong S, Koh ZX, Ong ME. EZ-IO in the ED: an observational, prospective study comparing flow rates with proximal and distal tibia intraosseous access in adults. Am J Emerg Med. 2012;30:1602–6.

Acute Liver Failure and Acute Decompensation of Chronic Liver Failure

15

Samantha L. Wood

Acute Liver Failure

Background/Epidemiology

Acute liver failure (ALF) is defined as new onset of hepatocellular dysfunction as reflected by coagulopathy (international normalized ratio [INR] > 1.5) and encephalopathy in the absence of preexisting liver disease. Acute liver failure is relatively rare, with 1–6 cases per million per year worldwide [1] and 2000–3000 cases per year in the United States [2]. Etiology varies by geography. Worldwide, infectious causes are the most common, followed by medication overdoses, idiosyncratic drug reaction, toxins, and metabolic causes. Globally hepatitis A and E are responsible for most infections causing acute liver failure. In the developed world, hepatitis vaccination has reduced prevalence of infectious etiologies. In the United States, acetaminophen toxicity is the most common cause of acute liver failure followed by indeterminate cause, drug related, hepatitis B, autoimmune disease, ischemia, hepatitis A, and Wilson's disease.

There are two primary classification systems that categorize patients by the timing of coagulopathy and encephalopathy and can be useful in pinpointing the most likely etiology of liver failure (Table 15.1).

Table 15.1 Acute liver failure classification systems by time from jaundice to encephalopathy

Berneau	0–14 days	14 days to 8 weeks	
	Fulminant	Acute	
O'Grady	0–7 days	8–28 days	29 days to 12 weeks
	Hyperacute	Acute	Subacute
	More likely due to acetaminophen or viral infection		More likely idiosyncratic, drug related, undetermined

Adapted from [1]

In pediatric patients, encephalopathy is difficult to evaluate and may appear late in the course or not at all; thus, the definition of ALF is based on the presence of coagulopathy [1]. The Pediatric Acute Liver Failure Study Group defined pediatric liver failure as biochemical evidence of acute liver injury plus coagulopathy defined as prothrombin time (PT) ≥ 15 seconds or INR ≥ 1.5 plus hepatic encephalopathy or PT ≥ 20 seconds, INR ≥ 2.0 regardless of encephalopathy in the absence of chronic liver disease [3].

In pediatric patients, metabolic diseases, such as neonatal hemochromatosis, Wilson's disease, and mitochondrial disorders are the most common causes of ALF, followed by infections (including herpes simplex virus, cytomegalovirus,

S. L. Wood (✉)
Emergency Department, Maine Medical Center, Portland, ME, USA
e-mail: WOODS@mmc.org

© Springer Nature Switzerland AG 2020
J. R. Shiber, S. D. Weingart (eds.), *Emergency Department Critical Care*, https://doi.org/10.1007/978-3-030-28794-8_15

and enterovirus), drug related, autoimmune disease, and hemophagocytic lymphohistiocytosis. However, the cause of acute liver failure in 32% of pediatric patients in one study was unknown [4] and no etiology was found in over half of patients in the pediatric ALF study group [5].

A large number of drugs can cause acute hepatic failure, most commonly phenytoin, carbamazepine, valproic acid, amiodarone, halothane, antibiotics, and antifungals. Over 1000 other medications have been reported to cause ALF [6]. Other less common causes of ALF include hyperthermia, Amanita mushroom poisoning, ischemia, Budd-Chiari syndrome, malignancy, pregnancy-associated syndrome of hemolysis, elevated LFTs, and low platelets (HELLP). In a significant percentage of patients, the cause of ALF is unknown (7–38%) [1].

Morbidity and mortality are high in ALF, with 33% mortality overall and 25% of patients requiring liver transplant [7]. In pediatric patients, 46% survived without transplant and 70% survived posttransplant [4]. Patients with hyperacute presentations are more likely to survive without liver transplant, perhaps because the cause is more commonly acetaminophen toxicity, which can be effectively treated.

Pathophysiology

The common pathway of acute liver failure is injury to hepatocytes that causes cell necrosis or apoptosis. In acetaminophen toxicity, an excess of the toxic metabolite N-acetyl-p-benzoquinone imine (NAPQI) overwhelms the ability of glutathione stores to bind and detoxify it, leading to cell damage. Viral hepatitis may cause direct cytotoxicity or as a result of immune response to the infection. Liver cell damage has a number of downstream effects including release of cell proteins such as lactate dehydrogenase (LDH), aspartate aminotransferase (AST), and alanine aminotransferase (ALT), impairment of bilirubin transport causing hyperbilirubinemia, and damage to Kupffer cells, which results in decreased clearance of endotoxin and increased risk of infection.

The pathophysiology of hepatic encephalopathy is not completely understood; however, two theories are favored as possible explanations [8]. The ammonia-glutamine hypothesis states that ammonia (which is elevated in liver failure because the liver's ability to metabolize the ammonia delivered via the portal circulation is diminished) is converted to glutamine by astrocytes and that this increased glutamine within astrocytes results in cell swelling and brain edema. The toxic liver or cerebral vasodilation hypothesis states that inflammatory cytokines released from the necrotic liver cause vasodilation and increased intracranial blood volume [2]. Based on studies of brain sections from patients with ALF, it appears that the blood-brain barrier is relatively well preserved and that cytotoxic edema predominates over vasogenic edema [9].

Cardiovascular effects of acute liver failure are due to increased portal pressure, which causes splanchnic pooling of blood and decreased venous return as well as systemic arterial vasodilation due to production of endogenous vasodilators.

Patient Presentation: Typical Complaints, Signs/Symptoms, and Physical Examination Findings

Patients in acute liver failure may have a wide range of presentations, from subtle complaints of fever, anorexia, fatigue, and abdominal pain to florid encephalopathy, cerebral edema, and hemodynamic collapse. A classic presentation includes hepatic dysfunction, abnormal liver function tests (LFTs), and coagulopathy with signs of encephalopathy.

Hepatic encephalopathy (HE) is graded on a scale with severity of encephalopathy correlating with likelihood of progression to cerebral edema and correlated with outcome (Table 15.2). In addition to clinical evaluation, bispectral index (BIS) monitoring can be useful to classify HE, as decreased BIS correlates well with increasing severity of HE [10]. Progression to cerebral edema should be suspected if there is progressive HE, new systemic hypertension, pupillary dila-

Table 15.2 Hepatic encephalopathy

Grade	Criteria	Progression to cerebral edema (%)	3-week transplant-free survival (%)	Overall survival (%)
Minimal	No clinical evidence of mental status change but abnormalities on psychometric or neuropsychological testing			
I	Trivial lack of awareness, euphoria or anxiety, shortened attention span, impairment of addition or subtraction	Rare	52	77
II	Lethargy or apathy, disorientation for time, obvious personality change, inappropriate behavior, dyspraxia, asterixis	Rare		
III	Somnolence to semistupor, responsive to stimuli, confused, gross disorientation, bizarre behavior	25–35	33	56
IV	Coma, unable to test mental state	65–75		

Adapted from [48, 73]

tion and/or decreased responsiveness, abnormal oculovestibular reflexes, or extensor posturing.

It is critical in the patient with suspected or confirmed ALF to obtain a thorough history with particular attention to medication history, herbals, foods, and travel. It is particularly important to identify acetaminophen-associated liver failure, whether from intentional overdose or therapeutic misadventure, as early treatment with N-acetylcysteine limits liver injury and improves prognosis. If there is any doubt about the possibility of acetaminophen toxicity, NAC should be administered while obtaining further information. Travel history to areas with endemic hepatitis is important to evaluate risk of infectious hepatitis.

Diagnostics

Initial laboratory studies should include liver function tests including aminotransferases, bilirubin, and alkaline phosphatase, coagulation tests (PT, PTT/INR), complete blood count, and chemistry panel. Acetaminophen levels are most useful in the setting of acute ingestion; however, acetaminophen levels should be drawn on all patients with ALF as this is the most common cause of ALF in the United States and there is an effective antidote [11]. Pregnancy history and testing should be obtained in women of childbearing age to evaluate for the possibility of HELLP syndrome. Additional testing for etiology of ALF can be undertaken (i.e., hepatitis panel, ceruloplasmin, autoimmune evaluation, etc.), but results are unlikely to change the emergent management of the patient. Additionally, if coexisting infection is suspected or if the diagnosis is uncertain, additional testing such as blood cultures should be obtained. Etiology-specific historical and diagnostic characteristics and treatment recommendations are shown in Table 15.3.

Head computed tomography (CT) is recommended for patients with grade III/IV hepatic encephalopathy or a change in mental status to evaluate for cerebral edema (as long as the patient is sufficiently stable for transport CT). It is also useful to rule out alternative causes of altered mental status (i.e., intracranial hemorrhage) in the altered patient. Transcranial Doppler may be useful to assess for hypoperfusion [12]. Magnetic resonance imaging is unlikely to contribute useful information and the travel and time required to obtain the study may be unsafe for an unstable patient.

Differential diagnosis in the patient with suspected ALF is broad and should include other causes of elevated LFTs, coagulopathy, and mental status change. Biliary tract obstruction, infiltrative hepatopathy, tumor, hepatic vein obstruction, acute exacerbation of chronic liver disease, sepsis, or warfarin ingestion should all be considered and evaluated.

Many different prognostic criteria have been proposed to predict outcome in patients with ALF and determine which patients should

Table 15.3 Causes of liver failure and treatments

	Diagnosis	Treatment
Amanita mushroom	History	Penicillin G and NAC List for transplant as this is often the only life-saving option
Hepatitis B	History Viral serologies	Nucleoside analogues
Other hepatitis	History Viral serologies	
VZV or HSV	Associated exam findings, PCR, biopsy	Acyclovir Consider transplant
Wilson disease	Presence of Kayser-Fleischer rings Serum ceruloplasmin Serum and urinary copper Liver biopsy Total bilirubin:alkaline phosphatase >2.0	Dialysis, plasma exchange Transplant
Autoimmune	Liver biopsy	Corticosteroids Transplant
HELLP syndrome, acute fatty liver of pregnancy	Pregnancy	Delivery
Ischemic	History of hypotension	Cardiovascular support
Budd-Chiari (acute hepatic vein thrombosis)	CT or Doppler ultrasonography	Transplant if underlying malignancy is excluded
Malignant infiltration	Imaging, biopsy	Treatment of underlying malignancy

undergo transplant. These include the King's criteria, Clichy's criteria, and the Model for End-stage Liver Disease (MELD) and Pediatric End-stage Liver Disease (PELD) score (see Table 15.4). However, all the scoring systems are imperfect and should not be relied on exclusively; clinical judgment remains important in prognostication and consideration of transplant [11].

Initial Stabilization: Time Critical Resuscitation

ABCs

As with all critically ill patients in the emergency department, initial stabilization of the patient with ALF begins with the ABCs. Intubation is indicated for hypoxic or hypercapnic respiratory failure, airway protection, agitation that impedes the ability to evaluate the patient, and if an intracranial pressure (ICP) monitor is necessary. In the patient with suspected elevated ICP, the emergency physician must be aware that laryngoscopy may transiently worsen ICP. The acute respiratory distress syndrome occurs in 21% of patients with ALF [13] and should be treated with lung protective ventilation strategies; however, the provider must also be aware that permissive hypercapnea may worsen ICP. High positive end-expiratory pressure may also increase ICP by increasing intrathoracic pressure and thus decreasing venous drainage from the brain; it can also decrease hepatic blood flow and thus should be avoided.

Hemodynamic stabilization relies primarily on intravenous fluids to correct hypovolemia. Crystalloids are generally preferred initially [11, 14]. If vasopressors are required, norepinephrine is recommended; ALF patients may exhibit reduced vasoconstriction in response to pure alpha agonists such as phenylephrine, and beta-adrenergic side effects of dopamine may limit its utility [14]. Vasopressin may be added but should play a secondary role as there is some concern that it could increase intracranial pressure [14]. A third of patients with liver failure have coexisting adrenal insufficiency [15]—consider a trial of hydrocortisone in refractory hypotension to intravenous fluids and vasopressors.

Table 15.4 Prognostic criteria for acute liver failure

	Definition		Comments
King's College Criteria: APAP	Arterial pH < 7.3 *OR* ALL the following: 1. PT > 100 seconds (INR > 6.5) 2. Creatinine > 3.4 mg/dL 3. Grade III/IV hepatic encephalopathy	Overall specificity 85.7%, sensitivity 48.3%. Specificity 92.4% in subset of patients with APAP overdose.	Calculated from laboratory values that are easily and rapidly obtained at presentation. Derived from a cohort treated for ALF in 1986–1987; however, high specificity value for mortality had been confirmed in independent cohorts since then. Poor sensitivity; not meeting the criteria does not ensure survival. May be less reliable in pediatric patients
King's College Criteria: non-APAP	PT > 100 seconds (INR > 6.5) *OR* Any three of the following: 1. Non-A, non-B viral hepatitis, drug, or halothane etiology 2. Jaundice to encephalopathy progression in >7 days 3. Age <10 or >40 years 4. PT > 50 seconds (INR > 3.5) 5. Bilirubin >17.4 mg/dL		
Clichy's Criteria	Presence of hepatic encephalopathy *AND* Factor V level <20% if patient <30 years old or <30% if patient ≥30 years old	Predictive accuracy approximately 60%	Less accurate that King's criteria Factor V level may take longer to obtain
MELD (Model for End-Stage Liver Disease)	3.78 × log*e*(bilirubin mg/dL) + 11.2 × log*e*(INR) + 9.57 × log*e* (creatinine mg/dL) + 6.4	MELD < 30 in APAP OD = high probability of survival MELD ≥30 in non = APA OD 81% PPV for mortality	Currently used in US for allocation of donor organs in patients awaiting liver transplant. Has not been shown to be more accurate than King's criteria
PELD (Pediatric End-stage Liver Disease Score)	PELD = 4.80(Ln serum bilirubin [mg/dL]) + 18.57(Ln INR) − 6.87(Ln albumin [g/dL]) + 4.36(<1 year old) + 6.67(growth failure)	Cut-off of 33 based on admission laboratory values is 81% specific and 86% sensitive for poor outcome	

Adapted from [18, 74] http://bestpractice.bmj.com/bestpractice/monograph/1010/diagnosis/criteria.html. Accessed 20 November 2014

Cerebral Edema

Elevated intracranial pressure is one of the most critical complications of ALF. Risk factors for cerebral edema include hyperacute liver failure (since astrocytes are unable to accommodate rapid increase in osmotic stress), degree of hyperammonemia, need for vasopressors, and renal failure [16]. A serum ammonia >150–200 μg/dL predicts development of intracranial hypertension and cerebral herniation, but the majority of patients who develop cerebral edema have ammonia levels lower than this [16, 17]. Grade III or IV hepatic encephalopathy is also a risk factor for progression to cerebral edema. Patients with serum ammonia <75 μg/dL and grades I–II hepatic encephalopathy rarely progress to cerebral edema [16]; however, close monitoring is indicated for any signs of deterioration; in these patients, sedation should be minimized to allow for neurologic examination, and the environment should be kept quiet to minimize agitation.

There is no evidence that ICP monitoring in patients with elevated ICP secondary to HE improves outcomes. However, monitoring is endorsed by the US Acute Liver Failure Study Group for patients at high risk of intracranial hypertension (ICH) including nontransplant candidates with higher rate of spontaneous survival (i.e., those with acetaminophen toxicity or hepatitis A) [18]. It should be considered in patients with grades III–IV hepatic encephalopathy and in patients awaiting liver transplant, though coagulopathy may complicate placement of a monitor.

Therapies are directed at maintaining intracranial pressure <20–25 mmHg and cerebral perfusion pressure >50 mmHg. First-line supportive measures include elevation of the head of bed to 30°, maintenance of a neutral neck position, and ensuring a quiet environment with limited stimulus and minimization of noxious stimuli such as chest physical therapy and suctioning.

Adequate sedation should be ensured. Propofol decreases cerebral blood flow and ICP in fulminant hepatic failure [19] and also has the benefit of a short recovery time which will allow frequent neurologic assessments; however, its use may be limited by hemodynamic effects. Morphine should be avoided in patients with renal failure because active metabolites accumulate. Avoid meperidine because it's metabolite, normeperidine, can cause neurotoxicity including hallucinations, tremors, and seixure.

Osmolar therapy is a cornerstone of treatment for elevated ICP. By increasing serum osmolarity, mannitol draws water out of neurons and thus reduces cerebral edema. Mannitol 0.5–1 g/kg is first line, but is contraindicated if serum osmolality is >320 or in patients with renal failure. There is limited experience with hypertonic saline for the treatment of elevated ICP in acute liver failure patients; however, one small study of 30 patients showed lower incidence of ICH when used prophylactically in patients with severe HE [20]. Based on this study, prophylactic use of hypertonic saline with a goal serum sodium of 145–155 mEq/L is recommended in patients with high risk for cerebral edema (those with serum ammonia >150 μg/dL, grade III/IV HE, acute renal failure [ARF], or requiring vasopressors) [11]. However, many liver failure patients are chronically hyponatremic, and rapid correction of their hyponatremia may lead to osmotic demyelination.

Strategies to reduce ammonia include lactulose and rifaximin; there is insufficient data to recommend these treatments for elevated ICP [18], but lactulose may be tried in patients with early-stage encephalopathy to reduce ammonia. Lactulose may cause gaseous distention, obscure the operative field for patients who undergo transplant, and can cause megacolon. It should not be administered to patients at risk of aspiration without intubating for airway protection. Patients must also be monitored for intravascular depletion. Neomycin can cause nephrotoxicity and is not recommended [18] to reduce ammonia.

Hyperventilation reduces pCO_2 thus causing cerebral vasoconstriction and temporarily reducing ICP. It can be used as short-term rescue therapy in patients with brain herniation or impending herniation, but is not recommended long term as vasoconstriction reduces cerebral oxygenation. It is not effective for prevention of brain edema in patients with liver failure [21]. In general, it is reasonable to keep pCO_2 30–40 mmHg.

Indomethacin has shown some positive effect as a "rescue therapy" for refractory intracranial hypertension; however, adverse effects including nephrotoxicity, platelet dysfunction, and GI bleeding are significant, and it is currently not recommended for routine use [22].

Seizures are common in patients with cerebral edema and are often subclinical or masked by sedative medications. Intermittent or continuous electroencephalography (EEG) is recommended for grade III/IV hepatic encephalopathy, sudden unexplained worsening of neurologic condition, myoclonus, and during titration of therapy in barbiturate coma [18]. Data regarding effectiveness of prophylactic anticonvulsant use is inconclusive [23, 24], and its use is not currently recommended [11].

Barbiturates may be considered for refractory elevated ICP; however, the provider must anticipate hypotension and markedly reduced clearance in the liver failure patient that will make it difficult to perform serial neurologic assessments.

Maintenance of normothermia is important because fever exacerbates intracranial hypertension. Animal studies suggest benefit with therapeutic hypothermia, and several small unrandomized studies have been suggestive of benefit in controlling ICP and as a bridge to transplant. However, harms of TH have not been defined, and there is no RCT at this time [23].

Steroids do not benefit cerebral edema secondary to ALF and are not recommended [11, 18].

Hypoglycemia

ALF patients are at high risk of developing hypoglycemia and glucose should be carefully monitored. Beware infusing hypotonic glucose-containing solutions as this may cause hyponatremia and worsen cerebral edema.

Infection

Bacterial infections (pneumonia, urinary tract infection, catheter associated, spontaneous bacteremia) occur in 80% of ALF patients and fungal infections in a third [25]. ALF patients often do not show signs of infection, so routine surveillance (daily blood and urine cultures and chest radiograph) are recommended since early intervention may improve outcome [18]. There is insufficient data for prophylactic antibiotics in all ALF patients, but guidelines recommend antibiotics if surveillance cultures are positive, if ≥2 systemic inflammatory response (SIRS) criteria are present, if there is refractory hypotension, in advanced hepatic encephalopathy (Grade III/IV), or if there is progression of hepatic encephalopathy. Antibiotics are also recommended in patients listed for liver transplant since development of infection can result in their removal from the list [7, 18]. Other authors recommend prophylactic antibiotics for all patients with coagulopathy plus organ failure, encephalopathy, and those for whom disease progression is thought likely [1]. Antibiotic choice should include broad-spectrum coverage of gram-positive and gram-negative organisms, and there should be a low threshold for antifungal coverage.

Coagulopathy

By definition patients with ALF have an associated coagulopathy. However, overall hemostasis may be "rebalanced" as hypocoaguable derangements including thrombocytopenia and decreased coagulation factors are offset by increased levels of von Willebrand factor, decreased protein C, protein S, and other anticoagulant substances, and low plasminogen [26]. Thromboelastography studies of the blood of patients with acute liver failure showed that most had normal hemostasis despite elevated INR [27]. Multiple studies have demonstrated that abnormal laboratory values in liver failure do not reflect gastrointestinal or procedure-related bleeding risk [28].

Spontaneous clinically significant bleeding in acute liver failure is rare (<5%) as is spontaneous ICH (<1%) [7]. Prophylactic treatment of the coagulopathy associated with acute liver failure in the patient without clinically significant bleeding is not indicated, and normalization of coagulation indices is generally not possible. Empiric administration of fresh frozen plasma (FFP) does not reduce bleeding, obscures the ability to monitor liver function by trending partial thromboplastin time (PTT), and can cause volume overload and transfusion-related acute lung injury. Empiric administration of platelets is generally not recommended unless platelet values are <10,000/mm^3; however some sources recommend a more conservative transfusion threshold of 15–20,000/mm^3. Liver failure patients often have risk factors for vitamin K deficiency and clinical or subclinical deficiency is found in about a quarter, so empiric administration of vitamin K is recommended in all ALF patients. It should be given parenterally, as oral absorption is unreliable in these patients [29]. Prophylactic administration of acid suppression medication (H2 blockers or proton pump inhibitor) is also indicated to reduce risk of gastrointestinal bleeding [30].

Clinically significant bleeding in ALF patient requires treatment. In the bleeding patient, platelets should be transfused for a goal of >50,000/mm^3 and fresh frozen plasma for a goal INR of close to 1.5. Factor VIIa may be preferable to FFP in the patient with volume overload, who has failed to correct with FFP, or prior to a very invasive procedure such as intraventricular catheter (IVC) placement; however, drawbacks include high cost and risk of thromboembolism. Cryoprecipitate is indicated in the bleeding ALF patient with low fibrinogen (<100 mg/dL) [9].

There is a lack of data regarding correction of coagulopathy for procedures. Risk of bleeding with placement of ICP monitor is generally low (5–7%) [31] and is proportional to the depth of the device [32]. Protocols differ regarding coagulopathy correction for ICP placement, though goals typically include target INR < 1.5 or 2, platelets >50 k/mm^3 [9], and fibrinogen <100 mg/dL. Diagnostic paracentesis is a very low-risk procedure with minimal risk of bleeding even in patients with abnormal coagulation studies [33], and prophylactic correction of coagulation abnormalities is not indicated [34]. Studies show that bleeding complications during central venous cannulation in patients with liver disease and coagulopathy are rare and suggest that elevated INR should not be considered a contraindication to the procedure in these patients [35, 36]. Overall there is no evidence that correction of laboratory abnormalities in the ALF patient for any procedure is beneficial.

Renal Failure

About 40–50% of patients with ALF will develop renal failure [2]. Possible causes include hepatorenal syndrome (HRS), prerenal state, acute tubular necrosis (ATN), and exposure to hepatotoxins that are also nephrotoxic. Nephrotoxic medications and contrast dye should be avoided if possible to avoid exacerbating renal injury. If dialysis is necessary, a continuous mode is theoretically preferable to minimize hemodynamic instability and reduce the risk of cerebral edema due to dialysis disequilibrium syndrome [11].

Etiology-Specific Treatment

Acetaminophen toxicity is effectively treated with N-acetylcysteine (NAC) if given within 8 hours after ingestion. Because NAC is effective and has minimal adverse effects, it should be given even if there is uncertainty about timing or dose of ingestion and should be given in cases where circumstances leading up to patient presentation are unknown but acetaminophen ingestion is possible, especially if aminotransferase levels are very high [11]. For additional information on acetaminophen ingestion, see Chap. 28.

N-Acetylcysteine has been shown to improve transplant-free survival when given to patients with acute liver failure and stage I or II hepatic encephalopathy due to causes other than acetaminophen [37]; its use should be considered in this patient population.

Other etiology-specific treatments for acute liver failure can be seen in Table 15.3.

Definitive Treatment

The American Association for the Study of Liver Diseases (AASLD) recommends that patients with ALF be hospitalized in a monitored setting, preferably an intensive care unit (ICU), and that contact with a transplant center should be made early in the process [11]. Management in an ICU setting with experience caring for patients with liver failure is indicated for patients with INR > 2 or grade II or greater hepatic encephalopathy, extremes of age (<10 or >45 years old), or etiology of liver failure that carries a poor prognosis [14].

Likelihood of recovery from ALF with medical therapy depends on the etiology. The majority of patients with acetaminophen-induced ALF will recover with early administration of NAC and supportive care, and only about 10% require liver transplant [38]; outcomes are worse in patients with liver failure due to other etiologies.

Decisions regarding listing a patient for transplant are complex. Transplant is indicated in ALF where prognostic indicators suggest a high likelihood of death [11]. However, prognostication of likelihood of death is not straightforward. Additionally, recipient age, illness severity, and presence of any contraindications such as sepsis, severe cardiorespiratory failure, ICH with low cerebral perfusion pressure, and extrahepatic malignancy must be considered. Given complexity of decision making and the extensive evaluation required to initiate this process, the most important intervention in the emergent setting is immediate involvement of a transplant team if available or early transfer of the patient to a transplant center.

Use of liver support systems (liver dialysis: Molecular Adsorbent Recirculating System (MARS)) remains an experimental approach and is currently not recommended outside clinical trials [11].

Acute Decompensation of Cirrhosis and Acute-on-Chronic Liver Failure

Introduction/Epidemiology

Chronic liver disease is common. It ranks as the 6th leading cause of death in the United States in people aged 25–44 and 5th in people aged 45–64 [39], though true incidence may be underestimated [40].

Acute decompensation of cirrhosis is defined as development of one or more of the complications of liver disease including ascites, encephalopathy, GI bleed, and bacterial infection in the setting of cirrhosis. It can be caused by either a hepatic or an extrahepatic precipitant. Hepatic causes of superimposed liver injury include acute alcoholic hepatitis, drug toxicity, viral hepatitis, portal vein thrombosis, or ischemia. Extrahepatic precipitants include trauma, surgery, variceal bleeding, and in particular infection.

A universally accepted definition of acute-on-chronic liver failure (ACLF) is lacking. In general, although specifics differ, the definitions of ACLF include (1) predisposition by chronic hepatitis/cirrhosis, (2) a precipitating event which may either be hepatic (alcoholic hepatitis, drug-induced liver injury, viral hepatitis, portal venous thrombosis, ischemic hepatitis) or extrahepatic (trauma, surgery, GI bleed, infection, or unrecognized), and (3) resultant liver necrosis and hepatic inflammation causing single or multiple organ failure (liver failure, renal failure, hepatic encephalopathy, cardiac collapse, coagulopathy). This condition is also in part identified by its high mortality rate—50% of patients with ACLF will die within 3 months [41]. Additional details of various definitions are included below. Regardless of the specific definition used, the emergency physician and intensivist must be able to identify and treat both precipitating events causing acute decompensation of cirrhosis and any associated organ failure with an appreciation for the high mortality of this condition.

Definitions of ACLF

- Acute decompensation plus either presence of 2+ organ failures, presence of kidney failure, or presence of single "nonkidney" organ failure plus kidney dysfunction [42].
- Acute hepatic insult manifesting as jaundice and coagulopathy, complicated within 4 weeks by ascites and/or encephalopathy in a patient with chronic liver disease (Asia Pacific Association for the Study of Liver Disease).
- A syndrome that defines a subgroup of patients who develop organ failure following hospital admission with or without an identifiable precipitating event and have increased mortality rates (EASL-AASLD).

Pathophysiology

Several pathophysiologic effects predispose patients with chronic liver disease to decompensation. Portal hypertension causes increased production of endogenous vasodilators [43] leading to dilation of the splanchnic arterial circulation. This leads to splanchnic blood "pooling" which decreases stimulus to stretch receptors in the carotids and aortic arch and causes inappropriate secretion of vasopressin, resulting in water retention and hyponatremia. Additionally underfilling of the arterial circulation results in compensatory renal vasoconstriction, decreased renal blood flow, and kidney injury. Bacterial translocation from gut lumen correlates with severity of liver disease [44] and leads to increased risk of infection as well as overproduction of inflammatory cytokines, which causes further dilation of splanchnic arterial vessels [43].

Causes of Acute Decompensation of Chronic Liver Failure

General

Many of the causes of decompensation in the chronic liver failure patient are interrelated. However, a primary cause for the decompensation must be sought; most commonly this cause is sepsis or another underlying infection.

Bacterial Infections

Approximately a third of patients admitted to the hospital with cirrhosis have a bacterial infection at admission or develop one during their hospital stay [45]. The most common infections include urinary tract infection, spontaneous bacterial peritonitis, pneumonia, spontaneous bacteremia, and cellulitis [46]. Spontaneous infections (i.e., those without an identifiable source such as spontaneous bacterial peritonitis [SBP], spontaneous bacterial empyema, and spontaneous bacteremia) are thought to be due to bacterial translocation from the gut lumen to the systemic circulation or ascitic/pleural fluid [47].

Infection should be suspected in the cirrhotic patient who meets two or more SIRS criteria, but there should also be a low threshold to work-up infection in the cirrhotic patient with unexplained encephalopathy, new renal failure, or other unexplained decompensation. Evaluation for source of infection should include blood cultures, urinalysis and urine culture, chest radiography, evaluation and culture of ascitic and pleural fluid, and careful skin examination for cellulitis or abscess. If spontaneous bacterial peritonitis is diagnosed or suspected as the cause in the stable patient, the recommended treatment is a third-generation cephalosporin; ceftriaxone is less preferable than cefotaxime or other choices for coverage of SBP because it is highly protein-bound, which may theoretically reduce penetration into ascites fluid [43]. In the septic patient or those with healthcare-associated infection, broad-spectrum coverage including methicillin-resistant *Staphylococcus aureus* and resistant gram-negative bacteria should be initiated while awaiting culture data. Patients with ascites may be receiving norfloxacin as SBP prophylaxis as an outpatient, so treatment with quinolones is not recommended if these patients develop infection as the pathogen is likely to be resistant.

Relative adrenal insufficiency is common in both critically ill patients with decompensated cirrhosis (76% of patients with septic shock [48] and 60% of patients with gastrointestinal hemorrhage [49]) and is also present in 26% of noncritical decompensated cirrhosis patients [50]. However, low-dose hydrocortisone therapy in patients with cirrhosis and septic shock did not improve mortality and increased adverse events [48].

Spontaneous Bacterial Peritonitis

SBP occurs in 30% of patients with ascites. Patients may present with abdominal pain, vomiting, and diarrhea; however, presentation is classically vague and bedside assessment will miss over a third of patients with SBP [51]. For this reason, diagnostic paracentesis is recommended in all patients with new onset moderate or large ascites, and in all patients hospitalized for worsening of ascites or any complication of cirrhosis [52].

SBP is diagnosed by ascitic fluid polymorphonuclear leukocyte (PMN) count of ≥250 cells/mL in a patient without an intra-abdominal source of infection (i.e., perforated viscus or abscess) or malignancy. Cultures are frequently negative; inoculation of culture bottles at the bedside is recommended to increase yield [47, 52]. Evaluation for other sources of infection should be undertaken simultaneously, especially blood cultures as a significant proportion of patients with SBP will also be bacteremic. If large volume of paracentesis is performed, then albumin (8 g/L of fluid removed) should be given to reduce the risk of circulatory dysfunction [34, 52].

SBP should be treated empirically with a third-generation cephalosporin to cover the three most common isolates (*Escherichia coli*, *Klebsiella*, and *Streptococcus pneumonia* [34]) while awaiting culture results. As discussed above, ceftriaxone may be less desirable in this setting than other 3rd generation cephalosporins. [43]. Administration of albumin to patients with SBP has been associated with improved mortality and less development of acute kidney injury (AKI) and is recommended in patients with Cr > 1 mg/dL, BUN > 30 mg/dL, or total bilirubin > 4 mg/dL [34, 53].

Acute Alcoholic Hepatitis

Acute alcoholic hepatitis may occur in chronic alcoholics or moderate drinkers after a period of binge drinking, and typically presents with fever, liver enlargement and tenderness, leukocytosis, hyperbilirubinemia, and impaired coagulation [54]. In severe cases, patients may manifest asterixis, hepatic encephalopathy, hepatorenal syndrome, liver failure, and multiorgan failure. Acute alcoholic hepatitis is clinically diagnosed in a chronic drinker or after an episode of binge drinking by liver enlargement, neutrophilic leukocytosis, increased AST and ALT with AST:ALT ratio >1, mixed hyperbilirubinemia, and increased prothrombin time [54].

Patients presenting with suspicion of acute alcoholic hepatitis should be risk stratified using the Maddrey discriminant function (MDF) (4.6 [patient's PT – control PT] + total bilirubin) and evaluation of the presence of hepatic encephalopathy. Patients with a MDF > 32 are considered to have severe alcoholic hepatitis and have high mortality. Corticosteroids or pentoxifylline therapy may improve outcomes in these patients and should be considered [55]. Abstinence from alcohol is the most critical therapeutic intervention for all patients with alcoholic hepatitis and, in addition to nutritional interventions and close monitoring, is the primary treatment for patients with lower-risk alcoholic hepatitis.

Portal Vein Thrombosis

Portal vein thrombosis in the acute phase typically presents with abdominal pain, fever, and nausea and may result in mesenteric ischemia with sepsis and infarction if the clot extends to the mesenteric circulation; it may also cause exacerbation of ascites or variceal bleed. Chronic portal vein thrombosis will typically present with symptoms of portal hypertension [56]. However, portal vein thrombosis frequently has nonspecific or absent symptoms and is frequently diagnosed at routine surveillance ultrasound in patients with cirrhosis [57].

Ultrasound with Doppler imaging of the portal vein is the test of choice for the diagnosis of portal vein thrombosis.

There is little clinical data to guide the use of anticoagulation in cirrhotic patients with PV thrombosis, and its use is not generally recommended [56].

Hepatic Hydrothorax

Hepatic hydrothorax occurs when ascites fluid passes through small defects in the diaphragm into the pleural space, causing a large, usually right-sided effusion. Thoracentesis is indicated for diagnostic or therapeutic reasons. However, placement of a chest tube carries a complication rate of up to 100% and mortality of 27–35% due to pneumothorax, empyema, and acute kidney injury and electrolyte disturbances caused by drainage of large amounts of protein-rich pleural fluid [58]. Chest tube placement in these patients is therefore contraindicated [34]. First-line treatment is diuretics and sodium restriction, with consideration of transjugular intrahepatic portosystemic shunt (TIPS) and liver transplantation if medical therapy is ineffective [59].

Variceal Bleed

Gastroesophageal varices are present in 50% of patients with cirrhosis; variceal hemorrhage is the most common lethal complication of cirrhosis [60]. Patients may present with hematemesis, which may be massive, melena, and hemodynamic instability. Treatment is focused on restoring blood volume and stopping hemorrhage.

Transfuse packed red blood cells (PRBCs) to maintain hemodynamic stability or to a hemoglobin goal of 8 g/dL as a higher goal may increase portal pressure and thus worsen bleeding [60]. Transfusion of FFP and platelets to correct coagulopathy should be considered. Patients with cirrhosis and acute variceal hemorrhage have high risk of development of bacterial infections and prophylactic antibiotics are recommended [34,

61]. Recommended prophylactic regimens include oral norfloxacin or ciprofloxacin, or IV ciprofloxacin or ceftriaxone [60].

Data regarding the use of splanchnic vasoconstrictors such as octreotide are variable. Some evidence exists that its use in addition to endoscopy improves control of bleeding [62, 63], but a Cochrane Review found a negligible effect [64]. However, guidelines recommend the use of pharmacologic agents in combination with esophagogastroduodenoscopy (EGD) and sclerotherapy for acute variceal hemorrhage [60].

EGD with banding or sclerotherapy should be performed within 12 hours in patients with variceal hemorrhage [60].

In the patient with uncontrolled bleeding and no immediate availability of definitive treatment, balloon tamponade may be used [60]. Emergent TIPS is effective in controlling bleeding that is refractory to medical therapy [59]. For additional discussion on GI bleed, see Chap. 14.

Renal Failure

Renal failure in the cirrhosis patient can be precipitated by any event that exacerbates splanchnic and systemic vasodilation (infection, large volume paracentesis, vasodilators) or depletes intravascular volume (overdiuresis, diarrhea, vomiting, gastrointestinal bleed) as well as by exposure to nephrotoxic drugs.

Renal failure in the cirrhotic patient is initially treated by withdrawal of diuretics and nephrotoxic medications, treatment of any underlying cause, and rehydration with IV fluids or albumin if the patient is thought to be volume depleted.

Hepatorenal syndrome (HRS) describes either an acutely worsening (type I) or chronic (type II) decrease in renal function in the absence of other causes of renal failure and is diagnosed based on the criteria seen below. Type I HRS carries a grave prognosis with only 15% of patients surviving more than 3 months [65]. Type I HRS should be treated with albumin resuscitation in conjunction with vasoconstrictors [66] (norepinephrine, vasopressin, or midodrine or octreotide), though high-quality data to support this intervention are lacking [67]. Use of terlipressin in this setting is associated with decreased mortality [68; however, this drug is not available in the United States. There is limited experience with TIPS in HRS patients; the only definitive treatment is liver transplant. Renal replacement therapy should be avoided in HRS unless there is thought to be an acute reversible cause of renal failure or liver transplantation is planned [66].

ATN should also be considered as the cause of renal failure in patients who have shock or have been exposed to nephrotoxins or contrast dye and those with granular or epithelial casts in the urine.

Diagnosis of HRS

- Chronic or acute hepatic disease with advanced hepatic failure and portal hypertension
- Serum Cr >1.5 mg/dL
- Absence of shock
- Absence of hypovolemia
  - Defined as no sustained improvement in renal function following 2 days of diuretic withdrawal and volume expansion with albumin (1 g/kg/day up to 100 g/day)
- No current or recent treatment with nephrotoxic drugs
- No parenchymal renal disease
  - Defined as proteinuria <0.5 g/d, no microhematuria, and normal renal ultrasound
- Type I HRS: rapidly progressive renal failure defined as doubling of serum creatinine to >2.5 mg/dL in <2 weeks
- Type II HRS: moderate renal failure (serum Cr >1.5 mg/dL) which follows a steady or slowly progressive course

Hepatic Encephalopathy

Hepatic encephalopathy in chronic liver disease presents with a range of symptoms from subtle derangements of memory and attention to sleep-wake disturbances, behavioral disturbances, confusion, and coma. Classic examination findings include asterixis (though this can be seen in other disease as well such as uremia), hypertonia and hyperreflexia, tremor, slow speech, and diminished movements.

Serum ammonia levels alone do not add additional diagnostic or prognostic information; however, they may be useful *if normal* to prompt reconsideration of the diagnosis of HE and for trending with ammonia reduction therapy [69]. Cerebral edema is less common in chronic liver failure patients than in acute liver failure; if it develops, it should be treated as described above.

Treatment of hepatic encephalopathy in the chronic liver failure patient is with lactulose, which should be titrated to a goal of 2–3 loose bowel movements per day. Rifaximin is an alternative choice and may be considered if there are complications from high stool output due to lactulose.

Hyponatremia

Hyponatremia is a challenging problem in the patient with advanced cirrhosis because symptoms can be similar to those of hepatic encephalopathy. Nonacute treatment includes water restriction and combination therapy with spironolactone and a loop diuretic. There are no guidelines specific to the treatment of hyponatremia in the liver failure patient; however, in general, patients with severe symptoms of hyponatremia (seizure, coma) should be treated with intravenous 3% saline (100 mL) over 10 minutes, repeated ×2 (if needed), with a goal of raising the serum Na by 4–6 mEq/L; patients with chronic liver disease and alcoholism are at high risk for osmotic demyelination; however, further correction should be very gradual at no more than 8 mEq/L total in a 24-hour period [70]

Hepatopulmonary Syndrome

The diffuse vasodilation that accompanies chronic liver disease can affect the pulmonary capillary beds and result in the hepatopulmonary syndrome. Patients classically present with hypoxia and orthodeoxia (worsening oxygenation upon moving from a laying down to a sitting position caused by worsening ventilation-perfusion mismatch). No effective medical treatments exist and liver transplant is the only therapeutic option [71].

Definitive Treatment

Evaluation for liver transplant in cirrhotic patients should be considered when an episode of decompensation results in a MELD score ≥15 [72]. Patients with end-stage liver disease secondary to alcoholic cirrhosis should be considered for liver transplant, with a 6-month abstinence period recommended prior to transplant and a thorough evaluation of likelihood of maintaining long-term abstinence [55]. Patients must also remain abstinent from tobacco consumption. Patients with renal failure should be evaluated for simultaneous liver and kidney transplant if they have end-stage renal disease, chronic kidney disease with GFR < 30 mL/minute, acute renal failure or hepatorenal syndrome with creatinine >2 mg/dL and dialysis for ≥ 8 weeks, or renal biopsy showing >30% glomerulosclerosis or >30% fibrosis [72]. Screening for appropriateness for liver transplant involves a complex evaluation of the patient's medical, social, psychological, nutritional, and financial circumstances; from the perspective of the emergency provider, the most critical step is early identification of a potential transplant candidate and engagement of the transplant team or transfer to a transplant center.

References

1. Bernal W, Wendon J. Acute liver failure. N Engl J Med. 2013;369(26):2525–34.
2. Sundaram V, Shaikh OS. Acute liver failure: current practice and recent advances. Gastroenterol Clin North Am. 2011;40(3):523–39.
3. Devictor D, Tissieres P, Durand P, Chevret L, Debray D. Acute liver failure in neonates, infants and children. Expert Rev Gastroenterol Hepatol. 2011;5(6):717–29.
4. Rajanayagam J, Coman D, Cartwright D, Lewindon PJ. Pediatric acute liver failure: etiology, outcomes, and the role of serial pediatric end-stage liver disease scores. Pediatr Transplant. 2013;17(4):362–8.

5. Squires RH Jr, Shneider BL, Bucuvalas J, Alonso E, Sokol RJ, Narkewicz MR, et al. Acute liver failure in children: the first 348 patients in the pediatric acute liver failure study group. J Pediatr. 2006;148(5):652–8.
6. Lat I, Foster DR, Erstad B. Drug-induced acute liver failure and gastrointestinal complications. Crit Care Med. 2010;38(6 Suppl):S175–87.
7. Stravitz RT. Critical management decisions in patients with acute liver failure. Chest. 2008;134(5):1092–102.
8. Mohsenin V. Assessment and management of cerebral edema and intracranial hypertension in acute liver failure. J Crit Care. 2013;28(5):783–91.
9. D'Agostino D, Diaz S, Sanchez MC, Boldrini G. Management and prognosis of acute liver failure in children. Curr Gastroenterol Rep. 2012;14(3):262–9.
10. Dahaba AA, Worm HC, Zhu SM, Bao FP, Salah A, Zakaria S, et al. Sensitivity and specificity of bispectral index for classification of overt hepatic encephalopathy: a multicentre, observer blinded, validation study. Gut. 2008;57(1):77–83.
11. Lee WM, Stravitz RT, Larson AM. Introduction to the revised American Association for the Study of Liver Diseases Position Paper on acute liver failure 2011. Hepatology. 2012;55(3):965–7.
12. Abdo A, López O, Fernández A, Santos J, Castillo J, Castellanos R, et al. Transcranial Doppler sonography in fulminant hepatic failure. Transplant Proc. 2003;35(5):1859–60.
13. Audimoolam VK, McPhail MJ, Wendon JA, Willars C, Bernal W, Desai SR, et al. Lung injury and its prognostic significance in acute liver failure. Crit Care Med. 2014;42(3):592–600.
14. Stravitz RT, Kramer DJ. Management of acute liver failure. Nat Rev Gastroenterol Hepatol. 2009;6(9):542–53.
15. O'Beirne J, Holmes M, Agarwal B, Bouloux P, Shaw S, Patch D, et al. Adrenal insufficiency in liver disease – what is the evidence? J Hepatol. 2007;47(3):418–23.
16. Bernal W, Hall C, Karvellas CJ, Auzinger G, Sizer E, Wendon J. Arterial ammonia and clinical risk factors for encephalopathy and intracranial hypertension in acute liver failure. Hepatology. 2007;46(6):1844–52.
17. Clemmeson JO, Larsen FS, Kondrup J, Hansen BA, Ott P. Cerebral herniation in patients with acute liver failure is correlated with ammonia concentration. Hepatology. 1999;29(3):648–53.
18. Stravitz RT, Kramer AH, Davern T, Shaikh AO, Caldwell SH, Mehta RL, et al. Intensive care of patients with acute liver failure: recommendations of the U.S. Acute Liver Failure Study Group. Crit Care Med. 2007;35(11):2498–508.
19. Wijdicks EF, Nyberg SL. Propofol to control intracranial pressure in fulminant hepatic failure. Transplant Proc. 2002;34(4):1220–2.
20. Murphy N, Auzinger G, Bernel W, Wendon J. The effect of hypertonic sodium chloride on intracranial pressure in patients with acute liver failure. Hepatology. 2004;39(2):464–70.
21. Ede RJ, Gimson AE, Bihari D, Williams R. Controlled hyperventilation in the prevention of cerebral oedema in fulminant hepatic failure. J Hepatol. 1986;2(1):43–51.
22. Raghavan M, Marik PE. Therapy of intracranial hypertension in patients with fulminant hepatic failure. Neurocrit Care. 2006;4(2):179–89.
23. Bhatia V, Batra Y, Acharya SK. Prophylactic phenytoin does not improve cerebral edema or survival in acute liver failure—a controlled clinical trial. J Hepatol. 2004;41(1):89–96.
24. Ellis AJ, Wendon JA, Williams R. Subclinical seizure activity and prophylactic phenytoin infusion in acute liver failure: a controlled clinical trial. Hepatology. 2000;32(3):536–41.
25. Rolando N, Philpott-Howard J, Williams R. Bacterial and fungal infection in acute liver failure. Semin Liver Dis. 1996;16(4):389–402.
26. Lisman T, Porte RJ. Rebalanced hemostasis in patients with liver disease: evidence and clinical consequences. Blood. 2010;116(6):878–85.
27. Stravitz RT, Lisman T, Luketic VA, Sterling RK, Puri P, Fuchs M, et al. Minimal effects of acute liver injury/acute liver failure on hemostasis as assessed by thromboelastography. J Hepatol. 2012;56(1):129–36.
28. Tripodi A, Mannucci PM. The coagulopathy of chronic liver disease. N Engl J Med. 2011;365(2):147–56.
29. Pereira SP, Rowbotham D, Fitt S, Shearer MJ, Wendon J, Williams R. Pharmacokinetics and efficacy of oral versus intravenous mixed-micellar phylloquinone (vitamin K1) in severe acute liver disease. J Hepatol. 2005;42(3):365–70.
30. Macdougall BR, Bailey RJ, Williams R. H2-receptor antagonists and antacids in the prevention of acute gastrointestinal haemorrhage in fulminant hepatic failure. Two controlled trials. Lancet. 1977;1(8012):617–9.
31. Karvellas CJ, Fix OK, Battenhouse H, Durkalski V, Sanders C, Lee WM, et al. Outcomes and complications of intracranial pressure monitoring in acute liver failure: a retrospective cohort study. Crit Care Med. 2014;42(5):1157–67.
32. Blei AT, Olafsson S, Webster S, Levy R. Complications of intracranial pressure monitoring in fulminant hepatic failure. Lancet. 1993;341(8838):157–8.
33. Lin CH, Shih FY, Ma MH, Chiang WC, Yang CW, Ko PC. Should bleeding tendency deter abdominal paracentesis? Dig Liver Dis. 2005;37(12):946–51.
34. Runyon BA. Aasld. Introduction to the revised American Association for the Study of Liver Diseases Practice Guideline management of adult patients with ascites due to cirrhosis 2012. Hepatology. 2013;57(4):1651–3.
35. Ferro D, Angelico F, Caldwell SH, Violi F. Bleeding and thrombosis in cirrhotic patients: what really matters? Dig Liver Dis. 2012;44(4):275–9.
36. Fisher NC, Mutimer DJ. Central venous cannulation in patients with liver disease and coagulopathy—a prospective audit. Intensive Care Med. 1999;25(5):481–5.

37. Lee WM, Hynan LS, Rossaro L, Fontana RJ, Stravitz RT, Larson AM, et al. Intravenous N-acetylcysteine improves transplant-free survival in early stage non-acetaminophen acute liver failure. Gastroenterology. 2009;137(3):856–64, 64.e1.
38. Lee WM. Etiologies of acute liver failure. Semin Liver Dis. 2008;28(2):142–52.
39. Heron M. Deaths: leading causes for 2010. Natl Vital Stat Rep. 2013;62(6):1–96.
40. Asrani SK, Larson JJ, Yawn B, Therneau TM, Kim WR. Underestimation of liver-related mortality in the United States. Gastroenterology. 2013;145(2):375–82.e1–2.
41. Jalan R, Gines P, Olson JC, Mookerjee RP, Moreau R, Garcia-Tsao G, et al. Acute-on chronic liver failure. J Hepatol. 2012;57(6):1336–48.
42. Moreau R, Jalan R, Gines P, Pavesi M, Angeli P, Cordoba J, et al. Acute-on-chronic liver failure is a distinct syndrome that develops in patients with acute decompensation of cirrhosis. Gastroenterology. 2013;144(7):1426–37, 37.e1–9.
43. Gordon FD. Ascites. Clin Liver Dis. 2012;16(2):285–99.
44. Wiest R, Lawson M, Geuking M. Pathological bacterial translocation in liver cirrhosis. J Hepatol. 2014;60(1):197–209.
45. Tandon P, Garcia-Tsao G. Bacterial infections, sepsis, and multiorgan failure in cirrhosis. Semin Liver Dis. 2008;28(1):26–42.
46. Fernandez J, Acevedo J, Castro M, Garcia O, de Lope CR, Roca D, et al. Prevalence and risk factors of infections by multiresistant bacteria in cirrhosis: a prospective study. Hepatology. 2012;55(5):1551–61.
47. Loo NM, Souza FF, Garcia-Tsao G. Non-hemorrhagic acute complications associated with cirrhosis and portal hypertension. Best Pract Res Clin Gastroenterol. 2013;27(5):665–78.
48. Arabi YM, Aljumah A, Dabbagh O, Tamim HM, Rishu AH, Al-Abdulkareem A, et al. Low-dose hydrocortisone in patients with cirrhosis and septic shock: a randomized controlled trial. CMAJ. 2010;182(18):1971–7.
49. Triantos CK, Marzigie M, Fede G, Michalaki M, Giannakopoulou D, Thomopoulos K, et al. Critical illness-related corticosteroid insufficiency in patients with cirrhosis and variceal bleeding. Clin Gastroenterol Hepatol. 2011;9(7):595–601.
50. Acevedo J, Fernandez J, Prado V, Silva A, Castro M, Pavesi M, et al. Relative adrenal insufficiency in decompensated cirrhosis: relationship to short-term risk of severe sepsis, hepatorenal syndrome, and death. Hepatology. 2013;58(5):1757–65.
51. Chinnock B, Afarian H, Minnigan H, Butler J, Hendey GW. Physician clinical impression does not rule out spontaneous bacterial peritonitis in patients undergoing emergency department paracentesis. Ann Emerg Med. 2008;52(3):268–73.
52. European Association for the Study of the Liver. EASL clinical practice guidelines on the management of ascites, spontaneous bacterial peritonitis, and hepatorenal syndrome in cirrhosis. J Hepatol. 2010;53(3):397–417.
53. Poca M, Concepcion M, Casas M, Alvarez-Urturi C, Gordillo J, Hernandez-Gea V, et al. Role of albumin treatment in patients with spontaneous bacterial peritonitis. Clin Gastroenterol Hepatol. 2012;10(3):309–15.
54. Ceccanti M, Attili A, Balducci G, Attilia F, Giacomelli S, Rotondo C, et al. Acute alcoholic hepatitis. J Clin Gastroenterol. 2006;40(9):833–41.
55. O'Shea RS, Dasarathy S, McCullough AJ, Practice Guideline Committee of the American Association for the Study of Liver Diseases, Practice Parameters Committee of the American College of Gastroenterology, et al. Hepatology. 2010;51(1):307–28.
56. Parikh S, Shah R, Kapoor P. Portal vein thrombosis. Am J Med. 2010;123(2):111–9.
57. Plessier A, Rautou P-E, Valla D-C. Management of hepatic vascular diseases. J Hepatol. 2012;56:S25–38.
58. Orman ES, Lok AS. Outcomes of patients with chest tube insertion for hepatic hydrothorax. Hepatol Int. 2009;3(4):582–6.
59. Boyer TD, Haskal ZJ, American Association for the Study of Liver Diseases. The role of transjugular intrahepatic portosystemic shunt (TIPS) in the management of portal hypertension: update 2009. Hepatology. 2010;51(1):306.
60. Garcia-Tsao G, Sanyal AJ, Grace ND, Carey W, Practice Guidelines Committee of the American Association for the Study of Liver Diseases, Practice Parameters Committee of the American College of Gastroenterology. Prevention and management of gastroesophageal varices and variceal hemorrhage in cirrhosis. Hepatology. 2007;46(3):922–38.
61. Fernandez J, Ruiz del Arbol L, Gomez C, Durandez R, Serradilla R, Guarner C, et al. Norfloxacin vs ceftriaxone in the prophylaxis of infections in patients with advanced cirrhosis and hemorrhage. Gastroenterology. 2006;131(4):1049–56; quiz 285.
62. Banares R, Albillos A, Rincon D, Alonso S, Gonzalez M, Ruiz-del-Arbol L, et al. Endoscopic treatment versus endoscopic plus pharmacologic treatment for acute variceal bleeding: a meta-analysis. Hepatology. 2002;35(3):609–15.
63. Corley DA, Cello JP, Adkisson W, Ko WF, Kerlikowske K. Octreotide for acute esophageal variceal bleeding: a meta-analysis. Gastroenterology. 2001;120(4):946–54.
64. Gotzsche PC, Hrobjartsson A. Somatostatin analogues for acute bleeding oesophageal varices. Cochrane Database Syst Rev. 2008;(3):CD000193.
65. Martin-Llahi M, Guevara M, Torre A, Fagundes C, Restuccia T, Gilabert R, et al. Prognostic importance of the cause of renal failure in patients with cirrhosis. Gastroenterology. 2011;140(2):488–96.. e4
66. Nadim MK, Kellum JA, Davenport A, Wong F, Davis C, Pannu N, et al. Hepatorenal syndrome: the 8th international consensus conference of the Acute Dialysis Quality Initiative (ADQI) Group. Crit Care. 2012;16(1):R23.

67. Verna EC, Wagener G. Renal interactions in liver dysfunction and failure. Curr Opin Crit Care. 2013;19(2):133–41.
68. Gluud LL, Christensen K, Christensen E, Krag A. Terlipressin for hepatorenal syndrome. Cochrane Database Syst Rev. 2012;(9):CD005162.
69. Vilstrup H, Amodio P, Bajaj J, Cordoba J, Ferenci P, Mullen KD, et al. Hepatic encephalopathy in chronic liver disease: 2014 Practice Guideline by the American Association for the Study of Liver Diseases and the European Association for the Study of the Liver. Hepatology. 2014;60(2):715–35.
70. Verbalis JG, Goldsmith SR, Greenberg A, Korzelius C, Schrier RW, Sterns RH, et al. Diagnosis, evaluation, and treatment of hyponatremia: expert panel recommendations. Am J Med. 2013;126(10 Suppl 1):S1–42.
71. Rodriguez-Roisin R, Krowka MJ. Hepatopulmonary syndrome—a liver-induced lung vascular disorder. N Engl J Med. 2008;358(22):2378–87.
72. Martin P, DiMartini A, Feng S, Brown R, Fallon M. Evaluation for liver transplantation in adults: 2013 practice guideline by the American Association for the Study of Liver Diseases and the American Society of Transplantation. Hepatology. 2014;59(3):1144–65.
73. Ostapowicz G, Fontana RJ, Schiodt FV, Larson A, Davern TJ, Han SH, et al. Results of a prospective study of acute liver failure at 17 tertiary care centers in the United States. Ann Intern Med. 2002;137(12):947–54.
74. Sanchez MC, D'Agostino DE. Pediatric end-stage liver disease score in acute liver failure to assess poor prognosis. J Pediatr Gastroenterol Nutr. 2012;54(2):193–6.

16 Vascular Emergencies

Michael T. McCurdy and Kami Hu

Acute Mesenteric Ischemia

Key Points

- Mortality in acute mesenteric ischemia (AMI) is high; early recognition is crucial to prevent bowel necrosis, sepsis, multiorgan failure, and death.
- Do *not* forget about the possibility of concomitant nonocclusive ischemia in your patients with shock from other causes, and do *not* forget abdominal compartment syndrome as a cause of hypotension and bowel ischemia.
- The mainstays of stabilization include fluid resuscitation, IV antibiotics, and, in occlusive AMI, a heparin drip. Avoid vasopressors in the under-resuscitated patient to avoid worsening splanchnic blood flow.
- Promptly involve vascular or interventional radiology consultants to obtain definitive treatment.

M. T. McCurdy (✉) · K. Hu
Departments of Medicine and Emergency Medicine, University of Maryland School of Medicine, Baltimore, MD, USA

Introduction

Although an uncommon disease, acute mesenteric ischemia (AMI) is associated with high mortality, largely due to diagnostic delays coupled with multiple medical comorbidities in the affected patient population [1]. Mortality rates remain high despite advances in medical technology and increased awareness [2, 3]. If identified within 24 hours of symptom onset, survival is around 50%. If the diagnosis is delayed, however, septic shock typically ensues and survival plummets to 30% or lower [2].

Pathophysiology

AMI can be broadly classified into occlusive and nonocclusive mesenteric ischemia (NOMI), with occlusive etiologies including arterial thromboembolism and venous thrombosis and nonocclusive causes including low-flow states, vasculitis, and abdominal compartment syndrome.

Arterial emboli, often from atrial fibrillation, are the most frequent cause of AMI and account for approximately half of cases [2, 4]. Other risk factors for cardiac thromboembolism are mechanical prosthetic valves, cardiomyopathy, or left ventricular dysfunction due to recent myocardial infarction or valvular disorders. Although emboli can certainly lodge anywhere downstream, the oblique angle of the superior mesen-

© Springer Nature Switzerland AG 2020
J. R. Shiber, S. D. Weingart (eds.), *Emergency Department Critical Care*,
https://doi.org/10.1007/978-3-030-28794-8_16

teric artery makes it the most common location of embolic obstruction [5, 6]. Paradoxical arterial emboli may arise from deep venous thromboses and pass into arterial circulation via a patent foramen ovale (PFO) or atrial septal defect (ASD).

Gradual atherosclerotic plaque buildup and subsequent plaque rupture at sites of atherosclerotic stenosis also cause arterial thrombosis. Due to gradual stenosis-induced collateral development, severe widespread chronic atherosclerotic occlusion generally must occur to cause AMI. Mesenteric venous thrombosis accounts for 15–20% of AMI cases [2]. Risk factors for mesenteric venous thrombosis include hypercoagulable states (e.g., malignancy, inherited), recent abdominal surgery, and local inflammation, such as pancreatitis or inflammatory bowel disease [7].

Nonocclusive acute mesenteric ischemia accounts for approximately a third of all AMIs and is mostly due to low-flow states such as cardiogenic shock, septic shock, or splanchnic vasoconstriction. Vasopressors may also contribute to AMI in the setting of low-flow states by further decreasing intestinal blood flow and oxygen delivery. Cocaine-induced vasospasm may also cause NOMI. Disease states in which diffuse bowel wall edema and/or intra-abdominal fluid cause increased abdominal pressures greater than 20 mmHg lead to abdominal compartment syndrome (ACS) in which blood flow to the gut is decreased via external compression of the mesenteric vessels and splanchnic vasculature. Alternatively, ACS may actually arise secondary to the edema and bowel wall distension that can be caused by an acute ischemic event. Thus, determining the true etiology of AMI in the setting of ACS can be challenging; the clinical picture may be cloudy, but without recognition of the disease processes at hand, the outcome remains dire.

Whatever the initial cause of AMI, patients with prolonged mesenteric ischemia have a high incidence of intestinal necrosis, which leads to multiorgan failure and death. Prolonged tissue hypoxia results in anaerobic metabolism-induced lactic acidosis, whereas ischemic injury caused by the mismatch of oxygen supply and demand rapidly progresses to transmural necrosis. Intestinal bacterial translocation into the peritoneum may trigger the release of inflammatory mediators into the lymphatic and systemic circulation, ultimately resulting in systemic inflammatory response syndrome (SIRS), acute respiratory distress syndrome (ARDS), shock, and multiorgan system failure [6].

Patient Presentation

The pathophysiological classification of AMI helps explain the differing clinical presentations related to each mechanism of ischemia. Acute mesenteric arterial occlusion presents more acutely, with sudden, severe, cramping abdominal pain that is poorly localized or elicited on examination, resulting in the classic "pain out of proportion" described in the literature. The patient also usually complains of nausea with or without nonbilious emesis and may experience forceful bowel evacuation and diarrhea. The nonspecific nature of these complaints contributes to the difficulty in obtaining an early diagnosis of bowel ischemia.

The atherosclerotic formation leading to arterial thrombosis requires longer periods of time to reach complete blockage, allowing the previously described collateral formation. These atherosclerotic vessels usually result in a subacute or chronic presentation of AMI in which the patient has abdominal pain only with increased intestinal metabolic demand, such as after meals. Such postprandial abdominal pain classically results in food fear and weight loss. Only if complete obstruction of the culprit artery and its collaterals develops, or alternatively, if an atherosclerotic plaque ruptures to cause sudden stenosis, does sudden severe abdominal pain typically occur.

Nonocclusive mesenteric ischemia can easily be missed in the ED, as a patient's primary illness, such as cardiogenic or septic shock, may cloud the clinical picture. For example, elderly patients with diffuse mesenteric atherosclerosis may only manifest symptoms of nonspecific abdominal pain and distension. Alternatively, NOMI may manifest as abdominal distension,

Table 16.1 Characteristics of acute mesenteric ischemia

Etiology	Acute mesenteric arterial thrombosis (AMAT)	Acute mesenteric arterial embolism (AMAE)	Mesenteric venous thrombosis (MVT)	Nonocclusive mesenteric ischemia (NOMI)
Incidence	25–30% [2]	40–50% [2, 4]	10–15% [2, 4, 6]	20–30% [2, 4]
Presentation	Gradual onset Generally present to ED after several days	Sudden onset Generally present to ED after several hours	Gradual onset Generally present to ED after several days	Gradual or sudden Often already hospitalized for other severe illnesses
Collateral blood supply	Usually present	Absent	Absent	Irrelevant (low flow affects entire blood supply)
Risk factors	Smoking Vasculitis Hyperlipidemia Atherosclerosis Diabetes mellitus Hypercoagulability	AFib PFO, ASD Recent MI Endocarditis Mechanical valve LV dysfunction	IBD Pancreatitis Hypercoagulability Trauma or major abdominal surgery Portal HTN	Hypotension Use of vasopressors Low cardiac output Cocaine, ergot, or digoxin use Vasculitis
Signs and symptoms	Postprandial abdominal pain Weight loss	Palpitations Other cardioembolic phenomena Severe abdominal pain	Abdominal pain Bloating GI bleed Nausea/vomiting	Hypotension Bloating Unexplained increase in lactate

elevated lactic acid levels, and septic shock refractory to vasopressors (Table 16.1).

After initial symptom onset, pain may occasionally abate for a period of 3–6 hours. This pain-free interval is thought to be due to hypoperfusion-induced downregulation of pain receptors in the bowel wall [8]. If the patient presents to the ED greater than 6 hours after initial symptom onset, other signs and symptoms related to underlying intestinal necrosis, peritonitis, and sepsis may exist (e.g., tachycardia, tachypnea, hypotension, poor skin turgor, abdominal distension with involuntary guarding, hematochezia, confusion), which should signal to the emergency provider the severity of the patient's illness.

Diagnostics

Laboratory Testing

The most common laboratory abnormalities seen in AMI are hemoconcentration and neutrophilic leukocytosis [1, 4, 9]. Although elevations in amylase, aspartate aminotransferase, and lactate dehydrogenase are common, they are neither sensitive nor specific enough to diagnose AMI. Despite its high sensitivity, D-dimer testing is unhelpful due to its low specificity and undefined clinical reference ranges for AMI. Lactate is both nonspecific and insensitive for early detection of AMI because, prior to any secondary injury, a well-functioning liver effectively clears lactic acid from the circulation [10].

Higher leukocyte counts and LDH concentrations correlate with higher mortality [9], and hyperkalemia and hyperphosphatemia indicate existing bowel necrosis [2]. Critically ill AMI patients exhibit hyperlactatemia and a high anion gap metabolic acidosis [2, 9, 10], among other laboratory derangements, consistent with their severity of illness.

Other biomarkers, such as intestinal fatty acid-binding protein (I-FABP), alpha glutathione S-transferase (GST), diamine oxidase (DAO), and citrulline, have been studied in the search for an early indicator of AMI; however, none have proven sufficient as stand-alone tests [9–14]; investigations into combined specificity and sensitivity are ongoing.

The ideal biomarker for AMI diagnosis must be highly sensitive and specific, but also must be released early enough in the disease course to enable an early diagnosis and thus earlier intervention to allow a good outcome. Because no current laboratory test has yet met those criteria, the purpose of blood work in AMI is to estimate the extent of damage and secondary organ dysfunction and to set aside blood products for transfusion in the case of surgery or coagulopathy. The emergency provider should obtain a CBC, CMP, phosphate level, coagulation panel, lactate, and type and screen.

Imaging

In general, the workup of suspected mesenteric ischemia should begin with a multidetector CT angiogram (CTA). With 96% sensitivity and 94% specificity [15, 16], its quick availability, noninvasiveness, and ability to make alternative diagnoses have made it the diagnostic test of choice over the historic gold-standard catheter-based angiogram. CT findings consistent with AMI include intraluminal filling defects, downstream lack of contrast enhancement, circumferential mural thickening, and, with severe hypoperfusion, transmural ischemia or infarction, bowel dilatation, pneumatosis, and portal venous gas [17].

If high suspicion for acute mesenteric ischemia exists but no signs of peritonitis (which requires immediate operative intervention) are present, the emergency provider can consider immediate consultation with the interventional radiologist or vascular surgeon for conventional angiography. An "angiography first" diagnostic algorithm permits immediate diagnosis with potential intervention and requires less overall contrast, benefits that must be balanced with the ease, speed, and availability of first utilizing a CTA [15].

Abdominal radiography is unhelpful in early AMI, although in the later stages it may demonstrate dilated loops of bowel with air-fluid levels, free air, pneumatosis, or portal venous gas. Doppler ultrasonography has some utility in the diagnosis and monitoring of chronic mesenteric ischemia [18], but is limited by the presence of bowel distension and is dependent on user experience and patient body habitus, and so should not be a cause for delayed CTA diagnosis.

Magnetic resonance angiography, while accurate [15, 19] and free of ionizing radiation, requires the patient to be away from the ED for an extended period and should not be ordered to diagnose AMI.

Other Considerations

Abdominal compartment syndrome (ACS), which manifests high extraluminal pressures that inhibit adequate splanchnic blood flow, may demonstrate the previously discussed image findings, especially marked bowel wall edema or dilatation. The diagnosis of ACS can be quickly made by (1) placement of a Foley and measurement of bladder pressure or (2) placement of a femoral central venous catheter and transduction of a central venous pressure (CVP); a pressure of >12 mmHg is indicative of intra-abdominal hypertension, and a pressure of >20 mmHg with evidence of end-organ dysfunction (e.g., high airway pressures, decreased urine output or worsening renal function, increased vasopressor requirement) is consistent with ACS.

Initial Stabilization

In the stable patient with suspected AMI, the most important steps for the emergency medicine physician are diagnosis, resuscitation, and early surgical consultation. Cardiac monitoring with frequent blood pressure assessments allows timely identification of instability while administering intravenous fluids.

In the unstable patient, standard resuscitative efforts should be initiated, including at least two large-bore IVs for rapid volume resuscitation, and avoidance of hypoxia with either supplemental oxygen or intubation to prevent tissue hypoxia. If the patient is in atrial fibrillation with rapid ventricular rate, calcium channel blockers may have the added benefit of theoretically vasodilating the splanchnic vasculature; digoxin, however, can worsen splanchnic vasoconstriction and should be avoided. To help decrease vasospasm, emergency physicians can start intravenous glucagon (up to 10 μg/kg/min as tolerated) [2] while awaiting definitive management. If the patient has an acute abdomen or continued hypotension, immediate surgical consultation should be obtained during resuscitative efforts.

Administer broad-spectrum antibiotics to cover gastrointestinal flora, such as ampicillin/sulbactam, piperacillin/tazobactam, or clindamycin with metronidazole. A portable abdominal x-ray can assess for perforation, and a bladder pressure should be obtained. If vasopressors *must* be used, low-dose dopamine (0.5–8 μg/kg/min) is preferred for its specific splanchnic vasodilatory properties via intestinal dopaminergic receptors [2, 20]. Similarly, lower doses of epinephrine (0.05–0.1 μg/kg/min) cause more beta than alpha receptor activation and, therefore, theoretically decreased splanchnic vasoconstriction [2, 20].

Except in cases of NOMI, a heparin bolus and continuous infusion should be started as soon as the diagnosis of AMI is made.

Definitive Treatment

As in other vascular emergencies, endovascular intervention has been increasingly used to treat acute arterial mesenteric ischemia in the past two decades. To date, no randomized controlled trial has compared endovascular and operative interventions, but some studies have reported decreased mortality, hospital length of stay, and need for bowel resection with endovascular repair as opposed to open repair [21–23].

Endovascular catheter-directed thrombolysis, thromboembolectomy, angioplasty, and stenting permit a less invasive procedure in a generally elderly patient population with a predominance of comorbidities; if endovascular approach fails, the intervention may be converted to an operative repair or bypass.

Emergent exploratory laparotomy is mandated in patients with bowel perforation and peritonitis (i.e., patients in whom bowel necrosis is highly suspected). After initial intraoperative revascularization and/or resection, most patients will be taken back to the operating room at 24–48 hours after the initial operation for a "second-look" exploration to reassess bowel viability.

Intra-arterial papaverine, an opium-derived phosphodiesterase inhibitor that dilates the vascular bed, is used as an adjunctive therapy in mesenteric ischemia. At the dose of 30–60 mg/kg, it provides symptomatic relief and, in early small studies, decreased mortality in conjunction with angiographic intervention [24, 25]. Because of its tendency to precipitate with heparin, papaverine should be used with caution in thromboembolism-induced AMI. It is, however, the only specific therapy for NOMI [26].

Because survival in AMI depends on early treatment, the emergency physician should initiate interhospital transfer for suspected AMI if no surgical consultant is immediately available to evaluate the need for a potential emergency intervention [27].

Acute Limb Ischemia

Key Points

- TIME IS LIMB. Start a heparin drip and immediately consult a vascular surgeon.
- Immediately place affected limb in a dependent position and prevent cold temperatures.
- Classification of acute limb ischemia (ALI) directs appropriate intervention (i.e., endovascular vs. open revascularization vs. amputation) and requires ABI measurement.
- For Stages I and IIa ALI, catheter-directed thrombolysis is the intervention of choice.
- Address underlying etiologies as appropriate (e.g., rate control in Afib).

Introduction

Acute limb ischemia (ALI) is caused by abrupt interruption of arterial blood flow to an extremity. In contrast to chronic limb ischemia, in which the limb vasculature is gradually compromised, allowing adaptation via collateral circulation, the limb in ALI has no other source of perfusion and therefore requires emergent action to remain viable. Tissue death commences at approximately

4 hours of ischemia, and irreversible necrosis occurs by hour 6. Lower extremity ischemia is more common than upper extremity ischemia, but both require prompt recognition and revascularization to decrease morbidity and need for amputation.

The incidence of ALI is reported to be 140 patients per million per year [28]. A recent Medicare data review revealed a hospitalization rate for ALI of 26 per 100,000 patients aged 65 years and older, with a 30-day and 1-year mortality of 19% and 42.5%, respectively [29]. Despite revascularization, overall amputation rate at 1 year in patients hospitalized for ALI is approximately 25%, and all-cause 1-year mortality remains near 20% [28, 30, 31].

Pathophysiology

Limb ischemia with symptom duration less than 14 days is considered acute, while longer symptomatology defines chronic limb ischemia. A patient with an embolic event generally presents to the ED within hours of a sudden, abrupt onset of pain, whereas one with a gradual expansion of an intra-arterial thrombus and resultant arterial occlusion presents several days after the start of slowly worsening symptoms.

The most common cause of upper extremity ALI is embolization of a cardiac thrombus, often developing in atrial fibrillation or low-flow states such as severe left ventricle dysfunction or following a myocardial infarction [30, 31]. Emboli can also originate from peripheral venous thrombi passing through an intracardiac shunt or directly from aortic plaque rupture, in vessel-to-vessel embolism [32, 33].

The most common etiology of lower extremity ALI is occlusive thrombosis within chronically stenosed arteries [28]. Atherosclerotic plaque rupture triggers downstream arterial occlusion, similar to the pathophysiology of acute coronary syndrome. Thrombi can also develop within aneurysms, especially of the popliteal artery [34], as well as at sites of vascular grafts, and spontaneously in patients with an underlying hypercoagulability. Rarely, venous thrombosis can cause edema-induced external arterial compression and subsequent ischemia, a condition called *phlegmasia cerulea dolens* (acute DVT will be discussed further in Chap. 7).

Less commonly, vasospasm, such as in Raynaud's, cocaine use, or vasculitis, can impede flow to distal extremities (especially the upper extremities) and cause acute ischemia. Buerger's disease (also called thromboangiitis obliterans) is a smoking-induced inflammatory disease strongly associated with critical ischemia of multiple extremities. Vasculitides most associated with acute limb ischemia include Takayasu's, giant cell arteritis, and Behcet's disease.

Proximal arterial dissection can cause distal limb ischemia by directing blood flow into the false lumen, which then obstructs flow through the true lumen. Traumatic arterial disruption (e.g., arterial dissection or laceration) can cause ALI, as can extrinsic arterial compression in trauma-induced compartment syndromes. Lastly, whether from trauma, tumor, repetitive strain, or congenital structural abnormalities such as a cervical rib, thoracic outlet syndrome can cause upper extremity arterial compression and resultant ischemia.

Patient Presentation

The sudden onset of severe limb pain in a patient with a cool extremity and decreased pulses is the cardinal presentation of acute limb ischemia. The limb may exhibit mottling, cyanosis, or dependent rubor. The classic findings of acute limb ischemia are "the 6 Ps": pain, pallor, poikilothermia, pulselessness, paresthesia, and paralysis. Importantly, however, the last three signs present late in the course of the disease and signify significant myonecrosis (Fig. 16.1).

Other findings may provide clues as to the inciting factors of ALI (e.g., chest or abdominal pain in proximal aortic or iliac artery dissection, an irregularly irregular rhythm in thromboembolism secondary to atrial fibrillation). The emergency physician must fully assess all extremities, noting color and temperature, and thoroughly examine pulses and neurologic function to identify the level

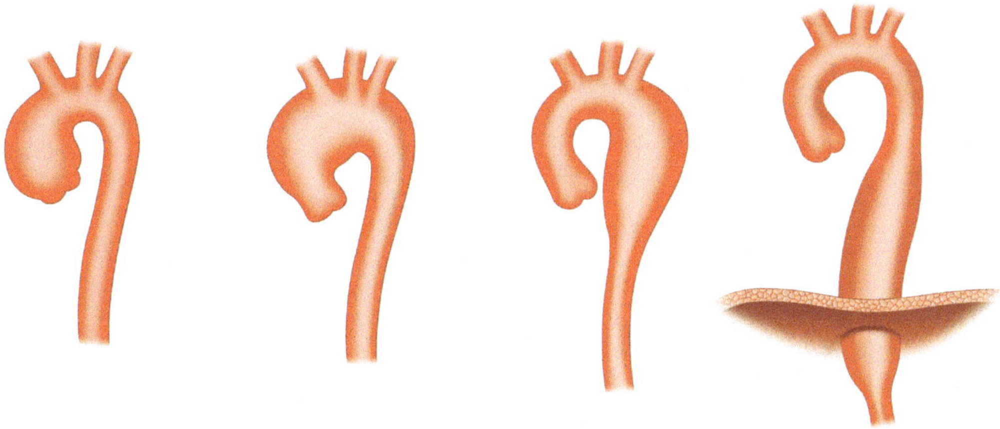

Fig. 16.1 Algorithm for management of acute limb ischemia. (Adapted from Tendera et al. [42])

Table 16.2 Rutherford Classification Chart

Class	Sensory loss	Muscle weakness	Doppler signals: Arterial	Doppler signals: Venous
(I) Viable *Not immediately threatened*	None	None	Audible	Audible
(IIa) Marginally threatened *Salvageable if promptly treated*	None or minimal (toes)	None	Inaudible	Audible
(IIb) Immediately threatened *Salvageable if immediately revascularized*	Mild to moderate	Mild to moderate	Inaudible	Audible
(III) Irreversible *Inevitable major tissue loss/nerve damage*	Profound to complete	Profound, paralyzed	Inaudible	Inaudible

Adapted from Rutherford et al. [35]

of ischemia and categorize its severity using the Rutherford Classification Chart [28, 35] (Table 16.2). Because the pulse may be difficult to palpate, a Doppler assessments of arterial signals and bilateral ankle-brachial indices (ABI) should be assessed, keeping in mind that noncompressible vessels due to atherosclerotic calcification may falsely elevate those numbers (Table 16.3).

$$\mathrm{ABI} = \frac{(\text{highest of dorsalis pedis or posterior tibial pressure on that side})}{(\text{highest of left or right brachial artery pressure})}$$

Diagnostics

Imaging

Digital subtraction angiography (DSA) is the preferred method of imaging for ALI because it enables immediate administration of catheter-directed therapy (CDT), such as thrombolytics, upon visualization of an occlusion. Despite its invasiveness and need for intravenous contrast, DSA should be immediately performed if it is available and deemed appropriate by Rutherford classification [36].

If DSA is unavailable, duplex ultrasonography (DUS) and computed tomography angiogram

Table 16.3 Ankle-brachial indices (ABI)

ABI value	Interpretation
0.91–1.3[a]	Normal
0.71–0.9	Mild disease
0.41–0.7	Moderate disease
≤ 0.4	Severe disease

[a]ABI >1.3 is abnormal and indicates calcified vessels resulting in an unreliable measure

(CTA) are viable diagnostic options. DUS is noninvasive, does not require contrast, and can be performed at the bedside. Compared to DSA in chronic occlusive disease, its specificity approaches 100%, but its sensitivity is as low as 80%, which is thought to be due to limited visualization of pelvic and infrageniculate vasculature [37–40]. CTA is quick, readily available, and accurate, with a sensitivity of 89–99% and specificity of 83–97% [40]. However, CTA exposes the patient to ionizing radiation and nephrotoxic contrast, which is not ideal because of the need for a further contrast load if endovascular treatment therapy is later pursued.

Contrast-enhanced magnetic resonance angiography (CE-MRI) is accurate [40] but time-consuming and frequently inaccessible after regular business hours. Despite its ability to diagnose chronic vaso-occlusive disease, it has no role in the acute setting.

Laboratory Work

No laboratory tests assist in diagnosing ALI, but basic blood work (e.g., CBC, BMP, type and screen, coagulation studies) may help with therapeutic and preoperative plans. Measurement of serum lactate, creatine kinase, and myoglobin levels can assist in diagnosing associated compartment syndromes or severity of limb malperfusion, guiding fluid resuscitation, and predicting the likelihood of postrevascularization reperfusion syndrome and need for fasciotomy.

Electrocardiogram (ECG)

An electrocardiogram may reveal a possible etiology of the patient's thromboembolism (e.g., atrial fibrillation, recent MI) and can help with preoperative risk assessment.

Initial Stabilization

The most immediate intervention in suspected acute limb ischemia is to place the affected extremity in a dependent position to assist with blood flow, avoiding pressure on areas distal to the suspected level of obstruction (e.g., heels, palms); this can easily be done during the initial history and physical examination.

An immediate vascular surgery consult is imperative. Depending on the hospital's available resources, transfer to a facility capable of the appropriate intervention may be necessary and the process should be initiated as soon as the diagnosis is suspected.

While awaiting the consultant, the patient should be given an aspirin (162 or 325 mg) and immediately initiated on a heparin drip [28, 41, 42]. Despite no RCTs indicating improved outcomes with its use in acute limb ischemia, aspirin has proven benefits in chronic critical limb ischemia [43] and in maintaining vessel patency post-revascularization [44] as well as an association with decreased mortality in the pathophysiologically similar acute coronary syndrome [45]. Although no RCTs exist to support heparin therapy in ALI, it is the mainstay of ALI treatment to help prevent further propagation of intra-arterial thromboembolism [46].

Intravenous hydration in anticipation of a contrast load or operative management is warranted. Additionally, avoiding temperature extremes, especially cold, helps prevent vasoconstriction and decreased flow to the affected limb. Adequate analgesia (e.g., narcotics) is usually necessary as well.

Definitive Treatment

Definitive therapy of ALI includes percutaneous endovascular revascularization (ER), operative revascularization (OR), or amputation. Vascular surgeons generally agree that the degree of ischemia should dictate the intervention employed, with earlier stage ischemia allowing for slower but less invasive reperfusion by ER and reserving amputation for the unsalvageable ischemic limb. ER techniques include embolectomy or thrombectomy, CDT, and endovascular stent deployment. Operative interventions include intraoperative thrombolysis, endarterectomy, angioplasty, bypass, associated fasciotomy, and, in cases of irreversible damage, amputation.

Several landmark studies can account for the increasing use of CDT in ALI. The STILE trial demonstrated decreased hospital length of stay and decreased amputation rates at 6 months in patients who underwent ER at presentation, but only in the subset of patients who presented with less than 2 weeks of symptoms [47]. Although more patients treated with initial lysis versus surgery required reintervention 1 year later, lytic therapy decreased the overall number of surgical interventions required, and no mortality difference existed between endovascular and operative treatment [48]. The TOPAS trial similarly found no difference between intra-arterial urokinase versus surgical revascularization in amputation rate or mortality at 6 months after intervention, although during initial hospitalization the urokinase group required less open surgical procedures or amputations and had a lower overall mortality [49].

More recent studies and a Cochrane Review have demonstrated no difference between initial treatment with thrombolysis versus OR in amputation rates or mortality at 1 year, although hemorrhagic complications are consistently more common in thrombolysis groups [30, 50]. For this reason, operative management should be utilized in patients who have a contraindication to thrombolysis (Table 16.4); otherwise, endovascular management is the initial intervention of choice in early ischemia, especially for patients with comorbidities precluding operative intervention [28, 42].

The current European Society of Cardiology (ESC) guidelines recommend endovascular intervention for Rutherford Class I–IIa ALI of <14 days' duration, or in whom comorbidities preclude operative intervention [42]. Both ESC and Trans-Atlantic Inter-Society guidelines state that patients with Rutherford IIb ischemia warrant immediate operative intervention, and patients with irreversible damage (Rutherford III) should undergo amputation [28, 42].

In some instances, patients with ALI may have comorbidities or a poor functional status that precludes operative intervention. If such patients also have contraindications to catheter-directed thrombolysis, conservative management with aspirin and heparin alone may be considered, but only after fully discussing all options and likely prognoses with both the vascular specialist and the patient and/or family members.

Table 16.4 Contraindications to thrombolysis[a]

Absolute	Relative major	Relative minor
Recent stroke[b] (<2 months)	Recent CPR (<10 days)	Hepatic failure with coagulopathy
Active bleeding diathesis	Recent major surgery or trauma (<10 days)	Bacterial endocarditis
Recent GI bleed (<10 days)	Uncontrolled HTN >180 mmHg systolic or >110 mmHg diastolic	Diabetic hemorrhagic retinopathy
Recent neurosurgery (<3 months)	Puncture of noncompressible vessel	Pregnancy
Recent intracranial trauma (<3 months)	Intracranial tumor Recent eye surgery	

Adapted from Norgren et al. [28]

CPR cardiopulmonary resuscitation, *GI* gastrointestinal, *HTN* hypertension

[a]Contraindications for *systemic* thrombolysis

[b]Excludes transient ischemic attacks

Special Considerations

Popliteal artery aneurysms carry a high rate of thromboembolism and subsequent limb ischemia [51, 52]. Because endovascular intervention of popliteal artery aneurysms is still relatively new and thought to be fraught with a high rate of post-procedural complications and need for reintervention [53], surgical repair is generally the treatment of choice [54]. However, recent studies indicate that endovascular repair may be a reasonable method of management [54–56]. Consulting the interventional radiologist for acute ischemia due to a popliteal artery thrombosis can be entertained, but the vascular surgeon should be called if the interventional radiologist is not comfortable with ER in this setting.

Emergency physicians at hospitals without the appropriate specialists should initiate transfer as soon as the diagnosis is suspected. Transfer should not be delayed for imaging such as CT angiography, but aspirin and heparin therapy must be initiated prior to transfer.

Aortic Aneurysm Rupture

Key Points

- Classic presentation of AAA is rare.
- Two large-bore IVs, CBC/INR/T&S
- A-line, Foley, hemodynamically stable RSI meds
- Clinical suspicion + positive bedside US for AAA → vascular consultation or STAT interhospital transfer
- CTA for suspected TAA, preoperative planning
- DDAVP, PCC, vitamin K, FFP as indicated for reversal of coagulopathy or poor/inhibited platelet function
- Delayed volume resuscitation to SBP 70–80s
- Crystalloid challenge → massive transfusion protocol (usually 1 unit PRBC: 1 unit FFP: 1 pack of platelets ratio)
- Broad-spectrum antibiotics for IAAs

Introduction

Although the overall rate of ruptured aortic aneurysm has decreased in the past decade, mortality after rupture remains high. In fact, aneurysmal disease is the 15th most common cause of death in the United States and the 10th leading cause of death in patients over 55 years of age [57]. Increased outpatient diagnosis and elective repair of abdominal aortic aneurysms (AAA) have decreased the rupture rate, but approximately 30% of patients with out-of-hospital rupture die before reaching the hospital [58], and the perioperative mortality rate is still 40–53% for those undergoing emergent repair [58–60]. Thoracic aortic aneurysms (TAA) occur less frequently but are also associated with high mortality [61] largely because as many as 95% are not diagnosed until rupture or dissection [62]. Emergency physicians must not only have a high suspicion for symptomatic aortic aneurysm to prevent progression to rupture, but must also know how to manage the critically ill patient immediately following rupture.

Pathophysiology

An aortic aneurysm is a focal outpouching of the aorta due to weakening of all three layers of the aortic wall (i.e., inner intima, media, outer adventitia). The exact mechanisms behind aneurysm formation are not fully understood and appear to differ slightly between thoracic and abdominal aortic aneurysms [63]. AAAs are thought to result from a complex interplay between inflammatory cells and mediators, oxidative stress, and matrix metalloproteinases that ultimately leads to extracellular matrix degradation, vascular smooth muscle cell apoptosis, and aortic wall breakdown [63–65]. Although still resulting in degenerative vascular wall breakdown, the process behind TAA formation involves less inflammation and more often has a significant underlying genetic basis. Of note, the renin-angiotensin system is highly activated in both thoracic and abdominal aortic aneurysm development [63].

Risk factors associated with the *development* of AAA (Table 16.5) include advanced age, smoking, hypertension, atherosclerosis, male sex, family history of aortic aneurysm, and presence of a connective tissue disease [65–67]. For specific subtypes of aneurysm, inflammatory illnesses and infection are the predisposing conditions. Surprisingly, the presence of diabetes is actually inversely related to aneurysm formation [67, 68].

Factors associated with AAA *rupture* (Table 16.5) include female sex, aneurysm diameter (≥6 cm in males, ≥5 cm in females), smoking, faster rate of aneurysm growth (≥1 cm/year or 0.5 cm/6 months) [70–72], a first-degree relative with AAA, coexisting diagnosis of chronic obstructive pulmonary disease or hypertension [68, 72], and history of cardiac or abdominal organ transplantation [74, 75].

Thoracic aortic aneurysms are classified into four types according to their relationship with the aortic

Table 16.5 Risk factors for abdominal aortic aneurysm development and rupture

Risk factors for AAA development [64–68]	Risk factors for AAA rupture [68–75]
Smoking	Female gender
Male gender	Aneurysm size (diameter)[a]
Advancing age	First degree relative with aortic aneurysm
Hypertension	Faster rate of aneurysm growth[b]
Hypercholesterolemia	Decreased FEV_1
Atherosclerosis[c]	Active smoking
Family history	Infected aneurysm
Inflammatory/infectious aortitis	History of abdominal organ transplant

[a]>6 cm in males, >5 cm in females
[b]Greater than 1 cm/year or >0.5 cm in 6 months
[c]Composite of coronary artery disease, cerebrovascular disease, and peripheral vascular disease

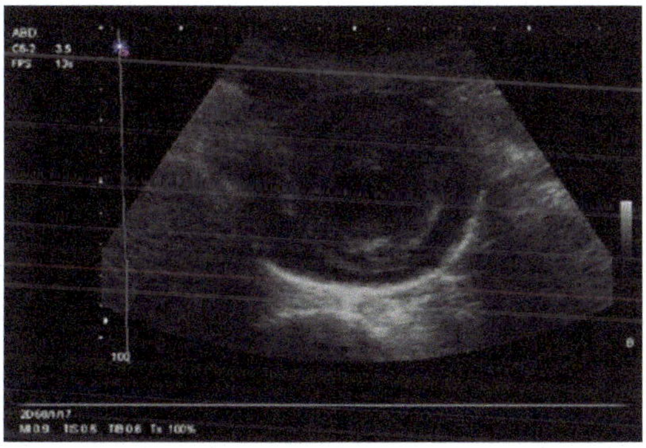

Fig. 16.2 Classification of thoracic aortic aneurysms

arch (Fig. 16.2): (1) ascending, (2) aortic arch, (3) descending, (4) thoracoabdominal aortic aneurysm (descending aneurysms that cross the diaphragm). The majority of TAAs are ascending, and overall, most TAAs are degenerative in nature, especially descending and thoracoabdominal aneurysms.

Twenty percent of TAAs are familial, associated with inherited genetic mutations and connective tissue disorders such as Marfan's, Ehlers-Danlos, and Loeys-Dietz syndrome [63], and most often affect the ascending aorta. Five percent are secondary to an inflammatory aortitis, most commonly giant cell and Takayasu's arteritis, although they have been reported in multiple other systemic autoimmune disorders [77, 78]. Although less common in the current age of antibiotics, infectious aneurysms carry a high risk of rupture and near 100% mortality without appropriate diagnosis and management [77]. Degenerative TAAs have the same risk factors as abdominal aortic aneurysms (i.e., older age, smoking, hypertension, atherosclerosis), although a higher female predominance exists for TAAs than for AAAs [62].

Patient Presentation

Diagnosing a symptomatic or ruptured AAA is a challenge because the classic triad of abdominal pain, hypotension, and pulsatile mass is only present in about a third of all patients presenting with ruptured aortic aneurysm [79, 80]. Patients with symptomatic AAA may manifest pain in various areas, including the back, buttock, leg, groin, and scrotum, often making the immediate diagnosis elusive. Additionally, palpating a pulsatile mass can be difficult in obese patients and in those with smaller aneurysms.

In some cases, the patient may present with symptoms of secondary complications, such as gastrointestinal bleed in patients with aortoenteric fistula, or a congestive picture with distended neck veins and lower extremity edema in aortovenous fistula. Patients with frank rupture can present with altered mental status and florid shock, which can be confused with sepsis in the elderly patient. Due to confounding presenting signs and symptoms, the emergency physician must maintain a wide differential and high clinical suspicion to avoid a potentially fatal misdiagnosis.

Up to 90–95% of patients with thoracic aortic aneurysms remain asymptomatic until rupture [63]. When present, the most classic symptoms are retrosternal chest pain (for ascending TAAs) radiating to the back between the scapulae (for descending TAAs). Rupture may cause hemothorax and respiratory distress, tamponade and hypotension, or aortic valve insufficiency, congestive heart failure, and flash pulmonary edema. Alternately, TAAs can present with symptoms related to the compression of or erosion into nearby structures, such as hoarseness due to laryngeal nerve compression, hemoptysis due to tracheobronchial erosion, or hematemesis due to aortoesophageal fistulization.

Diagnostics

Imaging

Plain films are insufficiently sensitive and specific for diagnosing aortic aneurysms. If performed as a part of a separate workup, x-rays may demonstrate mediastinal widening in the case of TAA, or widened aortic wall calcification or loss of a psoas shadow due to retroperitoneal hematoma in AAAs.

Bedside abdominal ultrasound has high sensitivity (99%) and specificity (98%) for diagnosing abdominal aortic aneurysm [81]. Additionally, its point-of-care assessment permits diagnosis without exposing the unstable patient to risky transport to locations where emergent care cannot be delivered (e.g., CT scanner). Transabdominal ultrasound is not sensitive enough to rule out rupture, however, as retroperitoneal AAA rupture is poorly visualized. Ultrasound accuracy is operator-dependent and can be limited in patients with large amounts of bowel gas, a tortuous aorta, or obesity (Figs. 16.3 and 16.4).

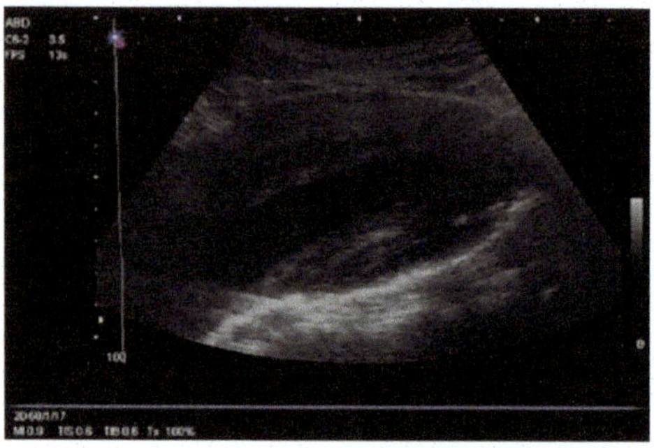

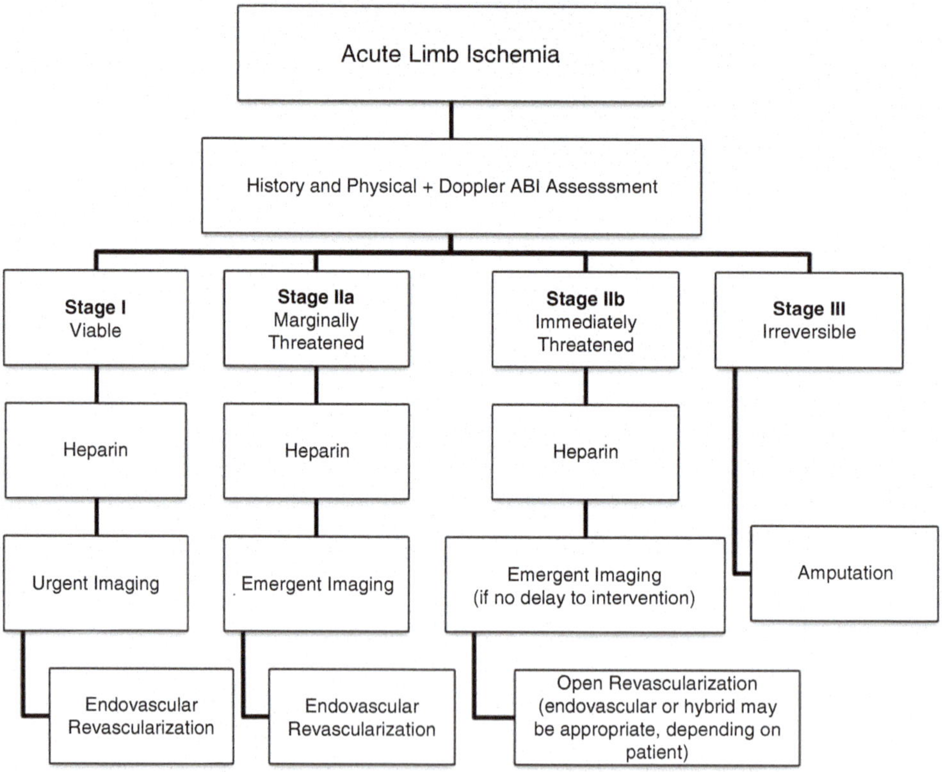

Figs. 16.3 and 16.4 Transverse and longitudinal ultrasound views of aortic aneurysm (Reprinted with permission from the *Encyclopedia of Intensive Care Medicine* (2012). Copyright 2012, Springer Science+Business Media)

Although readily available, bedside transthoracic echocardiography (TTE) has limited utility in diagnosing TAAs or their rupture due to its general poor visualization of the aortic root, aortic arch, and proximal descending aorta [76]. While transesophageal echocardiography (TEE) sufficiently evaluates the aortic root and proximal aorta, its imaging of the aortic arch and descending portions of the aorta is limited [82], and TEE requires sedation, a definitive airway, and, most importantly, a trained operator, which further limits its frequent use in the unintubated, critically ill ED patients. However, if the patient requires intubation and a skilled operator is present, TEE is an attractive option because of its ability to make a bedside diagnosis.

As previously mentioned, unstable patients, in whom the suspicion for ruptured aneurysm is high, should not be sent to the CT scanner. For stable patients with an unclear diagnosis, however, CT angiography (CTA) is helpful and is widely accepted as the imaging modality of choice to rule out aortic rupture. A study comparing CTA to intraoperative findings demonstrated 98% sensitivity and 94.9% specificity for aortic aneurysm rupture [83]. In addition, CTA provides information to guide therapeutic interventions such as endovascular versus operative repair, identifies the presence of concomitant aneurysms at other sites, assesses for the presence of infectious or inflammatory aortitis, and rules out alternate intrathoracic or intra-abdominal pathology. For patients with chronic kidney disease or severe iodinated contrast allergy, even a noncontrast-enhanced CT scan can detect most intrathoracic or retroperitoneal hemorrhage [84, 85]. Other noncontrast CT findings in aortic aneurysm rupture are listed in Table 16.6.

Laboratory Tests

No role for laboratory work exists for the diagnosis of aortic aneurysm rupture, but it is needed for operative planning and to assess secondary damage. Emergency providers should obtain a complete blood count (CBC) to evaluate extent of blood loss, a comprehensive metabolic panel (CMP) to assess renal and hepatic function and to provide information about acid-base status, type and cross for anticipated transfusion, coagulation studies for possible anticoagulation reversal or plasma transfusion, and a lactic acid level to measure the extent of systemic hypoperfusion. An electrocardiogram and cardiac troponin and/or natriuretic peptide level may be indicated, depending on patient presentation, to identify the presence of demand myocardial ischemia or coronary sinus involvement in proximal aortic aneurysm rupture.

Emergency providers should consider obtaining a thromboelastogram (TEG), if available, as soon as the diagnosis of ruptured aortic aneurysm is made or suspected, especially in patients with known coagulopathy or on anticoagulant therapy. Although unlikely to change acute management, erythrocyte sedimentation rate (ESR) and C-reactive protein (CRP) may be elevated in patients with vasculitis-associated aortitis and aneurysm such as Takayasu's or giant cell arteritis.

Initial Stabilization

Initial care of the patient with aortic aneurysm rupture mandates prompt adequate intravenous (IV) access, which may include at least two large-bore peripheral IVs or a large-bore central venous catheter capable of quickly infusing large volumes. The patient should have continuous cardiac monitoring, an arterial line for accurate hemodynamic monitoring, and a Foley catheter to monitor urine output. Endotracheal intubation should be reserved for patients unable to protect their airway or requiring rapid imaging or surgery. Because induction agents can precipitously lower an already tentative blood pressure, a hemodynamically stable sedative such as etomidate or ketamine should be used for induction and peri-intubation pressors should be readily available. In the case of ruptured TAA causing pericardial tamponade, intubation-induced decreases in venous return can cause PEA arrest. Intubation should, therefore, ideally be delayed until operative intervention.

For patients in whom impending rupture is suspected, reversal of any existing coagulopa-

Table 16.6 Signs of AAA rupture on noncontrast-enhanced CT [127–130]

Finding	Example	
1. Intraperitoneal/retroperitoneal hematoma adjacent to AAA *Images courtesy Department of Radiology, University of Maryland Medical Center, Baltimore MD*	*(Before rupture)* 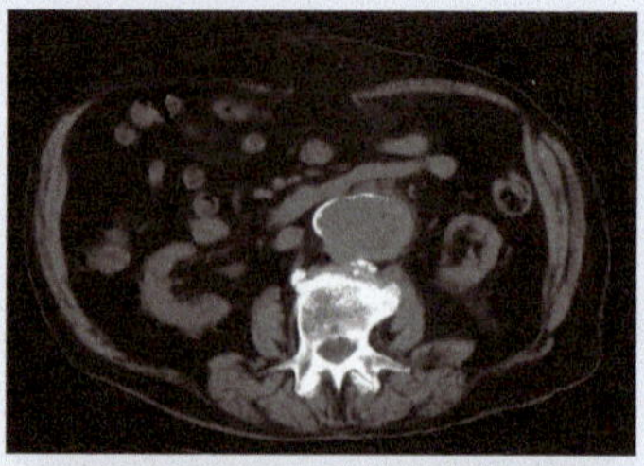	*(After rupture)* 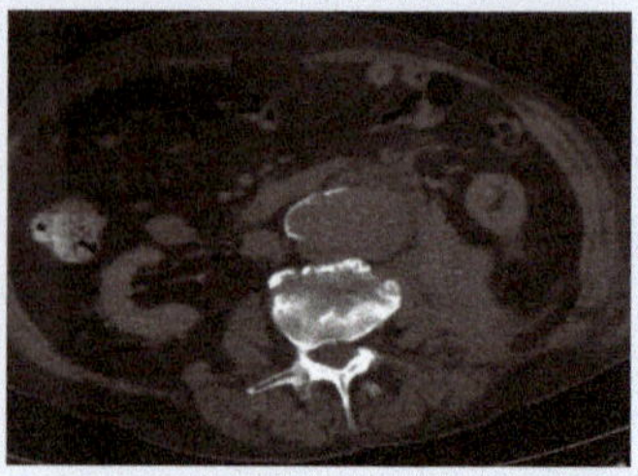
2. Deviation or focal disruption of circumferential aortic wall calcification [128] *Image reprinted with permission from Clinical Radiology (2013). Copyright 2013, Elsevier*	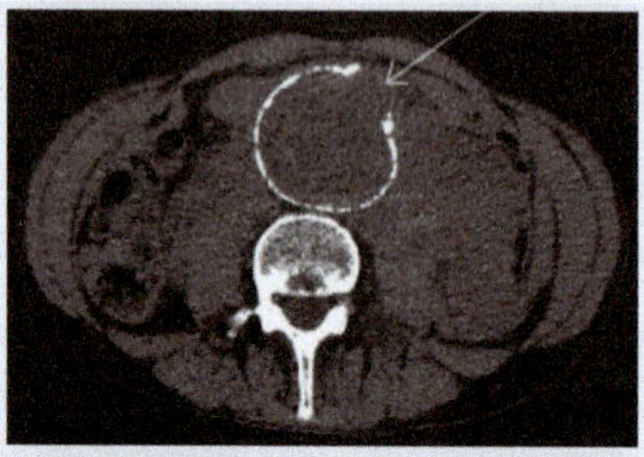	
3. "Draped aorta" sign – the posterior aortic wall is indistinct from adjacent structures or loses the regularity of its contour along adjacent structures (i.e., vertebral bodies) [129]. This example also shows disruption of aortic calcification *Image reprinted with permission from Abdominal Imaging (2008). Copyright 2008, Springer Science+Business Media, LLC*	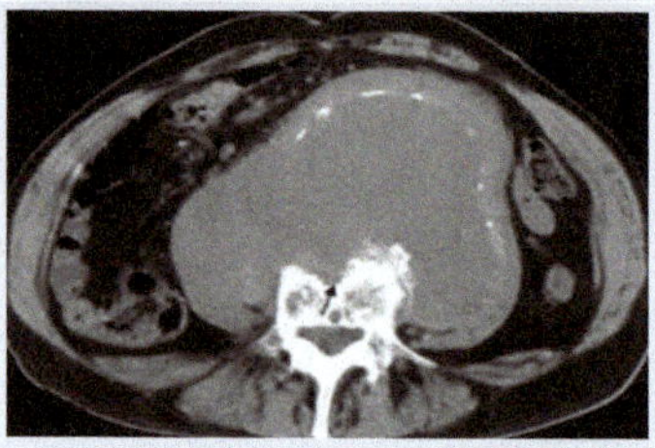	
4. "Hyperattenuated crescent" sign – a peripheral crescent that distinguishes the presence fresh blood (either dissection or hematoma) along the aneurysm wall or mural thrombus, in addition to an indistinct aortic wall [130] *Image A courtesy of Department of Radiology, University of Maryland Medical Center, Baltimore MD* *Image B reprinted with permission from Emergency Radiology (2013). Copyright 2013, Springer Science+Business Media, LLC*	*(A)* 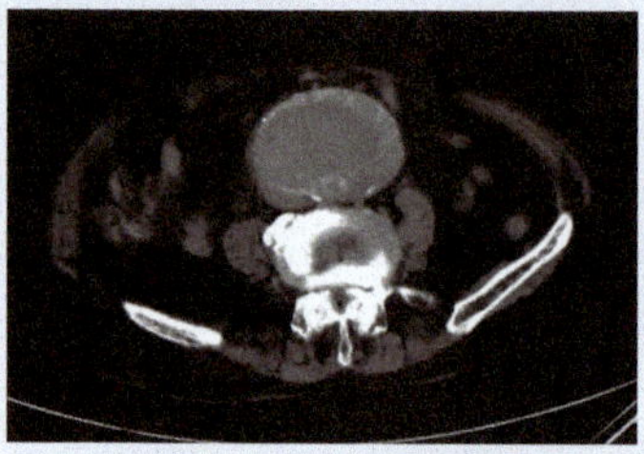	*(B)* 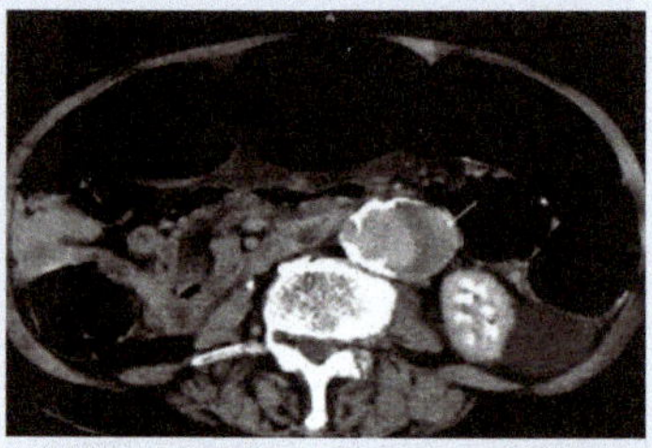

thies is imperative. Desmopressin (ddAVP) may be indicated for end-stage renal patients with uremic platelet dysfunction. Vitamin K, fresh frozen plasma, three-factor (II, IX, X) and four-factor (II, VII, IX, X) prothrombin complex concentrates (PCC), and recombinant activated factor VII (rVIIa) are all effective for the reversal of warfarin, though not all of them are readily available at all facilities and some are more effective than others [86, 87].

Direct antidotes for the newer anticoagulants dabigatran, rivaroxaban, and apixaban are still under investigation, including a monoclonal antibody against dabigatran [88] and both natural and recombinant factor Xa for the factor Xa inhibitors rivaroxaban and apixaban [89]. There is some evidence that four-factor PCC, more than FFP, improves bleeding times and laboratory parameters of coagulation when administered to reverse dabigatran [87, 90]. Similarly, use of pro-hemostatic agents rVIIa and factor VIII inhibitor bypassing activity (FEIBA), the only commercially available activated PCC (II, VIIa, IX, X), improves monitoring parameters, but no conclusive data demonstrate improved bleeding or mortality [87]. Less data exist for reversal of rivaroxaban and even less for apixaban, but rVIIa, four-factor PCC, and FEIBA are reasonable therapies in any patient on a novel anticoagulant with aortic aneurysm rupture [87, 90].

Permissive hypotension and delayed volume resuscitation, the practice of limiting volume resuscitation in patients with ruptured AAA until aortic hemostasis, is generally considered standard of care. The current European Society for Vascular Surgery (ESVS) guidelines include a level 4C recommendation for maintenance of systolic blood pressure (SBP) of 50–100 mmHg [91], while a narrower goal of 70–80 mmHg is more widely accepted [92–93].

Despite no randomized controlled trials directly investigating delayed volume resuscitation in patients with AAA rupture, several animal studies and trauma trials utilizing this practice demonstrate a survival benefit [92, 94–96]. Several retrospective studies link patient mortality to aggressive preoperative fluid resuscitation, including one by showing a 60% increase in relative risk of perioperative mortality for each additional liter of volume given per hour [97]. The concept behind these findings is that blood pressure normalization may dislodge tenuous clots and cause further blood and coagulation factor loss. Additionally, crystalloid infusion results in hemodilution, hypothermia, and acidosis, all of which promote coagulopathy and capillary leak [98, 99].

More recently, the IMPROVE trial found increased mortality among patients with a lowest recorded SBP < 70 mmHg. The prospective, randomized controlled trial looked at open versus endovascular repair in patients with ruptured AAA. Subanalysis showed no significant mortality difference based on the amount of fluids infused, and 30-day patient mortality was inversely proportional to systolic blood pressure, with every 10 mmHg increase in SBP correlating to a 13% increase in odds of survival [100]. With these findings, we recommend a general target SBP of 70–80 mmHg in younger patients with less comorbidities but caution that a higher SBP may be needed in older patients with less reserve and more inherent arterial resistance. The SBP goal is not necessarily a specific number but, rather, maintenance of adequate end-organ perfusion and that therapy titration should be guided by trends in such measurements (e.g., mentation, urine output, lactate clearance).

No guidelines exist to select the most appropriate resuscitation fluid in ruptured aortic aneurysms. However, we caution against overreliance on nonsanguinous products for the reasons listed above, and crystalloids should be reserved for short-term intravascular repletion until blood products are available. If appropriate SBP goals are not reached with 30 mL/kg of an initial balanced crystalloid infusion, utilization of blood transfusion is warranted. Some data indicate that patients with ruptured AAA have better outcomes with transfusion of plasma and platelets as compared to packed red blood cells alone [101, 102]. If transfusion is utilized, a 1:1:1 ratio of red blood cells, plasma, and platelets, with platelets ideally being given first [103], is recommended, per established evidence on massive transfusion [104, 105]. If available, however, a TEG can be used for goal-directed transfusion guidance. Few studies have examined TEG-directed transfusion in aortic aneurysm. Applying the evidence found in the trauma population, although TEG-guided transfusion results in a decreased total number of blood products given, no conclusive evidence demonstrates that it improves overall mortality [106]. It may result in decreased mortality compared to massive transfusion protocols (MTP) in the subset of patients requiring large-volume transfusion (≥10 units of packed red blood cells) [107].

Special Considerations

Infected Aortic Aneurysms

The possibility of a mycotic or infection-related aortic aneurysm (IAA) should be considered in any patient presenting with aortic aneurysm and fever; history of prior cardiac, aortic, or vertebral surgery; or signs of embolic phenomena on examination. The most common bacterial pathogens are *Staphylococcus*, *Streptococcus*, *Salmonella*, and *Klebsiella*, although a variety of pathogens have been documented in the literature [108, 109]. Tuberculous and syphilitic mycotic aneurysms are rare and usually involve the thoracic aorta. Fungal IAAs are also rare and usually result from systemic fungemia in immunosuppressed patients rather than focal infection. A contrast-enhanced CT, which is the diagnostic test of choice, may exhibit suggestive findings of an IAA, including reactive lymphadenopathy or an aneurysm with a multilobulated contour, adjacent soft tissue stranding, fluid collection, or gas [108]. Along with basic blood work, two sets of blood cultures, as well as fungal and acid-fast bacilli cultures, should be obtained and empiric antibiotic therapy should be started as soon as possible. Appropriate coverage includes intravenous vancomycin to cover methicillin-resistant *S. aureus* and gram-negative coverage with a third-generation cephalosporin, fluoroquinolone, or piperacillin/tazobactam. If there is reason to suspect a fungal mycotic aneurysm, such as a chronic indwelling catheter or total parenteral nutrition, an antifungal such as fluconazole or micafungin should be initiated as well. Immediate vascular surgery consultation should occur as soon as the diagnosis is suspected. Unfortunately, even with antibiotics and surgical intervention, persistent infection can be a problem and IAAs can have up to a 40% mortality rate [110, 111].

"Novel" Interventions

Percutaneous placement of a resuscitative endovascular intra-aortic balloon via the femoral artery in order to tamponade distal hemorrhage was first described in the literature in the early1950s, albeit not with great improvements in patient outcomes [62, 112, 113]. A brachial artery approach was also described for acute aortic rupture in 1964 [114] and a transaxillary approach was reported in 1972 [115]. In a 2003 study of 11 patients with ruptured AAA, Matsuda [116] demonstrated that brachially inserted intra-aortic balloons could be inserted in as little as 10 minutes from presentation and could yield significant improvements in systolic blood pressure. The authors suggested that insertion is something that could "be introduced during CPR in the emergency room" [116].

Most recently, Raux et al. [117] demonstrated via a retrospective comparison of 72 hemodynamically unstable patients with ruptured AAA who underwent either aortic cross-clamping or resuscitative endovascular balloon occlusion of the aorta (REBOA) that the preoperative use of balloon occlusion decreased intraoperative mortality (19% vs. 43%, $p = 0.31$), with more patients in the balloon occlusion group regaining hemodynamic stability (85% vs. 57%, $p = 0.014$), although these did not translate to improved in-hospital mortality or 30-day survival between the groups. Swine models undergoing balloon occlusion for 30, 60, and 90 minutes demonstrated an increase in the inflammatory marker IL-6 and a trend toward increased incidence of acute respiratory distress syndrome and requirement of vasopressor support with increasing occlusion times [118]. Although encouraging, the outcomes of REBOA use are not yet completely known.

A study out of R. Adams Cowley Shock Trauma Center [119] demonstrated the teachability of REBOA device placement to "novice interventionalists" (including a physician board certified in emergency medicine) utilizing an externally validated virtual reality simulator. All learners were able to perform the procedure quickly and effectively in a simulation environment, independent of endovascular experience in residency or residency type [119].

While no published data regarding the insertion of REBOA devices by emergency physicians currently exist, this procedure will likely be fully integrated into the emergency physician's scope of practice to temporize unstable patients with intra-abdominal hemorrhage in preparation for transport to the operating room or interhospital transfer.

Definitive Treatment

Historically, emergent open surgical repair was the standard of care for ruptured aortic aneurysms; however, multiple randomized controlled trials have demonstrated equal or better survival outcomes with endovascular aortic repair (EVAR) [120–123]. Although long-term survival did not differ, EVAR decreased perioperative mortality as compared to open surgical repair in one study [120]. Despite more postoperative complications, another demonstrated better 30-day and 5-year survival with EVAR [121].

Patients with symptomatic or suspected ruptured aortic aneurysm warrant immediate transfer if appropriate resources are unavailable at the presenting hospital. A recent expert consensus addressing patient eligibility for interhospital transfer agreed that the only contraindication to transfer should be patients with ruptured AAA presenting with cardiac arrest; this same group, comprising emergency physicians, vascular surgeons, and interventional radiologists, agreed that inotropic support, psychiatric institutionalization, moderate systemic disease, and fluctuating consciousness should *not* preclude transfer [124]. Additionally, they agreed that bedside ultrasound should be performed but transfer should not be delayed for CT scan confirmation, and that in-house consultation should not be mandated prior to arranging transfer unless particular concerns exist regarding a patient's suitability for intervention (e.g., preexisting terminal diagnosis or severe limitation in daily functioning, severe systemic disease) [124]. For hospitals without specialist services, streamlined protocols to expedite interhospital transfer have proven to decrease time to intervention and improve mortality [125].

Approximately 20% of patients transferred to another facility die before receiving the needed intervention at the second hospital [126], highlighting the importance of discussing this very real possibility with the patient and the family, while acknowledging the 100% mortality rate of rupture without repair.

References

Acute Mesenteric Ischemia

1. Wyers MC. Acute mesenteric ischemia: diagnostic approach and surgical treatment. Semin Vasc Surg. 2010;23(1):9–20.
2. Oldenburg WA, Lau LL, Rodenberg TJ, Edmonds HJ, Burger CD. Acute mesenteric ischemia: a clinical review. Arch Intern Med. 2004;164(10):1054–62.
3. Kassahun WT, Schulz T, Richter O, Hauss J. Unchanged high mortality rates from acute occlusive intestinal ischemia: six year review. Langenbecks Arch Surg. 2008;393:163–71.
4. Sise MJ. Acute mesenteric ischemia. Surg Clin N Am. 2014;94:165–81.
5. Acosta S, Ogren M, Sternby NH, et al. Clinical implications for the management of acute thromboembolic occlusion of the superior mesenteric artery: autopsy findings in 213 patients. Ann Surg. 2005;241:516–22.
6. Corcos O, Nuzzo A. Gastro-intestinal vascular emergencies. Best Pract Res Clin Gastroenterol. 2013;27(5):709–25.
7. Kohoutova D, Moravkova P, Kruzliak P, Bures J. Thromboembolic complications in inflammatory bowel disease. J Thromb Thrombolysis. 2015;39(4):489–98.
8. Klar E, Rahmanian PB, Bücker A, Hauenstein K, Jauch KW, Luther B. Acute mesenteric ischemia: a vascular emergency. Dtsch Arztebl Int. 2012;109(14):249–56.
9. Paladino NC, Inviati A, Di Paola V, Busuito G, Amodio E, Bonventre S, et al. Predictive factors of mortality in patients with acute mesenteric ischemia. A retrospective study. Ann Ital Chir. 2014;85(3):265–70.
10. Cudnik MT, Darbha S, Jones H, Macedo J, Stockton SW, Hiestand BC. The diagnosis of acute mesenteric ischemia: a systematic review and meta-analysis. Acad Emerg Med. 2013;20:1088–100.
11. Karabulut KU, Huseyin N, Gul M, Dundar ZD, Cander B, Girisgin S, et al. Diamine oxidase in diagnosis of acute mesenteric ischemia. Am J Emerg Med. 2013;31:309–12.
12. Reichert M, Hecker M, Hörbelt R, Lerner P, Höller J, Hecker CM, et al. [The role of biomarkers in the diagnosis of acute mesenteric ischemia]. Chirurg. 2015;86(1):47–55.
13. Chiu YH, Huang MK, How CK, Hsu TF, Chen JD, Chern CH, et al. D-dimer in patients with suspected acute mesenteric ischemia. Am J Emerg Med. 2009;27(8):975–9.
14. Acosta S, Nilsson T. Current status on plasma biomarkers for acute mesenteric ischemia. J Thromb Thrombolysis. 2012;33(4):355–61.
15. Oliva IB, Davarpanah AH, Rybicki FJ, Desjardins B, Flamm SD, Francois CJ, et al. ACR appropriateness criteria imaging of mesenteric ischemia. Abdom Imaging. 2013;38(4):714–9.

16. van den Heijkant TC, Aerts BA, Teijink JA, Buurman WA, Luyer MD. Challenges in diagnosing mesenteric ischemia. World J Gastroenterol. 2013;19(9):1338–41.
17. Turkbey B, Akpinar E, Cil B, Karçaaltincaba M, Akhan O. Utility of multidectector CT in an emergency setting in acute mesenteric ischemia. Diagn Interv Radiol. 2009;15(4):256–61.
18. Armstrong PA. Visceral duplex scanning: evaluation before and after artery intervention for chronic mesenteric ischemia. Perspect Vasc Surg Endovasc Ther. 2007;19(4):386–92.
19. Meaney JF, Prince MR, Nostrant TT, Stanley JC. Gadolinium-enhanced MR angiography of visceral arteries in patients with suspected chronic mesenteric ischemia. J Magn Reson Imaging. 1997;7:171–6.
20. Golan DE. Principles of pharmacology: the pathophysiologic basis of drug therapy. 2nd ed. Philadelphia: Lippincott Williams & Wilkins; 2008.
21. Beaulieu RJ, Arnaoutakis KD, Abularrage CJ, Efron DT, Scheider E, Black JH 3rd. Comparison of open and endovascular treatment of acute mesenteric ischemia. J Vasc Surg. 2014;59(1):159–64.
22. Arthurs ZM, Titus J, Bannazadel M, Eagleton MJ, Srivastava S, Sarac TP, et al. A comparison of endovascular revascularization with traditional therapy for the treatment of acute mesenteric ischemia. J Vasc Surg. 2011;53(3):698–704.
23. Block TA, Acosta S, Björck M. Endovascular and open surgery for acute occlusion of the superior mesenteric artery. J Vasc Surg. 2010;52(4):959–66.
24. Clark RA, Gallant TE. Acute mesenteric ischemia: angiographic spectrum. AJR. 1984;142(3):555–6.
25. Boley SJ, Spravregan S, Siegelman SS, Veith FJ. Initial results from an aggressive roentgenological and surgical approach to acute mesenteric ischemia. Surgery. 1977;82(6):848–55.
26. Klotz S, Vestring T, Rötker J, Schmidt C, Scheld HH, Schmid C. Diagnosis and treatment of nonocclusive mesenteric ischemia after open heart surgery. Ann Thorac Surg. 2001;72(5):1583–6.
27. Corcos O, Castier Y, Sibert A, Gaujoux S, Ronot M, Joly F, et al. Effects of a multimodal management strategy for acute mesenteric ischemia on survival and intestinal failure. Clin Gastroenterol Hepatol. 2013;11(2):158–65.

Acute Limb Ischemia

28. Norgren L, Hiatt WR, Dormandy JA, TASC II Working Group, et al. Inter-society consensus for the management of peripheral arterial disease (TASC II). J Vasc Surg. 2007;45(Suppl S):S5–67.
29. Baril DT, Ghosh K, Rosen AB. Trends in the incidence, treatment, and outcomes of acute lower extremity ischemia in the United States Medicare population. J Vasc Surg. 2014;60(3):669–772.
30. Berridge DC, Kessel DO, Robertson I. Surgery versus thrombolysis for initial management of acute limb ischaemia. Cochrane Database Syst Rev. 2013;(6):CD002784.
31. Fagundes C, Fuchs FD, Fagundes A, Poerschke RA, Vacaro MZ. Prognostic factors for amputation or death in patients submitted to vascular surgery for acute limb ischemia. Vasc Health Risk Manag. 2005;1(4):345–9.
32. Herity NA, Daizell GW. Venous thrombosis causing arterial embolization to the same limb through a patent foramen ovale. Clin Cardiol. 1997;20(10):893–6.
33. Saric M, Kronzon L. Aortic atherosclerosis and embolic events. Curr Cardiol Rep. 2012;14(3):342–9.
34. Kropman RH, Schriver AM, Kelder JC, Moll FL, de Vries JP. Clinical outcome of acute leg ischaemia due to thrombosed popliteal artery aneurysm: systematic review of 895 cases. Eur J Vasc Endovasc Surg. 2010;39:452–7.
35. Rutherford RB, Baker JD, Ernst C, Johnston KW, Porter JM, Ahn S, et al. Recommended standards for reports dealing with lower extremity ischemia: revised version. J Vasc Surg. 1997;26(3):517–38.
36. Gates J, Hartnell GG. Optimized diagnostic angiography in high-risk patients with severe peripheral vascular disease. Radiographics. 2000;39:452–7.
37. Ascher E, Hingorani A, Markevich N, Schutzer R, Kallakuri S. Acute lower limb ischemia: the value of duplex ultrasound arterial mapping (DUAM) as the sole preoperative imaging technique. Ann Vasc Surg. 2003;17(3):284–9.
38. Eiberg JP, Gronvall Rasmussen JB, Hansen MA, Schroeder TV. Duplex ultrasound scanning of peripheral arterial disease of the lower limb. Eur J Vasc Endovasc Surg. 2010;40(4):507–12.
39. Favaretto E, Pili C, Amato A, Conti E, Losinnot F, Rossi C, et al. Analysis of agreement between duplex ultrasound scanning and arteriography in patients with lower limb artery disease. J Cardiovasc Med (Hagerstown). 2007;8(5):337–41.
40. Collins R, Burch J, Cranny G, Aguiar-Ibáñez R, Craig D, Wright K, et al. Duplex ultrasonography, magnetic resonance angiography, and computed tomography angiography for diagnosis and assessment of symptomatic, lower limb peripheral arterial disease: systematic review. BMJ. 2007;334(7606):1257.
41. Sobel M, Verhaeghe R. Antithrombotic therapy for peripheral artery occlusive disease: American College of Chest Physicians Evidence-Based Clinical Practice Guidelines (8th edition). Chest. 2008;133(6 Suppl):815S–43S.
42. Tendera M, Aboyans V, Bartelink ML, Baumgartner I, Clément D, Collet JP, European Stroke Organisation, et al. ESC guidelines on the diagnosis and treatment of peripheral artery diseases: document covering atherosclerotic disease of extracranial carotid and vertebral, mesenteric, renal, upper and lower extremity arteries: the task force on the diagnosis and treatment of peripheral artery diseases of the European Society of Cardiology (ESC). Eur Heart J. 2011;32(22):2851–906.
43. Baigent C, Blackwell L, Collins R, Emberson J, Godwin J, Peto R, Antithrombotic Trialists' (ATT) Collaboration, et al. Aspirin in the primary and secondary prevention of vascular disease: collaborative

meta-analysis of individual participant data from randomised trials. Lancet. 2009;373(9678):1849–60.
44. Dörffler-Melly J, Koopman MM, Prins MH, Büller HR. Antiplatelet and anticoagulant drugs for prevention of restenosis/reocclusion following peripheral endovascular treatment. Cochrane Database Syst Rev. 2005;(1):CD002071.
45. Lewis HD Jr, Davis JW, Archibald DG, Steinke WE, Smietherman TC, Doherty JE 3rd, et al. Protective effects of aspirin against acute myocardial infarction and death in men with unstable angina: results of a Veterans Administration Cooperative Study. N Engl J Med. 1983;309(7):396–403.
46. Blaisdell FW, Steele M, Allen RE. Management of acute lower extremity ischemia due to embolism and thrombosis. Surgery. 1978;84:822–34.
47. The STILE Investigators. Results of a prospective randomized trial evaluating surgery versus thrombolysis for ischemia of the lower extremity. The STILE trial. Ann Surg. 1994;220(3):251–66.
48. Weaver FA, Comerota AJ, Youngblood M, Froelich J, Hosking JD, Papanicolaou G. Surgical revascularization versus thrombolysis for nonembolic lower extremity native artery occlusions: results of a prospective randomized trial. The STILE Investigators. Surgery versus Thrombolysis for Ischemia of the Lower Extremity. J Vasc Surg. 1996;24(4):513–21.
49. Ouriel K, Veith FJ, Sasahara AA. A comparison of recombinant urokinase with vascular surgery as initial treatment for acute arterial occlusion of the legs for the Thrombolysis or Peripheral Arterial Surgery (TOPAS) investigators. N Engl J Med. 1998;338:1105–11.
50. Taha AG, Byrne RM, Avgerinos ED, Marone LK, Majaroun MS, Chaer RA. Comparative effectiveness of endovascular versus surgical revascularization for acute lower extremity ischemia. J Vasc Surg. 2015;61(1):147–54.
51. Mousa AY, Beauford RB, Henderson P, Patel P, Earies PL, Flores L, et al. Update on the diagnosis and management of popliteal aneurysm and literature review. Vascular. 2006;14(2):103–8.
52. Robinson WP 3rd, Belkin M. Acute limb ischemia due to popliteal artery aneurysm: a continuing surgical challenge. Semin Vasc Surg. 2009;22(1):17–24.
53. Pulli R, Dorigo W, Fargion A, Pratesi G, Innocenti AA, Angiletta D, et al. Comparison of early and midterm results of open and endovascular treatment of popliteal artery aneurysms. Ann Vasc Surg. 2012;26(6):809–18.
54. Antonello M, Frigatti P, Battocchio P, Lepidi S, Cognolato D, Dall'Antonia A, et al. Open repair versus endovascular treatment for asymptomatic popliteal artery aneurysm: results of a prospective randomized study. J Vasc Surg. 2005;42:185–93.
55. Desai SS, DuBose JJ, Parham CS, Charlton-Ouw KM, Valdes J, Estrera AL, et al. Outcomes after endovascular repair of peripheral arterial trauma. J Vasc Surg. 2014;60(5):1309–14.
56. Huang Y, Gloviczki P, Oderich GS, Duncan AA, Kalra M, Fleming MD, et al. Outcomes of endovascular and contemporary surgical repairs of popliteal artery aneurysm. J Vasc Surg. 2014;60(3):631–8.

Aortic Aneurysm Rupture

57. Beckman JA. Aortic aneurysms: pathophysiology, epidemiology, and prognosis. In: Creager MA, Dzau VJ, Loscalzo J, editors. Vascular medicine. Philadelphia: Saunders Elsevier Inc; 2006.
58. Reimerink JJ, van der Laan MJ, Koelemay MJ, Balm R, Legemate DA. Systematic review and meta-analysis of population-based mortality from ruptured abdominal aortic aneurysm. Br J Surg. 2013;100(11):1405–13.
59. Hoornweg LL, Storm-Versloot MN, Ubbink DT, Koelemay MJ, Legemate DA, Balm R. Meta analysis on mortality of ruptured abdominal aortic aneurysms. Eur J Vasc Endovasc Surg. 2008;35:558–70.
60. Korhonen SJ, Ylonen K, Biancari F, Heikkinen M, Salenius JP, Lepäntalo M, Finnvasc Study Group. Glasgow Aneurysm Score as a predictor of immediate outcome after surgery for ruptured abdominal aortic aneurysm. Br J Surg. 2004;91:1449–52.
61. Johansson G, Markstrom U, Swedenborg J. Ruptured thoracic aortic aneurysms: a study of incidence and mortality rates. J Vasc Surg. 1995;21:985–8.
62. Elefteriades JA. Thoracic aortic aneurysm: reading the enemy's playbook. Curr Probl Cardiol. 2008;33:203–7.
63. Davis FM, Rateri DL, Daugherty A. Mechanisms of aortic aneurysm formation: translating preclinical studies into clinical therapies. Heart. 2014;100:1498–505.
64. Lindholt JS, Shi GP. Chronic inflammation, immune response, and infection in abdominal aortic aneurysms. Eur J Vasc Endovasc Surg. 2006;31:453–63.
65. Diehm N, Dick F, Schaffner T, Schmidli J, Kalka C, Di Santo S, et al. Novel insight into the pathobiology of abdominal aortic aneurysm and potential future treatment concepts. Prog Cardiovasc Dis. 2007;50(3):209–17.
66. Forsdahl SH, Singh K, Solberg S, Jacobsen BK. Risk factors for abdominal aortic aneurysms: a 7-year prospective study: the Tromso Study, 1994-2001. Circulation. 2009;119(16):2202–8.
67. Lederle FA, Johnson GR, Wilson SE, Chute EP, Littooy FN, Bandyk D, et al. Prevalence and associations of abdominal aortic aneurysm detected through screening. Aneurysm Detection and Management (ADAM) Veterans Affairs Cooperative Study Group. Ann Intern Med. 1997;126:441–9.
68. Chaikof EL, Brewster DC, Dalman RL, Makaroun MS, Illig KA, Sicard GA, et al. The care of patients with an abdominal aortic aneurysm: the Society for Vascular Surgery practice guidelines. J Vasc Surg. 2009;50(4):S2–S49.
69. Sweeting MJ, Thompson SG, Brown LC, Powell JT. Meta-analysis of individual patient data to examine factors affecting growth and rupture of small abdominal aortic aneurysms. Br J Surg. 2012;99(5):655–65.
70. Thompson SG, Brown LC, Sweeting MJ, Bown MJ, Kim LG, Glover MR, et al. Systematic review and meta-analysis of the growth and rupture rates of small abdominal aortic aneurysms: implications for surveillance intervals and their cost-effectiveness. Health Technol Assess. 2013;17(41):1–118.

71. Brewster DC, Cronenwett JL, Hallett JW Jr, Johnston KW, Krupski WC, Matsumura JS, et al. Guidelines for the treatment of abdominal aortic aneurysms. Report of a subcommittee of the Joint Council of the American Association for Vascular Surgery and Society for Vascular Surgery. J Vasc Surg. 2003;37:1106–17.
72. Brown PM, Zelt DT, Sobolev B. The risk of rupture in untreated aneurysms: the impact of size, gender, and expansion rate. J Vasc Surg. 2003;37(2):280–4.
73. Brown LC, Powell JT. Risk factors for aneurysm rupture in patients kept under ultrasound surveillance. UK Small Aneurysm Trial Participants. Ann Surg. 1999;230:289–97.
74. Cron DC, Coleman DM, Sheetz KH, Englesbe MJ, Waits SA. Aneurysms in abdominal organ transplant recipients. J Vasc Surg. 2014;59(3):594–8.
75. Englesbe MJ, Wu AH, Clowes AW, Zierler RE. The prevalence and natural history of aortic aneurysms in heart and abdominal organ transplant patients. J Vasc Surg. 2003;37(1):27–31.
76. Booher AM, Eagle KA. Diagnosis and management issues in thoracic aortic aneurysm. Am Heart J. 2011;162(1):38–46.
77. Gornik HL, Creager MA. Aortitis. Circulation. 2008;117(23):3039–51.
78. Pacini D, Leone O, Turci S, Camurri N, Giunchi F, Martinelli GN, et al. Incidence, etiology, histologic findings, and course of thoracic inflammatory aortopathies. Ann Thorac Surg. 2008;86:1518–23.
79. Marston WA, Ahlquist R, Johnson G Jr, Meyer AA. Misdiagnosis of ruptured abdominal aortic aneurysms. J Vasc Surg. 1992;16(1):17–22.
80. Kiell CS, Ernst CB. Advances in management of abdominal aortic aneurysm. Adv Surg. 1993;26:73–98.
81. Rubano E, Mehta N, Caputo W, Paladino L, Sinert R. Emergency department bedside ultrasonography for diagnosing suspected abdominal aortic aneurysm. Acad Emerg Med. 2013;20:128–38.
82. Meredith EL, Masani ND. Echocardiography in the emergency assessment of acute aortic syndromes. Eur J Echocardiogr. 2009;10(1):i31–9.
83. Biancari F, Paone R, Venermo M, D'Andrea V, Parala J. Diagnostic accuracy of computed tomography in patients with suspected abdominal aortic aneurysm rupture. Eur J Vasc Endovasc Surg. 2013;45(3):227–30.
84. Petridis A, Pilavaki M, Vafiadis E, Pälädas P, Finitsis S, Drevelegas A. CT of hemodynamically unstable abdominal trauma. Eur Radiol. 1999;9(2):250–5.
85. Bhalla S, Menias CO, Heiken JP. CT of acute abdominal disorders. Radiol Clin North Am. 2003;41:1153–69.
86. Chapman SA, Irwin ED, Abou-Karam NM, Rupnow NM, Hutson KE, Vestpa J, et al. Comparison of 3-factor prothrombin complex concentrate and low-dose recombinant factor VIIa for warfarin reversal. World J Emerg Surg. 2014;9:27.
87. Miller MP, Trujillo TC, Nordenholz KE. Practical considerations in emergency management of bleeding in the setting of target-specific oral anticoagulants. Am J Emerg Med. 2014;32(4):375–82.
88. Van Ryn J, Litzenburger T, Waterman A, Canada K, Hauel N, Kroe-Barrett R, et al. Dabigatran anticoagulant activity is neutralized by an antibody selective to dabigatran in in vitro and in vivo models. J Am Coll Cardiol. 2011;57:E1130.
89. Lu GP, Peng L, Hollenbach SJ, Abe K, DeGuzman FR, Siu G, et al. Reconstructed recombinant factor Xa as an antidote to reverse anticoagulation by factor Xa inhibitors. J Thromb Haemost. 2009;7:309.
90. Siegal DM, Crowther MA. Acute management of bleeding in patients on novel oral anticoagulants. Eur Heart J. 2013;34:489–500.
91. Moll FL, Powell JT, Fraedrich G, Verzini F, Haulon S, Waltham M, et al. Management of abdominal aortic aneurysms clinical practice guidelines of the European Society for Vascular Surgery. Eur J Vasc Endovasc Surg. 2011;41(Suppl 1):S1–S58.
92. Hamilton H, Constantinou J, Ivancev K. The role of permissive hypotension in the management of ruptured abdominal aortic aneurysms. J Cardiovasc Surg. 2014;55(2):151–9.
93. Roberts K, Revell M, Youssef H, Bradbury AW, Adam DJ. Hypotensive resuscitation in patients with ruptured abdominal aortic aneurysm. Eur J Vasc Endovasc Surg. 2006;31(4):339–44.
94. Crawford ES. Ruptured abdominal aortic aneurysm. J Vasc Surg. 1991;13:348e50.
95. Bickell WH, Wall MJ Jr, Pepe PE, Martin RR, Ginger VF, Allen MK, et al. Immediate versus delayed fluid resuscitation for hypotensive patients with penetrating torso injuries. N Engl J Med. 1994;331:1105–9.
96. Capone AC, Safar P, Stezoski W, Tisherman S, Peitzman AB. Improved outcome with fluid restriction in treatment of uncontrolled hemorrhagic shock. J Am Coll Surg. 1995;180:49e56.
97. Dick F, Erdoes G, Opfermann P, Eberle B, Schmidli J, von Allmen RS. Delayed volume resuscitation during initial management of ruptured abdominal aortic aneurysm. J Vasc Surg. 2013;57(4):943–50.
98. Hess J, Brohi K, Dutton R, Hauser CJ, Holcomb JB, Kluger Y, et al. The coagulopathy of trauma: a review of mechanisms. J Trauma. 2008;65:748–54.
99. Tieu BH, Holcomb JB, Schreiber MA. Coagulopathy: its pathophysiology and treatment in the injured patient. World J Surg. 2007;31(5):1055–64.
100. Powell JT, Hinchliffe RJ, Thompson MM, Sweeting MJ, Ashleigh R, Bell R, IMPROVE trial investigators, et al. Observations from the IMPROVE trial concerning the clinical care of patients with ruptured abdominal aortic aneurysm. Br J Surg. 2014;101(3):216–24.
101. Mell MW, O'Neil AS, Callcut RA, Acher CW, Hoch JR, Tefera G, et al. Effect of early plasma transfusion on mortality in patients with ruptured abdominal aortic aneurysm. Surgery. 2010;148(5):955–62.
102. Henriksson AE. The impact of blood component transfusion practices on patient survival after abdominal aortic aneurysm surgery. Vasc Endovasc Surg. 2013;47(1):38–41.
103. Holcomb JB, Tilley BC, Baraniuk S, Fox EE, Wade CE, Podbielski JM, PROPPR Study Group, et al. Transfusion of plasma, platelets, and red

blood cells in a 1:1:1 versus a 1:1:2 ratio and mortality in patients with severe trauma: the PROPPR randomized clinical trial. JAMA. 2015;313(5):471–82.

104. Holcomb JB, Wade CE, Michalek JE, Chisholm GB, Zarzabal LA, Schreiber MA, et al. Increased plasma and platelet to red blood cell ratios improves outcome in 466 massively transfused civilian trauma patients. Ann Surg. 2008;248(3):447–58.

105. Borgman MA, Spinella PC, Perkins JG, Grathwohl KW, Repine T, Beekley AC, et al. The ratio of blood products transfused affects mortality in patients receiving massive transfusions at a combat support hospital. J Trauma. 2007;63(4):805–13.

106. Da Luz LT, Nascimento B, Shankarakutty AK, Rizoli S, Adhikari NK. Effect of thromboelastography (TEG) and rotational thromboelastometry (ROTEM) on diagnosis of coagulopathy, transfusion guidance, and mortality in trauma: descriptive systematic review. Crit Care. 2014;18(5):518.

107. Tapia NM, Chang A, Norman M, Welsh F, Scott B, et al. TEG-guided resuscitation is superior to standardized MTP resuscitation in massively transfused penetrating trauma patients. J Trauma Acute Care Surg. 2013;74(2):378–85.

108. Leon LR Jr, Mills JL Sr. Diagnosis and management of aortic mycotic aneurysms. Vasc Endovasc Surg. 2010;44(1):5–13.

109. Revest M, Decaux O, Cazalets C, Verohye JP, Jégo P, Grosbois B. Thoracic infectious aortitis: microbiology, pathophysiology, and treatment. Rev Med Interne. 2007;28(2):108–15.

110. Jaffer U, Gibbs R. Mycotic thoracoabdominal aneurysms. Ann Cardiothorac Surg. 2012;1(3):417–25.

111. Kan CD, Lee HL, Yang YJ. Outcome after endovascular stent graft treatment for mycotic aortic aneurysm: a systematic review. J Vasc Surg. 2007;46(5):906–12.

112. Edwards WS, Salter PP Jr, Carnaggio VA. Intraluminal aortic occlusion as a possible mechanism for controlling massive intra-abdominal hemorrhage. Surg Forum. 1953;4:496–9.

113. Hughes CW. Use of an intra-aortic balloon catheter tamponade for controlling intra-abdominal hemorrhage in man. Surgery. 1954;36:65–8.

114. Heimbecker RO. An aortic tampon for emergency control of ruptured abdominal aneurysm. Can Med Assoc J. 1964;91:1024–5.

115. Smith FG. Emergency control of ruptured abdominal aortic aneurysm by transaxillary balloon catheter. Vasc Surg. 1972;6:79–84.

116. Matsuda H, Tanaka Y, Hino Y, Matsukawa R, Ozaki N, Okada K, et al. Transbrachial arterial insertion of aortic occlusion balloon catheter in patients with shock from ruptured abdominal aortic aneurysm. J Vasc Surg. 2003;38(6):1293–6.

117. Raux M, Marzelle J, Kobeiter H, Donnheur G, Allaire E, Cochennec F, et al. Endovascular balloon occlusion is associated with reduced intraoperative mortality of unstable patients with ruptured abdominal aortic aneurysm but fails to improve other outcomes. J Vasc Surg. 2015;61(2):304–8.

118. Morrison JJ, Ross JD, Markov NP, Scott DJ, Spencer JR, Rasmussen TE. The inflammatory sequelae of aortic balloon occlusion in hemorrhagic shock. J Surg Res. 2014;191(2):423–31.

119. Brenner M, Hoehn M, Pasley J, Dubose J, Stein D, Scalea T. Basic endovascular skills for trauma course: bridging the gap between endovascular techniques and the acute care surgeon. J Trauma Acute Care Surg. 2014;77(2):286–91.

120. Nedeau AE, Pomposelli FB, Hamdan AD, Wyers MC, Hsu R, Sachs T, et al. Endovascular vs open repair for ruptured abdominal aortic aneurysm. J Vasc Surg. 2012;56(1):15–20.

121. Mehta M, Byrne H, Darling RC 3rd, Paty PS, Roddy SP, Kreienberg PB, et al. Endovascular repair of ruptured infrarenal abdominal aortic aneurysm is associated with lower 30-day mortality and better 5-year survival rates than open surgical repair. J Vasc Surg. 2013;57(2):368–75.

122. Reimerink JJ, Hoornweg LL, Vahl AC, van den Broek TA, Legemate DA, Reekers JA, et al. Endovascular repair versus open repair of ruptured abdominal aortic aneurysms: a multicenter randomized controlled trial. Ann Surg. 2013;258:248–56.

123. Powell JT, Sweeting MJ, Thompson MM, Ashleigh R, Bell R, Gomes M, IMPROVE Investigators, et al. Endovascular or open repair strategy for ruptured abdominal aortic aneurysm: 30 day outcomes from IMPROVE randomised trial. BMJ. 2014;348:f7661.

124. Hinchliffe RJ, Ribbons R, Ulug P, Powell JT. Transfer of patients with ruptured abdominal aortic aneurysm from general hospital to specialist vascular centres: results of a Delphi consensus study. Emerg Med J. 2013;30(6):483–6.

125. Haveman JW, Karliczek A, Verhoeven ELG, Tielliu IF, de Vos R, Zwaveling JH, et al. Results of streamlined regional ambulance transport and subsequent treatment of acute abdominal aortic aneurysms. Emerg Med J. 2006;23(10):807–10.

126. Mell MW, Wang NE, Morrison DE, Hernandez-Boussard T. Interfacility transfer and mortality for patients with ruptured abdominal aortic aneurysm. J Vasc Surg. 2014;60(3):553–7.

127. Rakita D, Newatia A, Hines JJ, Siegel DN, Friedman B. Spectrum of CT findings in rupture and impending rupture of abdominal aortic aneurysms. Radiographics. 2007;27(2):497–507.

128. Ahmed MZ, Ling L, Ettles DF. Common and uncommon CT findings in rupture and impending rupture of abdominal aortic aneurysms. Clin Radiol. 2013;68(9):962–71.

129. Apter S, Rimon U, Konen E, Erlich Z, Guranda L, Amitai M, et al. Sealed rupture of abdominal aortic aneurysms: CT features in 6 patients and a review of the literature. Abdom Imaging. 2010;35(1):99–105.

130. Taheri MS, Haghighatkhah H, Pourghorban R, Hosseini A. Multidetector computed tomography findings of abdominal aortic aneurysm and its complications: a pictorial review. Emerg Radiol. 2013;20(5):443–51.

Renal Emergencies

17

Marie-Carmelle Elie, Charles Hwang, and Mark Segal

Basic Renal Physiology

Renal oxygen consumption occurs at a rate of 6–8 mL/min per 100 g. While the kidneys receive approximately 20–25% of cardiac output at rest, the kidneys use 7–10% of total oxygen uptake. The sodium-potassium ATPase pump utilizes approximately 2/3 of renal oxygen uptake [1]. Unlike other organs and tissues in which blood flow is determined by metabolic need, blood flow to the kidney is determined by metabolic need indirectly via sodium reabsorption and effects on the glomerular filtration rate. Additionally, as renal perfusion is autoregulated, changes in perfusion altering oxygen delivery are likely restricted in the kidney; this provides a basis for the production of erythropoietin in the presence of low tissue oxygen tension [2].

The kidneys represent a key component of homeostasis including the maintenance of blood volume and composition, and the regulation of blood pressure. Critical features include the regulation of the ion concentration in body fluids, sustaining the balance between water and electrolytes, and the filtration and elimination of wastes, byproducts, drugs, and toxins from the bloodstream. Blood pressure is regulated by the production of renin and the stimulation of red blood cell production in the bone marrow by producing erythropoietin [3].

Electrolyte Concentrations

The reabsorption of sodium (Na) along the nephron is powered by the Na-K ATPase pump. More than half of total Na reabsorption occurs along the proximal convoluted tubule and proximal straight tubule; another third is reabsorbed by the ascending portion of the loop of Henle; and approximately 10% is left to the distal collecting tubule and cortical and medullary collecting ducts. In the proximal tubule, Na reabsorption is dependent on the rate of filtration, known as glomerulotubular balance. By linking reabsorption and filtration, Na and fluid losses decrease as GFR increases and cessation of tubular flow is prevented with a decrease in GFR [1].

Phosphate plays an essential role in facilitating oxygen release from hemoglobin, nucleotide generation, the formation of cell membranes, protein regulation, bone formation, and enzymatic processes; thus, serum phosphorus is highly regulated by parathyroid hormone (PTH) and the kidney. Approximately 90% of plasma phosphate is filtered by the glomerulus, and then

M.-C. Elie (✉)
Department of Emergency Medicine, Critical Care, Hospice and Palliative Medicine, University of Florida, Gainesville, FL, USA

C. Hwang
Department of Emergency Medicine, UF Health, Levy County Department of Public Safety, Gainesville, FL, USA

M. Segal
Department of Medicine, University of Florida Health, Gainesville, FL, USA

© Springer Nature Switzerland AG 2020

J. R. Shiber, S. D. Weingart (eds.), *Emergency Department Critical Care*, https://doi.org/10.1007/978-3-030-28794-8_17

the proximal tubule reabsorbs approximately 90% of the filtered phosphate [4].

It is well known that in bone, PTH causes stimulation of receptor activator of nuclear factor kappa-β ligand (RANKL) by osteoblasts, leading to calcium and phosphate efflux. The kidney produces increased 1,25-dihydroxyvitamin D ($1,25(OH)_2D$), leading to increased intestinal reabsorption of both calcium and phosphate. To maintain serum balance, PTH decreases renal tubular phosphate reabsorption. In recent years, fibroblast growth factor 23 (FGF23) has been added to the bone-kidney axis. Bone secretes FGF23, which targets the kidneys to regulate phosphate and vitamin D metabolism. This axis with FGF23 appears to have at least two physiological functions: (1) for bone to provide an indicator to coordinate bone phosphate flux resulting from bone turnover and mineralization with kidney conservation of phosphate and (2) to provide a counterregulatory hormone that protects the organism from excessive vitamin D exposure. The main effects of FGF23 overexpression are hypophosphatemia, abnormal vitamin D metabolism, impaired growth, and rickets/osteomalacia; underexpression leads to hyperphosphatemia, excess $1,25(OH)_2D$, and calcium deposition in soft tissues [5].

Klotho is a type 1 membrane protein; structural analysis of FGF23 shows a possible klotho interaction site at the carboxy terminal of the FGF23 protein. Klotho expression has been found in the parathyroid gland, kidney, and brain. Experimental studies have shown that FGF23-klotho interaction can lead to decreased active vitamin D. In patients with chronic kidney disease, klotho levels are reduced making FGF23 nonfunctional. This reduced interaction decreases renal phosphate excretion in the urine and leads to elevated plasma levels of phosphate [6].

Volume Status

The kidneys are responsible for maintaining water balance within the body and are the major source through which water is eliminated from the body. To maintain balance, water influx into the body needs to match the elimination from the body; positive water balance exists if water influx is greater than elimination and negative water balance exists if elimination is greater than influx.

The kidneys regulate both tonicity and extracellular blood volume. Sodium balance regulates extracellular blood volume. Mechanisms directing extracellular blood volume and tonicity vary; however, there is some overlap in both physiological processes. While potassium does influence tonicity, the usual marker for tonicity is serum sodium concentration. As body water decreases, serum sodium concentration increases, and vasopressin is released by the posterior pituitary gland triggering thirst and decreased water excretion by the kidneys. As body water increases, serum sodium concentration decreases, and the kidneys increase water excretion by suppressing vasopressin [7].

Acid-Base Balance

Besides the kidney, acid-base balance is influenced by skeletal muscle (through exercise), the intestines (through the loss of bicarbonate or acid), bone (through the regulation of phosphate and carbonate), and diet. The kidney regulates acid-base balance through three mechanisms: acid or alkali excretion, the synthesis of ammonium and bicarbonate, and the reabsorption of filtered bicarbonate [8].

The proximal tubules reabsorb approximately 80% of filtered bicarbonate via the Na-bicarbonate cotransporter and the Na-hydrogen exchanger [9]. Classically, intercalated cells are present in the late convoluted tubule; type A intercalated cells secrete acid and non-type A cells excrete bicarbonate.

Pendrin is an anion exchanger expressed on the luminal membrane of non-type A intercalated cells. It is thought that in this location, pendrin regulates chloride/bicarbonate exchange by reabsorbing chloride and excreting bicarbonate into urine [8]. Jacques et al. created a mouse model in which intercalated cells overexpressed pendrin; this stimulated chloride reabsorption in the distal tubule, leading to hypertension (HTN) in the mice. This confirms previous studies that show the inability of sodium to raise blood pressure when chloride is replaced with another ion in a sodium salt; this conclusion has led some people to believe that salt-sensitive HTN is chloride-dependent [10].

Drug Elimination

Renal excretion of drugs in the urine involves three separate processes: glomerular filtration, active tubular secretion, and passive tubular reabsorption. The glomerular filtration rate determines the amount of drug or metabolite entering the tubular lumen; the ability of the drug/metabolite to bind to plasma proteins also influences the amount entering the lumen, as only unbound drugs are filtered. Various transporters located along the membrane function to secrete amphipathic anions, conjugated metabolites, and organic cations [11].

Alkalinization and acidification of urine influences drug elimination; the extent of the influence is determined by the degree of pH change and the role of pH-dependent passive reabsorption in the elimination of the drug [11]. In the tubules, passive reabsorption of nonionized weak acids and bases occurs. Passive reabsorption depends on the pH. If tubular urine is more alkaline, weak acids are mostly ionized and therefore more rapidly excreted and excreted to a larger extent. Excretion of acids is reduced if the tubular urine is more acidic.

Alterations in kidney function impact glomerular filtration, active tubular secretion, and passive tubular reabsorption, largely contributing to drug dosing recommendations. However, changes in kidney function also affect the metabolism of nonrenally metabolized drugs. Studies in rats show that uremia leads to decreased hepatic and intestinal activity of cytochrome P450 enzymes due to a reduction in gene and protein expression. Another mechanism through which uremia can affect nonrenal pharmacokinetics is via transporter function; it is thought that accumulated uremic toxins either modify transcription or translation or they directly alter proteins post-translation [12].

Blood Pressure Control

The kidneys regulate blood pressure by secreting hormones into circulation and through baroreceptor reflexes. Renovascular hypertension occurs with decreased renal perfusion. In the event of decreased blood flow to the kidneys, the juxtaglomerular apparatus releases renin [13]. The three mechanisms that lead to renin secretion are: (1) decreased sodium transport through the distal portion of the thick ascending limb of the loop of Henle, (2) decreased stretch or pressure in the afferent arteriole, and (3) direct stimulation of B_1 adrenoreceptors by the sympathetic nervous system [14]. Renin contributes to blood pressure regulation primarily through the production of angiotensin II. Angiotensin II then directly increases blood pressure via vasoconstriction and indirectly through the activation of aldosterone, leading to water retention [13].

The kidneys also play a role in several causes of secondary hypertension. In renal artery stenosis, the narrow lumen of the renal arteries leads to decreased renal perfusion, causing renin secretion and activation of the renin-angiotensin-aldosterone pathway. In primary hyperaldosteronism, the kidneys retain sodium; in this condition, because of elevated aldosterone levels, renin is inhibited through negative feedback; thus, aldosterone is elevated but renin is not. Additionally, certain renal tumors can produce excessive amounts of renin, activating the renin-angiotensin-aldosterone pathway and causing hypertension [13].

Erythropoietin Production

Erythropoietin (EPO) is an essential hormone in the production of red blood cells. In the fetal state, hepatocytes are primarily responsible for its production; however, fibroblasts from the renal cortex become the main producer of EPO following birth. When in circulation, EPO functions as an antiapoptotic agent for erythrocytic progenitors, mainly the colony-forming units – erythroid. Once stimulated by EPO, these cells differentiate into proerythroblasts and normoblasts [15].

EPO release is stimulated by hypoxia; its expression is activated when arterial partial pressure of oxygen declines or when oxygen affinity in the blood increases, such as in high-altitude settings. EPO values peak approximately 1–2 days following ascent to a higher altitude and then stabilize at approximately twice the level noted at sea level [15].

The critmeter hypothesis explains a theory where the kidney notes the relative volumes of red blood cell mass and plasma (the two components of hematocrit) through tissue oxygen pressure. If the relative volumes of the two components need to be coordinated, it would require the ratio be sensed and thus a signal would need to be present to generate the ideal hematocrit. In the kidney, this theory proposes that the tissue oxygen tension acts as the common factor in which afferent signals sensing the relative volumes converge. Afferent signals report total blood volume and efferent signals alter the plasma component via sympathetic, renin-angiotensin, and vasopressin systems. Additionally, it suggests that the renin-angiotensin-aldosterone system increases EPO production; this is supported by certain disease states in which hematocrit is maintained or elevated in the presence of elevated plasma renin [2].

Acute Renal Failure and Hemodialysis Emergencies

Introduction

Acute kidney injury (AKI), previously known as acute renal failure (ARF), is an important and common cause of morbidity and mortality for emergency department (ED) and critical care patients [16–21]. The disorder exposes patients to circulatory overload, acid-base disturbances, and life-threatening electrolyte disturbances including hyperkalemia, coagulopathy, and neurological complications [16, 22]. Despite advances in our understanding of the pathophysiology and management of AKI, many areas of this disease process still remain subject to controversy and lack of consensus [20]. This chapter aims to review the available evidence regarding the vast spectrum of AKI based on the level and type of renal impairment, the pathophysiology of AKI, and the management of these complex patients in the acute setting.

Definition

AKI is a broad term that refers to an abrupt, rapid (1–7 days), and sustained (>24 hours) decrease in renal excretory function, resulting in the retention of nitrogenous (urea and creatinine) and non-nitrogenous waste products [17, 20, 23–28]. AKI is best understood as a continuum; kidney injury exists well before any laboratory derangements can be measured as a result of decreased renal excretory function [17, 29]. Other clinical manifestations of AKI include decreased urine output, changes in fluid balance, acid-base disturbances, and metabolic derangements, including accumulation of organic acids and increase in serum potassium and phosphate concentrations [17, 24].

Until recently, an absence of consensus for the definition of AKI has resulted in wide variation in epidemiological estimates and difficulty in developing controlled trials or animal models [21, 22]. In fact, there are more than 60 definitions of AKI or ARF in the literature [20, 30, 31]. In 2002, the Acute Dialysis Quality Initiative (ADQI) [20] group proposed the RIFLE criteria, a consensus definition which embodies the AKI continuum [20, 21, 26, 31, 32]. Moreover, a new consensus definition from Kidney Disease: Improving Global Outcomes (KDIGO) has merged the RIFLE criteria and Acute Kidney Injury Network (AKIN) definitions [22, 30, 33–35].

The RIFLE criteria, a multilevel classification system, is an acronym that aims to provide a uniform definition of AKI; it identifies different stages along the complete spectrum of acute renal dysfunction: Risk of kidney dysfunction, Injury to the kidney, Failure of kidney function, Loss of

Table 17.1 RIFLE criteria for AKI: Risk, Injury, Failure, Loss of kidney function, and End-stage kidney disease (RIFLE) classification

Class	Glomerular filtration rate	Urine output
Risk	↑ SCr x 1.5 *or* ↓ GFR >25% *or* SCr ≥0.3 mg/dL	< 0.5 mL/kg/h × 6 h
Injury	↑ SCr × 2 *or* ↓ GFR >50%	< 0.5 mL/kg/h × 12 h
Failure	↑ SCr × 3 *or* ↓ GFR >75% *or* SCr ≥4 mg/100 mL (acute rise of ≥0.5 mg/dL) *or* initiation of renal replacement therapy	< 0.3 mL/kg/h × 24 h or anuria × 12 h
Loss of kidney function	Complete loss of kidney function >4 weeks	
End-stage kidney disease	Complete loss of kidney function >3 months	

GFR glomerular filtrate rate, *UO* urine output, *SCr* serum creatinine

kidney function, and End-stage kidney disease (see Table 17.1) [20, 21, 32]. The RIFLE classification is based on serum creatinine (SCr) and urine output (UO). It separates AKI into three severity classes (risk, injury, failure) and two outcome classes (loss of kidney function and end-stage kidney disease). A patient is classified using the either the SCR or UO criteria, whichever leads to the worse RIFLE classification [21, 32].

There are several limitations to the RIFLE classification. First, the RIFLE classification can be easily applied if a patient's baseline renal function is known. However, a significant number of patients may present with acute renal dysfunction where their baseline renal function is unknown; this is problematic for a classification system that is dependent on the change from baseline function for staging. In these situations, the theoretical baseline SCr should be calculated using the Modification of Diet in Renal Disease (MDRD) formula assuming a normal glomerular filtration rate (GFR) of approximately 75 mL min^{-1} per 1.73 m^2, and a relative change from baseline can be estimated for the patient [20, 21, 30, 32, 36, 37]. Second, the UO criteria have limited utility in the emergency department setting, since UO can only be accurately assessed in patients with a urinary catheter. Moreover, the sensitivity and specificity of UO is affected by diuretic use. Third, it is possible that the SCr and UO criteria for risk, injury, and failure do not directly correlate. The ADQI, which employs either of the criteria (SCr or UO), allows for the worse classification [21, 38, 39]. Lastly, RIFLE does not specify the etiology of AKI [21]. The use of biomarkers in the evaluation, prognostication, and management of AKI may help with these limitations and is discussed below.

Finally, we must consider scenarios of "acute-on-chronic" kidney injury. By definition, AKI refers to a decline in baseline renal function, but as we discussed previously, baseline renal function is frequently unknown. In a patient with pre-existing renal disease, the patient's actual GFR and SCr will be different from those predicted by the MDRD equation. Moreover, when applying the RIFLE criteria to patients with chronic kidney disease (CKD), the proportional changes required by RIFLE seem excessive [20, 33].

For example, a patient with a baseline creatinine of 1.0 mg/dL would fulfill the criteria of AKI with an increase to 1.5 mg/dL, while a perfectly matched patient for age, sex, and race with a baseline creatinine of 2.0 mg/dL would need to reach 3.0 mg/dL. Furthermore, the higher the baseline creatinine, the longer the duration required to reach the increased creatinine. Thus, a separate criterion for the diagnosis of acute-on-chronic kidney disease (acute rise of ≥0.3 mg/dL over 48 hours or less) helps to identify patients with AKI when their baseline creatinine is abnormal [20, 33].

Epidemiology

Epidemiological estimates of AKI vary significantly as widely disparate definitions have been used [20]. Nevertheless, AKI is common and remains a diagnostic and therapeutic challenge for clinicians.

The population-based incidence of AKI is estimated around 2147 cases per million people per year [40] or approximately 600,000 annual cases of AKI in the US population of 300 million. Some sources indicate the incidence ranges from more than 5000 cases per million people per year for nondialysis-requiring AKI to 295 cases per million people per year for dialysis-requiring AKI [41]. The disorder occurs in 1.9–16% of hospital inpatients [42–44] and in 1–25% of critically ill patients where it frequently accompanies multiorgan dysfunction syndrome [20, 24, 43, 45]. The prevalence increases to greater than 40% at admission to the intensive care unit if sepsis is also present [46]. The prevalence of AKI has even been estimated to be as high as 60% during intensive care unit admissions [39].

Furthermore, in-hospital AKI-related mortality has not changed significantly in the past 50 years [28]; the mortality rate in these populations remains unacceptably high, ranging from 28% to 90% [18, 20, 28, 43, 47]. After accounting for other factors, AKI is an independent risk factor for the future development of CKD and death [16, 18, 20–22, 25, 28, 38, 48–51]. Seven-day mortality for AKI is 10–12% in both high- and low-income countries [34]. Evidence suggests that even small changes in SCr are associated with increased inpatient mortality [21, 52]. Dialysis-requiring AKI is associated with a mortality of 40–70% [22].

Metnitz et al. found that AKI occurs in 19% of patients with moderate sepsis, 23% of patients with severe sepsis, and 51% of patients with septic shock when blood cultures were positive [53]. These statistics are even more sobering when one considers that 20% of patients with a diagnosis of acute tubular necrosis (ATN), a subset of AKI, progress to CKD stage IV within 18–24 months [54].

Pathophysiology

AKI is a complex syndrome that encompasses many different pathophysiological processes that occur simultaneously or in succession [55, 56]. The inflammatory pathway and antibody- and cell-mediated immune pathways are processes implicated in the development of AKI [17, 57, 58]; we will briefly consider several common and key processes.

Several clinical studies have demonstrated a significant correlation between the duration and severity of systemic hemodynamic instability with the development of AKI [59–66]. While the FINNAKI study showed that hypotensive episodes in the setting of severe sepsis were associated with development and progression of AKI [61], Martin et al. showed that restoration of perfusion and correction of hemodynamic stability had beneficial effects on renal function [62]. Izawa et al. demonstrated that cumulative hypotension duration was associated with AKI, especially in patients without sepsis [63].

Although global renal ischemia and hypoperfusion have been implicated in AKI, renal microcirculatory dysfunction plays a significant role in AKI development as well [67]. The two microvascular structures within each nephron, the glomeruli and the peritubular capillary network, play an integral role in the development and worsening of AKI. Even in the absence of global hypoperfusion, any change in the circulation of these capillary networks causes microvascular dysfunction, localized hypoperfusion, and microischemia. Inflammatory conditions, such as sepsis, can profoundly alter the local microvascular flow [68–70], resulting in local tissue hypoxia and ischemia, increased reactive oxygen species (ROS) generation [71–73], endothelial dysfunction with the upregulation of adhesion molecules causing increased leukocyte adherence [72–77], tubular cell injury [57, 73], upregulation of toll-like receptors [78], release of pro-inflammatory cytokines [72, 73, 79, 80], increased capillary permeability [72–74], increased tissue edema, microthrombi generation [72, 81], and increased distance that oxygen must diffuse.

Neurohormonal system activation in conditions such as sepsis, decompensated heart failure, and hepatorenal syndrome results in microcirculatory dysfunction. In these conditions, vasodilation results in arterial underfilling and baroreceptor activation. In an attempt to increase blood pressure and perfusion, the body activates the sympathetic system and increases renin-angiotensin-aldosterone and vasopressin activity, resulting in vasoconstriction, although this has deleterious effects on renal microcirculation [17].

Endothelial dysfunction is also implicated in inflammatory conditions such as glomerulonephritis and vasculitis through a separate mechanism. In these conditions, endothelial dysfunction results in increased permeability of the glomerular basement membrane, resulting in fibrin leakage, the formation of crescents, and the proliferation of cells within the Bowman's capsule. As the crescents enlarge, capillary function diminishes and glomerular function decreases [57].

As previously discussed, microcirculatory dysfunction can cause tubular cell damage. Another mechanism that damages tubular cells is direct exposure to certain filtered substances. Due to their inherent anatomic and physiologic placement, tubular cells have frontline exposure to filtered substances, such as drugs, cytokines, free hemoglobin, abnormal proteins (i.e., paraproteins), uric acid, calcium-phosphorus complexes, and inflammatory molecules [82]; exposure to these substances and subsequent injury result in apical membrane blebbing, loss of cellular polarity [83], cellular swelling and detachment from the basement membrane [24], and opening of tight junctions [57]. Moreover, mitochondrial damage results in generation of ROS and release of cytokines, furthering the progression of AKI [84]. Therefore, tubular cells are not merely damaged in AKI, but they also play an active role in propagating AKI as well.

AKI is complicated by metabolic and acid-base disturbances. Common electrolyte abnormalities include hyperkalemia and hyponatremia; loss of cellular polarity and tubular cell detachment from the basement membrane results in loss of Na+/K+-ATPase activity. AKI also causes the retention of nitrogenous waste products, hyperphosphatemia, hypocalcemia, and hypermagnesemia. Metabolic acidosis, hypofiltration, and decreased tubular secretion promotes potassium efflux from cells [27]. Fluid is retained systemically due to decreased GFR, further exacerbating hyponatremia [27, 58].

Mechanistic Pathways of AKI

AKI can be categorized into prerenal, intrinsic renal, and postrenal etiologies depending on the mechanistic pathway involved, so that the management of each category varies accordingly.

Prerenal AKI

The clinical syndrome of prerenal AKI is characterized by intact renal parenchymal function and renal hypoperfusion, either due to true hypovolemia (e.g., loss of blood volume from dehydration, fluid losses, hemorrhage, etc.) or relative hypovolemia (e.g., decreased cardiac output, fluid sequestration, systemic vasodilation, or intrarenal vasoconstriction, caused by obstructive shock, cardiogenic shock, distributive shock, etc.) [22, 24, 58, 85]. The body's primary defense against volume depletion occurs by a complex interplay between vasoconstriction and vasodilation of the afferent and efferent arterioles to maintain renal perfusion [58]. The physiological response to reduced intravascular volume and decreased renal perfusion is the activation of several reflexes and neurohumoral vasoconstrictive systems, including secretion of antidiuretic hormone (ADH), increased adrenergic, angiotensin II, and aldosterone secretion to increase reabsorption of water and urea, and the myogenic reflex and tubuloglomerular feedback [58]. Other mediators involved in maintaining renal perfusion include nitric oxide, endothelin, atrial natriuretic peptide (ANP), and dopamine [58, 85]. These neurohumoral vasoconstrictive systems attempt to maintain blood pressure, cerebral perfusion, and cardiac output [24, 85].

Renal autoregulation of blood flow occurs between systolic blood pressures of 80 mmHg and 150 mmHg [58]. When hypoperfusion is severe and occurs outside of this autoregulatory range, further incremental activation of the above systems overwhelms the compensatory mechanisms. In situations of marked hypoperfusion, angiotensin II promotes vasoconstriction of the efferent arteriole and prostaglandin (PG)E_2, which leads to vasodilation of the afferent arteriole, attempting to preserve GFR. Failure of autoregulation and further activation of compensatory systems result in a precipitous decline in GFR and AKI [85]. Additionally, since many patients are on angiotensin-converting enzyme inhibitors (ACEI) or angiotensin receptor blockers (ARB), which blocks the action of angiotensin II, and use nonsteroidal anti-inflammatory drugs (NSAIDs), which can block PGE_2, the full ability to maintain renal perfusion is impaired.

It is important to remember that renal injury occurs across a continuum. Mild ischemia leads to prerenal injury; if perfusion is restored, ischemia is reversed, and initial renal abnormalities quickly normalize. If more severe ischemia is present or reperfusion is delayed, renal tubular cells are injured; if perfusion is restored, renal function is eventually restored after renal reparation. In severe cases of ischemia, intrinsic renal injury in the form of acute tubular necrosis (ATN) and renal cortical necrosis occurs; fibrosis may follow incomplete repair and recovery, and CKD and ESRD may ensue [22, 58].

Prerenal failure is typically characterized by a high blood urea nitrogen (BUN) to SCr ratio (>15:1), low urine volume, increased specific gravity, and low urine sodium. Proteinuria, low serum albumin, or red blood cells in the urine are not features of prerenal failure in a person with no underlying kidney disease, but rather should prompt investigation to a more chronic intrinsic renal disease.

Intrinsic Renal Injury

Intrinsic renal disease is caused by tubulointerstitial injury, glomerular disease, or microvascular disease [22].

Tubulointerstitial disease is caused by ATN, which refers specifically to the histological finding of renal tubular cell necrosis [58]. ATN occurs secondary to ischemia, sepsis, nephrotoxins (i.e., aminoglycoside antibiotics, NSAIDs, ACEI, ARB, contrast-induced nephropathy, myoglobin), myeloma cast nephropathy, amyloidosis, or acute allergic interstitial nephritis (AIN) [86]. AIN is a rare, idiosyncratic reaction that is most commonly drug induced (i.e., NSAIDs, diuretics, penicillin antibiotics, proton pump inhibitors), although infectious and autoimmune disorders have been implicated as well [87].

The inflammatory pathway plays an integral part in intrinsic renal injury pathogenesis (from injury to propagation to repair). Anoxic injury to tubular cells and endothelial cells results in endothelial-erythrocyte interaction, sludging of erythrocytes, leukocyte adhesion, inability to regulate blood flow, and activation of innate and adaptive immunity. Natural killer (NK) cell activation, complement activation, toll-like receptor (TLR) upregulation, and pro-inflammatory cytokines (TNF-α, IL-6, IL-1b) have all been implicated in endothelial dysfunction. Mediators of tubular cell injury include reactive oxygen species (ROS) generation, intracellular influx of calcium, nitric oxide, phospholipase A2, TNF-α, complement, and cell-mediated immunity. Tubular cells are normally attached to the basement membrane; loss of cellular polarity can lead to detachment of the tubular cells from the basement membrane and sloughing of cells into the tubular lumen. The loss of Na+/K+-ATPase activity decreases sodium reabsorption and increases fractional excretion of sodium (FENa). The sloughing of tubular epithelial cells causes gaps in the tubular architecture, loss of tight junctions, denuded basement membrane, and tubular cast accumulation. Tubular filtrate leaks into the interstitium and is reabsorbed in the systemic circulation, decreasing GFR [27, 58].

Rapidly progressive glomerulonephritis (RPGN) causes the nephritic syndrome, consisting of hematuria, proteinuria, and AKI. Causes of glomerulonephritis include:

- Antiglomerular basement membrane (anti-GBM) antibody (Goodpasture syndrome if hemoptysis coexists)
- Lupus nephritis
- Post-streptococcal glomerulonephritis (recent group A β-hemolytic streptococcal infection or impetigo)
- Small vessel vasculitis (granulomatosis with polyangiitis [GPA]/Wegener's granulomatosis or microscopic polyangiitis [MPA])

Glomerulonephritides will typically demonstrate inflammatory glomerular crescents on immunohistological examination. Antiglomerular basement membrane antibody disease is characterized by linear deposition of IgG along the basement membrane. Lupus nephritis is characterized by "full-house" immune complex deposition.

Small vessel vasculitides are characterized by a "pauci-immune" pattern [86].

Finally, microvascular causes of intrinsic renal disease include hemolytic uremic syndrome (HUS), cholesterol emboli syndrome, malignant hypertension, and scleroderma [86].

Postrenal Failure

Postrenal failure occurs due to obstruction of the urinary tract [22]. Urinary obstruction can occur at any level from the tubules to the urethra, resulting in obstructive uropathy. Substances that are insoluble in urine (i.e., uric acid, methotrexate, acyclovir) may cause crystal formation within the tubules, resulting in urinary obstruction [88]. Other causes of obstruction include nephrolithiasis, bladder outflow obstruction from prostatic hypertrophy, neurogenic bladder, or urinary tract fibrosis.

In patients with suprapubic discomfort and a distended bladder with declining urine output, a urinary catheter should be temporarily placed to rule out bladder outlet obstruction [27].

Evaluation

Diagnostic

Clinically available variables that are useful in the diagnosis and evaluation of AKI include SCr, creatinine clearance, urea or blood urea nitrogen (BUN), urine output, and markers of tubular injury.

Creatinine Clearance and Serum Creatinine (SCr)

In the steady state, glomerular filtrate can be quantified by measuring 24-hour creatinine clearance. Patients with AKI, however, are not in steady state, as the GFR falls, creatinine secretion is increased, and thus the rise in SCr is less. Creatinine excretion is much greater than the filtered load, resulting in a potentially large overestimation of the GFR. Therefore, measured creatinine clearance reflects the upper limit of the GFR under steady-state conditions [20]. Clinicians, however, are interested in whether the renal function is stable, improving, or worsening, and this can be easily evaluated with the SCr alone [20].

SCr is an easily measured biomarker specific for renal function. It is formed from the nonenzymatic dehydration of creatine within the liver, and 98% of creatine is found in muscle. In the steady state, i.e., patients with normal renal function, creatinine excretion presumably equals creatinine production. Factors influencing creatinine production include hepatic dysfunction, markedly decreased muscle mass, trauma, fever, immobilization, and aging. The volume of distribution of creatinine also influences measured SCr levels as well [20].

SCr measurements, similar to creatinine clearance, will not accurately reflect GFR in the nonsteady state of AKI. SCr measurements will underestimate renal dysfunction as AKI evolves, while the opposite is true as renal function recovers. Nonetheless, the degree to which SCr changes from baseline will, to some degree, reflect the change in GFR [20]. To account for these changes, one can determine the kinetic GFR, an estimate of renal function dependent on the change in creatinine from one time point to another [89].

Urea or Blood Urea Nitrogen (BUN)

Urea or BUN is a nonspecific marker of renal function. A variety of nonrenal conditions can dramatically alter urea levels, making it a relatively poorer marker for AKI as compared to creatinine [20].

Urine Output (UO)

Urine output (UO) is one of the criteria used in the RIFLE classification. Although changes in UO often occur before biochemical changes are able to be measured, oliguria is neither sensitive nor specific [17]; severe AKI can exist in the setting of normal UO [20]. Therefore, UO is not helpful in diagnosing the etiology of AKI, but it plays an important role for directing management and for predicting outcome [27]. Kellum notes that patients meeting both SCr and UO criteria for AKI have dramatically worse outcomes when compared to patients who meet only one RIFLE criteria; he concludes that UO assessment is an "absolute necessity" for AKI staging [30].

Other Markers

Urine analysis may be helpful in identifying and managing specific conditions. Abnormal urinary sediment suggests intrarenal cause of AKI. For example, urine eosinophils indicate allergic interstitial nephritis (AIN) and red cell casts are indicative of glomerulonephritis. A patient with ATN frequently has "dirty" brown, opaque urine with "muddy brown" tubular casts.

Biochemical analysis of urine can help evaluate the functional integrity of the renal tubules. The fractional excretion of sodium (FENa) is defined as

$$\text{FENa} = \frac{\text{Urine Na} \times \text{Plasma Cr}}{\text{Urine Cr} \times \text{Plasma Na}} \times las.$$

Generally speaking, the FENa is <1.0% in prerenal azotemia and is usually >1.0% in ATN, although the ratio has poor sensitivity and specificity. The FENa can be inaccurate in patients with diuretics, burns, contrast nephropathy, liver disease, or glomerulonephritis, and for this reason, the FENa should not be used alone in assessing the etiology of AKI [27]. Importantly, since everyone in the steady state has a FENa of <1%, FENa is only useful when the creatinine is increasing.

Outside of these specific disease entities, the routine use of urine analysis and urine biochemical analysis in evaluating and managing AKI often has poor sensitivity and does not lead to a change in clinical course, prognosis, or management [17, 20, 27].

Biomarkers

Delay in diagnosis of AKI can further deteriorate renal function and progress to CKD or end-stage kidney disease. Identification of patients with kidney damage at an early stage enables prompt intervention and prognosis.

The diagnosis of AKI and CKD is based primarily on surrogate markers of GFR, such as SCr and UO, although these clinical data points remain imperfect. Unfortunately, SCr is a suboptimal marker of renal dysfunction in both conditions for several reasons. First, SCr can be elevated in prerenal azotemia when there is no tubular injury [28]. Second, SCr is influenced by many nonrenal factors, such as body weight, volume of distribution, muscle mass, diet and nutrition, protein intake, gender, race, age, muscle metabolism, presence of gastrointestinal bleeding, and drugs [17, 25, 28, 32]. For example, patients with AKI are frequently edematous, diluting SCr levels and confounding the clinical picture, potentially delaying recognition of AKI [19, 32]. Third, in AKI, the utility of SCr is worse; changes in SCr lag behind renal injury [25, 28]. Therefore, increases in SCr are often not able to be measured until 48–72 hours after the initial renal injury, thereby decreasing its sensitivity to detect early AKI. Moreover, significant renal disease can occur with minimal change to SCr due to enhanced tubular creatinine secretion and renal reserve, among other factors [10, 13]. Other markers such as fractional excretion of sodium or urea may be affected by diuretic use or volume status [28].

At the onset of kidney injury, biological and molecular changes induce cellular signaling molecules to be upregulated or downregulated, ultimately evolving into cellular damage. These signaling molecules can be measured and used as a surrogate marker, a biomarker, for renal injury. Biomarkers are defined as parameters of structural, biochemical, physiological, or genetic changes that indicate the presence, severity, or progress of a disease [90]. Ideally, the development of a renal-specific biomarker that is noninvasive, undetectable when there is no disease, detectable early once the disease develops, easily measured, precise and accurate, highly sensitive and specific, correlates with disease severity, able to be measured serially to monitor disease progression, and unaffected by other factors is a top priority of the American Society of Nephrology [25, 28, 90–93].

In patients who develop AKI, some biomarker levels have been shown to change earlier than SCr concentrations [17, 22]. Early diagnostic biomarkers of AKI include plasma and urine neutrophil gelatinase-associated lipocalin (NGAL), urinary cystatin C, urinary kidney injury molecule (KIM-1), urinary interleukin-18 (IL-18), and glutathione S-transferase (GST), which have been shown to be present approximately 48 hours before AKI develops [25, 28, 94]. Insulin-like growth factor-binding protein 7 (IGFBP7) and tissue inhibitor of metalloproteinases-2 (TIMP-2) are cycle arrest biomarkers that induce G_1 cell cycle arrest; they are novel markers of AKI that have performed better than any other biomarker to date [28, 30]. Biomarkers are also useful in determining the clinical course of AKI, including severity, duration, hospital length of stay, mortality, and likelihood of renal recovery; prognostic biomarkers include plasma NGAL, *N*-acetyl-ß-(D)-glucosaminidase (NAG), urinary KIM-1, and urinary IL-18. In particular, urinary NGAL has been shown to be highly sensitive (90%) and specific (99%) for AKI, as well as distinguishing AKI versus CKD and identifying different causes of AKI [25, 28].

With respect to CKD, NGAL is a promising biomarker for CKD progression, along with cystatin C for CKD progression, renal function, and cardiovascular risk [95]. Increased levels of asymmetric dimethylarginine (ADMA) have been associated with rapid renal function loss and may cause renal dysfunction from glomerular hypertension and endothelial damage [92, 93].

Renal biomarkers have potential diagnostic and prognostic value for AKI and CKD, although, currently, there is insufficient evidence regarding their role in clinical decision-making [25, 28]. One significant limitation regarding the use of biomarkers is that renal disease follows a continuum and is not separated into distinct entities, making it difficult to set a threshold or discriminatory zone separating AKI from CKD [28]. In addition, AKI increases the risk of CKD development, and CKD is a risk factor for AKI [16, 18, 25, 96–99]. As would be expected, AKI and CKD share biomarkers, reflecting the continuous nature of renal disease. Many other questions remain. What management should be implemented if biomarkers are positive? At what biomarker threshold should we initiate dialysis? Does early intervention decrease morbidity and mortality? What is the temporal relationship between the collection of the biomarker and the diagnosis of AKI? Are these biomarkers consistent across subgroups of patients (i.e., sepsis, postkidney transplant, etc.)? Future studies need to address these and many other questions [25, 28].

Imaging

Renal ultrasonography is useful in identifying either small kidneys providing evidence of chronic kidney disease or medical renal disease, or hydronephrosis suggesting an obstructive process [17, 22, 30]. Whenever urinary tract obstruction is considered in the differential diagnosis, ultrasonography provides a readily available, noninvasive, accurate, reliable, cost-effective, and reproducible radiologic evaluation of the renal and urinary systems [27]; findings may include ureteral and renal pelvis dilatation. In intrinsic renal disease, ultrasonography may show increased echogenicity of the renal parenchyma, although this is neither sensitive nor specific [27].

Computed tomography (CT) or magnetic resonance imaging (MRI) may identify an obstructive process or parenchymal renal disease, although they are of limited value and generally do not provide additional information [27].

Dialysis

Given, as discussed above, that an emergency department assessment of GFR is generally one time point, often without the benefit of the knowledge of baseline SCr values, renal replacement therapy should only be instituted for an emergent indication. Although there are some studies that suggest that earlier initiation, AKIN stage 2, of renal replacement therapy (RRT) may improve outcomes, other studies suggest earlier initiation does not improve outcomes and no study has studied AKI in the emergency department. Thus, the conventional indications for renal replacement therapy are:

1. Volume overload unresponsive to diuretic therapy
2. Hyperkalemia refractory to medical management

3. Metabolic acidosis refractory to medical management
4. Uremia with symptoms of encephalopathy, pericarditis, or uremic bleeding
5. Intoxication with a drug that can be removed with dialysis

In addition, a broader clinical context which includes general severity of illness, number of failed nonrenal organs, presence of oliguria and fluid overload, whether patient is recovering or deteriorating, and AKI with severe multiorgan dysfunction may benefit from early initiation of RRT.

Volume Overload

Volume overload is an indication for initiation for RRT in 2% of AKI [100], in those individuals not responsive to diuretic therapy. Interestingly, in a patient with AKI, being nonresponsive to diuretics is associated with worse outcomes. This concept was formalized by the "furosemide stress test" [101]. In this test, critically ill subjects with early AKI who responded to a single dose of 1.0 or 1.5 mg/kg, depending on prior furosemide exposure, with less than 200 mL of urine output during the next 2 hours were more likely to have progression of the AKI.

Given the role of kidney ischemia in worsening AKI, it is important if dialysis is being initiated for volume overload to remove volume in a manner that does not worsen the blood pressure. However, while RRT can be limited to solitary fluid removal (ultrafiltration), conventional dialysis should be performed as well if volume overload is associated with metabolic abnormalities.

Hyperkalemia

Hyperkalemia is an indication for initiation for RRT in ~22% of AKI [100], in those individuals not responsive to medical therapy. However, over the past 2 years, an additional treatment has been added to the traditional medical management of insulin and D50, albuterol, sodium polystyrene sulfonate, and/or diuretics, and patiromer [102] and sodium zirconium cyclosilicate [103] are the novel potassium binders. While these treatments are not FDA approved for emergent treatment of hyperkalemia, 8.4–25.2 g of oral patiromer reliably will reduce potassium within 7 hours.

It is recommended that patients who take patiromer should avoid taking other oral medications at least 3 hours before or 3 hours after other oral medications (Veltassa [patiromer for oral suspension] prescribing information: Relypsa Inc., Redwood City, CA).

Relypsa Inc. FDA approves supplemental new drug application for Veltassa removing boxed warning regarding drug-drug interactions. Press release 27 November 2016.

While RRT will reliably reduce potassium, using a potassium dialysate <2 mEq/L has been associated with increased risk of arrhythmias and sudden cardiac death in dialysis units [104, 105].

Metabolic Acidosis

Metabolic acidosis is an indication for initiation for RRT in ~29% of AKI [100], in those individuals not responsive to medical therapy. Treatment of metabolic acidosis is the replacement with sodium bicarbonate. However, in cases of severe ongoing lactic acidosis or in cases were severe volume overload limits the ability to administer sodium bicarbonate, RRT is indicated.

Uremia

While BUN is the easily measurable uremic toxin, uremia has been associated with an increase in dozens of solutes affected by kidney insufficiency [106], and thus uremia as an emergent indication of dialysis should not be determined by a sole urea value alone. Rather, the constellation of uremic symptoms such as early morning nausea, pruritis, sleep reversal, loss of appetite, and difficulty concentrating should all be considered in diagnosing uremia. Emergent uremic indication for RRT would be pericarditis, encephalopathy, or bleeding thought to be secondary to uremia.

Intoxications

The emergency department is the primary site for diagnosis of toxic ingestions, and hemodialysis has been demonstrated to be an effective treatment of toxic alcohol ingestion (such as methanol or ethanol glycol), salicylate overdose, severe valproic acid toxicity, metformin overdose, and lithium poisoning. In the case of alcohol ingestions, the indications would be as discussed above, severe metabolic acidosis, worsening AKI and target organ damage, such as retinal toxicity in the case of methanol intoxication [107] and AKI in the case of ethylene glycol toxicity [108].

The efficacy of dialysis to remove toxins in general is dependent on a number of different factors. A knowledge of how different toxins and medications are cleared and their volume of distribution, protein binding, and molecular weight all help to determine the potential benefit of utilizing renal replacement therapy and determining the optimal type of RRT for any toxin or medication. When the clearance of a toxin, drug, or metabolite is dependent on renal clearance, in the setting of AKI, RRT may be considered. Since removal of a toxin, drug, or metabolite by dialysis is dependent on the substance passing through the pores of a membrane, large molecular weight medications are less effectively cleared than lower molecular weight substances. Also, substances that have a high protein binding are also removed less efficiently by RRT than substances that are water soluble. Finally, medications with a large volume of distribution will take longer to clear than medications that have a smaller volume of distribution.

Methanol

Methanol is found in rocket fuels and as a general solvent in many household products such as windshield washers, paint removers, carburetor cleaners, and deicing fluids. The diagnosis of methanol intoxication should be considered in those patients with an anion gap acidosis and who have an osmolar gap. Classic findings of methanol intoxication are hyperemic optic disks and putamen swelling which occur when methanol is metabolized to formic acid. While fomepizole is considered first-line treatment of a methanol ingestion (see Chap. 28), hemodialysis should be considered for severe metabolic acidosis, renal failure, electrolyte disturbance unresponsive to conventional therapy, visual symptoms, deteriorating vital signs despite intensive care, and plasma methanol concentration ≥50 mg/dL (15.6 mmol/L) [109, 110].

Ethylene Glycol

Like methanol, ethylene glycol ingestion is also associated with an anion gap and an osmolar gap. The primary source of ethylene glycol ingestion is due to automotive antifreeze ingestion. The classic findings with ethylene glycol ingestion are flank pain, hematuria, and glycolate-induced damage to tubules. Similar to methanol, fomepizole is considered first-line treatment of an ethylene glycol ingestion. Hemodialysis should be considered for severe metabolic acidosis, renal failure, electrolyte imbalances unresponsive to conventional therapy, and deteriorating vital signs despite intensive, supportive care. While initial serum glycolic acid >8 seems to be a good criterion for the initiation of hemodialysis, dialysis is not necessary regardless of ethylene glycol level, specifically when glycolic acid is ≤8 mmol/L, or in patients receiving fomepizole [111] when glycolic acid levels are not readily available.

Unlike methanol and ethylene glycol, isopropyl alcohol does not cause an elevated anion gap acidosis, retinal toxicity (as does methanol), or renal failure (as does ethylene glycol). The hallmark of isopropyl alcohol is an increase in the serum osmolality as well as ketonemia and ketonuria, since isopropanol is metabolized by alcohol dehydrogenase to acetone, a terminal ketone. While metabolic acidosis is usually absent, the hypotension associated with isopropyl alcohol could be severe enough to produce lactic acidosis. Isopropyl alcohol is found in rubbing alcohol, hand sanitizers, and certain cleaning products and supportive measures are often sufficient.

However, if hypotension is present along with coma, then initiation of hemodialysis has been recommended. Given the effectiveness of dialysis in removing isopropanol and the safety of this procedure, it seems reasonable to initiate hemodialysis in the presence of severe coma, hypotension, or serum isopropanol levels >200 mg/dL.

Salicylate

Hemodialysis is the most efficient way to eliminate salicylate and normalize salicylate-induced acid-base and electrolyte imbalances [112]. Indications for hemodialysis include serum salicylate level greater than 120 mg/dL acutely or greater than 100 mg/dL 6 h postingestion, renal insufficiency, severe pulmonary edema, altered mental status, deteriorating vital signs, and severe acid-base disturbance or clinical deterioration despite treatment [113, 114]. In chronic overdose, hemodialysis may be required for a symptomatic patient with a serum salicylate level greater than 60 mg/dL.

Although charcoal hemoperfusion has a slightly higher rate of drug clearance than hemodialysis, dialysis is recommended because of its ability to correct for fluid and electrolyte disorders and to remove salicylates. Peritoneal dialysis is only 10–25% as efficient as hemoperfusion or hemodialysis and is not even as efficient as renal excretion.

Options for RRT

No study has convincingly demonstrated that one type of RRT is more advantageous than another, and thus the availability of different modalities and staff familiarity with a particular modality are usually the deciding factors with regard to what type of RRT is performed.

Hemodialysis

With regard to hemodialysis, the filter used determines whether high efficiency or high flux verse standard dialysis is performed. In both modalities, the clearance is diffusion with the major difference being the pore size of the membrane, membrane type, and dialysis flow. The pore size in high-flux dialysis is generally as large as 20 kDa.

Continuous Renal Replacement Therapy (CRRT)

CRRT either in a convective mode by effecting mass transport across the membrane or in a diffusive mode is routinely used in patients with AKI. Studies using sieving coefficients have clearly demonstrated that there is a higher clearance of larger molecular weight molecules and higher protein membrane mediations when convective clearance is used [115]. Therefore, if CRRT is to be used for intoxications, the focus should be predominantly on a convective modality. A large disadvantage of CRRT is that it is less efficient and the patient has less mobility as compared to hemodialysis (HD) [116].

Peritoneal Dialysis (PD)

The most likely reason to encounter PD in the emergency room is peritonitis. Peritonitis should be suspected in all patients with a PD catheter who presents to the emergency department with gastrointestinal or intra-abdominal symptoms. These include, but are not limited to, pain localized or generalized over abdomen; nausea, vomiting, or diarrhea; fever; and/or a cloudy PD effluent.

Abdominal examination of patient suspected of PD peritonitis should include examination of the exit site which should be performed in a sterile manner. The PD catheter tunnel assessment should include an examination for focal tenderness or exudate for evidence of occult catheter-associated hernia or focal intra-abdominal process. If a focal or intra-abdominal pathology is suspected, further evaluation may be required including CT of the abdomen and a possible surgical consult. However, routine CT for PD peritonitis is not indicated.

Ideally the PD catheter should be manipulated and accessed only by a trained dialysis provider. In order to diagnose or rule out peritonitis, peritoneal fluid needs to be obtained. If the patient presents to the ED with a dialysis dwell that is greater than 2 hours but less than 24 hours old, the dialysis provider can drain that fluid directly and send it for the PD fluid cell count, Gram stain, and cultures. If the patient has a dry abdomen and PD peritonitis is suspected, the patient should receive his or her regular dwell volume following lavage, and PD fluid cell count, Gram stain, and culture should be sent only after a dwell of 4 hours (minimum of 2 hours).

Once the PD fluid cell count, Gram stain, and cultures are sent, intraperitoneal (IP) administration of antibiotics can proceed. If the dialysate is cloudy or the peritoneal WBC is greater than 100 with over 50% PMS, peritonitis should be assumed and antibiotics for gram-positive and/or gram-negative organisms should be initiated based on the Gram stain and clinical circumstance. For coverage of Gram-positive organisms, Ancef 1–1.5g IP daily or vancomycin 1–1.5 g IP every 5–7 days should be initiated, and for gram-negative organisms, ceftazidime 1–1.5g IP daily or cefepime 1 g IP daily should be initiated. Importantly, intraperitoneal administration of antibiotics is the preferred route for the treatment of PD peritonitis since many, if not all, antibiotics compatible with the intraperitoneal administration have excellent systemic bioavailability (e.g., vancomycin, ceftazidime, cefazolin, cefepime, ampicillin, fluconazole, etc.).

A stable, uncomplicated PD peritonitis patient usually does not require hospitalization and can be treated with outpatient therapy. Common indications for hospitalizations for a suspected PD peritonitis include uncontrolled/severe abdominal pain not relieved despite abdominal lavage; intractable/severe GI symptoms; suspected intra-abdominal causes such as complicated hernia, diverticulitis, perforations, and cholecystitis; or the presence of systemic inflammatory response syndrome (SIRS) or sepsis with hypotension.

References

1. Palmer LG, Schnermann J. Integrated control of Na transport along the nephron. Clin J Am Soc Nephrol. 2015;10(4):676–87.
2. Dunn A, Lo V, Donnelly S. The role of the kidney in blood volume regulation: the kidney as a regulator of the hematocrit. Am J Med Sci. 2007;334(1): 65–71.
3. Rizzo JD, et al. Erythropoietin: a paradigm for the development of practice guidelines. Hematol Am Soc Hematol Educ Program. 2001;2001:10–30.
4. Gattineni J, Baum M. Regulation of phosphate transport by fibroblast growth factor 23 (FGF23): implications for disorders of phosphate metabolism. Pediatr Nephrol. 2010;25(4):591–601.
5. Martin A, David V, Quarles LD. Regulation and function of the FGF23/klotho endocrine pathways. Physiol Rev. 2012;92(1):131–55.
6. Razzaque MS. Bone-kidney axis in systemic phosphate turnover. Arch Biochem Biophys. 2014;561C:154–8.
7. George AL, Neilson EG. Cellular and molecular biology of the kidney. In: Fauci A, editor. Harrison's principles of internal medicine. New York: McGraw-Hill; 2015.
8. Wagner CA, et al. Regulated acid-base transport in the collecting duct. Pflugers Arch. 2009;458(1): 137–56.
9. Nakamura M, et al. Roles of renal proximal tubule transport in acid/base balance and blood pressure regulation. Biomed Res Int. 2014;2014:504808.
10. Jacques T, et al. Overexpression of pendrin in intercalated cells produces chloride-sensitive hypertension. J Am Soc Nephrol. 2013;24(7):1104–13.
11. Buxton IO, Benet LZ. Goodman & Gilman's the pharmacological basis of therapeutics. In: Brunton LL, editor. Goodman & Gilman's the pharmacological basis of therapeutics. New York: McGraw-Hill; 2011.
12. Nolin TD, et al. Emerging evidence of the impact of kidney disease on drug metabolism and transport. Clin Pharmacol Ther. 2008;83(6):898–903.
13. Lote CJ, editor. Principles of renal physiology. 5th ed. New York: Springer; 2012.
14. Kotchen TA, Guthrie GP Jr. Renin-angiotensin-aldosterone and hypertension. Endocr Rev. 1980;1(1):78–99.
15. Jelkmann W. Regulation of erythropoietin production. J Physiol. 2011;589(Pt 6):1251–8.
16. Chawla LS, et al. The severity of acute kidney injury predicts progression to chronic kidney disease. Kidney Int. 2011;79(12):1361–9.
17. Bellomo R, Kellum JA, Ronco C. Acute kidney injury. Lancet. 2012;380(9843):756–66.
18. James MT, et al. Glomerular filtration rate, proteinuria, and the incidence and consequences of acute kidney injury: a cohort study. Lancet. 2010;376(9758):2096–103.

19. Star RA. Treatment of acute renal failure. Kidney Int. 1998;54(6):1817–31.
20. Bellomo R, et al. Acute renal failure – definition, outcome measures, animal models, fluid therapy and information technology needs: the second international consensus conference of the Acute Dialysis Quality Initiative (ADQI) Group. Crit Care. 2004;8(4):R204–12.
21. Ricci Z, Cruz D, Ronco C. The RIFLE criteria and mortality in acute kidney injury: a systematic review. Kidney Int. 2008;73(5):538–46.
22. Lameire NH, et al. Acute kidney injury: an increasing global concern. Lancet. 2013;382(9887):170–9.
23. Barasch J, Zager R, Bonventre JV. Acute kidney injury: a problem of definition. Lancet. 2017;389(10071):779–81.
24. Lameire N, Van Biesen W, Vanholder R. Acute renal failure. Lancet. 2005;365(9457):417–30.
25. Coca SG, et al. Biomarkers for the diagnosis and risk stratification of acute kidney injury: a systematic review. Kidney Int. 2008;73(9):1008–16.
26. Mehta RL, Chertow GM. Acute renal failure definitions and classification: time for change? J Am Soc Nephrol. 2003;14(8):2178–87.
27. Kaul A, Ruhela V. Approach to a patient with acute kidney injury. Clin Queries Nephrol. 2012;1(1):6–12.
28. Wasung ME, Chawla LS, Madero M. Biomarkers of renal function, which and when? Clin Chim Acta. 2015;438:350–7.
29. Vanmassenhove J, et al. Management of patients at risk of acute kidney injury. Lancet. 2017;389(10084):2139–51.
30. Kellum JA. Diagnostic criteria for acute kidney injury: present and future. Crit Care Clin. 2015;31(4):621–32.
31. Kellum JA, et al. Developing a consensus classification system for acute renal failure. Curr Opin Crit Care. 2002;8(6):509–14.
32. Lopes JA, Jorge S. The RIFLE and AKIN classifications for acute kidney injury: a critical and comprehensive review. Clin Kidney J. 2013;6(1):8–14.
33. Mehta RL, et al. Acute Kidney Injury Network: report of an initiative to improve outcomes in acute kidney injury. Crit Care. 2007;11(2):R31.
34. Sawhney S, Fraser SD. Epidemiology of AKI: utilizing large databases to determine the burden of AKI. Adv Chronic Kidney Dis. 2017;24(4):194–204.
35. Group, T.K.D.I.G.O.K.W. Definition and classification of acute kidney injury. Kidney Int. 2012;Suppl 2:19–36.
36. Manjunath G, Sarnak MJ, Levey AS. Prediction equations to estimate glomerular filtration rate: an update. Curr Opin Nephrol Hypertens. 2001;10(6):785–92.
37. National Kidney Foundation. K/DOQI clinical practice guidelines for chronic kidney disease: evaluation, classification, and stratification. Am J Kidney Dis. 2002;39(2 Suppl 1):S1–266.
38. Cruz DN, et al. North East Italian Prospective Hospital Renal Outcome Survey on Acute Kidney Injury (NEiPHROS-AKI): targeting the problem with the RIFLE criteria. Clin J Am Soc Nephrol CJASN. 2007;2(3):418–25.
39. Hoste EA, et al. RIFLE criteria for acute kidney injury are associated with hospital mortality in critically ill patients: a cohort analysis. Crit Care. 2006;10(3):R73.
40. Ali T, et al. Incidence and outcomes in acute kidney injury: a comprehensive population-based study. J Am Soc Nephrol. 2007;18(4):1292–8.
41. Hsu CY, et al. Community-based incidence of acute renal failure. Kidney Int. 2007;72(2):208–12.
42. Liangos O, et al. Epidemiology and outcomes of acute renal failure in hospitalized patients: a national survey. Clin J Am Soc Nephrol CJASN. 2006;1(1):43–51.
43. Nash K, Hafeez A, Hou S. Hospital-acquired renal insufficiency. Am J Kidney Dis. 2002;39(5):930–6.
44. Sawhney S, et al. Intermediate and long-term outcomes of survivors of acute kidney injury episodes: a large population-based Cohort Study. Am J Kidney Dis. 2017;69(1):18–28.
45. de Mendonca A, et al. Acute renal failure in the ICU: risk factors and outcome evaluated by the SOFA score. Intensive Care Med. 2000;26(7):915–21.
46. Bagshaw SM, George C, Bellomo R. Early acute kidney injury and sepsis: a multicentre evaluation. Crit Care. 2008;12(2):R47.
47. Cosentino F, Chaff C, Piedmonte M. Risk factors influencing survival in ICU acute renal failure. Nephrol Dial Transplant. 1994;9(Suppl 4):179–82.
48. Liano F, Pascual J. Epidemiology of acute renal failure: a prospective, multicenter, community-based study. Madrid Acute Renal Failure Study Group. Kidney Int. 1996;50(3):811–8.
49. Ahlstrom A, et al. Comparison of 2 acute renal failure severity scores to general scoring systems in the critically ill. Am J Kidney Dis. 2006;48(2):262–8.
50. Bell M, et al. Optimal follow-up time after continuous renal replacement therapy in actual renal failure patients stratified with the RIFLE criteria. Nephrol Dial Transplant. 2005;20(2):354–60.
51. Uchino S, et al. An assessment of the RIFLE criteria for acute renal failure in hospitalized patients. Crit Care Med. 2006;34(7):1913–7.
52. Chertow GM, et al. Acute kidney injury, mortality, length of stay, and costs in hospitalized patients. J Am Soc Nephrol. 2005;16(11):3365–70.
53. Metnitz PG, et al. Effect of acute renal failure requiring renal replacement therapy on outcome in critically ill patients. Crit Care Med. 2002;30(9):2051–8.
54. Amdur RL, et al. Outcomes following diagnosis of acute renal failure in U.S. veterans: focus on acute tubular necrosis. Kidney Int. 2009;76(10):1089–97.
55. Bellomo R, et al. Acute kidney injury in sepsis. Intensive Care Med. 2017;43(6):816–28.
56. Sharfuddin AA, Molitoris BA. Pathophysiology of ischemic acute kidney injury. Nat Rev Nephrol. 2011;7(4):189–200.
57. Ostermann M, Liu K. Pathophysiology of AKI. Best Pract Res Clin Anaesthesiol. 2017;31(3):305–14.

58. Kumar J. Pathophysiology of ischemic acute tubular necrosis. Clin Queries Nephrol. 2012;1(1):18–26.
59. Post EH, et al. Renal perfusion in sepsis: from macro- to microcirculation. Kidney Int. 2017;91(1):45–60.
60. Raimundo M, et al. Low systemic oxygen delivery and BP and risk of progression of early AKI. Clin J Am Soc Nephrol CJASN. 2015;10(8):1340–9.
61. Poukkanen M, et al. Hemodynamic variables and progression of acute kidney injury in critically ill patients with severe sepsis: data from the prospective observational FINNAKI study. Crit Care. 2013;17(6):R295.
62. Martin C, et al. Renal effects of norepinephrine used to treat septic shock patients. Crit Care Med. 1990;18(3):282–5.
63. Izawa J, et al. Early-phase cumulative hypotension duration and severe-stage progression in oliguric acute kidney injury with and without sepsis: an observational study. Crit Care. 2016;20(1):405.
64. Sun LY, et al. Association of intraoperative hypotension with acute kidney injury after elective noncardiac surgery. Anesthesiology. 2015;123(3):515–23.
65. Wesselink EM, et al. Intraoperative hypotension and the risk of postoperative adverse outcomes: a systematic review. Br J Anaesth. 2018;121(4):706–21.
66. Walsh M, et al. Relationship between intraoperative mean arterial pressure and clinical outcomes after noncardiac surgery: toward an empirical definition of hypotension. Anesthesiology. 2013;119(3):507–15.
67. Prowle J, Bagshaw SM, Bellomo R. Renal blood flow, fractional excretion of sodium and acute kidney injury: time for a new paradigm? Curr Opin Crit Care. 2012;18(6):585–92.
68. Bougle A, Duranteau J. Pathophysiology of sepsis-induced acute kidney injury: the role of global renal blood flow and renal vascular resistance. Contrib Nephrol. 2011;174:89–97.
69. Bellomo R, et al. Septic acute kidney injury: the glomerular arterioles. Contrib Nephrol. 2011;174:98–107.
70. Ergin B, et al. The renal microcirculation in sepsis. Nephrol Dial Transplant. 2015;30(2):169–77.
71. Legrand M, et al. Renal hypoxia and dysoxia after reperfusion of the ischemic kidney. Mol Med. 2008;14(7–8):502–16.
72. Verma SK, Molitoris BA. Renal endothelial injury and microvascular dysfunction in acute kidney injury. Semin Nephrol. 2015;35(1):96–107.
73. Zarbock A, Gomez H, Kellum JA. Sepsis-induced acute kidney injury revisited: pathophysiology, prevention and future therapies. Curr Opin Crit Care. 2014;20(6):588–95.
74. Sutton TA. Alteration of microvascular permeability in acute kidney injury. Microvasc Res. 2009;77(1):4–7.
75. Versteilen AM, et al. Rho-kinase inhibition reduces early microvascular leukocyte accumulation in the rat kidney following ischemia-reperfusion injury: roles of nitric oxide and blood flow. Nephron Exp Nephrol. 2011;118(4):e79–86.
76. Kwon O, Hong SM, Ramesh G. Diminished NO generation by injured endothelium and loss of macula densa nNOS may contribute to sustained acute kidney injury after ischemia-reperfusion. Am J Physiol Renal Physiol. 2009;296(1):F25–33.
77. Kato N, et al. The E-selectin ligand basigin/CD147 is responsible for neutrophil recruitment in renal ischemia/reperfusion. J Am Soc Nephrol. 2009;20(7):1565–76.
78. Pulskens WP, et al. Toll-like receptor-4 coordinates the innate immune response of the kidney to renal ischemia/reperfusion injury. PLoS One. 2008;3(10):e3596.
79. Chawla LS, et al. Elevated plasma concentrations of IL-6 and elevated APACHE II score predict acute kidney injury in patients with severe sepsis. Clin J Am Soc Nephrol CJASN. 2007;2(1):22–30.
80. Thurman JM. Triggers of inflammation after renal ischemia/reperfusion. Clin Immunol. 2007;123(1):7–13.
81. Molitoris BA, Sandoval RM. Kidney endothelial dysfunction: ischemia, localized infections and sepsis. Contrib Nephrol. 2011;174:108–18.
82. Gomez H, et al. A unified theory of sepsis-induced acute kidney injury: inflammation, microcirculatory dysfunction, bioenergetics, and the tubular cell adaptation to injury. Shock. 2014;41(1):3–11.
83. Zuk A, et al. Polarity, integrin, and extracellular matrix dynamics in the postischemic rat kidney. Am J Physiol. 1998;275(3 Pt 1):C711–31.
84. Agarwal A, et al. Cellular and molecular mechanisms of AKI. J Am Soc Nephrol. 2016;27(5):1288–99.
85. Blantz RC. Pathophysiology of pre-renal azotemia. Kidney Int. 1998;53(2):512–23.
86. Kanagasundaram NS, Arunachalam C. Assessment and initial management of acute kidney injury. Medicine. 2015;43(8):440–5.
87. Jeloka TK. Pathophysiology of acute interstitial nephritis. Clin Queries Nephrol. 2012;1(1):27–8.
88. Perazella MA. Renal vulnerability to drug toxicity. Clin J Am Soc Nephrol CJASN. 2009;4(7):1275–83.
89. Chen S. Retooling the creatinine clearance equation to estimate kinetic GFR when the plasma creatinine is changing acutely. J Am Soc Nephrol. 2013;24(6):877–88.
90. Schiffl H, Lang SM. Update on biomarkers of acute kidney injury: moving closer to clinical impact? Mol Diagn Ther. 2012;16(4):199–207.
91. American Society of Nephrology. American Society of Nephrology renal research report. J Am Soc Nephrol. 2005;16(7):1886–903.
92. Khan Z, Pandey M. Role of kidney biomarkers of chronic kidney disease: an update. Saudi J Biol Sci. 2014;21(4):294–9.
93. Breit M, Weinberger KM. Metabolic biomarkers for chronic kidney disease. Arch Biochem Biophys. 2016;589:62–80.
94. Herget-Rosenthal S, et al. Early detection of acute renal failure by serum cystatin C. Kidney Int. 2004;66(3):1115–22.

95. Fassett RG, et al. Biomarkers in chronic kidney disease: a review. Kidney Int. 2011;80(8):806–21.
96. Ishani A, et al. Acute kidney injury increases risk of ESRD among elderly. J Am Soc Nephrol. 2009;20(1):223–8.
97. Lo LJ, et al. Dialysis-requiring acute renal failure increases the risk of progressive chronic kidney disease. Kidney Int. 2009;76(8):893–9.
98. Uchino S, et al. Acute renal failure in critically ill patients: a multinational, multicenter study. JAMA. 2005;294(7):813–8.
99. Mehta RL, et al. Spectrum of acute renal failure in the intensive care unit: the PICARD experience. Kidney Int. 2004;66(4):1613–21.
100. Vaara ST, et al. Timing of RRT based on the presence of conventional indications. Clin J Am Soc Nephrol. 2014;9(9):1577–85.
101. Chawla LS, et al. Development and standardization of a furosemide stress test to predict the severity of acute kidney injury. Crit Care. 2013;17(5):R207.
102. Weir MR, et al. Patiromer in patients with kidney disease and hyperkalemia receiving RAAS inhibitors. N Engl J Med. 2015;372(3):211–21.
103. Packham DK, et al. Sodium zirconium cyclosilicate in hyperkalemia. N Engl J Med. 2015;372(3):222–31.
104. Pun PH, et al. Modifiable risk factors associated with sudden cardiac arrest within hemodialysis clinics. Kidney Int. 2011;79(2):218–27.
105. Karnik JA, et al. Cardiac arrest and sudden death in dialysis units. Kidney Int. 2001;60(1):350–7.
106. Duranton F, et al. Normal and pathologic concentrations of uremic toxins. J Am Soc Nephrol. 2012;23(7):1258–70.
107. Schep LJ, et al. Diethylene glycol poisoning. Clin Toxicol (Phila). 2009;47(6):525–35.
108. Barceloux DG, et al. American Academy of clinical toxicology practice guidelines on the treatment of ethylene glycol poisoning. Ad Hoc Committee. J Toxicol Clin Toxicol. 1999;37(5):537–60.
109. Hovda KE, et al. Methanol and formate kinetics during treatment with fomepizole. Clin Toxicol (Phila). 2005;43(4):221–7.
110. Barceloux DG, et al. American Academy of Clinical Toxicology practice guidelines on the treatment of methanol poisoning. J Toxicol Clin Toxicol. 2002;40(4):415–46.
111. Porter WH, et al. Ethylene glycol toxicity: the role of serum glycolic acid in hemodialysis. J Toxicol Clin Toxicol. 2001;39(6):607–15.
112. Magness JL, Murray JB. Treatment of salicylate intoxication using extracorporeal hemodialysis. J Lancet. 1961;81:253–4.
113. McGuigan MA. A two-year review of salicylate deaths in Ontario. Arch Intern Med. 1987;147(3):510–2.
114. Murray PT, Brady HR, Hall JB. Clinical toxicology. In: Intensive care in nephrology. London; New York: Taylor and Francis; 2005.
115. Messer J, Mulcahy B, Fissell WH. Middle-molecule clearance in CRRT: in vitro convection, diffusion and dialyzer area. ASAIO J. 2009;55(3):224–6.
116. Kim Z, Goldfarb DS. Continuous renal replacement therapy does not have a clear role in the treatment of poisoning. Nephron Clin Pract. 2010;115(1):c1–6.

Acid-Base and Electrolyte Disorders in Emergency Critical Care

18

Sage P. Whitmore and Kyle J. Gunnerson

Normal Acid-Base Physiology and Definitions

Acid-base balance contributes to normal cellular function, with normal serum pH falling between 7.35 and 7.45 [1]. Acid*emia* is defined as a decrease in serum pH below 7.35 and alkal*emia* a rise above 7.45; the terms acid*osis* and alkal*osis* refer to primary pathologic processes regardless of the overall pH. These processes may be acute, chronic, or a combination thereof, depending on the underlying disease state(s).

The major determinants of blood pH are as follows: (1) the partial pressure of carbon dioxide (PCO_2), (2) the balance of strong ions such as sodium (Na+) and chloride (Cl−), and (3) the presence of weak organic acids [2]. Carbohydrate and fat metabolism produces CO_2, a volatile acid excreted via alveolar ventilation. Protein metabolism produces phosphate, sulfur, and nitrogen waste, nonvolatile weak acids which are excreted by the kidney. Bicarbonate (HCO_{3-}) ion concentration changes as a result of acid-base conditions and is a measurable marker of acid-base disorders.

The carbonic anhydrase equation offers a simplistic conceptualization of the balance of volatile and nonvolatile acids in the body [3]:

$$H^+ + HCO_3^- \leftrightarrow H_2O + CO_2 \leftrightarrow \text{alveolar ventilation}$$

Alveolar hypoventilation will increase PCO_2 and cause acidosis (right-to-left shift in the equation); adding nonvolatile acid (H+) to the system will result in rapid buffering and conversion of bicarbonate (HCO_3^-) to water and CO_2, which requires increased alveolar ventilation to balance the pH (left-to-right shift of the equation).

Nonvolatile acids are elegantly managed by the kidneys. These protein byproducts are buffered by sodium bicarbonate ($NaHCO_3$) and become sodium salts; they are converted to ammonia (NH4+) in the kidney, and with the assistance of carbonic anhydrase enzymes, H+ is excreted while HCO_{3-} is reabsorbed [3]. In response to acidosis, the net renal acid excretion must increase: ammoniagenesis increases with increased NH4+ excretion and $NaHCO_3$ reabsorption, and increased mineralocorticoid activity in response to acidosis increases Na + reabsorption in exchange for H (and K+) excretion in the distal tubule.

In the acute response to metabolic acidosis, respiratory centers within the brainstem will increase minute ventilation via increased tidal volume and respiratory rate in an attempt to unload CO_2; this response occurs within minutes [2]. In the case of a metabolic alkalosis, acute compensation

S. P. Whitmore (✉)
Department of Emergency Medicine, Division of Emergency Critical Care, Ann Arbor, MI, USA
e-mail: swhitmor@med.umich.edu

K. J. Gunnerson
Emergency Medicine, Anesthesiology, and Internal Medicine, University of Michigan Health Center, Ann Arbor, MI, USA

© Springer Nature Switzerland AG 2020
J. R. Shiber, S. D. Weingart (eds.), *Emergency Department Critical Care*,
https://doi.org/10.1007/978-3-030-28794-8_18

is again a respiratory phenomenon, with decreased alveolar ventilation and CO_2 retention. Importantly, compensatory mechanisms mitigate pH changes but do not overcorrect or normalize pH.

Compensation for respiratory acid-base disturbances occurs mostly via renal mechanisms, which take several days to come fully online [4]. During acute respiratory acidosis, pH will drop briskly and the kidneys will attempt to retain HCO_3^-, increasing over 24–48 hours to blunt the acidemia. During acute respiratory alkalosis, the kidney begins to excrete HCO_3^-, again becoming more efficient after 24–48 hours. Table 18.1 demonstrates the typical compensation patterns for various primary acid-base disturbances. Acid-base compensation may be dangerously inadequate in patients with neurologic, pulmonary, and renal comorbidities, requiring direct medical intervention such as mechanical ventilation or bicarbonate infusion.

Table 18.1 Summary of compensatory changes in acid-base disorders

Primary disorder	Expected compensation
Metabolic acidosis	$PCO_2 = 1.5\ (HCO_3) + 8$
Metabolic alkalosis	$PCO_2 = 0.9\ (HCO_3) + 15$
Acute respiratory acidosis	$\Delta\ HCO_3 = 0.1\ (\Delta\ PCO_2)$
Chronic respiratory acidosis	$\Delta\ HCO_3 = 0.35\ (\Delta\ PCO_2)$
Acute respiratory alkalosis	$\Delta\ HCO_3 = 0.2\ (\Delta\ PCO_2)$
Chronic respiratory alkalosis	$\Delta\ HCO_3 = 0.5\ (\Delta\ PCO_2)$

Physiologic Effects of Acidemia and Alkalemia

The clinical significance of acid-base disorders varies greatly depending on acuity, individual host factors, and the underlying disease(s). Extreme derangements in pH may manifest as central nervous system dysfunction and cardiovascular collapse; however, in vivo studies demonstrate a wide range of compensatory and adaptive responses to acidemia in particular. Table 18.2 summarizes important physiologic effects of acid-base disturbances.

It is generally thought that a pH <7.2 exerts deleterious effects on end-organ function [5]. These effects are widespread and may include cerebral

Table 18.2 Important physiologic effects of acid-base disturbances

Body system	Acidemia	Alkalemia
CNS	Cerebral edema Altered mental status Coma	Agitation Seizure Cerebral vasoconstriction/ischemia
Cardiovascular	*Mild acidosis* Increased contractility Increased cardiac output Increased catecholamine response Decreased afterload *Severe acidosis* Decreased contractility[a] Decreased cardiac output Decreased catecholamine response	Coronary vasoconstriction Cardiac ischemia Systemic vasoconstriction Increased LV afterload Malignant arrhythmias
Pulmonary	Increased pulmonary vascular resistance Increased RV afterload RV dysfunction Decreased diaphragm contractility	Decreased pulmonary vascular resistance
Metabolic	Increased serum potassium Increased ionized calcium Increased phosphorus Insulin resistance	Decreased serum potassium Decreased ionized calcium Decreased free magnesium Decreased phosphorus
Peripheral tissues	Vasodilation Oxy-Hgb curve shifts right Increased O_2 delivery to tissues	Vasoconstriction Oxy-Hgb curve shifts left Decreased O_2 delivery to tissues

[a]Lactic acidosis associated with relatively less negative inotropy and diaphragm dysfunction compared to respiratory acidosis

edema, decreased cardiac contractility, hemodynamic changes and altered response to catecholamines, predisposition to arrhythmias, electrolyte abnormalities, insulin resistance, inhibition of anaerobic glycolysis and glucose metabolism, and changes in immune system function [5, 6].

In vitro studies have demonstrated that cardiac contractility and intracellular function, including calcium signaling, suffer in low pH [7–9]; however, a number of in vivo animal and human studies demonstrate that the cardiovascular system responds quite well to modest acidemia (pH ≥7.1). For example, sympathetic tone, cardiac output, blood pressure and flow, and QT interval may hold steady or even improve [10–14]. In response to permissive hypercapnia for acute respiratory distress syndrome, an acute pH drop from 7.4 to around 7.25 resulted in increased cardiac index, decreased systemic vascular resistance, and improved systemic perfusion with no drop in blood pressure [15]. In particular, lactic acidosis does not appear to result in the same negative inotropy seen in respiratory or hyperchloremic acidosis [16].

Acidemia does however significantly affect the right ventricle and diaphragm function. Pulmonary vascular resistance increases in acidemic conditions, worsening right ventricular afterload and contractility [13–15, 17]. Acute respiratory acidosis appears to inhibit diaphragm contractility, and lactic acidosis may suppress diaphragm function when pH <6.9 [17–21].

Tissue perfusion and oxygen delivery are affected by low pH. Acidemia has been shown to increase nitric oxide products and result in arterial hypotension [12]; however, there may be vasodilation within the tissue bed. When combined with a shift of the oxyhemoglobin curve to the right (known as the Bohr effect), oxygen delivery to the tissues may be enhanced; thus, acidemia during hypoxemia may be tissue-protective [15, 17, 22, 23].

It is unclear to what extent acidemia contributes directly to mortality. Cohort studies are contradictory, one illustrating an association between acidemia (particularly lactic acidosis) and mortality; while a second shows no correlation even down to a pH of 6.8 [24, 25]. This implies that it is the underlying disease, not the pH, which is responsible for mortality.

Alkalemia has also been associated with increased mortality [26]. Alkalemia causes decreased cerebral blood flow and cerebral ischemia, systemic arteriolar vasoconstriction and increased left ventricular afterload, coronary vasoconstriction with resultant myocardial ischemia, and decreased threshold for malignant arrhythmias [27]. It may be the multiple associated electrolyte shifts—particularly hypokalemia and hypocalcemia—that are responsible for much of the symptomatology. Oxygen delivery is impeded as the oxyhemoglobin curve shifts to the left [22]. Metabolic alkalosis may impair respiratory drive and interfere with ventilator triggering or weaning in patients with chronic lung disease [28].

Diagnosis of Acid-Base Disorders

The purpose of evaluating a patient's acid-base status is to formulate a differential diagnosis in order to tailor workup and treatment. There are multiple methods used clinically to evaluate and diagnose acid-base disorders, including the Henderson-Hasselbalch method, the Stewart method, and the standard base excess [2]. When used correctly, there is no difference between these methods in identifying and quantifying acid-base disorders [29]. The following steps are suggested using the Henderson-Hasselbalch method. Arterial blood gas (ABG) values are presented as pH/PCO_2.

Step 1: Analyze the ABG for primary disorders.
Step 2: Evaluate serum HCO_3 and test for respiratory compensation.
Step 3: Calculate the anion gap.
Step 4: Calculate the "Gap Rise" to the "Bicarb Drop" ("delta-delta").
Step 5: Calculate the osmolar gap.

Analysis of the Arterial Blood Gas

Analysis of acid-base status begins with arterial pH and PCO_2 (Fig. 18.1). A pH <7.35 confirms a primary acidosis, and a pH >7.45 confirms a primary alkalosis. If the PCO_2 has changed in the *same direction* as the pH, a primary *meta-*

ABG (pH/PCO2)	Pattern	Rules
7.40/40	Normal	
7.24/24	Metabolic acidosis	pH ↓, PCO2 ↓; *change in the **same** direction*
7.24/60	Respiratory acidosis	pH ↓, PCO2 ↑; change in the ***opposite** direction*

ABG (pH/PCO2)	Pattern	Rules
7.24/24	Primary metabolic acidosis, with adequate respiratory compensation	pH ↓, PCO2 ↓; change in the same direction. *PCO2 is **similar** to last two digits of pH*
7.18/34	Primary metabolic acidosis, ***plus*** primary respiratory acidosis	pH ↓, PCO2 ↓; change in the same direction. *However, PCO2 is **much higher** than last two digits of pH*
7.32/18	Primary metabolic acidosis, ***plus*** primary respiratory alkalosis	pH ↓, PCO2 ↓; change in the same direction. *However, PCO2 is **much lower than** last two digits of pH*

ABG (pH/PCO2)	Pattern	Rules
7.24/60	Respiratory acidosis, ***Acute***	Satisfies the **"10-to-0.08 Rule"** *PCO2 ↑ by 20 (2 x **10**); pH ↓ by 0.16 (2 x **0.08**)*
7.34/60	Respiratory acidosis, ***Chronic***	Satisfies the **"10-to-0.03 Rule"** *PCO2 ↑ by 20 (2 x **10**); pH ↓ by 0.06 (2 x **0.03**)*

Fig. 18.1 Examples of acid-base disorders diagnosed by arterial blood gas (ABG)

bolic process is present. If the PCO_2 has changed in the *opposite direction* as the pH, a primary *respiratory* process is present. For example, a patient with an ABG showing 7.30/32 has *primary metabolic acidosis;* a patient with an ABG showing 7.30/54 has a *primary respiratory acidosis.*

If a primary *metabolic* acidosis is identified on the ABG, a rough idea of respiratory compensation can be derived (Fig. 18.1). In a well-compensated metabolic acidosis, the PCO_2 and the *last two digits* of the pH should be roughly the same, and a large disparity may signify poor respiratory compensation (*additional* primary respiratory acidosis) or relative hyperventilation (*additional* primary respiratory alkalosis). For example, an ABG showing 7.24/26 demonstrates adequate respiratory compensation for a primary metabolic acidosis. An ABG showing 7.12/30 demonstrates inadequate respiratory compensation, with an inappropriately high PCO_2 relative to the pH.

If a primary *respiratory* acidosis is identified on the ABG, clues regarding acuity versus chronicity may be gleaned from the ratio of PCO_2 rise to pH drop (Fig. 18.1). In an *acute* respiratory acidosis, the pH will drop by 0.08 for every 10 mmHg rise in the PCO_2; in a chronic respiratory acidosis, the pH only drops by 0.03 for the same rise in PCO_2 because of increased renal HCO_{3-} reabsorption.

Much controversy has surrounded the accuracy of venous blood gas (VBG) measurements in analyzing acid-base derangements. In a mixed ICU population, as well as in studies of patients with diabetic ketoacidosis, arterial and venous pH differ by only about 0.03 [30, 31], and in hemodynamically stable patients, arterial to venous (A-V) PCO_2 measurements differ by about 5 mmHg [32]. However, the disparity between A-V pH and PCO_2 grows in conditions of low cardiac output; venous pH may be 0.1–0.25 lower than arterial pH, and venous PCO_2 may up to be 20 mmHg higher than arterial PCO_2 [27, 32, 33]. It has been demonstrated that an A-V PCO_2 gap >6 correlates closely with significantly reduced cardiac index and lactate clearance [34]. During cardiac arrest or profound cardiogenic shock, the VBG and ABG may be completely different, the VBG reflecting tissue level acidosis and the ABG showing a "pseudo-respiratory alkalosis" (Fig. 18.2).

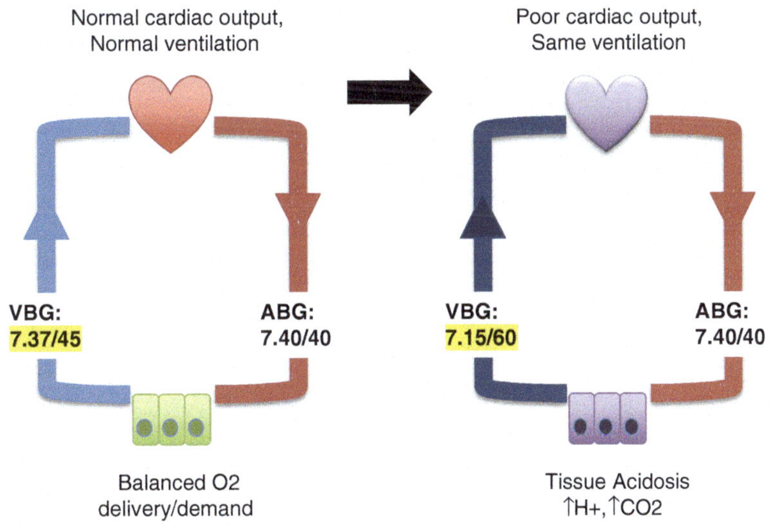

Fig. 18.2 Cardiac output and the arterial-venous PCO_2 difference

Therefore, in a patient with *normal* hemodynamics, a *normal* VBG is likely reflective of a normal ABG; however, in the critically ill patient with *abnormal* hemodynamics and an *abnormal* VBG, it will require measurement of an ABG to differentiate a true respiratory acidosis from poor cardiac output and tissue level acidosis. We recommend obtaining both for a complete assessment.

Analysis of Serum Bicarbonate and Respiratory Compensation

An abnormal HCO_3 on a chemistry panel is diagnostic of a metabolic acid-base disorder, regardless of pH; HCO_3 <22 mEq/L indicates a metabolic acidosis, and HCO_3 >26 mEq/L indicates a metabolic alkalosis [1]. Whether these metabolic processes are primary or secondary (compensatory) depends on the agreement between pH and the bicarbonate. For example, a *low pH* with a *low HCO_3* indicates a *primary* metabolic acidosis; a *low pH* with an *elevated HCO_3* indicates a *compensatory* metabolic alkalosis, usually in response to a chronic respiratory acidosis.

If a primary metabolic disorder is uncovered, the next step is to evaluate the patient's respiratory compensation using the following formulae [4]:

For an acute metabolic acidosis: Expected $PCO_2 = 1.5(HCO_{3-}) + 8 +/- 2$

For an acute metabolic alkalosis: Expected $PCO_2 = 0.9(HCO_{3-}) + 15 +/- 2$

If the arterial PCO_2 is within 1–2 of the expected (calculated) value, the patient would be described as having adequate respiratory compensation [35]. If the PCO_2 is significantly higher than expected, the patient is suffering hypercapnic respiratory failure, *even if* the patient's PCO_2 is still within a "normal" range; if the PCO_2 is significantly lower than expected, an additional primary respiratory alkalosis exists. Figure 18.3 contains several examples of assessing respiratory compensation based on serum bicarbonate.

Calculate the Anion Gap

Regardless of serum pH and HCO_3, always calculate the anion gap (AG):

$$AG = Na^{+} - Cl^{-} - HCO_3^{-}$$

The AG represents unmeasured anions balanced by measured cations (mostly sodium) in serum. As depicted in Fig. 18.4, the AG is largely made up of serum albumin and phosphorus, along with organic acids, lactate, and ketoacids. A normal AG is anywhere between 6 and 16 (we use 12 as the upper limit of normal). The "normal"

ABG, Serum HCO3	Primary Disorder	Check for respiratory compensation: Metabolic Acidosis: *Expected PCO2 = 1.5 (HCO3) + 8 +/- 2* Metabolic Alkalosis: *Expected PCO2 = 0.9 (HCO3) + 15 +/- 2*	Additional Respiratory Disorder?
7.19/21, **8 mEq/L**	Primary metabolic acidosis	Expected PCO2 = 1.5 (8) + 8 +/- 2 = 20 +/- 2	None; Normal compensation
7.10/28, **6 mEq/L**	Primary metabolic acidosis	Expected PCO2 = 1.5 (6) + 8 +/- 2 = 17 +/- 2 *Actual PCO2 is > Expected PCO2*	*Additional* primary respiratory acidosis
7.32/16, **10 mEq/L**	Primary metabolic acidosis	Expected PCO2 = 1.5 (10) + 8 +/- 2 = 23 +/- 2 *Actual PCO2 is < Expected PCO2*	*Additional* primary respiratory alkalosis
7.43/45, **33 mEq/L**	Primary metabolic alkalosis	Expected PCO2 = 0.9 (33) + 15 +/- 2 = 45 +/1 2	None; Normal compensation
7.41/64, **39 mEq/L**	Primary metabolic alkalosis	Expected PCO2 = 0.9 (39) + 15 +/- 2 = 51 +/- 2 *Actual PCO2 is > Expected PCO2*	*Additional* primary respiratory acidosis

Fig. 18.3 Examples of acid-base disorders and respiratory compensation diagnosed by arterial blood gas (ABG) and serum bicarbonate (HCO_3)

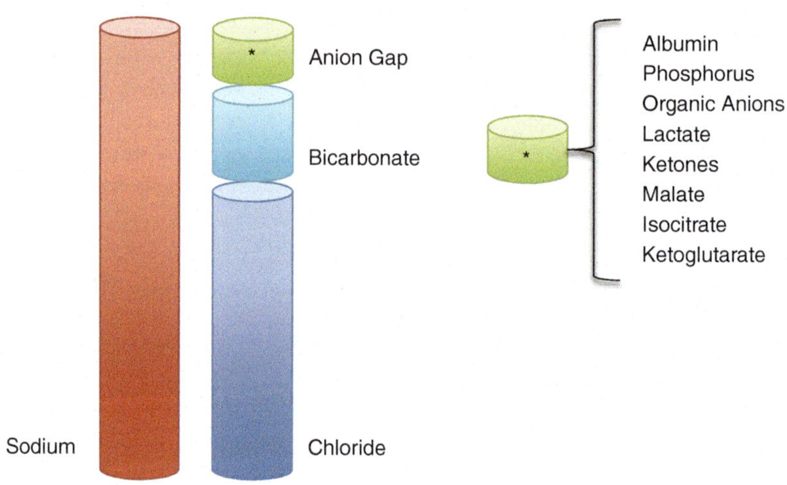

Fig. 18.4 The anion gap

value for a given patient depends on their albumin concentration [36, 37]. Thus, to increase the detection of a subtly elevated AG in a hypoalbuminemic patient, add a correction factor of 2.5 for every gram drop in albumin below the normal value of 4 g/dL (Fig. 18.5):

$$\text{Corrected AG} = \left(\text{Na}^+ - \text{Cl}^- - \text{HCO}_3^-\right) + \left(2.5 \times \left[4.0 - \text{Albumin}\right]\right)$$

An elevated AG ("AG metabolic acidosis" [AGMA]) signifies the presence of pathologic levels of organic acids and/or ketoacids in the blood (i.e., lactic acid, beta-hydroxybutyric acid, salicylic acid) (Table 18.3a). Conversely, an abnormally narrowed or negative AG signifies pathologic levels of positively charged molecules in the blood (i.e., paraproteins, myeloma or amyloid, protein, lithium) [37] (Table 18.3b). A primary metabolic acidosis with a normal AG is termed a "non-AG metabolic acidosis" (NAGMA) (Table 18.3c). Be aware that an elevated AG is not sensitive enough to substitute for directly measuring serum lactate, nor is it specific for any particular disease process; it has been shown that critically ill patients may have an elevated AG without discernable cause due to the presence of intermediary metabolites, such as isocitrate, ketoglutarate, malate, and D-lactate [38, 39].

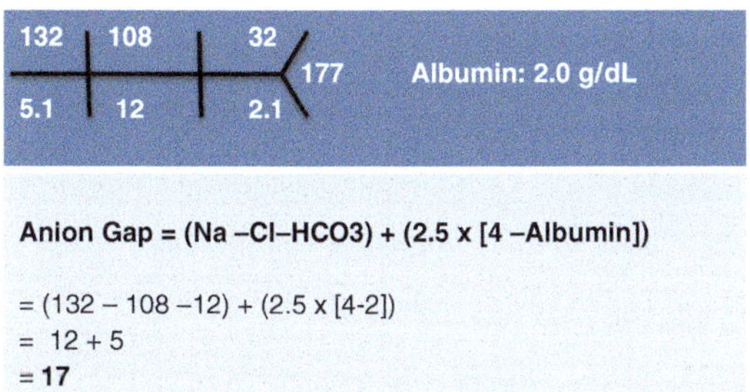

Fig. 18.5 Calculation of the anion gap

Table 18.3a Causes of elevated anion gap

	Mnemonic: "MUKTPILES"	Contributing acid
M	Methanol	Formic acid
U	Uremia	Nitrogen and sulfate waste, others
K	Ketoacidosis (diabetic, alcoholic, starvation)	Beta-hydroxybutyric acid, acetoacetic acid
T	Toluene	Benzoic acid, hippuric acid
P	Paracetamol (acetaminophen)	Pyroglutamic acid, lactic acid
	Propylene glycol (intravenous lorazepam, diazepam)	Lactic acid
	Propofol infusion syndrome	Lactic acidosis due to mitochondrial poisoning
I	Iron	Lactic acidosis due to hypovolemia, GI hemorrhage, and mitochondrial poisoning
	Isoniazid	Lactic acidosis due to seizure
L	Lactic acidosis	*See* Table 18.3a
E	Ethylene glycol	Oxalic acid, glycolic acid
S	Salicylate	Acetylsalicylic acid, lactic acid

Table 18.3b Causes of narrowed or negative anion gap

Toxins	Lithium Iodine Bromide
Paraproteinemia	Multiple myeloma Amyloidosis

Table 18.3c Causes of non-AG (hyperchloremic) metabolic acidosis

	Mnemonic: "HARD-UPs"	Scenario
H	Hyperalimentation	High chloride load in feeding formula or parenteral nutrition
A	Adrenal crisis	Hyponatremia, hyperkalemia, hypoglycemia
	Acetazolamide	
R	Renal tubular acidosis	Type I (distal): decreased H+ secretion Type II (proximal): decreased HCO_3– reabsorption Type IV (diabetes, renal failure, NSAID use, aldosterone deficiency or resistance): decreased ammoniagenesis
D	Diarrhea	GI bicarbonate losses
U	Ureteral diversion	Ileal conduit absorbs urinary substrates
P	Pancreatic/biliary loss	Pancreatic or biliary drains, fistulas
S	Saline	Resuscitation with chloride-rich fluids such as 0.9% saline

Compare the "AG Rise" to the "HCO_3 Drop" to Find Hidden Metabolic Disorders

If an AGMA is detected (AG >12), the next step is to evaluate for any additional NAGMA or metabolic alkalosis. These "hidden disorders" are uncovered by comparing the magnitude of elevation of the AG (the "AG Rise") to the magnitude of fall of HCO_3 (the "HCO_3 Drop"), also termed the "delta-delta" (Fig. 18.6).

$$\text{AnionGapRise} = \text{AG} - 12$$

$$HCO_3^- \text{ Drop} = 24 - HCO_3$$

In a pure AGMA with no hidden disorder, the AG Rise and HCO_3 Drop should be within about 2 points of each other. If the HCO_3 Drop is *greater* than the AG Rise, an additional primary NAGMA is present; if the HCO_3 Drop is *less* than the AG Rise, an additional primary metabolic alkalosis is present.

Calculate the Osmolar Gap

A complete analysis involves ancillary studies to narrow the differential. At a minimum, one should measure the serum osmolality and lactate in any critically ill patient with an acid-base disorder. Calculation of the osmolar gap (OG) allows for the detection of osmotically active substances not accounted for on standard chemistries [40]. Further testing for ethanol, toxic alcohols, ingested substances such as acetaminophen, acetylsalicylic acid (ASA), illicit drugs, and co-oximetry for carboxyhemoglobin and methemoglobin is prudent in patients with unexplained acid-base abnormalities.

$$\text{Calculated Serum Osmolality} = (2 \times \text{Na}) + (\text{BUN}/2.8) + (\text{Glucose}/18) + (\text{EtOH}/3.7)$$

$$\text{OG} = \text{measured osmolality} - \text{calculated osmolality}$$

Na | Cl | BUN < Gluc; K | HCO3 | Creat	What is the anion gap? *AG = Na – Cl – HCO3*	"AG ↑" versus "HCO3 ↓" *"Anion Gap ↑" = AG – 12* *"HCO3 ↓" = 24 – HCO3*	Hidden Disorder
140 | 104 | 20 < 76; 3.6 | 11 | 1.6	*AG = 140 –104 – 11 = 25* *AG Acidosis*	AG ↑ = 25 –12 = 13 HCO3 ↓ = 24 – 11 = 13 *AG ↑ = HCO3 ↓*	None
134 | 88 | 25 < 622; 2.8 | 16 | 1.4	*AG = 134 – 88 – 16 = 30* *AG Acidosis*	AG ↑ = 30–12 = 18 HCO3 ↓ = 24 – 16 = 8 *AG ↑ > HCO3 ↓*	Additional primary **metabolic alkalosis**
142 | 115 | 20 < 55; 3.0 | 5 | 1.6	*AG = 142 – 115 – 5 = 22* *AG Acidosis*	AG↑ = 22 – 12 = 10 HCO3 ↓ = 24 – 5 = 19 *AG ↑ < HCO3 ↓*	Additional primary non-AG **metabolic acidosis**
146 | 122 | 43 < 188; 5.5 | 12 | 4.0	*AG = 146 – 122 – 12 = 12* *Non-AG acidosis*	N/A	N/A

Fig. 18.6 Examples of acid-base disorders diagnosed by anion gap and "AG rise" versus "Bicarb Drop" ("delta-delta") calculations

Table 18.4 Causes of an elevated osmolar gap

Toxins	Methanol Ethylene glycol Isopropyl Propylene glycol
Ketones	Beta-hydroxybutyrate Acetoacetate Acetone

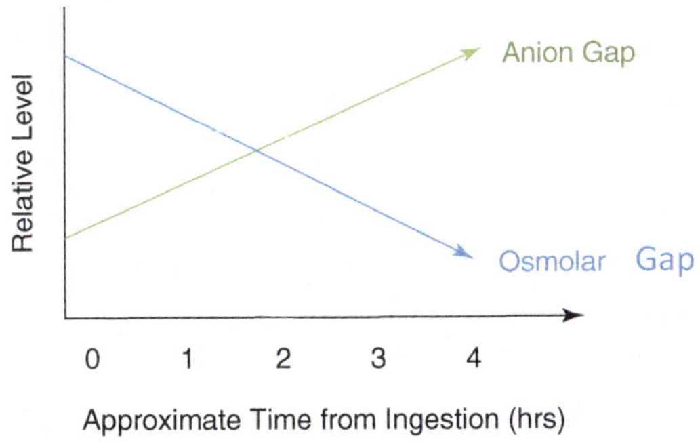

Fig. 18.7 Temporal relationship between the osmolar gap and anion gap after toxic alcohol ingestion

An OG >10 suggests the presence of osmotic substances in the blood, such as toxic alcohols (methanol, ethylene glycol, propylene glycol, isopropyl alcohol), ketones bodies (acetone or beta-hydroxybutyrate), or other metabolites (Table 18.4) [41]. In clinical practice, an OG <10 has high sensitivity and negative predictive value to rule out toxic alcohol ingestions that would require emergent therapy, but *not* 100%; nor is an elevated OG specific to toxic ingestion, as patients with alcoholic ketoacidosis or lactic acidosis may also have elevated serum osmolality [41, 42]. It is also critical to realize that as toxic alcohols are metabolized in the hours after ingestion, the OG will normalize and obscure the diagnosis (Fig. 18.7).

Differential Diagnosis of Acid-Base Disturbances

An organized acid-base analysis may trigger additional workup or initiation of life-saving therapies in clinical scenarios that may have otherwise gone unnoticed (i.e., early respiratory failure, salicylate toxicity, toxic alcohol ingestion). Tables 18.3a, 18.3b, 18.3c, 18.4, 18.5a, 18.5b, 18.5c, and 18.5d describe the dif-

Table 18.5a Causes of respiratory acidosis

CNS	Primary brain injury Opiate or depressant overdose Central apnea Hypothermia
Neuromuscular	Myasthenia gravis Guillain-Barre Severe hypokalemia, hypophosphatemia
Chest wall mechanics	Morbid obesity Chest wall trauma or burns Massive ascites Abdominal compartment syndrome Severe kyphoscoliosis
Pulmonary	Obstructive lung disease Severe upper airway obstruction
Metabolic	Hyperpyrexia Rigors, shivering Muscle rigidity (malignant hyperthermia, agitation, seizure) Sodium bicarbonate infusion Carbohydrate-rich nutrition

Table 18.5b Causes of respiratory alkalosis

CNS	Primary brain injury Meningoencephalitis Status epilepticus Hepatic encephalopathy Agitation, anxiety, pain
Hypoxemia	Pulmonary diseases Shunt physiology High altitude
Toxic/metabolic	Salicylate toxicity Sepsis Thyrotoxicosis
Pseudo-respiratory alkalosis	Hyperventilation + poor cardiac output (i.e., severe cardiogenic shock or cardiac arrest)
Physiologic	Pregnancy

Table 18.5c Causes of lactic acidosis

Type A lactic acidosis (related to poor oxygen delivery)	Shock Mesenteric ischemia Compartment syndrome Microcirculatory dysfunction Severe anemia Carbon monoxide poisoning
Type B lactic acidosis (independent of oxygen delivery)	Liver dysfunction Drugs/toxins (cyanide, metformin, salicylates, nitroprusside, propofol, antivirals, iron toxicity) Catecholamines (shunting of pyruvate → lactate) Hematologic malignancy (hypermetabolic cells) Metabolic deficiencies (thiamine, carnitine) Bacterial overgrowth

Table 18.5d Causes of metabolic alkalosis

Chloride depletion (*Chloride responsive*)	Endocrine/renal (*Chloride unresponsive*)
Hypovolemia	Conn syndrome (hypoaldosteronism)
Vomiting, nasogastric suction	Cushing syndrome (hypercortisolism)
Loop diuretics	Mineralocorticoids/glucocorticoids
Posthypercapnia/chronic respiratory acidosis	Renal artery stenosis
Sodium bicarbonate infusion	Liddle's syndrome
Sodium lactate load (i.e., lactated Ringer's)	Bartter's syndrome
Citrate load (i.e., massive transfusion)	Gitelman's syndrome
Acetate load (i.e., parenteral nutrition)	

ferential diagnoses of various acid-base disturbances [5, 27, 35, 37, 43–48].

Treatment of Acid-Base Disorders

The treatment of acid-base disorders centers on supportive care and management of the underlying disease process(es) once uncovered. At times, emergent management may require control of the airway, mechanical ventilation, and use of intravenous buffers or other medications. While describing the detailed management of individual disease states is beyond the scope of this chapter, key management points for various acid-base disorders are summarized in Table 18.6 [5, 27, 45, 49], and broad principles are outlined below.

Tight pH Control Versus Permissive Hypercapnia

Permissive hypercapnia (pH 7.20–7.30) in acute respiratory failure is commonplace. Within the pH ranges of 7.20–7.60, most patients will not suffer serious consequences, but there are notable exceptions. The following are the five distinct patient populations who will not tolerate marked deviation of pH and/or PCO_2 (see Table 18.7) and will need careful attention to ensuring adequate ventilation and more liberal use of intravenous sodium bicarbonate: (1) brain-injured patients, especially those with mass effect at risk of elevated intracranial pressure (with the exception of rescue from impending brain herniation, strict eucapnia (pH 7.35–7.40) is recommended [50]), (2) patients with severe left ventricular dysfunction and/or ischemic myocardium who will lose

Table 18.6 Summary of treatment for select acid-base disorders

Scenario	Acute treatments
Respiratory acidosis	Provide adequate oxygenation Naloxone or other reversal agent Noninvasive ventilation in select cases Intubation/mechanical ventilation *Avoid sodium bicarbonate*
Respiratory alkalosis	Provide adequate oxygenation Analgesia, anxiolysis, sedation Decrease tidal volume and/or respiratory rate Neuromuscular blockade if severe
Lactic acidosis with shock	Resuscitation of shock Disease-specific treatment Consider bicarbonate infusion, especially if AKI
DKA	IV fluids, potassium replacement, insulin infusion *Avoid sodium bicarbonate*
Alcoholic ketoacidosis	IV fluids, thiamine, folate, dextrose *Avoid sodium bicarbonate*
Methanol, ethylene glycol	IV 4-methylpyrazole (fomepizole), thiamine, folate, dextrose, hemodialysis if severe
Salicylate overdose	Sodium bicarbonate for urinary alkalinization, potassium replacement, hemodialysis if severe
Renal failure, renal tubular acidosis	Sodium bicarbonate replacement, hemodialysis
Non-AG acidosis	Balanced resuscitation fluids (i.e., lactated Ringer's) Sodium bicarbonate replacement
Metabolic alkalosis + Hypovolemia	0.9% saline resuscitation Potassium replacement
Metabolic alkalosis + Volume overload	Potassium chloride, acetazolamide, hemodialysis, hydrochloric acid infusion if severe symptoms
Metabolic alkalosis + Hypokalemia	Potassium chloride, acetazolamide, amiloride

Table 18.7 Patients requiring tight pH control

Population	pH or $PaCO_2$ target	Reasoning
Brain injury	$PaCO_2$ 35–40	Acidemia → increased intracranial pressure Alkalemia → cerebral vasoconstriction and ischemia
Left ventricular failure	pH 7.3–7.4	Acidemia → decreased contractility Alkalemia → hypokalemia, arrhythmias, coronary vasospasm, ischemia
Pulmonary hypertension	pH ~7.4	Acidemia → increased pulmonary vascular resistance, increased RV afterload, RV failure
Tricyclic overdose, salicylate overdose	pH 7.5–7.55	Serum alkalinization → reduced sodium channel blocker binding Urine alkalinization → enhanced excretion of salicylate
Pregnancy	$PaCO_2$ 32–35	Acidemia → fetal CO_2 retention and acidosis

contractility and response to catecholamines as pH drops below normal [8], (3) patients with pulmonary hypertension and/or right ventricular failure who do not tolerate acidemia (low pH or acutely elevated PCO_2 causes pulmonary vasoconstriction, increased right ventricular afterload, decreased right ventricular function, and it may lead to right heart failure and cardiovascular collapse [13, 14, 17]), (4) patients with certain overdoses, such as tricyclic or salicylate toxicity, requiring alkalemia and urinary alkalinization to treat the toxidrome [51, 52], and (5) the pregnant patient requiring a respiratory alkalosis (target PCO_2 32–35) to maintain a gradient for fetal CO_2 off-loading; if the mother's PCO_2 is elevated, fetal acidemia may rapidly develop [53, 54, 55].

Choice of Resuscitation Fluid

A growing body of literature suggests that the chloride content and pH of resuscitation fluid may impact patient outcome. When compared to balanced intravenous fluids such as Hartmann's

Table 18.8 Preferred uses of 0.9% saline

0.9% saline preferred	Balanced solution (e.g., LR) preferred
Brain injury	General ICU population
Cerebral edema	Septic shock
Metabolic alkalosis	Hemorrhagic shock
Adrenal crisis	Surgical abdomen
Hypercalcemia	Severe pancreatitis
Hyperphosphatemia	

solution or Plasma-Lyte, 0.9% normal saline (NS) appears to result in decreased renal blood flow and renal perfusion, decreased urine output, increased third spacing, and prolonged hyperchloremic acidosis [56, 57]. NS is also associated with increased duration of systemic inflammation in acute pancreatitis and increased blood transfusion requirements and renal replacement therapy in patients with major abdominal surgery [58–60]. A large cross-over trial and a recent randomized trial of critically ill adults show the use of NS is associated with an increased incidence of acute kidney injury and need for renal replacement therapy [58, 61, 62]. Balanced solutions, however, are relatively hypotonic and should not be used in patients with cerebral edema or elevated intracranial pressure [50]. NS may also be preferred in the treatment of patients with contraction alkalosis, hypochloremia, and certain endocrine or electrolyte disorders [63]. Table 18.8 summarizes recommendations for the use of NS versus balanced fluids.

Sodium Bicarbonate

Supplementing base in the form of sodium bicarbonate is the mainstay of treatment for NAGMA (also known as "hyperchloremic" acidosis), especially in the presence of acute kidney injury, as these processes are essentially "bicarbonate wasting" disorders [5, 64]. Sodium bicarbonate is also appropriate in the treatment of salicylate overdose and sodium channel blocker overdose. Bicarbonate replacement for critically ill patients in shock and/or respiratory failure with a pH <7.20, even with a component of lactic acidosis or AGMA, has been shown to significantly reduce the need for renal replacement therapy and may

Table 18.9 Pitfalls of sodium bicarbonate administration

May not improve blood pressure in shock
Increased $PaCO_2$/respiratory acidosis
Intracellular and CNS acidosis
Oxy-Hgb curve shift to left, decreased tissue O_2 delivery
Decreased O_2 utilization by tissues
Increased lactate production
Delayed ketone clearance
Hypernatremia
Volume overload

even improve mortality in those patients with acute kidney injury [65]. Except in cardiovascular collapse where rapid pushes are needed, it should be given as an isotonic solution (150 mEq of sodium bicarbonate in 1 L of sterile water or 5% dextrose) in the form of a bolus or maintenance rate [5], or a slow infusion of concentrated (1 mEq/mL) straight bicarbonate at 20–30 mL/hr.

The use of sodium bicarbonate to treat other types of AGMA, lactic acidosis, or respiratory acidosis may have adverse effects (Table 18.9). When bicarbonate is given intravenously, it is converted rapidly into CO_2 and water; CO_2 freely diffuses across cell membranes causing a paradoxical intracellular and central nervous system acidosis [64, 66]. If bicarbonate is given, it is critical to account for this increase in CO_2 production and ensure adequate alveolar ventilation, particularly in a sedated, ventilated patient. Other effects demonstrated include decreased O_2 delivery and utilization by the heart and other tissues, hypocalcemia, decreased ketone clearance, increased lactate production, and it may not reliably increase blood pressure, even in patients with a starting pH <7.20 or in patients with poor cardiac contractility [67–71]. In the absence of specific indications, bicarbonate infusion should not be used simply to target a "normal" pH [66].

Sodium and Water Homeostasis

Overlapping neuroendocrine mechanisms tightly regulate sodium, water, and intravascular volume. Total body water (TBW), about 0.5 × ideal body weight (IBW) for adult women and about 0.6 × IBW for adult men, is roughly 30–40 L [72]. Approximately 60% of TBW is contained intracellularly (ICF), and 40% remains extracellular (ECF) [73]. About 25% of ECF is intravascular—about 3.5–4.5 L.

Water diffuses freely across cell membranes, but osmotically active substances (sodium being the most important) cannot [72]; therefore, movement of water between compartments is determined by the relative tonicity within each compartment (Fig. 18.8). When sodium is added to the intravascular compartment, water diffuses out of cells into the vasculature; conversely, if water is added to the vascular compartment and dilutes the sodium content, it will diffuse into the cells causing cellular edema. When *isotonic* fluid such as 0.9% saline (NS) is infused into the vascular space, the water equilibrates throughout the ECF compartment, leaving only about ¼ of the infused volume in the vasculature with no net water movement in or out of cells.

Sodium and water are handled in response to two main variables: tonicity (largely dependent on sodium concentration) and intravascular volume status (referred to as effective arterial blood volume [EABV]) (Fig. 18.9) [72, 74, 75]. In response to free water losses or increased sodium concentration (dehydration), osmoreceptors within the hypothalamus stimulate thirst and secretion of antidiuretic hormone (ADH, also known as arginine vasopressin) from the posterior pituitary. ADH acts primarily on the distal renal tubules via upregulation of aquaporins, resulting in free water reabsorption and the excretion of small volumes of concentrated urine. As free water and/or intravascular volume are replaced, ADH activity subsides resulting in diuresis of large volumes of dilute urine.

When hypotension or low EABV is sensed by vascular baroreceptors, the renin-angiotensin cascade is activated, as well as thirst and ADH release. Angiotensin is responsible for vasoconstriction and stimulation of aldosterone release, which leads to increased renal salt and water reabsorption. ADH leads to direct vasoconstriction and stimulation of glucocorticoid and mineralocorticoid production, in addition to increasing water reabsorption in the distal tubules [72]. When EABV and sodium concentration increase, these mechanisms are suppressed, and natriuretic peptide is released from the

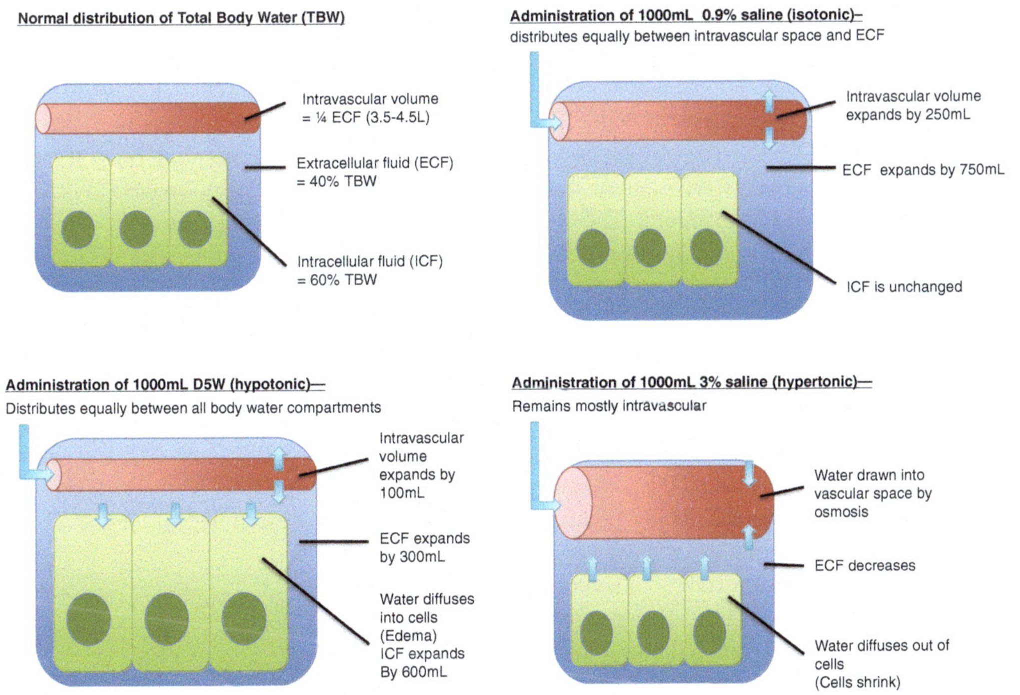

Fig. 18.8 Body water compartments and effects of administration of isotonic, hypotonic, and hypertonic intravenous fluids

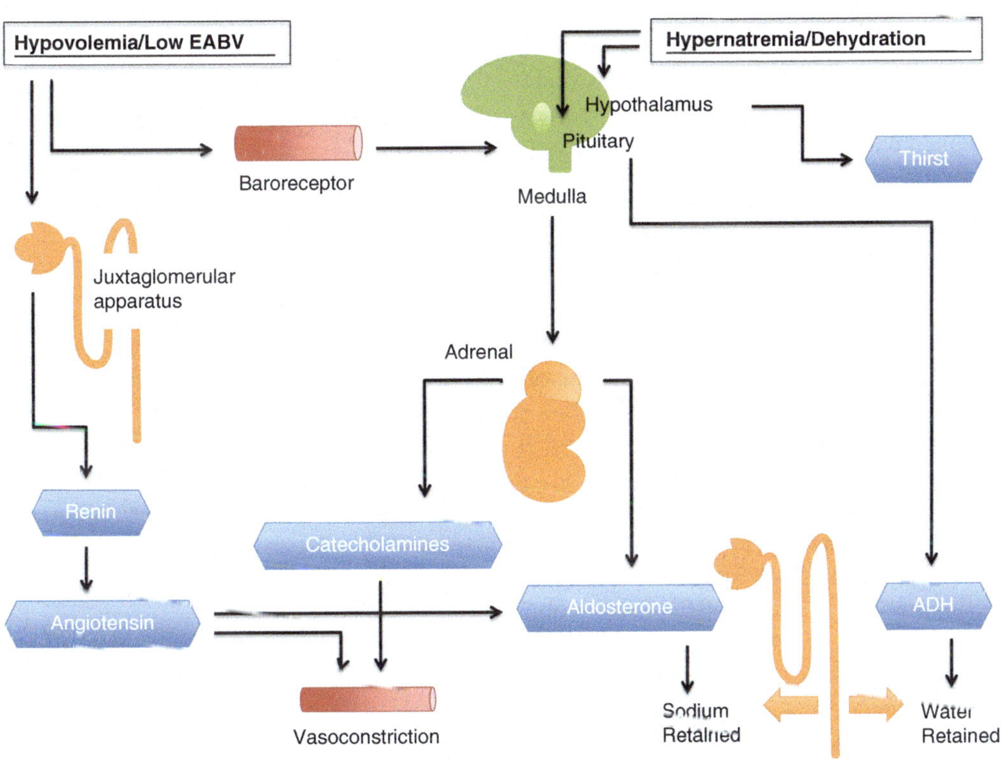

Fig. 18.9 Summary of homeostatic mechanisms in hypovolemia and dehydration

brain to facilitate renal sodium excretion and increased urine output (natriuresis). Importantly, the response to low EABV is more potent than the response to decreased sodium concentration [74]; for example, high ADH activity will persist in a hypovolemic patient even as the sodium drops, leading to hypovolemic hyponatremia. Therefore, volume status must be addressed when treating hyponatremia.

Hyponatremia

Hyponatremia is defined as a serum sodium concentration less than 136 mEq/L [72]. When the sodium concentration in the ECF is low relative to ICF, water diffuses into cells by osmosis [74]. In the CNS, this can cause cerebral edema and increased intracranial pressure, with symptoms including headache, confusion, vomiting, ataxia, seizures, and finally coma, cerebral herniation, and death. Over about 48 hours, neurons adapt to these conditions by transporting sodium, potassium, and other organic osmolytes out of the cell to restore osmotic equilibrium across the membrane [73, 74]. Rapid normalization of sodium into the ECF compartment then pulls water out of the vulnerable neurons, leading to a devastating neurologic syndrome known as osmotic demyelination syndrome (ODS), also called central pontine myelinolysis (CPM) [74]. Symptoms of ODS include the delayed onset of cognitive impairment, loss of motor strength and tone, or even coma days to weeks after rapid correction of hyponatremia. Patients with malnutrition, alcoholism, liver disease, and those with concomitant hypokalemia are at increased risk for this adverse event [73, 74].

Discerning the cause of hyponatremia requires several clinical and laboratory assessments of blood and urine [73]. Typically, clinicians are taught to differentiate hyponatremia in terms of volume status, i.e., "hypovolemic" vs "euvolemic" vs "hypervolemic," but this is difficult. Except for obvious cases like hypovolemic shock with massive enteral losses or the anasarcic cirrhotic or heart failure patient, laboratory data is more important. First, look for elevated serum glucose and triglycerides, which can cause pseudohyponatremia. Second, make sure urine osmolality is >100 mOsm/kg; below this threshold, look for water intoxication, polydipsia, or beer potomania. Third, make sure the kidney is responding appropriately to hyponatremia: the normal renal response is to let very little sodium pass into the urine (urine Na <30 mEq). If this is the case, a low EABV state is likely present; look for true hypovolemia, cirrhosis, hepatorenal syndrome, nephrotic syndrome, heart failure, etc. If the urine Na is >30 mEq/L, the kidneys are not properly responding; look for intrinsic renal disease, diuretic use (especially thiazides), medications such as SSRIs, adrenal failure, hypothyroidism, syndrome of inappropriate ADH (SIADH), etc. A relatively low serum BUN and uric acid support a diagnosis of SIADH. See Table 18.10 for a suggested diagnostic algorithm [73].

Table 18.10 Causes of hyponatremia

Step 1. Rule out iso- or hyper-osmolar state (serum Osm)	
If serum Osm >280 mOsm/hg, consider: Hyperglycemia (i.e., DKA, HHS) Pseudohyponatremia (i.e., hypertriglyceridemia, hyperlipidemia) Iatrogenic osmotic load (i.e., mannitol, contrast dye)	
Step 2. Rule out water intoxication (urine Osm)	
If urine Osm <100 mOsm/kg, consider: Psychogenic polydipsia Beer potomania Acute water intoxication	
Step 3. Evaluate renal response to hyponatremia (urine Na)	
If urine Na <30 mEq/L, consider:	If urine Na >30 mEq/L, consider:
Low EABV state Hypovolemia Cirrhosis Nephrotic syndrome Heart failure	Inappropriate renal Na handling Intrinsic renal disease, AKI, CKD Diuretics (*thiazides*) Medications (*SSRI, antipsychotics, antiepileptics, etc.*) Adrenal insufficiency (*ACTH stim*) Hypothyroidism (*TSH*) SIADH (*low uric acid and BUN*) Cerebral salt wasting

Osm osmolality (mOsm), *DKA* diabetic ketoacidosis, *HHS* hyperglycemic hyperosmolar syndrome, *UNa* urinary sodium (mEq/L), *EABV* effective arterial blood volume, *AKI* acute kidney injury, *CKD* chronic kidney disease, *SSRI* serotonin reuptake inhibitor, *ACTH stim* adrenocorticotropic hormone stimulation test, *TSH* thyroid-stimulating hormone, *SIADH* syndrome of inappropriate antidiuretic hormone, *BUN* blood urea nitrogen

The treatment of hyponatremia depends on three critical factors: (1) the presence of severe neurologic sequelae, (2) the presence of hemodynamic instability, and (3) the acuity of onset (< or >48 hours). Severe neurologic complications such as seizures, motor deficits, or coma typically appear with serum sodium less than 120 mEq/L and constitute a true emergency. An easy treatment strategy is to administer 3% hypertonic saline in boluses of 2 mL/kg, repeating up to three times as needed, to cause an acute rise of 3–5 mEq/L [72–74]. If the patient is already volume overloaded, a loop diuretic should be administered as well to enhance renal sodium clearance and prevent further hypervolemia [73].

Second, in the case of true hemodynamic instability (tachycardia, hypotension, signs of hypoperfusion), isotonic crystalloid such as LR or NS should be given as a bolus to restore perfusion [73, 74]. Do not bolus large amounts of fluid to "fill up the tank" on the *assumption* of hypovolemic hyponatremia—this may lead to rapid overcorrection, which will be signaled by a sudden jump in the output of large quantities of dilute urine. Boluses are reserved for the unstable patient!

Third, unless hyponatremia can be proven to be acute (e.g., lab results from the day before, a healthy runner with seizures during a marathon), assume the patient has been hyponatremic for >48 hours and aim for slow, controlled correction of no more than 6–8 mEq/L per 24-hour period (~0.3 mEq/hr) [74]. This rate is fast enough to resolve symptoms but below the lowest correction rate reported to lead to ODS. The method of correction depends upon the underlying disorder (Table 18.11). The formula below estimates the change in serum sodium (ΔNa) after 1 L of any given fluid depending on the sodium concentration of the fluid and the patient's weight. Taking 0.3 divided by the calculated ΔNa gives the desired fluid rate per hour (Fig. 18.10) [73]. Note that adding potassium replacement will further increase serum Na and *significantly LOWER* the safe rate of fluid administration:

$$\Delta \mathrm{Na} = \left(\mathrm{infusate}\left[\mathrm{Na}\right] + \mathrm{infusate}\left[\mathrm{K}\right] - \mathrm{serum}\left[\mathrm{Na}\right]\right)$$

Table 18.11 Summary of treatments for hyponatremia

Na <120 mEq/L + Neurologic emergency	3% hypertonic saline, 2 mL/kg over 10 minutes Repeat if still symptomatic, increase Na by 3–4 mEq/L Loop diuretic if hypervolemic
Hemodynamically unstable	Isotonic crystalloid bolus (NS or LR) until stable
Suspected hypovolemia	Slow fluid replacement with *gentle hourly rate* *Avoid fluid bolus,* may lead to rapid overcorrection Calculate fluid rate per Fig. 18.10
Suspected euvolemia	Free water restriction 3% hypertonic saline infusion if severe or SIADH suspected Thyroid or corticosteroid replacement as indicated
Suspected hypervolemia	Free water restriction Loop diuretics Consider renal replacement therapy
Rapid overcorrection (ΔNa trajectory >10 mEq/24 hr)	Stop all Na-containing fluids Start D5W infusion at 100–200 mL/hr Consult with nephrologist Consider desmopressin 2 mcg IV

Follow urine output q1h
Check sodium q4h
Sodium correction goal for all cases is no more than 6–8 mEq per 24-hour period

Age: **52**
Sex: **Male**
Weight: **80kg**

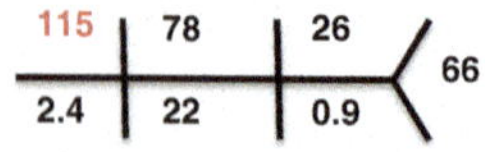

Sodium composition of common fluids (mEq/L)
3% hypertonic saline: **513**
0.9% saline: **154**
Ringer's lactate: **130**
0.45% saline: **77**
D5W: **0**

1. Estimate Total Body Water *TBW = 0.6 x Wt (male)* *TBW = 0.5 x Wt (female)*	2. Estimate ΔNa for given fluid *ΔNa per liter= $(Na_{infused} + K_{infused} - Na_{serum})$ / (TBW + 1)*	3. Divide hourly correction goal by ΔNa *Neurologic Emergency: 3-4mEq acutely* *Non-emergent: 0.3mEq/hr*
TBW = **0.6 x 80** = **48 liters**	**ΔNa** for 1 liter of ***3% hypertonic saline*** = (**513** + 0 – **115**) / (**48** + 1) = **8.12**mEq/L	Neurologic Emergency: (**3**mEq) / (**8.12**mEq/L) = 0.369L, or **370mL bolus** Non-emergent correction: (**0.3**mEq/hr) / (**8.12**mEq/L) = 0.037, or **37mL/hr**
	ΔNa for 1 liter of ***0.9% saline*** = (**154** + 0 – **115**) / (**48** + 1) = **0.8**mEq/L	Non-emergent correction: (**0.3**mEq/hr) / (**0.8**mEq/L) = 0.375, or **37mL/hr**
	ΔNa for 1 liter of ***0.9% saline + 40mEq KCl*** = (**154** + **40** – **115**) / (**48** + 1) = **1.61**mEq/L	Non-emergent correction: (**0.3**mEq/hr) / (**1.61** mEq/L) = 0.186, or **186mL/hr**

Fig. 18.10 Examples of correcting hyponatremia with hypertonic saline, and 0.9% saline, including the effect of supplementing potassium chloride

In hypovolemic patients, such as those with vomiting, diarrhea, diabetic ketoacidosis, or heat-related illness, intravascular volume should be replaced with LR or NS at an hourly rate rather than large boluses. In stable euvolemic or hypervolemic patients (renal failure, congestive heart failure, SIADH, and others), free water restriction is generally indicated. In patients with SIADH, treatment with 0.9% isotonic saline may perpetuate hyponatremia because water will be perpetually reabsorbed in excess of sodium, and hypertonic saline may be needed initially [74]. Vasopressin receptor antagonists such as tolvaptan may be used in patients with congestive heart failure or SIADH in later, stable phases of illness. Patients with hyponatremia related to hypothyroidism or adrenal insufficiency will require hormone replacement. In patients with renal failure, intermittent hemodialysis may result in too rapid a correction rate of serum sodium, and continuous renal replacement therapy may be advantageous [72]. Patients with neurologic injury, especially subarachnoid hemorrhage, may suffer inappropriate natriuresis due to cerebral salt wasting, which leads to hypovolemia. Fluid restriction is *contraindicated* in these patients; instead, gentle hypertonic saline infusions should be used to correct hyponatremia in the brain-injured patient.

Despite careful calculation, it is common to see an abrupt overcorrection, especially in hypovolemia and with concomitant hypokalemia; therefore, it is critical to monitor hourly urine output and labs every 4 hours during the first 24 hours. In the event that the patient begins to diurese, large amounts of dilute urine and serum sodium levels are on trajectory to exceed 9–10 mEq/L over 24 hours, and it is necessary to take corrective action such as stopping isotonic fluids, starting a D5W infusion, and possibly administering desmopressin 2 mcg IV, in consultation with a nephrologist [73].

Hypernatremia

Hypernatremia is defined as serum sodium in excess of 145 mEq/L [72] and is usually due to a loss of free water relative to sodium (dehydration) (Table 18.12). As ECF sodium concentration increases, water is initially drawn out of CNS cells via osmosis, causing a shrinking of the brain relative to the intracranial space [72, 75]. Other widespread effects of hypernatremia include insulin resistance and hyperglycemia, systemic inflammation, increased risk of venous thrombosis, rhabdomyolysis, and renal failure [75]. Symptoms are similar to those of hyponatremia, including lethargy, confusion, agitation, vomiting, and progression to coma, as well as cramps and muscle weakness. Over time, intracellular machinery with the CNS will begin to produce idiogenic osmoles, and osmotically active molecules are retained within the cells that act to balance the elevated sodium externally, pulling water back into the cells and restoring water balance. If the ECF compartment is rapidly flooded with a hypotonic fluid, water would rush into the cells leading to cerebral edema with further neurologic sequelae including cerebral herniation and death [76].

Patients with hypernatremia are categorized by underlying conditions, assessment of volume status, as well urine osmolality urine sodium, each category representing an important differential diagnosis.

The cornerstones of treatment of hypernatremia are the restoration of intravascular volume followed by free water replacement (Table 18.13). Based on clinical assessment, if the patient is hypovolemic to the point of shock or poor perfusion, gently administer isotonic crystalloids regardless of the serum sodium concentration before attempting to specifically correct the sodium [75]. Once the patient is deemed stable, correct the free water deficit with hypotonic fluids in a slow and carefully monitored fashion to prevent the development of cerebral edema. Unless there is strong evidence that the patient developed acute hypernatremia within a 24–48-hour time span, the safe upper limit of sodium correction is no more than 0.5 mEq/hr acutely, or about 8–10 mEq/L over the first 24 hours (Fig. 18.11) [72, 75–77]. The ΔNa equation can again be used to predict the change in sodium after administering 1 L of a particular fluid [76].

Special cases of hypernatremia, such as diabetes insipidus (DI) related to brain injury, congestive heart failure, or oliguric/anuric renal failure, will not respond to hypotonic fluids alone. Desmopressin, a synthetic arginine vasopressin analogue, will increase free water reabsorption in the distal renal tubules and suppress free water diuresis in cases of central DI. Patients with congestive heart failure will need loop diuretics to promote renal sodium excretion. In patients with oliguric/anuric renal failure, intermittent hemodialysis may correct serum sodium too rapidly, and continuous renal replacement therapy may be more appropriate [72]. Check serum Na levels

Table 18.12 Causes of hypernatremia

Hypovolemic	Euvolemic/hypervolemic
Immobility and poor access to water	Conn syndrome (hyperaldosteronism)
GI losses	Cushing syndrome (hypercortisolism)
Insensible losses – sweat, respiratory	Sodium bicarbonate infusion
Osmotic diuresis (i.e., DKA)	Hypertonic saline infusion
Loop diuretics	
DI	

DI diabetes insipidus, *DKA* diabetic ketoacidosis

Table 18.13 Summary of treatments for hypernatremia

Hypernatremia + Hypovolemia	Isotonic crystalloid bolus if hemodynamically unstable Hypotonic crystalloid infusion (0.45% saline) if hypovolemic but clinically stable Desmopressin (DDAVP) for suspected central DI
Hypernatremia + Euvolemia	Enteral free water replacement Desmopressin (DDAVP) for suspected central DI Thiazide diuretic or amiloride for nephrogenic DI
Hypernatremia + Hypervolemia	Enteral free water replacement Loop diuretics Consider hemodialysis if severe

Check sodium q2-4h
Sodium correction goal for all cases is no more than 8–10 mEq per 24-hour period
DI diabetes insipidus

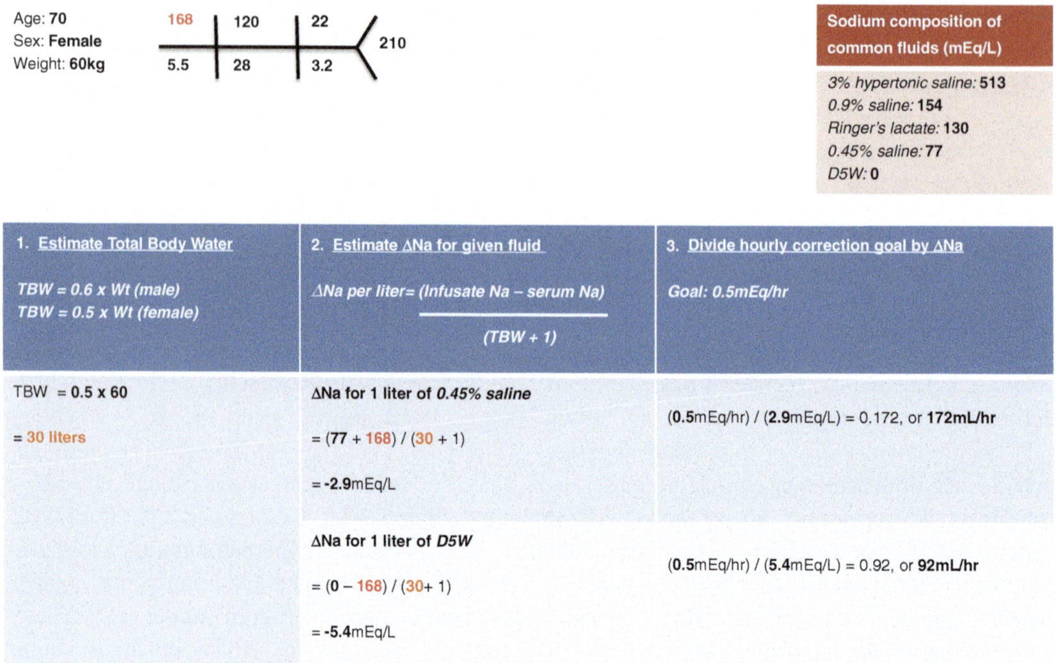

Fig. 18.11 Examples of correcting hypernatremia with 0.45% saline and 5% dextrose in water

every 2 hours initially, then every 4 hours when a stable trajectory is reached, to ensure that the rate of correction is in line with the treatment goal.

Hypokalemia

Hypokalemia is defined as serum potassium less than 3.5 mEq/L. Low serum potassium measurements are usually reflective of a large whole body potassium deficit; for every 0.1 mEq/L drop in serum potassium, there may be an estimated total body deficit of 30 mEq or more [78]. Hypokalemia may occur via several mechanisms, including poor dietary intake, gastrointestinal losses, endocrinopathy, renal losses (usually iatrogenic), or intracellular shift due to alkalemia, beta-agonists, or insulin (Table 18.14).

Table 18.14 Causes of hypokalemia

Poor intake	Malnutrition, alcoholism
GI losses	Vomiting, diarrhea, pancreatic/biliary losses
Renal losses	Osmotic diuresis (i.e., DKA), loop diuretics, sodium bicarbonate infusion, renal artery stenosis, distal RTA, Liddle's syndrome, Bartter's syndrome, Gitelman's syndrome
Endocrinopathy	Conn syndrome (hyperaldosteronism), Cushing syndrome, elevated renin/angiotensin/aldosterone state
Intracellular shift	Insulin, alkalemia, catecholamines, re-feeding

RTA renal tubular acidosis

The major effect of hypokalemia is on cardiac conduction, resulting in repolarization abnormalities. Common ECG findings include prolonged QT, diffuse ST segment depression and T-wave flattening, as well as the appearance of U waves (Fig. 18.12) [79]. These repolarization abnormalities, particularly a QT prolongation greater than 500 msec, increase the risk of malignant dysrhythmias, including ventricular tachycardia or torsades de pointes [80]. Arrhythmias typically are not seen with potassium levels above 3 mEq/L; however, in patients with myocardial infarction, the risk of ventricular ectopy rises substantially when serum potassium drops below 4 mEq/L [78, 81]. Low serum potassium may also cause muscle cramps, rhabdomyolysis at levels below 2.5 mEq/L, and weakness including

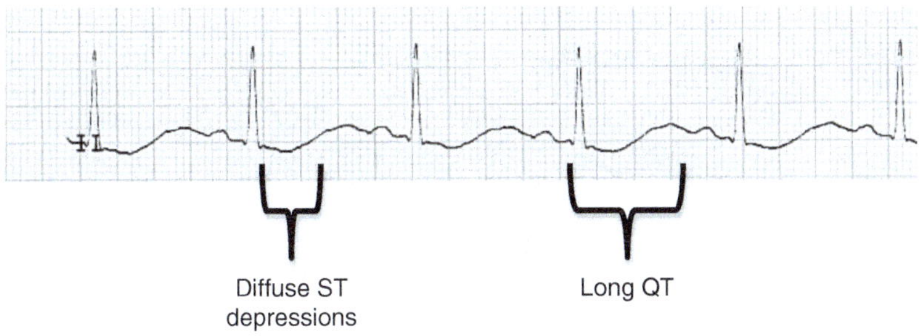

Fig. 18.12 ECG changes in hypokalemia

acute flaccid paralysis and respiratory failure below levels of 2.0 mEq/L [78].

Treatment of mild-to-moderate cases of hypokalemia without serious cardiac or musculoskeletal symptoms consists of oral supplementation of 40–60 mEq of potassium chloride every few hours [82, 83]. For more urgent cases or when enteral supplementation is not tolerated, intravenous potassium chloride is necessary at a rate of 10–20 mEq/hr; on average, 20 mEq of potassium replacement will increase serum potassium by 0.25 mEq/L [84, 85]. For patients with myocardial infarction, ischemic heart disease, or cardiomyopathy, consider initiating potassium replacement at serum potassium levels less than 4 mEq/L. In patients with diabetic ketoacidosis, potassium replacement should begin as soon as the patient's serum potassium descends below 5 mEq/L, provided the patient is making urine. For patients with refractory ventricular tachycardia due to severe hypokalemia, consider a slow intravenous push of 5 mEq KCl along with 2 g of magnesium sulfate.

Of critical importance is to empirically treat hypomagnesemia when hypokalemia is diagnosed. Hypokalemia and hypomagnesemia occur in parallel, and serum magnesium levels are notoriously unreliable [86, 87]. Without magnesium repletion, renal wasting of potassium will persist and hypokalemia will be more difficult to treat [78]. Furthermore, magnesium sulfate may improve QT prolongation and stabilize the myocardium in cases of ventricular ectopy. Table 18.15 summarizes the treatment of hypokalemia.

Table 18.15 Summary of treatments for hypokalemia

Potassium replacement	
Mild	Oral KCl, 40–60 mEq every 4–6 hours
Moderate/severe	IV KCl, 10 mEq/hr
Arrhythmia/severe symptoms	IV KCl, 20 mEq/hr via central line
Refractory Vtach/Vfib arrest	IV KCl, 5 mEq as a slow push
Magnesium replacement	
Stable patient	IV Magnesium sulfate, 500 mg/hr
Long QT	IV Magnesium sulfate, 2 g over 1 hour
Stable arrhythmia	IV Magnesium sulfate, 2 g over 10 minutes
Cardiac arrest	IV Magnesium sulfate, 2 g IV push

KCl potassium chloride

Hyperkalemia

Hyperkalemia is defined as a serum potassium level greater than 5 mEq/L. There are numerous causes of hyperkalemia, the most common of which is the spurious elevation of potassium in a blood sample that has hemolyzed during handling. True hyperkalemia can be viewed in five mechanistic categories: renal failure, drug effects, cell lysis, endocrinopathies, and cellular shifts (Table 18.16).

The major effect of hyperkalemia is cardiotoxicity. The electrocardiogram (ECG) is the preferred method for assessing for these effects. There are five key patterns to recognize, including peaked T waves, loss of P waves, widening of

Table 18.16 Causes of hyperkalemia

Renal failure	Acute renal failure, chronic kidney disease, oliguria/anuria, missed hemodialysis
Iatrogenic	Succinylcholine, ACE inhibitor/ARB, NSAIDs, trimethoprim-sulfa antibiotics, beta-blocker overdose, spironolactone, amiloride, acute digoxin toxicity, tacrolimus
Extracellular shift	Acidemia, ischemia-reperfusion (i.e., laparotomy for abdominal compartment syndrome, reperfusion of ischemic limb)
Cell lysis	Rhabdomyolysis, tumor lysis syndrome, massive hemolysis, massive transfusion, crush injury
Endocrinopathy	Addison disease (hypoaldosteronism), adrenal insufficiency, type IV RTA

ACE angiotensin-converting enzyme, *ARB* angiotensin receptor blocker, *NSAID* nonsteroidal anti-inflammatory drug, *RTA* renal tubular acidosis

the QRS, the "sine wave," or an unexplained narrow-complex junctional bradycardia (Fig. 18.13). It is important to note that the emergence of peaked T waves, widened QRS, and sine wave do not reliably correlate to any given potassium level, and any ECG finding may herald rapid progression to cardiac arrest in a seemingly stable patient [79, 88–90].

The treatment strategy for hyperkalemia depends most importantly on the presence of ECG changes. If hyperkalemia is suspected, an ECG should be obtained immediately while a serum potassium level is checked. In the absence of ECG findings, the serum potassium level should be rechecked before treatment is instituted, so as not to induce hypokalemia in case of a false positive. There are three steps in the acute management of hyperkalemia: stabilize cardiac membranes, promote intracellular potassium shifts, and enhance potassium elimination (Table 18.17).

In any patient with signs of QRS widening in the context of suspected hyperkalemia, the cardiac membrane must be stabilized emergently with intravenous calcium, preferably 1 g of calcium chloride as a slow push through a large proximal intravenous line or central line over several minutes. We advise *not* waiting for central access to use this medication in an emer-

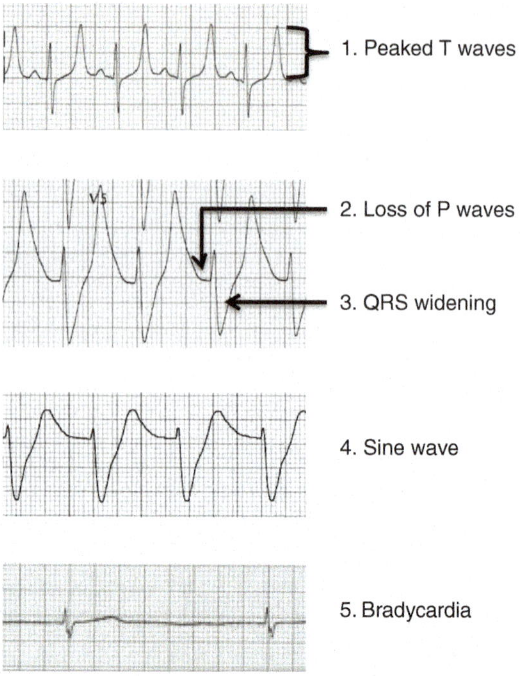

Fig. 18.13 ECG changes of hyperkalemia

gency, as delays may be life threatening. The effects of intravenous calcium may be as brief as 10–20 minutes, and it may need to be redosed. Calcium gluconate is commonly used to prevent venous sclerosis with small peripheral intravenous lines [91], but consider that only 1/3 of the calcium ions are freely available in this solution. It has been taught that intravenous calcium is contraindicated in hyperkalemia due to acute digoxin overdose, but evidence for the dreaded "stone heart" is lacking. Calcium appears to neither help nor harm in this situation, and emergent administration of digoxin immune Fab fragments (DigiBind) is indicated for any patient on digoxin with evidence of hyperkalemia even prior to laboratory results [92–94]. Because calcium chloride may cause sudden tachyarrhythmias and severe hypertension, it should not be pushed quickly unless for cardiac arrest, and it should not be used for isolated peaked T waves unless the patient has rapidly progressive hyperkalemia such as rhabdomyolysis, massive hemolysis, or sudden reperfusion of ischemic tissues (i.e., laparotomy for abdominal compartment syndrome or reperfusion of an ischemic or crushed limb).

Table 18.17 Summary of treatments for hyperkalemia

Phase	Treatment	Details
Stabilize the cardiac membrane	1 g calcium chloride, or 2–3 g calcium gluconate; slow IV push	Indicated for widened QRS (or any EKG changes in a rapidly progressive condition, i.e., rhabdomyolysis, ischemia-reperfusion)
Shift potassium intracellularly	10 units regular insulin, plus 2 amps D50; IV push	Monitor serum phosphorus
	Albuterol 10–20 mg/hr inhaled	Monitor heart rate and rhythm
	Sodium bicarbonate: 150 mEq in 1 L D5W; bolus or infusion	Only indicated if acidemic
Remove potassium from the body	Normal saline infusion	In patients who make urine
	Loop diuretics	Hypervolemic patients who make urine
	Hemodialysis	Oliguric/anuric renal failure or refractory cardiac arrest
Special situations	*Digoxin toxicity*—administer digoxin Fab fragments (Digibind ®) as soon as the diagnosis is suspected	

After stabilizing the cardiac membranes, attention should be turned to shifting potassium intracellularly. There are three methods to accomplish this: intravenous insulin with dextrose, inhaled albuterol, and the administration of sodium bicarbonate if severe metabolic acidosis is present. We advise using 10 units of insulin along with 50 g of dextrose to prevent hypoglycemia. Continuous nebulized albuterol can be given at a rate up to 20 mg/h, which is effective in lowering serum potassium by nearly 1 mEq/L within 30 minutes, and safe despite tachycardia [95, 96]. Combining insulin and albuterol will lower serum potassium by as much as 1.2 mEq/L acutely [97]. Caution must be exercised in the use of sodium bicarbonate: it is only effective in the presence of severe acidosis, and even then, the effect is negligible unless combined with other methods [89, 98, 99]. Furthermore, the large sodium load may be harmful in patients with volume overload. Keep in mind that these treatments also shift phosphorus intracellularly, which may result in muscle weakness, respiratory insufficiency, or rhabdomyolysis in severe cases.

Finally, efforts are focused on removing potassium from the body. In patients who make urine, this may be accomplished by providing normal saline to increase urine output. Furosemide may be added if the patient is euvolemic or hypervolemic. Hemodialysis is the definitive treatment for hyperkalemia in patients with oliguric or anuric renal failure, and it should be instituted urgently. Hemodialysis will lower potassium by 2 mEq/L within 3 hours [95, 96, 98]. Intra-arrest hemodialysis has been used successfully for severe hyperkalemia and resulted in neurologically intact survival despite prolonged down time [100]. Cation exchange resins given enterally, such as sodium polystyrene (Kayexalate), do not appear to decrease serum potassium levels acutely and should not be used in isolation [101].

Hypocalcemia

Hypocalcemia is defined as a serum ionized calcium level below 1.1 mmol/L [102]. Calcium is a unique divalent cation with widespread physiologic responsibilities, including the electrical conduction properties of nerves and cardiac myocytes, sarcomere shortening for contraction of cardiac and vascular smooth muscle, activation and linkage of platelets and coagulation factors in clot formation, and cell signaling cascades such as insulin release from pancreatic beta cells [102, 103]. Calcium is tightly regulated by endocrine and renal mechanisms [103]. In response to low serum calcium levels, parathyroid hormone (PTH) and calcitonin activity are increased, leading to increased active vitamin D, increased renal and gastrointestinal absorption of calcium, and release of calcium from bone. In the blood, nearly half of calcium is bound to proteins (predominantly albumin), while the remaining free ionized calcium exerts its effects [103]. Albumin binding is acutely affected by serum pH, phosphate, bicarbonate, lipids, propofol, free fatty acids, and other sub-

Table 18.18 Causes of hypocalcemia

Poor intake	Malnutrition, alcoholism
Free calcium sequestration	Alkalemia, hyperventilation, rhabdomyolysis, tumor lysis syndrome, blood product transfusion, lipid infusion, hydrofluoric acid toxicity
Endocrinopathy	Hypoparathyroidism, hypomagnesemia, hypermagnesemia, postparathyroidectomy ("hungry bone syndrome"), overtreatment of hyperparathyroidism
Saponification	Severe pancreatitis
Renal losses	Loop diuretics, ethylene glycol toxicity

stances; therefore, ionized calcium levels are required to diagnose calcium disorders in the critically ill [103–106]. Causes of hypocalcemia may be categorized as poor intake, free calcium sequestration, saponification, endocrinopathies, and renal losses (Table 18.18). Hypocalcemia for unclear reasons is common in patients with critical illness and is likely multifactorial [103].

Hypocalcemia results in myriad clinical abnormalities, the most important of which are cardiovascular and neuromuscular. In mild cases, hypocalcemia can cause perioral paresthesia, cramps, and irritability [104], but in more severe cases (ionized calcium much less than 0.9 mmol/L), hypocalcemia may lead to reduced cardiac output, reversible cardiomyopathy, malignant arrhythmias, vasoplegia, hypotension, and reduced platelet and clotting factor activity [102, 107–110]. Muscle tetany may also occur, and in severe cases, altered mental status and seizures may follow. The primary ECG finding of hypocalcemia is a prolonged QT segment, which makes patients prone to ventricular ectopy [105, 111].

Calcium replacement is the mainstay of therapy for hypocalcemia. In mild cases with no or mild symptoms, oral calcium can be given. If marked hypocalcemia is verified by ionized calcium measurement and the patient demonstrates hemodynamic instability, arrhythmia, muscle weakness or tetany, or seizures, they must receive intravenous calcium gluconate or calcium chloride. With the exception of cardiac arrest, calcium should be pushed slowly or given by intravenous piggyback over several minutes, as it may cause severe hypertension and tachydysrhythmias including ventricular tachycardia. Calcium chloride is preferentially given via central line, but it can certainly be given in a large proximal peripheral IV in an emergency. It is important to recognize that in calcium gluconate solution, only 1/3 of the calcium ions are freely available versus the same volume of calcium chloride, and thus, multiple doses of calcium gluconate may be necessary. If respiratory alkalosis is the cause of hypocalcemia, corrective action such as analgesia, anxiolysis, and sedation to decrease minute ventilation will improve ionized calcium levels. Use caution when administering calcium to dialysis patients with hyperphosphatemia, as peripheral tissue deposition of calcium phosphate crystals may occur; the goal is to maintain a calcium phosphate product ([Ca] mg/dL × [Phos] md/dL) less than 55 mg^2/dL [2, 103, 104]. Hypocalcemia and hypomagnesemia are often seen in concert, and supplementation with intravenous magnesium sulfate may increase calcium levels [105].

Hypercalcemia

Hypercalcemia is defined as a rise in serum ionized calcium above 1.3 mmol/L. There are multiple causes of hypercalcemia, such as severe hypovolemia, endocrinopathies, malignancy and paraneoplastic syndromes, granulomatous disease, and iatrogenic factors (Table 18.19). Hypovolemia may cause or worsen hypercalcemia, as calcium is reabsorbed along with sodium in renal efforts to maintain EABV [105]. Mild hypercalcemia may be asymptomatic, whereas severe hypercalcemia typically presents as a constellation of nonspecific findings, including hypertension, confusion and mood changes, lethargy, polyuria with hypovolemia, abdominal pain with nausea and vomiting, constipation, myalgias, and bony pain [112]. ECG findings are uncommon but may include QT segment shortening, typically without arrhythmia [105].

The treatment of hypercalcemia starts with replacement of intravascular volume. Normal saline should be started at a rate between 100 and

Table 18.19 Causes of hypercalcemia

Hypovolemia	Increased renal reabsorption of sodium and calcium
Endocrinopathy	Hyperparathyroidism, hyperthyroidism
Malignancy	Lung cancer, breast cancer, multiple myeloma, bone metastasis
Granulomatous disease	Tuberculosis, sarcoidosis, histoplasmosis
Iatrogenic	Thiazide diuretics, lithium, hypervitaminosis D

Table 18.20 Summary of treatments for hypercalcemia

All patients	0.9% saline infusion
Hypervolemic	Add loop diuretic
Hyperparathyroidism or malignancy	Consider calcitonin nasal spray
Granulomatous disease	Consider steroids
Oliguric/anuric renal failure	Hemodialysis

300 mL/hr, which will correct intravascular volume, increase urine output, and lower serum total calcium levels by as much as 1–2 mg/dL [105, 112]. Problematic medications such as lithium, digoxin, and thiazides should be discontinued. Furosemide may be used to increase urinary calcium excretion and block reabsorption; however, this should only be used if the patient is developing signs of volume overload [112]. Patients with oliguric or anuric renal failure will require hemodialysis [105]. Exogenous calcitonin can be given as an injection or nasal spray and will decrease serum calcium within a few hours, and it may be useful when combined with normal saline for severe hypercalcemia [112]. Corticosteroids have been used to reduce the effects of vitamin D in states of hypervitaminosis or granulomatous diseases [105]. Bisphosphonates such as pamidronate inhibit osteoclast activity, but take about 48 hours to work and should not be used in patients with renal insufficiency [112]. Table 18.20 summarizes the treatment of hypercalcemia.

Disorders of Magnesium

Magnesium is primarily an intracellular cation with multiple enzymatic and cellular functions; it is a cofactor for the sodium-potassium-ATPase pump and other ATP-dependent processes, regulates intracellular calcium, and augments cardiac and smooth muscle function [113]. Magnesium intake is dietary; storage is predominantly in the bone, soft tissue, and muscle; and the kidney plays a major homeostatic role in excreting or reabsorbing magnesium depending on a host of endocrine and local factors.

Table 18.21 Causes of hypo- and hypermagnesemia

Causes of hypomagnesemia	Causes of hypermagnesemia
Poor intake—malnutrition, alcoholism *GI losses*—vomiting, diarrhea, proton pump inhibitors *Renal losses*—diabetes, loop diuretics *Endocrinopathy*—hyperparathyroidism, hyperthyroidism, hyperaldosteronism, diabetes *Intracellular shifts*—alkalemia, insulin, refeeding, catecholamines, postparathyroidectomy ("hungry bone syndrome")	*Oliguria/anuria*—renal failure *Iatrogenic*—magnesium infusion for preeclampsia, severe asthma, magnesium antacids or cathartics *Extracellular shifts*—acidemia

Total magnesium levels are specific but not sensitive for true total body or intracellular magnesium depletion [113, 114]. Therefore, disease states associated with magnesium imbalance must be recognized in order to prompt treatment. Hypomagnesemia is defined as a serum magnesium level less than 1.7 mg/dL [115] and is associated with several broad categories of disease, such as malnutrition, alcoholism, gastrointestinal losses, renal magnesium wasting, endocrinopathies, and intracellular shifts [116]. Hypermagnesemia is defined as a serum magnesium level above 2.4 mg/dL and is almost always iatrogenic via intravenous administration of magnesium for severe asthma or preeclampsia, or enterally in the form of antacids or cathartics. Magnesium clearance is compromised in renal failure [113]. See Table 18.21 for a summary of the causes of magnesium disorders.

Hypomagnesemia, because of the interplay between magnesium and calcium, has unique cardiovascular and neuromuscular implications—specifically, magnesium depletion causes increased excitability of neurons and muscles

[113]. Symptoms and signs include headache, fatigue, weakness, seizures, tremors or fasciculations, tetany, myalgias, ileus, prolonged QT segment and arrhythmias, and hypertension due to increased vascular tone. Hypomagnesemia can directly cause both hypokalemia and hypocalcemia via renal wasting and decreased PTH activity, respectively [113, 114]. Hypomagnesemia also frequently complicates digoxin toxicity.

Because of the difficulty in using serum magnesium levels to predict true hypomagnesemia, we recommend liberal magnesium replacement in populations with risk factors or symptoms, such as patients with hypokalemia, alcoholism, diarrhea, malnutrition, prolonged QT, and/or ventricular ectopy. Dosing is typically 1–2 g of magnesium sulfate intravenously over 1–2 hours in the acute phase followed by up to 250–500 mg per hour for the first day or longer [114, 115]. For ventricular arrhythmias, the dose is 1–2 g over 10 minutes [115]. Enteral magnesium causes diarrhea and should not be used.

Signs and symptoms of hypermagnesemia are the opposite of hypomagnesemia, with overall decreased neuromuscular tone. Patients present with decreased deep tendon reflexes, diffuse muscle weakness, hypoventilation, vasodilation with flushed skin and hypotension, decreased inotropy, and cardiac dysrhythmias. Hypermagnesemia also inhibits PTH release and can lead to hypocalcemia [113]. In severe hypermagnesemia, intravenous calcium is used to antagonize the effects of magnesium. Giving 100–1000 mg of calcium chloride as a slow push or piggyback infusion will quickly reverse the effects of magnesium, and insulin with glucose can be used to shift magnesium intracellularly; hemodialysis may be necessary for patients in renal failure [113, 114].

Disorders of Phosphorus

Phosphorus is a predominantly intracellular anion with critical functions, including proper cellular membrane composition and function, numerous enzymatic functions, and energy storage as adenosine triphosphate (ATP) [117]. Dietary consumption is the main source of phosphorus, and the majority is stored in bone and soft tissues. Phosphorus is excreted or reabsorbed in the kidney, with vitamin D contributing to reabsorption and PTH activity contributing to excretion.

Hypophosphatemia is defined as a serum phosphorus level less than 2.7 mg/dL [118]. Like magnesium levels, serum phosphorus levels are not necessarily an accurate reflection of true hypophosphatemia or phosphorus depletion, and careful attention must be paid to high-risk patients with possible symptoms of hypophosphatemia [117, 118]. Causes of hypophosphatemia include malnutrition and poor intake, gastrointestinal losses such as vomiting, renal losses due to diuretics or overaggressive dialysis, endocrinopathy such as hyperparathyroidism, and intracellular shifts such as with insulin, refeeding, and alkalosis (Table 18.22). Patients with DKA, COPD, malignancy, malnutrition, alcoholism, and sepsis are particularly prone to hypophosphatemia [117]. Severe hypophosphatemia can have serious consequences, from myalgias and malaise to weakness of skeletal and respiratory muscles, frank ventilatory failure, rhabdomyolysis, hemolysis, cardiac dysfunction including arrhythmias and decreased contractility, confusion, and seizures [117, 118].

Patients with symptomatic hypophosphatemia, critically ill patients with levels below normal, or any patient with levels below 1.5 mg/dL should be treated [117, 118]. Two main options exist for intravenous phosphate replacement:

Table 18.22 Causes and treatment of hypophosphatemia

Causes of hypophosphatemia	Treatment of hypophosphatemia
Poor intake—malnutrition, alcoholism *GI losses*—vomiting *Renal losses*—diuretics, over dialysis *Endocrinopathy*—hyperparathyroidism *Intracellular shifts*—alkalemia, insulin, refeeding	*If potassium <4.0 mEq/L:* IV potassium phosphate, 15–30 mmol over 2–4 hours (contains 1.47 mEq of potassium per mmol of phosphate) *If potassium >4.0 mEq/L:* IV sodium phosphate, 15–30 mmol over 2–4 hours (contains 1.33 mEq of sodium per mmol of phosphate) Monitor for hypocalcemia

potassium phosphate, which contains approximately 1.47 mEq of potassium per mmol of phosphate, and sodium phosphate, which contains about 1.33 mEq of sodium per mmol of phosphate [118]. The typical dose for either is 15–30 mmol of the phosphate component, at a rate of 7 mmol/hr [118]. Potassium phosphate infusion at a rate of 15 mmol/hr (about 22 mEq of potassium per hour) has been administered safely in critically ill patients with severe hypophosphatemia, but may result in hyperkalemia and should be reserved for patients with concomitant hypokalemia and normal renal function [119]; otherwise, sodium phosphate should be used. Because phosphate and ionized calcium tend to bind together, be aware that the administration of intravenous phosphate may lead to rapid hypocalcemia with resultant hypotension, tetany, and arrhythmias [120]. Table 18.22 summarizes the causes and treatment of hypophosphatemia.

Hyperphosphatemia is defined as a serum phosphorus level greater than 4.5 mg/dL and is most commonly caused by renal failure; other causes include cell lysis, cellular shifts during acidemia, endocrinopathies such as hypervitaminosis D, and iatrogenic overuse of phosphate replacement or certain laxatives [118]. Because of calcium-phosphate binding, the symptoms of hyperphosphatemia are really those of hypocalcemia. Treatment for severe hyperphosphatemia begins with using normal saline to ensure euvolemia and promote adequate urine output. Enteral calcium-containing phosphorus binders have delayed effects and are not appropriate for acute treatment. Hemodialysis is required for severe cases with concomitant hypocalcemia and renal failure [117]. Caution is advised when confronted with hyperphosphatemia and hypocalcemia in patients with renal failure: administration of calcium may promote widespread deposition of calcium phosphate crystals in the tissues. This can be avoided so long as the calcium phosphate product ([Ca] mg/dL × [Phos] md/dL) is maintained at less than 55 mg^2/dL [2] [104]. Table 18.23 summarizes the causes and treatment of hyperphosphatemia.

Table 18.23 Causes and treatment of hyperphosphatemia

Causes of hyperphosphatemia	Treatment of hyperphosphatemia
Renal failure *Cell lysis*—rhabdomyolysis, tumor lysis syndrome, hemolysis *Iatrogenic*—phosphorus containing laxatives, over supplementation *Endocrinopathy*—hypervitaminosis D *Extracellular shifts*—acidemia	*If hypovolemic:* 0.9% saline *If hypocalcemic:* Supplement calcium cautiously to keep [Ca (mg/dL) × Phos (mg/dL) <55] *Renal failure and/or severe hypocalcemia:* Renal replacement therapy Enteral phosphate binders (i.e., sevelamer)

References

1. Kellum JA. Chapter 12: Acid-base disorders. In: Vincent JL, Abraham E, et al., editors. Textbook of critical care medicine. 6th ed. Philadelphia: Elsevier Saunders; 2011. p. 43–52.
2. Kellum JA. Determinants of blood pH in health and disease. [Review]. Crit Care. 2000;4:6–14.
3. Koeppen BM. The kidney and acid-base regulation. Adv Physiol Educ. 2009;33(4):275–81.
4. Schlichtig R, Grogono A, et al. Human $PaCO_2$ and standard base excess compensation for acid-base imbalance. Crit Care Med. 1998;26(7):1173–9.
5. Androgue HJ, Madias NE. Management of life-threatening acid-base disorders: first of two parts. N Engl J Med. 1998;338(1):26–34.
6. Lardner A. The effects of extracellular pH on immune function. J Leukoc Biology. 2001;69(2):522–30.
7. Orchard CH, Kentish JC. Effects of the changes of pH on the contractile function of cardiac muscle. Am J Physiol. 1990;258(6 Pt 1):967–81.
8. Schotola H, Toischer K, Popov AF, Renner A, Schmitto JD, Gummert J, et al. Mild metabolic acidosis impairs the beta-adrenergic response in isolated human failing myocardium. Crit Care. 2012;16(4):R153.
9. Bountra C, Vaughan-Jones RD. Effect of intracellular and extracellular pH on contraction in isolated, mammalian cardiac muscle. J Physiol. 1989;418:163–87.
10. Rocamora JM, Downing SE. Preservation of ventricular function by adrenergic influences during metabolic acidosis in the cat. Circ Res. 1969;24:373–81.
11. George AK, Shih A, Regan TJ. Effect of acute ketoacidosis on the myocardium in diabetes. Am J Med Sci. 1996;311(2):61–4.
12. Pedoto A, Caruso JE, Nandi J, Oler A, Hoffmann SP, Tassiopoulos AK, et al. Acidosis stimulates nitric oxide production and lung damage in rats. Am J Respir Crit Care Med. 1999;159(2):397–402.

13. Stengle M, Ledvinova L, Chvojka J, Benes J, Jarkovska D, Holas J, et al. Effects of clinically relevant acute hypercapnic and metabolic acidosis on the cardiovascular system: an experimental porcine study. Crit Care. 2013;17(6):R303.
14. Balanos GM, Talbot NP, Dorrington KL, Robbins PA. Human pulmonary vascular response to four hours of hypercapnia and hypocapnia measured using Doppler echocardiography. J Appl Physiol. 2003;94:1543–51.
15. Thorens JB, Jolliet P, et al. Effects of rapid permissive hypercapnia on hemodynamics, gas exchange, and oxygen transport and consumption during mechanical ventilation for the acute respiratory distress syndrome. Intensive Care Med. 1996;22:182–91.
16. Berger DS, Fellner SK, Robinson KA, Vleasica K, Godoy IE, Shroff SG. Disparate effects of three types of extracellular acidosis on left ventricular function. Am J Physiol. 1999;276(2 Pt 2):582–94.
17. Ijland MM, Heunks LM, van der Hoeven JG. Bench-to-bedside review: hypercapnic acidosis in lung injury–from 'permissive' to 'therapeutic. Crit Care. 2010;14(6):237.
18. Esau SA. Hypoxic, hypercapnic acidosis decreased tension and increased fatigue in hamster diaphragm muscle in vitro. Am Rev Respir Dis. 1989;139(6):1410–7.
19. Jaber S, Jung B, Sebbane M, Ramonatxo M, Capdevila X, Mercier J, et al. Alteration of the piglet diaphragm contractility in vivo and its recovery after acute hypercapnia. Anesthesiology. 2008;108(4):651–8.
20. Juan G, Calverley P, Talamo C, Schnader J, Roussos C. Effect of carbon dioxide on diaphragmatic function in human beings. N Engl J Med. 1984;310(14):874–9.
21. Coast JR, Shanely RA, Lawler JM, Herb RA. Lactic acidosis and diaphragmatic function in vitro. Am J Respir Crit Care Med. 1995;152(5 Pt 1):1648–52.
22. Refsum HE, Opdahl H, Leraand S. Effect of extreme metabolic acidosis on oxygen delivery capacity if the blood: an in vitro investigation of changes in the oxyhemoglobin dissociation curve in blood with pH values of approximately 6.30. Crit Care Med. 1997;25(9):1497–501.
23. Heijnen BHM, Elkhakoufi Y, et al. Influence of acidosis and hypoxia on liver ischemia and reperfusion injury in an in vivo rat model. J Appl Physiol. 2002;93(1):319–23.
24. Gunnerson KJ, Saul M, et al. Lactate versus non-lactate metabolic acidosis: a retrospective outcome evaluation of critically ill patients. Crit Care. 2006;10(1):R22.
25. Paz Y, Zegerman A, Sorkine P, Matot I. Severe acidosis does not predict fatal outcomes in intensive care unit patients: a retrospective analysis. J Crit Care. 2014;29(2):210–3.
26. Anderson LE, Henrich WL. Alkalemia associated morbidity and mortality in medical and surgical patients. South Med J. 1987;80:729–33.
27. Androgue HJ, Madias NE. Management of life-threatening acid-base disorders: second of two parts. N Engl J Med. 1998;338(2):107–11.
28. Banga A, Khilnani GC. Post-hypercapnic alkalosis is associated with ventilator dependence and increase ICU stay. J COPD. 2009;6(6):437–40.
29. Dubin A, Menises M, et al. Comparison of three different methods of evaluation of metabolic acid-base disorders. Crit Care Med. 2007;35(5):1264–70.
30. Middleton P, Kelly AM, et al. Agreement between arterial and central venous values for pH, bicarbonate, base excess, and lactate. Emerg Med J. 2006;23:622–4.
31. Brandenburg MA, Dire DJ. Comparison of arterial and venous blood gas values in the initial emergency department evaluation of patient with diabetic ketoacidosis. Ann Emerg Med. 1998;31(4):459–65.
32. Androgue HJ, Rashad MN, et al. Assessing acid-base status in circulatory failure: differences between arterial and central venous blood. N Engl J Med. 1989;320:1312–6.
33. Weil MH, Rackow EC, et al. Difference in acid-base state between venous and arterial blood during cardiopulmonary resuscitation. N Engl J Med. 1986;315:153–6.
34. Vallee F, Mathe O, et al. Central venous-to-arterial carbon dioxide difference: an additional target for goal-directed therapy in septic shock? Intensive Care Med. 2008;34:2218–25.
35. Gunnerson KJ, Venkataraman R, Kellum JA. Chapter 20: Acid-base disorders. In: Murray PT, et al., editors. Intensive care in nephrology. Oxford: Tyler & Francis; 2006. p. 438–56.
36. Figge J, Jabor A, Kazda A, Fancle V. Anion gap and hypoalbuminemia. Crit Care Med. 1998;26(11):1807–10.
37. Kraut JA, Madias NE. Serum anion gap: its uses and limitations in clinical medicine. Clin J Am Soc Nephrol. 2007;2(1):162–74.
38. Levraut J, Bounatirou T, et al. Reliability of anion gap as an indicator of blood lactate in critically ill patients. Intensive Care Med. 1997;23(4):417–22.
39. Forni LG, McKinnon W, et al. Circulating anions usually associated with the Krebs cycle in patients with metabolic acidosis. Crit Care. 2005;9(5):R591–5.
40. Purrsell RA, Pudek M, et al. Derivation and validation of a formula to calculate the contribution of ethanol to the osmolal gap. Ann Emerg Med. 2001;38(6):653–9.
41. Schelling JR, Howard RL, Winter SD, Linas SL. Increased osmolar gap in alcoholic ketoacidosis and lactic acidosis. An Intern Med. 1990;113(8):580–2.
42. Lynd LD, Richardson KJ, et al. An evaluation of the osmole gap as a screening test for toxic alcohol poisoning. BMC Emerg Med. 2008;8(5)
43. Jurado RL, del Rio C, Nassar G, Navarette J, Pimental JL. Low anion gap. South Med J. 2008;91(7):624–9.

44. Garcia-Alvarez M, Marik P, et al. Sepsis-associated hyperlactatemia. Crit Care. 2014;18:503.
45. Soifer JT, Kim HT. Approach to metabolic alkalosis. Emerg Med Clin North Am. 2014;32:453–63.
46. Luke RG, Galla JH. It is chloride depletion alkalosis, not contraction alkalosis. J Am Soc Nephrol. 2012;23(2):204–7.
47. Wilson KC, Reardon C, Theodore AC, et al. Propylene glycol toxicity: a severe iatrogenic illness in ICU patients receiving IV benzodiazepines; a case series and prospective, observational pilot study. Chest. 2005;128(3):1674–81.
48. Diedrich DA, Brown DR. Analytic reviews: propofol infusion syndrome in the ICU. J Intensive Care Med. 2011;26(2):59–72.
49. Peixoto AJ, Alpern RJ. Treatment of severe metabolic alkalosis in a patient with congestive heart failure. Am J Kidney Dis. 2013;61(5):822–7.
50. Brain Trauma Foundation. Guidelines for the management of severe traumatic brain injury. J Neurotrauma. 2007;24(1):S1–106.
51. Proudfoot AT, Krenzelok EP, et al. Position paper on urine alkalinization. Clin Toxicol. 2004;42(1):1–26.
52. Bradberry SM, Thanacoody HKR, et al. Management of the cardiovascular complications of tricyclic antidepressant poisoning. Toxicol Rev. 2005;24(3):195–204.
53. Hanka R, Lawn L, et al. The effects of maternal hypercapnia on foetal oxygenation and uterine blood flow in the pig. J Physiol. 1975;247(2):447–60.
54. Walker AM, Oakes GK, et al. Effects of hypercapnia on uterine and umbilical circulations in conscious pregnant sheep. J Appl Physiol. 1976;41(5 Pt. 1):727–33.
55. Meschia G. Fetal oxygenation and maternal ventilation. Clin Chest Med. 2011;32(1):15–9.
56. Reid F, Lobo DN, et al. (Ab)normal saline and physiological Hartmann's solution: a randomized double-blind crossover study. Clin Sci. 2003;104:17–24.
57. Chowdhury AH, Cox EF, et al. A randomised, controlled, double-blind crossover study on the effects of 2-L infusions of 0.9% Saline and PLasma-Lyte 148 on renal blood flow velocity and renal cortical tissue perfusion in healthy volunteers. Ann Surg. 2012;256(1):18–24.
58. Wu BU, Hwang JQ, et al. Lactated Ringer's solution reduces systemic inflammation compared with saline in patients with acute pancreatitis. Clin Gastroenterol Hepatol. 2011;9:710–717.e1.
59. Waters JH, Gottlieb A, et al. Normal saline versus lactated Ringer's solution for intraoperative fluid management in patients undergoing abdominal aortic aneurysm repair: an outcome study. Anesth Analg. 2001;93:817–22.
60. Shaw AD, Bagshaw SM, et al. Major complications, mortality, and resource utilization after open abdominal surgery: 0.9% saline compared to Plasma-Lyte. Ann Surg. 2012;255:821–9.
61. Yunos NM, Bellomo R, et al. Association between a chloride-liberal vs chloride-restrictive intravenous fluid administration strategy and kidney injury in critically ill adults. JAMA. 2012;308:1566–2.
62. Semler MW, Self WH, Wanderer JP, et al. Balanced crystalloids versus saline in critically ill adults. N Engl J Med. 2018;378:829–39.
63. Ince C, Groeneveld ABJ, et al. The case for 0.9% NaCl: is the undefendable, defensible? Kidney Int. 2014;86:1087–95.
64. Forsythe SM, Schmidt GA. Sodium bicarbonate for the treatment of lactic acidosis. Chest. 2000;117:260–7.
65. Jaber S, Paugam C, Futier E, et al. Sodium bicarbonate therapy for patient with severe metabolic acidemia in the intensive care unit (BICAR-ICU): a multicenter, open label, randomized controlled phase 3 trial. Lancet. 2018;392:31–40.
66. Nakashima K, Yamashita T, et al. The effect of sodium bicarbonate on CBF and intracellular pH in man: stable Xe-CT and 31-P-MRS. Acta Neurol Scand. 1996;166:96–8.
67. Bellingham AJ, Detter JC, et al. Regulatory mechanisms of hemoglobin oxygen affinity in acidosis and alkalosis. J Clin Invest. 1971;50:700–6.
68. Cooper DJ, Walley KR, et al. Bicarbonate does not improve hemodynamics in critically ill patients who have lactic acidosis: a prospective, controlled clinical study. Ann Intern Med. 1990;112(7):492–8.
69. Mathieu D, Neviere R, et al. Effects of bicarbonate therapy on hemodynamics and tissue oxygenation in patients with lactic acidosis: a prospective, controlled clinical study. Crit Care Med. 1991;19(11):1352–6.
70. Okuda Y, Androgue HJ, et al. Counterproductive effects of sodium bicarbonate in diabetic ketoacidosis. J Clin Endocrinol Metab. 1996;81(1):314–20.
71. Bersin RM, Chatterjee K, et al. Metabolic and hemodynamic consequences of sodium bicarbonate administration in patients with heart disease. Am J Med. 1989;87:7–14.
72. Pokaharel M, Block CA. Dysnatremia in the ICU. Curr Opin Crit Care. 2011;17:581–93.
73. Spasovski G, Vanholder R, Allolio B, et al. Clinical practice guidelines on diagnosis and treatment of hyponatremia. Nephrol Dial Transplant. 2014;29:ii1–39.
74. Sterns RH, Hix JK, et al. Management of hyponatremia in the ICU. Chest. 2013;144(2):672–9.
75. Lindner G, Funk GC. Hypernatremia in critically ill patients. J Crit Care. 2013;28:216e11–20.
76. Adrogue HJ, Madias NE. Hypernatremia. N Engl J Med. 2000;342(20):1493–9.
77. Fang C, Mao J, et al. Fluid management of hypernatraemic dehydration to prevent cerebral oedema: a retrospective case control study of 97 children in China. J Paediatr Child Health. 2010;46(6):301–3.

78. Gennari FJ. Hypokalemia. N Engl J Med. 1998;339(7):451–8.
79. Slovis C, Jenkins R. ABC of clinical electrocardiography: conditions not primarily affecting the heart. BMJ. 2002;324(7349):1320–3.
80. Krahn LE, Lee J, Richardson JW, et al. Hypokalemia leasing to torsades de pointes. Munchausen's disorder or bulimia nervosa? Gen Hosp Psychiatry. 1997;19:370–7.
81. Nordrehaug JE, Johannessen KA, Von Der Lippe G. Serum potassium concentration as a risk factor of ventricular arrhythmias early in acute myocardial infarction. Circulation. 1985;71:645–9.
82. Graham DY. Effectiveness and tolerance of "solid" vs. "liquid" potassium replacement therapy. In: Cameron JS, Glussock RL, Whelton A, editors. Kidney disease. New York: Marcel Dekker Inc; 1986.
83. Melikian AP, Cheng LK, Wright GJ, et al. Bioavailability of potassium from three dosage forms: suspension, capsule, and solution. J Clin Pharmacol. 1988;28:1046–50.
84. Hamill RH, Robinson LM, Wexler GJ, et al. Efficacy and safety of potassium infusion therapy in hypokalemic critically ill patients. Crit Care Med. 1991;19:613–7.
85. Kruse JA, Carlson RW. Rapid correction of hypokalemia using concentrated intravenous potassium chloride infusions. Arch Intern Med. 1990;150(3):613–7.
86. Whang R, Oei TO, Aikawa JK, et al. Predictors of clinical hypomagnesemia: hypokalemia, hypophosphatemia, hyponatremia, and hypocalcemia. Arch Intern Med. 1984;144:1794–6.
87. Whang R, Whang DD, Ryan MP. Refractory potassium repletion: a consequence of magnesium deficiency. Arch Intern Med. 1992;152:40–5.
88. Alfonzo AV, Isles C, Geddes C, et al. Potassium disorders–clinical spectrum and emergency management. Resuscitation. 2006;70:10–25.
89. Allon M, Shanklin N. Effect of bicarbonate administration on plasma potassium in dialysis patients: interactions with insulin and albuterol. Am J Kidney Dis. 1996;28:508–14.
90. Parham WA, Mehdirad AA, Biermann KM, et al. Hyperkalemia revisited. Tex Heart Inst J. 2006;33(1):40–7.
91. Ahmed J, Weisberg LS. Hyperkalemia in dialysis patients. Semin Dial. 2001;14:348–56.
92. Fenton F, Smally AJ, Laut J. Hyperkalemia and digoxin toxicity in a patient with kidney failure. An Emerg Med. 1996;28(4):440–1.
93. Hack JB, Woody JH, Lewis DE, et al. The effect of calcium chloride in treating hyperkalemia due to acute digoxin toxicity in a porcine model. J Toxicol Clin Toxicol. 2004;42(4):337–42.
94. Van Deusen SK, Birkhahn RH, Gaeta TJ. Treatment of hyperkalemia in a patient with unrecognized digitalis toxicity. J Toxicol Clin Toxicol. 2003;41(4):373–6.
95. Allon M, Dunlay R, Copkney C. Nebulized albuterol for acute hyperkalemia in patients on hemodialysis. Ann Intern Med. 1989;110(6):426–9.
96. Mahoney BA, Smith WA, Lo DS, et al. Emergency interventions for hyperkalemia. Cochrane Database Syst Rev. 2005;(2):CD003235.
97. Allon M, Copkney C. Albuterol and insulin for treatment of hyperkalemia in hemodialysis patients. Kidney Int. 1990;38:869–72.
98. Blumberg A, Weidmann P, Shaw S, et al. Effect of various therapeutic approaches on plasma potassium and major regulating factors in terminal renal failure. Am J Med. 1988;85(4):507–12.
99. Carvalhana V, Burry L, Lapinsky SE. Management of severe hyperkalemia without hemodialysis: case report and literature review. J Crit Care. 2006;21(4):316–21.
100. Lin JL, Lim PS, Leu ML, et al. Outcomes of severe hyperkalemia in cardiopulmonary resuscitation with concomitant hemodialysis. Intensive Care Med. 1994;20(4):287–90.
101. Gruy-Kapral C, Emmett M, Santa Ana CA, et al. Effect of single dose resin-cathartic therapy on serum potassium concentration in patients with end-stage renal disease. J Am Soc Nephrol. 1998;9(10):1924–30.
102. Lier H, Krep H, Schroeder S, et al. Preconditions of hemostasis in trauma: a review; the influence of acidosis, hypocalcemia, anemia, and hypothermia on functional hemostasis in trauma. J Trauma. 2008;65:951–60.
103. Carlstedt F, Lind L. Hypocalcemic syndromes. Crit Care Clin. 2001;17(1):139–53.
104. Wei M, Taskapan H, Esbaei K, Jassal SV, Bargman JM, Oreopoulos DG. K/DOQI guideline requirements for calcium, phosphate, calcium phosphate product, and parathyroid hormone control in dialysis patients: can we achieve them? Int Urol Nephrol. 2006;39(3–4):739–49.
105. Ariyan CE, Sosa JA. Assessment and management of patients with abnormal calcium. Crit Care Med. 2004;32(4):S146–54.
106. Slomp J, Van Der Voort PHJ, Gerritsen RT, et al. Albumin adjusted calcium is not suitable for diagnosis of hyper- and hypocalcemia in the critically ill. Crit Care Med. 2003;31(5):1389–93.
107. Newman DB, Fidahussein SS, Kashiwagi DT, et al. Reversible cardiac dysfunction associated with hypocalcemia: a systematic review and meta-analysis of individual patient data. Heart Fail Rev. 2014;19:199–205.
108. Hurley K, Baggs D. Hypocalcemic cardiac failure in the emergency department. J Emerg Med. 2005;28(2):155–9.
109. Chavan CB, Sharada K, Rao HB, et al. Hypocalcemia as a cause of reversible cardiomyopathy with ventricular tachycardia. Ann Intern Med. 2007;147(7):541–2.
110. Desai T, Carlson R, Thill-Baharozian M, et al. A direct relationship between ionized calcium and arterial pressure among patients in an intensive care unit. Crit Care Med. 1988;16(6):578–82.
111. RuDusky B. ECG abnormalities associated with hypocalcemia. Chest. 2001;119:668–9.

112. Maier JD, Levine SN. Hypercalcemia in the intensive care unit: a review of pathophysiology, diagnosis, and modern therapy. J Intensive Care Med. 2013;30(5):235–52.
113. Swaminathan R. Magnesium metabolism and its disorders. Clin Biochem Rev. 2003;24:47–110.
114. Ayuk J, Gittoes NJ. How should hypomagnesaemia be investigated and treated? Clin Endocrinol (Oxf). 2011;65(6):743–6.
115. Tong GM, Rude RK. Magnesium deficiency in critical illness. J Intensive Care Med. 2005;20(1):3–17.
116. Noronha JL, Matuschak GM. Magnesium in critical illness: metabolism, assessment, and treatment. Intensive Care Med. 2002;28(6):667–79.
117. Shiber JR, Mattu A. Serum phosphate abnormalities in the emergency department. J Emerg Med. 2002;23(4):395–400.
118. Kraft MD, Btaiche IF, Sacks GS, et al. Treatment of electrolyte disorders in adult patients in the intensive care unit. Am J Health-Syst Pharm. 2005;62:1663–82.
119. Charron T, Bernard F, Skrobik Y, et al. Intravenous phosphate in the intensive care unit: more aggressive repletion regimens for moderate and severe hypophosphatemia. Intensive Care Med. 2003;29(8):1273–8.
120. Suzuki S, Egi M, Schneider AG, et al. Hypophosphatemia in critically ill patients. J Crit Care. 2013;28(4):536e9–19.

19 Sepsis and Septic Shock

Gina Hurst, Jayna Gardner-Gray,
Jacqueline Pflaum-Carlson, Brad A. Johnson,
Lauren N. Rodriguez, and Emanuel P. Rivers

Introduction

The diagnosis, treatment, and management of infectious processes are a daily occurrence in emergency departments (ED) across the world. Sepsis and septic shock can arise from any seemingly simple infection and lead to significant morbidity and mortality.

As stated by the Surviving Sepsis Campaign in 2018 [1], sepsis is defined as life-threatening organ dysfunction caused by a dysregulated host response to infection, and septic shock is defined as underlying circulatory, cellular and metabolic dysfunction associated with a higher risk of mortality (Table 19.1).

Sepsis is associated with an in-hospital mortality ranging from 15% to 49% [2] and while present in less than 1 out of every 12 US hospitalizations, it contributes up to nearly 17–40% of hospital deaths [2–7]. Sepsis is not only a cause of great mortality, but has also been associated with substantial morbidity, as pulmonary, renal, neuromuscular, psychiatric, and cardiovascular dysfunction is of great socioeconomic burden in many survivors [8, 9]. Long-term follow-up studies show that even after surviving one episode of sepsis, the survivor's mortality risk continues to be increased and quality of life is reduced [10]. Patients admitted for sepsis are one-half as likely

Table 19.1 Definitions of SIRS, sepsis and septic shock

SIRS (systemic inflammatory response syndrome)	Two or more of the following: Temperature >38° C or <36° C Heart rate >90 bpm Respiratory rate >20 or $PaCo_2$ <32 mmHg White blood cell count >12,000 cells/mm³ or <4000 cells/mm³ or bandemia >10%
Sepsis	Infection with organ dysfunction and/or tissue hypoperfusion
Septic shock	Sepsis with ongoing hypotension despite adequate fluid resuscitation or lactate >4 mmol/L

G. Hurst (✉) · J. Gardner-Gray · J. Pflaum-Carlson
Department of Emergency Medicine and
Division of Pulmonary and Critical Care,
Henry Ford Hospital, Wayne State University,
Detroit, MI, USA
e-mail: ghurst1@hfhs.org

B. A. Johnson
Department of Anesthesiology,
University of Iowa Hospital,
Iowa City, IA, USA

L. N. Rodriguez
Department of Emergency Medicine,
Kaiser Moanalua Medical Center,
Honolulu, HI, USA

E. P. Rivers
Department of Emergency Medicine and Department
of Surgery, Henry Ford Hospital, Wayne State
University, Detroit, MI, USA

© Springer Nature Switzerland AG 2020
J. R. Shiber, S. D. Weingart (eds.), *Emergency Department Critical Care*,
https://doi.org/10.1007/978-3-030-28794-8_19

to be discharged home, twice as likely to be transferred to another short-term care facility, and three times as likely to be discharged to long-term care institutions [4].

Unfortunately, the incidence of sepsis has increased by 83% and two-thirds of the patients affected are over the age of 65 years [4, 11–15]. In accordance with a rising incidence, the occurrence of hospital admissions for sepsis has increased by over 100% (11.6 per 10,000 to 24.0 per 10,000) [16]. With our ever-aging population, it is likely that we will continue to observe a rise in the diagnosis of sepsis and its related complications.

As the prevalence of this disease continues to soar, it is imperative to identify and provide early treatment. It has been observed that early intervention and protocol-driven therapy of patients with sepsis lead to a significant decrease in mortality and sepsis-related morbidity [17–20]. Accordingly, it is paramount that ED providers are able to differentiate simple infection from those complicated by sepsis. Throughout this chapter, we will discuss how to identify, stabilize, and care for patients with this disease.

Pathophysiology

Sepsis is associated with significant organ dysfunction in the presence of an identified infection. This end-organ dysfunction is the result of an inflammatory cascade which, when unregulated, results in altered microcirculation including a shift toward thrombosis, impaired oxygen delivery, and global tissue hypoxia. This tissue hypoxia may result in mild organ injury to overt shock and multi-organ system failure (Fig. 19.1).

In models of early sepsis, tissue hypoxia results from hemodynamic disturbances that cre-

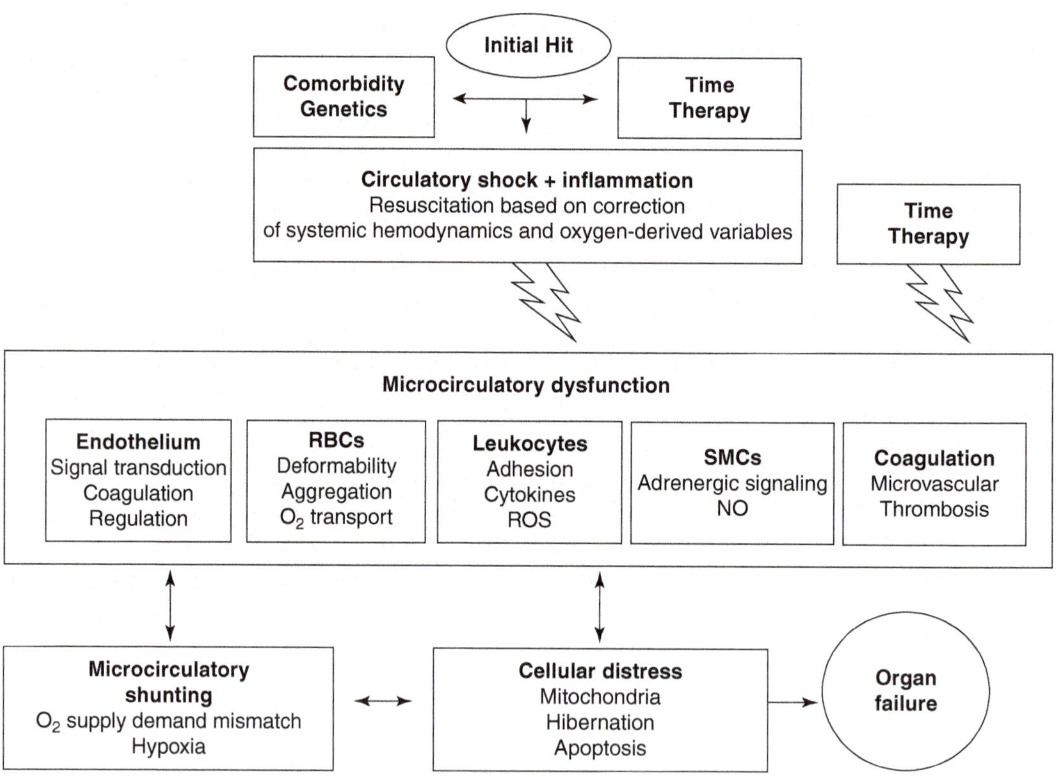

Fig. 19.1 Microcirculation and organ failure in sepsis

ate an imbalance between systemic oxygen delivery and demands. These perturbations can include hypovolemia, decreased vasomotor tone, decreased arterial oxygen content, decreased cardiac output (CO) from myocardial suppression, increased metabolic demands, and microcirculatory or mitochondrial derangements [21–24]. A critical decrease in oxygen delivery is followed by an increase in the systemic oxygen demands resulting in a decrease in central venous ($ScvO_2$) or mixed venous oxygen saturation (SvO_2) [25]. Anaerobic metabolism ensues when the limits of this compensatory mechanism cannot maintain systemic oxygen consumption (VO_2) most often leading to lactate production [26]. As the inflammatory cascade continues, the latter stage is an impairment of systemic oxygen utilization secondary to microcirculatory defects or impaired cellular respiration, often followed by worsening hemodynamic instability, organ failure, and death.

Patient Presentation

Sepsis is a disease process that resides on a continuum (Fig. 19.2). It can range from mild organ dysfunction to multiple organ system failure and severe hemodynamic instability. The presentation of a patient to the emergency department will vary based on where a patient lies on this continuum.

Often, patients will present with symptomatology suggestive of an underlying infection such as fever, rigors, cough, etc. (Table 19.2). Sepsis may then be classified by first diagnosing an infection and subsequently identifying underlying organ dysfunction. This presentation occurs commonly, however is quite idyllic. Many patients with sepsis or septic shock are unable to provide an adequate history and instead present to the emergency department with altered mental status, malaise, hemodynamic instability, or even cardiac arrest. Thus, the diagnosis of sepsis should also be enter-

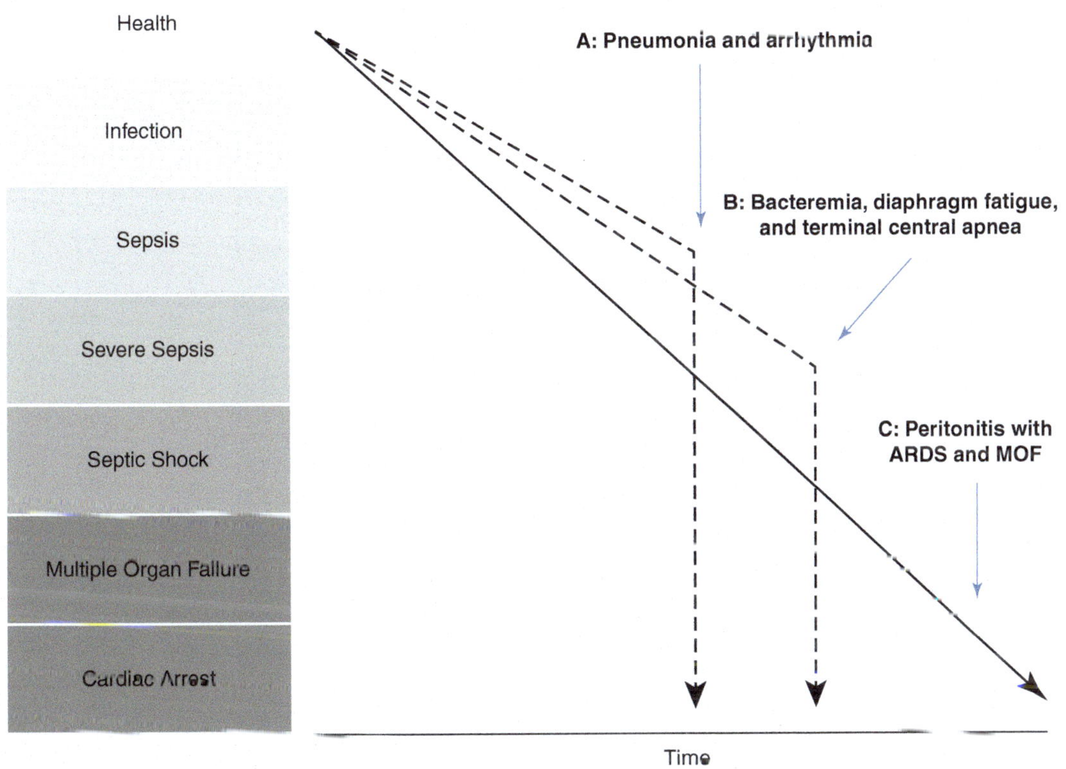

Fig. 19.2 Sepsis continuum

Table 19.2 Indicators based on history and exam that can help suggest the idea of early sepsis or infection are dependent on the system and include

Respiratory*	History: productive cough, fevers, chills, shortness of breath, rhinorrhea, congestion, sinus, throat, and ear pain. Exam findings: hypoxia, tachypnea, exudative tonsillitis, sinus tenderness, tympanic membrane injection, and crackles or dullness on lung auscultation.
Gastrointestinal**	History: location of pain, last bowel movement, nausea/vomiting, diarrhea, hematemesis, melena, hematochezia, oral intake, prior surgeries. Exam findings: signs of peritoneal irritation, abdominal tenderness, and hyperactive or hypoactive bowel sounds, Murphy's sign indicating cholecystitis, pain at McBurney's point indicating appendicitis, left lower quadrant pain suggesting diverticulitis, or rectal examination revealing a rectal abscess or prostatitis.
Neurologic	History: lethargy, altered mentation, or headache, focal weakness. Exam consistent with nuchal rigidity, fevers, neurologic deficits, and change in consciousness or low glasgow coma scale (GCS). Keep in mind that lethargy or altered mentation may also be signs of hypoperfusion to the brain or metabolic dysfunction. Septic encephalopathy has been reported between 10% and 70%. The mortality rate in patients with septic encephalopathy is higher than that in septic patients without significant neurologic involvement.
Cardiovascular	History: often indolent with fever, chills, malaise, suspect with intravenous drug use, dialysis, or indwelling catheters. Exam consistent with splinter hemorrhages, Roth's spots, Janeway lesions.
Genitourinary	History: flank pain, dysuria, polyuria, discharge, Foley catheter placement, genitourinary instrumentation, and a sexual history. Exam: costovertebral angle tenderness, external genitalia for ulcers, discharge, and penile or vulvar lesions, assessing for a tender, boggy prostate, a red and friable cervix, cervical discharge, or cervical motion or adnexal tenderness
Skin/soft tissue/ musculoskeletal	History of pain, swelling, and redness of a particular area. Exam: redness, swelling, warmth, and tenderness of specific area. Important to expose all patients in order to fully assess.

* Most common source of infection
** Second most common source

tained when a patient presents with significant hemodynamic instability or organ dysfunction that is without apparent cause.

The systemic inflammatory response syndrome (SIRS) was developed as a clinical aide to direct the clinician to entertain the diagnosis of infection. It comprises two of the following four items:

1. Temperature >38 °C or <36.0 °C
2. Heart rate >90 beats/min
3. Respiration rate >20 breaths/min, or PaCO2 < 32 mmHg
4. White blood cell (WBC) count >12,000 or <4000/mm^3, or >10% increased bands or immature cells

Extremes of age and concomitant medical conditions and medications can often mask these normal physiologic responses making the use of SIRS and diagnosis of sepsis more challenging. Because of these truths, as well as the significant burden of delay in diagnosis, it is important that we consider factors that increase the risk of developing sepsis (Table 19.3).

Table 19.3 Sepsis risk factors

Factors that further increase the risk of sepsis
Advanced age >65
Immunosuppression
Diabetes and comorbid disease
Cancer
Community-acquired pneumonia
Previous hospitalizations, nursing home, or rehabilitation residents

Despite their common use, SIRS can be present with many disease processes as these abnormalities are the manifestation of a pro-inflammatory cascade. It is important to

Table 19.4 Hemodynamic profile of sepsis

Hemodynamic picture	CVP	CO	Lactate	$ScvO_2$
Hypovolemia	↓	↑	↑	↓
Myocardial suppression	↑	↓	↑	↓
Resuscitated or compensated	Normal	↑	Normal or ↑	↑
Impaired oxygen Utilization	Normal	↑	↑	↑

understand that this is one of the several responses that patients mount when reacting to infection. Described by *Bone* in 1997, SIRS is not the only consequence of the massive cytokine release that is present in the setting of sepsis. Following an initial pro-inflammatory cascade, an anti-inflammatory cascade may occur. This can result in downregulation of inflammatory mediators and immune suppression referred to as a compensatory anti-inflammatory response syndrome or a mixed antagonist response syndrome. This loss of regulatory balance potentiates organ dysfunction and immune homeostasis [27].

Just as there are varied immune responses to sepsis, there are also differing hemodynamic profiles (Table 19.4). The development of these profiles is multifactorial and often related to time course of disease, severity of illness, and patient's underlying comorbid conditions. The typical presentation of sepsis and related shock is a result of systemic vasodilation and volume depletion. In response to the pro-inflammatory state, the systemic vascular resistance (SVR) decreases, resulting in low central venous pressure (CVP) and subsequent increased cardiac output. Mean arterial pressure (MAP) is a product of cardiac output (CO) and systemic vascular resistance. In early sepsis, compensatory increases in systemic vascular resistance secondary to catecholamine surges may maintain MAP, while CO or systemic oxygen delivery decreases to the tissues and the microcirculation. In this setting, the host may be warm, flushed, and with bounding pulses [28, 29]. When the limit of this compensatory mechanism (oxygen extraction ratio >50%) is reached, anaerobic metabolism ensues leading to lactate production [26]. In this oxygen-dependent phase, lactate concentrations begin to increase as oxygen delivery (DO_2) and central venous oxygen saturation ($ScvO_2/SvO_2$) decrease [22]. Without intervention, oxygen supply and demand continues to be mismatched, hypovolemia persists, acidosis worsens, and compensatory mechanisms will fail leading to systemic hypotension. As hypoperfusion persists, patient may transition from warm shock to cool and clammy due to redirection of blood flow to core organs. As shock state advances, the host will become lethargic, mottled, and cyanotic due to severe tissue hypoxia.

The heart is particularly vulnerable to these early compensatory mechanisms because it already has an increased rate of oxygen use under normal states [30]. A further increase in myocardial oxygen extraction in early sepsis will induce anaerobic metabolism quickly. This is exacerbated in patients with preexisting limited coronary blood flow. There is also a direct impairment of myocardial function from sepsis. As a result, markers of myocardial dysfunction or distress, such as increased troponin, B-type natriuretic peptide (BNP), heart rate variability, and atrial fibrillation, are associated with increased mortality [31–36].

Understanding the hemodynamic profile of a patient upon evaluation in the ED is key to appropriate and individualized resuscitation efforts. Diagnostic efforts should aim to not only evaluate end-organ hypoperfusion, but also to assess hemodynamic parameters and their surrogates.

Diagnosis

The diagnostic landscape of sepsis is continuously evolving. Sepsis was once considered a disease diagnosed only in the intensive care unit (ICU), however, we now realize that earlier detection and diagnosis of this disease process lead to significantly lower morbidity and mortality [37]. Thus, efforts are needed to enhance clinician awareness of diagnostic sepsis tools to better identify and risk stratify patients who present to the ED with this potentially deadly condition [38].

A plethora of tests have been suggested to improve diagnostic decision-making in the clinical setting of infection. As the differential diagnosis of SIRS is extremely broad, these tests can aid in eliminating unlikely diagnoses. The lack of sensitivity and specificity of SIRS for sepsis is reflected in the fact that more than two-thirds of intensive care unit patients, and a substantial number of patients on general medical units, at some point during their hospitalization have at least two SIRS criteria [39, 40] as well as almost one in five patients admitted with infection from the ED will have an alternative diagnosis at hospital discharge.

The gold standard of diagnosis in the setting of sepsis is identifying a causative microorganism. Paracentesis for ascitic fluid evaluation, lumbar punctures for cerebrospinal fluid (CSF) evaluation, and sinus and soft tissue aspirations are among the many invasive techniques that should be performed when clinically appropriate. Any purulent discharge or sputum and potentially infected bodily fluids, such as CSF, urine, or stool, should be sent for microbiologic culture. Tissue biopsies of an affected area should also be arranged when clinically indicated. Blood cultures are an additional important part of the diagnostic evaluation. Because rapid sterilization of blood cultures can occur within a few hours after the first antimicrobial dose, obtaining blood cultures before therapy (if possible without delaying administration by >60 min) is essential to confirm infection, identify the responsible pathogens, and to allow de-escalation of antimicrobial therapy. Two or more blood cultures are recommended [41].

Various imaging studies are often needed for localizing potential sources of infection. Chest radiograph is the modality that is most frequently used for diagnosis of pulmonary infections. Interestingly, some studies show chest radiograph alone may miss up to 20% of community-acquired pneumonias [42] and has been demonstrated to be an insensitive method with relatively low accuracy in this clinical scenario [43, 44]. Subsequently, computer-assisted tomography (CT) and magnetic resonance imaging (MRI) are being increasingly utilized as primary imaging techniques for the diagnosis of various infections ranging from intra-abdominal processes to osteomyelitis. This is due to the high sensitivity and specificity of these imaging techniques for identifying infectious processes. Such imaging is vital for providing specific diagnostic clues such as locating foreign bodies or abscesses requiring respective removal or drainage. When using these imaging modalities, consideration should be given to the risk of patient exposure to the toxicities of contrast agents as well as the risk of radiation exposure.

A diagnostic imaging modality not associated with the above-mentioned risks and rapidly growing in popularity is the use of ultrasonography. Focused ultrasonography is a diagnostic technique to consider as part of hemodynamic assessment during the care of select patients with severe sepsis and septic shock. Ultrasonography is recommended for the prompt recognition of complicating physiology such as hypovolemia or cardiogenic shock as well as a tool to assess volume responsiveness. A 2010 consensus documented by the American Society of Echocardiography and the American College of Emergency Physicians recommends that "focused ultrasonography may assist in early shock diagnosis and alert clinicians to underlying physiologic disturbance" [45]. However, there are no randomized controlled trials to date testing ultrasonography in sepsis or its application in clinical practice (grade C evidence – expert opinion), so these recommendations should be used with caution.

Sepsis

Patients with sepsis who develop organ dysfunction represent approximately 25% of those who initially present to the ED with sepsis [46]. The mortality of severe sepsis and septic shock increases with delay in each of these respective diagnoses [47]. One study describes a 20% higher absolute hospital mortality among septic patients who develop shock later in their hospital course compared to those who are diagnosed earlier in their clinical course [48]. Prompt recognition of sepsis and septic shock involves understanding the pathophysiology and subsequent clinical manifestations of affected patients as well as obtaining specific laboratory values that suggest organ dysfunction (See Table 19.5).

Table 19.5 Clinical findings and laboratory markers in sepsis

Transient sepsis-induced hypotension
Lactate above upper limits laboratory normal (>2 mmol/L)
Urine output <0.5 mL/kg/hr for more than 2 hours, despite adequate fluid resuscitation
Acute lung injury with PaO_2/FiO_2 <250 in the absence of pneumonia as infection source
Acute lung injury with PaO_2/FiO_2 <200 in the presence of pneumonia as infection source
Creatinine >2.0 mg/dL (176.8 μmol/L)
Bilirubin >2 mg/dL (34.2 μmol/L)
Platelet count <100,000 μL
Coagulopathy (international normalized ratio >1.5)

Though many signs of end-organ damage manifest themselves clinically, some require laboratory testing. Clinical findings, suggestive of sepsis, include neurologic sequelae leading to mental status changes, hypotension with systolic blood pressure (SBP) <90 mmHg, responsiveness to intravenous (IV) fluids, and decreased urine output <0.5 mL/kg/hr. Laboratory tests that should be obtained on a patient suspected of having sepsis or septic shock should include but not be limited to a complete blood count (CBC) with differential, coagulation studies including prothrombin time (PT) and the activated partial thromboplastin time (aPTT), complete metabolic profile, blood cultures, and an arterial or venous blood gas with lactic acid.

Septic Shock

The transition from sepsis to septic shock is diagnosed when the host is persistently hypotensive, despite adequate volume resuscitation. There are no overt laboratory abnormalities to differentiate the two states, except perhaps for lactate elevation. A lactate level ≥4 mmol/L meets the diagnostic criteria for septic shock, as it suggests ongoing tissue hypoperfusion. The disturbances of lactate metabolism in sepsis are probably more complex than an isolated defect of cellular oxygenation [49]. However, it remains established that a lactate value greater than or equal to 4 mM/L on hospital admission is associated with a mortality between 20% and 50% [50–54]. It is important not to overrely on lactate, as it is still considered a very complicated biomarker that is not fully understood and can be normal in up to 30% of patients with septic shock as well as elevated in many other conditions [55].

Initial Stabilization

In patients with uncomplicated sepsis, IV fluid administration and antibiotic therapy along with control of the infectious source may be the only treatment required. However, once organ injury or hypotension has developed, early stabilization and aggressive intervention of the patient is key to reducing mortality and sepsis-related organ dysfunction. Due to the significant benefit of early intervention, the Centers for Medicare and Medicaid Services (CMS) have adopted quality measures for management of sepsis and septic shock (Table 19.6). Given the complexity of the pathophysiology of the septic patient, a standardized protocol-driven approach is recommended (Fig. 19.3).

Table 19.6 CMS criteria for sepsis resuscitation

Surviving sepsis campaign resuscitation bundle
To be completed within 3 hours of time of presentation[a]:
Measure *lactate* level
Obtain *blood cultures* prior to administration of antibiotics
Administer *broad-spectrum antibiotics*
Administer 30 ml/kg crystalloid for hypotension or lactate ≥4 mmol/L
To be completed within 6 hours of time of presentation:
Apply *vasopressors* for hypotension refractory to volume resuscitation
Reassess volume status and tissue perfusion and document findings (if persistent hypotension after fluids, or if initial lactate ≥4)
Repeat focused exam: vital signs, cardiopulmonary, capillary refill, pulse, and skin findings
OR
Two of the following
Measure central venous pressure
Measure central venous oxygen saturation
Bedside cardiovascular ultrasound
Dynamic assessment of fluid responsiveness with passive leg raise or fluid challenge
Remeasure lactate if initial lactate is elevated.

[a]"Time of presentation" is defined as the time of triage in the emergency department or, if presenting from another care venue, from the earliest chart annotation consistent with all elements of severe sepsis or septic shock ascertained through chart review

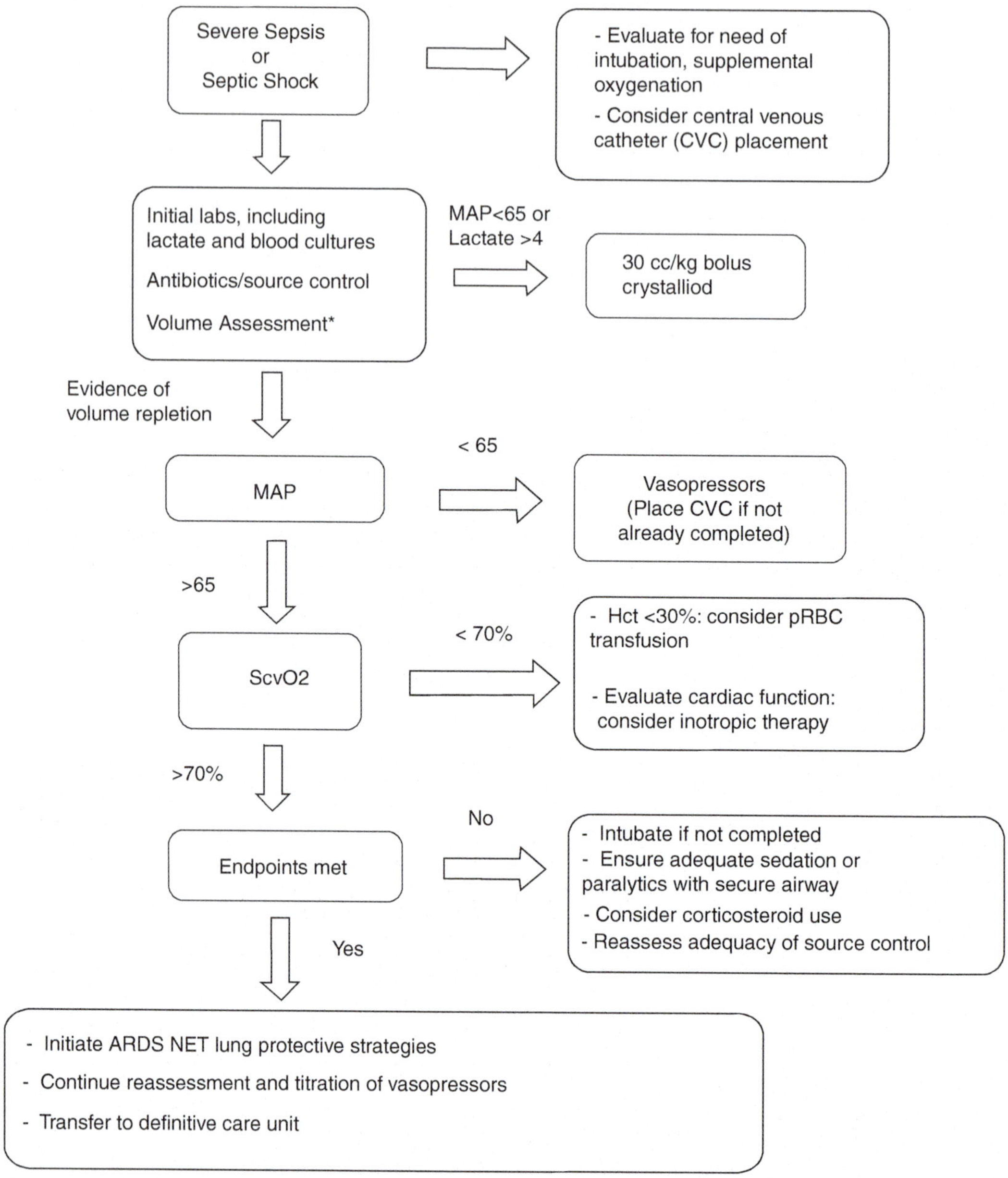

Fig. 19.3 Protocol-driven approach to severe sepsis/septic shock management

Intubation or Supplemental Oxygenation

Optimizing the central venous saturation and improving hemodynamics require improvements in oxygenation. The increased work of breathing in septic patients can increase oxygen consumption up to 20% [56], and reducing this consumption via intubation can preserve available oxygen supplies for other vital organs in critical demand. It is important to note, however, that intubation and mechanical ventilation are often associated with an increase in intrathoracic pressure and a consequential decrease in preload that can result in critical hypotension. Additionally, the agents used for rapid sequence intubation can blunt sympathetic response and cause venodilation. Appropriate volume resuscitation can help combat this effect, but providers should be prepared for postintubation hypotension.

Alternatively, if a patient has increased oxygen demands but does not meet overt clinical need for intubation or care facility lacks ability to intubate, supplemental oxygen in the form of nasal cannula, nonrebreather mask, or high flow nasal cannula may be considered an adjunct to improve oxygen delivery. The use of supplemental oxygen, although potentially increasing oxygen delivery, will not reliably reduce oxygen consumption.

Volume Resuscitation

Early and aggressive fluid resuscitation with crystalloid solutions is associated with decreases in systemic inflammation and vasopressor use, as well as improved outcomes [57]. Surviving Sepsis Campaign recommends a 30 cc/kg initial bolus to combat hypotension or for lactate ≥4 mmol/L. Late aggressive fluid therapy is associated with increased mortality. Isotonic crystalloid solutions, such as normal saline or the "balanced" plasmalyte-A or lactated ringers, are favored [58]. Albumin has not consistently been proven effective; however, there is some evidence for diminished vasopressor requirements and mortality reduction in the subset of patients with septic shock [59].

Antibiotic Administration

International consensus guidelines recommend administering broad-spectrum antibiotics within the first hour of recognizing severe sepsis and septic shock. Mortality can increase up to 7.6% for each hour delay in antibiotic administration after the onset of hypotension or shock [60]. Although a direct correlation between delayed antibiotic administration and mortality is well known, many septic patients do not receive antibiotics until after hospital admission and frequently with inadequate coverage [61]. Some recent trials have recently called into question the strength of the association between hourly delays in antibiotic administration and mortality in septic shock patients [62]. However, multiple prospective observation studies have shown that antibiotic administration is most beneficial in the first 6 hours and does reduce healthcare costs [17, 60, 63–66].

Broad-spectrum antibiotics, aimed at managing the suspected infectious source, should be initiated early as inappropriate antibiotic choice has shown to increase mortality [67, 68]. If source is unknown, empiric therapy to cover gram positives, gram negatives, and anaerobes should be initiated. Common regimens include vancomycin and piperacillin/tazobactam or vancomycin with cefepime and metronidazole. Despite initial benefit of broad antibiotic therapy, reevaluation once bacterial source is confirmed is needed as de-escalation of antibiotics is strongly associated with improved outcomes [69].

Volume Assessment

Volume repletion in the management of sepsis and septic shock may seem somewhat trivial, as we assume the majority of patients will require large volume resuscitation. However, studies have shown that volume overload in the setting of renal injury has been associated with increased mortality [70, 71]. Accordingly, judicious volume replacement is highly relevant to improvement of resuscitation strategies and reassessment of volume status after initial and subsequent boluses should occur.

The original early goal-directed therapy (EGDT) study by Rivers et al. recommended early placement of central venous catheter (CVC) and measuring the central venous pressure (CVP) to achieve a goal pressure of 8–12 mmHg as an endpoint of adequate volume resuscitation. CVP is useful when at extremes of measurement; however, its ability to assess volume responsiveness continues to be debated. CVP monitoring can be erroneously interpreted by inappropriate positioning and conditions that increase right atrial pressure, pulmonary artery pressure, or cardiac compliance. While there is still use for CVC placement, advancements in diagnostics have allowed for alternative adjuncts to assess for volume responsiveness.

Other tools include evaluation of stroke volume variation (SVV), in which a value of greater than 10% is highly sensitive (84%) for prediction of volume responsiveness. This, however, is dependent on the patient being mechanically ventilated and in sinus rhythm [72, 73]. Esophageal Doppler monitors can adjust for the presence of nonsinus tachyarrythmias and assess cardiac output in response to fluid resuscitation but requires training, familiarity with the equipment, and is not often available in the emergency department [74].

Perhaps, the easiest and most available assessment of volume responsiveness is with point-of-care ultrasound for assessment of the inferior vena cava (IVC) diameter. The determination of an IVC size less than 1.2 cm in diameter correlates with hypovolemia [75]. This technique is valid both on the intubated and on nonintubated patients and can be completed prior to, or during the placement of, more invasive monitoring. Further evaluation of distensibility in the mechanically ventilated, and collapsibility in the patient spontaneously breathing, can also be used [76, 77]. The caveat to this evaluation is that cardiac structure and function are presumed to be normal.

Based on this short review, it is clear that each of these modalities has its own unique limitations. With this in mind, simultaneous use of multiple assessment tools as well as the patient's clinical picture in response to volume is likely the most reliable form of evaluation.

Vasopressors

Even with adequate fluid administration, vasodilation and a loss of autoregulation often lead to the necessitation of starting vasopressor therapy. Current guidelines recommend initiation of vasopressors if MAP is less than 65 and the patient has been appropriately volume resuscitated [78–81]. Norepinephrine is considered the vasopressor of choice [82]. Epinephrine can be used as a second line alternative to norepinephrine or as an additive agent in the event that additional vasopressors are needed (Table 19.7). Although this practice has not been adequately proven effective, studies show no increase in mortality when compared [83, 84]. Vasopressin, dopamine, and phenylephrine are not generally favorable choices, as they have no evidence of improved outcomes and the latter two are associated with possible harm [85–87]. Dopamine can be considered when the heart rate is inappropriately low, as it will increase the heart rate, while phenylephrine may be useful when there is already tachycardia or a tachyarrhythmia since it has no beta-stimulating effects of the heart.

Table 19.7 Vasopressor agents

Agent	Mechanism	Effects	Dose range	Adverse effects
Norepinephrine	α_1, α_2, β_1, some β_2	↑BP, HR, SVR	Start: 8–12 mcg/min WBD[a]: 0.01–3 mcg/kg/min	Can increase lactate, increase myocardial demand
Epinephrine	α_1, α_2, β_1, β_2	↑BP, HR, SVR	Start: 5–35 mcg/min WBD: 0.1–0.5mcg/kg/min	No studied benefit in sepsis
Vasopressin	Vascular smooth muscle contraction	↓/↔HR, ↑SVR, BP	Fixed: 0.04 U/min	Increased risk of arrhythmias and increased O_2 demand
Phenylephrine	Primarily α_1,some α_2	↓/↔HR, ↑SVR, BP ↔CO	Start: 25–180 mcg/min WBD: 0.5 mcg/kg/min	Impaired splanchnic blood flow, decrease in O_2 delivery

[a]*WBD* weight-based dosing

Inotropes

After volume repletion and treatment of hypotension (with or without vasopressor therapy), the combination of a low $ScvO_2$, increased CVP, and increased lactate is indicative of hemodynamically significant myocardial dysfunction [88]. If this hemodynamic profile is present, evaluation of cardiac function should take place. This can be achieved with point-of-care ultrasound, Fick equation, or use of other monitoring devices such as a pulmonary artery (PA) catheter or arterial pulse-contour wave analysis (eg. EV1000). Myocardial dysfunction can be present in up to 15% of patients in septic shock [89–91], and patients with cardiovascular comorbidities are more likely to have an impaired ability to increase oxygen delivery. If ongoing hypoperfusion is attributed to poor cardiac output, dobutamine or milrinone should be considered to improve inotropic function of the heart when the intravascular volume and MAP goals have already been reached.

Blood Transfusion

As frequently alluded to throughout this chapter, resuscitation from severe sepsis and septic shock is directly related to oxygen delivery. It follows that the host's ability to carry oxygen in the form of hemoglobin molecules will play a role in resuscitation. Various targets have been proposed for optimal hemoglobin and research has found that a higher threshold value of hemoglobin is not proven superior [92]. However, in the setting of low $ScvO_2$ after resuscitation and in the absence of significant myocardial dysfunction, blood transfusion may be useful to aid in improvement of oxygen delivery. While there are many publications that suggest RBC transfusions are associated with increased morbidity and mortality [93], observational studies show no increase in mortality [94] and even a decrease in mortality in large observational cohorts [95, 96]. Others have observed that RBC transfusion may increase $ScvO_2$ but does not improve mortality [97]. Based on the transfusion requirements in septic shock (TRISS) trial by Holst, most clinicians would agree that transfusion for hemoglobin less than 7 or $ScvO_2$ less than 69.5% is advisable. However, it is clear that this topic is up for ongoing debate, and clinical judgment for individual transfusion needs is necessary.

Corticosteroids

There are two major populations where stress dose steroids should be considered in the management of severe sepsis and septic shock. The apparent cases are those involving patients who are steroid dependent, either due to adrenal insufficiency or due to chronic steroid use. Another population who may benefit are patients with hypotension refractory to vasopressor therapy. Refractory to vasopressor therapy has been defined as persistent hypotension, despite adequate volume resuscitation and vasopressor support for more than 60 minutes [98]. Hydrocortisone when administered in "stress doses" (50 mg q6 hr) diminishes vasopressor requirements, duration, and total dose [99]. While the impact of steroids on mortality draws continued debate, recent evidence suggests that early treatment (within 9 hours) decreases vasopressor requirement and positively impacts outcome, especially in patients of higher illness severity [100]. Despite significant individual clinician variation, the overall outcome benefits continue to support the use of steroids in refractory septic shock.

Definitive Treatment

The goal in the management of septic patients is to treat early and aggressively in an attempt to limit morbidity and mortality. By using physiologic end points in conjunction with early identification of high-risk patients, appropriate cultures, source control, and appropriate antibiotic administration, this goal can be achieved.

Source Control

It is paramount to identify the anatomical source of a patient's infection. This key component of sepsis management may include drainage of infected fluids, debridement of soft tissue infection, removal of infected devices or foreign bodies, and/or management of intra-abdominal causes of infection. Source control should occur as rapidly as possible, ideally, within the first 12 hours of diagnosis [1]. The process of source control involves appropriate radiographic imaging interpretation, removal of the infectious focus, and early intervention with the least possible physiologic stress on the patient.

Every hour of delay from admission to surgery is associated with an adjusted 2.4% decreased probability of survival or a 16% reduction in mortality if no source control is achieved within 6 hours [101].

1. Drainage: The removal of fluid through the opening of an abscess is performed either by incision and drainage or by insertion of a drain. This converts a closed abscess into a controlled sinus or fistula. The drainage of an abscess can be performed surgically or percutaneously.
   Examples:
   Incision and drainage of a perirectal abscess
   Percutaneous drainage of a diverticular abscess
   Open surgical drainage of multiple intra-abdominal abscesses
2. Debridement: The removal of devitalized or infected solid tissue from the patient.
   Examples:
   Excision of gangrenous soft tissue or intestine
   Surgical excision of infected pancreatic necrosis
   Wet-to-dry dressings of an infected surgical wound
3. Device Removal: The removal of a prosthetic device or foreign body that has become colonized by microorganisms living in a biofilm.
   Examples:
   Removal of infected venous or urinary catheter
   Excision of an infected vascular graft
4. Restoration of Anatomy and Function: Other inventions performed to remove a focus of infection and to restore optimal function and quality of life.
   Examples:
   Phlegmonous appendix requiring removal
   Perforated gastric ulcer in need of repair

Lactate Clearance

The initial serum lactate is associated with mortality, independent of clinically apparent organ dysfunction and shock in patients diagnosed with sepsis. Both intermediate and high serum lactate levels are associated with increased mortality [53]. Studies have shown that lactate clearance over the first 6 hours is associated with a significant decrease in inflammation, improved organ function, and reduced mortality [102]. When using this endpoint, we must be aware of the subset of patients in septic shock that may have a normal lactate level (alactemic septic shock), which is associated with increased mortality [55]. Also, lactate clearance can be confounded by certain medications such as metformin, packed red blood cells (RBCs), as well as certain disease processes such as cirrhosis which impair lactate clearance. Lactate clearance should be used in conjunction with $ScvO_2$ as resuscitation endpoints.

Central Venous Oxygen Saturation

The clinical utility of $ScvO_2$ is based on its diagnostic ability to detect early imbalances of oxygen delivery (DO_2) to oxygen consumption (VO_2), particularly in the early phase of sepsis where vital signs and lactate can be normal [103]. During the early phase of sepsis, the patient is in an oxygen-dependent phase. This is evidenced by a low SVO_2/$Scvo_2$ saturation. When this deficit is recognized, therapeutic maneuvers to increase oxygen delivery (DO_2) or decrease oxygen consumption (VO_2) should be undertaken to prevent tissue hypoxia, further inflammation, lactate generation, myocardial dysfunction, and ultimately increased mortality. Effective maneuvers work to increase DO_2, decrease VO_2, or both (Table 19.8). Normalization of $ScvO_2$ has been shown to positively impact mortality [104, 105]. Thus, resuscitation using this parameter as an endpoint is encouraged.

Table 19.8 Oxygen supply and demand

	Clinical problem	Therapeutic intervention
Oxygen supply	Decreases DO_2 Hypoxemia Anemia Myocardial dysfunction	Increases DO_2 Increase supplemental oxygen Red blood cell transfusion Inotropic support
Oxygen demand	Increases VO_2 Anxiety Pain Hyperthermia Shivering Work of breathing	Decreases VO_2 Anxiolytics Analgesia Antipyretics Sedation/paralytics Ventilator synchrony

Conclusion

Sepsis identification, classification, and management are a necessary skill for emergency medicine providers. Early recognition and intervention reduces organ dysfunction and saves lives. The treatment strategies delineated in this chapter are aimed at infectious source control and improvement of oxygen delivery. While sepsis bundles and protocols are useful guidelines, considering the patient's individual hemodynamic profile can help to deliver specialized critical care in the emergency department.

Critical Points

- Sepsis spectrum is caused by dysregulated host response leading to impaired oxygen delivery or uncontrolled oxygen consumption
- Identify infectious source – so it can be controlled
- Check lactate, CBC, electrolytes, liver function tests (LFTs), and coagulation profile for extent of organ failure
- Fluid bolus at least 30 cc/kg of crystalloid for hypotension or lactate > 4
- Antibiotic administration - broad empiric therapy, as early as possible (no later than 3 hours)
- Evaluate and reassess volume and perfusion status frequently using a combination of modalities (i.e. CVP, ultrasound, $ScvO_2$, etc.)
- Vasopressors for persistent hypotension after fluid resuscitation
- For persistent hypotension after 1 hour of vasopressor therapy, give 50 mg of hydrocortisone every 6 hours
- Consider inotropic therapy if cardiac output or index is reduced

References

1. Rhodes A, Evans L, Alhazzani W, Levy MM, et al. Surviving Sepsis Campaign: international guidelines for management of sepsis and septic shock, 2018. Intensive Care Med. 2017;43(3):304–77.
2. Angus DC, Linde-Zwirble WT, Lidicker J, Clermont G, Carcillo J, Pinsky MR. Epidemiology of severe sepsis in the United States: analysis of incidence, outcome, and associated costs of care. Crit Care Med. 2001;29(7):1303–10.
3. Kumar G, Kumar N, Taneja A, Kaleekal T, Tarima S, McGinley E, et al. Nationwide trends of severe sepsis in the 21st century (2000--2007). Chest. 2011;140(5):1223–31.
4. Hall MJ, Williams SN, DeFrances CJ, Golosinskiy A. Inpatient care for septicemia or sepsis: a challenge for patients and hospitals. NCHS Data Brief. 2011;62:1–8.
5. Wang HE, Shapiro NI, Angus DC, Yealy DM. National estimates of severe sepsis in United States emergency departments. Crit Care Med. 2007;35(8):1928–36.
6. Liu V, Escobar GJ, Whippy A, Angus DC, Iwashyna TJ. Sepsis contributes to nearly half of all hospital deaths in the US [abstract]. Am J Respir Crit Care Med. 2014;189(Meeting Abstracts):A2188.
7. Reed K, May R. The first annual HealthGrades emergency medicine in American hospitals study. Health Grades, Inc: Golden; 2010.
8. Davydow DS, Hough CL, Langa KM, Iwashyna TJ. Symptoms of depression in survivors of severe sepsis: a prospective cohort study of older Americans. Am J Geriatr Psychiatry. 2013;21(9):887–97.
9. Shen HN, Lu CL, Li CY. Do physicians have lower risk of severe sepsis and associated mortality? A matched cohort study. Crit Care Med. 2014;42(4):816–23.
10. Winters BD, Eberlein M, Leung J, Needham DM, Pronovost PJ, Sevransky JE. Long-term mortality and quality of life in sepsis: a systematic review. Crit Care Med. 2010;38(5):1276–83.

11. Lagu T, Lindenauer PK, Rothberg MB, Nathanson BH, Pekow PS, Steingrub JS, et al. Development and validation of a model that uses enhanced administrative data to predict mortality in patients with sepsis. Crit Care Med. 2011;39(11):2425–30.
12. Lemay AC, Anzueto A, Restrepo MI, Mortensen EM. Predictors of long-term mortality after severe sepsis in the elderly. Am J Med Sci. 2014;347(4):282–8.
13. Wichmann MW, Inthorn D, Andress HJ, Schildberg FW. Incidence and mortality of severe sepsis in surgical intensive care patients: the influence of patient gender on disease process and outcome. Intensive Care Med. 2000;26(2):167–72.
14. de Montmollin E, Tandjaoui-Lambiotte Y, Legrand M, Lambert J, Mokart D, Kouatchet A, et al. Outcomes in critically ill cancer patients with septic shock of pulmonary origin. Shock. 2013;39(3):250–4.
15. Bateman BT, Schmidt U, Berman MF, Bittner EA. Temporal trends in the epidemiology of severe postoperative sepsis after elective surgery: a large, nationwide sample. Anesthesiology. 2010;112(4):917–25.
16. Seymour CW, Iwashyna TJ, Cooke CR, Hough CL, Martin GS. Marital status and the epidemiology and outcomes of sepsis. Chest. 2010;137(6):1289–96.
17. Gaieski DF, Mikkelsen ME, Band RA, Pines JM, Massone R, Furia FF, et al. Impact of time to antibiotics on survival in patients with severe sepsis or septic shock in whom early goal-directed therapy was initiated in the emergency department. Crit Care Med. 2010;38(4):1045–53.
18. Rivers EP, Kruse JA, Jacobsen G, Shah K, Loomba M, Otero R, et al. The influence of early hemodynamic optimization on biomarker patterns of severe sepsis and septic shock. Crit Care Med. 2007;35(9):2016–24.
19. Rivers EP, Katranji M, Jaehne KA, Brown S, Abou Dagher G, Cannon C, et al. Early interventions in severe sepsis and septic shock: a review of the evidence one decade later. Minerva Anestesiol. 2012;78(6):712–24.
20. Cannon CM, Holthaus CV, Zubrow MT, Posa P, Gunaga S, Kella V, et al. The GENESIS project (GENeralized Early Sepsis Intervention Strategies): a multicenter quality improvement collaborative. J Intensive Care Med. 2013;28(6):355–68.
21. Rackow EC, Astiz ME. Pathophysiology and treatment of septic shock. JAMA. 1991;266(4):548–54.
22. Rosario AL, Park M, Brunialti MK, Mendes M, Rapozo M, Fernandes D, et al. SvO(2)-guided resuscitation for experimental septic shock: effects of fluid infusion and dobutamine on hemodynamics, inflammatory response, and cardiovascular oxidative stress. Shock. 2011;36(6):604–12.
23. Conti-Patara A, de Araujo CJ, de Mattos-Junior E, de Carvalho HS, Reinoldes A, Pedron BG, et al. Changes in tissue perfusion parameters in dogs with severe sepsis/septic shock in response to goal-directed hemodynamic optimization at admission to ICU and the relation to outcome. J Vet Emerg Crit Care (San Antonio). 2012;22(4):409–18.
24. Correa TD, Vuda M, Blaser AR, Takala J, Djafarzadeh S, Dunser MW, et al. Effect of treatment delay on disease severity and need for resuscitation in porcine fecal peritonitis. Crit Care Med. 2012;40(10):2841–9.
25. von Seth M, Sjolin J, Larsson A, Eriksson M, Hillered L, Lipcsey M. Effects of tigecycline and doxycycline on inflammation and hemodynamics in porcine endotoxemia: a prospective, randomized, and placebo-controlled trial. Shock. 2015;43(6):604–11.
26. Kasnitz P, Druger GL, Yorra F, Simmons DH. Mixed venous oxygen tension and hyperlactatemia. Survival in severe cardiopulmonary disease. JAMA. 1976;236(6):570–4.
27. Bone RC, Grodzin CJ, Balk RA. Sepsis: a new hypothesis for pathogenesis of the disease process. Chest. 1997;112(1):235–43.
28. De Backer D, Creteur J, Preiser JC, Dubois MJ, Vincent JL. Microvascular blood flow is altered in patients with sepsis. Am J Respir Crit Care Med. 2002;166(1):98–104.
29. Trzeciak S, Dellinger RP, Parrillo JE, Guglielmi M, Bajaj J, Abate NL, et al. Early microcirculatory perfusion derangements in patients with severe sepsis and septic shock: relationship to hemodynamics, oxygen transport, and survival. Ann Emerg Med. 2007;49(1):88–98.e1–2.
30. Miwa K, Fujita M, Ejiri M, Sasayama S. Biphasic changes (initial increase and late decrease) in coronary sinus venous oxygen saturation during anginal attacks induced by intracoronary acetylcholine in patients with variant angina. Cardiology. 1992;81(4–5):221–32.
31. Rivers EP, McCord J, Otero R, Jacobsen G, Loomba M. Clinical utility of B-type natriuretic peptide in early severe sepsis and septic shock. J Intensive Care Med. 2007;22(6):363–73.
32. Klouche K, Pommet S, Amigues L, Bargnoux AS, Dupuy AM, Machado S, et al. Plasma brain natriuretic peptide and troponin levels in severe sepsis and septic shock: relationships with systolic myocardial dysfunction and intensive care unit mortality. J Intensive Care Med. 2014;29(4):229–37.
33. Ahmad S, Ramsay T, Huebsch L, Flanagan S, McDiarmid S, Batkin I, et al. Continuous multiparameter heart rate variability analysis heralds onset of sepsis in adults. PLoS One. 2009;4(8):e6642.
34. Walkey AJ, Greiner MA, Heckbert SR, Jensen PN, Piccini JP, Sinner MF, et al. Atrial fibrillation among Medicare beneficiaries hospitalized with sepsis: incidence and risk factors. Am Heart J. 2013;165(6):949–55.e3.
35. Salman S, Bajwa A, Gajic O, Afessa B. Paroxysmal atrial fibrillation in critically ill patients with sepsis. J Intensive Care Med. 2008;23(3):178–83.

36. Walkey AJ, Wiener RS, Ghobrial JM, Curtis LH, Benjamin EJ. Incident stroke and mortality associated with new-onset atrial fibrillation in patients hospitalized with severe sepsis. JAMA. 2011;306(20):2248–54.
37. Rivers E, Nguyen B, Havstad S, Ressler J, Muzzin A, Knoblich B, et al. Early goal-directed therapy in the treatment of severe sepsis and septic shock. N Engl J Med. 2001;345(19):1368–77.
38. Brown T, Ghelani-Allen A, Yeung D, Nguyen HB. Comparative effectiveness of physician diagnosis and guideline definitions in identifying sepsis patients in the emergency department. J Crit Care. 2015;30(1):71–7.
39. Marshall JC. SIRS and MODS: what is their relevance to the science and practice of intensive care? Shock. 2000;14(6):586–9.
40. Vincent JL. Dear SIRS, I'm sorry to say that I don't like you. Crit Care Med. 1997;25(2):372–4.
41. Weinstein MP, Reller LB, Murphy JR, Lichtenstein KA. The clinical significance of positive blood cultures: a comprehensive analysis of 500 episodes of bacteremia and fungemia in adults. I. Laboratory and epidemiologic observations. Rev Infect Dis. 1983;5(1):35–53.
42. Hagaman JT, Rouan GW, Shipley RT, Panos RJ. Admission chest radiograph lacks sensitivity in the diagnosis of community-acquired pneumonia. Am J Med Sci. 2009;337(4):236–40.
43. Hayden GE, Wrenn KW. Chest radiograph vs. computed tomography scan in the evaluation for pneumonia. J Emerg Med. 2009;36(3):266–70.
44. Lim WS, Baudouin SV, George RC, Hill AT, Jamieson C, Le Jeune I, et al. BTS guidelines for the management of community acquired pneumonia in adults: update 2009. Thorax. 2009;64 Suppl 3:iii1–55.
45. Labovitz AJ, Noble VE, Bierig M, Goldstein SA, Jones R, Kort S, et al. Focused cardiac ultrasound in the emergent setting: a consensus statement of the American Society of Echocardiography and American College of Emergency Physicians. J Am Soc Echocardiogr. 2010;23(12):1225–30.
46. Glickman SW, Cairns CB, Otero RM, Woods CW, Tsalik EL, Langley RJ, et al. Disease progression in hemodynamically stable patients presenting to the emergency department with sepsis. Acad Emerg Med. 2010;17(4):383–90.
47. Shapiro NI, Wolfe RE, Moore RB, Smith E, Burdick E, Bates DW. Mortality in Emergency Department Sepsis (MEDS) score: a prospectively derived and validated clinical prediction rule. Crit Care Med. 2003;31(3):670–5.
48. Sakr Y, Vincent JL, Schuerholz T, Filipescu D, Romain A, Hjelmqvist H, et al. Early- versus late-onset shock in European intensive care units. Shock. 2007;28(6):636–43.
49. James JH, Luchette FA, McCarter FD, Fischer JE. Lactate is an unreliable indicator of tissue hypoxia in injury or sepsis. Lancet. 1999;354(9177):505–8.
50. Broder G, Weil MH. Excess lactate: an index of reversibility of shock in human patients. Science. 1964;143(3613):1457–9.
51. Cady LD Jr, Weil MH, Afifi AA, Michaels SF, Liu VY, Shubin H. Quantitation of severity of critical illness with special reference to blood lactate. Crit Care Med. 1973;1(2):75–80.
52. Aduen J, Bernstein WK, Khastgir T, Miller J, Kerzner R, Bhatiani A, et al. The use and clinical importance of a substrate-specific electrode for rapid determination of blood lactate concentrations. JAMA. 1994;272(21):1678–85.
53. Mikkelsen ME, Miltiades AN, Gaieski DF, Goyal M, Fuchs BD, Shah CV, et al. Serum lactate is associated with mortality in severe sepsis independent of organ failure and shock. Crit Care Med. 2009;37(5):1670–7.
54. Shapiro NI, Howell MD, Talmor D, Nathanson LA, Lisbon A, Wolfe RE, et al. Serum lactate as a predictor of mortality in emergency department patients with infection. Ann Emerg Med. 2005;45(5):524–8.
55. Jones AE. Lactate clearance for assessing response to resuscitation in severe sepsis. Acad Emerg Med. 2013;20(8):844–7.
56. Manthous CA, Hall JB, Kushner R, Schmidt GA, Russo G, Wood LD. The effect of mechanical ventilation on oxygen consumption in critically ill patients. Am J Respir Crit Care Med. 1995;151(1):210–4.
57. Lee SJ, Ramar K, Park JG, Gajic O, Li G, Kashyap R. Increased fluid administration in the first three hours of sepsis resuscitation is associated with reduced mortality: a retrospective cohort study. Chest. 2014;146(4):908–15.
58. Yunos NM, Bellomo R, Hegarty C, Story D, Ho L, Bailey M. Association between a chloride-liberal vs chloride-restrictive intravenous fluid administration strategy and kidney injury in critically ill adults. JAMA. 2012;308(15):1566–72.
59. Caironi P, Tognoni G, Masson S, Fumagalli R, Pesenti A, Romero M, et al. Albumin replacement in patients with severe sepsis or septic shock. N Engl J Med. 2014;370(15):1412–21.
60. Ferrer R, Martin-Loeches I, Phillips G, Osborn TM, Townsend S, Dellinger RP, et al. Empiric antibiotic treatment reduces mortality in severe sepsis and septic shock from the first hour: results from a guideline-based performance improvement program. Crit Care Med. 2014;42(8):1749–55.
61. Filbin MR, Arias SA, Camargo CA Jr, Barche A, Pallin DJ. Sepsis visits and antibiotic utilization in U.S. emergency departments. Crit Care Med. 2014;42(3):528–35.
62. Ryoo SM, Kim WY, Sohn CH, Seo DW, Koh JW, Oh BJ, et al. Prognostic value of timing of antibiotic administration in patients with septic shock treated with early quantitative resuscitation. Am J Med Sci. 2015;349(4):328–33.
63. Natanson C, Danner RL, Reilly JM, Doerfler ML, Hoffman WD, Akin GL, et al. Antibiotics versus cardiovascular support in a canine model of human septic shock. Am J Physiol. 1990;259(5 Pt 2):H1440–7.

64. Levy MM, Dellinger RP, Townsend SR, Linde-Zwirble WT, Marshall JC, Bion J, et al. The Surviving Sepsis Campaign: results of an international guideline-based performance improvement program targeting severe sepsis. Crit Care Med. 2010;38(2):367–74.
65. Kumar A, Ellis P, Arabi Y, Roberts D, Light B, Parrillo JE, et al. Initiation of inappropriate antimicrobial therapy results in a fivefold reduction of survival in human septic shock. Chest. 2009;136(5):1237–48.
66. Siddiqui S, Razzak J. Early versus late pre-intensive care unit admission broad spectrum antibiotics for severe sepsis in adults. Cochrane Database Syst Rev. 2010;(10):CD007081.
67. Carbajal-Guerrero J, Cayuela-Dominguez A, Fernandez-Garcia E, Aldabo-Pallas T, Marquez-Vacaro JA, Ortiz-Leyba C, et al. Epidemiology and long-term outcome of sepsis in elderly patients. Med Intensiva. 2014;38(1):21–32.
68. Oshima T, Kodama Y, Takahashi W, Hayashi Y, Iwase S, Kurita T, et al. Empiric antibiotic therapy for severe sepsis and septic shock. Surg Infect (Larchmt). 2016;17(2):210–6.
69. Vogel L. EMR alert cuts sepsis deaths. CMAJ. 2014;186(2):E80.
70. Payen D, de Pont AC, Sakr Y, Spies C, Reinhart K, Vincent JL. A positive fluid balance is associated with a worse outcome in patients with acute renal failure. Crit Care. 2008;12(3):R74.
71. Zhang L, Chen Z, Diao Y, Yang Y, Fu P. Associations of fluid overload with mortality and kidney recovery in patients with acute kidney injury: a systematic review and meta-analysis. J Crit Care. 2015;30(4):860.e7–13.
72. Marik PE, Cavallazzi R, Vasu T, Hirani A. Dynamic changes in arterial waveform derived variables and fluid responsiveness in mechanically ventilated patients: a systematic review of the literature. Crit Care Med. 2009;37(9):2642–7.
73. Michard F. Changes in arterial pressure during mechanical ventilation. Anesthesiology. 2005;103(2):419–28.
74. Monnet X, Rienzo M, Osman D, Anguel N, Richard C, Pinsky MR, et al. Esophageal Doppler monitoring predicts fluid responsiveness in critically ill ventilated patients. Intensive Care Med. 2005;31(9):1195–201.
75. Jue J, Chung W, Schiller NB. Does inferior vena cava size predict right atrial pressures in patients receiving mechanical ventilation? J Am Soc Echocardiogr. 1992;5(6):613–9.
76. Barbier C, Loubieres Y, Schmit C, Hayon J, Ricome JL, Jardin F, et al. Respiratory changes in inferior vena cava diameter are helpful in predicting fluid responsiveness in ventilated septic patients. Intensive Care Med. 2004;30(9):1740–6.
77. Nagdev AD, Merchant RC, Tirado-Gonzalez A, Sisson CA, Murphy MC. Emergency department bedside ultrasonographic measurement of the caval index for noninvasive determination of low central venous pressure. Ann Emerg Med. 2010;55(3):290–5.
78. Dunser MW, Takala J, Ulmer H, Mayr VD, Luckner G, Jochberger S, et al. Arterial blood pressure during early sepsis and outcome. Intensive Care Med. 2009;35(7):1225–33.
79. Thooft A, Favory R, Salgado DR, Taccone FS, Donadello K, De Backer D, et al. Effects of changes in arterial pressure on organ perfusion during septic shock. Crit Care. 2011;15(5):R222.
80. Varpula M, Tallgren M, Saukkonen K, Voipio-Pulkki LM, Pettila V. Hemodynamic variables related to outcome in septic shock. Intensive Care Med. 2005;31(8):1066–71.
81. Asfar P, Meziani F, Hamel JF, Grelon F, Megarbane B, Anguel N, et al. High versus low blood-pressure target in patients with septic shock. N Engl J Med. 2014;370(17):1583–93.
82. De Backer D, Biston P, Devriendt J, Madl C, Chochrad D, Aldecoa C, et al. Comparison of dopamine and norepinephrine in the treatment of shock. N Engl J Med. 2010;362(9):779–89.
83. Levy B, Bollaert PE, Charpentier C, Nace L, Audibert G, Bauer P, et al. Comparison of norepinephrine and dobutamine to epinephrine for hemodynamics, lactate metabolism, and gastric tonometric variables in septic shock: a prospective, randomized study. Intensive Care Med. 1997;23(3):282–7.
84. Annane D, Vignon P, Renault A, Bollaert PE, Charpentier C, Martin C, et al. Norepinephrine plus dobutamine versus epinephrine alone for management of septic shock: a randomised trial. Lancet. 2007;370(9588):676–84.
85. Russell JA, Walley KR, Singer J, Gordon AC, Hebert PC, Cooper DJ, et al. Vasopressin versus norepinephrine infusion in patients with septic shock. N Engl J Med. 2008;358(9):877–87.
86. De Backer D, Aldecoa C, Njimi H, Vincent JL. Dopamine versus norepinephrine in the treatment of septic shock: a meta-analysis*. Crit Care Med. 2012;40(3):725–30.
87. Morelli A, Ertmer C, Rehberg S, Lange M, Orecchioni A, Laderchi A, et al. Phenylephrine versus norepinephrine for initial hemodynamic support of patients with septic shock: a randomized, controlled trial. Crit Care. 2008;12(6):R143.
88. Ander DS, Jaggi M, Rivers E, Rady MY, Levine TB, Levine AB, et al. Undetected cardiogenic shock in patients with congestive heart failure presenting to the emergency department. Am J Cardiol. 1998;82(7):888–91.
89. Parrillo JE. Cardiovascular dysfunction in septic shock: new insights into a deadly disease. Int J Cardiol. 1985;7(3):314–21.
90. Grissom CK, Morris AH, Lanken PN, Ancukiewicz M, Orme JF Jr, Schoenfeld DA, et al. Association of physical examination with pulmonary artery catheter parameters in acute lung injury. Crit Care Med. 2009;37(10):2720–6.

91. Kumar A, Haery C, Parrillo JE. Myocardial dysfunction in septic shock. Crit Care Clin. 2000;16(2):251–87.
92. Holst LB, Haase N, Wetterslev J, Wernerman J, Guttormsen AB, Karlsson S, et al. Lower versus higher hemoglobin threshold for transfusion in septic shock. N Engl J Med. 2014;371(15):1381–91.
93. Marik PE, Corwin HL. Efficacy of red blood cell transfusion in the critically ill: a systematic review of the literature. Crit Care Med. 2008;36(9):2667–74.
94. Perner A, Smith SH, Carlsen S, Holst LB. Red blood cell transfusion during septic shock in the ICU. Acta Anaesthesiol Scand. 2012;56(6):718–23.
95. Park DW, Chun BC, Kwon SS, Yoon YK, Choi WS, Sohn JW, et al. Red blood cell transfusions are associated with lower mortality in patients with severe sepsis and septic shock: a propensity-matched analysis. Crit Care Med. 2012;40(12):3140–5.
96. Vincent JL, Sakr Y, Sprung C, Harboe S, Damas P. Are blood transfusions associated with greater mortality rates? Results of the sepsis occurrence in acutely Ill patients study. Anesthesiology. 2008;108(1):31–9.
97. Sadaka F, Trottier S, Tannehill D, Donnelly P, Griffin M, Bunaye Z, et al. 1082: Early resuscitation of septic shock patients: is RBC transfusion necessary? Crit Care Med. 2013;41(12 Suppl):A273.
98. Briegel J, Forst H, Haller M, Schelling G, Kilger E, Kuprat G, et al. Stress doses of hydrocortisone reverse hyperdynamic septic shock: a prospective, randomized, double-blind, single-center study. Crit Care Med. 1999;27(4):723–32.
99. Gordon AC, Mason AJ, Perkins GD, Stotz M, Terblanche M, Ashby D, et al. The interaction of vasopressin and corticosteroids in septic shock: a pilot randomized controlled trial. Crit Care Med. 2014;42(6):1325–33.
100. Katsenos CS, Antonopoulou AN, Apostolidou EN, Ioakeimidou A, Kalpakou GT, Papanikolaou MN, et al. Early administration of hydrocortisone replacement after the advent of septic shock: impact on survival and immune response. Crit Care Med. 2014;42(7):1651–7.
101. Buck DL, Vester-Andersen M, Moller MH. Surgical delay is a critical determinant of survival in perforated peptic ulcer. Br J Surg. 2013;100(8):1045–9.
102. Nguyen HB, Rivers EP, Knoblich BP, Jacobsen G, Muzzin A, Ressler JA, et al. Early lactate clearance is associated with improved outcome in severe sepsis and septic shock. Crit Care Med. 2004;32(8):1637–42.
103. Rady MY, Rivers EP, Nowak RM. Resuscitation of the critically ill in the ED: responses of blood pressure, heart rate, shock index, central venous oxygen saturation, and lactate. Am J Emerg Med. 1996;14(2):218–25.
104. Boulain T, Garot D, Vignon P, Lascarrou JB, Desachy A, Botoc V, et al. Prevalence of low central venous oxygen saturation in the first hours of intensive care unit admission and associated mortality in septic shock patients: a prospective multicentre study. Crit Care. 2014;18(6):609.
105. Bracht H, Hanggi M, Jeker B, Wegmuller N, Porta F, Tuller D, et al. Incidence of low central venous oxygen saturation during unplanned admissions in a multidisciplinary intensive care unit: an observational study. Crit Care. 2007;11(1):R2.

Severe Skin and Soft Tissue Infections

20

Catherine Gogela Carlson and Alan C. Heffner

Complicated Soft Tissue Infections

Introduction

Complicated soft tissue infections encompass a wide spectrum of life-threatening bacterial infections including necrotizing cellulitis, necrotizing fasciitis, and myonecrosis. These differ from the milder, more superficial soft tissue infections by clinical presentation, risk for major tissue destruction, systemic manifestations, and therapeutic management. Several distinct soft tissue infections with unique pathogenesis share the hallmarks of life-threatening rapid progression. Essential management focuses on early recognition, cardiovascular support, and source control. The importance of radical surgical debridement, complete resection of all necrotic tissues, and early limb amputation has been well described in the surgical literature. In contrast, one-time surgical debridement and limited incision and drainage as monotherapy have been shown to be ineffective and do not result in a decrease in morbidity or mortality [6]. General treatment principles and unique clinical syndromes of complicated soft tissue infection are reviewed in this chapter [8, 9].

Pathophysiology

The skin and associated soft tissues are divided into the epidermis and dermis, the subcutaneous tissues (containing the nerve and blood vessels), and the fascia and muscle. Although any of these layers may be involved in a skin/soft tissue infection, more severe infections tend to be associated with deep tissue invasion [16]. The normal intact epidermis provides robust natural protection against infection. The development of bacterial infection is determined by a point of entry past the epidermis, host defense, and immune response to microbial invasion as well as the pathogenic properties of the microorganism. Rarely, hematogenous spread of bacteria from the circulation may seed acute soft tissue infection [12].

Patient Presentation

Complicated soft tissue infections differ from more superficial infections by clinical presentation and coexisting systemic manifestations. Necrotizing soft tissue infections classically manifest with rapid onset, progressive local

C. G. Carlson (✉)
Department of Critical Care Medicine, Department of Emergency Medicine, Carolinas Medical Center, Charlotte, NC, USA
e-mail: Catherine.carlson@carolinas.org

A. C. Heffner
Department of Internal Medicine, Department of Emergency Medicine, Carolinas Medical Center, Charlotte, NC, USA

© Springer Nature Switzerland AG 2020
J. R. Shiber, S. D. Weingart (eds.), *Emergency Department Critical Care*, https://doi.org/10.1007/978-3-030-28794-8_20

symptoms with pain disproportionate to clinical exam findings. Palpation of the effected tissue might reveal extreme pain and/or crepitus, even in the absence of advanced skin changes. As the infection progresses, visual signs often become apparent as the affected area develops edema and erythema. Bullae progression with hemorrhagic transformation indicates dermal necrosis. Paradoxical improvement in pain can also occur due to anesthesia stemming from infarction of superficial nerves. Although unreliable as a marker of complicated infection, palpable crepitus may stem from deep facial inflammation or microbial gas formation [10, 11].

Systemic manifestations including general toxicity, remote end-organ dysfunction, or shock are critical features of complicated soft tissue infection. These signs, representing severe sepsis, may occur early during clinical infection and coincide with deceptively benign local signs of infection. Bacteremia complicates approximately two-thirds of patients with necrotizing soft tissue infections [17].

Differential diagnostic considerations should include superficial cellulitis, drug eruption such as erythema multiforme, Stevens–Johnsons syndrome or toxic epidermal necrolysis (TEN), deep vein thrombosis, warfarin-induced skin necrosis, envenomations, cutaneous infiltration with underlying malignancy, chemotherapy or radiation-induced vasculitis, Sweet syndrome, and graft-vs-host disease in allogenic transplant recipients.

Complicated Soft Tissue Infection Syndromes

Complicated soft tissue infections are categorized into two distinct bacteriologic patterns:

Type I necrotizing fasciitis is a polymicrobial infection involving a combination of aerobic and anaerobic organisms most commonly associated with trauma, surgery, bowel perforation, and parenteral drug abuse including "skin popping." Complicated head and neck and genitourinary tract infections are also frequently polymicrobial. Affected patients are commonly immunocompromised either by age or by comorbid illness such as diabetes, malignancy, or end-stage liver disease.

Fournier's gangrene is a variant of necrotizing soft tissue infection which involves the scrotum and penis or vulva. The majority of effected patients have significant medical comorbidities or immunosuppression. They may present with acute or insidious symptoms and are frequently unaware of advanced skin changes. For this reason, physical examination of this site is important in patients with occult sepsis.

Type II necrotizing fasciitis is a monomicrobial soft tissue infection which is typically community acquired. The most common monomicrobial causes of rapidly progressive skin and soft tissue infections include group A streptococcus (GAS), *Clostridium perfringens*, *Pasteurella* spp., *Aeromonas hydrophila*, and *Vibrio* spp. [16] Other micoorganisms have been reported such as methicillin-resistant *Staphylococcus aureus* (MRSA), Enterobacteriaceae, and *Pseudomonas*. Group B streptococcus (GBS) has also been isolated in postpartum females and neonates.

GAS Necrotizing Fasciitis

The absence of subcutaneous emphysema in type II infections can occur, particularly in group A streptococcal infections. Necrotizing fasciitis caused by M protein types 1 and 3 is most common and approximately 50% of cases are associated with streptococcal toxic shock syndrome [15]. Most of these community-acquired infections present in the extremities, with approximately two-thirds of cases in the lower extremities [13]. Patients typically have underlying diabetes, arteriosclerotic vascular disease, or venous insufficiency with edema.

Necrotizing Myositis

Necrotizing myositis is a relatively rare but aggressive necrotizing infection of skeletal muscle caused by GAS or other beta-hemolytic streptococci. Victims are typically healthy and initial misdiagnosis of benign musculoskeletal conditions is common.

Clostridial myonecrosis, or gas gangrene, is a rapidly progressive infection caused by the Gram-positive, anaerobic, spore-forming rod *Clostridium* species including *C. perfringens* and *C. septicum*. Deep skeletal muscle infection most commonly occurs after penetrating trauma with gross contamination. Postsurgical disease including minor trauma is also recognized. Parenteral injections, including intracutaneous injection of black heroin, have resulted in local outbreaks [13]. In contrast to traumatic gangrene, spontaneous gangrene can develop in normal tissue as a result of hematogenous seeding from the gastrointestinal tract, classically stemming from a colonic malignancy in patients with neutropenia.

Necrotizing cellulitis includes anaerobic infection (both clostridial and nonclostridial species) and Meleney's synergistic gangrene, which is a rare infection that occurs in postoperative patients resulting from a synergistic interaction between *Staphylococcus aureus* and microaerophilic streptococci…….

Non-Necrotizing/Purulent Soft Tissue Infections

Pyomyositis is the presence of pus within individual muscle groups rather than gangrenous necrosis as in necrotizing myositis. It is primarily caused by *Staphylococcus aureus*. Due to geographical distribution, pyomyositis is often referred to as "tropical myositis," although it also occurs in more temperate climates. Classic clinical signs include localized pain in a single muscle group, muscle tenderness, and fever. The infection typically occurs in an extremity, but any muscle group may be involved, including the psoas or trunk muscles. In advanced cases, the bulging abscess is palpable in the muscle. Abscess drainage is required for definitive treatment. Fluid aspirated from abscess should be sent for Gram stain and culture. With the emergence of MRSA, knowing antimicrobial susceptibility is important to guide antimicrobial therapy.

Furnacle/carbuncle/abscess. Severe purulent infections are defined in patients who have failed incision and drainage plus oral antibiotics or those with systemic signs of infection such as temperature >38 °C, tachycardia (heart rate > 90 beats per minute), tachypnea (respiratory rate >24 breaths per minute) or abnormal white blood cell count (<12,000 or <400 cells/μL), or immunocompromised patients [13].

Patient Management

Early Recognition

Early recognition of complicated soft tissue infections is crucial to minimize morbidity and mortality. Unfortunately, distinguishing cellulitis from early necrotizing fasciitis or myonecrosis is difficult. Early local signs are rarely diagnostic. Physical features such as disproportionate pain or tenderness, bullous skin changes, accompanying wound, or crepitance suggest deep infection requiring surgical intervention. Remember that local skin changes are frequently attenuated in immunocompromised hosts and that early deep atraumatic infections may have a deceptively normal surface appearance. Although sepsis may stem from superficial cellulitis, the presence of early severe sepsis or shock, regardless of local findings, warrants strong consideration for complicated deep infection.

Clinical Pitfalls

Surface exam findings may be limited in patients with atraumatic deep soft tissue infection and symptoms such as pain disproportionate to local exam findings should be appreciated.

Acute encephalopathy and critically illness limit localization and sources may remain concealed due to deep location or inadequate physical exam, especially for Fournier's gangrene.

Labs

Laboratory findings are rarely diagnostic. Abnormalities noted might include leukocytosis with left shift, elevated serum creatine phosphokinase (CPK), and elevation in serum creatinine concentration. Hematologic values at the time of hospital admission have been used to predict mortality such as serum lactate and sodium levels. However, the diagnosis of necrotizing soft tissue infection cannot be reliably made based exclusively on laboratory data but must be used in combination with clinical assessment and patient risk factors/comorbidities. Laboratory data have been used to guide ongoing therapy. One study suggests that use of a procalcitonin ratio on postoperative day 1 to day 2 can also be a valuable tool in determining whether the source of infection was eliminated with surgical intervention or if the initial treatment was not radical enough to eradicate the infectious focus [7].

LRINEC score

The LRINEC (Laboratory Risk Indicator for Necrotizing Fasciitis) score is used to detect even clinically early cases of necrotizing fasciitis and attempts to distinguish necrotizing fasciitis from severe cellulitis. The variables used include the following: C-reactive protein (CRP), whole-blood glycosylation (WBG), hemoglobin (Hgb), serum sodium, creatinine clearance, and glucose. Patients with a LRINEC score of ≥6 should be carefully evaluated for the presence of necrotizing fasciitis. This tool was developed retrospectively, but has been validated prospectively. The scoring system has a positive predictive value of 92.0% and a negative predictive value of 96.0% [17–19] (Table 20.1).

Table 20.1 LRINEC score for necrotizing soft tissue infection

CRP (mg/L)	<150	0 points
	≥150	+ 4 points
WBC (per mm^3)	<15	0 points
	15–25	+ 1 point
	>25	+ 2 points
HgB (g/dL)	>13.5	0 points
	11–13.5	+ 1 point
	<11	+ 2 points
Serum Na^+	≥135	0 points
	<135	+ 2 points
Creatinine	≤1.6 mg/dL	0 points
	>1.6 mg/dL	+ 2 points
Glucose	≤180 mg/dL	0 points
	>180 mg/dL	+ 1 point

Diagnostic Imaging

Although radiographic imaging studies might be useful for distinguishing cellulitis from a necrotizing soft tissue infection, these studies should not delay surgical intervention in patients with a high pretest probability for necrotizing infection. Imaging studies are most helpful if subcutaneous emphysema is identified. Computed tomography (CT) is an imaging study of choice as it can define the extent of disease and can potentially identify a source of infection while aiding in surgical planning. In the case of Fournier's gangrene, gas in the scrotal wall on ultrasonographic evaluation is considered the sonographic hallmark for the disease. Magnetic resonance imaging (MRI) is the recommended diagnostic study for pyomyositis [20].

Source Control

Antibiotics

Early administration of parenteral antibiotics directed at the most likely pathogen(s) is a fundamental part of early resuscitation (Table 20.2). Attention to acute imaging and surgical consultation should not delay antimicrobial therapy as bacteremia complicates two-thirds of necrotizing soft tissue infections [17]. Empiric antibiotic therapy should be intentionally broad, even in community-acquired disease, in order to avoid missing the primary pathogen. In cases of MRSA, it should be assumed that the microorganism is resistant pending culture results and sensitivities. Fifty percent of methicillin-resistant *S. aureus* (MRSA) strains have inducible or constitutive clindamycin resistance [13, 21, 22].

Surgical Intervention

If there is a high clinical suspicion for necrotizing soft tissue infection, early surgical evaluation is imperative, as surgery is the only definitive diagnostic modality. Intraoperative findings consistent with necrotizing fasciitis might include the following: the presence of grayish necrotic

Table 20.2 Antimicrobial treatment of necrotizing soft tissue infections

Organism	Drug of choice	Alternatives
Polymicrobial infection	Vancomycin 15–20 mg/kg IV PLUS Piperacillin/Tazobactam 4.5 g IV PLUS Clindamycin 600–900 mg IV	Meropenem 1 g IV OR PCN G 4 million U IV AND Clindamycin 600–900 mg IV OR Imipenem/Cilastatin 500 mg IV
Streptococcus spp.	Clindamycin 600–900 mg IV AND PCN 4 million U IV	
MRSA	Vancomycin 15–20 mg/kg IV Q8-12h	Daptomycin 4 mg/kg IV QD OR Linezolid 600 mg IV BID OR Ceftaroline 600 mg IV BID OR Telavancin 10 mg/kg IV QD
MSSA	Nafcillin 1–2 g IV Q4h	Cefazolin 1 g IV Q8h OR Clindamycin 600–900 mg IV
Clostridium spp.	Clindamycin 600–900 mg IV AND PCN 4 million U IV	
Aeromonas hydrophila	Ceftriaxone 1–2 g IV Q24h	Doxycycline 100 mg Q12h PLUS Ciprofloxacin 500 mg IV Q12h
Vibrio vulnificus	Cefotaxime 2 g IV TID	Doxycycline 100 mg IV Q12h PLUS Ceftriaxone 1 g QID

fascia, lack of resistance of normally adherent muscular fascia to blunt dissection, lack of bleeding of the fascia during dissection, and the presence of foul-smelling pus. Histopathological features often include soft tissue necrosis, vasculitis, and thrombosis of perforating veins. Source control is prioritized and should be considered a component of early resuscitation. Delays in the initiation of appropriate antibiotics and surgical debridement are both associated with adverse outcomes [2, 6]. In patients with necrotizing soft tissue infections who do not exhibit hemodynamic instability or end-organ failure, studies have concluded that early surgical intervention should be as prompt as possible [6]. While aggressive goal-oriented resuscitation is paramount for patients with shock, prolonged resuscitation with expectation for shock resolution should not delay early surgical intervention [2].

At the time of surgical evaluation, samples should be obtained for Gram stain and for histopathological examination to confirm the diagnosis. Surgical debridement with subsequent reexplorations is typically necessary. Even with early aggressive surgical intervention, mortality rates are in the range of 30–40%.

Adjunctive Therapies

Intravenous immunoglobulin (IVIG) contains neutralizing antibodies against some streptococcal superantigens and clostridial toxins. Though data on the efficacy of IVIG as adjunctive therapy for necrotizing soft tissue infections are limited, for cases of necrotizing fasciitis due to GAS complicated by streptococcal toxic shock syndrome, the use of IVIG is suggested [1].

Hyperbaric oxygen therapy (100% at 3 atm) (HBOT) has been recommended for perioperative use for clostridial myonecrosis based on in vitro evidence that it inhibits bacterial growth and toxin production. Animal models have suggested a mortality benefit when used in addition to surgery and antibiotic therapy. One of the physiologic effects of HBOT is that it increases tissue oxygen tension in the wounds of patients with necrotizing fasciitis, thereby salvaging the critically ischemic penumbra of tissue. In addition, hyperoxia is thought to potentiate antibiotic efficiency, improve white blood cell killing efficacy, and is anti-inflammatory.

Critical Points

- Complicated soft tissue infections are characterized by fulminant tissue destruction, systemic signs of toxicity, and high mortality rates.
- Necrotizing soft tissue infections and myonecrosis can be associated with subcutaneous emphysema such as in polymicrobial necrotizing fasciitis and clostridial myonecrosis. However, the absence of subcutaneous emphysema does not necessarily exclude the diagnosis, as it is not typically seen in monomicrobial infections such as group A streptococcal infections.
- Physical exam findings suggestive of a potentially severe deep soft tissue infection include: [1] pain out of proportion to physical exam findings, [2] cutaneous hemorrhage, [3] violaceous bullae, [4] skin sloughing, [5] localized anesthesia, [6] gas in the tissue, and [7] rapid progression of symptoms.
- Early identification and surgical exploration are imperative in diagnosis and management of necrotizing soft tissue infections.
- The use of IVIG as adjunctive therapy for cases of necrotizing fasciitis due to GAS complicated by streptococcal toxic shock syndrome can be considered.
- HBOT can be considered for perioperative use in cases of clostridial myonecrosis but should not delay more definitive surgical interventions.

Toxic Shock Syndromes

Introduction

Cutaneous infections with Gram-positive bacteria are an important source of morbidity and mortality as these bacteria can produce toxins which can lead to the development of syndromes such as the toxic shock and scalded skin syndromes. Toxic shock syndromes (TSS) are caused by superantigenic toxins whereas the scalded skin syndromes are the result of exfoliative toxins.

Pathophysiology

Staphylococcal Toxic Shock Syndrome

Toxic shock syndrome is an inflammatory response to staphylococcal toxin. The most common staphylococcal toxin associated with toxic shock syndrome (TSS) is TSS toxin-1 and is the primary toxin associated with the use of highly absorbent tampons in menstruating women. Other types of toxic shock syndrome can be associated with sinusitis, postsurgical wounds, osteomyelitis, IV drug abuse, burn wounds, and influenza. These are typically caused by staphylococcal enterotoxins A–C.

Diagnostic criteria (Fig. 20.1).

Streptococcal Toxic Shock Syndrome

Invasive GAS and GBS infection may be associated with rapidly progressive shock and multi-organ failure (Fig. 20.2). The clinical syndrome occurs as a result of capillary leak and tissue damage caused by the release of inflammatory cytokines induced by streptococcal toxins. Streptococcal toxic shock syndrome is similar to staphylococcal TSS, but is caused by invasive group A streptococcus. The most common types of infections associated with streptococcal TSS are wounds, though in many cases, the route of infection cannot be determined. Streptococcal TSS is well described as a complication of varicella and influenza A infection. The primary toxins responsible for this clinical syndrome are the streptococcal pyrogenic exotoxins A and C.

Clinical Criteria

An illness with the following clinical manifestations:

- Fever: temperature greater than or equal to 102.0°F (greater than or equal to 38.9°C)
- Rash: diffuse macular erythroderma
- Desquamation: 1-2 weeks after onset of rash
- Hypotension: systolic blood pressure less than or equal to 90 mm Hg for adults or less than fifth percentile by age for children aged less than 16 years
- Multisystem involvement (three or more of the following organ systems):
  - Gastrointestinal: vomiting or diarrhea at onset of illness
  - Muscular: severe myalgia or creatine phosphokinase level at least twice the upper limit of normal
  - Mucous membrane: vaginal, oropharyngeal, or conjunctival hyperemia
  - Renal: blood urea nitrogen or creatinine at least twice the upper limit of normal for laboratory or urinary sediment with pyuria (greater than or equal to 5 leukocytes per high-power field) in the absence of urinary tract infection
  - Hepatic: total bilirubin, alanine aminotransferase enzyme, or asparate aminotransferase enzyme levels at least twice the upper limit of normal for laboratory
  - Hematologic: platelets less than 100,000/mm^3
  - Central nervous system: disorientation or alterations in consciousness without focal neurologic signs when fever and hypotension are absent

Laboratory Criteria for Diagnosis

Negative results on the following tests, if obtained:

- Blood or cerebrospinal fluid cultures blood culture may be positive for *Staphylococcus aureus*)
- Negative serologies for Rocky Mountain spotted fever, leptospirosis, or measles

Fig. 20.1 2011 CDC (Center for Disease Control and Prevention) definition of staphylococcal toxic shock syndrome

Patient Presentation

The signs and symptoms of toxic shock syndrome may develop rapidly in otherwise healthy individuals. Patients with toxic shock syndrome may have fever, hypotension and skin manifestations, and eventually signs of multisystem involvement (Figs. 20.1 and 20.2).

Definitive Treatment

The treatment of toxic shock syndrome is supportive and focused on eradicating the primary bacteria. Beta-lactamase-resistant, antistaphylococcal antibiotics have historically been used to treat these infections. Concomitant clindamycin, which can inhibit bacterial toxin production, is often used as well. Due to increasing incidence of methicillin-resistant staphylococci, vancomycin is often recommended. In addition, IV immunoglobulin (IVIG), which presumably acts partly by neutralizing antibodies against toxins, has been used with some promising results. Although there is evidence for the role of extracellular streptococcal toxins in shock, organ failure, and soft tissue destruction, different batches of IVIG contain variable amounts of neutralizing antibodies to some of these toxins and definitive evidence for use of IVIG is lacking [14]. Contraindications to IVIG include hypersensitivity to immunoglobulin or immunoglobulin A (IgA) deficiency. Systemic stress dose corticosteroids are unlikely to provide any benefit since superantigen-mediated immune cell activation has been associated with corticosteroid resistance.

- Hypotension defined by a systolic blood pressure less than or equal to 90 mm Hg for adults or less than the fifth percentile by age for children aged less than 16 years.
- Multi-organ involvement characterized by two or more of the following:
  - Renal impairment: Creatinine greater than or equal to 2 mg/dL (greater than or equal to 177 μmol/L) for adults or greater than or equal to twice the upper limit of normal for age. In patients with preexisting renal disease, a greater than twofold elevation over the baseline level.
  - Coagulopathy: Platelets less than or equal to 100,000/mm^3 (less than or equal to 100 x 10^6/L) or disseminated intravascular coagulation, defined by prolonged clotting times, low fibrinogen level, and the presence of fibrin degradation products.
  - Liver involvement: Alanine aminotransferase, aspartate aminotransferase, or total bilirubin levels greater than or equal to twice the upper limit of normal for the patient's age. In patients with preexisting liver disease, a greater than twofold increase over the baseline level.
  - Acute respiratory distress syndrome: defined by acute onset of diffuse pulmonary infiltrates and hypoxemia in the absence of cardiac failure or by evidence of diffuse capillary leak manifested by acute onset of generalized edema, or pleural or peritoneal effusions with hypoalbuminemia.
  - A generalized erythematous macular rash that may desquamate.
  - Soft-tissue necrosis, including necrotizing fasciitis or myositis, or gangrene.

Fig. 20.2 2010 CDC definition of streptococcal toxic shock syndrome (STSS)

For Streptococcal toxic shock syndrome, cellulitis associated with necrotizing fasciitis and myositis with streptococcal invasion into the bloodstream can develop. For cases associated with necrotizing fasciitis or myositis, rapid identification and surgical debridement are imperative to improve morbidity and mortality.

References

1. Barry W, Hudgins L, Donta ST, Pesanti EL. Intravenous immunoglobulin therapy for toxic shock syndrome. JAMA. 1992;267:3315.
2. Boyer A, et al. Influence of surgical treatment timing on mortality from necrotizing soft tissue infections requiring intensive care management. Intensive Care Med. 2009;35:847–53.
3. Chapnick EK, Abter EI. Necrotizing soft-tissue infection. Inf Dis Clin N Am. 1996;10:835–55.
4. Childers BJ, et al. Necrotizing fasciitis: a fourteen-year retrospective study of 163 consecutive patients. Am Surg. 2002;68:109–16.
5. Darenberg J, et al. Molecular and clinical characteristics of invasive group A streptococcal infection in Sweden. Clin Infect Dis. 2007;45:450.
6. Elliott DC, Kufera JA, Myers RAM. Necrotizing soft tissue infections. Risk factors for mortality and strategies for management. Ann Surg. 1996;224:672–83.
7. Friederichs J, et al. Procalcitonin ratio as a predictor of successful surgical treatment of severe necrotizing soft tissue infections. Am J Surg. 2013.
8. Centers for Disease Control and Prevention. 2011. Toxic Shock Syndrome (Other Than Streptococcal)|2011 Case Definition. [online]. Available at: http://wwwn.cdc.gov/nndss/script/casedef.aspx?CondYrID=869&DatePub=1/1/2011%2012:00:00%20AM. [Accessed 26 Jun 2019].
9. Mulla ZD, Leaverton PE, Wiersma ST. Invasive group A streptococcal infections in Florida. South Med J. 2003;96:968–73.
10. Rajan S. Skin and soft-tissue infections: classifying and treating a spectrum. Cleve Clin J Med. 2012;79(1):57–66.
11. Sarani B, Strong M, Pascual J, et al. Necrotizing fasciitis: current concepts and review of the literature. J Am Coll Surg. 2008;208:279–88.
12. Swartz MN. Clinical practice. Cellulitis. N Engl J Med. 2004;350:904–12.
13. Stevens DL, Bisno AL, Chambers HF, et al. Practice guidelines for the diagnosis and management of skin and soft tissue infections. CID. 2005;41:1373–406.
14. Stevens DL. Dilemmas in the treatment of invasive *Streptococcus pyogenes* infections. Clin Infect Dis. 2003;37:341–3.
15. Stevens DL, et al. Severe group A streptococcal infections associated with a toxic shock-like syndrome and scarlet fever toxin. N Engl J Med. 1989;321(1):1.

16. Vinh D, Embil J. Rapidly progressive soft tissue infections. Lancet. 2005;5:501–13. http://infection.thelancet.com. [Accessed 26 Jun 2019].
17. Wolff K, et al. Fitzpatrick's dermatology in general medicine. 7th ed. New York: McGraw Hill; 2008. p. 1689.
18. Wong CH, Chang HC, Pasupathy S, et al. Necrotizing fasciitis: clinical presentation, microbiology and determinants of mortality. J Bone Joint Surg Am. 2003;85:1454.
19. Wong CH, Khin LW, et al. The LRINEC (Laboratory Risk Indicator for Necrotizing Fasciitis) score: a tool for distinguishing necrotizing fasciitis from other soft tissue infections. Crit Care Med. 2004;32(7):1535–41.
20. Young JM. Necrotising fasciitis. Lancet. 1994;343:1427.
21. Young LM, Price CS. Community-acquired MRSA emerging as an important cause of necrotizing fasciitis. Surg Infect. 2008;9:469–74.
22. Zimbelman J, Palmer A, Todd J. Improved outcome of clindamycin compared with beta-lactam antibiotic treatment for invasive *Streptococcus pyogenes* infection. Pediatr Infect Dis J. 1999;18:1096–100.

Stroke: Ischemic and Hemorrhagic

21

Kimberly Boswell

Introduction

Epidemiology

Every 40 seconds, someone in the United States has a stroke. Approximately 87% of all strokes are ischemic in nature while the remaining 13% are hemorrhagic, divided between intracerebral and subarachnoid hemorrhage. According to the American Heart Association 2015 statistics, there are nearly 800,000 strokes annually in the United States with three-quarters of those being a patient's first stroke [1]. The rates of stroke are decreasing among high-income countries, but continue to increase in other parts of the world. Interestingly, stroke is common in younger men, but even more common in older women. Stroke occurs more frequently in blacks and Hispanics than whites and is one of the leading causes of disability and death in the world [2, 3]. It is estimated that approximately 6.6 million Americans, over the age of 20, have had a stroke. This number is expected to increase by approximately 3.5 million by the year 2030, which will reflect a 20% increase from 2012. As a result, it should be treated aggressively in hopes to limit its negative effects and associated morbidity and mortality.

K. Boswell (✉)
University of Maryland School of Medicine, Baltimore, MD, USA
e-mail: Kboswell2@umm.edu

Pathophysiology

Ischemic Stroke

Reduction or occlusion of blood flow through arterial vasculature within the brain results in hypoperfusion or complete lack of perfusion to a specific vascular territory [4]. This change in perfusion leads to ischemia and ultimately, to the manifestation of clinical symptoms that a patient will develop.

The vast majority of ischemic strokes are due to thrombus, emboli, or small vessel ischemia. Thrombus is usually the result of atherosclerotic disease, but is a localized process that occurs directly within the lumen of the affected vessel. Acute platelet aggregation at the site of the plaque or gradual narrowing over time due to progression of the plaque growth (worsening of atherosclerosis) are two common etiologies for thrombosis that lead to strokes.

Embolic strokes are the result of extracranial material traveling to the brain and causing occlusion and ischemia. The etiology of the emboli is numerous, but most commonly include cardiac sources (valvular calcifications, pieces of vegetation(s) from endocarditis, clot caused by atrial fibrillation or ventricular thrombus), air, amniotic, or fat emboli. Occasionally, in the presence of a patent foramen ovale (PFO) a patient can have an embolic stroke from venous clot. Consider adding vessel-to-vessel source of

© Springer Nature Switzerland AG 2020
J. R. Shiber, S. D. Weingart (eds.), *Emergency Department Critical Care*,
https://doi.org/10.1007/978-3-030-28794-8_21

emboli such as from aortic arch or internal carotid artery (ICA) disease/plaque.

Lacunar infarcts are due to chronic small vessel disease. The smaller vasculature, penetrating vessels, are at greater risk when considering the effect of hypertension. Long-term hypertension eventually leads to thickening of the tunica media and therefore overall narrowing of the small vessel's lumen. Over time, the narrowing progresses, and finally ischemia results. Like thrombotic strokes, lacunar infarcts can also be caused by atherosclerotic disease on a microscopic level.

Hemorrhagic Stroke

There are classically two types of hemorrhagic strokes: intracerebral hemorrhage (ICH) and subarachnoid hemorrhage (SAH). Intracerebral hemorrhage is most commonly a result of uncontrolled hypertension, but many etiologies exist. Tumors, coagulopathies, bleeding diathesis, amyloid angiopathy, vascular malformations, hemorrhagic conversion at site of prior ischemic injury, mycotic aneurysms, vasculitis, and Moyamoya are alternative causes of ICH. Typically, the hemorrhage originates from smaller arteries and arterioles and bleeding occurs directly into the parenchyma creating a hematoma, which slowly enlarges over time as bleeding, continues [5]. There is some evidence to support the presence of "microbleeds" in patients, which are subclinical arterial leaks that can be precursors to larger hemorrhages and have been seen on susceptibility and T2-weighted magnetic resonance imaging (MRI) [6]. These microbleeds are believed to be the result of pseudoaneurysm formation, likely due to chronic hypertension, but are also seen in patients who are on antithrombotic or antiplatelet medications. Patients on warfarin have been noted to have increased areas of microbleeding on MRI, compared to those not on warfarin, but it is unclear if this predisposes them to clinically significant warfarin-associated hemorrhage [7].

Patient Presentation

Presentations of stroke symptoms can vary widely, but there are often patterns of symptoms that can be recognized which allow a physician to quickly identify the geographical location of a stroke. The following is a limited compilation of some of the more common and recognizable ischemic stroke patterns (See Table 21.1)

- The middle cerebral artery supplies a significant portion of the brain. When ischemia occurs in this distribution, symptoms are dependent on whether the ischemia is affecting the dominant or nondominant hemisphere. In the dominant hemisphere, patients will present with aphasia, motor and/or sensory deficits typically in the face and both the upper and lower extremities. [Ischemia of the nondominant hemisphere will manifest as neglect, motor and/or sensory deficits consistent with the dominant hemisphere.] Unclear – you may mead of the dominant side of body?

Table 21.1 Cerebral artery distribution and stroke symptoms

Vessel involved	Symptom patterns
Middle cerebral artery	*Dominant hemisphere* Motor/sensory deficits (face/arm > leg) Hemiplegia possible Aphasia *Nondominant hemisphere* Hemineglect Motor/sensory deficits (face/arm > leg) Homonymous hemianopsia
Anterior cerebral artery	Motor/sensory deficits (leg > arm/face) Apraxic gait Loss of volition/"Frontal" behavior
Posterior circulation (Vertebral and posterior cerebral artery)	Visual symptoms (diplopia, homonymous hemianopsia) Cranial nerve deficits/palsy Vertibrobasilar symptoms (dizziness, vomiting) Ataxic gait Coma
Lacunar and small arteries	"Pure" sensory or motor deficits Hemiparesis possible Dysarthric speech

- Anterior cerebral artery strokes involve symptoms of motor and sensory deficits usually more pronounced in the affected lower extremity, but can also be noted in the face and upper extremity as well. An apraxic gait and a loss of volition can also be appreciated.
- Ischemia of the posterior circulation presents with symptoms involving vision and balance. Cranial nerve deficits are also common findings.
- Lacunar infarcts, or ischemia involving smaller arteries or vascular distributions, can be identified as "pure" strokes. These commonly exhibit a pure sensory or motor deficit. Dysarthria and ataxia can also be seen.

Presentations of hemorrhagic strokes are dependent on the type. They usually occur in the setting of routine activity, but can be precipitated with physical exertion or an emotionally stressful circumstance. Subarachnoid hemorrhages typically fit the "thunderclap" headache picture reaching maximal intensity at its onset, or very shortly thereafter. A short loss of consciousness can occur, and is not uncommon, with the onset of the headache. Ruptured arterial aneurysms remain the most common cause of nontraumatic SAH and it is important to recognize that no focal findings may be present on neurologic examination as the majority of these bleeds do not occur into the brain tissue, but rather, remain within the cerebral spinal fluid (CSF).

ICH, on the other hand, evolves and gradually worsens as the bleed increases in size. Physical symptoms mimic this gradual nature and over the course of minutes to hours, the neurologic deficits increase. The presence of blood within the brain results in physical pain in the form of a headache and can cause nausea and vomiting, although this combination of headache and vomiting is far more common in SAH [8]. Meningismus can be, but is not always present. The initial neurologic symptoms exhibited are dependent upon the location of the bleeding.

Initial Stabilization and Early Resuscitation

Initial emergent management of stroke is based on standard emergency medicine practice. A patient presenting with acute stroke symptoms should be assessed rapidly and with immediate attention directed toward the ABCs: airway, breathing, and circulation.

Establishing the patient's level of consciousness, ability to maintain and protect their own airway and determining the likelihood of rapid decompensation should be a physician's initial steps. Patients with elevated intracranial pressure (ICP) due to bleeding or ischemia can present with a complete spectrum of mental statuses. A Glasgow coma scale (GCS) less than 8 should generally *(patient may localize but be nonverbal and not open eyes, so that is a GCS of 7 and be fine with a natural airway)* facilitate immediate intubation. If any concern exists about a patient's ability to swallow, oxygenate, or protect their airway from aspiration, even with a GCS greater than 8, the patient should be intubated in safe and controlled fashion.

An important goal for the emergency physician should be to limit secondary injury. The primary injury is the stroke itself and its effects on the surrounding brain tissue. Secondary injury is an event that occurs following the stroke, which can contribute to, or worsen the brain injury and potentially worsen prognosis. Examples of secondary injury include hypoxia, hypercapnia, profound hypotension (in the setting of ischemic stroke), and hypertension (in the setting of hemorrhagic stroke). It is important to ensure adequate oxygenation and ventilation in these patients, to ensure, if and when intubated, that peri-induction hemodynamic changes are minimized.

Ensuring hemodynamic stability in an acute stroke patient can be difficult as many present to the emergency department hypertensive. Correction of any acute abnormalities that could be contributing to the patient's symptoms should be addressed immediately and corrected if possible. These factors may include, but are not limited to: metabolic derangements, hypercapnia, hypoxia, electrolyte aberrations, hypoglycemia, or hyperglycemia.

A thorough and precise history and physical examination should be performed as time in the setting of hemorrhage or ischemia is of the essence. The history can offer clues as to the etiology (hemorrhagic or thromboembolic) in addition to providing vital information as to alternative diagnoses including stroke mimics or alternative diagnosis like seizures, syncope, aortic dissection, drug overdose, or hypoglycemia.

While obtaining the history and performing the physical examination, the physician should also be gathering information about the time of the onset of symptoms, the patient's comorbidities, and use of anticoagulants, in order to assist in determining if the patient is a thrombolytic candidate or if he/she is experiencing an ischemic event.

The physical examination should be head-to-toe in nature. An overall assessment to ensure there are no signs of traumatic injury, which could explain some or all of the presenting symptoms, should be done. If head trauma exists and the patient has an altered level of consciousness, a hard cervical collar should be placed and computed tomography (CT) imaging of the cervical spine should be considered. A pupillary exam should be performed. Asymmetric pupils, sluggish or nonreactive pupils should be concerning to the physician and can be an indicator of elevated intracranial pressure. A cardiac examination to document the presence or absence of murmurs or irregular rhythms should be performed. Lungs should be auscultated for the evidence of heart failure or fluid overload. Peripheral examination of the extremities for edema, asymmetric or not, skin findings concerning endocarditis, hemorrhage, or thrombocytopenia should be evaluated.

Neurologic evaluation should be extensive and rapid. Full assessment of motor, sensory, cranial nerve function, and speech should be completed. Every emergency physician should be familiar with the National Institutes of Health Stroke Scale (NIHSS), which is composed of 11 elements, each of which contributes to a total score of 0–42. The higher the score, the more significant the stroke symptoms, with a score of 20 or greater constituting a "severe stroke" and "minor stroke" (NIHSS less than or equal to 3) [9]. This scale is a widely used and validated scale and should be used to determine severity, but the score has also been linked to outcomes. Use of the scale also provides a clear, concise, and well-understood way to communicate your findings in the emergency room when discussing the patient's care with neurology and/or neurosurgical colleagues. In 2005, Goldstein and Simel found that there were three physical examination findings that, if present, could improve diagnostic reliability, which included facial paresis, pronator drift, and speech impairment [10].

Diagnostics

Laboratory Evaluation

Samples should be drawn and sent to the laboratory as quickly as possible. Specific treatment options, specifically Alteplase (tPA), will be dependent upon some laboratory results, so that expedited processing should be requested. Finger-stick blood glucose should be done immediately on presentation to ensure symptoms are not due to hypo- or hyperglycemia.

Basic laboratory tests including a complete blood count (CBC) to assess hemoglobin and platelet counts, complete metabolic panel (CMP) including liver function studies, coagulation studies (PT/INR/aPTT) to assess for underlying coagulopathy, urinalysis (UA), toxicology screen, cardiac enzymes, specifically, a troponin should be performed on all patients presenting with stroke-like symptoms. A urine or serum pregnancy test should be sent for every female of childbearing age. If concern for hypercapnia or hypoxia exists, consider an arterial blood gas (ABG) for further assessment (see Table 21.2).

An electrocardiogram (EKG) should be done to evaluate the patient's cardiac rhythm. Abnormal rhythms like atrial fibrillation should be considered a potential etiology of embolic/ischemic stroke. It is not uncommon to note acute

Table 21.2 Initial laboratory evaluation of the suspected stroke patient

Initial laboratory evaluation of the suspected stroke patient
CBC
CMP
Coagulation Studies (PT/INR/aPTT)
Troponin
UA
Toxicology screen
Things to consider adding
Blood or urine cultures
Pregnancy test
ABG

EKG changes in a person with increased ICP and commonly in patients with SAH.

Additional laboratory tests to consider include blood or urine cultures in the setting of a fever.

Imaging

A chest radiograph should be performed and is obligatory in the setting of intubation or to rule out infectious causes of altered mental status.

The primary goal of imaging in the evaluation of acute stroke symptoms is primarily to exclude hemorrhage and to evaluate for evidence of stroke mimics. As quickly as the history and physical examination is completed, the patient should be evaluated with imaging to determine the nature of the stroke. A patient who has signs or symptoms, a history or physical examination findings consistent with increased intracranial pressure, or acute hemorrhagic stroke should be imaged with a noncontrast CT scan as quickly as possible. Acute hemorrhage on CT dictates vastly different management in almost every aspect, both in additional diagnostics and emergent interventions than ischemic findings. A patient with a history and physical examination findings more suggestive of ischemia should receive an emergent CT scan or MRI to assess for evidence of early stroke. Positive imaging demonstrating ischemia in a territory consistent with physical examination findings should precipitate a rapid evaluation to determine if the patient is a candidate for thrombolytic therapy, consultation with neurology and, if available, interventional radiology. Diffusion-weighted MRI (DWI) is more sensitive in the hyperacute phase of stroke to detect evidence of ischemia. It is important to appreciate the difference in time needed to obtain CT versus MRI imaging. If concern for hemorrhage exists, it is likely more prudent to obtain a CT first, as the longer duration of study with MRI utilizes valuable minutes in which emergent interventions can take place.

Definitive Treatment

Acute Ischemic Stroke

After initially stabilizing a patient with signs and symptoms concerning for acute stroke, aiming treatment directed and improving outcomes and limiting secondary injury should be started. There are many issues that are directly related to the management of strokes that will be discussed. Patients diagnosed with acute stroke, hemorrhagic or ischemic, should be admitted to an intensive care unit (ICU) for close monitoring as neurologic decompensation can occur.

Blood Pressure Management

Blood pressure management is an important issue in patients having acute strokes, but the goals are markedly different depending on whether the stroke is hemorrhagic or ischemic. In ischemic strokes, patients are dependent on increased perfusion pressures to maintain whatever minimal amount of blood supply may still be perfusing ischemic areas. Watershed areas, which may not be actively ischemic, may nevertheless be at risk if a patient were to become normo- or hypotensive. Therefore, in the event of ischemic strokes, blood pressure goals are rather liberal and patients are "allowed" to remain hypertensive, deemed, permissive hypertension [11]. As noted above, many patients who are having acute strokes will present hypertensive. It is believed this is due to several possible factors such as acute pain, chronic, uncontrolled hypertension, stroke-mediated events, or possibly even a stress response. Regardless of the etiology, the blood pressure should not be aggressively controlled in the first 24 hours. Several studies have shown a direct association with blood pressure reduction in the first 24 hours of stroke and poor outcomes [12, 13]. Blood pressure for patients with acute, ischemic stroke who are not going to receive thrombolytics should only be treated if, extreme, persistent hypertension is noted. This is commonly defined as a systolic blood pressure (SBP) greater than 220 mmHg or a diastolic blood pressure (DBP) greater than 120 mmHg. Several exceptions to these guidelines exist and include patients with active cardiac ischemia, decompensated heart failure, evidence of other end-organ hypoperfusion (acute renal insufficiency/injury/failure), pregnancy with evidence of preeclampsia or eclampsia, or in the setting of acute aortic dissection. If needed, intravenous (IV) medications should be used to control blood pressure, preferably short-acting ones. The current American Heart Association (AHA) guidelines from 2013 suggest Labetalol and Nicardipine as first-line choices [14].

Blood pressure goals are going to differ if a patient is a thrombolytic candidate. In the acute setting, immediately after presentation, and while determining if a patient meets criteria for thrombolytics, blood pressure is important. One of the exclusion criteria to receiving tPA includes blood pressure parameters. A patient must maintain a SBP less than 185 and diastolic blood pressure less than 110. Bolused IV medications can be used, if needed, and included in the 2013 AHA is the allowance for a nicardipine drip to be used to sustain blood pressures at goal. If tPA is given, it is imperative that the patient's blood pressure is maintained with SBP <185 and DBP <105 for 24 hours after administration to prevent complications. Again, the use of IV medications is the preferred means to control hypertension in this group of patients.

Fluids

Intravenous fluids should be initiated at the time of IV placement. The majority of stroke patients will be in need of some volume resuscitation, will have their oral intake restricted as an aspiration precaution, some will require anesthesia for intubation, and some will simply be dehydrated depending upon their presentation. Avoidance of hypotonic solutions is important, as it can contribute to worsening cerebral edema and increase intracranial pressure. Normal saline or plasma-Lyte is an appropriate choice for initial volume resuscitation.

Hyperglycemia

Most patients presenting with acute stroke have some degree of hyperglycemia, regardless of a history of diabetes. It appears that not only can this be simply a result of stress, but it is also believed to be a result of the stroke itself causing abnormal glucose metabolism [15]. Aggressive glucose control should be initiated to maintain euglycemia, as many studies have demonstrated that hyperglycemia after acute stroke, both hemorrhagic and ischemic, can portend a poor prognosis [16, 17]. Current AHA guidelines suggest keeping the serum blood sugar between 140 mg/dL and 180 mg/dL. Insulin drips are not necessary as long as the patient's blood sugar can be controlled with sliding scale insulin. Consider including that hypoglycemia must be avoided.

Fever

Fever is not uncommon in the setting of brain injury and therefore can be and is often seen in acute stroke. Many studies have clearly demonstrated worse outcomes and increased mortality associated with fevers *Temperature >38° C* [18, 19]. Not only did the height of the fever but also the duration of the fever (in days) play a role in the associated increase in mortality [20]. Although it is clear that fevers have a negative impact on stroke prognosis, it is unclear what they should be treated with to control them. Studies have been done which demonstrate no benefit in using medications or external cooling devices to control temperature, but more studies are needed to determine if active control to achieve euthermia will ultimately result in improved outcomes [21, 22].

Fibrinolytic Therapy

The use of IV tPA in the setting of acute ischemic stroke is reserved for those with known time of symptom onset. Patients who present within 4.5 hours of symptom onset should be rapidly assessed to determine if they are candidates for tPA administration (See Table 21.2). Once the patient's initial assessment, history, and physical examination have been performed, airway concerns and hemodynamics addressed, neurologic consultants should be involved. The patient should receive imaging (either CT or MRI, whichever can be obtained more expediently) and the decision to give fibrinolytics, or withhold, should be made. The current recommendation is to give OFFER? tPA to any patient who meets criteria and *agrees or consents* to treatment. The AHA guidelines recommend that every attempt should be made by the treating emergency physician to give tPA within 60 minutes of the patient presenting to the emergency room (ER).

In response to many clinicians' concerns about ambiguity of initial guidelines presented by the exclusion criteria for tPA, a taskforce was convened to clarify some of these issues. Specifically, The Re-examining Acute Eligibility for Thrombolysis (TREAT) group of investigators addressed the utility and safety of administering IV tPA to acute stroke patients who demonstrate "rapidly improving stroke symptoms." Overall, the consensus of the group was that in patients whose neurologic examination was improving at the time of assessment, but demonstrated persistent and "potentially disabling" neurologic deficits, tPA is safe and should be administered in the absence of other clear exclusion criteria. The particular deficits identified include severe aphasia, motor weakness preventing sustained effort against gravity, any deficit totaling an NIHSS score of greater than 5, visual deficits (complete hemianopia, visual extinction), or any residual deficit that the patient, patient's family, or the physician would consider possibly disabling [23].

The possibility of treating a patient with evidence of neurologic deficit with tPA without an actual ischemic stroke should be of utmost concern for any emergency physician. There are many conditions in which stroke-like symptoms are the presenting complaint and these are referred to as "stroke mimics" and include conditions like complicated migraines, seizures, and conversion disorders. Studies have shown that even when patients presenting with stroke mimics are treated with IV tPA, no significant complications, related to thrombolytic therapy, occur [24].

Intracranial Hemorrhage after tPA

Intracerebral hemorrhage following tPA administration is the most concerning and life-threatening complication of thrombolysis. Other possible complications include bleeding (not intracranial) from other sites and angioedema, and although are complications, tend to be more manageable. Prospective observational studies have demonstrated that the risk of intracerebral hemorrhage following tPA ranges from approximately 5 to 8% [25–27]. The data support the use of IV tPA for those that meet eligibility criteria with a low symptomatic intracerebral hemorrhage rate of complication following administration.

If symptomatic intracerebral hemorrhage occurs following tPA, discontinuation and reversal of anticoagulation should immediately take place. Options for reversal are discussed in detail below and include Prothrombin Complex Concentrate (PCC), blood products (FFP, platelets and cryoprecipitate, and Tranexamic acid (TXA)) depending on coagulation profiles at the time of bleeding. Neurosurgical consultation should be obtained urgently for evaluation of possible evacuation if hemorrhage is amenable.

Intra-arterial Thrombolysis

Although still considered an investigational therapy, intra-arterial tPA is gaining momentum and clinical studies are actively being done to clarify its efficacy. Intra-arterial therapies are an endovascular technique, which offers the benefit of direct visualization and removal of the thromboembolic burden while administering tPA directly to the occlusion. In addition, direct visualization allows for an appreciably smaller dose of thrombolytic to be required and consequently allows this therapy to be an option for some patients who are not candidates for systemic thrombolysis [28].

Acute Hemorrhagic Stroke

Medical Management

Initial management of patients with hemorrhagic strokes is similar to ischemic strokes. Treatment of hyperglycemia, fever, and volume status is important and unchanged from the above recommendations. There are several important differences in the management of acute ICH with respect to blood pressure, reversal of anticoagulation, and involvement of surgical colleagues.

Blood Pressure Management

Similar to ischemic stroke, many patients with acute ICH present with elevated blood pressure. However, unlike the treatment of ischemic stroke, allowing for liberal blood pressure management, elevated blood pressure in the setting of hemorrhage can precipitate bleeding and worsen outcomes. The complicating issue of tight blood pressure control in these patients revolves around the fact that many patients with spontaneous ICH have chronic, uncontrolled hypertension and too rapid a decrease in the mean arterial pressure (MAP) can result in ischemic stroke or cerebral hypoperfusion.

The current guidelines for the management of hypertension in the setting of acute ICH are from the AHA 2010 [29]. They are as follows:

- Aggressive blood pressure management for any patient with a SBP >200 mmHg or MAP >150 mmHg using continuous IV infusions and frequent blood pressure monitoring.
- In patients with evidence of elevated ICP or concern for increased ICPs who have a SBP >180 mmHg or MAP >130 mmHg, blood pressure should be reduced to maintain cerebral perfusion pressures (CPP) between 61 and 80 mmHg. This implies that ICP monitoring should be strongly considered. Intermittent or continuous IV medications are recommended.
- In patients without evidence of, or concern for, elevated ICPs, but with a SBP >180 mmHg or MAP >130 mmHg, a more conservative reduction in blood pressure is suggested with a goal MAP of 110 mmHg or total blood pressure of 160/90 mmHg. Again, intermittent bolused or continuous infusions of antihypertensives can be used.

Regardless of the therapy or aggressiveness of blood pressure management utilized, frequent, repeated neurologic examinations should be performed. Taking these current guidelines into account, the Intensive Blood Pressure Reduction in Acute Cerebral Hemorrhage Trial 2 (INTERACT2) found that aggressively lowering the SBP to 140 mmHg in patients presenting with SBP 150–200 mmHg is likely safe and did not increase the risk of death or severe disability in the population studied [30].

Reversal of Anticoagulants

Individuals who present with spontaneous ICH while taking anticoagulants or antiplatelet medications present a more complicated and highly morbid situation. It is imperative that every attempt at reversal of the anticoagulant or antiplatelet be undertaken and done so emergently. It is important to note that no therapy that reverses anticoagulation is without potential complication whether pro-thrombotic itself, known to cause anaphylaxis, or related to the product volume required to make the treatment effective. Each option has risks and benefits that need to be evaluated based on the patient's history, clinical picture, and individual risks.

Warfarin-associated ICH carries a significant morbidity and mortality when compared to spontaneous hemorrhage. Patients with ICH while on warfarin have been found to have greater expansion of the hemorrhage and, likely as a result, have a great mortality than those with spontaneous ICH and not taking anticoagulation [31].

Warfarin is a vitamin K antagonist and therefore affects clotting factors II, VII, IX, and X from functioning properly. Bleeding can be reversed using several options including fresh frozen plasma (FFP), PCC, vitamin K, and recombinant factor VIIa. Fresh frozen plasma is widely used and readily available to almost all emergency physicians. In comparison to the alternative reversal agents, like factor VIIa and PCC, FFP is inexpensive and can quickly, and fully, reverse the international normalized ratio (INR). Unfortunately, the total volume of FFP required to fully reverse the effects of warfarin can sometimes be prohibitory. This is especially true when taking care of patients with a history of cardiac disease of heart failure. The blood bank needs time to crossmatch and thaw FFP before it can start infusing, this time is often critical and can allow for hemorrhage expansion. Increasingly available is PCC, which is a complex of the vitamin-K-dependent factors in addition to some small amounts of proteins C and S. Prothrombin complex concentrate is available in three- and four-factor formulations. The three-factor formulation contains very little, if any, factor VII and is often given with two units of FFP because of this. Four-factor is thus preferred if available. Kcentra is the only four-factor PCC available in the United States at this time and was approved by the FDA in 2013. PCC can normalize the INR within minutes of infusion and does not require crossmatch or thawing time like its alternative, FFP. PCC dosing is based on initial INR and the patient's weight. For a standard, therapeutic INR (2 to <4), the dose of four-factor PCC is 25 units/kg with a maximum dose of 2500 units. Although, not well studied, literature suggests that administration of PCC is a generally well-tolerated event with few complications [32].

Recombinant factor VIIa is a better-studied reversal agent, but is not currently recommended for the reversal of warfarin-associated ICH due to significant concerns about the risk of thrombosis after treatment. In addition, a large multicenter randomized trial demonstrated no improved survival benefit of functional outcome following the administration of factor VIIa [33].

Vitamin K should be given to nearly every patient on warfarin, despite concurrent treatment with PCC or FFP as the normalization of the INR from these treatments is a transient event. Intravenous vitamin K (10 mg) should be given as soon as possible in the emergency department and infused slowly due to the possibility of anaphylaxis when infused at faster rates. Doses can be repeated as often as every 12 hours until INR remains normalized.

Protamine should be given as quickly as possible when a heparin-associated ICH is identified. If available at the time of initial laboratory investigation, and if it is known or suspected that a patient may be on heparin or heparin products, a heparin concentration should be sent to assist in determining the appropriate dose of protamine necessary to completely reverse the heparin effect.

The use of novel oral anticoagulants (direct oral anticoagulants), including dabigatran, rivaroxaban, and apixaban, has introduced a more complicated picture when discussing the reversal of anticoagulation. Currently, dabigatran is the only oral anticoagulant that has a reversal agent also available. Idarucizumab is the reversal agent for dabigatran and can completely reverse the effects within minutes [34]. Idarucizumab should not be given in combination with any other reversal agent, like PCC, given an increased risk of thrombosis. Approximately, one-half of the circulating volume of dabigatran can also be removed via hemodialysis if its reversal agent is unavailable.

Patients presenting with acute ICH while taking one of these medications should have the same laboratory evaluation as any other patients. A full coagulation profile should be sent and the emergency physician should consider a fibrinogen level as well. These oral anticoagulants can be treated, to a degree, with the PCC. If significant or recent ingestion has occurred, oral activated charcoal can be considered if the patient has a protected airway or is awake, alert, and able to protect his own airway without any concern for aspiration.

Seizures and Seizure Prophylaxis

The occurrence of hemorrhage- related seizures is cited as anywhere between 4 and 29% of patients. It is important to note that nonconvulsive seizures can occur in up to half of patients with acute hemorrhagic stroke and most seizures are in patients with cortical bleeds [35]. The current recommendation for treatment of seizures, should they occur, is fosphenytoin or phenytoin [36, 37]. It is important to consider each patient individually as well as possible contraindications and special circumstances when selecting an antiepileptic medication. The 2010 AHA guidelines recommend against the routine prophylaxis of seizures in the acute hemorrhagic stroke patient. There are no current data to strongly support or refute the use of prophylaxis at this time.

Intracerebral Pressures

Patients with acute hemorrhage can present alert, oriented, and without significant focal deficits, or they can present profoundly obtunded and unresponsive depending on the severity and location of the bleeding. Elevated ICPs are an important concern and should be monitored in specific patients. Patients with minimal symptoms or no evidence of elevated ICP can be monitored closely with frequent neurologic examinations. Those patients presenting with a depressed GCS of <8, those with transtentorial herniation on examination or hydrocephalus on imaging, or those who have significant ICH should have invasive ICP monitoring placed [29]. Once the monitoring is placed, the goal CPP is between 50 and 70 mmHg.

Alternatives to invasive monitoring and likely more useful to the emergency physician include positioning, ventilatory, and pharmacologic interventions that can result in rapid decreases in ICP. There are several acute interventions, which can be beneficial in a patient who is declining due to elevated ICPs. Simply positioning the patient with the head of bed at 30 degrees can improve cerebral venous outflow. Treating a patient's pain, agitation, or anxiety can assist in both decreasing blood pressure and ICP. Using osmotic diuretics or hypertonic solutions like mannitol and hypertonic saline, respectively, is an option available in most emergency departments. Osmotic agents work by increasing the plasma's oncotic pressure and therefore drawing fluid out of the parenchyma. An initial dose of 1g/kg of mannitol is standard and its effects are usually seen within minutes of administration. Hypertonic saline comes in various concentrations from 3% to 23.4%. If multiple aliquots of hypertonic saline are given, central venous access should be considered. A 2011 meta-analysis evaluated the efficacy of mannitol versus hypertonic saline for elevated ICP management and it concluded that hypertonic saline is likely a better choice to control ICP acutely. [38]. The use of osmotic diuretics or hypertonic fluids warrants frequent assessments of serum osmolality, sodium, chloride, and potassium levels. It is also imperative when using mannitol (or any diuretic) to monitor a patient's volume status to prevent hypovolemia. Hyperventilation with a goal $PaCO_2$ of 25–30 mmHg can produce profound and brisk cerebral vasoconstriction, rapidly and effectively lowering the ICP. This effect is temporary and should only be utilized in the setting of imminent herniation (Tables 21.3 and 21.4).

Barbiturates and paralytics are typically reserved for use in the ICU, but can be considered if control of ICPs is proving to be difficult and other measures have failed. Consultation with neurologic and neurosurgical colleagues

Table 21.3 Initial diagnostic evaluation of the suspected stroke patient

Initial diagnostic evaluation of the suspected stroke patient
CT head (without contrast)
EKG
Chest X-ray
MRI brain
Things to consider adding
EEG if concerned for seizures
MRA head and neck
CTA brain/neck

Table 21.4 Contraindications for tPA

Contraindications for tPA
Absolute:
<18 years old
>4.5 hours since symptom onset *OR* unknown symptoms onset with last known "normal" time being >4.5 hours
Prior IC hemorrhage
Current ICH
Recent spinal or cranial surgery
Known brain AVM, aneurysm, or mass
Arterial puncture at noncompressible site in prior 7 days
Relative:
Current use of anticoagulation
Improving stroke symptoms/neuro exam.
Recent history of GI or GU bleeding (within 3 weeks)
>80 years old
Pregnancy
Myocardial infarction within the past 3 months
Major surgery in prior 14 days
Significant trauma in prior 2 weeks
Platelet <100,000; INR >1.7; PT >15 seconds

Table 21.5 ICP management

ICP Management
Position
Head of bed 30 degrees
Pain control/sedation
Oversedation can cloud neuro exam
Propofol
Osmotic diuretics
Mannitol 1g/kg, initial dose
Hypertonic saline
3% to 23.4%
Monitor serum Osm, Na, Cl, K
Paralytics/barbiturates
Hyperventilation
Goal $PaCO_2$ 25–30 mmHg
Reserved for imminent herniation
Avoid rebound, slowly normalize $PaCO_2$

should be sought prior to intitiating these therapies (Table 21.5).

Surgical Interventions

Indications for surgery in acute hemorrhagic stroke are dependent upon the location of the hemorrhage. Surgical evacuation of hemorrhage in the supratentorial region is, at best, controversial and without clear indication. Patients should be evaluated on a case-by-case basis for intervention. Patient characteristics that are associated with improved outcomes include fewer comorbid conditions, younger age, nondominant hemisphere involvement, hemorrhage near the surface of the brain, and recent bleed. Patients who are continuing to decline clinically, despite maximal medical treatment, should also be considered for surgical intervention. Cerebellar hemorrhage carries a notable risk and neurosurgical colleagues should be consulted emergently. The infratentorial/posterior region is a smaller, closed compartment that, with increased pressure or space occupying lesion, will result in brainstem compression and possible herniation more rapidly than hemorrhage within the supratentorial space. Hemorrhage of >3 cm in diameter, continued decline on neurologic examination, evidence of brainstem compression, or hydrocephalus due to ventricular obstruction on CT should be emergently assessed for surgical evacuation of the hemorrhage [37].

Subarachnoid Hemorrhage

There are several issues specific to the diagnosis and management of subarachnoid hemorrhage which should be addressed as it can be easily misdiagnosed even when clinically suspected, and results can be erroneously interpreted. Well known is the acute onset, "worst headache of my life" usually associated with nausea, vomiting, occasionally syncope, seizures, and/or meningismus. However, approximately 10–15% of patients who suffer from ruptured aneurysm and SAH will die prior to reaching the hospital. Interestingly, approximately 10–40% of patients will experience a sudden, severe headache several days prior to the subarachnoid hemorrhage by 1–3 weeks [39].

The vast majority of nontraumatic subarachnoid hemorrhages are due to aneurysms. The remainder can be due to vascular malformations, arterial dissections, or perimesencephalic hemorrhage. For many of these patients, a definitive diagnosis is never obtained.

Subarachnoid hemorrhage is associated with a high mortality rate. It has been observed that the mortality rate can be as high as 51% [40].

Diagnosis

The diagnosis of subarachnoid hemorrhage starts with the clinical suspicion of the physician. A patient with a presentation concerning for subarachnoid hemorrhage should be evaluated until all aspects of the evaluation are negative. The initial imaging should be a noncontrast CT scan to assess for clear evidence of SAH. CT is most sensitive in the first 6–12 hours of onset and if within the first 6 hours nears 100% sensitivity [41]. If the CT is negative and the clinical suspicion exists, a lumbar puncture should be considered obligatory. The lumbar puncture should be done, opening pressures should be measured (often elevated in SAH), and the CSF should be collected. Cell counts should be performed on tubes 1 and 4, but declining red blood cell (RBC) counts should not be considered a way to rule out SAH. Xanthochromia is the classic finding associated with SAH on lumbar puncture and is the result of hemoglobin breakdown and can last for up to 2 or more weeks [42].

Once the diagnosis is made, additional studies should be obtained to determine the cause, treatment, and prognosis needed.

Imaging

CT angiography (CTA) is typically the initial radiographic modality after the diagnosis of SAH is made. CTA, in addition to magnetic resonance angiography (MRA), is highly sensitive for aneurysms 3 mm and larger and CTA is highly sensitive for the detection of ruptured aneurysms. The use of multidetector CT scanners increases the sensitivity and specificity to >97% [43]. If CTA is negative, then digital subtraction angiography should be used to aid in the diagnosis. The gold standard for diagnosis remains, traditional angiography.

Complications

There are several potential complications of SAH that can occur in the acute to subacute period of SAH. As emergency department overcrowding and length of stay are increasing, we often find ourselves caring for critically ill patients for longer than we are accustomed to. It is important to be aware of the complications that can occur during the subacute period in which these patients may remain in our care.

Rebleeding of the aneurysm occurs in between 8 and 23% of all aneurysmal SAHs and usually this occurs within the first 24–72 hours after the initial event [44]. It is usually diagnosed as the result of a sudden clinical or neurologic change in a patient. There are several factors that are considered to increase the likelihood of rebleed in a particular individual. These factors include delay in the presentation from the onset of symptoms, elevated blood pressure at the time of presentation, history of sentinel headache, and ventriculostomy placement prior to intervention for aneurysm treatment [45–47].

Pulmonary edema and cardiac arrhythmias are relatively common in patients with SAH, occurring in 25 and 35% of people, respectively [48]. Cardiac arrhythmias and EKG changes are common. Deep, symmetric T-wave inversions, ST depressions, and evident U-waves are all frequent findings. The frequency of cardiac arrhythmias and left ventricular dysfunction (or Frank heart failure) is associated with increased severity of SAH [49].

The development of increased ICP is most likely the result of hydrocephalus (due to obstruction of CSF flow) or increasing volume of hemorrhage. Hydrocephalus is seen in about 15% of all patients with SAH, nearly half of which were symptomatic [50]. If symptomatic or severe, a ventriculostomy drain may need to be placed for acute management.

Vasospasm and delayed cerebral ischemia (DCI) are common complications in SAH. Usually occurring no sooner than 3 days after symptom onset and achieving a peak risk at days 7–8, symptomatic vasospasm is associated with poorer prognosis. DCI is believed to likely be the result of vasospasm and can be clinically silent or manifest as a new or worsened neurologic deficit or changes in a patient's level of consciousness. It is estimated that 20–30% of all patients with aneurysmal SAH will have symptomatic ischemia. Nimodipine is the medication of choice for the prevention of vasospasm and DCI. The goal is to begin this medication within 4 days of SAH, sooner being preferred. The mechanism by which nimodipine has its effect on preventing cerebral vasospasm is unclear and no angiographic evidence exists to support its effectiveness, but studies have demonstrated improved outcomes, including a trend toward decreased mortality and lower rates of vasospasm and evidence of infarction on imaging, with its use and therefore it is currently the standard of care [51, 52].

References

1. Mozaffarian D, Benjamin EJ, Go AS, Arnett DK, Blaha MJ, Cushman M, et al. Heart disease and stroke Statistics-2016 update: a report from the American Heart Association. American Heart Association statistics committee and stroke statistics subcommittee. Circulation. 2016;133(4):e38–e360. Epub 2015 Dec 16.
2. Schneider AT, Kissela B, Woo D, Kleindorfer D, Alwell K, Miller R, et al. Ischemic stroke subtypes: a population-based study of incidence rates among blacks and whites. Stroke. 2004;35(7):1552.
3. Morgenstern LB, Smith MA, Lisabeth LD, Risser JM, Uchino K, Garcia N, et al. Excess stroke in Mexican Americans compared with non-Hispanic whites: the

brain attack surveillance in Corpus Christi project. Am J Epidemiol. 2004;160(4):376.
4. Caplan LR. Basic pathology, anatomy, and pathophysiology of stroke. In: Caplan's stroke: a clinical approach. 4th ed. Philadelphia: Saunders Elsevier; 2009. p. 22.
5. Caplan LR. Intracerebral haemorrhage. Lancet. 1992;339(8794):656.
6. Cheng AL, Batool S, McCreary CR, Lauzon ML, Frayne R, Goyal M, et al. Susceptibility-weighted imaging is more reliable than T2*-weighted gradient-recalled echo MRI for detecting microbleeds. Stroke. 2013;44(10):2782.
7. Lovelock CE, Cordonnier C, Naka H, Al-Shahi Salman R, Sudlow CL, Sorimachi T, Werring DJ, Gregoire SM, Imaizumi T, Lee SH, Briley D, Rothwell PM, Edinburgh Stroke Study Group. Antithrombotic drug use, cerebral microbleeds, and intracerebral hemorrhage: a systematic review of published and unpublished studies. Stroke. 2010;41(6):1222.
8. Gorelick PB, Hier DB, Caplan LR, Langenberg P. Headache in acute cerebrovascular disease. Neurology. 1986;36(11):1445.
9. Goldstein LB, Samsa GP. Reliability of the National Institutes of Health Stroke Scale. Extension to non-neurologists in the context of a clinical trial. Stroke. 1997;28(2):307.
10. Goldstein LB, Simel DL. Is this patient having a stroke? JAMA. 2005;293(19):2391.
11. Aiyagari V, Gorelick PB. Management of blood pressure for acute and recurrent stroke. Stroke. 2009;40(6):2251–6. Epub 2009 Apr 23.
12. Oliveira-Filho J, Silva SC, Trabuco CC, Pedreira BB, Sousa EU, Bacellar A. Detrimental effect of blood pressure reduction in the first 24 hours of acute stroke onset. Neurology. 2003;61(8):1047.
13. Castillo J, Leira R, García MM, Serena J, Blanco M, Dávalos A. Blood pressure decrease during the acute phase of ischemic stroke is associated with brain injury and poor stroke outcome. Stroke. 2004;35(2):520.
14. Jauch EC, Saver JL, Adams HP Jr, Bruno A, Connors JJ, Demaerschalk BM, Khatri P, PW MM Jr, Qureshi AI, Rosenfield K, Scott PA, Summers DR, Wang DZ, Wintermark M, Yonas H. American Heart Association Stroke Council, Council on Cardiovascular Nursing, Council on Peripheral Vascular Disease, Council on Clinical Cardiology. Guidelines for the early management of patients with acute ischemic stroke: a guideline for healthcare professionals from the American Heart Association/American Stroke Association. Stroke. 2013;44(3):870.
15. Dave JA, Engel ME, Freercks R, Peter J, May W, Badri M, et al. Abnormal glucose metabolism in non-diabetic patients presenting with an acute stroke: prospective study and systematic review. QJM. 2010;103(7):495.
16. Weir CJ, Murray GD, Dyker AG, Lee KR. Is hyperglycaemia an independent predictor of poor outcome after acute stroke? Results of a long-term follow up study. BMJ. 1997;314(7090):1303.
17. Béjot Y, Aboa-EbouléC HM, Jacquin A, Osseby GV, Rouaud O, et al. The deleterious effect of admission hyperglycemia on survival and functional outcome in patients with intracerebral hemorrhage. Stroke. 2012;43(1):243.
18. Saini M, Saqqur M, Kamruzzaman A, Lees KR, Shuaib A, VISTA Investigators. Effect of hyperthermia on prognosis after acute ischemic stroke. Stroke. 2009;40(9):3051.
19. Prasad K, Krishnan PR. Fever is associated with doubling of odds of short-term mortality in ischemic stroke: an updated meta-analysis. Acta Neurol Scand. 2010;122(6):404–8.
20. Phipps MS, Desai RA, Wira C, Bravata DM. Epidemiology and outcomes of fever burden among patients with acute ischemic stroke. Stroke. 2011;42(12):3357–62. Epub 2011 Oct 6.
21. Den Hertog HM, van der Worp HB, van Gemert HM, Algra A, Kappelle LJ, van Gijn J, Koudstaal PJ, Dippel DW, PAIS Investigators. The Paracetamol (Acetaminophen) In Stroke (PAIS) trial: a multicentre, randomised, placebo-controlled, phase III trial. Lancet Neurol. 2009;8(5):434.
22. Den Hertog HM, van der Worp HB, Tseng MC, Dippel DW. Cooling therapy for acute stroke. Cochrane Database Syst Rev. 2009.
23. Levine SR, Khatri P, Broderick JP, Grotta JC, Kasner SE, Kim D, Meyer BC, Panagos P, Romano J, Scott P, lRe-examining Acute Eligibility for Thrombolysis (TREAT) Task Force, NINDS rt-PA Stroke Trial Investigators. Review, historical context, and clarifications of the NINDS rt-PA stroke trials exclusion criteria: part 1: rapidly improving stroke symptoms. Stroke 2013;44(9):2500–2505. . Epub 2013 Jul 11.
24. Tsivgoulis G, Zand R, Katsanos AH, Perren F, Saqqur M, Rubiera M, et al. Safety of intravenous thrombolysis in stroke mimics: prospective 5-year study and comprehensive meta-analysis. Stroke. 2015;46(5):1281–7. Epub 2015 Mar 19.
25. Albers GW, Bates VE, Clark WM, Bell R, Verro P, Hamilton SA. Intravenous tissue-type plasminogen activator for treatment of acute stroke: the standard treatment with Alteplase to reverse stroke (STARS) study. JAMA. 2000;283(9):1145.
26. LaMonte MP, Bahouth MN, Magder LS, Alcorta RL, Bass RR, Browne BJ, et al. A regional system of stroke care provides thrombolytic outcomes comparable with the NINDS stroke trial. Emergency Medicine Network of the Maryland Brain Attack Center. Ann Emerg Med. 2009;54(3):319.
27. Hill MD, Buchan AM, Canadian Alteplase for Stroke Effectiveness Study (CASES) Investigators. Thrombolysis for acute ischemic stroke: results of the Canadian Alteplase for Stroke Effectiveness Study. CMAJ. 2005;172(10):1307.
28. Meyers PM, Schumacher HC, Higashida RT, Barnwell SL, Creager MA, Gupta R, et al. Indications for the performance of intracranial endovascular neurointerventional procedures: a scientific statement from the American Heart Association Council on

Cardiovascular Radiology and Intervention, Stroke Council, Council on Cardiovascular Surgery and Anesthesia, Interdisciplinary Council on Peripheral Vascular Disease, and Interdisciplinary Council on Quality of Care and Outcomes Research. Circulation. 2009;119(16):2235.
29. Morgenstern LB, Hemphill JC 3rd, Anderson C, Becker K, Broderick JP, Connolly ES Jr, Greenberg SM, Huang JN, RL MD, MesséSR MPH, Selim M, Tamargo RJ, American Heart Association Stroke Council and Council on Cardiovascular Nursing. Guidelines for the management of spontaneous intracerebral hemorrhage: a guideline for healthcare professionals from the American Heart Association/American Stroke Association. Stroke. 2010;41(9):2108.
30. Anderson CS, Heeley E, Huang Y, Wang J, Stapf C, Delcourt C, Lindley R, Robinson T, Lavados P, Neal B, Hata J, Arima H, Parsons M, Li Y, Wang J, Heritier S, Li Q, Woodward M, Simes RJ, Davis SM, Chalmers J. INTERACT2 investigators. Rapid blood-pressure lowering in patients with acute intracerebral hemorrhage. N Engl J Med. 2013;368(25):2355–65. Epub 2013 May 29.
31. Cucchiara B, Messe S, Sansing L, Kasner S, Lyden P. CHANT Investigators. Hematoma growth in oral anticoagulant related intracerebral hemorrhage. Stroke. 2008;39(11):2993.
32. Bershad EM, Suarez JI. Prothrombin complex concentrates for oral anticoagulant therapy-related intracranial hemorrhage: a review of the literature. Neurocrit Care. 2010;12(3):403–13.
33. Mayer SA, Brun NC, Begtrup K, Broderick J, Davis S, Diringer MN, Skolnick BE, Steiner T, FAST Trial Investigators. Efficacy and safety of recombinant activated factor VII for acute intracerebral hemorrhage. N Engl J Med. 2008;358(20):2127.
34. Pollack CV Jr, Reilly PA, Eikelboom J, Glund S, Verhamme P, Bernstein RA, et al. Idarucizumab for dabigatran reversal. N Engl J Med. 2015;373(6):511.
35. Claassen J, JettéN CF, Green R, Schmidt M, Choi H, et al. Electrographic seizures and periodic discharges after intracerebral hemorrhage. Neurology. 2007;69(13):1356.
36. Manno EM. Update on intracerebral hemorrhage. Continuum (Minneap Minn). 2012;18(3):598–610.
37. Broderick J, Connolly S, Feldmann E, Hanley D, Kase C, Krieger D, et al. Guidelines for the management of spontaneous intracerebral hemorrhage in adults: 2007 update: a guideline from the American Heart Association/American Stroke Association stroke council, high blood pressure research council, and the quality of care and outcomes in research interdisciplinary working group. Stroke. 2007;38(6):2001–23.
38. Kamel H, Navi BB, Nakagawa K, Hemphill J, Claude MAS 3rd, Ko N. Hypertonic saline versus mannitol for the treatment of elevated intracranial pressure: a meta-analysis of randomized clinical trials. Crit Care Med. 2011;39(3):554.
39. Polmear A. Sentinel headaches in aneurysmal subarachnoid haemorrhage: what is the true incidence? A systematic review. Cephalalgia. 2003;23(10):935.
40. Hop JW, Rinkel GJ, Algra A, van Gijn J. Case-fatality rates and functional outcome after subarachnoid hemorrhage: a systematic review. Stroke. 1997;28(3):660.
41. Perry JJ, Stiell IG, Sivilotti ML, Bullard MJ, Emond M, Symington C, et al. Sensitivity of computed tomography performed within six hours of onset of headache for diagnosis of subarachnoid haemorrhage: prospective cohort study. BMJ. 2011;343:d4277.
42. Vermeulen M, Hasan D, Blijenberg BG, Hijdra A, van Gijn J. Xanthochromia after subarachnoid haemorrhage needs no revisitation. J Neurol Neurosurg Psychiatry. 1989;52(7):826.
43. Menke J, Larsen J, Kallenberg K. Diagnosing cerebral aneurysms by computed tomographic angiography: meta-analysis. Ann Neurol. 2011;69(4):646.
44. Inagawa T, Kamiya K, Ogasawara H, Yano T. Rebleeding of ruptured intracranial aneurysms in the acute stage. Surg Neurol. 1987;28(2):93.
45. Naidech AM, Janjua N, Kreiter KT, Ostapkovich ND, Fitzsimmons BF, Parra A, et al. Predictors and impact of aneurysm rebleeding after subarachnoid hemorrhage. Arch Neurol. 2005;62(3):410.
46. Bederson JB, Connolly ES Jr, Batjer HH, Dacey RG, Dion JE, Diringer MN, Duldner JE Jr, Harbaugh RE, Patel AB, Rosenwasser RH. American Heart Association. Guidelines for the management of aneurysmal subarachnoid hemorrhage: a statement for healthcare professionals from a special writing group of the Stroke Council, American Heart Association. Stroke. 2009;40(3):994.
47. Beck J, Raabe A, Szelenyi A, Berkefeld J, Gerlach R, Setzer M, et al. Sentinel headache and the risk of rebleeding after aneurysmal subarachnoid hemorrhage. Stroke. 2006;37(11):2733.
48. Solenski NJ, Haley EC Jr, Kassell NF, Kongable G, Germanson T, Truskowski L, et al. Medical complications of aneurysmal subarachnoid hemorrhage: a report of the multicenter, cooperative aneurysm study. Participants of the Multicenter cooperative aneurysm study. Crit Care Med. 1995;23(6):1007–17.
49. Hravnak M, Frangiskakis JM, Crago EA, Chang Y, Tanabe M, Gorcsan J 3rd, et al. Elevated cardiac troponin I and relationship to persistence of electrocardiographic and echocardiographic abnormalities after aneurysmal subarachnoid hemorrhage. Stroke. 2009;40(11):3478.
50. Graff-Radford NR, Torner J, Adams HP Jr, Kassell NF. Factors associated with hydrocephalus after subarachnoid hemorrhage. A report of the Cooperative Aneurysm Study. Arch Neurol. 1989;46(7):744.
51. Barker FG 2nd, Ogilvy CS. Efficacy of prophylactic nimodipine for delayed ischemic deficit after subarachnoid hemorrhage: a metaanalysis. J Neurosurg. 1996;84(3):405.
52. Dorhout Mees SM, Rinkel GJ, Feigin VL, Algra A, van den Bergh WM, Vermeulen M, et al. Calcium antagonists for aneurysmal subarachnoid haemorrhage. Cochrane Database Syst Rev. 2007.

Seizures and Status Epilepticus

22

Kabir Rezvankhoo and Munish Goyal

Critical Points

- Seizures occur on a continuum. Most seizures stop within 1 minute. The longer a seizure lasts, the more difficult it is to terminate.
- Status epilepticus (SE) leads to death from a combination of hyperpyrexia, acidosis, hypoxemia, and ultimately cerebral ischemia. Halting seizure activity, protecting the airway, and administering adequate supplemental oxygen are the cornerstones of therapy.
- The goal is to treat early with an aggressive, multireceptor approach. Simultaneous first-line and second-line therapies are the best approaches.
- First-line antiepileptic drug (AED) for SE is midazolam (0.2 mg/kg up to 10 mg) given intramuscularly (IM) or lorazepam (0.1 mg/kg up to 4 mg) given intravenously (IV).
- Second-line AEDs for SE include phenytoin (20 mg/kg), fosphenytoin (20 mg PE/kg), and valproate sodium (20–40 mg/kg).
- Consider nonconvulsive SE (NCSE) in patients who remain persistently altered or comatose after overt motor activity stops.
- Refractory SE (RSE) is defined as patients who are in either convulsive or NCSE, despite adequate therapy with first -and second-line AEDs.
- Patients with RSE should be endotracheally intubated and placed on continuous midazolam (0.05–2 mg/kg/h) or propofol (30–200 μg/kg/min) infusions.
- All of these patients will need continuous EEG (cEEG) monitoring in the intensive care unit (ICU).

Introduction

Seizures are defined as sudden abnormal electrical activity involving cortical, subcortical, and thalamic neuronal networks, which may cause a change in mental status and possible convulsive motor activity. They are categorized as generalized or focal, convulsive (involving rhythmic muscle contraction and relaxation) or nonconvulsive, provoked or unprovoked and based on duration. They are common, with 11% of the population having a seizure at some

K. Rezvankhoo (✉)
New York-Presbyterian Hospital Columbia University Medical Center, New York, NY, USA
e-mail: kr2293@columbia.edu

M. Goyal
MedStar Washington Hospital Center, Washington, DC, USA

© Springer Nature Switzerland AG 2020
J. R. Shiber, S. D. Weingart (eds.), *Emergency Department Critical Care*,
https://doi.org/10.1007/978-3-030-28794-8_22

point in life and resulting in 1 million ED visits annually [30]. The terminology used to categorize seizures is not standardized. In this chapter, status epilepticus (SE) refers to generalized convulsions lasting greater than 5 minutes or repeated seizures without a return to baseline cognitive state. Refractory SE (RSE) refers to generalized convulsions that do not resolve after administration of two or more antiepileptic drugs (AEDs). Nonconvulsive SE (NCSE) refers to seizure activity in the absence of motor findings, usually confirmed by EEG.

Most seizures are brief and self-limited. Among patients who present to the ED with seizures, most do not have SE and are discharged home. The objective of this chapter is to provide an evidence-based review of the pathophysiology and current therapeutic approaches to manage SE. In the past 35 years, results of critical trials have allowed us to establish our current standards of practice; however, the current body of work pertaining to seizures and SE is inadequate to definitively answer many clinical questions. Part of this chapter will provide an in-depth review of the pathophysiology of SE to help guide the clinician when first-line therapies are ineffective. We feel this is important, as an early aggressive multireceptor approach should be taken when it comes to treating patients with SE [2, 3].

Status Epilepticus – An Evolving Definition

Status epilepticus (SE) is either witnessed seizure activity lasting greater than 5 minutes or repeated seizures without a return to baseline cognitive state. The seizure duration that defines SE has evolved throughout the years and remains controversial. Classically, the America's Working Group on Status Epilepticus in 1993 defined SE as seizure activity lasting for 30 minutes [6]. Seizure duration was reduced to 10 minutes in the 1998 Veterans Affairs Status Epilepticus Cooperative Study. [7] The timeline changed again to 5 minutes in 2001 when Alldredge and colleagues published their landmark study comparing the efficacy of halting seizures with lorazepam vs. diazepam vs. placebo.

The past 35 years of basic science research has attempted to shed light on SE and its underlying neurophysiology. Although still incomplete, we now have more insight into what makes patients prone to have seizures, how AEDs function, and why certain patients develop refractory SE. The theory of pharmacoresistance, first described by Wasterlain and colleagues [11, 12], is the most practical explanation of the importance of early aggressive multireceptor approach to treating SE. This theory will be discussed in detail below and helps us understand why delayed treatment of SE can lead to decreased efficacy of benzodiazepines and ultimately lead to increased morbidity and mortality [1, 8–10].

Status Epilepticus – Etiology

Status epilepticus is a heterogeneous disease process that encompasses not only people with underlying epilepsy, but also those with acute neurologic and systemic illnesses. The average duration of generalized tonic–clonic seizures is only 1 minute in humans based on video EEG studies; thus, convulsions lasting longer than 5 minutes are a clear marker of abnormal seizure activity [5]. From a practical standpoint, the majority of SE cases are due to subtherapeutic AED levels or due to a known trigger. Other etiologies of SE include alcohol use and withdrawal, metabolic encephalopathy, trauma, cerebrovascular accident (CVA), hypoxemia, and anoxia. There have been a handful of both prospective and retrospective US-based population studies that describe the underlying cause and associated mortality in patients with SE. The results of four of these studies are summarized in Fig. 22.1 [23–26].

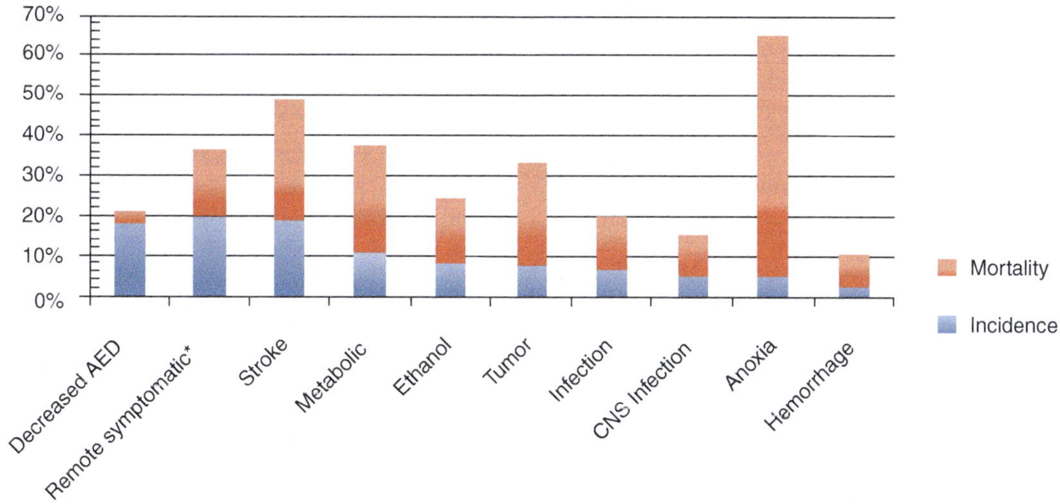

Fig. 22.1 Associated underlying etiology of SE and its corresponding mortality based on the studies of US population [23–26]. (*Remote symptomatic is a classification described in the Richmond Study by DeLorenzo et al., in which an acute cause of SE could not be found; however the patient has a history of prior stroke, meningitis, congenital malformation, hydrocephalus, arteriovenous malformation (AVM), or genetic disease)

Status Epilepticus – Pathophysiology and Current Concepts

Seizures involve abnormally synchronized electrical activity involving cortical, subcortical, and thalamic neuronal networks. The start of a generalized tonic–clonic seizure begins with excitation of susceptible epileptic cerebral neurons, which leads to synchronous discharges that can progressively recruit larger cortical networks and ultimately lead to the clinical manifestation of seizure activity. Why seizures don't stop (known as self-sustaining SE), when the stimulus is withdrawn, is central to the theory of why SE develops.

In a series of studies with a rodent model designed to mimic SE, Mazarati and colleagues used bipolar stimulating electrodes to directly induce SE [11, 31]. When brain stimulation was withdrawn in as little as 15 minutes, the rodents continued to seize. They demonstrated that benzodiazepines lose efficacy in prolonged SE and are most effective when given prior to seizure onset. Similarly, Kapur and McDonald showed that the potency of diazepam decreases >20-fold within 30 minutes of self-sustaining SE in a rat model [13]. These data suggest that seizure mechanisms evolve as seizures continue.

Naylor and colleagues used a similar rat model where self-sustaining SE (SSE) was induced chemically and immunocytochemical studies were performed on hippocampal slices. They demonstrated that after approximately 1 hour of SSE, there was a 50% decrease in the number of physiologically active gamma-aminobutyric acid type A (GABAA) receptors, with subsequent increase of gamma-aminobutyric acid (GABA) receptor subunit uptake from the synaptic membrane to the cytoplasm by endocytosis [12]. Interestingly, glutamate receptors appear to be upregulated in SE. Mathern and colleagues found that patients with autopsy evidence of temporal lobe epilepsy (hippocampal sclerosis) have a significantly higher level of glutamate receptor density per dentate granule cell [17]. Other studies have also shown a significant increase in gene transcription of *N*-methyl-D aspartate (NMDA) glutamate receptor subunits in hippocampal tissue from humans with chronic temporal lobe epilepsy compared to nonepilepsy humans [18, 19]. These studies have shed light on the concept of the plasticity of GABA receptors and development of pharmacoresistance, which is the underlying biochemical explanation for what causes refractory SE in humans (Fig. 22.2) [14–16].

Continuous SE leads to cell injury and neuronal death secondary to excess release of glutamate causing intracellular hypercalcemia and the development of an "excitotoxic" state [20]. This excess presynaptic activity activates glutamate

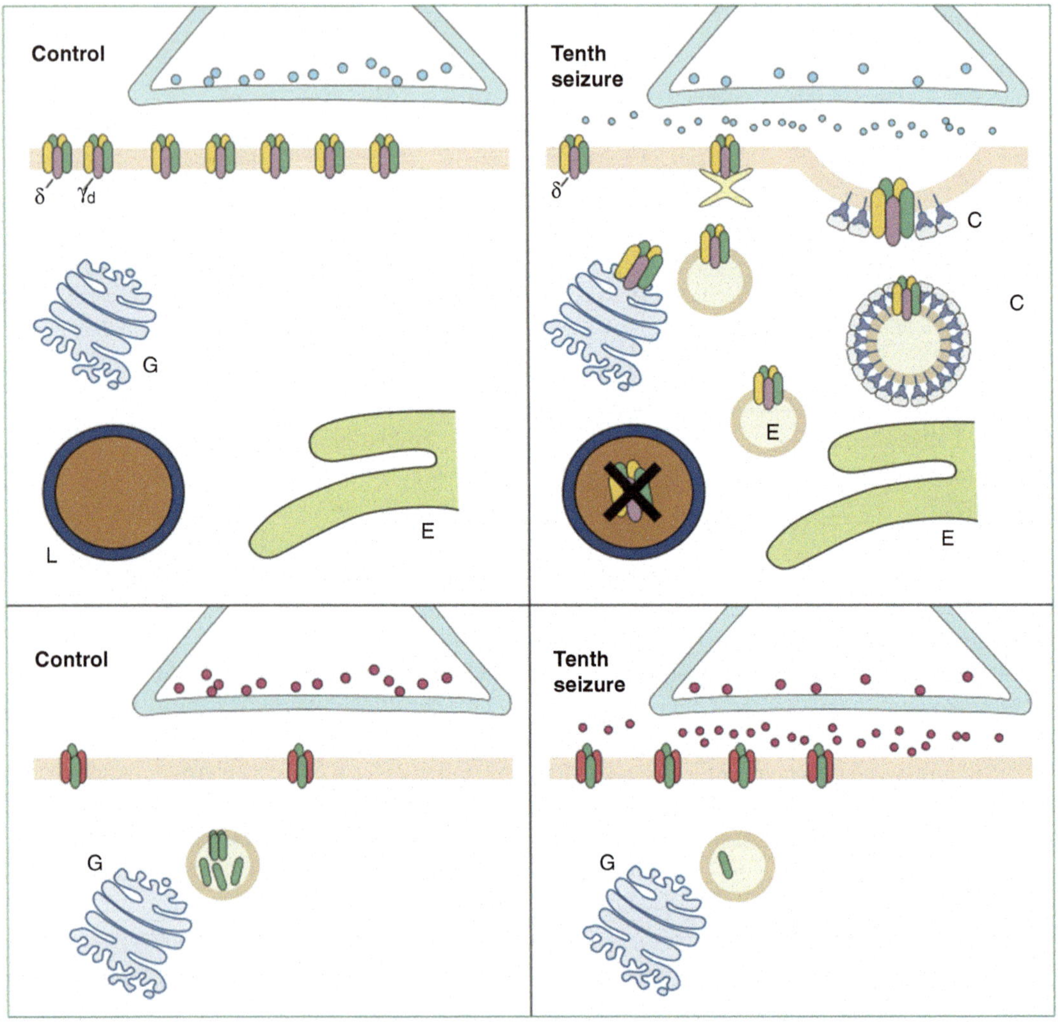

Fig. 22.2 After repeated seizures, the synaptic membrane containing the gamma-aminobutyric acid type A (GABAA) receptors forms clathrin-coated pits, which internalize as clathrin-coated vesicles (C). These vesicles develop into endosomes (E), which can deliver the receptors to lysosomes (L) to be destroyed, or to the Golgi apparatus (G) to be recycled back to the membrane. Bottom: during status epilepticus, *N*-methyl-d-aspartate (NMDA) receptor subunits are mobilized to the synaptic membrane and assembled into additional receptors. As a result, the number of functional NMDA receptors per synapse increases whereas the number of functional GABAA receptors decreases [12]. (Reprinted from, Chen JW, Wasterlain CG. Status epilepticus: patho-physiology and management in adults. The Lancet Neurology. 2006;5(3):246–256, Copyright 2006, with permission from Elsevier and Dr. Wasterlain.)

release, which binds to various NMDA and non-NMDA glutamate receptors within the postsynaptic neuron causing intracellular hypercalcemia. On the cellular level, once SE is initiated, it can transition into what is called a maintenance phase of SE, which is believed to be secondary to maladaptive changes by various mechanisms such as receptor trafficking, activation of neuropeptides, and apoptosis signaling pathways, which are beyond the scope of this chapter. Ultimately, prolonged SE causes an excitotoxic state from unopposed glutamate receptor activation in the postsynaptic membrane causing intracellular hypercalcemia, which then activates multiple pathways leading to cellular apoptosis, neuronal injury, release of cytokines, and neuronal death [4, 21].

Status Epilepticus – Diagnostic Studies

The 2012 Neurocritical Care Society clinical guidelines for initial diagnostic workup for patients with SE include checking fingerstick glucose, basic blood work including the complete blood count (CBC) and chemistries, noncontrast computed tomography (CT), and AED levels if appropriate (Fig. 22.3). This diagnostic approach is practical, given the three most prevalent etiologies of SE which are acute stroke, subtherapeutic AED levels, and remote symptomatic causes (i.e., no acute precipitating event but with history of previous central nervous system (CNS) insult, injury, or malformation) [22].

Status Epilepticus – Treatment

Benzodiazepines, specifically lorazepam (IV) and most recently midazolam (IM), have always been the cornerstones for treating SE because of their efficacy and safety profile (Table 22.1). Figure 22.4 is a graph showing the results of four landmark randomized controlled trials (RCTs) that were done in both prehospital and in-hospital settings.

It is important to recognize that although benzodiazepines are first-line therapy, there is a 30–40% failure rate for termination of SE. The Veterans Affairs Epilepticus Cooperative Study by Treiman et al. showed that patients with subtle SE had a higher mortality compared to overt SE (64.7% versus 27%, respectively). They defined subtle SE as comatose patients with ictal discharges on EEG with or without subtle convulsive movements in the arms, legs, trunk, facial muscles, tonic eye deviation, or eye jerking. This brings out the importance of maintaining high suspicion of ongoing seizures if a patient does not return to their baseline mental status and of an early aggressive multireceptor approach to treating SE with the goal of emergently stopping both clinical and electrographic seizure activities. Basic measures should be taken as always to manage airway, breathing, and circulation which should be done simultaneously while treating the patient and screening for the underlying etiology of SE.

Refractory Status Epilepticus – Definition

Refractory status epilepticus is defined as the SE that fails to respond to first- and second-line therapies. Some studies use a time criterion of up to 60 minutes with the requirement of continuous EEG making it a phenomenon that is seen only in the ICU [27]. This is a clinical scenario that is usually seen in the ICU, however, it can also be seen in the ED. An example would be the clinical scenario where a patient is brought to the ED by Emergency Medical Services (EMS) with active seizures in the field that is continuing to have tonic–clonic seizures, despite multiple doses of benzodiazepines and a phosphenytoin load. Less commonly, a comatose patient who was treated adequately and no longer exhibits active convulsions however their mental status cannot be simply explained by a postictal period or somnolence secondary to AED use. Our usual clinical intuition correctly guides us to proceed with orotracheal intubation and deep sedation with either propofol or midazolam infusions.

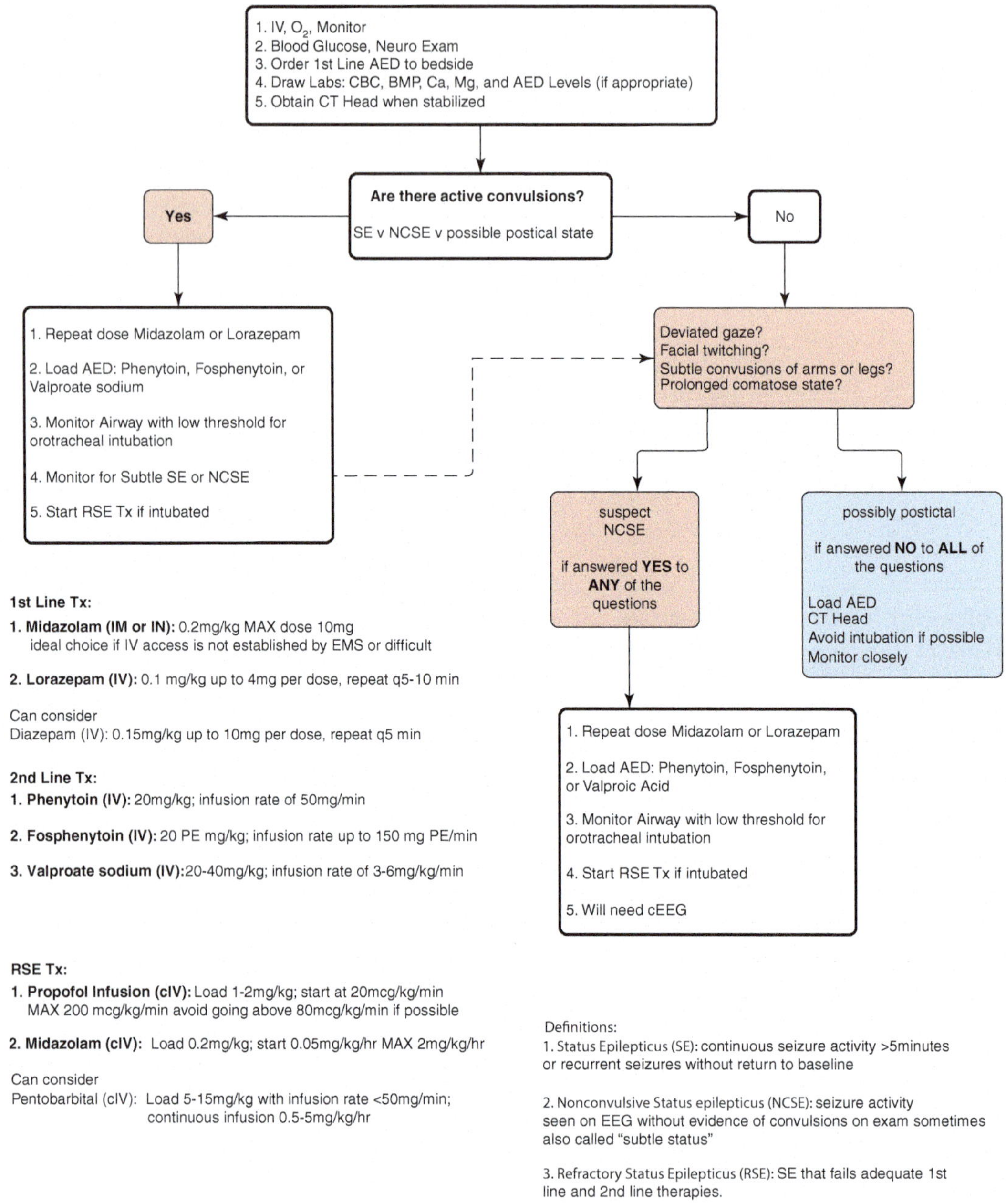

Fig. 22.3 Status epilepticus

It is important to remember that patients can continue to have seizure activity without obvious movements of the extremities; thus, continuous EEG monitoring is crucial to determine the efficacy of AEDs in patients who have an altered mental status or who are already intubated. Occasionally however, there are some subtle clinical signs of continued seizure activity that one may pick up if clinically suspecting RSE. The results of the Veterans Affairs Cooperative Study had an overall incidence of subtle SE that ranged between 7.7 and 24.2% in patients with verified

Table 22.1 Status epilepticus – treatment

Drug	Class/level of evidence	Loading dose	Side effects	Special considerations
Midazolam (IM)	Class I, Level A	0.2 mg/kg Max 10 mg	Respiratory depression Hypotension	Ideal agent if IV access is not available
Lorazepam (IV)	Class I, Level A	0.1 mg/kg up to 4 mg Repeat in 5–10 min	Respiratory depression Hypotension	Contains propylene glycol
Diazepam (IV)	Class IIa, Level A	0.1 mg/kg up to 10 mg Repeat in 5 min	Respiratory depression Hypotension	Contains propylene glycol
Phenytoin (IV)	Class IIb, Level A	20 mg/kg Max infusion rate of 50 mg/min	Hypotension Prolong QT/arrhythmia Purple glove syndrome	Contains propylene glycol
Fosphenytoin (IV)	Class IIb, Level A	20 mg PE/kg Max infusion rate of 150 mg PE/kg	Hypotension Prolong QT/ arrhythmia	
Phenobarbital (IV)	Class IIb, Level A	20 mg/kg Infusion rate of 50–100 mg/min	Respiratory depression Hypotension	Contains propylene glycol Avoid in hepatic disease
Valproate sodium (IV)	Class IIb, Level A		Hepatotoxicity Hyperammonemia Thrombocytopenia Pancreatitis	Less sedating than phenytoin Avoid in hepatic disease
Levetiracetam (IV)	Class IIb, Level C	1000–3000 mg Infusion rate of 2–5 mg/kg/min		Minimal side effects

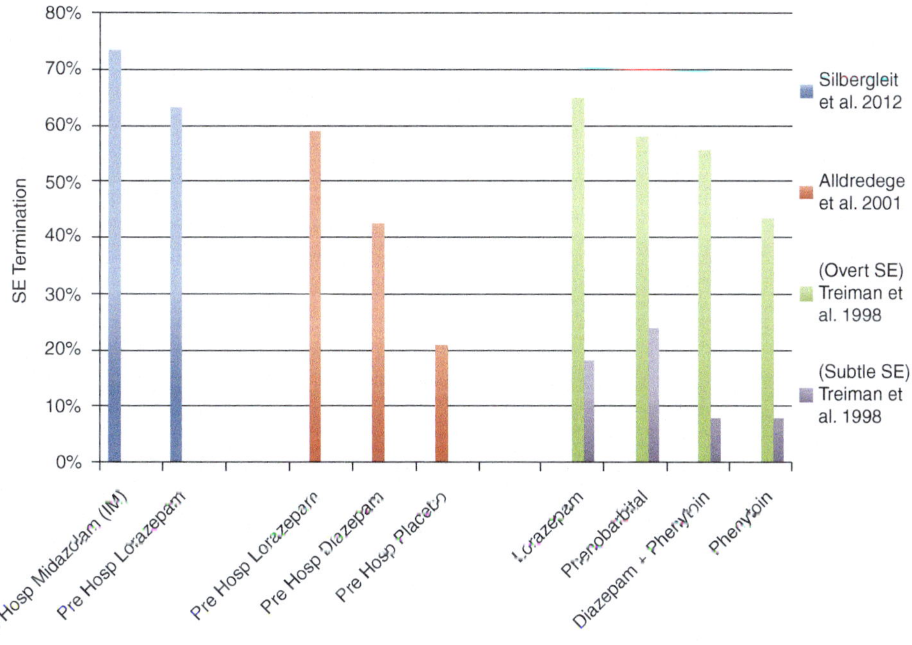

Fig. 22.4 Efficacy of benzodiazepines on the termination of status epilepticus in randomized controlled trials (RCTs). RCT by Alldredge et al. was the first RCT that studied the administration of lorazepam, diazepam, or placebo in the prehospital setting, which found that the number needed to treat (NNT) is 3 to avoid one mortality at discharge. Silbergleit et al. studied the application of midazolam (IM) compared to lorazepam (IV) in the prehospital setting and found a higher efficacy of successful SE termination

diagnosis of SE. [7] Subtle SE was considered present when patients had coma and ictal discharges on EEG, with or without subtle convulsive motor movements such as rhythmic twitching of extremities and face or eye deviation. First-line AEDs were less effective in this subset of patients.

Mayer and colleagues found that 31% of patients admitted to the neuro-ICU who were initially presumed to have SE and were adequately treated with both a benzodiazepine and loaded with a second-line agent such as phenytoin did in fact have RSE which was defined as EEG evidence of seizure activity lasting greater than 60 minutes [27]. These patients were less likely to present with generalized convulsive SE and had a higher incidence of nonconvulsive status epilepticus (NCSE) in the ICU. There are various subtypes of NCSE that are beyond the scope of this chapter, but for all practical purposes, NCSE refers to seizure activity in the absence of motor findings. This would likely manifest as a comatose patient who appears to have an abnormally prolonged postictal period. It is also important to note that nonconvulsive status (NCS) and NCSE are commonly seen in myriad of pathology such as epilepsy-related seizures, subarachnoid hemorrhage, intracerebral hemorrhage (ICH), hypoxic-ischemic encephalopathy, and CNS infections [32, 33].

The majority of emergency departments are unable to have spot EEG or continuous EEG monitoring immediately available for this subgroup of patients and it would be prudent to assume that patients are in RSE if they continue to have an altered mental state and the decision point would be to either proceed with repeat doses of benzodiazepines or continue with more aggressive therapies. The 2012 Neurocritical Care Society Guidelines recommend continued treatment of these patients immediately [22].

Refractory Status Epilepticus – Treatment

There is variable practice among emergency physicians, intensivists, and neurologists when it comes to choosing second- and third-line agents for SE. This is due to a lack of robust evidence evaluating the efficacy of second-line agent antiepileptics such as valproate sodium, levetiracetam, and phenytoin. The 2012 Neurocritical Care Society Guidelines also provided an evidence-based review of the literature along with expert opinion in the management of SE, which was partly incorporated into ACEP 2014 Clinical Policy. Still no enough data are available to support a standardized regimen, and treatment algorithms must be decided based on individual practitioners and the available resources [28].

Basic care should include orotracheal intubation and initiation of a continuous infusion such as midazolam or propofol. In 2002, Claassen et al. showed that barbiturates may be more efficacious compared to propofol and midazolam in a systematic review; however, the use of pentobarbital infusion in the emergency department is not practical, as there is a higher incidence of hypotension leading to the use of vasopressors [29, 34]. An alternative approach would be to load the patient with a second AED, such as valproate sodium or levetiracetam, if there is a high clinical suspicion for RSE. Prior to the escalation of AED, however, it would be necessary to maximize all initial therapies including continuous infusion of either propofol or midazolam. It is important to note that you should anticipate the patient to become hypotensive in such a setting and bring the importance of optimizing preload with adequate crystalloids well in advance (Table 22.2).

Table 22.2 Refractory status epilepticus – treatment

Drug	Initial dose	Continuous infusion	Serious adverse effects
Midazolam	0.2 mg/kg	0.05–2 mg/kg/h; can increase the rate by 0.05–0.1 mg/kg/h every 3–4 h	Hypotension; respiratory depression
Propofol	1–2 mg/kg	30–200 μg/kg/min	Hypotension; respiratory depression; propofol infusion syndrome (PRIS)
Pentobarbital	5–15 mg/kg; Infusion rate <50 mg/min	0.5–5 mg/kg/h	Hypotension; respiratory depression; IV contains propylene glycol

References

1. Alldredge BK, Gelb AM, Isaacs SM, et al. A comparison of lorazepam, diazepam, and placebo for the treatment of out-of-hospital status epilepticus. N Engl J Med. 2001;345:631–7.
2. Clinical Policy: Critical issues in the evaluation and management of adult patients presenting to the emergency department with seizures. Ann Emerg Med. 2004;43:605–25.
3. Silbergleit RDVLDCRPAPYBWftNI. Intramuscular versus intravenous therapy for prehospital status epilepticus. N Engl J Med. 2012;366:591–600.
4. Wasterlain CG, Chen JW. Mechanistic and pharmacologic aspects of status epilepticus and its treatment with new antiepileptic drugs. Epilepsia. 2008;49(Suppl 9):63–73.
5. Theodore WH, Porter RJ, Albert P, et al. The secondarily generalized tonic-clonic seizure: a videotape analysis. Neurology. 1994;44:1403–7.
6. Bone RM. Treatment of convulsive status epilepticus. Recommendations of the Epilepsy Foundation of America's working group on status epilepticus. JAMA. 1993;270:854–9.
7. Treiman DM, Meyers P, Walton N, Collins J, Colling C, Rowan J, Handforth A, Faught E, Calabrese V, Uthman B, Ramsay E, Mamdani M, The Veterans Affairs Status Epilepticus Cooperative Study Group. A Comparison of four treatments for generalized convulsive status epilepticus. N Engl J Med. 1998;339:792–8.
8. DeLorenzo RJ, Garnett LK, Towne AR, et al. Comparison of status epilepticus with prolonged seizure episodes lasting from 10 to 29 minutes. Epilepsia. 1999;40:164–9.
9. Meldrum BS. The revised operational definition of generalised tonic-clonic (TC) status epilepticus in adults. Epilepsia. 1999;40:123–4.
10. Lowenstein DH, Bleck T, Macdonald RL. It's time to revise the definition of status epilepticus. Epilepsia. 1999;40:120–2.
11. Mazarati AB, Baldwin RA, Sankar R, Wasterlain C. Time-dependent decrease in the effectiveness of antiepileptic drugs during the course of self-sustaining status epilepticus. Brain Res. 1998; 814:179.
12. Naylor DE, Liu H, Wasterlain CG. Trafficking of GABA(A) receptors, loss of inhibition, and a mechanism for pharmacoresistance in status epilepticus. J Neurosci. 2005;25:7724–33.
13. Kapur J, Macdonald R. Rapid Seizure-Induced reduction of benzodiazepine and Zn21 sensitivity of hippocampal dentate granule cell GABAA receptors. J Neurosci. 1997;17:7532–40.
14. Hsieh CY, Sung PS, Tsai JJ, Huang CW. Terminating prolonged refractory status epilepticus using ketamine. Clin Neuropharmacol. 2010;33:165–7.
15. Kramer AH. Early ketamine to treat refractory status epilepticus. Neurocrit Care. 2012;16:299–305.
16. Pruss H, Holtkamp M. Ketamine successfully terminates malignant status epilepticus. Epilepsy Res. 2008;82:219–22.
17. Mathern GW, Leite JP, Babb TL, et al. Aberrant hippocampal mossy fiber sprouting correlates with greater NMDAR2 receptor staining. Neuroreport. 1996;7:1029–35.
18. Mathern GW, Pretorius JK, Mendoza D, et al. Hippocampal N-methyl-D-aspartate receptor subunit mRNA levels in temporal lobe epilepsy patients. Ann Neurol. 1999;46:343–58.
19. Neder L, Valente V, Carlotti CG Jr, et al. Glutamate NMDA receptor subunit R1 and GAD mRNA expression in human temporal lobe epilepsy. Cell Mol Neurobiol. 2002;22:689–98.
20. Olney JW. Excitatory transmitters and epilepsy-related brain-damage. Int Rev Neurobiol. 1985;27:337–62.
21. Fujikawa DG. Prolonged seizures and cellular injury: understanding the connection. Epilepsy Behav. 2005;(7 Suppl):3:S3–11.
22. Brophy GM, Bell R, Claassen J, et al. Guidelines for the evaluation and management of status epilepticus. Neurocrit Care. 2012;17:3–23.
23. DeLorenzo RJ, Hauser WA, Towne AR, et al. A prospective, population-based epidemiologic study of status epilepticus in Richmond, Virginia. Neurology. 1996;46:1029–35.
24. DeLorenzo RJ, Kirmani B, Deshpande LS, et al. Comparisons of the mortality and clinical presentations of status epilepticus in private practice community and university hospital settings in Richmond, Virginia. Seizure: J Br Epilepsy Assoc. 2009;18:405–11.
25. Rossetti AO, Hurwitz S, Logroscino G, Bromfield EB. Prognosis of status epilepticus: role of aetiology, age, and consciousness impairment at presentation. J Neurol Neurosur Ps. 2006;77:611–5.
26. Wu YW, Shek DW, Garcia PA, Zhao S, Johnston SC. Incidence and mortality of generalized convulsive status epilepticus in California. Neurology. 2002;58:1070–6.
27. Mayer SA, Claassen J, Lokin J, Mendelsohn F, Dennis LJ, Fitzsimmons BF. Refractory status epilepticus: frequency, risk factors, and impact on outcome. Arch Neurol. 2002;59:205–10.
28. Huff JS, Melnick ER, Tomaszewski CA, et al. Clinical policy: critical issues in the evaluation and management of adult patients presenting to the emergency department with seizures. Ann Emerg Med. 2014;63:437–47 e15.
29. Balosso S, Ravizza T, Pierucci M, et al. Molecular and functional interactions between tumor necrosis factor-alpha receptors and the glutamatergic system in the mouse hippocampus: implications for seizure susceptibility. Neuroscience. 2009;161:293–300.
30. Pallin DJ, Goldstein JN, Moussally JS, Pelletier AJ, Green AR, Camargo CA Jr. Seizure visits in US emergency departments: epidemiology and potential disparities in care. Int J Emerg Med. 2008;1(2):97–105.

31. Sankar R, Shin D, Mazarati AM, Liu H, Wasterlain CG. Ontogeny of self-sustaining status epilepticus. Dev Neurosci. 1999;21(3–5):345–51.
32. Claassen J, Mayer SA, Kowalski RG, Emerson RG, Hirsch LJ. Detection of electrographic seizures with continuous EEG monitoring in critically ill patients. Neurology. 2004;62(10):1743–8.
33. Laccheo I, Sonmezturk H, Bhatt AB, Tomycz L, Shi Y, Ringel M, DiCarlo G, Harris D, Barwise J, Abou-Khalil B, Haas KF. Non-convulsive Status Epilepticus and Non-convulsive Seizures in Neurological ICU Patients. Neurocrit Care. 2014 (online).
34. Claassen J, Hirsch LJ, Emerson RG, Mayer SA. Treatment of refractory status epilepticus with pentobarbital, propofol, or midazolam: a systematic review. Epilepsia. 2002;43(2):146–53.

Spinal Cord Injuries

23

William A. Knight IV and Natalie P. Kreitzer

Introduction

The annual incidence of spinal cord injuries (SCI) in the United States is 40 patients per million, which represents 12,000 new cases per year [1]. Though it was classically thought to be a disease of younger patients, recent studies depict a bimodal distribution, with the first peak in adolescents and young adults, and a second peak in the elderly population aged >65 years [2]. A recent observational study demonstrated that the incidence of cervical spinal cord injury in a general population is 11.8/100,000 per year. This study also found that 68% of patients with cervical spinal cord injuries were male [3]. Other demographics show an increased risk of cervical spine injuries in the elderly and Caucasian groups [4]. In the United States, the incidence is between 28 and 55 per million people each year that sustain a traumatic spinal cord injury, with 10,000 new cases reported each year [5]. The male-to-female ratio is 4:1 [6, 7].

The most common causes of SCI include automobile crashes (31.5%) and falls (25.3%). Gunshot wounds, motorcycle crashes, diving accidents, and medical/surgical complications also cause a large number of SCIs [8]. Spinal cord injuries related to medical diagnostic procedures and treatment specifically caused 4.3% of injuries in the United States based on data from the National SCI Database (NSCID) and National Shriners SCI Database (NSSCID).

The life expectancy for a patient who sustains a SCI is significantly lower than that of the general population due to complications caused by the injury [8]. Health care costs are also tremendously higher with the average lifetime cost for a patient with a SCI ranging from almost US $4,400,000 for a 25-year-old patient with high tetraplagia to US $1,000,000 for a 50-year-old patient with an incomplete injury at any level [9]. Very few patients experience a complete neurologic recovery following a SCI [8], and these lifetime costs are not only staggering to patients with SCI, but also pose a significant burden to their families and society [8]. Rehospitalization in patients with spinal cord injuries is high. Approximately 55% of patients sustaining a SCI are hospitalized again within the same year and then 37% each subsequent year. The leading causes of rehospitalization are respiratory illness (including pneumonia) in patients with tetraplegia, diseases of the genitourinary tract, and pressure ulcers [10]. There is a higher mortality risk in patients with a higher neurologic level of injury, complete spinal cord injury, and older age at injury [11].

W. A. Knight IV
Emergency Medicine and Neurosurgery, University of Cincinnati, Cincinnati, OH, USA
e-mail: knightwa@ucmail.uc.edu

N. P. Kreitzer (✉)
Emergency Medicine, Neurovascular Emergencies and Neurocritical Care, University of Cincinnati, Cincinnati, OH, USA
e-mail: kreitzne@ucmail.uc.edu

© Springer Nature Switzerland AG 2020
J. R. Shiber, S. D. Weingart (eds.), *Emergency Department Critical Care*,
https://doi.org/10.1007/978-3-030-28794-8_23

Pathophysiology

Injuries to the spine tend to occur at areas of maximal mobility, thus, cervical spine injuries are the most common [2]. Most spine fractures involve the lower cervical (29%) or thoracolumbar junction (21%) [12]. Fifty percent of patients with a spine injury have an isolated injury, but nearly 25% have concomitant brain, chest, or major extremity injuries [12]. Patients with thoracic and lumbar fractures have more associated nonspine injuries compared to those with lower cervical spine fractures [12]. An injury severity score > 15 is associated with a cervical spinal injury [13].

Patient Presentation

When patients present following a trauma, the airway, breathing, and circulation (ABC) must first be addressed. A brief neurologic exam should follow, accompanied by the decision of who may or may not require spinal imaging. After these issues have been addressed, if there is concern for spinal cord injury, a full neurologic examination should be performed. Sensory and motor levels should be determined (Tables 23.1 and 23.2).

The physical exam findings of a patient with spinal cord injuries are typically categorized by the American Spinal Injury Association (ASIA) impairment scale. This scale was first described in 1969 by Frankel and is described in Table 23.3 [14]. Patients are stratified into five groups, ASIA A through E, with ASIA A being the worst with no sensory or motor function, even in the sacral segments. ASIA B describes patients who have sensory function below the neurologic level including sacral segments, but no motor function greater than three levels below the motor level on either side. ASIA C describes patients who have motor function below the neurologic level, with more than half of the muscles having a grade less than 3/5 strength. ASIA D patients demonstrate motor function below the neurologic level, and at least half of the muscles below the level of injury have a muscle grade greater than 3/5 strength. ASIA E patients have normal sensory and motor function in all segments. ASIA E is reserved for patients who had prior deficits, such that a person who does not have a spinal cord injury does not receive an ASIA grade.

A rectal examination should be performed to determine sacral root involvement. The sacral roots are considered spared if there are any rectal motor

Table 23.1 Motor strength scale

0: No contraction or movement
1: Minimal movement
2: Active movement, but not against gravity
3: Active movement against gravity
4: Active movement against resistance
5: Active movement against full resistance

Table 23.2 Important muscle groups to test to determine neurologic level

C4: Diaphragm
C5: Elbow flexors
C6: Wrist extensors
C7: Elbow extensors
C8: Long finger flexors
T1: Small finger abductors
L2: Hip flexors
L3: Knee extensors
L4: Ankle dorsiflexors
L5: Long toe extensors
S1: Ankle plantar flexors

Table 23.3 American Spinal Injury Association Impairment (ASIA) Scale (Modified from Frankel) [14, 15]

A = *Complete*. No sensory or motor function is preserved in the sacral segments S4–S5
B = *Sensory incomplete*. Sensory but not motor function is preserved below the neurologic level and includes the sacral segments S4–S5, and no motor function is preserved more than three levels below the motor level on either side of the body
C = *Motor incomplete*. Motor function is preserved below the neurologic level, and more than half of key muscle functions below the single neurologic level of injury (NLI) have a muscle grade less than 3 (Grades 0–2)
D = *Motor incomplete*. Motor function is preserved below the neurologic level, and at least half (half or more) of key muscle functions below the NLI have a muscle grade > 3
E = *Normal*. If sensation and motor function are graded as normal in all segments, and the patient had prior deficits, then the AIS grade is E. Someone without a SCI does not receive an AIS grade

or sensory findings present on exam. The following elements should be documented: perineal sensation, bulbocavernosus reflex (S3 and S4), anal wink (S5), rectal tone, urinary retention or incontinence, and priapism in males. Spinal injuries are defined in terms of the ASIA classification, which has been modified from the Frankel classification (Table 23.3). A thorough rectal exam should be performed on patients with a suspected spinal cord injury, not necessarily on all trauma patients.

Diagnostics

To avoid unnecessary radiation exposure, patients who have low or moderate pretest probability of cervical spine injury should undergo evaluation with a clinical decision rule prior to imaging [2]. Emergency departments in the United States and Canada annually treat more than 13 million patients at risk for cervical spine injury, but very few of these patients will actually have a cervical spine fracture, as the C-spine is injured in only 3% of major trauma patients [16, 17]. The two most frequently utilized clinical decision rules include the National Emergency X-Radiography Utilization Study (NEXUS) and Canadian C-spine criteria. However, no decision instrument is ever 100% sensitive [18]. Approximately, 20%–30% of patients with a C-spine fracture will have normal plain films [19, 20].

As opposed to the cervical spine, there are no validated decision rules to help guide whether to obtain imaging of the thoracic or lumbar spines [2]. High-risk mechanism, tenderness, and neurologic findings should be used to help guide imaging of these patients as they have demonstrated an increased likelihood of a T- or L-spine fracture [21]. In a retrospective review of a level 1 trauma center with 1485 patients, routine imaging of the thoracic and lumbar spine is recommended for patients who have midline spinal tenderness, fall from height of 10 feet or more, ejection from a motorcycle or Motor Vehicle Collision (MVC) at 50 mph or more, a Glasgow Coma Scale (GCS) of 8 or less, or a neurologic deficit [21]. These findings increased sensitivity to 100% for thoracolumbar fractures. Interestingly, in this study, 40% of patients did not have pain associated with their thoracolumbar fracture. The Eastern Association for the Surgery of Trauma (EAST) guidelines recommend that all trauma patients do not need "routine screening" computed tomography (CT) scans of the thoracolumbar spines (TLS). They further delineate that patients who have altered mentation or a significant mechanism of trauma may require imaging of the thoracic and lumbar spines. If this is performed, EAST recommends that these patients have multidetector CT imaging as the modality of choice. Patients who have normal mentation or do not have a significant mechanism of injury should not ever require a "screening" CT scan of the thoracic and lumbar spines. Patients who have a gross neurologic deficit or who have concerning clinical exam findings ultimately require a magnetic resonance imaging (MRI) and a spinal surgery consult according to EAST level 1 recommendation based on Class II data [22]. It is currently recommended that patients undergo CT imaging as opposed to plain imaging when evaluating the spinal column [23]. This is further recommended by the American College of Radiology (ACR) Appropriateness Criteria [24]. The drawback of CT scanning is that it has been historically poorly sensitive for purely ligamentous injuries, but trauma registry data are somewhat conflicting on this point. Woodring et al. evaluated 216 consecutive trauma patients with cervical spine injuries and demonstrated that only 54% of the sublaxations and dislocations were picked up by CT [25]. Although patients who have neurologic abnormalities should definitely have an MRI, it is unclear which patients who have a normal neurologic exam need further imaging with MRI after a negative CT. Schuster et al. prospectively collected registry data for 2854 blunt trauma patients, 93 of whom had a normal neurologic exam, a negative CT, and persistent C-spine pain. These 93 patients all got an MRI, and the MRI was negative in all patients for a clinically significant injury. However, the argument could also be made that since no clinically significant injuries were detected by MRI there was no need at all for further imaging studies [26]. In patients with one vertebral column fracture, the presence of a second nonadjoining fracture is estimated to approach 15%. Thus, when one fracture is identified it is recommended that the entire spinal column undergo imaging to evaluate for a concomitant fracture [27]. Examples of CT confirmed spinal fractures are demonstrated below in Figs. 23.1 and 23.2.

Patients who present with an incomplete injury may regain some useful function and might be spared the progression to complete injury with rapid diagnosis of fracture fragments,

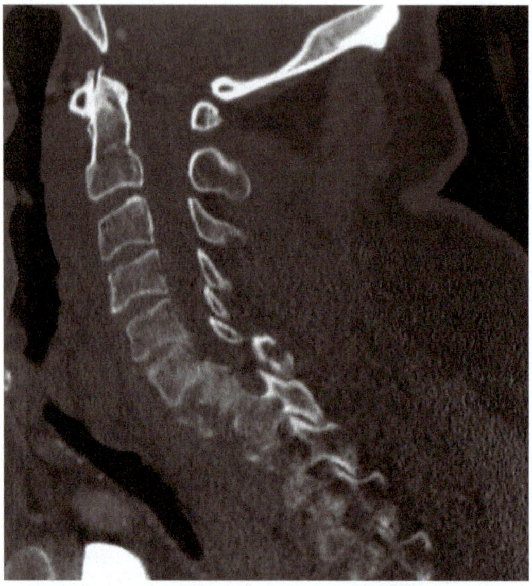

Fig. 23.1 C7 burst fracture with retropulsion of fracture fragments and spinous process fracture of C6

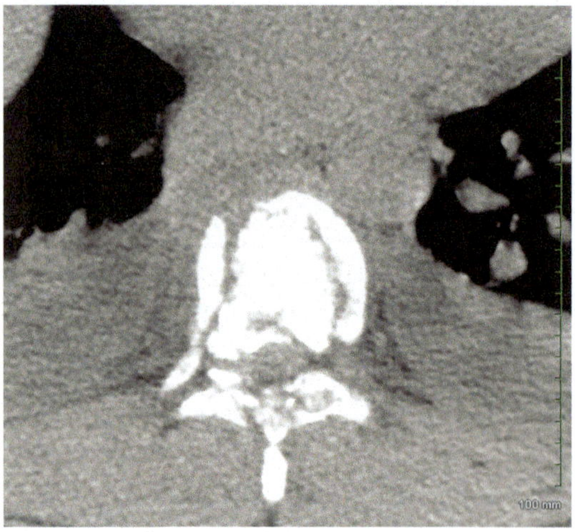

Fig. 23.2 Burst fracture of T7

hematomas, or other lesions that compress the spinal cord. Imaging is required in these patients to confirm the exact location and nature of the injury [28].

For patients whose spines cannot be clinically cleared or patients who have a possible C-spine injury may need to have an MRI to clear their cervical spine. A meta-analysis of patients with possible C-spine injuries or patients who were unable to be cleared clinically revealed no false negatives with MRI. This resulted in a negative predictive value of 100% [29]. This study concluded that MRI should be the gold standard in patients whose C spines could not be cleared clinically. In patients who do not have high impact trauma and a normal mental status, CT of the C spine alone may be sufficient to clear the C spine [30].

Symptomatic patients with normal plain films and CTs are labeled as spinal cord injury without radiographic abnormality (SCIWORA). These patients usually show abnormalities with MRI, which correlates to their physical exam findings; however, in the age of MRI, SCIWORAs are defined as having a negative MRI [31, 32].

Initial Stabilization

Prehospital

Prehospital personnel must assume that a patient has a spinal column injury until proven otherwise. Spinal immobilization should be obtained on scene. A fitted cervical collar should be placed on the patient if there is any suspicion for a spinal fracture and transferred on a backboard. Within the EMS literature, there is current controversy as to whether or not all blunt trauma patients require spine immobilization. Traditionally, EMS has assumed a potential cervical spine injury in trauma patients who have an appropriate mechanism of injury. However, there has been a movement recently to develop more sensitive and specific prehospital protocols for cervical spine immobilization, such that patients selected for cervical spine immobilization are treated appropriately [33].

Emergency Department Initial Evaluation/Stabilization

Once a patient arrives to the emergency department, the immediate evaluation of a patient with a potential spine injury is no different from any other blunt trauma patient. The ABCs in the primary survey are the first priority, and the diagnosis and treatment of most spine injuries are deferred if hemorrhage or airway compromise is suspected, but spine immobilization should be maintained [2]. The disability portion of the initial assessment will pick up gross neurologic deficits, and this can be obtained by doing a thorough Glasgow Coma Scale (GCS), pupil size and reactivity, and ability to move all four extremities [2].

During the secondary survey, the entire spinal column must be examined for deformity and palpated for areas of focal tenderness. Again, spinal precautions must be maintained at all times [2]. During the secondary survey, the rigid EMS collar may be carefully exchanged for a soft collar, as rigid collars have demonstrated to be most effective for restricting spinal movement [34].

After the primary or secondary survey, patients should be moved off the backboard as quickly as possible. Skin breakdown may start to occur within 1 hour of being placed on a backboard, and those at highest risk are elderly patients, obese patients, and those with hypotension [35].

Airway

Respiratory complications are the top cause of morbidity and mortality in the acute phase of SCI, and the incidence of respiratory complications is estimated between 36% and 83% [36]. Patients with high cervical and thoracic injuries are at highest risk [36]. One third of patients with cervical spinal cord injuries require intubation in the first 24 hours after injury [37]. The diaphragm, the major muscle of inspiration, receives innervation from the third, fourth, and fifth cervical spinal segments [36]. Thus, patients who exhibit injury at a level equal to or higher than C5 will almost always require ventilator support [38], and elective intubation is recommended [36]. High cervical lesions of C3 and higher are incompatible with life, unless respiratory support is begun immediately following injury. Cervical lesions below C5 have preserved neural control of the diaphragm, but ventilation is significantly compromised and ventilatory failure is common within days following the acute injury [36].

Signs that may be present in patients who require intubation following spinal cord injury include an increased respiratory rate, decreased forced vital capacity, increasing pCo_2 (or continuous waveform capnography), and declining pO_2 [39, 40]. Factors associated with tracheostomy are increased age (69 years of age or older), severe neurologic impairment determined by using the ASIA impairment scale, low forced vital capacity ($\leq$ 500 mL), and low percentage of vital capacity to the predicted value [41].

When there is doubt with whether or not to intubate a patient with a cervical SCI, it is best to perform the intubation early to prevent morbidity [42]. Patients typically develop worsening from their primary injury shortly after presentation due to cord edema, so routine, nonemergent intubations may prevent complications associated with hypoxia [2]. These patients are at risk of prevertebral soft tissue swelling from their cervical spine injury, which may also contribute to their respiratory distress. Patients who have sustained a major trauma may also have associated chest wall injuries and may require intubation for these purposes as well. Three independent risk factors are associated with need for intubation: injury severity score >16 (calculated post hoc), cord injury C5 or higher, and complete quadriplegia. The combination of the two latter risk factors resulted in intubation in 95% of patients studied [42].

Endotracheal intubation may be difficult in the patient with SCI. Advanced airway management frequently needs to occur before the presence or location of an injury is confirmed. Thus, all patients who require intubation following trauma must be approached as though they have a cervical spine injury. The ultimate goal of intubation is to secure the airway with little movement of the cervical spine [38].

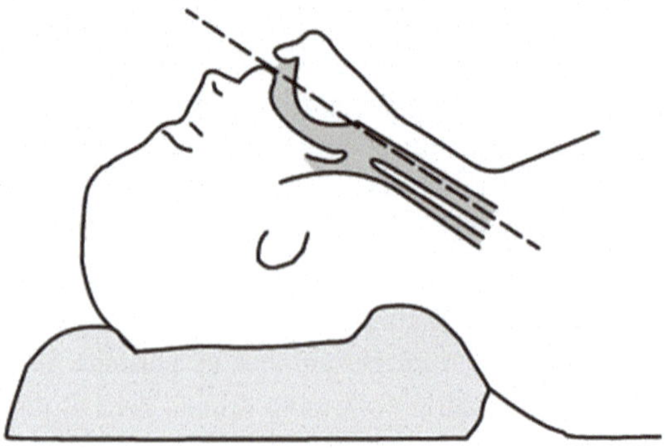

Fig. 23.3 The angle that is most optimal for intubation is depicted. Note that the cervical spine is significantly extended in this picture

Various intubation techniques have been advocated as the most appropriate for patients suspected of having a spine injury. The sniffing position involves near-full extension of the atlanto-occipital and atlantoaxial joints and flexion of the lower cervical spine as demonstrated in Fig. 23.3 [43]. An awake fiberoptic intubation may be preferred in a cooperative patient without impending respiratory failure, as this can be accomplished with minimal to no movement of the cervical spine and the neurologic exam is preserved immediately after the procedure [36–38, 44, 45]. Although there are case reports that secondary injury may have been incurred during the intubation of patients with unstable cervical spines, it is unclear whether these patients would have worsened regardless, as data collected have suggested that secondary neurologic injury associated with airway management is actually exceedingly rare [45]. This has led to discordant opinion in the literature regarding the optimal means of securing the airway in patients with C-spine injuries [45]. Endotracheal intubation in suspected SCI is most commonly performed with removal and subsequent replacement of the anterior portion of the cervical collar, while inline manual stabilization is maintained [43]. Our recommendation is that providers should intubate patients in the manner in which they are most skilled with as little cervical spine manipulation as possible during the procedure. The use of video laryngoscopy may also be beneficial in these patients, as the neck does not need to be manipulated to achieve an adequate view of the vocal cords.

It should be noted that in patients with SCI, the cardiovascular responses to laryngoscopy and intubation are different from those without a SCI. In patients with an intact spinal cord, the pressor response to intubation leads to hypertension and tachycardia. This is blunted in patients with high SCIs, since the sympathetic preganglionic neurons to the heart exit the spinal cord between T1 and T4, to the vascular beds from T1 to L2, and to the adrenal medulla from T3 to L3. Thus, quadriplegics lose all sympathetic outflow, and may exhibit pronounced bradycardia and hypotension during intubation [46].

Ventilation

Patients with SCI may exhibit paradoxical movement of the abdomen, in that it retracts during inspiration and protrudes during expiration. This leads to an increase in the work of breathing and may contribute to respiratory muscle fatigue [36].. This can contribute to significant ventilation problems, even without hypoxia, and it is recommended that spinal cord injured patients be placed on continuous end-tidal capnography in addition to pulse oximetry.

Patients who have a cervical SCI have a high likelihood of experiencing bronchospasm. This is thought to be secondary to the autonomic changes and a predominance of vagal nerve tone. Bronchodilators are recommended before bronchospasm is apparent [36], as it has been documented that even asymptomatic patients with SCI exhibit bronchospasm on spirometry during the acute injury phase [47]. The increased parasympathetic tone during acute spinal cord injury also causes some patients to develop production of excessive and tenacious bronchial mucus. These factors predispose the patient to atelectasis, pneumonia, and potential respiratory failure [36].

Blood Pressure

Patients with a SCI require early appropriate fluid resuscitation without becoming fluid overloaded. However, the appropriate resuscitation end point and optimal mean arterial blood pressure to

Table 23.4 How to differentiate neurogenic shock from hemorrhagic shock

Neurogenic shock will only take place in spinal cord injury above T6
Without a neurologic deficit, neurogenic shock is highly unlikely
Hypotension in neurogenic shock is usually mild and may be associated with bradycardia. The etiology is due to the absence of peripheral vasoconstriction, whereas patients with hemorrhagic shock tend to have an increased peripheral vascular resistance
Patients in neurogenic shock may have warm extremities and good urine output due to their decreased peripheral vascular resistance

maintain spinal cord perfusion are not known [38]. Despite the fact that there is little evidence to support it, current recommendations include the use of vasopressors to achieve a mean arterial pressure of 85–90 mmHg for a minimum of 7 days in order to deter ischemia and secondary insults [48].

Neurogenic shock was first described over 160 years ago [49]. Unfortunately, the etiology and pathophysiology of neurogenic shock are still poorly understood. It may be due to a loss of peripheral vascular resistance, decreased vascular capacitance, and cardiogenic shock or a combination of these etiologies [50]. Neurogenic shock clinically consists of hypotension and bradycardia [51]. It is likely caused by a lack of sympathetic control and unopposed parasympathetic control [52]. Cardiac dysrhythmias, most commonly bradycardia rhythms, are present in the acute phase, and in the first few weeks, may be lethal [52]. Thirty-five of patients with ASIA A or B spinal cord injuries ultimately require vasopressors [53]. Emergency physicians should be cautious not to attribute hypotension to neurogenic shock in a patient who could potentially be suffering from hemorrhagic shock (Table 23.4).

Definitive Treatment

Intensive care unit (ICU) monitoring is recommended for all patients with deficits resulting from a spinal cord injury. In particular, patients with C-spine injuries, and especially those with severe deficits, ultimately require ICU monitoring [54]. Patients should be transferred to an institution with spine surgery capabilities. All patients with confirmed spinal cord injury require a spine surgery consult. Patients with spinal cord injuries have many immediate and long-term complications (Table 23.5), and patients should be admitted to a center equipped at managing these complex patients.

Table 23.5 Complications from spinal cord injury

Deep venous thrombosis/pulmonary embolism (highest between 72 hours and 2 weeks)
Urinary tract infections
Decubitus ulcers
Autonomic hyperreflexia
Spasticity
Depression
Osteoporosis
Pain
Pneumonia

Five prospective randomized controlled studies have been performed to evaluate the potential benefit of high dose steroids in patients with confirmed spinal cord injuries. In all five of these studies, there was no significant difference or improvement in ASIA classification. Within these studies, there was a trend toward harmful complications associated with high dose steroid administration including sepsis, pulmonary emboli, and pneumonia [55–60]. Our recommendation is that steroids should not be given to patients who have sustained a spinal cord injury.

A retrospective analysis of the trauma data bank demonstrated that the timing of decompression in isolated spinal cord injuries does not change outcome [61]. However, there are proponents of early surgery for spinal fractures. Those who cite reasons to perform early surgery report that it can decrease the duration of hospital stay, reduce pulmonary complications, and decrease the number of ventilator days per patient [62]. Surgery should be immediate when a patient is having a progressive neurologic decline [63].

References

1. Spinal Cord Injury Facts. (Accessed 12/1/2014, at http://www.fscip.org/facts.htm.)

2. Stein DM, Roddy V, Marx J, Smith WS, Weingart SD. Emergency neurological life support: traumatic spine injury. Neurocrit Care. 2012;17(Suppl 1):S102–11.
3. Fredo HL, Rizvi SA, Lied B, Ronning P, Helseth E. The epidemiology of traumatic cervical spine fractures: a prospective population study from Norway. Scand J Trauma Resusc Emerg Med. 2012;20:85.
4. Lowery DW, Wald MM, Browne BJ, Tigges S, Hoffman JR, Mower WR. Epidemiology of cervical spine injury victims. Ann Emerg Med. 2001;38:12–6.
5. McDonald JW, Sadowsky C. Spinal-cord injury. Lancet. 2002;359:417–25.
6. McIntosh TK, Juhler M, Wieloch T. Novel pharmacologic strategies in the treatment of experimental traumatic brain injury: 1998. J Neurotrauma. 1998;15:731–69.
7. Ackery A, Tator C, Krassioukov A. A global perspective on spinal cord injury epidemiology. J Neurotrauma. 2004;21:1355–70.
8. Chen Y, Tang Y, Vogel LC, Devivo MJ. Causes of spinal cord injury. Topics in spinal cord injury rehabilitation. 2013;19:1–8.
9. DeVivo MJ, Krause JS, Lammertse DP. Recent trends in mortality and causes of death among persons with spinal cord injury. Arch Phys Med Rehabil. 1999;80:1411–9.
10. Cardenas DD, Hoffman JM, Kirshblum S, McKinley W. Etiology and incidence of rehospitalization after traumatic spinal cord injury: a multicenter analysis. Arch Phys Med Rehabil. 2004;85:1757–63.
11. Frankel HL, Coll JR, Charlifue SW, et al. Long-term survival in spinal cord injury: a fifty year investigation. Spinal Cord. 1998;36:266–74.
12. Saboe LA, Reid DC, Davis LA, Warren SA, Grace MG. Spine trauma and associated injuries. J Trauma. 1991;31:43–8.
13. Clayton JL, Harris MB, Weintraub SL, et al. Risk factors for cervical spine injury. Injury. 2012;43:431–5.
14. Frankel HL, Hancock DO, Hyslop G, et al. The value of postural reduction in the initial management of closed injuries of the spine with paraplegia and tetraplegia. I Paraplegia. 1969;7:179–92.
15. Waters RL, Adkins RH, Yakura JS. Definition of complete spinal cord injury. Paraplegia. 1991;29:573–81.
16. Crim JR, Moore K, Brodke D. Clearance of the cervical spine in multitrauma patients: the role of advanced imaging. Semin Ultrasound CT MR. 2001;22:283–305.
17. Stiell IG, Clement CM, McKnight RD, et al. The Canadian C-spine rule versus the NEXUS low-risk criteria in patients with trauma. N Engl J Med. 2003;349:2510–8.
18. Hoffman JR, Mower WR, Wolfson AB, Todd KH, Zucker MI. Validity of a set of clinical criteria to rule out injury to the cervical spine in patients with blunt trauma. National Emergency X-radiography utilization study group. N Engl J Med. 2000;343:94–9.
19. Woodring JH, Lee C. Limitations of cervical radiography in the evaluation of acute cervical trauma. J Trauma. 1993;34:32–9.
20. Griffen MM, Frykberg ER, Kerwin AJ, et al. Radiographic clearance of blunt cervical spine injury: plain radiograph or computed tomography scan? J Trauma. 2003;55:222–6; discussion 6–7.
21. Frankel HL, Rozycki GS, Ochsner MG, Harviel JD, Champion HR. Indications for obtaining surveillance thoracic and lumbar spine radiographs. J Trauma. 1994;37:673–6.
22. Sixta S, Moore FO, Ditillo MF, et al. Screening for thoracolumbar spinal injuries in blunt trauma: an eastern Association for the Surgery of trauma practice management guideline. The journal of trauma and acute care surgery. 2012;73:S326–32.
23. Como JJ, Diaz JJ, Dunham CM, et al. Practice management guidelines for identification of cervical spine injuries following trauma: update from the eastern association for the surgery of trauma practice management guidelines committee. J Trauma. 2009;67:651–9.
24. Daffner RH, Hackney DB. ACR appropriateness criteria on suspected spine trauma. Journal of the American College of Radiology: JACR. 2007;4:762–75.
25. Woodring JH, Lee C. The role and limitations of computed tomographic scanning in the evaluation of cervical trauma. J Trauma. 1992;33:698–708.
26. Schuster R, Waxman K, Sanchez B, et al. Magnetic resonance imaging is not needed to clear cervical spines in blunt trauma patients with normal computed tomographic results and no motor deficits. Archives of surgery (Chicago, Ill: 1960). 2005;140:762–6.
27. Holmes JF, Miller PQ, Panacek EA, Lin S, Horne NS, Mower WR. Epidemiology of thoracolumbar spine injury in blunt trauma. Acad Emerg Med. 2001;8:866–72.
28. Parizel PM, van der Zijden T, Gaudino S, et al. Trauma of the spine and spinal cord: imaging strategies. European spine journal: official publication of the European Spine Society, the European Spinal Deformity Society, and the European Section of the Cervical Spine Research. Society. 2010;19(Suppl 1):S8–17.
29. Muchow RD, Resnick DK, Abdel MP, Munoz A, Anderson PA. Magnetic resonance imaging (MRI) in the clearance of the cervical spine in blunt trauma: a meta-analysis. J Trauma. 2008;64:179–89.
30. Tan LA, Kasliwal MK, Traynelis VC. Comparison of CT and MRI findings for cervical spine clearance in obtunded patients without high impact trauma. Clin Neurol Neurosurg. 2014;120:23–6.
31. Mohanty SP, Bhat NS, Singh KA, Bhushan M. Cervical spinal cord injuries without radiographic evidence of trauma: a prospective study. Spinal Cord. 2013;51:815–8.
32. Yucesoy K, Yuksel KZ. SCIWORA in MRI era. Clin Neurol Neurosurg. 2008;110:429–33.
33. Hong R, Meenan M, Prince E, et al. Comparison of three prehospital cervical spine protocols for missed injuries. West J Emerg Med. 2014;15:471–9.
34. Tescher AN, Rindflesch AB, Youdas JW, et al. Range-of-motion restriction and craniofacial tissue-interface pressure from four cervical collars. J Trauma. 2007;63:1120–6.

35. Gefen A. How much time does it take to get a pressure ulcer? Integrated evidence from human, animal, and in vitro studies. Ostomy Wound Manage. 2008;54:26–8, 30-5.
36. Galeiras Vazquez R, Rascado Sedes P, Mourelo Farina M, Montoto Marques A, Ferreiro Velasco ME. Respiratory management in the patient with spinal cord injury. Biomed Res Int. 2013;2013:168757.
37. Gardner BP, Watt JW, Krishnan KR. The artificial ventilation of acute spinal cord damaged patients: a retrospective study of forty-four patients. Paraplegia. 1986;24:208–20.
38. Early acute management in adults with spinal cord injury: a clinical practice guideline for health-care professionals. J Spinal Cord Med. 2008;31:403–79.
39. Stevens RD, Bhardwaj A, Kirsch JR, Mirski MA. Critical care and perioperative management in traumatic spinal cord injury. J Neurosurg Anesthesiol. 2003;15:215–29.
40. Ball PA. Critical care of spinal cord injury. Spine. 2001;26:S27–30.
41. Yugue I, Okada S, Ueta T, et al. Analysis of the risk factors for tracheostomy in traumatic cervical spinal cord injury. Spine. 2012;37:E1633–8.
42. Velmahos GC, Toutouzas K, Chan L, et al. Intubation after cervical spinal cord injury: to be done selectively or routinely? Am Surg. 2003;69:891–4.
43. Austin N, Krishnamoorthy V, Dagal A. Airway management in cervical spine injury. International journal of critical illness and injury science. 2014,4:50–6.
44. Avitsian R, Lin J, Lotto M, Ebrahim Z. Dexmedetomidine and awake fiberoptic intubation for possible cervical spine myelopathy: a clinical series. J Neurosurg Anesthesiol. 2005;17:97–9.
45. Crosby ET. Airway management in adults after cervical spine trauma. Anesthesiology. 2006;104:1293–318.
46. Yoo KY, Jeong CW, Kim SJ, et al. Altered cardiovascular responses to tracheal intubation in patients with complete spinal cord injury: relation to time course and affected level. Br J Anaesth. 2010;105:753–9.
47. Spungen AM, Dicpinigaitis PV, Almenoff PL, Bauman WA. Pulmonary obstruction in individuals with cervical spinal cord lesions unmasked by bronchodilator administration. Paraplegia. 1993;31:404–7.
48. Levi L, Wolf A, Belzberg H. Hemodynamic parameters in patients with acute cervical cord trauma: description, intervention, and prediction of outcome. Neurosurgery 1993;33:1007–16; discussion 16-7.
49. Hall M. On the diseases and derangements of the nervous system: in their primary forms and in their modifications by age, sex, constitution, hereditary predisposition, excesses, general disorder, and organic disease: H. Baillière; 1841.
50. Summers RL, Baker SD, Sterling SA, Porter JM, Jones AE. Characterization of the spectrum of hemodynamic profiles in trauma patients with acute neurogenic shock. J Crit Care. 2013;28:531.e1–5.
51. Popa C, Popa F, Grigorean VT, et al. Vascular dysfunctions following spinal cord injury. J Med Life. 2010;3:275–85.
52. Krassioukov AV, Karlsson AK, Wecht JM, Wuermser LA, Mathias CJ, Marino RJ. Assessment of autonomic dysfunction following spinal cord injury: rationale for additions to International Standards for Neurological Assessment. J Rehabil Res Dev. 2007;44:103–12.
53. McKinley W, Garstang S, Wieting J, et al. Cardiovascular concerns in spinal cord injury. Cord Injury: eMedicine Specialties/Physical Medicine and Rehabilitation/Spinal. 2006.
54. Management of acute central cervical spinal cord injuries. Neurosurgery. 2002;50:S166–72.
55. Bracken MB, Shepard MJ, Hellenbrand KG, et al. Methylprednisolone and neurological function 1 year after spinal cord injury. Results of the National Acute Spinal Cord Injury Study. J Neurosurg. 1985;63:704–13.
56. Bracken MB, Shepard MJ, Collins WF, et al. A randomized, controlled trial of methylprednisolone or naloxone in the treatment of acute spinal-cord injury. Results of the second national acute spinal cord injury study. N Engl J Med. 1990;322:1405–11.
57. Bracken MB, Shepard MJ, Collins WF Jr, et al. Methylprednisolone or naloxone treatment after acute spinal cord injury: 1-year follow-up data. Results of the second National Acute Spinal Cord Injury Study. J Neurosurg. 1992;76:23–31.
58. Bracken MB, Shepard MJ, Holford TR, et al. Administration of methylprednisolone for 24 or 48 hours or tirilazad mesylate for 48 hours in the treatment of acute spinal cord injury. Results of the third National Acute Spinal Cord Injury Randomized Controlled Trial. National Acute Spinal Cord Injury Study. JAMA. 1997;277:1597–604.
59. Petitjean ME, Pointillart V, Dixmerias F, et al. Medical treatment of spinal cord injury in the acute stage. Annales francaises d'anesthesie et de reanimation. 1998;17:114–22.
60. Pointillart V, Petitjean ME, Wiart L, et al. Pharmacological therapy of spinal cord injury during the acute phase. Spinal Cord. 2000;38:71–6.
61. Sacks GD, Panchmatia JR, Marino M, Hill C, Rogers SO Jr. The effect of operative timing on functional outcome after isolated spinal trauma. J Trauma. 2011;71:1668–72.
62. O'Boynick CP, Kurd MF, Darden BV 2nd, Vaccaro AR, Fehlings MG. Timing of surgery in thoracolumbar trauma: is early intervention safe? Neurosurg Focus. 2014;37:E7.
63. Heary RF, Kumar S. Decision-making in burst fractures of the thoracolumbar and lumbar spine. Indian journal of orthopaedics. 2007;41:268–76.

Traumatic Brain Injury

24

William A. Knight IV and Natalie P. Kreitzer

Critical Points

- Avoid hypoxia and hypotension
- Assume concomitant systemic trauma and cervical spine injuries. Maintain full spinal precautions until radiographic or clinical clearance is achieved. Treat other traumatic injuries simultaneously
- Attention to appropriate ventilator management to avoid prophylactic or inadvertent hyper- or hypo-ventilation.
- The patient with a severe traumatic brain injury should be transported to a Level I trauma center as soon as possible
- Aggressively resuscitate shock, while searching for likely etiologies (hemorrhagic, neurogenic etc). The use of Isotonic crystalloids or balanced intravenous fluids and blood products should follow institutional guidelines.
- Steroids are contraindicated for the treatment of severe traumatic brain injury
- Basic treatment of suspected elevated intracranial pressure includes head of bed >30°, appropriate sedation and analgesia, targeted pCO_2 35-45 mmHg, and hyperosmolar therapy
- A patient with a severe TBI who is systemically anticoagulated should be aggressively reversed as soon as possible, if a reversal agent exists.
- Non-contrast head CT is the recommended first-line imaging modality given its efficiency and sensitivity to detect traumatic brain injury

W. A. Knight IV (✉)
Emergency Medicine and Neurosurgery, University of Cincinnati, Cincinnati, OH, USA
e-mail: knightwa@ucmail.uc.edu

N. P. Kreitzer
Emergency Medicine, Neurovascular Emergencies and Neurocritical Care, University of Cincinnati, Cincinnati, OH, USA
e-mail: kreitzne@ucmail.uc.edu

Introduction

Traumatic brain injury is one of the leading causes of death and long-term disability in the United States. TBI is a spectrum of disease, ranging from mild to severe. Recent military conflicts, as well as concussions to high profile athletes in professional and collegiate sports have brought increased attention to the overall spectrum of disease. In the United States, over 1.3 million cases of TBI are treated in emergency departments

© Springer Nature Switzerland AG 2020

J. R. Shiber, S. D. Weingart (eds.), *Emergency Department Critical Care*,
https://doi.org/10.1007/978-3-030-28794-8_24

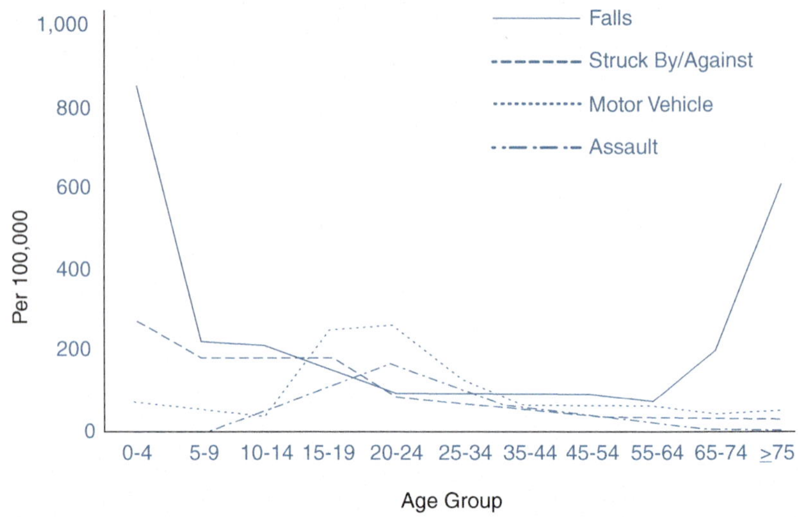

Fig. 24.1 Etiology of TBI related presentations by age group to EDs in the United States, 2002–2006 [1]. (Image courtesy of William A. Knight IV, MD)

(ED), with 275,000 patients hospitalized, and 52,000 deaths each year [1].

The long-term neurologic disabilities, as well as the significant financial and societal impacts are overwhelming. In the United States in 2000, direct medical costs and indirect costs of TBI, such as lost productivity, were an estimated $60 billion [2].

The incidence of TBI is highest in children aged 0–4 years, adolescents/young adults aged 15–24 years, and adults aged 65 years and older [1]. Falls cause the majority of TBIs in young children and older adults, and non-accidental trauma is the leading cause of death in children less than 2 years of age [1, 3]. Motor vehicle accidents are the leading cause of TBI-related mortality, highest in adults aged 20–24 years of age [1] (Fig. 24.1).

Nearly half of the mortalities from TBI die in the first 2 hours after injury, highlighting the role of the EP in the early management [4]. The pathophysiology of severe TBI is complicated. The initial primary injury occurs at impact, and is irreversible and immediately present. Secondary injuries occur after the initial impact and evolve. Secondary injury is potentially preventable and represents targeted end-points for goal directed resuscitation and research.

The neurologic exam can rapidly fluctuate during the initial management and resuscitation of a patient with a severe TBI. It is important to have an effective method to evaluate and define dynamic exams. The Glasgow Coma Scale (GCS) [5], AVPU (Alert, verbal stimulus, painful stimulus, unresponsive) and the FOUR score (Full Outline of UnResponsiveness) [6] are 3 such methods to facilitate communication. Regardless of the method chosen, it should be easily applied across EMS, nursing, and multiple physician specialties, and widely adopted in a particular setting.

Table 24.1 Traumatic brain injury [8]

	GCS	Incidence (%)
Mild	13–15	80
Moderate	9–12	10
Severe	3–8	10

In addition to the aggregate score, the GCS should be followed by each individual score; ex – GCS 8 (E2 V2 M4). This allows providers to better understand the complexity of the injury. In order to score a "4" for eye opening, the patient should regard the examiner in order to convey the higher level of cerebral functioning the score intends. In order to award a "6" for motor, the patient must follow commands. For a "5," the patient should cross midline to address noxious stimuli. Older terms such as "decerebrate" and "decorticate" posturing should be avoided, with focus on physiologic descriptions such as "flexion," "extension," or "withdrawal" [7] (Table 24.1).

Condensed scores have the potential to oversimplify and potentially replace a detailed neurologic exam, which was not the initial intent. These scores are limited by physiologic and pharmacologic parameters such as intoxication, confounding injuries, hypotension, acidosis, paralysis, and sedation among others. A single score does not adequately explain the severity of injury after trauma, and although can be associated with outcomes, has no prognostic value [9, 10].

Pathophysiology

The disease that is "TBI" is made up of several different, distinct and unique diseases that together make up the parent definition. Each of these "subcategories" can have different treatment options, and often several are present in a single patient. This makes the management of not only the primary injury difficult, but also the prevention and treatment of secondary injuries. The most common primary injuries include subdural hematomas, epidural hematomas, traumatic subarachnoid hemorrhages, cerebral contusions, intraventricular hemorrhage, diffuse axonal injuries and penetrating injuries.

Despite the anatomic and cellular differences of the various primary injuries of severe TBI, there are similar sequelae shared by all. The initial clinical management in the ED is directed at minimizing the damage from the primary injury, recognizing immediate surgical candidates and preventing secondary injury [7] (Fig. 24.2) (Table 24.2).

Subdural hematomas (SDH) are the most common injury related to blunt trauma, and often the result of the tearing of bridging cortical veins (Fig. 24.3). The appearance of SDH) on CT is of a concave or crescent shape with irregular borders, which can cross bony suture lines, but does not cross the falx to the contralateral hemisphere as the blood collects below the dura and directly on brain parenchyma. Blood can be seen bilaterally, but this represents 2 separate injuries, rather than one that extends to both sides. This can lead to cerebral compression, mid-line shift, and increased intracranial pressure, as well as contribute to an increased risk for seizures, delayed cerebral ischemia, and cerebral vasoconstriction. Surgical and medical options vary based on the patient's neurologic exam, the acuity of the hematoma, and concomitant injuries, but in gen-

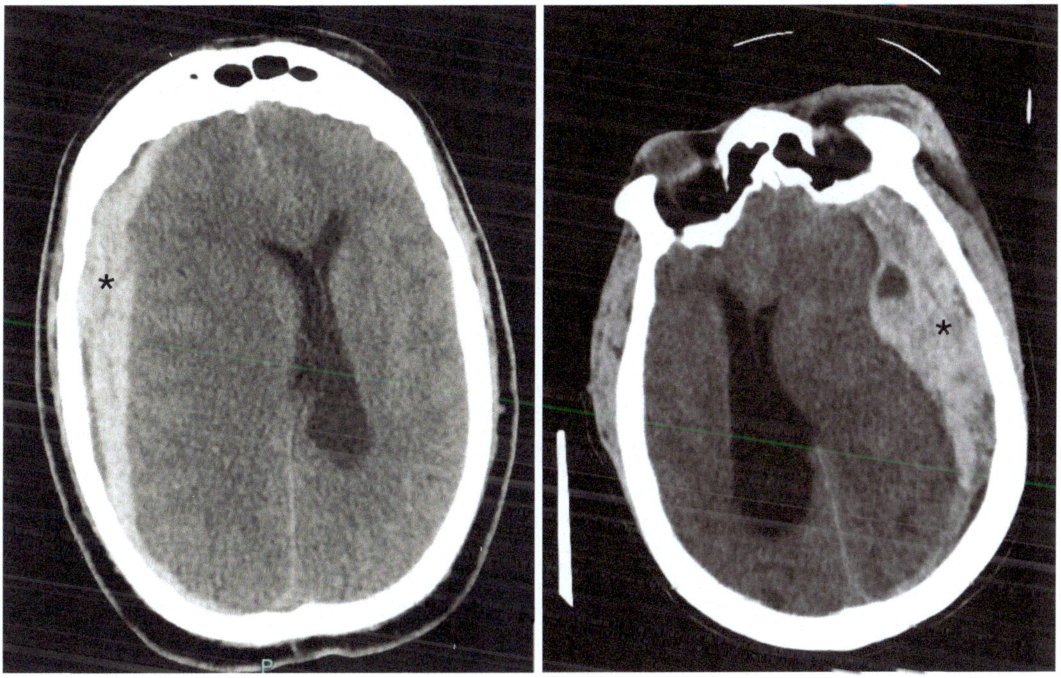

Fig. 24.2 Subdural hematoma. (Image courtesy of William A. Knight IV, MD)

Table 24.2 Secondary injury [7]

Systemic	Central nervous system
Hypoxia	Hematoma
Hypotension	Brain edema Cytotoxic Vasogenic
Anemia	Brain herniation
Hyperthermia	Seizures
Hyper/hypocarbia	Hydrocephalus
Fluid imbalance	Ischemia
Sepsis	Infection

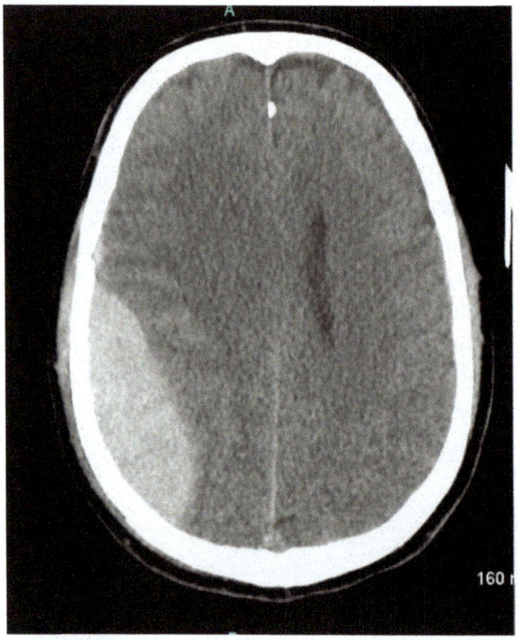

Fig. 24.3 Epidural hematoma. (Image courtesy of William A. Knight IV, MD)

eral, it is recommended that acute SDHs greater than 1 cm or with an associated 5 mm of mid-line shift be evacuated regardless of the patient's GCS [11]. Patients with chronic hematomas and favorable neurologic exams may have surgical intervention delayed to allow for the breakdown of the clotted, septated blood [12].

Epidural hematomas (EDH) (Fig. 24.4) are caused by the often-rapid accumulation of blood between the dura and the skull (blood is not directly on brain parenchyma), giving a CT appearance of a smooth, lenticular or convex shape, which do not cross bony suture lines. They are more common in younger patients [13]. The most common cause of an EDH is a side head impact, with associated skull fracture. The middle meningeal artery is the classically described culprit, but veins can often be the source of bleeding as well. These patients often undergo rapid surgical decompression and hematoma removal (depending on location and size), and if accomplished rapidly, these patients have lower rates of mortality than other categories of severe TBI [14].

Traumatic subarachnoid hemorrhage (tSAH)) (Fig. 24.5) is caused by damage to small arteries in the potential space under the arachnoid mater. The amount of blood measured on CT has clinical and prognostic significance; likely related to both direct parenchymal injury and/or the tSAH blood itself [15]. Secondary injuries are common with tSAH, including hydrocephalus (via obstruction of arachnoid villi and increased cerebral venous pressure), and decreased cerebral perfusion. Delayed ischemia related to tSAH vasospasm is increasingly recognized as a cause of delayed cerebral infarction, but should not be a source of concern in the ED [16].

Intraparenchymal hemorrhages (ie. cerebral contusions) (Fig. 24.6) are caused by direct injury to the brain parenchyma. The equivalent of an ecchymosis to the brain, this injury is an accumulation of blood within the brain tissue and appears hyperdense on CT. The frontal and temporal lobes are the most common locations for contusions due to the adjacent and irregular bony structures. As with all TBIs, practitioners should consider repeat imaging between 6 and 24 hours to assess for evolution and growth of hematomas, edema and midline shift. These complications are more common in patients who abuse alcohol, who have end-stage renal disease, or use anticoagulant or antiplatelet therapy [17].

Diffuse axonal injury (DAI)) often has a benign CT appearance, with either small, randomly distributed punctate areas of hyper-acute blood, cerebral edema, or most commonly, a normal CT (Fig. 24.7). DAI can occur anywhere in the brain, but especially in the brainstem, corpus collosum, deep grey matter, and cortical white matter. DAI is the result of severe acceleration-deceleration and rotational forces, which cause stretching and

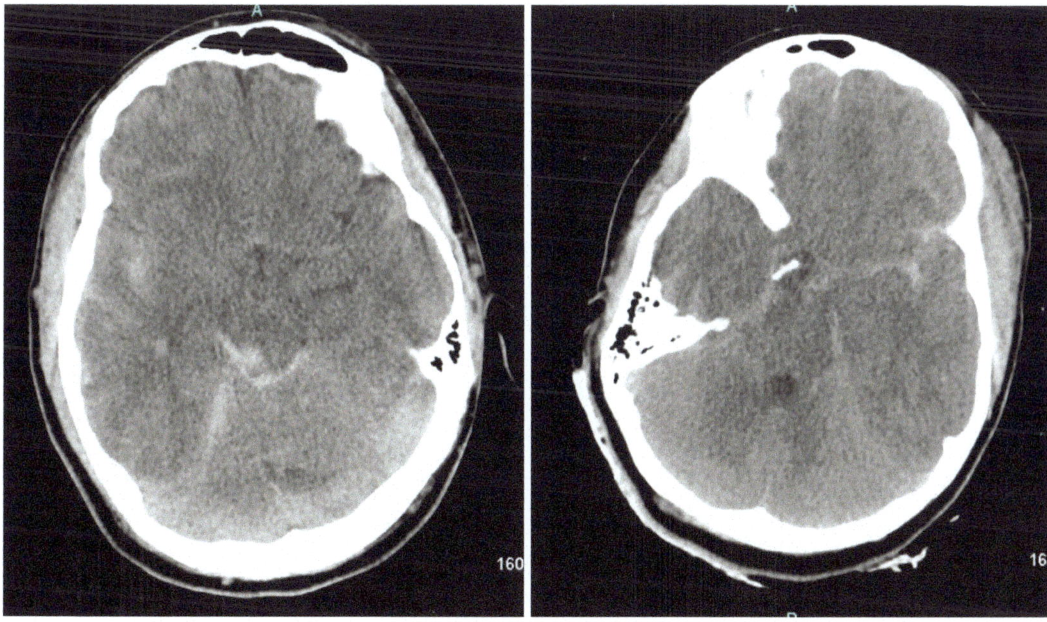

Fig. 24.4 Traumatic subarachnoid hemorrhage. (Image courtesy of William A. Knight IV, MD)

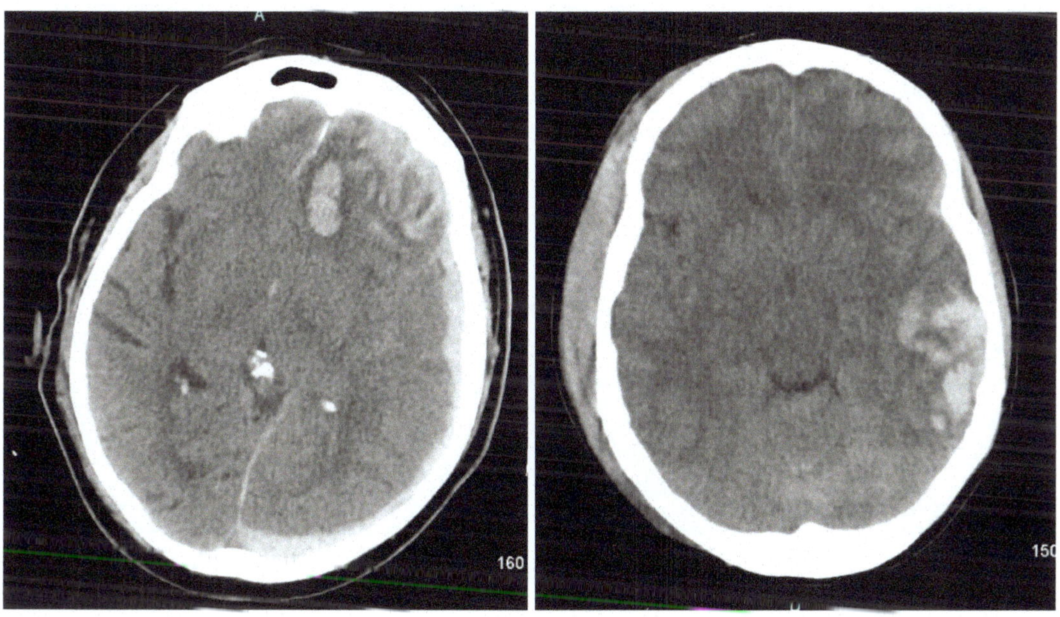

Fig. 24.5 Cerebral contusions. (Image courtesy of William A. Knight IV, MD)

disruption of axons. This leads to a biochemical cascade of events that ultimately ends in neuronal death [18]. This damage is widespread, irreversible and a significant contribution to the morbidity and mortality of severe TBI. Patients with DAI are especially susceptible to secondary injuries from hypotension and hypoxia, given cell level injury of the neurons [18].

Penetrating TBI is not as common as blunt TBI, but accounts for a disproportionate rate of mortality. The morbidity and mortality from penetrating TBI depends on the characteristics of the

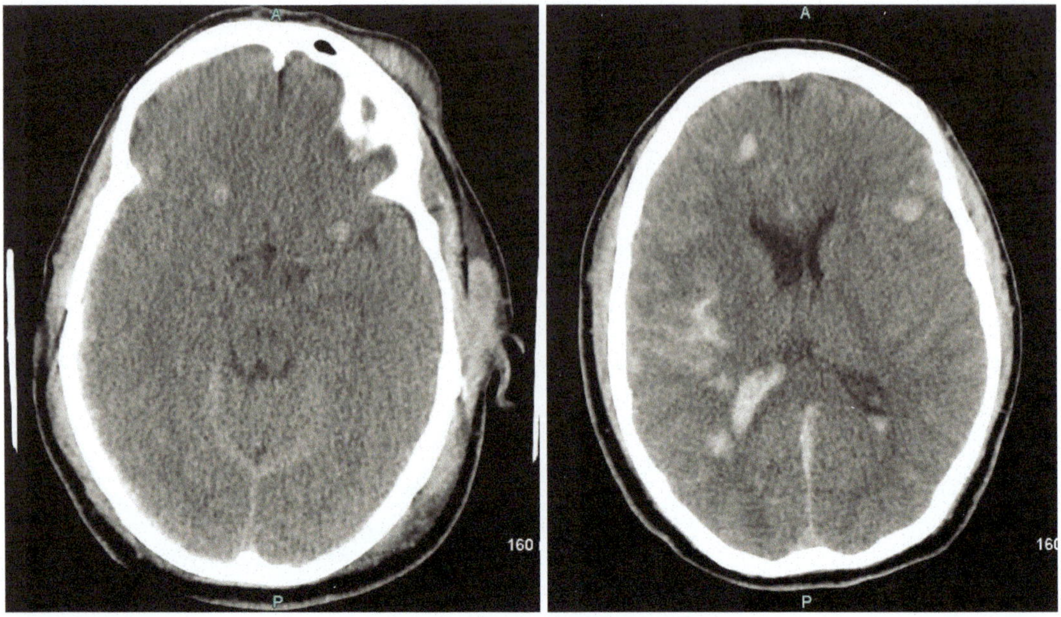

Fig. 24.6 Diffuse axonal injury (DAI). (Image courtesy of William A. Knight IV, MD)

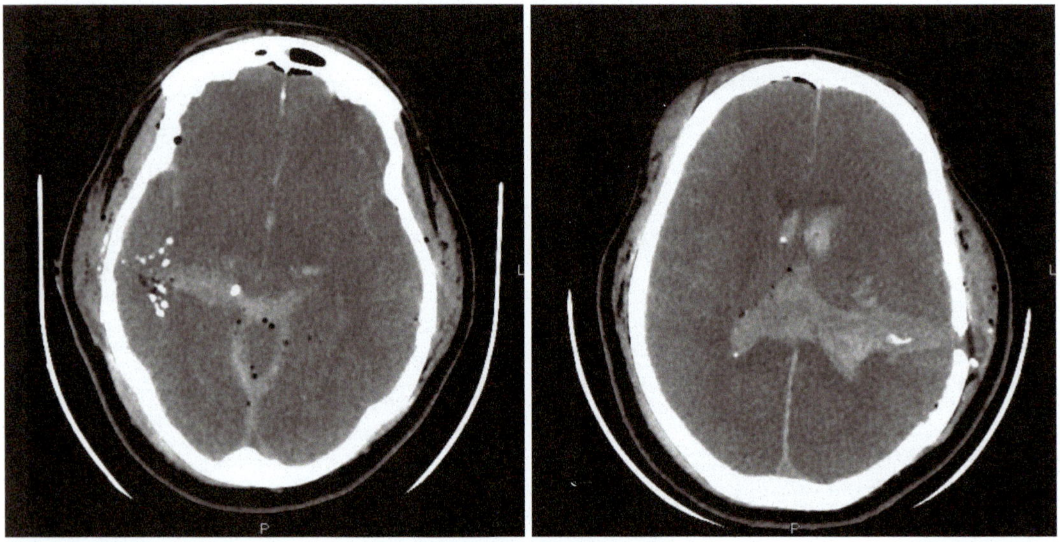

Fig. 24.7 Penetrating injury. (Image courtesy of William A. Knight IV, MD)

weapon or projectile, the trajectory and location of the injury, and the energy of the impact [19]. In addition to the physical damage from the penetrating TBI, a high velocity missile also has damaging properties from the resultant pressure waves and rotational forces of the projectile. These cause stretching or tearing of cerebral tissue and often create cavities larger than the missile itself. Penetrating injuries are also more susceptible to a systemic release of thromboplastin by disrupting cerebral parenchyma, potentially causing a profound coagulopathy, hemorrhage and resultant shock [20]. The most common secondary injury after penetrating TBI is infection [21]. Although the overall outcome of missile penetrating TBI (GSW) has historically been poor, patient outcomes from the Iraq and Afghanistan conflicts suggest a possible role for early, aggressive medical and surgical management [22].

Patient Presentation

Initial ED resuscitation of a patient with a suspected severe TBI should focus on the tenets of airway, ventilation and circulation. Care should include maintenance of in-line cervical spine immobilization and evaluation for concomitant traumatic injuries [7]. Even isolated episodes of hypoxia and hypotension contribute to worse outcomes in a patient with severe TBI [23]. When both hypotension and hypoxia occur in a single patient, there is significant morbidity and mortality. This occurs by increasing neuronal death and contributing to worsened motor deficits [24]. The practitioner should focus on physiologic homeostasis, avoiding supra or sub-therapeutic values in both vital signs and labs

Diagnostics

Imaging

Non-contrast computed tomography (CT) of the head is the preferred initial imaging for a patient with a suspected TBI. CT is highly sensitive to detect acute hemorrhage and bony pathology (fractures, mass, erosion). In addition, CT is sensitive for detecting sequelae and secondary injury after trauma, such as cerebral edema, mass effect, mid-line shift, and hydrocephalus. It is important to note that some patients with severe TBI can have an initially normal or underwhelming CT due to diffuse axonal injury (DAI). This is one of the biggest limitations of CT with TBI diagnosis.

Additional imaging modalities do not have much of a role in the initial diagnosis and workup of TBI in the ED. Table 24.3 demonstrates appropriate indications and limitations [7]. All patients with severe TBI should have appropriate imaging of the cervical spine. These patients are unable to be clinically cleared, and there are a significant percentage of patients with concomitant traumatic brain injuries and cervical spine fractures.

Table 24.3 Imaging modalities in severe TBI

	Indications	Limitations
Computed tomography	1. Initial modality choice for traumatic brain injury in the ED 2. Non-contrast	1. Not sensitive for DAI 2. Limited for early anoxic or ischemic changes
CT-angiography	1. Penetrating trauma with concern for violation of cerebral sinus or carotid canal 2. Skull or cervical spine fractures a. Carotid canal	1. Nephrotoxic contrast 2. Often indicated after patient has received contrast for body imaging for other traumatic injuries
Magnetic resonance imaging	1. Late management a. Occult injuries (DAI) b. Assist with prognosis	1. No role in acute management 2. Less sensitive than CT for bony fractures and acute hemorrhage 3. Not universally available 4. Longer time for acquisition 5. Challenges for monitoring acute, critically ill patients

Lab Tests

Local trauma protocol may guide the selection of the initial laboratory evaluation. A point of care blood glucose should be performed on every patient who presents with altered mental status, as hypoglycemia is a common and easily reversible condition [25]. A blood alcohol and/or toxicology screen (blood or urine) may be of assistance in identifying contributing causes to altered mental status, but should not change the clinical management of a patient with a suspected severe TBI. Patients with a severe TBI should have coagulation studies evaluated, especially international normalized ratio (INR). Pertinent history should guide the need for additional studies such as prothrombin time (PT), partial thromboplastin time (PTT), or factor Xa level. A thromboelastogram (TEG) can help with overall resuscitation by providing specific guidance as to the particular aspect of the coagulopathy defect, such as platelet dysfunction, plasma components, fibrinogen, or even the presence of novel oral anticoagulants (NOACs) [26]. If the patient is taking a medication that is monitored with a common laboratory therapeutic profile, those should be monitored as well (digoxin, lithium, phenytoin, valproic acid, etc.).

Initial Stabilization

Pre-hospital Management

The association between prehospital hypoxia (SpO2 < 90%) and/or hypotension (SBP < 90 mmHg) and increased mortality in severe TBI has been well described [24, 27] EMS providers should focus on normoxia and normotension during prehospital management and transport. There is likely a benefit to prehospital RSI for severe TBI patients under the following circumstances [28–30]:

1. Patients with an inability to protect their airway or maintain oxygenation.
2. When being transported by aeromedical providers.
3. Patients with ground transport times of greater than 10 minutes and being performed by providers with regular intubation experience and advanced critical care and RSI training.

End-tidal CO_2 should be used on all ventilated patients to target eucapnea (35–40 mmHg). There is an association between both prehospital hypercapnia or hypocapnia and poor outcomes in both intubated and non-intubated patients [27, 31, 32]. Hypercarbia causes cerebral arterial vasodilatation, which initially produces an increase in CBF as well as an increase in ICP, a subsequent decrease in CPP, and the potential expansion of hemorrhagic lesions [33]. Hypercarbic systemic acidosis may comprise cardiac output as well as coagulation mechanisms, further reducing CPP and promoting the expansion of intracranial hematomas.

Table 24.4 Indications for therapeutic hyperventilation in TBI

1. Dilated and unreactive pupils (<1 mm response)
2. Asymmetric pupils in the setting of coma (>1 mm difference)
3. Flexor or extensor posturing to painful stimulus
4. No motor response to pain (not caused by spinal cord injury)
5. Decrease in 2 points on the GCS when the best initial score was <9

If the patient is well oxygenated, normotensive and any of the below signs of herniation are present, hyperventilation (goal $ETCO_2$ of 30–35 mmHg) is recommended Table 24.4 [34]. Hyperventilation causes a reduction of $PaCO_2$, which leads to cerebral vasoconstriction, a reduction in cerebral blood flow and ultimately ICP by 25% [35]. This can be a valuable short-term maneuver during an acute deterioration or herniation, but can cause further ischemia and increased morbidity if utilized prophylactically [8]. It is important to note that end-tidal CO2 can be falsely lower in patients who are in shock, and one should never decrease the respiratory rate to target 45-40 mmHg in this situation.

Emergency Department Evaluation/Stabilization

Airway

A patient with a severe TBI should be intubated when there is a failure to oxygenate, a failure to ventilate, a failure to protect the airway, or for an anticipated clinical course (air medical transport, operation, need for cross-sectional imaging, etc). The decision regarding the need for endotracheal intubation should be considered on a case-by-case basis. Historically, practitioners have been taught that patients with a GCS GCS ≤ 8, regardless of disease pathology, require intubation and mechanical ventilation.

The GCS was never designed or validated for this indication, and has significant limitations when used as the sole indication for airway management. Many patients with a GCS ≤ 8 have adequate oxygenation and ventilation in the ED, further confounding appropriate patient selection for intubation [36]. The GCS can be also be particularly misleading in patients who are in shock or intoxicated.

While providing the positive benefit of definitive airway protection, endotracheal intubation also carries a significant risk of contributing to secondary injury through hypoxia, hypotension and increased ICP. Patients should be pre-oxygenated and appropriate pharmacologic agents that avoid hypotension should be selected. The recently described apneic oxygenation technique is particularly beneficial for severe TBI patients. These patients have oxygen delivered via nasal cannula throughout the induction and intubation period, contributing to a potentially longer apneic period with adequate oxygenation [37].

Laryngoscopy with subsequent laryngeal manipulation and tracheal intubation can lead to elevated ICP through a reflexive sympathetic response. This response leads to tachycardia and hypertension, which can contribute to pathologic increases in ICP in a patient who has lost cerebral autoregulation due to severe traumatic injury. Patients with severe TBI often have occult cervical spine injuries, and in-line cervical spine immobilization should be maintained throughout intubation. Fiberoptic or video-assisted intubation is recommended, if available, to minimize potential manipulation of the cervical spine. Once the endotracheal tube (ETT) is in place, manipulation of the tube with tracheal irritation can cause a direct cough reflex with resultant ICP spikes.

Sedation and Induction

There are a number of different sedation/induction agents that can be used prior to paralysis for endotracheal intubation. Even with coma, it is important that patients receive a sedative prior to administration of a paralytic. Appropriate sedation helps positively affect ICP, blood pressure, heart rate and amnesia of the intubation procedure. The ideal pharmacologic agent is rapid in onset, provides deep sedation to facilitate amnesia, and maintains hemodynamic stability. The most important characteristic of any selected pharmacologic agent is the practitioner's familiarity with its desired effects, as well as any potential adverse side effects. Unfortunately, there is no perfect, single recommended agent for patients who have sustained a TBI, especially when considering different medical histories, presenting shock, concomitant injuries, etc. [38]. Choices and doses selected in the ED have downstream ramifications in the ICU, especially with medications selected for continuous infusion.

Breathing

Once a patient is placed on mechanical ventilation, the practitioner must focus on both oxygenation as well as ventilation ($PaCO_2$), as inappropriate ventilator settings can be lethal. Hypoxia ($PaO_2 < 60$ mmHg or $SpO_2 < 90\%$) must be avoided at all costs in a patient with a severe TBI [23]. Although most patients will be intubated and mechanically ventilated, supplemental oxygen should be administered for the patients who do not require mechanical ventilation, or who are about to be intubated. Continuous end-tidal CO_2 monitoring should be employed to allow for real-time ventilator adjustments [39].

Initial ventilator settings should focus on lung protective ventilation with goal tidal volumes of 6–8 cc/kg based on ideal body weight. High tidal volume ventilation is associated with acute lung injury (ALI) and adult respiratory distress syndrome (ARDS) in patients with severe TBI, and should not be utilized [40]. Normal physiologic parameters should be the rule, and the ventilator should be adjusted for a normal PaO_2 (80–120 mmHg) and $PaCO_2$ (35-45 mmHg). The fractionated inspired concentration of oxygen

(FiO_2) should be reduced (<60%) once the airway is secured and adequate oxygenation is demonstrated, to prevent both pulmonary and cerebral oxygen toxicity [41].

Prophylactic hyperventilation is associated with increased morbidity and mortality and is not indicated [42]. Cerebral blood flow can be significantly lowered in the first hours after a TBI due to a loss of auto-regulation [43]. The beneficial lowering of elevated ICP during a herniation event is short-lived, and deleterious rebound ICP elevation can be seen as the patient equilibrates. If hyperventilation is used for an acute herniation, it should be a temporizing, life-saving maneuver (goal $PaCO_2$ = 30 mmHg) until more definitive interventions can be employed (sedation, hyperosmolar therapy, decompressive hemicraniectomy, etc.) [35].

Circulation

It has been well described that one episode of hypotension (systolic blood pressure < 90 mmHg) doubles mortality rates and worsens neurologic outcome [39, 44]. The optimal resuscitation fluid has not been defined in the literature, but isotonic solutions (normal saline, Plasmalyte-A normosol, etc) are preferred if hemorrhagic shock is not present. Lactated Ringer's is occasionally used, but the practitioner should be aware that LR is a somewhat hypotonic solution with an osmolarity of 273 mmol, and sodium content of 130 g/dL. Dextrose containing fluids should be avoided, as there is a theoretical risk of osmotic fluid shifts, contributing to increased cerebral edema. Albumin is contraindicated for use in patients with severe TBI, as one study demonstrated increased mortality [45]. There is no literature to support the use of blood products as a resuscitation fluid for TBI, and their use should be guided by local trauma protocol. The use of hyperosmolar agents (mannitol, hypertonic saline, etc) should be reserved for patients with evidence of acute herniation or signs of elevated ICP in the ED. Hypoosmolar (free water, half-normal saline) should not be used in the acute management phase of any patient with a suspected TBI.

The optimal blood pressure in the ED is difficult to determine in the ED without ICP monitoring, as the target should support the ideal cerebral perfusion pressure (CPP). ICP monitoring will rarely, if ever, be available in the ED. The optimal CPP is between 50-70 mmHg, with an ICP less than 20 mmHg, but some patients will need their values targeted individually, based on cerebral parameters [35]. The focus in the ED must be on euvolemia and prevention of hypotension and hypoxia. Induced hypertension is not recommended due to an increased risk of acute lung injury (ALI) or acute respiratory distress syndrome (ARDS), but pressors are encouraged for correction of hypotension if the provider is confident that the patient is euvolemic [39, 40, 46]. If a patient is hypertensive, the provider should not attempt to lower the blood pressure unless the MAP > 120 mmHg. During a traumatic brain injury, there is often a loss of cerebral autoregulation, and pharmacologic management of blood pressure can directly affect the cerebral perfusion pressure. If malignant hypertension is present, the provider should investigate an underlying medical condition and use short acting agents until an ICP monitor can be placed.

ICP Management

The initial management of the patient with a severe TBI is complex and challenging. Traditionally, management of a patient has been a step-wise process with pharmacologic and procedural interventions. Focusing solely on individual parameters such as CPP or ICP is likely not effective, and may be harmful. ICP monitoring is often not immediately available in the ED, but providers must be aware of the indications to help facilitate transfer to appropriate centers and/or ICU's. ICP should be monitored in all salvageable patients with a severe TBI and an abnormal CT scan. ICP monitoring is indicated in patients with a normal CT scan if 2 of the following are present: age > 40, motor posturing, or hypotension (SBP < 90) [35]. There are multiple options to monitor ICP, but the ideal monitor is a ventriculostomy, as it can provide both diagnostic ICP values, as well as a therapeutic option (CSF drainage) [47]. If ICP monitoring is available, treatment of ICP should be considered when the pressure exceeds 20 mmHg or with evidence of herniation. Many of the therapies recommended in the ED are directed towards prevention of elevated ICP and optimization of CPP.

The head of the bed should be elevated to 30° to help facilitate cerebral venous drainage and CSF drainage. Almost all patients will be in spinal precautions until they can be clinically or radiographically cleared per local protocol. In these cases, reverse trendelenberg position can be used instead of head elevation. The cervical immobilization collar must be sized appropriately to avoid unnecessary pressure on the neck, causing jugular venous congestion, decreased venous return and elevated ICP.

Sedation and analgesia have been shown to decrease ICP and optimize CPP [35]. The optimal sedative has a rapid onset and short duration, so that the patient's neurologic status can be examined on a regular basis. It is imperative to avoid medication-induced hypotension with adequate dosing and volume resuscitation. Most commonly used sedatives do not have analgesic properties, and an appropriate concomitant analgesic agent is warranted, even if the patient is comatose. Sedation and analgesia goals in the ED should focus on physiologic targets such as heart rate, blood pressure, respiratory rate, ventilator tolerance, facial grimace, diaphoresis and motor agitation. Paralytic use is not recommended in the ED other than the peri-intubation period. If necessary, one should strongly consider ICP monitoring prior to paralysis since the patient's neurologic exam will be masked. The initial ED resuscitation of the severe TBI patient is a dynamic process, and it is important to regularly assess the patient's neurologic and physical exams.

Fever is an independent predictor of poor outcome in most neurologic injuries, including TBI [48], and providers should be aggressive in the temperature management of patients with severe TBI. There is no evidence to suggest that any particular method, technology or device is superior to another in maintenance of euthermia or neurologic outcome, and local practice should be guided by consensus protocols. Antipyretics should be administered in the event of fever, favoring acetaminophen [4]. NSAIDs should be avoided given the theoretical anti-platelet effect. Shivering should be controlled, as this can contribute to increased cerebral metabolism and elevated ICP. Shivering can often be effectively managed medically with skin counter warming with a convection blanket, sedation, analgesia, and acetaminophen. In difficult cases, buspirone, magnesium sulfate, meperidine and dexmedetomidine have been recommended [49].

Definitive Treatment

The initial management of a patient with a severe TBI should focus on normal physiologic values, particularly blood pressure and oxygenation, as well as searching for concomitant injuries. If the patient neurologically deteriorates, the focus should be on aggressively optimizing CPP and implementing ICP lowering therapies. The head of the bed should be raised to 30°, or placed in reverse trendelenberg if necessary. The patient should receive adequate sedation and analgesia. If a herniation event is suspected, the provider can hyperventilate the patient to a goal end-tidal CO2 of 30–35 mm Hg and administer hyperosmolar therapy. If the patient is suspected to be on anti-coagulants, reversal agents should be expeditiously provided. TEG should be considered if available, as it can provide valuable information regarding individualized management of coagulopathy.

If a patient herniates from a confirmed or suspected expanding epidural or subdural hematoma and there is an expected delay or inability to transfer the patient to neurosurgical care, skull trephination [50] or burr hole decompression can be considered. This is best performed in communication with Neurosurgery. Limited reports suggest this is a procedure that can be performed by an emergency physician and may improve patient outcomes [50].

Reversal of Anticoagulation

The population is aging, and there is a growing use of anticoagulation agents for various medical conditions. Patients with a severe TBI who are therapeutically anticoagulated have higher mortality and worse neurologic outcomes when compared to patients who are not anti-coagulated [51, 52]. Studies have demonstrated benefit in reversing anticoagulation in patients with spontaneous intracranial hemorrhage, and it is reasonable and logical to do the same in patients with severe TBI.

The development of novel oral anticoagulants introduced additional medications that do not require frequent monitoring, yet have similar (or possibly better) efficacy with less bleeding complications and fewer food and medication interactions. Unfortunately, they do not have readily available and approved reversal agents [53]. *Apixaban* and *Rivaroxaban* are oral, lipophilic, reversible competitive antagonists of activated factor X (Xa) and *Dabigatran* is an oral, lipophilic, direct reversible competitive antagonist of thrombin (factor IIa). There are currently no reversal agents or antidotes available for these agents, and their anticoagulant effects will not be reversed by administration of vitamin K or plasma. Dabigatran can theoretically be partially reversed with hemodialysis, but this is often not practical in an emergent setting for patients with a severe TBI. Similarly, rivaroxaban and apixaban may be amenable to reversal with 4-factor prothrombin, but additional research is needed.

Tranexamic Acid (TXA)

Primary fibrinolysis is integral in the development of the acute coagulopathy of trauma. The use of antifibrinolytic agents for trauma patients with acute hemorrhage has been investigated as a treatment option. Tranexamic acid (TXA) is an antifibrinolytic agent that acts by binding to plasminogen and blocking the interaction of plasminogen to fibrin, preventing dissolution of a fibrin clot. It is currently FDA approved as an injection for hemophiliacs during tooth extraction and as an oral agent for cyclic heavy menstrual bleeding. TXA has promise in the treatment algorithm for the management of severe TBI if given early in the disease course. Studies have suggested a reduction in hematoma growth, focal cerebral ischemia and mortality in those administered TXA, but the results have not been statistically significant in a small patient population [54, 55]. Use of TXA in patients with severe TBI would be an off-label indication and not recommended at this time. One exception would be the consideration of TXA if evidence of fibrinolysis were present via the elevation of the Lysis30 on thromboelestrography. Additional research is necessary to determine the optimal indication, if any, for the use of TXA in TBI.

Hyperosmolar Therapy

Hyperosmolar therapy is commonly used to manage elevated ICP in severe TBI, but the optimal agent remains unclear. Mannitol has the most evidence and clinical experience with its utilization. Hypertonic saline has shown promise, but does not have strong evidence to support its routine use and/or recommendation. If advanced intracranial monitoring is available in the ED, hyperosmolar therapy is part of a more complicated discussion and treatment algorithm.

Mannitol is a sugar alcohol that functions as a potent osmotic diuretic by not being resorbed by the renal tubule and causing excretion of free water and sodium [56]. Mannitol causes a shift of free water out of the cerebral tissue and therefore a reduction of edema and overall brain mass [57]. Due to similar fluid shifts from the interstitium to the vascular space throughout the body, there is a transient increase in cardiac output just prior to the free water excretion. Mannitol indirectly reduces the hematocrit and blood viscosity temporarily, which leads to increased cerebral blood flow and oxygen delivery. Mannitol decreases cerebral spinal fluid (CSF) production, further reducing intracranial contents and decreasing ICP. In patients with a disrupted blood brain barrier, mannitol can cross into the cerebral tissue and cause a delayed rebound increased ICP. This negative effect of the osmotic gradient draws free water back into the brain, causing increased edema [57]. Mannitol is dosed 0.5 g – 1.0 g/kg as a bolus, and there is no role for "high-dose" mannitol or a constant infusion. It can be given every

2–8 hours, but should not be used in a hypovolemic or under-resuscitated patient, as hypotension and decreased cerebral perfusion can occur. The provider should consider placing a urinary catheter to record strict urine output and replace diuresed volume with an isotonic solution to help avoid hypovolemia.

Hypertonic saline (HTS) ranges from 2% to 30% normal saline, and its use should be guided by clearly defined protocols, as dosing regimens and preferences for use vary widely amongst practitioners. HTS functions as a plasma expander, rather than a diuretic like mannitol. HTS functions by causing an osmolar gradient to draw free water from the tissues into the vasculature. HTS is more likely to stay in the vasculature and maintain an elevated osmolality than mannitol, contributing to a robust intravascular resuscitation, while minimizing the possibility of a rebound elevation in ICP [58]. Several trials have suggested that HTS has improved ICP control and contributes to higher brain tissue oxygenation than mannitol, but definitive reduction in mortality and/or neurologic improvement have not been demonstrated [58].

Osmotic agents should be reserved for clinical evidence of acute herniation or neurologic deterioration unexplained by any other cause. Mannitol and 2% NS can be given through a peripheral intravenous line. Concentrations 3% and higher of hypertonic saline should be given through central venous access, except for during emergencies. Protocols for the use of hyperosmolar agents should be developed in collaboration between Emergency Medicine, Neurosurgery and Trauma Surgery.

Disposition

Neurosurgery should be promptly consulted and/or the patient should be immediately transferred to a facility with neurosurgical and/or trauma surgery capabilities. If consultation is not readily available, the EP should quickly stabilize the patient and arrange transfer to a facility capable of managing severe TBI. Advanced ICP lowering therapies, such as barbiturates or hypothermia, and invasive management, such as ICP monitors, ventriculostomy, craniotomy, or craniectomy are best carried out in consultation with Neurosurgery, Trauma Surgery, and/or Neurocritical Care specialists.

Patients who are operative candidates should not be delayed en route to the operating room. All severe TBI patients should be managed in an intensive care unit (ICU) by practitioners familiar with current management guidelines. Special consideration should be given to managing these patients in a Neurologic Intensive Care Unit by neurointensivists or intensivists with experience managing neurologic disorders [7].

Summary

Severe traumatic brain injury remains a devastating cause of death and disability, with adjusted mortality rates near 25%. Primary injury is permanent and irreversible, while the prevention and treatment of secondary injuries is critical to reducing long-term neurologic morbidity and mortality. The emergency practitioner should focus on early aggressive resuscitation, targeting normal physiologic goals (blood pressure and oxygenation) and disposition to physicians and centers with neurologic, trauma and critical care expertise. All attempts at neurologic prognosis should be avoided for the first 24 hours to allow for maximal resuscitation, even when confronted with an apparently devastating injury.

References

1. Faul M, et al. Traumatic brain injury in the United States: emergency department visits, hospitalizations and deaths 2002–2006. Atlanta: Centers for Disease Control and Prevention, National Center for Injury Prevention and Control; 2010. http://www.cdc.gov/traumaticbraininjury/pdf/tbi_blue_book_external-cause.pdf.
2. Finkelstein EA, Corso PS, Miller TR. Incidence and economic burden of injuries in the United States. New York. Oxford University Press; 2006.
3. Kochanek P, et al. Inflicted childhood neurotrauma: new insight into the detection, pathobiology, preven-

tion, and treatment of our youngest patients with traumatic brain injury. J Neurotrauma. 2007;24(1):1–4.
4. Chesnut R. Care of central nervous system injuries. Surg Clin North Am. 2007;87(1):119–56, vii.
5. Teasdale G, Jennett B. Assessment of coma and impaired consciousness. A practical scale. Lancet. 1974;2(7872):81–4.
6. Wijdicks EFM, Bamlet WR, Maramattom BV, Manno EM, McClelland RL. Validation of a new coma scale: the FOUR score. Ann Neurol. 2005;58:585–93.
7. Zammit C, Knight WA. Severe traumatic brain injury in adults. Emerg Med Pract. 2013;15(3):1–28.
8. Heegaard W, Biros M. Traumatic brain injury. Emerg Med Clin North Am. 2007;25(3):655–78, viii.
9. Teasdale G, Jennett B. Assessment and prognosis of coma after head injury. Acta Neurochir. 1976;34(1–4):45–55.
10. Narayan RK, et al. Improved confidence of outcome prediction in severe head injury. A comparative analysis of the clinical examination, multimodality evoked potentials, CT scanning, and intracranial pressure. J Neurosurg. 1981;54(6):751–62.
11. Bullock MR, et al. Surgical management of acute subdural hematomas. Neurosurgery. 2006;58(3 Suppl):S16–24; discussion Si-iv.
12. Cenic A, Bhandari M, Reddy K. Management of chronic subdural hematoma: a national survey and literature review. Can J Neurol Sci. 2005;32(4):501–6.
13. Greenberg M. Handbook of neurosurgery. Lakeland: Greenberg Graphics; 1997.
14. Cooper DJ, et al. Decompressive craniectomy in diffuse traumatic brain injury. N Engl J Med. 2011;364(16):1493–502.
15. Servadei F, et al. Traumatic subarachnoid hemorrhage: demographic and clinical study of 750 patients from the European brain injury consortium survey of head injuries. Neurosurgery. 2002;50(2):261–7; discussion 267-9.
16. Oertel M, et al. Posttraumatic vasospasm: the epidemiology, severity, and time course of an underestimated phenomenon: a prospective study performed in 299 patients. J Neurosurg. 2005;103(5):812–24.
17. Oertel M, et al. Progressive hemorrhage after head trauma: predictors and consequences of the evolving injury. J Neurosurg. 2002;96(1):109–16.
18. Iwata A, et al. Traumatic axonal injury induces proteolytic cleavage of the voltage-gated sodium channels modulated by tetrodotoxin and protease inhibitors. J Neurosci. 2004;24(19):4605–13.
19. Stuehmer C, et al. Influence of different types of guns, projectiles, and propellants on patterns of injury to the viscerocranium. J Oral Maxillofac Surg. 2009;67(4):775–81.
20. Feldman Z, Narayan RK, Robertson CS. Secondary insults associated with severe closed head injury. Contemp Neurosurg. 1992;14(4):1–8.
21. Antibiotic prophylaxis for penetrating brain injury. J Trauma. 2001;51(2 Suppl):S34–40.
22. Martin EM, et al. Traumatic brain injuries sustained in the Afghanistan and Iraq wars. Am J Nurs. 2008;108(4):40–7; quiz 47-8.
23. Stocchetti N, Furlan A, Volta F. Hypoxemia and arterial hypotension at the accident scene in head injury. J Trauma. 1996;40(5):764–7.
24. Chi JH, et al. Prehospital hypoxia affects outcome in patients with traumatic brain injury: a prospective multicenter study. J Trauma. 2006;61(5):1134–41.
25. Brady WJ, et al. Hypoglycemia in multiple trauma victims. Am J Emerg Med. 1999;17(1):4–5.
26. Windelov NA, et al. The prognostic value of thrombelastography in identifying neurosurgical patients with worse prognosis. Blood Coagul Fibrinolysis. 2011;22(5):416–9.
27. Davis DP, et al. The impact of hypoxia and hyperventilation on outcome after paramedic rapid sequence intubation of severely head-injured patients. J Trauma. 2004;57(1):1–8; discussion 8-10.
28. Winchell RJ, Hoyt DB. Endotracheal intubation in the field improves survival in patients with severe head injury. Trauma Research and Education Foundation of San Diego. Arch Surg. 1997;132(6):592–7.
29. Davis DP, et al. The effect of paramedic rapid sequence intubation on outcome in patients with severe traumatic brain injury. J Trauma. 2003;54(3):444–53.
30. Bernard SA, et al. Prehospital rapid sequence intubation improves functional outcome for patients with severe traumatic brain injury: a randomized controlled trial. Ann Surg. 2010;252(6):959–65.
31. Brorsson C, et al. Severe traumatic brain injury: consequences of early adverse events. Acta Anaesthesiol Scand. 2011;55(8):944–51.
32. Dumont TM, et al. Inappropriate prehospital ventilation in severe traumatic brain injury increases in-hospital mortality. J Neurotrauma. 2010;27(7):1233–41.
33. Marion DW, et al. Effect of hyperventilation on extracellular concentrations of glutamate, lactate, pyruvate, and local cerebral blood flow in patients with severe traumatic brain injury. Crit Care Med. 2002;30(12):2619–25.
34. Badjatia N, et al. Guidelines for prehospital management of traumatic brain injury 2nd edition. Prehosp Emerg Care. 2008;12(Suppl 1):S1–52.
35. The Brain Trauma Foundation. The American Association of Neurological Surgeons. The Joint Section on Neurotrauma and Critical Care. Guidelines for the management of severe traumatic brain injury. J Neurotrauma. 2007;24(Suppl 1):S14–20.
36. Davis DP, et al. The association between field Glasgow Coma Scale score and outcome in patients undergoing paramedic rapid sequence intubation. J Emerg Med. 2005;29(4):391–7.
37. Weingart SD, Levitan RM. Preoxygenation and prevention of desaturation during emergency airway management. Ann Emerg Med. 2012;59(3):165–75.
38. Roberts DJ, et al. Sedation for critically ill adults with severe traumatic brain injury: a systematic review

of randomized controlled trials. Crit Care Med. 2011;39(12):2743–51.
39. Chesnut RM, et al. The role of secondary brain injury in determining outcome from severe head injury. J Trauma. 1993;34(2):216–22.
40. Mascia L, et al. High tidal volume is associated with the development of acute lung injury after severe brain injury: an international observational study. Crit Care Med. 2007;35(8):1815–20.
41. Davis DP, et al. Early ventilation and outcome in patients with moderate to severe traumatic brain injury. Crit Care Med. 2006;34(4):1202–8.
42. Muizelaar JP, et al. Adverse effects of prolonged hyperventilation in patients with severe head injury: a randomized clinical trial. J Neurosurg. 1991;75(5):731–9.
43. Sioutos PJ, et al. Continuous regional cerebral cortical blood flow monitoring in head-injured patients. Neurosurgery. 1995;36(5):943–9; discussion 949-50.
44. Fearnside MR, et al. The Westmead head injury project outcome in severe head injury. A comparative analysis of pre-hospital, clinical and CT variables. Br J Neurosurg. 1993;7(3):267–79.
45. Myburgh J, et al. Saline or albumin for fluid resuscitation in patients with traumatic brain injury. N Engl J Med. 2007;357(9):874–84.
46. Contant CF, et al. Adult respiratory distress syndrome: a complication of induced hypertension after severe head injury. J Neurosurg. 2001;95(4):560–8.
47. Fakhry SM, et al. Management of brain-injured patients by an evidence-based medicine protocol improves outcomes and decreases hospital charges. J Trauma. 2004;56(3):492–9; discussion 499-500.
48. Jones PA, et al. Measuring the burden of secondary insults in head-injured patients during intensive care. J Neurosurg Anesthesiol. 1994;6(1):4–14.
49. Choi HA, Ko SB, Presciutti M, et al. Prevention of shivering during therapeutic temperature modulation: the Columbia anti-shivering protocol. Neurocrit Care. 2011;14(3):389–94.
50. Nelson JA. Local skull trephination before transfer is associated with favorable outcomes in cerebral herniation from epidural hematoma. Acad Emerg Med. 2011;18(1):78–85.
51. Pieracci FM, et al. Degree of anticoagulation, but not warfarin use itself, predicts adverse outcomes after traumatic brain injury in elderly trauma patients. J Trauma. 2007;63(3):525–30.
52. Huttner HB, et al. Hematoma growth and outcome in treated neurocritical care patients with intracerebral hemorrhage related to oral anticoagulant therapy: comparison of acute treatment strategies using vitamin K, fresh frozen plasma, and prothrombin complex concentrates. Stroke. 2006;37(6):1465–70.
53. Battinelli EM. Reversal of new oral anticoagulants. Circulation. 2011;124(14):1508–10.
54. Crash-2 Collaborators. Effect of tranexamic acid in traumatic brain injury: a nested randomised, placebo controlled trial (CRASH-2 intracranial bleeding study). BMJ. 2011;343:d3795.
55. Shakur H, et al. Effects of tranexamic acid on death, vascular occlusive events, and blood transfusion in trauma patients with significant haemorrhage (CRASH-2): a randomised, placebo-controlled trial. Lancet. 2010;376(9734):23–32.
56. Wakai A, Roberts I, Schierhout G. Mannitol for acute traumatic brain injury. Cochrane Database Syst Rev. 2005;4:CD001049.
57. Kaufmann AM, Cardoso ER. Aggravation of vasogenic cerebral edema by multiple-dose mannitol. J Neurosurg. 1992;77(4):584–9.
58. Vialet R, et al. Isovolume hypertonic solutes (sodium chloride or mannitol) in the treatment of refractory posttraumatic intracranial hypertension: 2 mL/kg 7.5% saline is more effective than 2 mL/kg 20% mannitol. Crit Care Med. 2003;31(6):1683–7.

Evaluation and Management of Polytrauma Patients

25

Jay Menaker and Kimberly Boswell

Unintentional injury remains the leading cause of death for those between the ages of 1 and 44 [1]. For those between the ages of 45 and 64, it is the third leading cause of death, only behind malignancy and heart disease [1]. It results in 2.8 million hospitalizations and 29 million emergency department visits annually in the United States [2]. The estimated annual cost in the United States for medical expenses and lost productivity resulting from injury is $355 billion [2]. As a result, many efforts of injury prevention including juvenile delinquent therapy programs, automobile safety belts, child safety seats, bicycle helmets, and gun control have evolved. These efforts have been shown to reduce medical costs and save lives [3].

Despite all this, critically ill trauma patients continue to present to the emergency room requiring timely evaluation and intervention in order to improve outcome. All critically injured patients' evaluation should begin with airway, breathing, and circulation. Advanced Trauma Life Support (ATLS) guidelines are well established and provide a specific organization for the evaluation of a trauma patient. The concept of primary and secondary survey should be familiar to all emergency physicians and should be followed for every trauma patient. When trauma patients present in shock, resuscitation should begin immediately and occur simultaneously with the evaluation. Patients with polytrauma may have more than one source of shock (hemorrhagic, cardiogenic, neurogenic, obstructive) leading to hemodynamic instability. This necessitates the emergency physician to be able to quickly and effectively assess the situation and implement appropriate resuscitation and hemorrhage control as quickly as possible.

The concept of resuscitation is not as simple as one may think. Traditional teaching states that 1–2 liters of a crystalloid solution should be given prior to administration of blood products for the acutely injured patient [4]. Infusions of crystalloid in a patient with ongoing hemorrhage cause a dilution effect and worsen bleeding by aggravating the lethal triad of acidosis, hypothermia, and coagulopathy [5, 6]. Recent data suggest that high volume crystalloid infusion is associated with increased morbidity including the development of acuter respiratory distress syndrome (ARDS), increased ventilator days, increased intensive care unit (ICU) days as well as increased incidence of multisystem organ failure [6, 7]. As a result, many institutions have begun to give blood products, through a warmer if possible, earlier in the resuscitation of a patient

J. Menaker (✉)
Program in Trauma, R Adams Cowley Shock Trauma Center, University of Maryland School of Medicine, Baltimore, MD, USA
e-mail: jmenaker@umm.edu

K. Boswell
University of Maryland School of Medicine, Baltimore, MD, USA

© Springer Nature Switzerland AG 2020

J. R. Shiber, S. D. Weingart (eds.), *Emergency Department Critical Care*,
https://doi.org/10.1007/978-3-030-28794-8_25

with ongoing hemorrhage. The appropriate administration ratio of blood products has not been elucidated. There has been considerable amount of research in both civilian and military situation trying to determine the ideal ratio. The PROPPR (Pragmatic Randomized Optimal Platelet and Plasma Ratios) trial, a multicenter randomized trial comparing blood product ratios, has recently been completed [8]. The authors demonstrated that for patients with severe trauma and major bleeding, there was no significant difference in mortality at 24 hours when comparing a 1:1:1 ratio versus a 1:1:2 ratio of plasma, platelets, and red blood cells. However, those patients receiving the 1:1:1 ratio had a lower rate of death from hemorrhage in the first 24 hours. Additionally, the 1:1:1 group had significantly higher rate of hemostasis achieved. Finally, there was no difference in complications between the two groups.

The ideal resuscitation fluid for patients who are not actively bleeding remains unknown. Many prehospital providers have traditionally used lactated ringers. At our institution, we use Plasmalyte (Baxter International), which is slightly more physiologic than lactated ringers and significantly more than normal saline. The concern with large amounts of normal saline is that it can cause a hyperchloremic metabolic acidosis (See Table 25.1).

Some institutions used colloids in their resuscitation. Studies have suggested that crystalloid solution use after injury may have a mortality benefit; however, the numbers are too small to demonstrate a definitive advantage [9, 10]. Other centers use hypertonic saline (3% NaCl solution) as a resuscitative fluid. It is believed to increase and improve perfusion by acting as a volume expander [11]. Animal models have demonstrated that hypertonic solutions minimize the inflammatory response after injury [11–13]; however, no trials have shown benefit for the resuscitation of the hypovolemic patient in shock after injury [14]. Empiric use of hypertonic saline as a resuscitative fluid for patients with traumatic brain injury theoretically should be beneficial, but to date no study has demonstrated a mortality benefit [15].

Table 25.1 Fluids

	Normal saline	Lactated ringers	Plasmalyte
pH	5.0	6.5	7.4
Sodium	154	130	140
Potassium	0	4	5
Chloride	154	109	98
Acetate	0	0	27
Lactate	0	28	0

Chest

Injuries to the chest are common after both penetrating and blunt injuries. Up to 25% of deaths following trauma have been attributed to chest trauma [16]. As a result, rapid evaluation and intervention is required. Primary survey should help identify any life-threatening issues including external hemorrhage, tension pneumothorax, and pericardial tamponade. For those that require imaging, either bedside ultrasound or portable chest X-ray should be the imaging modality of choice. Although chest X-ray has been the traditional screening imaging, recent data suggest that for the diagnosis of pneumothorax following injury, thoracic ultrasound has a higher sensitivity and negative predictive value than chest X-ray [17].

In most large volume trauma centers, including ours, stable patients will proceed to CT scan following initial evaluation and imaging. Some centers suggest that if a chest CT is obtained following injury, then a plain chest X-ray in a stable asymptomatic patient is not required [18]. Others, however, argue the opposite and suggest if a stable asymptomatic patient has a normal chest X-ray, a chest CT is unwarranted because it does not alter treatment [19]. While other authors still recommend a chest CT even if the chest X-ray is normal as the CT has a higher diagnostic value and results in treatment differences in a substantial number of patients [20]. A 2010 study by Brink and colleagues identified nine predictors of chest injury on CT scan [21] (Table 25.2). The one injury that many believe cannot be ruled out by a normal chest X-ray is a traumatic aortic injury (TAI). As many as 44% of patients with a normal chest X-ray may have a TAI and thus in the correct clinical setting, any patient who is at risk for a TAI must have a CT scan to rule out the injury [22–25].

Management of chest trauma is best divided into blunt and penetrating. Patients who present to the emergency department following blunt trauma and are hemodynamically unstable require rapid evaluation in the organized fashion described in ATLS. Table 25.3 shows an effective algorithm for the initial evaluation and management of those hemodynamically unstable patients.

For those that are hemodynamically stable, patients at a minimum should have a focused abdominal sonography for trauma (FAST) exam and a chest X-ray done. Depending on the mechanism of injury and the index of suspicion for a TAI, the need for a CT scan can be determined. Table 25.4 represents a comparison from speed to equivalent height, which may help in determining a patient's risk for TAI There are a number of abnormalities on chest X-ray that are indicative of a TAI (Table 25.5). Any patient who has a high index of suspicion for TAI warrants immediate medical treatment, even prior to radiographic confirmation. Blood pressure and heart rate control are paramount to preventing worsening of the injury. Although no specific targets for blood pressure and heart rate are well studied, Fabian and colleagues suggested a systolic blood pressure on <100 mmHg (<120 mmHg in the elderly) and heart rate <100 beats per minute to decrease in-hospital rupture [26]. This author typically titrates heart rate to the 70s if possible. One must be cautious in patients who have concomitant traumatic brain injury. Clinicians need to attempt to maintain cerebral perfusion pressure while trying to minimize progression of a TAI until definitive therapy is possible. Once confirmed by CT scan, TAIs are typically treated with an endovascular stent as opposed to an open repair (Figs. 25.1, 25.2, and 25.3).

Other blunt chest injuries include rib fractures, pulmonary contusions, sternal fractures, and cardiac contusions. Isolated rib fractures in a young

Table 25.2 Risk factors for chest injury on CT following injury [21]

1. Age ≥55 years
2. Abnormal chest physical exam
3. Altered level of consciousness
4. Abnormal thoracic spine exam
5. Abnormal chest X-ray
6. Abnormal thoracic spine X-ray
7. Abnormal pelvic x-ray/FAST exam
8. Base deficit < -3 mmol/L
9. Hemoglobin <6 mmol/L

Table 25.3 Hemodynamically unstable blunt chest trauma

Inspection
- Open pneumothorax ->large (≥36 French) bore chest tube

Auscultation
- Absent breath sounds ->large (≥36 French) bore chest tube

FAST exam
- Positive for pericardial fluid (very rare in blunt trauma)
  - Resuscitation
  - Surgical/Cardiac surgical consult
  - Emergency department thoracotomy if indicated

Portable chest X-ray/Ultrasound
- Pneumothorax/Hemothorax
  - Large (≥36 french) bore chest tube

CT scan
- If hemodynamics improve and there is no indication for operative exploration

Table 25.4 Speed versus height comparison

Speed	Equivalent height
10 mph	3.5 feet
15 mph	7.5 feet
20 mph	13 feet
25 mph	21 feet
30 mph	30 feet
35 mph	41 feet
40 mph	54 feet

Table 25.5 Chest X-ray findings concerning for traumatic aortic injury (TAI)

1. Widened mediastinum
2. Indistinct aortic knob
3. Left pleural effusion/hemothorax
4. Apical cap
5. 1st/2nd rib fractures
6. Tracheal deviation to the right
7. Depressed left main stem bronchus
8. Nasogastric tube deviation to the right

person, who is hemodynamically stable and not hypoxic, can be managed with adequate pain control and be discharged home from the emergency department. The use of an incentive spirometer should be highly encouraged. If patients do not meet all these criteria, they should either be admitted or transferred to a trauma center. The situation is not the same for the elderly. Rib fractures in the elderly can be lethal. Many studies have demonstrated this increased mortality in the elderly following isolated rib fractures [27–29]. Additionally, as the number of rib fractures increases so does mortality [27, 28]. Isolated pulmonary contusions should be managed very similarly to that of rib fractures. The young otherwise healthy person who is hemodynamically stable, not hypoxic, and has adequate analgesia can be discharged home. Pulmonary contusions in the elderly should be admitted for observation.

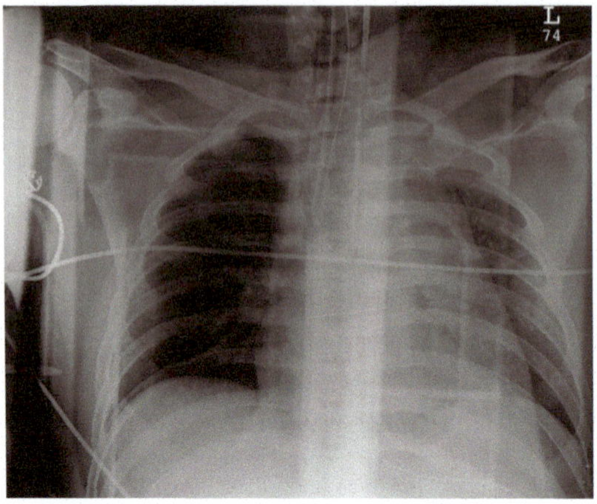

Fig. 25.1 Widened mediastinum concerning traumatic aortic injury

Management of sternal fractures and blunt cardiac injury (BCI) is a bit more unclear. The Eastern Association for the Surgery of Trauma (EAST) has developed guidelines for the management of both BCI and sternal fractures [30] (Table 25.6).

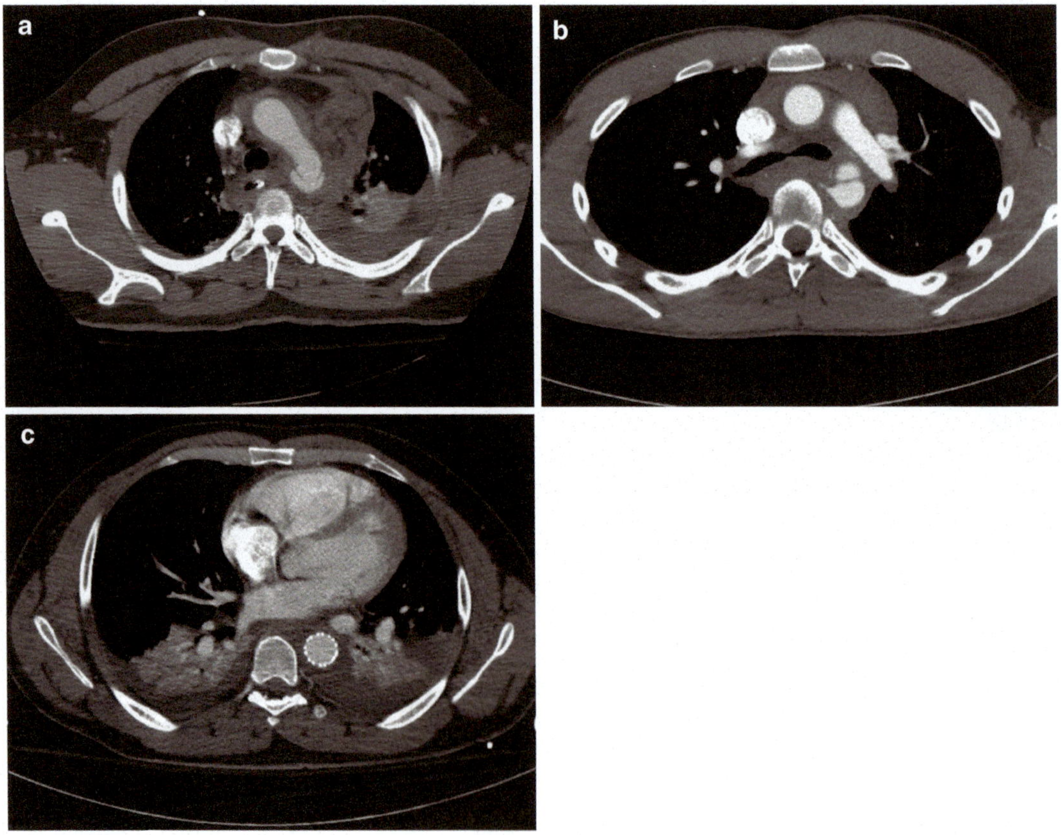

Fig. 25.2 (**a**) CT scan of traumatic aortic injury. (**b**) CT scan of traumatic aortic injury. (**c**) CT scan of traumatic aortic injury after stent placement

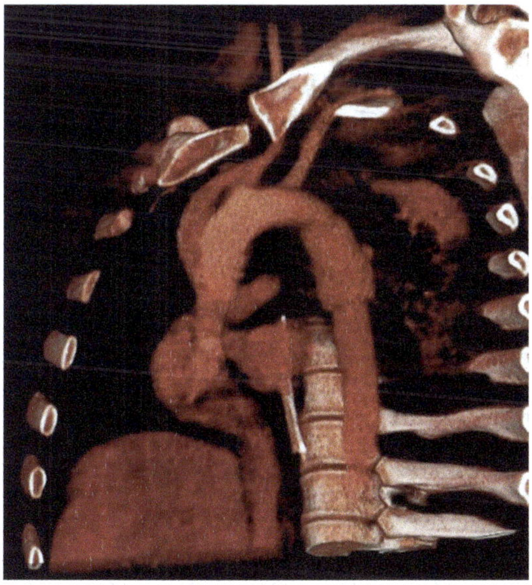

Fig. 25.3 Reconstructed CT images of traumatic aortic injury

Table 25.6 Eastern Association for the Surgery of Trauma (EAST) guidelines for the management of BCI and sternal fractures

Suspicion of blunt cardiac injury
Admission electrocardiogram (EKG) and troponin I should be obtained
If admission EKG reveals new abnormality (arrhythmia, ST changes, ischemia, heart block), then patients should be admitted for continuous monitoring
If admission EKG is normal and admission troponin I is normal, then BCI is ruled out
Hemodynamic instability or persistent new arrhythmia warrants an echocardiogram and admission
Cardiac CT scan or MRI can be used to help differentiate acute myocardial infarction and BCI in patients with abnormal EKG, cardiac enzymes, and/or echocardiogram
Sternal fracture alone does not predict the presence of BCI
CK or CK–MB should not be used in the evaluation for BCI
Nuclear medicine tests add little when compared to echocardiography and should not be routinely performed
Isolated sternal fracture
Not a marker for BCI with or without a retrosternal hematoma
Can be discharged if hemodynamically stable with normal chest X-ray and EKG

Regarding isolated sternal fractures, despite the EAST guideline stating that no echocardiogram is required, it is the routine practice of our faculty to obtain an echocardiogram of all patients with a sternal fracture to evaluate for a retrosternal hematoma and any cardiac dysfunction. The presence of the hematoma typically warrants admission at our facility for 24 hours of cardiac monitoring.

Most patients with penetrating thoracic trauma do not require operative intervention. Those that present with hemodynamic instability should have a bedside clinical exam, FAST exam, and portable chest X-ray done immediately. Absent or decreased breath sounds warrant immediate chest tube placement. If the FAST exam is positive for pericardial fluid, the emergency physician should adequately resuscitate the patient while arranging for either transport to the operating room or transfer to a trauma center. If the patient decompensates, emergency department thoracotomy (EDT) is indicated. Over the years, there have been many suggested indications for EDT following penetrating chest trauma [4, 31–35] (Table 25.7).

Patients who are hemodynamically stable following penetrating thoracic trauma should have a full evaluation. The management of patients with isolated thoracic stab wounds is variable. Patients at a minimum should have a chest X-ray and FAST exam performed. If both are negative, then practice varies among institutions. Traditionally, patients would have a repeat chest X-ray after 6 hours of observation, and if negative and patients remained stable they would be discharged [36, 37]. Newer studies have demonstrated that 3-hour follow-up films demonstrated all delayed findings, thus shortening the time of

Table 25.7 Indications for emergency department thoracotomy following penetrating chest trauma

1. Penetrating thoracic injuries of patients who arrive pulseless with myocardial activity should undergo immediate EDT [4]
2. Penetrating chest trauma and <15 minutes of prehospital cardiopulmonary resuscitation [32]
3. Patients with signs of life who do not respond to fluids and losing vital signs in the ED [30]

Table 25.8 Indications for operative exploration after chest tube placement for hemothorax

1. Initial output >1500 ml
2. Ongoing output >200 cc/hr for 2–4 hours
3. Persistent transfusion requirements

observation [38–40]. A 2013 study by Berg and colleagues has suggested that repeat chest X-ray as early as 1 hour may be sufficient to exclude any clinically significant injury [41]. Despite the existing literature, many centers, including our own, have a tendency to perform a chest CT scan on all hemodynamically patients following penetrating chest trauma.

Patients who have a hemothorax after penetrating chest trauma require tube thoracostomy. For those who have a retained hemothorax (RH) due to inadequate drainage additional procedures, including additional chest tube placement, may be required (Table 25.8). Adequate drainage is important because the RH is associated with high rates of empyema and pneumonia [42]. Some patients will have a large output after chest tube placement. Additionally, the blood can be and should be autotransfused from the pleurovac to the patient.

Abdomen/Pelvis

Blunt

Injuries to the abdominal cavity can occur from both blunt and penetrating mechanisms. Diagnostic peritoneal lavage (DPL) was the traditional test used to diagnose intraabdominal injury/hemorrhage. However, with the now widespread use of both ultrasound and CT scan, DPL has become virtually obsolete. Ultrasound (FAST) is now the accepted initial imaging of choice for intraabdominal injury. It is a rapid, portable test that can be easily repeated if necessary. It has high sensitivity and specificity in hypotensive patients following both penetrating precordial trauma and blunt trauma [43, 44].

Figure 25.4 is adapted from the algorithm used at our institution for patients who present the following blunt trauma. The use of oral contrast is no longer used when ordering a CT scan of the abdomen and pelvis. A 1999 study by Stafford and colleagues suggested that oral contrast did not add in the diagnosis of hollow viscous injury following blunt trauma. In 2004, Stuhlfaut and colleagues demonstrated that oral contrast is not needed to accurately identify bowel and mesenteric injuries [45–47]. Stable patients with a negative CT scan and no other injuries or indications for hospitalization can be discharged from the emergency department. Patients, who were selected to have a repeat physical exam and FAST exam at 6 hours, can also be discharged if both exams were negative and the patient remains hemodynamically stable [48].

Patients with positive CT scans will need to be managed accordingly. The spleen is the most commonly injured organ after blunt trauma [49, 50] (Fig. 25.5). The American Association for the Surgery of Trauma's (AAST) Organ Injury Scaling Committee created a grading scale for splenic injuries. The scale is graded from 1 to 5 and is based on radiographic and operative findings [51]. Traditionally, splenic injuries were managed operatively with splenectomy. However, with the discovery of overwhelming postsplenectomy sepsis (OPSS), practice patterns have changed. Despite the low incidence (0.05–2.0%) [52] of OPSS, the management of splenic injuries evolved from partial splenectomy, to splenorrhaphy and now to nonoperative management (NOM). NOM has the advantages of shorter hospital length of stay, decreased hospital costs, decreased blood transfusions, and decreased intraabdominal complications [53, 54]. NOM has evolved into using angio-embolization as adjunctive therapy for higher-grade injuries. Many studies have demonstrated that NOM decreased the need for laparotomy. However, as the grade of injury increased, so did the failure rate of NOM. As the amount of literature on NOM of the spleen continues to grow, along with newer technology and treatment technique, there is no standard for the NOM treatment of splenic injuries. Figure 25.6 is adapted from our institution's practice guideline for the management of blunt splenic injuries.

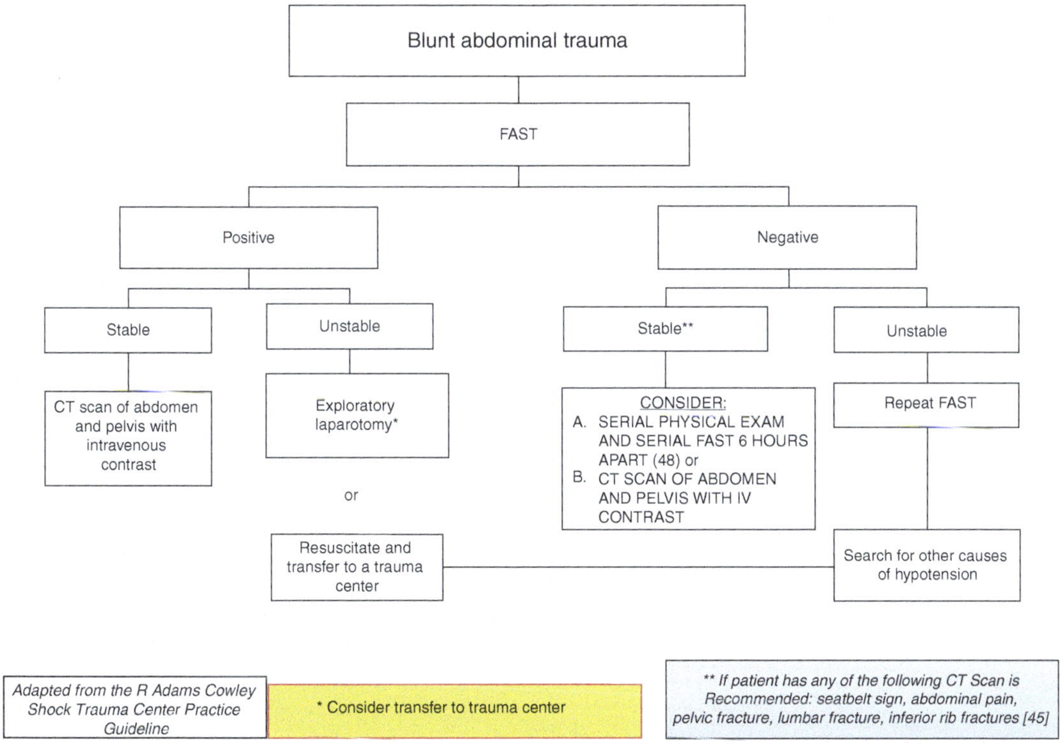

Fig. 25.4 Algorithm for blunt abdominal trauma

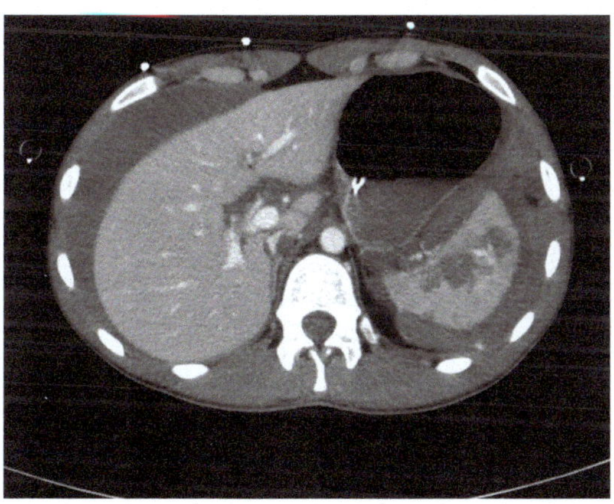

Fig. 25.5 Splenic injury with active extravasation

The diagnostic workup for blunt liver injuries is similar to that of the spleen. An AAST grading system exists for liver injuries as well [51] (Fig. 25.7). Exploratory laparotomy was once the accepted treatment for blunt liver injuries, but since many injuries were found to be very minor with minimal bleeding, practice paradigms have changed [55, 56]. A large body of literature now supports the use of NOM for blunt liver injuries in patients who are hemodynamically stable [56–58]. Unstable patients should be taken to the operating room for surgical exploration or arranged to be transported to a trauma center. Stable patients with low-grade injuries can be managed with observation and serial laboratory evaluation. Higher-grade injuries without active extravasation can also be managed with observation as long as patients remain hemodynamically stable. Those patients who have active extravasation on the CT scan warrant angiographic evaluation [58]. Angiographic embolization has been shown to be a successful adjunct in the management of these patients [57, 59–61]. However, as with any intervention, angio-embolization has been associated with a number of complications including major hepatic necrosis, abscess formation, gall bladder necrosis, and bile leak [62–64].

Genitourinary injuries are somewhat less common. Patients with blood at the meatus

a

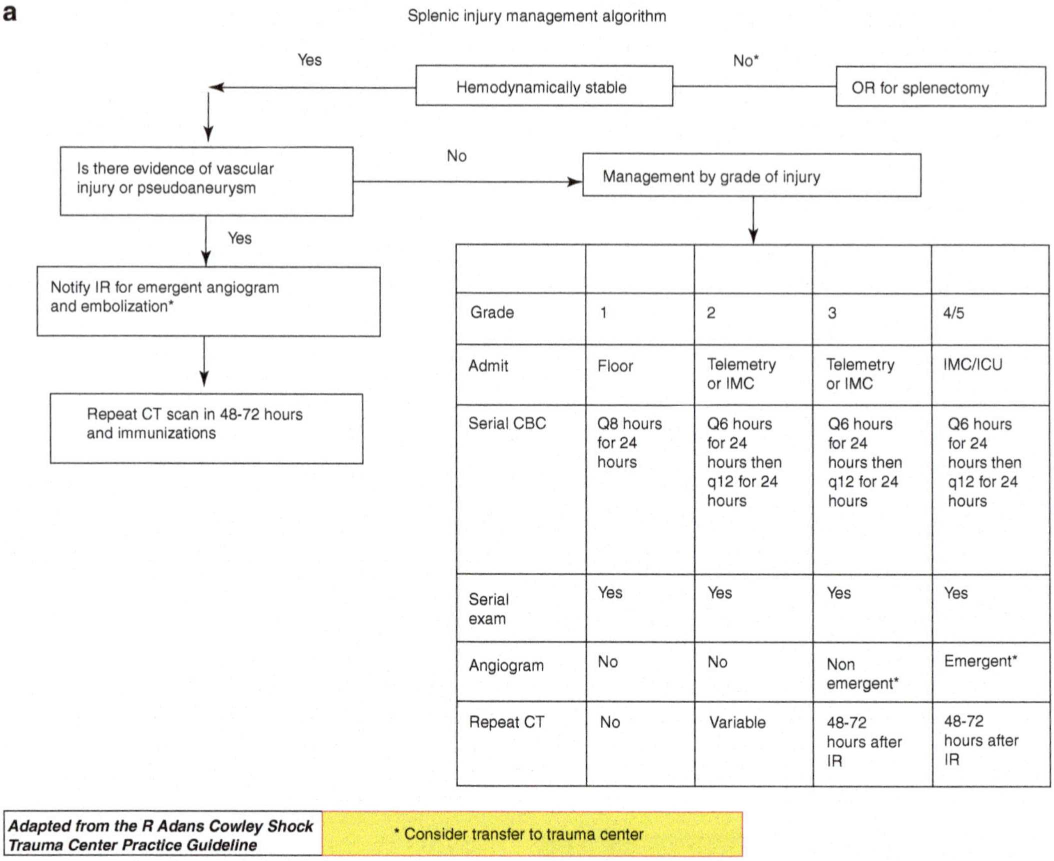

Grade	1	2	3	4/5
Admit	Floor	Telemetry or IMC	Telemetry or IMC	IMC/ICU
Serial CBC	Q8 hours for 24 hours	Q6 hours for 24 hours then q12 for 24 hours	Q6 hours for 24 hours then q12 for 24 hours	Q6 hours for 24 hours then q12 for 24 hours
Serial exam	Yes	Yes	Yes	Yes
Angiogram	No	No	Non emergent*	Emergent*
Repeat CT	No	Variable	48-72 hours after IR	48-72 hours after IR

b

Splenic injury:

Grade I	Subcapsular hematoma <10% surface area; capsular tear <1 cm in depth
Grade II	Subcapsular hematoma, non-expanding 10-50% surface area; intraparenchymal hematoma, non-expanding <2 cm in diameter
Grade III	Subcapsular hematoma >50% surface area or expanding intraparenchymal hematoma >2 cm and/or laceration >3 cm in depth or involving trabecular vessels.
Grade IV	Ruptured intraparenchymal hematoma with active bleeding; laceration involving segmental or hilar vessels producing major devascularization (>25% of spleen).
Grade V	Shattered spleen, hilar vascular injury that devascularizes spleen

Fig. 25.6 Algorithm for blunt splenic injury

should be considered to have a urethral injury until proven otherwise. Although traditionally practiced to avoid placing a Foley in these patients, at the author's institution, a single attempt by the most experienced care provider is the common practice. Any resistance warrants immediate cessation and requires a suprapubic catheter placement. Once a patient has completed his/her evaluation and is hemodynamically stable, a retrograde urethrogram can be formed. Bladder injuries are classified as intraperitoneal and extraperitoneal. Extraperitoneal bladder injuries only require Foley decompression for initial treatment. Intraperitoneal bladder ruptures require operative fixation in addition to Foley decompression. As a result, patients with intraperitoneal bladder ruptures should be transferred to a trauma center.

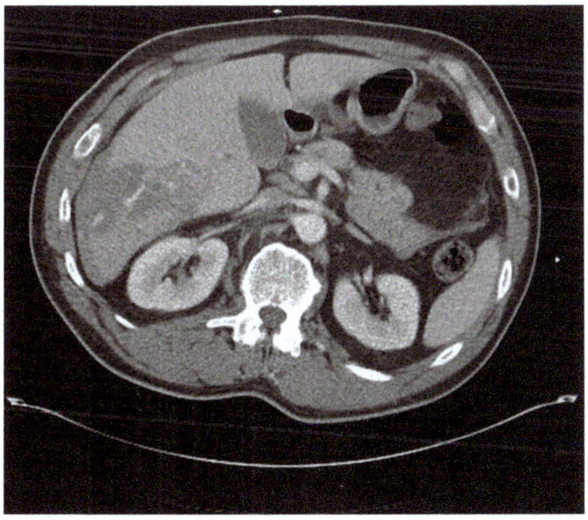

Fig. 25.7 Liver injury with active extravasation

Injuries to the kidney occur in up to 10% of patients [65]. An AAST grading system exists for the kidney as with the liver and spleen [51]. Most injuries to the kidney are minor and can be managed conservatively without follow-up imaging [66]. Management of higher-grade injuries is an area of debate [67, 68]. Although angio-embolization for *hemorrhage control* has been used for renal salvage, success rates vary in the literature [67–70].

Penetrating

The initial management of a patient with penetrating abdominal/flank trauma should be focused on airway breathing and circulation. Any unstable patient with penetrating injury requires immediate operative exploration. If the hospital does not have the appropriate surgical capabilities, expedited transfer to a trauma center is warranted. While awaiting transport the patient should be appropriately resuscitated. *Although no ideal systolic blood pressure (SBP) goal is known, the author's institution routinely resuscitates these patients to a SBP ~ 90 mmHg. A landmark study by Bickell and colleagues demonstrated that hypotensive patients with penetrating torso trauma have improved outcome if fluid resuscitation is delayed until patients are in the operating room* [71]. *Once operative intervention has begun aggressive resuscitation with blood products should be aimed at reversing the patient's shock state.* Stable patients can be managed with serial abdominal exams, local wound exploration (LWE), ultrasound, diagnostic peritoneal lavage, or CT scan. Numerous studies of both anterior stab wounds and gunshot wounds have demonstrated that serial physical exam alone can identify injuries that require surgical intervention [72–76].

Local wound exploration is an option for anterior abdominal stab wounds. The wound must be sufficiently extended allowing for clear visualization of the wound tract and fascia [77]. Probing the wound does not exclude peritoneal violation and this practice should be discouraged [78]. After an appropriate LWE, if the fascia is not violated the patients can be discharged with local wound care [79]. Ultrasound (FAST) is probably the most widely used method for initial evaluation of stable patient with penetrating anterior abdominal wounds. It has a high specificity and positive predictive value; however, it has a relatively low sensitivity [44, 79–82]. Patients with a positive FAST should proceed to the operating room, unless a solid organ injury is believed to be the sole injury. Stable patients with a negative FAST should proceed to either CT scan or serial exams (See Fig. 25.8).

For those who elect to proceed with CT scan, triple contrast (oral, intravenous, and rectal) has become the standard practice. Many studies over the past 30 years have demonstrated its accuracy in diagnosing peritoneal violation and the need for laparotomy with high sensitivity and specificity [83–85]. Patients who do not have peritoneal violation or other injuries can be safely discharged from the emergency department [79]. Some authors believe that intravenous contrast alone is sufficient to determine which patients require a laparotomy following penetrating injury [86, 87]. However, the authors of this article support the use of triple contrast in any penetrating torso trauma.

Penetrating injuries to the back and flank require a special consideration. As with any unstable patient with penetrating injury, immediate operative exploration or appropriate resuscitation and transfer to a trauma center is warranted.

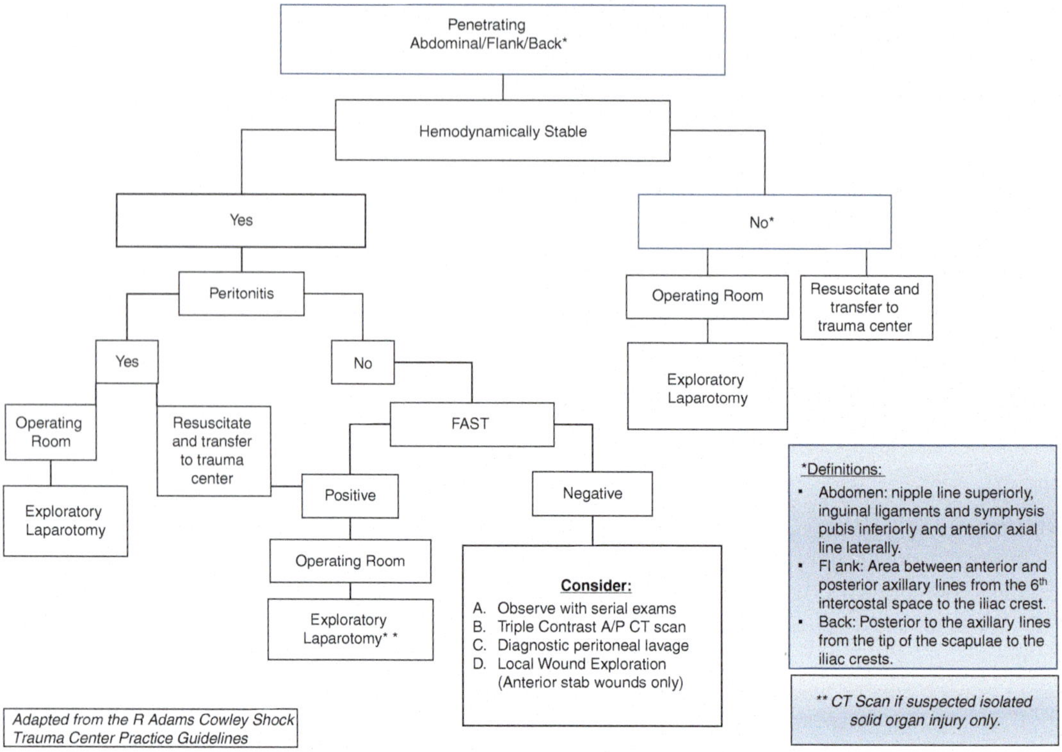

Fig. 25.8 Algorithm for hemodynamically stable patients with penetrating abdominal/flank/back trauma

Unlike anterior abdominal wounds, both the FAST exam and DPL may not be helpful [79]. Additionally, LWE *is not recommended* for the back and flank wounds, as the facial planes are not well defined and often wounds have self-tamponaded [79]. LWE can dislodge clots and cause significant hemorrhage, which can be very difficult to control in the emergency department [79]. Thus for stable patients who require further evaluation, triple contrast CT scan is the imaging modality of choice [83–85].

Boney Pelvic Trauma

Overall mortality of patients with pelvic fractures is 6% [88, 89]. As many as 50% of patients with pelvic fractures may have concomitant intraabdominal injury including major vascular injuries [88, 90, 91]. The Young and Burgess classification is what our center uses in describing the fracture pattern [92, 93]. It is based on the vector of force involved and classified as lateral compression (LC), anteroposterior compression (APC), vertical shear (VS), and combined [93]. Lateral compression fractures are characterized as oblique fractures through the rami *as well as disruption of the posterior elements*. They are subtyped I, II, and III with increasing severity of injury. APC fractures are characterized or often described as "open book" pelvis. These involve widening of the pubic symphysis and are often associated with hemorrhage. APC are also subtyped I, II, and II with increasing severity of injury. Vertical shear fractures, sometimes referred to as Malgaigne fractures, often occur as a result of fall from height onto lower limbs. It is associated with fractures through the rami as well as posterior fractures of the sacroiliac complex or the sacrum. Additionally, there is superior displacement of lateral part of the pelvis. As a result, there may be shortening of the leg on the side of injury [88].

Initial management as usual should focus on airway breathing and circulation. Unstable patients should be resuscitated and set up to be transferred to a trauma center. Initial imaging for patients with suspected pelvic fractures should begin with a pelvic X-ray (PXR). Unfortunately, PXR can miss up to 50% of fractures, as compared to CT scan [94]. Many authors have demonstrated the superiority of CT scan to PXR for diagnosing injury, and believe that it is the gold standard [94–96]. For the emergency medicine physician, the key points are to know which patients are at risk of bleeding from their pelvic fracture. Typically, patients with lateral compression fractures have a low likelihood of having clinically significant hemorrhage. This, however, is not true for patients over the age of 55 and clinicians should have a heightened awareness in these patients [97]. Both APC and VS fractures have a much higher likelihood of bleeding. Patients with APC fractures should have a binder applied immediately. This can be as simple as a bedsheet or as elaborate as premanufactured binders. The key point is placement of the binder. Binders should be placed over the greater trochanter of the femur and then tightened. A common mistake is to place the binder over the iliac wings which when tightened actually widens the pubic symphysis. When appropriately applied, the pressure will decrease the widened pubic symphysis and create a tamponade effect by decreasing the pelvic diameter. Once in place binders should only be removed by the orthopedic surgeons (Figs. 25.9a, b). Figures 25.10 and 25.11 provide algorithms for unstable and stable patients with pelvic fractures, respectively. Most of these patients will require transfer to a trauma center for *operative fixation and angiographic evaluation for hemorrhage control.*

Extremity Trauma

Vascular injury and compartment syndrome are two key concepts of extremity trauma that are critical for the emergency medicine physician to be able to recognize and treat in the emergency department. Vascular injuries can occur following fractures, dislocations, or penetrating trauma. It is often difficult to palpate a pulse in a patient in shock or difficult to hear using a Doppler in a busy loud emergency department. If any hard signs of vascular injury are present, they mandate immediate surgical intervention or transfer to trauma center as quickly as possible [98] (Table 25.9). Additionally, any soft sign of vascular injury warrants admission and observation, but not mandatory exploration [98] (Table 25.10).

In 2012, the Eastern Association for the Surgery of Trauma (EAST) updated their practice guidelines for penetrating lower extremity trauma [99]. As stated above if any hard signs exist, immediate operative exploration is mandated. For centers that do not have this capability, timely transfer to a trauma center is required. Direct pressure or application of a tourniquet

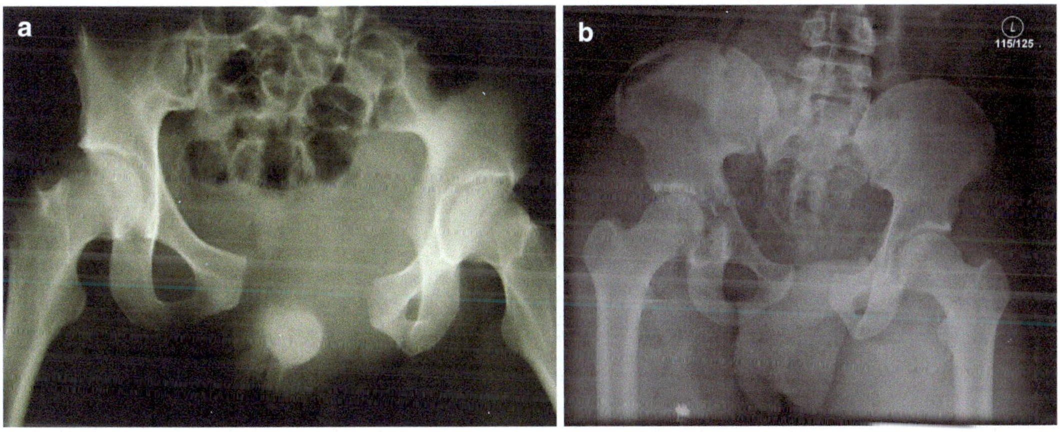

Fig. 25.9 (**a**) Open book pelvis. (**b**) Open book pelvis after the binder is applied

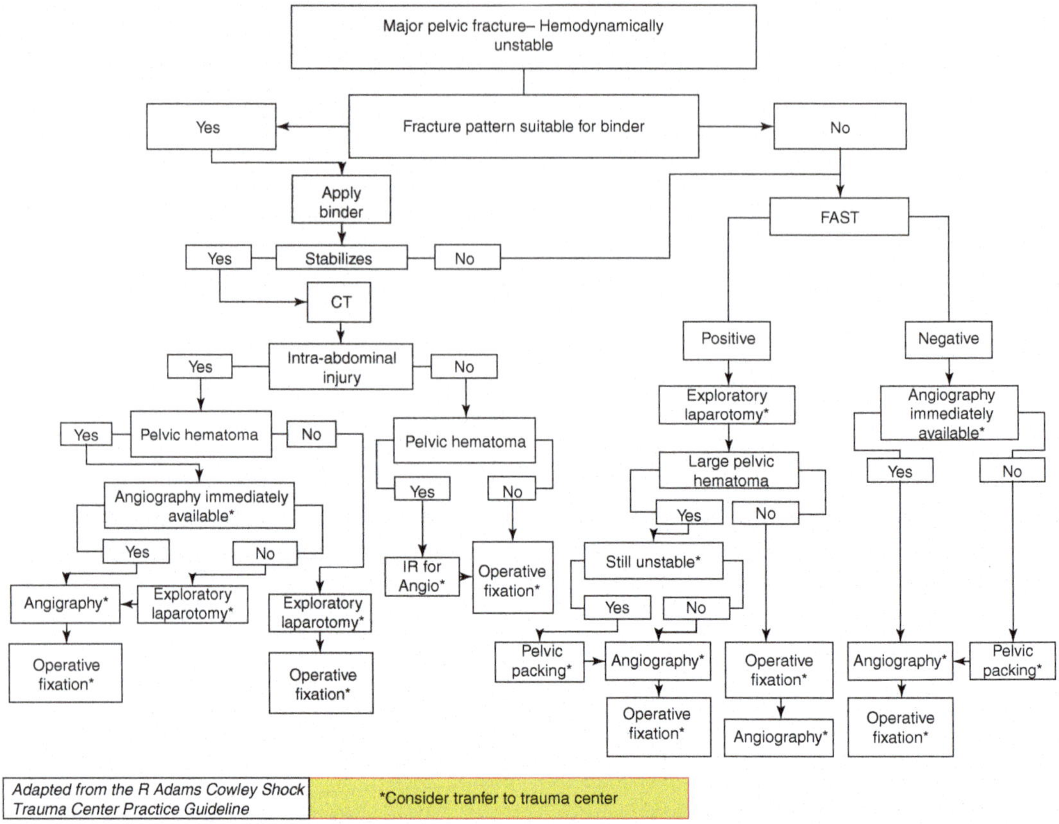

Fig. 25.10 Algorithm for hemodynamically unstable patients with major pelvic trauma

may be used as temporary hemorrhage control until definitive repair [99]. The committee's key findings are shown in Table 25.11.

Blunt vascular injury without fracture or dislocation is rare. Patients with lower extremity fractures who do not have a palpable pulse equal to the ipsilateral extremity warrant further evaluation. Computed tomography angiogram (CTA) has been shown to be the diagnostic imaging of choice in these patients [100]. Additionally for patients with a dislocation and an absent pulse, relocation of the joint as quickly as possible is warranted. Following relocation if pulses are equal, no additional imaging is often required. For those that remain with a pulse deficit, CTA should be obtained.

Emergency medicine physicians need to have a high index of suspicion for knee *(tibial-femoral)* dislocations as some may spontaneously relocate prior to arrival in the emergency department. As a result, the incidence of knee dislocations may have been historically underreported [101]. The incidence of vascular injury associated with knee dislocations had been reported to be as high as 64%; however, recent literature suggest only as high as 14% [101]. The traditional dictum of emergency medicine has always mandated evaluation of the popliteal artery following a knee dislocation. The diagnostic test of choice has been challenged. Although angiography is the gold standard, CTA is a less invasive alternative with a high sensitivity and specificity [101]. Other alternatives include serial physical exams, ankle–brachial indexes (ABIs), and *arterial duplex*; however, the author's institution's standard is to obtain a CTA of the extremity to rule out a vascular injury in any patient suspected of having a knee dislocation. *Of note, isolated patella dislocations do not warrant a workup for vascular injury.*

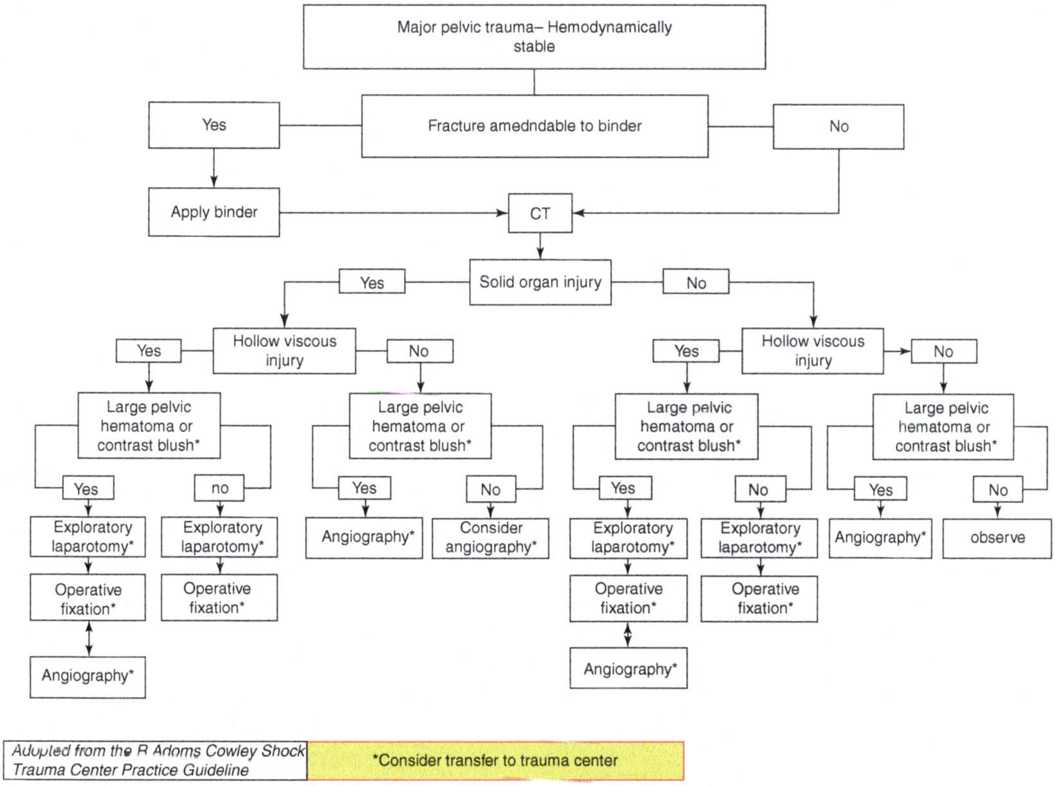

Fig. 25.11 Algorithm for hemodynamically stable patients with major pelvic trauma

Table 25.9 Hard signs of vascular injury

1. Pulsatile bleeding
2. Expanding hematoma
3. Absent distal pulses
4. Cold pale limb
5. Palpable thrill
6. Audible bruit

Table 25.10 Soft signs of vascular injury

1. Peripheral nerve deficit
2. Large blood loss at scene
3. Reduced but palpable pulse
4. Injury proximity to major blood vessel

Compartment syndrome (CS) can result following a vascular injury or as a result of fractures alone. Pain with passive motion and pain out of proportion to exam are often the earliest signs. Additionally, paresthesias occur early while pallor, paralysis, and pulselessness are late findings. Compartment pressures are usually less than 8 mmHg; however, when pressures *become*

Table 25.11 Eastern Association for the Surgery of Trauma (EAST) guidelines for lower extremity penetrating injury [99]

1. Patients without hard signs who have an abnormal exam or ankle–brachial index (ABI) <0.9 should have further evaluation
2. Computed tomography angiogram (CTA) is the primary diagnostic study for those requiring imaging
3. Patients without hard signs with normal physical exams and ABI >0.9 can be discharged
4. Tourniquets can be applied for temporary hemorrhage control until definitive surgical repair

greater than 20 mmHg, fasciotomies are often required. If left untreated, CS can lead to tissue necrosis, rhabdomyolysis, renal failure, and loss of limb. Thigh compartment syndrome is rare; however, up to 20% of closed tibia fractures can develop compartment syndrome [102]. Fractures of the tibia diaphysis have higher rates of developing compartment syndrome than do those of the more proximal or distal portions [103]. Additionally, fractures of the tibia and fibula associated with ballistic fragments have a higher incidence of developing CS than other ballistic associated fractures [104]

Conclusion

Management of trauma to the chest abdomen and pelvis and extremities can often be very challenging. It is imperative to evaluate and treat life-threatening injuries rapidly. Although the concepts of trauma care have remained unchanged over time, technology and the resources available have significantly improved leading to better outcomes. Goal-directed resuscitation and a paradigm shift in using blood products rather than large volume crystalloid and colloid have significantly altered the way in which we care for patient following injury. Although the ideal ratio of blood product transfusion remains *unknown*, it is clear that massive crystalloid infusion is detrimental to patient outcomes.

As the use of ultrasound expands, the quality of CT scan continues to improve and the use of catheter-based technique evolving immediate operative exploration is no longer mandatory for all trauma patients. It is imperative that the emergency physician be skilled at managing life-threatening injuries, implementing appropriate resuscitation measures and if needed advising rapid transfer to a trauma center. Although the future remains unknown, techniques such as resuscitative endovascular balloon occlusion of the aorta (REBOA) for temporary hemorrhage control may soon be a realistic option for the emergency physician and can be life saving for the bleeding trauma patient [105–107].

Critical points

1. Hemodynamically unstable polytrauma patients can have more than one source of shock and require rapid evaluation and treatment
2. High volume crystalloid resuscitation is associated with worse outcomes after injury
3. Early administration of blood products for hemorrhagic shock after injury improves outcome, although the ideal ratio of products remains unknown
4. Nonoperative management and catheter-based interventions are becoming standards in care for appropriately selected trauma patients.

References

1. Centers for Disease Control and Prevention. Injury prevention and control: data & statistics (WISQARS™). http://www.cdc.gov/injury/wisqars/LeadingCauses.html. Accessed 2 Jan 2015.
2. Centers for Disease Control and Prevention (CDC). CDC grand rounds: evidence-based injury prevention. MMWR Morb Mortal Wkly Rep. 2014;62(51–52):1048–50.
3. Miller TR, Levy DT. Cost-outcome analysis in injury prevention and control: eighty-four recent estimates for the United States. Med Care. 2000;38(6):562–82.
4. American College of Surgeons. Shock. In: American College of Surgeon – Committee on Trauma, editor. ATLS advanced trauma life support for doctors. 8th ed. Chicago: American College of Surgeons; 2008. p. 10–1.
5. Kasotakis G, Sideris A, Yang Y, et al. Aggressive early crystalloid resuscitation adversely affects outcomes in adult blunt trauma patients: an analysis of the Glue Grant database. J Trauma Acute Care Surg. 2013;74:1215–22.
6. Moore FA, McKinley BA, Moore EE. The next generation in shock resuscitation. Lancet. 2004;363:1988–96.
7. Duchesne JC, Heaney J, Guidry C, et al. Diluting the benefits of hemostatic resuscitation: a multi-institutional analysis. J Trauma Acute Care Surg. 2013;75:76–82.
8. Holcomb JB, Tilley BC, Baraniuk S, Fox EE, Wade CE, Podbielski JM, et al. Transfusion of plasma, platelets, and red blood cells in a 1:1:1 vs a 1:1:2 ratio and mortality in patients with severe trauma: the PROPPR randomized clinical trial. JAMA. 2015;313:471–82.
9. Choi PT, Yip G, Quinonez LG, Cook DJ. Crystalloids vs. colloids in fluid resuscitation: a systematic review. Crit Care Med. 1999;27:200–10.
10. Finfer S, Bellomo R, Boyce N, French J, Myburgh J, Norton R, SAFE Study Investigators, et al. N Engl J Med. 2004;350:2247–56.
11. Pieracci FM, Biffl WL, Moore EE. Current concepts in resuscitation. J Intensive Care Med. 2012;27:79–96.

12. Junger WG, Coimbra R, Liu FC, et al. Hypertonic saline resuscitation: a tool to modulate immune function in trauma patients? Shock. 1997;8:235–41.
13. Coimbra R, Hoyt DB, Junger WG, et al. Hypertonic saline resuscitation decreases susceptibility to sepsis after hemorrhagic shock. J Trauma. 1997;42:602–6.
14. Bulger EM, May S, Kerby JD, Emerson S, Stiell IG, Schreiber MA, et al. Out-of-hospital hypertonic resuscitation after traumatic hypovolemic shock: a randomized, placebo controlled trial. Ann Surg. 2011;253:431–41.
15. Bulger EM, May S, Brasel KJ, Schreiber M, Kerby JD, Tisherman SA, Newgard C, et al. Out-of-hospital hypertonic resuscitation following severe traumatic brain injury: a randomized controlled trial. JAMA. 2010;304:1455–64.
16. Livingston DH, Hauser CJ. Trauma to the chest wall and lung. In: Feliciano DV, Mattox KL, Moore EE, editors. Trauma. 5th ed. New York: McGraw-Hill; 2004. p. 507–38.
17. Nagarsheth K, Kurek S. Ultrasound detection of pneumothorax compared with chest X-ray and computed tomography scan. Am Surg. 2011;77:480–4.
18. Wisbach GG, Sise MJ, Sack DI, Swanson SM, Sundquist SM, Paci GM, Kingdon KM, Kaminski SS. What is the role of chest X-ray in the initial assessment of stable trauma patients? J Trauma. 2007;62:74–8.
19. Kea B, Gamarallage R, Vairamuthu H, Fortman J, Lunney K, Hendey GW, Rodriguez RM. What is the clinical significance of chest CT when the chest x-ray result is normal in patients with blunt trauma? Am J Emerg Med. 2013;31:1268–73.
20. Deunk J, Dekker HM, Brink M, van Vugt R, Edwards MJ, van Vugt AB. The value of indicated computed tomography scan of the chest and abdomen in addition to the conventional radiologic work-up for blunt trauma patients. J Trauma. 2007;63:757–63.
21. Brink M, Deunk J, Dekker H, Edwards MJ, Kool DR, van Vugt AB, van Kuijk C, Blickman JG. Criteria for the selective use of chest computed tomography in blunt trauma patients. Eur Radiol. 2010;20:818–28.
22. Woodring JH. The normal mediastinum in blunt traumatic rupture of the thoracic aorta and brachiocephalic arteries. J Emerg Med. 1990;8:467–76.
23. Exadaktylos AK, Sclabas G, Schmid SW, Schaller B, Zimmermann H. Do we really need routine computed tomographic scanning in the primary evaluation of blunt chest trauma in patients with "normal" chest radiograph? J Trauma. 2001;51:1173–6.
24. Demetriades D, Gomez H, Velmahos GC, Asensio JA, Murray J, Cornwell EE 3rd, Alo K, Berne TV. Routine helical computed tomographic evaluation of the mediastinum in high-risk blunt trauma patients. Arch Surg. 1998;133:1084–8.
25. Plurad D, Green D, Demetriades D, Rhee P. The increasing use of chest computed tomography for trauma: is it being overutilized? J Trauma. 2007;62:631–5.
26. Fabian TC, Davis KA, Gavant ML, Croce MA, Melton SM, Patton JH Jr, et al. Prospective study of blunt aortic injury: helical CT is diagnostic and antihypertensive therapy reduces rupture. Ann Surg. 1998;227:666–76.
27. Bulger EM, Arneson MA, Mock CN, Jurkovich GJ. Rib fractures in the elderly. J Trauma. 2000;48:1040–6.
28. Sharma OP, Oswanski MF, Jolly S. Perils of rib fractures. Am Surg. 2008;74:310–4.
29. Cameron P, Dziukas L, Hadj A, Clark P, Hooper S. Rib fractures in major trauma. Aust N Z Surg. 1996;66:530–4.
30. Clancy K, Velopulos C, Bilaniuk JW, Collier B, Crowley W, Kurek S, et al. Screening for blunt cardiac injury: an Eastern Association for the Surgery of Trauma practice management guideline. J Trauma Acute Care Surg. 2012;73:S301–6.
31. Rhee PM, Acosta J, Bridgeman A, Wang D, Jordan M, Rich N. Survival after emergency department thoracotomy: review of published data from the past 25 years. J Am Coll Surg. 2000;190:288–98.
32. Working Group, Ad Hoc Subcommittee on Outcomes, American College of Surgeons. Committee on Trauma. Practice management guidelines for emergency department thoracotomy. J Am Coll Surg. 2001;193:303–9.
33. Powell DW, Moore EE, Cothren CC, Ciesla DJ, Burch JM, Moore JB, et al. Is emergency department resuscitative thoracotomy futile care for the critically injured patient requiring prehospital cardiopulmonary resuscitation? J Am Coll Surg. 2004;199:211–5.
34. Cothren CC, Moore EE. Emergency department thoracotomy. In: Feliciano DV, Mattox KL, Moore EE, editors. Trauma. 6th ed. New York: McGraw-Hill; 2008.
35. Moore EE, Knudson MM, Burlew CC, Inaba K, Dicker RA, Biffl WL, et al. Defining the limits of resuscitative emergency department thoracotomy: a contemporary Western Trauma Association perspective. J Trauma. 2011;70:334–9.
36. Weigelt JA, Aurbakken CM, Meier DE, Thal ER. Management of asymptomatic patients following stab wounds to the chest. J Trauma. 1982;22:291–4.
37. Kerr TM, Sood R, Buckman RF, Gelman J, Grosh J. Prospective trial of the six hour rule in stab wounds of the chest. Surg Gynecol Obstet. 1989;169:223–5.
38. Kiev J, Kerstein MD. Role of three hour roentgenogram of the chest in penetrating and nonpenetrating injuries of the chest. Surg Gynecol Obstet. 1992;175:249–53.
39. Shatz DV, de la Pedraja J, Erbella J, Hameed M, Vail SJ. Efficacy of follow-up evaluation in penetrating thoracic injuries:3- vs. 6-hour radiographs of the chest. J Emerg Med. 2001,20:281284.
40. Seamon MJ, Medina CR, Pieri PG, Fisher CA, Gaughan JP, Bradley KM, et al. Follow-up after

asymptomatic penetrating thoracic injury: 3 hours is enough. J Trauma. 2008;65:549–53.
41. Berg RJ, Inaba K, Recinos G, Barmparas G, Teixeira PG, Georgiou C, et al. Prospective evaluation of early follow-up chest radiography after penetrating thoracic injury. World J Surg. 2013;37:1286–90.
42. DuBose J, Inaba K, Demetriades D, Scalea TM, O'Connor J, Menaker J, et al. Management of post-traumatic retained hemothorax: a prospective, observational, multicenter AAST study. J Trauma Acute Care Surg. 2012;72:11–22.
43. Rozycki GS, Ballard RB, Feliciano DV, Schmidt JA, Pennington SD. Surgeon-performed ultrasound for the assessment of truncal injuries: lessons learned from 1540 patients. Ann Surg. 1998;228:557–67.
44. Udobi KF, Rodriguez A, Chiu WC, Scalea TM. Role of ultrasonography in penetrating abdominal trauma: a prospective clinical study. J Trauma. 2001;50:475–9.
45. Chiu WC, Cushing BM, Rodriguez A, Ho SM, Mirvis SE, Shanmuganathan K, et al. Abdominal injuries without hemoperitoneum: a potential limitation of focused abdominal sonography for trauma (FAST). J Trauma. 1997;42:617–23.
46. Stafford RE, McGonigal MD, Weigelt JA, Johnson TJ. Oral contrast solution and computed tomography for blunt abdominal trauma: a randomized study. Arch Surg. 1999;134:622–6.
47. Stuhlfaut JW, Soto JA, Lucey BC, Ulrich A, Rathlev NK, Burke PA, et al. Blunt abdominal trauma: performance of CT without oral contrast material. Radiology. 2004;233:689–94.
48. Scalea TM, Rodriguez A, Chiu WC, Brenneman D, Fallon W, Kazuyoshi K, et al. Focused assessment with sonography for trauma (FAST): results from an international consensus conference. J Trauma. 1999;45:466–72.
49. Peitzman AB, Heil B, Rivera L, Federle MB, Harbrecht BG, Clancy KD, et al. Blunt splenic injury in adults: multi-institutional study of the Eastern Association for the Surgery of Trauma. J Trauma. 2000;49:177–87.
50. Cogbill TH, Moore EE, Jurkovich GJ, Morris JA, Mucha P Jr, Shackford SR, et al. Nonoperative management of blunt splenic trauma: a multicenter experience. J Trauma. 1989;29:1312–7.
51. Moore EE, Cogbill TH, Malangoni MA, Jurkovich GJ, Shackford SR, Champion HR, et al. Organ injury scaling. Surg Clin North Am. 1995;75:293–303.
52. Shatz DV. Vaccination practices among North American trauma surgeons in splenectomy for trauma. J Trauma. 2002;53:950–6.
53. Sartorelli KH, Frumiento C, Rogers FB, Osler TM. Non-operative management of hepatic, splenic, and renal injuries in adults with multiple injuries. J Trauma. 2000;49:56–61.
54. Pachter HL, Guth AA, Hofstetter SR, Spencer FC. Changing patterns in the management of splenic trauma. Ann Surg. 1998;227:708–19.
55. Carrillo EH, Platz A, Miller FB, Richardson JD, Polk HC Jr. Non-operative management of blunt hepatic trauma. Br J Surg. 1998;85:461–8.
56. Croce MA, Fabian TC, Menke PG, Waddle-Smith L, Minard G, Kudsk KA, et al. Nonoperative management of blunt hepatic trauma is the treatment of choice for hemodynamically stable patients. Results of a prospective trial. Ann Surg. 1995;221:744–55.
57. Stein DM, Scalea TM. Nonoperative management of spleen and liver injuries. J Intensive Care Med. 2006;21:296–304.
58. Velmahos GC, Toutouzas K, Radin R, Chan L, Rhee P, Tillou A, et al. High success with nonoperative management of blunt hepatic trauma: the liver is a sturdy organ. Arch Surg. 2003;138:475–01.
59. Hagiwara A, Murata A, Matsuda T, et al. The efficacy and limitations of transarterial embolization for severe hepatic injury. J Trauma. 2002;52:1091–6.
60. Hagiwara A, Yukioka T, Ohta S, et al. Nonsurgical management of patients with blunt hepatic injury: efficacy of transcatheter arterial embolization. AJR Am J Roentgenol. 1997;169:1151–6.
61. Carrillo EH, Spain DA, Wohltmann CD, et al. Interventional techniques are useful adjuncts in nonoperative management of hepatic injuries. J Trauma. 1999;46:619–24.
62. Dabbs DN, Stein DM, Scalea TM. Major hepatic necrosis: a common complication after angioembolization for treatment of high-grade liver injuries. J Trauma. 2009;66:621–7.
63. Misselbeck TS, Teicher EJ, Cipolle MD, et al. Hepatic angioembolization in trauma patients: indications and complications. J Trauma. 2009;67:769–73.
64. Mohr AM, Lavery RF, Barone A, et al. Angiographic embolization for liver injuries: low mortality, high morbidity. J Trauma. 2003;55:1077–81.
65. Coburn M. Genitourinary trauma. In: Feliciano DV, Mattox KL, Moore EE, editors. Trauma. 6th ed. New York: McGraw-Hill; 2008. p. 789–824.
66. Malcolm JB, Derweesh IH, Mehrazin R, et al. Nonoperative management of blunt renal trauma: is routine early follow-up imaging necessary? BMC Urol. 2008;8:11.
67. Boswell K, Menaker J. Assessment and treatment of the trauma patient in shock. Emerg Med Clin North Am. 2014;32:777–95.
68. Menaker J, Joseph B, Stein DM, et al. Angiointervention: high rates of failure following blunt renal injuries. World J Surg. 2011;35:520–7.
69. van der Wilden GM, Velmahos GC, Joseph DK, et al. Successful nonoperative management of the most severe blunt renal injuries: a multicenter study of the research consortium of New England Centers for Trauma. JAMA Surg. 2013;148:924–31.
70. Sarani B, Powell E, Taddeo J, et al. Contemporary comparison of surgical and interventional arteriography management of blunt renal injury. J Vasc Interv Radiol. 2011;22:723–8.
71. Bickell WH, Wall MJ Jr, Pepe PE, Martin RR, Ginger VF, Allen MK, Mattox KL. Immediate

versus delayed fluid resuscitation for hypotensive patients with penetrating torso injuries. N Engl J Med. 1994;331(17):1105–9.
72. Alzamel HA, Cohn SM. When it is safe to discharge asymptomatic patients with abdominal stab wounds? J Trauma. 2005;58:523–5.
73. Demetriades D, Rabinowitz B. Indications for operation in abdominal stab wounds. A prospective study of 651 patients. Ann Surg. 1987;205:129–32.
74. Navsaria PH, Berli JU, Edu S, Nicol AJ. Non-operative management of abdominal stab wounds--an analysis of 186 patients. S Afr J Surg. 2007;45:128–30.
75. Demetriades D, Charalambides D, Lakhoo M, Pantanowitz D. Gunshot wounds of the abdomen: role of selective conservative management. Br J Surg. 1991;78:220–2.
76. Demetriades D, Velmahos G, Cornwell E 3rd, Berne TV, Cober S, Bhasin PS, et al. Selective nonoperative management of gunshot wounds of the anterior abdomen. Arch Surg. 1997;132:178–83.
77. Thompson JS, Moore EE, Van Duzer-Moore S, Moore JB, Galloway AC. The evolution of abdominal stab wound management. J Trauma. 1980;20:478–83.
78. Rosenthal RE, Smith J, Walls RM, Chen H, Kline PP, Shesser RF, et al. Stab wounds to the abdomen: failure of blunt probing to predict peritoneal penetration. Ann Emerg Med. 1987;16:172–4.
79. Menaker J, Scalea TM. Penetrating thoraco-abdominal injury. Trauma Rep. 2010;11:1–12.
80. Soffer D, McKenney MG, Cohn S, Garcia-Roca R, Namias N, Schulman C, et al. A prospective evaluation of ultrasonography for the diagnosis of penetrating torso injury. J Trauma. 2004;56:953–7.
81. Kirkpatrick AW, Sirois M, Ball CG, Laupland KB, Goldstein L, Hameed M, et al. The hand-held ultrasound examination for penetrating abdominal trauma. Am J Surg. 2004;187:660–5.
82. Boulanger BR, Kearney PA, Tsuei B, Ochoa JB. The routine use of sonography in penetrating torso injury is beneficial. J Trauma. 2001;51:320–5.
83. Phillips T, Sclafani SJ, Goldstein A, Scalea T, Panetta T, Shaftan G. Use of the contrast-enhanced CT enema in the management of penetrating trauma to the flank and back. J Trauma. 1986;26:593–601.
84. Shanmuganathan K, Mirvis SE, Chiu WC, Killeen KL, Scalea TM. Triple-contrast helical CT in penetrating torso trauma: a prospective study to determine peritoneal violation and the need for laparotomy. AJR Am J Roentgenol. 2001;177:1247–56.
85. Shanmuganathan K, Mirvis SE, Chiu WC, Killeen KL, Hogan GJ, Scalea TM. Penetrating torso trauma: triple contrast helical CT in peritoneal violation and organ injury--a prospective study in 200 patients. Radiology. 2004;231:775–84.
86. Ramirez RM, Cureton EL, Ereso AQ, Kwan RO, Dozier KC, Sadjadi J, et al. Single-contrast computed tomography for the triage of patients with penetrating torso trauma. J Trauma. 2009;67:583–8.
87. Salim A, Sangthong B, Martin M, Brown C, Plurad D, Inaba K, et al. Use of computed tomography in the anterior abdominal stab wound: results of a prospective study. Arch Surg. 2006;141:745–50.
88. Uzcategui M, Menaker J. Blunt pelvic trauma. Trauma Rep. 2014;15:1–10.
89. Scalea TM, Stein DM, O'Toole RV. Pelvic fractures. In: Feliciano DV, Mattox KL, Moore EE, editors. Trauma. 6th ed. New York: McGraw Hill; 2008. p. 759–87.
90. Cryer HM, Miller FB, Evers BM, Rouben LR, Seligson DL. Pelvic fracture classification: correlation with hemorrhage. J Trauma. 1988;28:973–80.
91. Ben-Menachem Y, Coldwell DM, Young JW, Burgess AR. Hemorrhage associated with pelvic fractures: causes, diagnosis, and emergent management. AJR Am J Roentgenol. 1991;157:1005–14.
92. Dalal SA, Burgess AR, Siegel JH, Young JW, Brumback RJ, Poka A, et al. Pelvic fracture in multiple trauma: classification by mechanism is key to pattern of organ injury, resuscitative requirements, and outcome. J Trauma. 1989;29:981–100.
93. Burgess AR, Eastridge BJ, Young JW, Ellison TS, Ellison PS Jr, Poka A, et al. Pelvic ring disruptions: effective classification system and treatment protocols. J Trauma. 1990;30:848–56.
94. Guillamondegui OD, Pryor JP, Gracias VH, Gupta R, Reilly PM, Schwab CW. Pelvic radiography in blunt trauma resuscitation: a diminishing role. J Trauma. 2002;53:1043–7.
95. Berg EE, Chebuhar C, Bell RM. Pelvic trauma imaging: a blinded comparison of computed tomography and roentgenograms. J Trauma. 1996;41:994–8.
96. Obaid AK, Barleben A, Porral D, Lush S, Cinat M. Utility of plain film pelvic radiographs in blunt trauma patients in the emergency department. Am Surg. 2006;72:951–4.
97. Henry SM, Pollak AN, Jones AL, Boswell S, Scalea TM. Pelvic fracture in geriatric patients: a distinct clinical entity. J Trauma. 2002;53:15–20.
98. Brohi K. Peripheral vascular trauma. http://www.trauma.org/archive/vascular/PVTdiag.html. Accessed 5 Feb 2015.
99. Fox N, Rajani RR, Bokhari F, Chiu WC, Kerwin A, Seamon MJ, et al. Evaluation and management of penetrating lower extremity arterial trauma: an Eastern Association for the Surgery of Trauma practice management guideline. J Trauma Acute Care Surg. 2012;73(5 Suppl 4):S315–20.
100. Patterson BO, Holt PJ, Cleanthis M, Tai N, Carrell T, Loosemore TM, London Vascular Injuries Working Group. Imaging vascular trauma. Br J Surg. 2012;99:494–505.
101. Howells NR, Brunton LR, Robinson J, Porteus AJ, Eldridge JD, Murray JR. Acute knee dislocation: an evidence based approach to the management of the multiligament injured knee. Injury. 2011;42:1198–204.
102. Wheeless' textbook of orthopedics. Compartment syndrome resulting from Tibial Frx. http://www.

wheelessonline.com/ortho/compartment_syndrome_resulting_from_tibial_frx. Accessed 5 Feb 2015.
103. Park S, Ahn J, Gee AO, Kuntz AF, Esterhai JL. Compartment syndrome in tibial fractures. J Orthop Trauma. 2009;23:514–8.
104. Meskey T, Hardcastle J, O'Toole RV. Are certain fractures at increased risk for compartment syndrome after civilian ballistic injury? J Trauma. 2011;71:1385–9.
105. Brenner ML, Moore LJ, DuBose JJ, Tyson GH, McNutt MK, Albarado RP, et al. A clinical series of resuscitative endovascular balloon occlusion of the aorta for hemorrhage control and resuscitation. J Trauma Acute Care Surg. 2013;75:506–11.
106. Brenner M, Hoehn M, Pasley J, Dubose J, Stein D, Scalea T. Basic endovascular skills for trauma course: bridging the gap between endovascular techniques and the acute care surgeon. J Trauma Acute Care Surg. 2014;77:286–91.
107. Brenner M, Hoehn M, Stein DM, Rasmussen TE, Scalea TM. Central pressurized cadaver model (CPCM) for resuscitative endovascular balloon occlusion of the aorta (REBOA) training and device testing. J Trauma Acute Care Surg. 2015;78:197–200.

26 Endocrine Emergencies in the ICU

Beranton Whisenant

Critical Points

- In the United States, autoimmune cell-mediated cytotoxicity is the most common cause of primary adrenal gland destruction and failure.
- Immune checkpoint inhibitors are associated with adverse side effects of adrenalitis, thyroiditis causing hyper- and hypothyroidism, hypohysitis, diabetes mellitus, and diabetes insipidus.
- In thyrotoxicosis or thyroid storming, the patient should be given PTU over preference to methimazole because PTU prevents the peripheral conversion of T4 to T3.
- Myxedema coma is rare, but when present the mortality is high up to 36% even with appropriate treatment. Altered mental status and not coma is the most important clinical findings.
- The most common cause of severe diabetic ketoacidosis in African American and Hispanics is a new disease entity called Flatbush diabetes, *ketosis-prone Type 2 DM*. This variant of DM was initially described in Flatbush Bronx, New York among ethnic groups that had presented with severe DKA but are type 2 DM.
- Hypoglycemia is occurring with increased frequency in the emergency department as a side effect of weight reduction surgeries. The emergency physician should be familiar with the diagnostic work-up of patients presenting with hypoglycemia.
- Patients often present to the emergency department with polyuria, and it is important for the emergency physician to differentiate forms of diabetes insipidus.
- Euglycemic DKA is a recently recognized disorder associated with the use of sodium-glucose cotransporter 2 inhibitors, dapagliflozin, canagliflozin, and empagliflozin, for glycemic control in type 1 and type 2 diabetic patients.

Adrenal Emergencies

All emergency medicine physician must be familiar with the diagnosis and treatment of adrenal insufficiency (AI). Once believed to be a rare disorder, it is more common than anticipated. AI

B. Whisenant (✉)
Emergency Department, University of Florida Health – Jacksonville, Jacksonville, FL, USA
e-mail: beranton.whisenant@jax.ufl.edu

© Springer Nature Switzerland AG 2020
J. R. Shiber, S. D. Weingart (eds.), *Emergency Department Critical Care*,
https://doi.org/10.1007/978-3-030-28794-8_26

represents a true medical emergency that is fatal if it is not recognized or treated promptly with fluid resuscitation and stress dose hydrocortisone administration [1, 2]. The major pathophysiological defect in AI is an absolute or relative deficiency in the synthesis of glucocorticoids [1–8]. In primary adrenal insufficiency (PAI), there is destruction or failure of the adrenal gland in the production of glucocorticoid and mineralocorticoid hormones or secondary due to failure of the pituitary gland to release adrenocortical tropic hormone (ACTH) which stimulates the adrenal gland to produce glucocorticoid. Tertiary AI is due to the impaired release of corticotrophin-releasing hormone (CRH) from the hypothalamus [1, 5, 10].

The most common cause of primary adrenal failure in the United States is autoimmune adrenalitis. Antibodies are generated against 21-hydroxylase and are detected in 90% of patients with Addison's disease but not in other causes of adrenal insufficiency [1–4, 6]. The pathogenesis of auto-immune Addison's disease is believed to be due to environmental and genetic predisposition [5]. Certain HLA genotypes DR3-DQ2/DRB1 are specific for the development autoimmune adrenitis [5]. *Mycobacterium tuberculosis* is the most common causes of primary adrenal insufficiency in the world outside of the Western industrialized countries [6]. Other causes of primary adrenal gland insufficiency [1, 7] are outlined in Table 26.1.

Table 26.1 Common causes of primary adrenal insufficiency [11]

Primary adrenal insufficiency Autoimmune adrenalitis	Type II polyglandular autoimmune syndrome *Isolated autoimmune adrenalitis*
Acute adrenal hemorrhage	Anticoagulation, Overwhelming sepsis: *Staphylococcus*, *Pseudomonas*, Meningococcal sepsis, Anti-phospholipids syndrome
Infections	Disseminated *Mycobacteria tuberculosis* MAC, HIV infection, CMV, PJP Fungal infections: Histoplasmosis Cryptococcus Toxoplasmosis Candidiasis
Infiltrative disorders	Sarcoidosis, Amyloidosis, hemochromatosis, Metastatic cancer: Lung, Breast, Kidney
Drugs	HIV meds, ketoconazole, dilantin, rifampin, Etomidate
Surgery and trauma	Adrenal trauma, adrenalectomy
Associated endocrinopathies`	Hypoparathyroidism, Type I DM, hypothyroidism, hypogonadism, hepatitis

In patients with advanced HIV/AIDS, the prevalence of adrenal insufficiency is 33–88%. Opportunistic infectious etiologies infiltrating the adrenal gland are believed to be the mechanism of the relative glucocorticoid deficiency seen in this disorder [7]. A number of medications such as etomidate carbamazepine, ketoconazole, and rifampin directly impair steroid synthesis or may the adrenal gland impervious to stimulation in the genesis and release of glucocorticoids [1, 8–14].

Secondary adrenal insufficiency is caused by disorders that affect the hypothalamo-pituitary axis causing an absolute or relative deficiency of adrenocorticotropic hormone (ACTH) [10]. Severe head injury, cerebral vascular accidents, anoxic encephalopathy, brain neoplasms, and surgery for pituitary macroadenoma are some causes of secondary adrenal insufficiency, but the most common cause is abrupt withdrawal of corticosteroids after prolonged therapy [1, 10, 12] (see Table 26.2). These neoplastic and infiltrate lesions also cause hormonal deficiencies involving other endocrine glands and multiple endocrine disorders [1, 2, 5, 14–17].

Patients with advance solid and hematological malignancies are increasingly being seen in the ED due to advanced and effective anticancer therapies, specifically immunotherapies. Immune checkpoint inhibitors such as (ICPI) ipilimumab, nivolumab, and pembrolizumab are programmed cell-death receptors antibodies and used to treat a number of advanced cancers such as refractory non-small cell lung cancers, and metastatic mela-

Table 26.2 Causes of secondary adrenal insufficiency

HPA axis dysfunction	Examples
Corticosteroid cessation after prolonged (most common)	Prolonged steroid use: COPD Asthma
Pituitary or metastatic tumor	Macroadenoma, meningioma, craniopharyngioma
Medications	Opioids effects diurnal release of cortisol Progestin binds to GCR, ↓ACTH responsiveness
Pituitary surgery and/ or irradiation Head trauma involving pituitary gland	↓ ACTH production
Pituitary necrosis or bleeding	Postpartum pituitary necrosis (Sheehan syndrome)
Infiltrative diseases	Sarcoidosis, amyloidosis, hemochromatosis, Langerhans giant cell arteritis, lymphoma, mets
Empty sella syndrome	

noma that a few years ago were incurable [14, 15]. Recently, use of these new immunotherapy drugs has resulted in life-threatening side effects mainly endocrinopathies of primary and secondary AI, thyroiditis and diabetes mellitus and diabetes insipidus [14–17]. Initial presentation is general one of adrenal crisis and/or multi-organ system failure and shock. The signs and symptoms of adrenalitis due to these ICPI and PDL-1 are the same as other causes of adrenal crisis. One exception is visual field defects and headaches due to pituitary axis involvement with associated edema. The risk of developing these endocrinopathies is greatest with combination therapies CTLA-4 combined with PD-1 at the start of treatment and for the first 6 months. The pituitary and thyroid glands are the most affected endocrine organs with thyroid gland in the form of transient hyperthyroidism that is followed by overt hypothyroidism that is permanent. To date, there has been no emergency medicine or critical care specialist society recommendations on the management of these side effects. We will give our recommendations based on the current available data [14–18].

Clinical Symptoms and Signs of Adrenal Insufficiency

Adrenal insufficiency presents with a number of nonspecific symptoms and signs (see Table 26.3). In primary AI, symptoms and signs are results of deficiency of all adrenocortical hormones synthesized in the outer most layer of the adrenal gland with general preservation of catecholamine synthesized in the adrenal medulla [1, 5–8] (see Fig. 26.1). Patients often present with weight loss, fatigue, weakness, dehydration, nausea, vomiting, diarrhea, muscle pain and cramps, abdominal pain, fever, obtundation, coma, orthostatic hypotension [5, 6, 17].

The common signs and symptoms of secondary AI are vague and nonspecific and listlessness, fatigue, joint pain, myalgia, which often delay diagnosis and treatment [10]. Some patients may present with headache, fatigue, and rarely visual field defects that are suggestive of hypophysitis or pituitary axis deficiency [5, 16, 17].

In the emergency department and ICU environment, adrenal crisis may be the initial presentation with symptoms and signs of severe abdominal pain simulating an acute abdomen, nausea, vomiting, musculoskeletal pain and weakness, syncope, fever, fatigue, obtundation, coma; Or the initial presentation maybe one of profound hypotension and shock that is refractory to iv fluid resuscitation and vasopressors [9, 11, 12].

Common Laboratory Findings

Patients with primary adrenal insufficiency typically show hyponatremia, hyperkalemia, hypoglycemia, mild hypercalcemia, and prerenal failure. These abnormalities are due to infiltration and destruction of zones of the adrenal gland that produce both glucocorticoids and mineralocorticoid hormones [9].

In secondary adrenal insufficiency, the electrolyte disturbance is mild due to the ability of the gland to continue to make mineralocorticoids, and there is no hyperpigmentation since ACTH levels are not elevated [1, 9].

Table 26.3 Common symptoms and signs of adrenal insufficiency

Symptoms	Signs
Gastrointestinal symptoms (nausea, vomiting, abdominal pain)	Weight loss Orthostatic hypotension
Weakness, fatigue	Hyperpigmentation, Vitiligo
Orthostatic hypotension	Confusion
Salt craving	Cardiovascular collapse

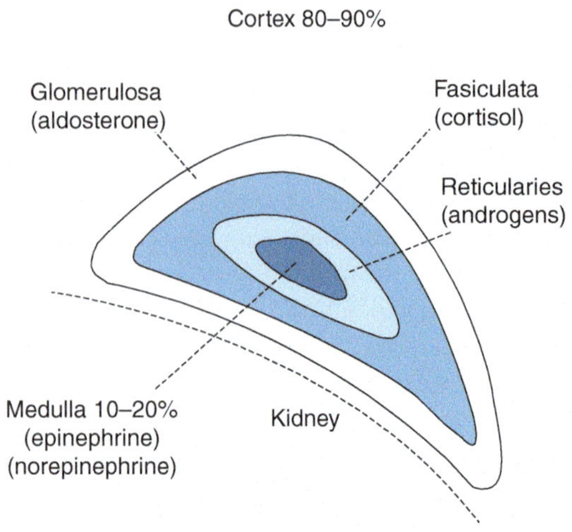

Fig. 26.1 Illustrative drawing of the adrenal gland. (Adapted from Nussey SS, Whitehead SA: The Adrenal Gland Endocrinology: an integrated approach. See text for details). When the outermost layer of the adrenal gland is destroyed by autoimmune process or infiltrative disorder, zona glomerulosa and zona fasciculate, both glucocorticid and mineralocorticoid are decreased or absent and are fatal if untreated

Eosinophilia counts, defined as >3% of total leukocyte count in severe septic shock and refractory hypotension, may be useful as biomarkers in identifying patient with impaired adrenocortical function [12]. This relative eosinophilia has been demonstrated to be present 2 days prior to the onset of septic shock. Seventy-five percent of these patient with septic shock and eosinophilia who are nonresponder to fluid and vasopressors were found to have absolute or relative adrenal insufficiency [12]. Treatment of these septic shock patients with corticoid steroid results in the hemodynamic stability and the early withdrawal of vasopressor therapy within 24 h. The mechanism behind the responsiveness of septic shock patients is due to an eosinophilic product, macrophage inhibitor factor (MIF), and its counter-regulator role in glucocorticoid biochemical action and as a mediator of septic shock perpetuating the inflammatory response. For patient with sepsis and eosinophilia, a cosyntropin stimulation test may be indicated [9, 11–13].

Diagnosis

An ACTH stimulation test is used to detect almost all cases of acute or chronic insufficiency [41].

For adrenal crisis, following the establishment of intravenous assess, blood is drawn for electrolytes, glucose, creatinine and BUN, CBC cortisol, and ACTH chest X-ray. Pan cultures are performed for the evaluation of sepsis and infection. Treatment is initiated immediately without waiting for the return of results of diagnostic studies.

If AI is suspected in a patient who is hemodynamically stable, a random cortisol is drawn for the determination of cortisol and ACTH, aldosterone and renin, blood pressure and orthostatic or postural blood pressure, electrolytes, glucose cultures of blood, and urine. The patient is treated with replacement glucocorticoids without waiting for lab results [1–6, 8–17].

If secondary adrenal insufficiency is suspected and/or the patient is receiving immunotherapy with checkpoint inhibitors, then collect sufficient blood for pituitary hormonal studies: prolactin, ACTH, TSH, estradiol, testosterone, LH/FSH, IGF-1 in males; LH, FSH, estradiol in premenopausal female [14–17].

For clinically and hemodynamically stable patients: [1, 3, 5, 9]

- If cortisol is <3 mcg/dL, the diagnosis is confirmed and no further testing is indicated.
- A rapid cosyntropin ACTH stimulation test is performed for cortisol levels <18 mcg/dL.
- The patient is given synthetic ACTH 250 ug IV, and cortisol and simultaneous ACTH levels are measured at 30 and 60 min.
- A cortisol level <18 ug/dL or an increase of cortisol <9 mcg/dL confirm AI.

During severe illness, patients who are febrile, hypovolemic, hypotensive, and hypoxic with SIRS, sepsis, multi-trauma have cortisol level >23 mcg/dL. Thus, a random serum cortisol level of 18 ug/dL is inappropriately low for such major and intense stressors, and a diagnosis of relative AI is highly suggestive of AI [12].

To distinguish primary and secondary AI, low-dose cosyntropin (LD cosyntropin) and high-dose cosyntropin (HD cosyntropin) are used [1, 9, 12].

- Patients with primary AI with ACTH levels <25 ug/dL will not increase their serum cortisol level with either LD or HD corticotrophin stimulation.
- Patients with secondary AI with baseline cortisol <25 ug/dL will increase their cortisol level above 25 ug/dL.

These are not diagnostic studies that are required or necessary to be performed in the emergency department setting.

CT scan of the adrenal glands or head may help in determining the cause of acute or chronic AI [14]. If secondary AI diagnosis is established, then MRI of the pituitary should be obtained to rule out pituitary adenoma or lesions, hemorrhage, or infarction [10, 16, 17].

Another entity associated with adrenal insufficiency is critical illness-related corticosteroid insufficiency. This syndrome is defined as inadequate glucocorticoid levels relative to the degree of stress. It is most often seen in sepsis and septic shock and acute lung injury. A serum cortisol level <20 mcg/dL following a corticotropin stimulation test or <9 mcg/dL level of increase over baseline represents an inadequate adrenal response [2, 12]. The most recent guidelines for the treatment of critical illnesses indicated a random cortisol level <18 mcg/dL in a patient with sepsis shock and likely AI is an indication to initiate steroid therapy [3, 8–10, 17].

There is an opioid epidemic in the United States with more than 25 million Americans receiving opioids for management of chronic pain. Heroin use is also on the rise due to restriction of access to prescription narcotics and is associated with AI. Emergency physicians frequently encounter patients using long-term opioid treatment. It is important to be able to recognize the endocrinopathy associated with its use [9, 13]. Opioid-induced adrenal insufficiency (OIAI) is an undiagnosed side effect of prolonged opioid use [9, 13]. OIAI has a prevalence of up to 29% with chronic administration and is associated with increased mortality and mortality [13]. Opioids exert their effects on μ, δ, and κ receptors in the hypothalamus and pituitary glands causing inhibition of the HPA axis with resulting secondary adrenal insufficiency. Chronic opioid users who present to the ED with signs and symptoms of AI should be screened for AI with a baseline serum cortisol level and/or CTS [9, 13].

Management

Adrenal insufficiency is a medical emergency that must be recognized and treated immediately with steroids, intravenous fluids, and vasopressors if indicated. Outlined is one clinical guideline to the management of adrenal crisis and symptomatic adrenal insufficiency [8–10, 13] (see Table 26.4).

Empiric antibiotics should be given until an infectious process is ruled out.

Thyroid Storm

Introduction

Thyroid storm is an acute life-threatening exacerbation of thyrotoxicosis that is due to hypermetabolic response of all organ systems of the body to elevated production of thyroid hormone [19, 20].

It is commonly seen in patients with undiagnosed Graves' disease or partially or untreated hyperthyroidism who undergoes some stressful event. The most common stressful event is infectious etiologies with pneumonia with URI being the most common. Precipitating factors for thyroid storm are: [19, 20, 24]

Table 26.4 A Suggestive management of adrenal crisis: profound hypotension/shock [1–5, 8–16]

Establish airway and breathing
Place on continuous ECG monitoring with oximetry
Establish a central line and/or two large bore IV for blood draw and iv fluid hydration
Give 20–30 ml/kg bolus of 0.9% NaCl as determined by state of dehydration; urine output may need 4 liters over the next 24 h
For significant hyponatremia, do not raise serum Na greater than 8–10 mEq/dL in 24 h to avoid osmotic demyelination.
D_{10} may be needed for hypoglycemia and ongoing treatment of adrenal crisis
If diagnosis is confirmed, give hydrocortisone 100 mg iv stat and then 50 mg IV every 6 h.
Check pH, electrolytes, and glucose every 2 h
For moderate dehydration and hypotension
Place on continuous ECG monitoring and monitoring of vital signs, oximetry
Give 1000 ml fluid boluses until circulation volume is restored
Give the remaining fluid deficit evenly over 24 h using D_5 NS
Give steroid hydrocortisone 100 mg iv bolus, then 50 mg hydrocortisone every 6 h IV or continuous infusion of 200–300 mg hydrocortisone over 24 h
Repeat point-of-care (POC) electrolytes, glucose, and venous pH every 2 h.
For mild hydration normotensive
D5 NS at 125–150 ml/h over 24 h
Check glucose, electrolytes every 4–6 h for 24 h
Give hydrocortisone 100 mg IV bolus and 50 mg iv every 6–8 h.

- DKA or hyperglycemic hyperosmolar syndrome
- Nonthyroidal surgeries
- Sepsis, gastroenteric infections, UTI
- CVA
- MI, anesthetic agents, acute iodide load

The most common cause of hyperthyroidism is Graves' disease, multi-nodular goiter, toxic solitary adenoma, and subacute thyroiditis [19]. Graves' disease typically occurs in the third and fourth decade and is 10 times more common in women [22]. Toxic multinodular goiter is more common among women and older age group in the fifth and seventh decade [22, 26].

The pathophysiologic mechanism for the development of thyroid storm from noncomplicated thyrotoxicosis is not known. It appears to be related to a hyperadrenergic hyperactive response of multiple organs to the altered interaction of thyroid hormone and catecholamines resulting in the generation of high metabolic rate, fever, and dysregulation of hypothalamus in temperature regulation [19, 20].

Clinical Symptoms and Signs of Thyroid Storm

Thyroid storm is a clinical diagnosis and that cannot be distinguished on biochemical basis from thyrotoxicosis. The initial signs of thyroid storm are elevated temperature out of proportion to infection and heart rate that does not correlate with disturbance with resting heart rates sustained at 80s to 90s and up to >200 bpm. Profuse diaphoresis, agitation, hyperdefecation, and diarrhea are early symptoms and signs of impending thyroid storm. If this early stage of presentation is not recognized and treated, then multiple organ system will decompensate from the constant stimulus of thyroid hormone (TH) and tip over into congestive heart failure, refractory pulmonary edema, circulatory shock state, coma, and death [18, 20, 24]. The cardiovascular manifestations of thyroid storm are the most important and the leading cause of death; however, neurological complications are present in >90% of patients [19, 20]. In elderly patients, the manifestation of thyroid crisis may take a different form referred to as apathetic storm with weakness, emotional apathy, absence of fever, delirium, and coma [20]. See Table 26.5 for symptoms and signs of thyroid storm.

Table 26.5 Clinical signs and symptoms of thyroid storm

Symptoms	Signs
Diaphoresis, heat intolerance	Hyperthermia
Palpitation	Tachydysrhythmias: ST, AF
Nervousness	Systolic hypertension
Weight loss	Wide pulse pressure
Angina pectoris	Signs of CHF
Difficulty concentrating	Mental status change
Generalized weakness	Muscle wasting and atrophy

Common Laboratory Findings

Elevated T4 and T3 with low TSH are common findings, but the degree of elevation is not different from clinically stable thyrotoxicosis. A mild leukocytosis is usual with increase in red blood cell mass. Routine studies that need to be drawn on presentation to the ED are CBC, creatinine, electrolytes, cortisol, liver function studies, serum calcium, thyroid function studies with total T4, T3, free T4, and T3 levels with TSH, chest X-ray, and EC. There are no laboratory studies that will confirm or refute the diagnosis of thyroid storm. It is a clinical diagnosis [20, 22].

Diagnosis

The clinical symptoms and signs of thyrotoxicosis and that of thyroid storm are nonspecific and the patient may present with the symptoms of severe sepsis, illicit substance ingestion, or coma, and thyroid storm may be masked and go undiagnosed, untreated, and succumb to multiorgan decompensation and death [19]. If there is a delay in the diagnosis and treatment of thyroid storm for more than 24 h, the multiorgan dysfunction, usually cardiovascular disorder, may be irreversible.

The diagnosis is clinical and is based on the presence of known precipitant, hypothalamic temperature dysregulation, and dysfunction of cardiovascular, CNS, and gastrointestinal systems with temperature out of proportion to an existing infection process being the most important in making a diagnosis. The Burch and Wartofsky diagnostic point scoring scale uses precise clinical criteria to aid in the diagnosis of thyroid storm. A score of <25 is unlikely to be thyroid storm, while a score of >45 is highly likely [19, 24]. The Japanese Association diagnostic system is another recent developed diagnostic criteria based on the five BWPS diagnostic criteria plus thyrotoxicosis. Definite diagnosis of thyroid storm includes CND dysfunction plus one other manifestation or three manifestations other than CNS. The two systems, BWPS and JTA, may be used together to facilitate an accurate diagnosis of TS.

Management [18–20, 24]

Thyroid storm is a life-threatening medical condition that is 100% fatal if left untreated and management must be conducted in an ICU (see Box 26.1).

A multifacet approach is used for the treatment of TS which involves:

Box 26.1 Proposed Management of Thyroid Storm [10, 14, 15]

Supportive care
- Sedative bed-rest IV hydration and electrolyte replacement
- Antipyretics, cooling blankets
- Antibiotics for infectious etiology

Specific measures
- Propranolol 0.5–1 mg IV initially, and if no hypotension or bradycardia, 2–3 mg over 15 min. Oral propranolol 40–80 mg every 6 h.
- PTU 400 mg initial and then 200 mg every 4 h or 1200 mg daily in divided dose or methimazole 15–25 mg every 6 h.
- After 2 h, give 5 drops of potassium iodide every 6 h.
- Hydrocortisone 100 mg every 8 h or decadron 2 mg every 6 h.

Alternative measures
- Lithium 300 mg every 6 h
- Ipodate 500 mg daily or twice a day
- Esmolol if propranolol is not tolerated or cardiac decompensation

For resistant cases of thyroid storm
- Plasma exchange, plasmapheresis, or dialysis

- Supportive measures: antipyretics, cooling blankets, and IV fluids for dehydration, and antibiotics for infectious etiology [14]
- Antithyroid drugs to reduce synthesis of thyroid hormones (T4 and T3) in 60–120 min
  - PTU 150–250 mg Q 6 h DOC
  - Methimazole 20 mg Q 6 h (safer than PTU)
- Blockage of action and peripheral conversion of T4 to T3
  - Propranolol 0.5–1 mg IV loading dose, then 1 mg over 10 min hourly for heart rate control
  - Propranolol 60–80 mg Q 4–6 h
  - Esmolol 50 mcg bolus, then 50–100 mcg/kg/min for HR control for critically ill in shock states
  - Glucocorticoids-hydrocortisone 300 mg iv load, then 100 mg Q 8 h or dexamethasone 2 mg Q 6 h
- Treatment of cardiac decompensation: CHF, hypovolemic shock
- Treatment of precipitants: DKA, sepsis, CVA

If patient remains hypermetabolic following the above intervention, the ion-exchange resin 20–30 mg daily can be used to block recirculation of T4 and T3. With continued failure of convention therapy to control TS and then dialysis, plasma exchange or AV ECMO will be life saving [20, 24].

Treatment includes supportive measures with antipyretics, IV hydration, cooling blankets, treatment of tachycardia (atrial fibrillation), congestive heart failure, sedation, and antibiotics for precipitating infectious etiology [19, 20].

Nonselective beta blocker (BB), propranolol, is the drug of choice in the management of TS, but if there is a contraindication to the use of nonselective BB (Asthma, COPD, CHF), then either a selective BB, esmolol drip, atenolol, or calcium block may be used to treat the adrenergic hyperresponsiveness [20].

Myxedema Coma [21–24]

Introduction

Myxedema coma is defined as a severe manifestation of hypothyroidism due to decreased secretion of thyroid hormones that results from decompensation of adaptive mechanisms in maintaining body's homeostasis. This condition is rare in occurrence and is seen during the winter months among women >60 years of age after a prolonged history of hypothyroidism [16–19]. This medical condition occurs in patients with severe untreated hypothyroidism due to autoimmune thyroiditis, Hashimoto thyroiditis, thyroidectomy resulting in decrease secretion of thyroid hormones. Pituitary macroadenomas or hypothalamic lesions through lack of stimulation of the thyroid gland may cause decreased TH in the circulation. The syndrome is usually precipitated by an acute concurrent illness such as UTI, pulmonary infection, CHF, myocardial infarction, exposure to cold weather, or drugs such as amiodarone, opiates, and sedates. The mortality rate is high (40–60%) even with treatment [24].

Clinical Symptoms and Signs of Myxedema Coma

The signs and symptoms of hypothyroidism and myxedema coma are similar but more exaggerated in myxedema. The three cardinal features of myxedema coma are altered mental status, hypothermia, and a precipitating event. In myxedema patients, altered mental status is the most prominent presenting symptom with the patient manifesting depression, decline in intellectual function. Coma is a very rare occurrence. Hypothermia in myxedema is usually less than 95.9 F, the low the temperature the worse the prognosis. Physical examination generally reveals bradycardia, hypotension, and hypoventilation that may deteriorate to hypercapnic respiratory failure, macroglossia, and deepening of voice.

Table 26.6 Suggested clinical features in myxedema coma [16–20]

Symptoms	Signs
Intolerance to cold	Hypothermia
Confusion	Bradycardia, low cardiac output
Lethargy	Dry coarse skin
Dry coarse skin	Central hypoventilation syndrome
Myalgia, leg cramps, fatigue	Macroglossia
Constipation	Alopecia
	Hyporeflexia
	Obtundation, stupor
	Puffy facies
	Diastolic hypertension
	Narrow pulse pressure
	Low cardiac output, cardiogenic shock
	Pleural effusion, hypoxia, hypercarbia

Table 26.7 Treatment of myxedema coma [16–18]

Airway management with mechanical ventilation until altered mental state and respiratory depression resolves
Levothyroxine iv loading dose 300–500 ug[a]
Levothyroxine maintenance dose 100 ug daily iv or 1.6 ug/kg iv[a]
Hydrocortisone 100 mg iv every 8 h
D5NS for euglycemia if necessary
Management of hyponatremia with fluid restriction and/or conivaptan for elevated SIADH associated with myxedema
Prophylactic antibiotics until infection as precipitating cause can be rule out
Passive rewarming with blankets to avoid vasodilation-induced hypotension

[a]Caution: For patients with risk factors for tachyarrhythmia or coronary artery disease, CVA use 50–100 ug of levothyroxine as loading and maintenance dosing along with cardiac monitoring

See Table 26.6 for clinical findings in myxedema coma [23, 24].

Common Laboratory Findings

Most patients have low T4 and T3 with elevated TSH levels, but TSH may be normal or low due to secondary causes of hypothyroidism [3–24]. Hyponatremia is usually present and will resolve with the replacement of thyroid hormones.

Management

Patients presenting to the ED with myxedema coma usually have depressed sensorium, and protection of the airway is paramount in the initial management [20–22].

Table 26.7 outlines the treatment of myxedema coma.

The replacement doses of levothyroxine are discussed in Table 26.7. There has been no control trials of the appropriate replacement dose of levothyroxine, but T4 is initially given IV at a dose of 200–500 mcg IV in the first 24 h and then 100 mcg followed by 100 mcg daily [20–24].

If the patient with myxedema coma has low serum albumin and/or cardiac disease, use 200 mcg loading dose of levothyroxine, and 50–100 mcg of levothyroxine can be added for several hours while monitoring patient for signs of myocardial ischemia. Give hydrocortisone 100 mg iv to avoid clinical deterioration from occult adrenal insufficiency [22].

Despite early and aggressive management, the prognosis of patients with myxedema is poor and still has a high mortality rate [23, 24].

Diabetic Ketoacidosis

Diabetic ketoacidosis (DKA) and hyperglycemic hyperosmolar state, formerly called hyperosmolar nonketotic coma (HONK), are commonly seen and managed in the emergency departments on a regular basis. Our physiologic understanding is that DKA occurs most commonly in type I DM, which represents an absolute deficiency of insulin. Hyperglycemic hyperosmolar state (HHS)] occurs in type 2 DM, which is due to a relative deficiency of insulin [25–28, 30–33]. These traditional learned physiologic principles of complication of diabetes have come into question with the recognized clinical entity of atypical DKA referred to as Flatbush DM, ketosis-prone DM, or ketosis type 2 DM [29]. In African-American and Hispanic populations, there is a new and increasingly recognized entity, referred to as Flatbush diabetes mellitus, also called ketosis-prone type 2 diabetes mellitus (K2DM). This form of diabetes accounts for 50–64% of African-American and Hispanic individuals diagnosed with new-onset DKA. It has also been recently recognized in Indians, Asians, and sub-Saharan Africans. A distinguishing feature of Flatbush diabetes is that patients present with unprovoked precipitating cause of DKA compared with type 1 and type 2 DM [29].

U.S. Food and Drug Administration (FDA) in 2014 approved sodium-glucose cotransporter 2 (SGLT2) inhibitors as a antihyperglycemic agent to treat T2D for glycemic control [35]. It is used off-labeled for the management of T1D due to its enhancement of glycemic control, weight loss, and avoidance of hypoglycemia. There are three SGLT-2 inhibitors in the US market. They lower serum glucose by noninsulin-dependent mechanism preventing the reabsorption of glucose from the proximal renal tubules, promoting glycosuria making them useful adjuncts in diabetes management [34]. The glucouria suppressed the release of insulin from pancreatic beta cells and leads to a cascade of ketogenesis with increased fatty acid metabolism and formation of ketone body production with mild to normal serum glucose. eDKA is a rare disorder that every emergency medicine physician must be able to recognize and manage [34–37].

Hyperglycemia of DKA and HHS develops from gluconeogenesis, glycogenolysis, and decreased glucose utilization by predominately skeletal muscles due to lack of insulin or increase in insulin resistance. DKA is defined as a clinical triad of hyperglycemia with glucose >250 mg/dL, anion gap >12, metabolic acidosis with pH < 7.3, and ketonemia and positive ketone in the urine. The oxidation and utilization of fatty acids as an energy source lead to the accumulation of ketones that are converted to an equilibrium of acetoacetate, and β- hydroxybutyrate in a ratio of 1:4 to 1:12. The marked elevated serum glucose in HHS and to a lesser extent in DKA leads to osmotic diuresis with dehydration, a hyperosmolarity state, and impaired consciousness. The large solute load that is presented to the kidneys leads to a further decline in renal function, decreased GFR, electrolyte loss, worsening hyperglycemic and hyperosmolarity state, and impaired consciousness [28–30]. See Fig. 26.2 for pathophysiologic mechanism of DKA/HHS.

The pathophysiologic mechanism of ketosis prone DKA is not known. It is considered to be

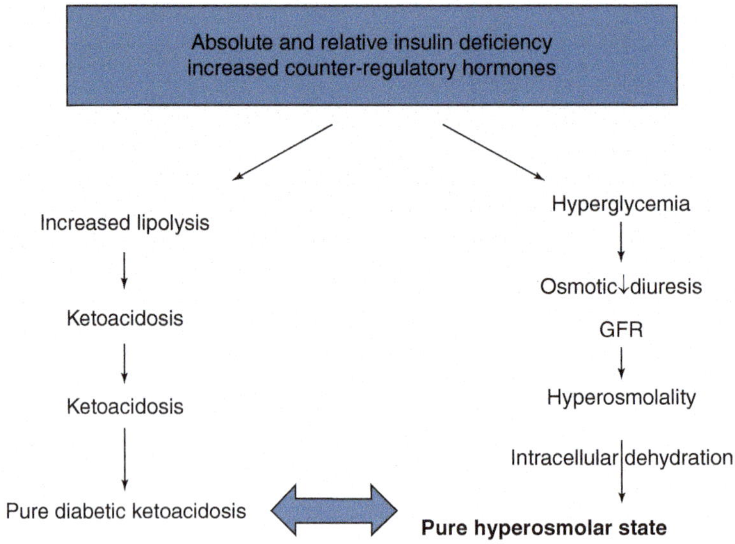

Fig. 26.2 Pathophysiology of DKA/HHS

an atypical presentation of classic DKA or an extreme form of T2DM [29].

Precipitating Factors for DKA and HHS

The most common precipitating factors in the development of DKA or HHS are noncompliance and infections [28, 30–33]. Other factors that are associated with the precipitation of DKA and HHS are myocardial infarction, CVA, urosepsis, gastrointestinal bleed, pneumonia, pulmonary embolic, severe stress, sepsis, pancreatitis, and hyperthyroidism. A diligent search for site of infections should be initiated for any patient presenting with DKA or HHS particularly if they have an elevated temperature and/or leukocytosis [28, 30–33]. Precipitating factors for the development of EDKA in patients on SGLT-2 [34–36] are decreased insulin or secretagogue dose, decreased oral intake of carbohydrates, fasting state, acute illness, marathon participation, insulin pump failure, alcohol and cocaine use, and pregnancy. The clinical presentation of African Americans, Afro-Caribbean, as well as other ethnic groups is DKA without an apparent cause [29]. Its initial presentation is new onset severe hyperglycemia and ketoacidosis in middle-aged, modestly obese individuals of color [29]. The metabolic derangement and insulin requirement resolves after several months of euglycemic control. These patients can be managed by diet alone or diet and an oral hypoglycemic agent [29].

Common Laboratory Findings

Initial laboratory studies should include a basic metabolic profile with Mg++, Ca++, and phosphorus, CBC with differential, UA, venous pH, and/or ABG, β hydroxybutyrate, urinalysis, urine ketone, ECG, and chest X-ray. Additional studies that may be indicated are pregnancy test, HbA1C, and lipase and lipid profile to rule out pancreatitis. Blood, urine, and sputum cultures should also be obtained to look for infection [25–32]. For eDKA, detection of the presence of ketones in the blood and/or urine is helpful in leading to the diagnosis.

Diagnosis of DKA and HHS

Diagnostic criteria for DKA and HHS are presented in Table 26.8.

Table 26.8 Diagnostic criteria and typical body deficits of water and electrolytes in DKA and HHS

DKA				
Diagnostic criteria	Mild	Moderate	Severe	HHS
Plasma glucose mg/dL	>250 mg/dL	>250 mg/dL	>250 mg/dL	>600 mg/dL
pH	7.25–7.30	7.00 – <7.25	<7.00	>7.30
HCO3-	15–18	10–15	<10	>15
Urine ketone	Positive	Positive	Positive	Small
Serum ketone	Positive	Positive	Positive	small
Serum osmolality	Variable	Variable	Variable	>320 mOsm/kg
Anion gap	>10	>12	>12	<12
Mental status	Alert	Alert/drowsy	Stuporous/coma	Coma
Typical deficits				
Water	6 liters			9 liters
Na	100			100
K	7–10			5–13
PO4	3–5			3–5
Mg	5–7			3–7
	1–2			1–2

Patients with DKA usually presents to the ED with abdominal pain, polyuria, polydipsia, nausea, vomiting, and weight loss. With worsening ketonemia and acidosis, the patient develops Kussmaul respirations, tachycardia, hypotension, and sometimes shock [25, 28–30].

HHS hallmark is a marked elevated serum glucose, glucose greater than 600 hyperosmolality usually 320 mOsm or greater, and may be associated with ketones formation though mild. The diagnosis of eDKA is the same as standard DKA except the serum glucose is not elevated. There may be a history of SGLT2 inhibitor use along with insulin or oral hypoglycemic agents, alone with the precipitating factors of reduced food intake, inadvertent discontinuation of insulin or cocaine or alcohol intoxication [28]. KPD is diagnosed by the lack of finding precipitating factors and the absence of autoimmune antibodies against pancreatic β-islet cells and glutamic acid decarboxylase [38–40].

Management of DKA and HHS

When the diagnosis of DKA and HHS has been confirmed, aggressive fluid resuscitation with normal saline is instituted to reestablish intravascular volume status and improve organ perfusion and lower serum glucose, hyperosmolality state, and ketones levels.

Normal saline is the fluid of choice. The initial 1–3 liters of 0.9% saline is given over 2–3 h, and then 0.9% NS alternating with 0.5% NS can be used based on state of dehydration and serum sodium [20, 21]. Due to concerns with hyperchloremic acidosis, a number of studies have advocated the use of plasmalyte infusion for volume resuscitation as opposed to normal saline. There is improved renal function, and metabolic acidosis resolves sooner. The average patient has a 7–9 liter free water deficit, and 50% of this is replaced in the first 12 h with the remaining deficit replaced over the next 24 h. In HHS, fluid replacement is more important than insulin compared to DKA where insulin is the primary treatment and fluids are an adjunct [25–28, 30, 34] (see Box 26.2).

Box 26.2 Management of Adults with DKA and HONK and Adults with Ketosis-Prone Type 2 DM [23–26]

Biochemistry Studies

- Upon Emergency Department Presentation: CBC with differential complete metabolic profile, ABG or venous pH, and serum β-hydroxybutyrate.
- Perform POC glucose every hour, and every 2 h check basic metabolic profile, venous pH, and phosphorus until DKA resolves.

IV Fluids

- Hydration Status Assessment:
  - Mildly hypotensive and dehydration: evaluate corrected [Na] and give 0.9% NaCl or 0.45% NaCl at 250–500 ml/h based [Na].
  - For Orthostatic Hypotension and/or Shock: give 1 liter NaCl over 1–2 h; then 0.45% NaCl with 20–30 mEq/L of KCl at 500–250 ml/h.
  - Replace 50% of free H2O deficits in first 12 h and the second 50% over 12–24 h (usual free deficit is 6–9 liters for DKA).
  - When blood glucose is <250 mg/dL, change IV fluids to D50. 45% NaCl at 150–250 ml/h until plasma osmolarity is <320 mOsm/kg.

Insulin

- Give regular insulin, IV bolus 0.1 units/kg. The continuous infusion at 0.1 units/kg/h may need second IV bolus of insulin if glucose fails to ↓ by 10%. In the first hour of starting infusion (50 mg/dL), give 0.14 units of insulin and continue infusion at same rate.
- Keep serum glucose at 150–200 mg/dL and ↓ insulin rate to 0.05 units/kg/h until DKA (venous pH) is resolved.
- Check venous pH every 3–4 h until normal, and give NPH 2 h prior to dis-

continuing IV insulin infusion. Long-acting insulin detemir or glargine can be given to provide basal insulin coverage.

Potassium

- If K+ is between 3.3 mEq/l and ≤ 5.0 mEq/L, add 20 mEq K+ to each liter of IV fluid to keep serum K+ at 4–5 mEq/L.
- If K+ is <3.3 mEq/L, give 40 mEq and consider holding insulin for HONK or mild DKA but not moderate-severe DKA until K+ >3.3 mEq/L.

For patients who present to the emergency department with mild to moderate DKA, an alternative to continuous insulin can be given with rapid-acting insulin lispro or aspart.

In two prospective randomized, open-label studies, subcutaneous insulin lispro administered subcutaneously was found to be feasible and cost-effective in the treatment of uncomplicated DKA, but larger studies need to be performed [25–28]. See Table 26.9 for subcutaneous insulin regimen for selected mild to moderate DKA.

The management of patient presenting with eDKA is the same as DKA with the exception of administrating D5NS with IV insulin therapy to avoid iatrogenic hypoglycemia [46]. Insulin should be infused at 0.1 u/kg/h without an insulin bolus until the Ag closes on two consecutive lab draw [25–30, 33, 42].

Hypoglycemia [43–48]

Hypoglycemia is one of the most common endocrine emergencies seen in the ED. It is common in individuals being treated for diabetes and rare in those without diabetes who are apparently healthy appearing. ED visits and hospitalization due to insulin-related hypoglycemia is more common in older patients >45 and highest among patients >80 years. Based on CDC statistics, there are approximately 300,000 ED visits annually for hypoglycemic episodes. Nondiabetic hypoglycemia is rare and may be diagnostic challenge for the busy ED physician in determining the cause. The inadvertent administration of insulin or oral hypoglycemic agent is the most common cause of hypoglycemia in patients who do not have diabetes [43]. The clinical diagnosis of hypoglycemia is based on Whipple triad: symptoms of hypoglycemia, documenting serum glucose <55 mg/dL and resolution of symptoms after administration of glucose [46–48] (see Table 26.10).

Table 26.9 Subcutaneous insulin regimen for mild to moderate DKA

Lispro or aspart insulin			
Insulin	Onset of action	Time to peak	Duration
Regular	30–60 min	2–3 h	8–10 h
Aspart	5–15 min	30–90 min	4–6 h
Lispro	5–15 min	30–90 min	4–6 h
Glulisine	5–15 min	30–90 min	5.3 h
NPH	2–4 h	4–10 h	12–18 h
Emergency department observation unit admission for DKA management			
Hours	Fluids		
1st	1 liter		
30 min – h	1 liter		
2nd hour	500 ml–1 L		
3rd hour	500 ml–1 L		
4th hour			
Replace 50% free H2O in first 12 h			
Second half over 12 h			

Initial loading dose – 0.2 IU/kg SC or IM followed by 0.1 IU/kg every hour until blood glucose is 250 mg/dL

For insulin resistance individuals or obese, give an initial dose of 0.3 IU/kg SC and 0.2 IU/kg every 2 h while BG remains >250 mg/dl

When blood glucose is <250 mg/dL, the SC insulin dose is ↓ to 0.05 IU/kg every 1–2 h until acidosis resolves.

Give intermediate or long-acting insulin when HCO3 is >18 mEq/L, AG normal, pH > 7.3

30% basal insulin

70% rapid acting insulin

Or

Usual home dose of insulin

Table 26.10 Clinical manifestation of hypoglycemia [31]

Sympathoadrenal	Neuroglycopenia
Diaphoresis	Dizziness, blurred vision
Hunger	Weakness, drowsiness
Palpitations, tremors	Difficulty concentrating,
Nervousness, anxiety	Seizure, coma, or death

Modified from Ref. [30]

Pathophysiology of Hypoglycemia

Serum glucose levels are maintained in a narrow range for homeostasis. The brain requires a constant fuel source of glucose and can only store glucose for a few minutes and has limited glycogen stores. If serum glucose drops less than 55 mg/dL, this signals the release of glucagon as the first sign of defense against hypoglycemia. If glucose levels are not raised and continue to decline, then epinephrine, norepinephrine growth hormone, and cortisol released are triggered to increase glucose production by inhibiting the peripheral utilization of glucose and increase gluconeogenesis and glycogenolysis in the liver and proteolysis from protein breakdown for the synthesis of glucose. In T1DM and longstanding T2DM, these counter-regulatory mechanism are ineffective and result in hypoglycemia [30–32].

Signs and Symptoms

Symptoms and signs are classified as neuroglycopenic as a result of brain glucose deprivation and neurogenic symptoms derived from sympathoadrenal autonomic nerve discharge manifested as tremor, palpitations, anxiety/arousal, diaphoresis, and hunger. The neuroglycopenic symptoms are fatigue, weakness, confusion, seizures, coma, and brain death [46–48].

Diagnostic Approach to Hypoglycemia [46]

The most common cause of hypoglycemia is insulin-induced from failure to adjust the insulin dose based on the caloric intake particularly in patients <30 years of age, and the concomitant use of alcohol is the most common cause in all age groups. Hypoglycemia is particularly common in critically ill patients due to worsening renal function, with impaired insulin metabolism, and clearance of oral hypoglycemic agents [44–48]. The oral hypoglycemic agent, glyburide, causes the most hypoglycemic episode of any other oral hypoglycemic agent, and it should be discontinued in critically ill patients [43]. It has a long duration of action and may lead to refractory hypoglycemia requiring cortisol, D10 infusion for correction [43]. Factors that predispose to hypoglycemia are listed in Table 26.11 [47, 48]. In diabetics, drugs are a common cause of hypoglycemia while in nondiabetics, renal, hepatic failure, and infection are common causes of hypoglycemic episodes.

Diagnosis

The first step in the evaluation of a patient with a history suggestive of hypoglycemia is to perform a concise history and physical examination and determine if the patient has diabetes, appears well with no preexisting disease, or is ill appear-

Table 26.11 Conditions and drugs associated with hypoglycemia

Well-appearing patient	Ill-appearing patients
DM type 1 and 2 inappropriate insulin or oral agent dose ETOH	Sepsis, renal failure, liver failure Congestive heart failure Trauma, Burns
Insulinoma Non-islet cell tumors	Endocrinopathies: hypoadrenalism, hypopituitarism
Drug use: salicylate, haldol, indomethacin, quinine, angiotensin receptor antagonist, ciprofloxacin, bactrim, heparin, lithium, pentamidine	Starvation, anorexia nervosa Topical salicylates in renal failure
Factitious use of insulin or sulfonyl urea	Large non β cell tumors: fibroma, sarcoma
Insulin antibodies, insulin receptor antibodies	
Post gastric bypass hypoglycemia	

ing with comorbid conditions. The diagnostic work-up is entirely different if there is no history of diabetes [29, 31]. It is important to document a low plasma glucose level (<55 mg/dL) when the patient is symptomatic and it resolves when the glucose level is raised (Whipple's triad). After hypoglycemia has been established, the next step is to determine the mechanism, if it is insulin mediated versus noninsulin mediated (Fig. 26.3).

Laboratory studies that should be sent simultaneously with the blood glucose are [48]:

- Plasma glucose
- Alcohol level
- Sulfonylurea
- Proinsulin
- C-peptide
- Insulin level
- Beta hydroxybutyrate

The diagnostic approach to a patient presenting to the ED with documented hypoglycemia is confirmation of Whipple's triad and biochemical testing. Table 26.12 provides a guide to those patients that will require hospitalization for a formal 72-h fasting protocol [45–48].

Hypoglycemic episodes due to inadvertent insulin overdose or oral hypoglycemia agents have insulin levels >100 μU/ or 600 μU/ml and low C-peptide levels. Insulin level in insulinoma rarely exceeds 100 μU/ml and is not suppressed

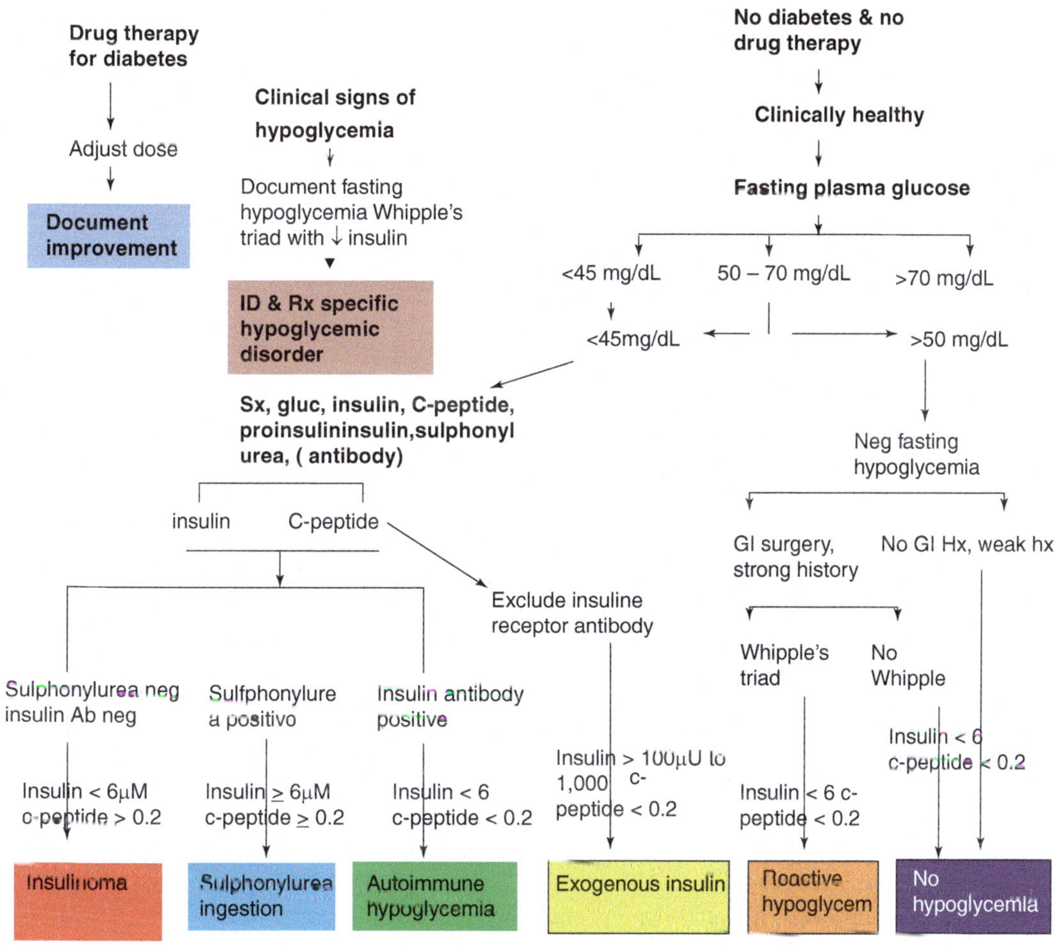

Fig. 26.3 Clinical pathway for the diagnostic evaluation of hypoglycemia [33]

Table 26.12 Interpretation of biochemical tests for hypoglycemia

	Insulin	C-peptide	Proinsulin	B-OH butyrate	Sulfonylurea
Normal	↓	↓	↓	↑	No
exogenous insulin	↑↑	↓	↓	↓	No
Non-β cell-mediated hypoglycemia	↓	↓	↓	↑	No
Insulinoma	↑↑	↑↑↑	↑↑	↓	No
Sulfonylurea-induced hypoglycemia	↑↑	↑↑	↑↑	↓	Yes

by low glucose. The C-peptide in insulinoma is also not suppressed.

A new designated hypoglycemic disorder in adults who have hypersecretion of insulin 2–4 h after ingestion of a meal is referred to as noninsulinoma pancreatogenous hypoglycemia syndrome (NIPHS). Unlike insulinoma, it occurs primarily in males. Further specialized testing is necessary to differentiate this disorder from insulinoma.

Management of Hypoglycemia [45, 46, 48]

For symptomatic patients with mild hypoglycemia, the ingestion of 15 grams of simple carbohydrate substances in the form of glucose tablets, lifesavers candy, fruit juices, or drinks can raise the serum glucose above 60 mg/dL. The patient is then given a well-balanced meal consisting of protein, complex carbohydrates, and fat to prevent the return of the hypoglycemia [10, 14].

For hypoglycemic-induced coma from long-acting insulin or oral hypoglycemic agents, these patients should receive aggressive treatment of their hypoglycemia with glucagon 1 mg IV and 25 g of glucose with ampule of D50 infusion or 100 ml of D10 until the hypoglycemia resolves (Box 26.3) [10, 14]. Diabetic patients with end-stage liver disease on oral hypoglycemic agents may experience prolonged refractory hypoglycemic episodes. This is due to depleted hepatic glycogen stores and impaired glucose production by the liver. In this situation, the patient will require ICU management with infusion of D10 and/or D20 and octreotide subcutaneous or IV bolus or continuous infusion every 6 h until serum glucose remains >60 mg/dL. An alternative treatment modality may be the constant infusion of D10W with hydrocortisone 100 mg IV and/or glucagon 1 mg IV in 1000 ml of D10W [45–48].

Box 26.3 Management of Life-Threatening Hypoglycemia [10, 14, 29, 31]

- Constant infusion of glucose D10 with repeat glucose testing every 20–30 min until persistently mild hyperglycemic.
- If blood glucose fails to remain >200 mg/dL, then an alternative method of treatment needs to be initiated for refractory hypoglycemia.
- For hypoglycemia refractory to D10 infusion (blood glucose persistently <200 mg/dL give:
  - 100 mg hydrocortisone and 1 mg glucagon per 1 liter of D10.
  - Give diazoxide in D5W infuse over 30 min and repeat every 4 h until glucose is >20 mg/dL.
  - When glucose is >200 mg/dL, then can stop glucagon, hydrocortisone, and diazoxide and decrease infusion of D10.
  - Octreotide infusion 50 ug every 6–8 h for refractory hypoglycemia.

For insulinoma that are non-resectable:

- Diazoxide 3–8 mg/kg/d tid (drug of choice)
- Thiazide diuretics
- Propranolol
- 5-Fluorouracil and streptozotocin combination chemotherapy

Diabetes Insipidus [49–53]

Diabetes insipidus (DI) is defined and characterized as the excretion of large volume of urine 3 liters per day or > 50 ml/kg/24 h with a urine osmolarity <300 mOsm/kg [34]. It is a consequence of inadequate synthesis or secretion of (ADH) from the hypothalamus or the posterior pituitary gland (central DI) or insensitivity of the nephron to the action of ADH (nephrogenic DI). The manifestations of these disorders are polyuria, nocturia, and polydipsia

In the emergency department, central DI (neurogenic DI) is commonly seen in patients who have sustained severe head injuries. It is more commonly seen in basilar skull fractures, penetrating brain trauma, and transphenoidal approach to pituitary surgeries. It can also be seen in patients with suprasellar or intrasellar tumors and lung and breast cancer metastatic lesions. Other causes of central DI are listed in Box 26.4.

Box 26.4 Causes of Central Diabetes Insipidus [34]

- Head Trauma
- Primary brain tumors: meningioma, pituitary adenoma, craniopharygioma
- Metastatic cancer: Breast, lung
- Intracerebral hemorrhage
- Postanoxic/ischemic injury
- Infectious etiology
- Idiopathic

Central DI may be categorized as complete or partial depending if the lesion is in the hypothalamic neurohypophyseal tract. The etiologies of central DI are numerous and include CNS infections: meningitis, encephalitis, anoxic brain injuries, granulomatous infiltration: Langerhans cell histiocytosis and congenital disorders. An MRI should be used to locate the anatomic structure that is damaged, either the pituitary stalk or infiltrative lesions [34–36].

Nephrogenic DI is due to insensitivity of the renal collecting tubules to ADH. Common causes of nephrogenic DI are tubulointerstitial disease such as sarcoidosis, sickle cell anemia, medullary sponge kidney disease, drugs: lithium, ofloxacin, hypokalemia, and hypercalcemia. Other causes of nephrogenic DI are listed in Box 26.5 [49, 51].

Box 26.5 Causes of Nephrogenic Diabetes Insipidus [37]

Drugs: Lithium, cisplatin, amphotericin B, aminoglycosides

Postobstructive, uropathy, renal transplant, chronic renal failure

Pyelonephritis, acute tubular necrosis (ATN)

Sickle cell disease

Metabolic derangements (hypercalcemia, hypokalcmia)

Sarcoidosis, amyloidosis

Genetics: V2-receptor mutation, Aquaporin-2 mutation

Psychogenic polydipsia is a form of DI that must be differentiated from CDI and NDI. It is due to medullary interstitial solute wash-out and presents with voiding of large amount of dilute urine.

Clinical Symptoms and Signs of DI

Patients with central DI present with sudden onset of urinary output greater than 3 liters/day, polydipsia, urinary frequency, and nocturia. Patients are found to have mildly elevated serum osmolality, 295 mOsm, elevated sodium concentration 145 mEq/dL, urine osmolality <200, and specific gravity <1.005 and present with severe dehydration if there is limitation of access to water [34 36].

Diagnostic Evaluation of Polyuria [49–51]

To distinguish DI from other forms of polyuria, urinalysis, urine osmolality, specific gravity, electrolytes, and plasma ADH should be sent. If the patient has hypernatremia and inappropriately low urine osmolality or a low ADH level, the diagnosis of diabetes insipidus is made and additional testing is needed only to distinguish between central and nephrogenic DI [36].

The water deprivation test helps to determine the causes of polyuria. The differential diagnosis of polyuria includes psychogenic polydipsia, diabetes mellitus, and drug use: corticosteroids, lithium, or aminoglycosides (see Table 26.13).

For critically ill patients, a provocation water deprivation test is not necessary and can cause hemodynamic instability and hypovolemia. They were generally mild volume depleted and have hypernatremia. If the urine osmolality is low, an inappropriate response than the diagnosis of DI is likely. Measurement of serum AVP at the time of mild hypernatremia in these patients will confirm the diagnosis if serum AVP is low <2 pg/ml or nondetectable. For patients seen in the ED who are critically ill or at risk of hemodynamic instability, a water deprivation test should be performed.

For water deprivation test, under direct supervision, all fluids are withheld and urine samples are collected hourly for measurement of specific gravity and osmolality. Serum electrolytes and osmolality are collected at the start of the test and every 2 h thereafter. When the serum sodium is >145 mEq/dL or urine osmolality is >800 mOsm/kg, this represents a normal response and the test is terminated [35, 36].

In central DI with water deprivation, desmopressin is given and the urine is collected 60 min afterward and the test is terminated. In normal patients, the urine will be maximally concentrated following the water deprivation test with specific gravity of >1.025 or urine osmolality of >700. In CDI, the patient's urine osmolality does not exceed plasma osmolality but they able to increase their urine osmolality by >50% to 100% after the administration of DDAVP. In partial CDI, they are able to concentrate their urine above serum osmolality but only have a partial concentrating response to desmopressin of 50% increase or less. NDI urine osmolality is lesser than plasma osmolality and has no response to DDAVP [14–17, 49–53].

In patients with acute psychogenic polydipsia, they are able to concentrate their urine during the water deprivation test. If there is medullary wash from chronic excessive water ingest, then the response to deprivation and DDAVP are similar to NDI. Determination of serum basal vasopressin concentration will be low in psychogenic polydipsia [50, 51, 53].

Management [49–51]

The drug of choice for central DI is desmopressin or DDAVP (vasopressin analog desamino-D-arginine-8-vasopressin) . See Table 26.14 for treatment of central and nephrogenic DI [33, 35–37].

The usual dose for the treatment of central DI is 1–2 mcg DDAVP q 12 h IV or subcutaneously with careful monitoring of electrolytes and serum osmolarity determinations [35].

Aqueous AVP can be used but has a vasoconstrictive component on V1 receptors and may precipitate ischemic events or cardiac arrhythmias. DDAVP is a V2 receptor analog and has no vasoconstrictive effect, has a T1/2 of 8–12 h, and is safer to use

Table 26.13 Diagnostic approach to polyuria [36]

	Water restrict test Urine osmolality	Desmopressin Urine osmol	Desmopressin test Plasma osmolality	Desmopressin test Urine volume
Primary Polydipsia	↑↑	(–)	(–)	(–)
Central DI	↑	↑↑	↓	↓
Partial DI	↑	↑	↓↓	
Nephrogenic DI	↑	↔	↔	↔

Table 26.14 Drug therapy for diabetes insipidus [33–37]

Disorder	Drugs	Dose
Central DI:	Desmopressin (DDAVP)	5–40 mcg IV
	Aqueous vasopressin	1–4 mcg
	Carbamazepine	200–600 mg daily
	Diabinese	100–500 mg daily
	Clofibrate	500 mg every 6 h
	Thiazide diuretics	25 mg daily
Nephrogenic DI	Amiloride	2.5–10 mg daily
	Thiazide diuretics	25 mg daily
	Indomethacin	20–40 mg BID or TID
	High dose DDAVP may be tried. Usually will not work [33]	10–20 mcg IV [33]

For nephrogenic DI, the most effective treatment is discontinuation of all medication that could be associated with the disorder. Thiazide and sodium restriction are used to treat nephrogenic DI [33, 36].

Thiazide works in DI by producing volume contraction by decreasing GFR and increasing proximal tubule reabsorption of sodium and water. Thiazide also increases the aquaporin expression on the principle cells of the collecting tubules in lithium-induced nephrogenic DI [36].

In the treatment of patients with diabetes insipidus, if there is impaired enteric intake of fluids, then hypotonic iv fluid may be given avoiding rapid correction of hypernatremia and inducing hyponatremia and cerebral edema particularly in neurosurgical postoperative patients [49–51].

References

1. Arlt W, Allolio B. Adrenal insufficiency. Lancet. 2003;361:1881–93.
2. Bornstein SR. Predisposing factors for adrenal insufficiency. N Engl J Med. 2009;360:2328–39.
3. Charmandari E, Nicholaides N, Chrousos GP. Adrenal insufficiency. Lancet. 2014;383:2152–67.
4. Neary N, Neiman L. Adrenal insufficiency: etiology, diagnosis and treatment. Curr Opin Endocrinol Diabetes Obes. 2010;17(3):217–23.
5. Oelkers W. Adrenal insufficiency. N Engl J Med. 1996;335:1206–12.
6. Erichsen MM, Lovas K, Skinningsrud B, et al. Clinical, immunological and genetic features of autoimmune primary adrenal insufficiency: observations from a Norwegian registry. J Clin Endocrinol Metab. 2009;94:4882–90.
7. Kelestimur F. The endocrinology of adrenal tuberculosis: the effects of tuberculosis on the Hypothalamo-pituitary-adrenal axis and adrenocortical function. J Endocrinol Investig. 2004;27:380–6.
8. Nicolaides NC, Charmandari E, Chrousos GP. Adrenal insufficiency. www.endotext.org, http://www.endotext.org/adrenal/adrenal13/adrenalframe13.htm.
9. Grossman A, Naziat A. Adrenal insufficiency July 12, 2012. http://www.endotext.org/adrenal.
10. Paragliola R. Salvatore M Corsello secondary adrenal insufficiency: from the physiopathology to the possible role of modified-release hydrocortisone treatment. Minerva Endocrinol. 2018;43(2):183–97.
11. Mouloudi E, Katsanoulas K, Aslanidis T, Lampiri C, Papageorgiouch C, Tholioti T, Vrochides D. Eosinophilia: an early marker of adrenal insufficiency in critically ill patients with septic shock? Eur J Perioper Med. 2018;17(a):61–70.
12. Beishuizen A, Vermes I, Hylkcnia BS, Haanen C. Relative eosinophilia and functional adrenal insufficiency in critical ill patients. Lancet. 1999;353:1675–6.
13. Diane D, Bancos I. Opioid-induced adrenal insufficiency. Mayo Clin Proc. 2018;93(7):937–44.
14. Stefan R, Allolio B, Arlt W, Barthel A, Don-Wauchope A, Hammer GD, Husebye ES, Merke DP, Murad MH, Stratakis CA, Torpy DJ. Diagnosis and treatment of primary adrenal insufficiency: an endocrine society clinical practice guideline. J Clin Endocrinol Med. 2016;10(2):364–89.
15. Gonzalez-Rodriquez E, Rodriguez-Abreu D. Immune checkpoint inhibitors: review and management of endocrine adverse events. Oncologist. 2016;21:804–16.
16. Higham CE, Olsson-Brown A, et al. Acute management of the endocrine complication of checkpoint inhibitor therapy. 2018. p. 1–7. www.endocrineconnections.org.
17. F Castinetti, Albareli F, et al. French Endocrine Society Guidance on endocrine side effect of immunotherapy. Bioscientifica Ltd; 2019. p. 1–18.
18. Varon J, Acosta P. Handbook of critical and intensive care medicine. 2nd ed. New York: Springer; 2012.
19. DeGoot L, Bartalena L. Thyroid storm. 2012. www.endotext.org/thyroid.
20. Ringel MD. Management of hypothyroidism and hyperthyroidism in the intensive care unit. Crit Care Clin. 2001;17:59–74.
21. Wiersinga WM. Myxedema and coma (severe hypothyroidism). 2012. www.thyroidmanager.org.

22. Klubo-Gwiezdzinska J, Wartosfsky L. Thyroid emergencies. Med Clin N Am. 2012;96:385–403.
23. Mathew V, Misgar R, Ghosh S, et al. Myxedema coma: a new look into an old crisis. J Thyroid Res. 2011;2011:493462.
24. Mills L, Lim S. Identifying and treating thyroid storm and myxedema coma in the emergency department. Emerg Med Pract+ Em Pract Guidel Updat. 2009;11(8):1–22.
25. Gosmanov AR, Gosmanova EO, Dillard-Cannon E. Management of adult diabetes ketoacidosis. Diabetes Metab Syndr Obes: Target Ther. 2014;7:255–64.
26. Golberg PA, Inzucchi SE. Critical issues in endocrinology. Clin Chest Med. 2003;24:583–606.
27. Westerberg DP. Diabetic ketoacidosis evaluation and treatment. Am Fam Physician. 2013;87(5):337–46.
28. Kitabchi AE, Umpierrez GE, Miles JM, Fisher JN. Hyperglycemic crisis in adult patients with diabetes. Diabetes Care. 2009;32(7):1336.
29. Umpierrez GE, Smiley D, Kitabchi AE. Narrative review: ketosis-prone type 2 diabetes mellitus. Ann Intern Med. 2006;144:350–7.
30. Nematollahi LR, Kitabchi AE. Hyperglycemia crises: diabetic ketoacidosis (DKA), and hyperglycemic hyperosmolar state (HHS). 2012. p. 1–43. www.endotext.org/diabtebets.
31. Joint British Societies Inpatient Care Group. The management of ketoacidosis in adults. 2nd ed. 2013. p. 1–44. http://www.diabetologists-abcd.org.uk/JBDS/JBDS.htm
32. Laine C, Turner BJ, Williams S. In the clinic diabetic ketoacidosis. Ann Intern Med. 2010;152:ITCH1.
33. Feingold KR, Anawalt B, Boyce A, et al., editors. South Dartmouth (MA): MDText.com, Inc.; 2000.
34. Peters AL, Buschur EO, Buse JB, Cohan P, Diner JC, Hirsch IB. Euglycemic diabetic ketoacidosis: potential complication of treatment with sodium-glucose cotransporter 2 inhibition diabetes care. Diabetes Care. 2015;38(9):1687–93.
35. US Food and Drug Administration Communication. FDA warns that SDLT2 inhibitors for diabetes may result in serious condition too much acid in the blood. Besthesda: US.FDA; 2016.
36. Chou YM, Seak CJ, Goh ZN, Seak JC, Seak CK, Lin CC. Euglycemic diabetes ketoacidosis caused by dapagliflozin. Medicine. 2018;97:25e.
37. Handelsman Y, et al. American Association of Clinical Endocrinologists and American College of Endocrinology position statement on the association of SGLT-2 inhibitors and diabetic ketoacidosis. Endocr Pract. 2016;22(6):753–62.
38. Qiu H, Novikov A, Vallon V. Ketosis and diabetic ketoacidosis in response to SGLT2 inhibitors: basic mechanisms and therapeutic perspectives. Diabetes/Metab Res Rev. 2017;33(5):e2886.
39. Watts W, Edge J. How can cerebral edema during treatment of diabetic ketoacidosis be avoided? Pediatr Diabetes. 2014;15:271–6.
40. Chou YM, Seak CJ, ZNL G, Seak JC, Seak CK, Lin CC. Euglycemic diabetic ketoacidosis caused by dapagliflozin: a case report. Medicine (Baltimore). 2018;97(25):e11056.
41. Rosenstock J, Ferrannini E. Euglycemic diabetic ketoacidosis: a predictable, detectable, and preventable safety concern with SGLT2 inhibitors. Diabetes Care. 2015;38:1638–42.
42. Yu X, Zhang S, Zhang L. Newer perspectives of mechanisms for euglycemic diabetic ketoacidosis. Int J Endocrinol Hindawi. 2018;2018:1–8.
43. Klein-Schwartz W, Stassinos G, Ishister G. Treatment of sulfonylurea and insulin overdose. Br J Clin Pharmacol. 2016;8(3):496–504.
44. Le Roith D. Tumor-induced hypoglycemia. N Engl J Med. 1999;341:757–8.
45. Desimone M, Weinstock RS. Hypoglycemia. 2012. 1–6. www.endotext.org.
46. Hanna Amir Hypoglycemic Disorders. 2003:3. www.endocrinologyrounds.ca.
47. Service FJ. Hypoglycemic disorders. N Engl J Med. 1995;332:1144–51.
48. Agarwal A, Singula S, Agarwal N, Kumar A. Approach to as case of hypoglycemia. J Indian Acad Clin Med. 2007;8(1):12–22.
49. Khardori R, Griffing G. www.emedicine.medscape.com.
50. Makaryus A, McFarlane S. Diabetes insipidus: diagnosis and treatment of a complex disease. Cleve Clin J Med. 2006;73(1):65–71.
51. Saifan C, Nasi R, Metha S, Sharma P, Acharya P, Perrera I. Review article diabetes insipidus: a challenging diagnosis with new drug therapies. ISRN Nephrol. 2013;2013:797620.
52. Sands J, Bichet D. Nephrogenic diabetes insipidus. Ann Intern Med. 2006;144:186–94.
53. Shapiro M, Weiss J. Diabetes insipidus. A review. J Diabetes Metab. 2012;S:8.

Environmental Emergencies

27

Jason Cohen and Evie Marcolini

Anaphylaxis

First described in dogs repeatedly injected with sea anemone toxin, anaphylaxis and anaphylactoid reactions are one of the few medical conditions that can progress from onset to death in minutes. There is no universally agreed-upon clinical definition for anaphylaxis. Fortunately, the precise definition is not necessary for treatment. The European Academy of Allergology and Clinical Immunology Nomenclature Committee has proposed a rather general definition: "Anaphylaxis is a severe, life-threatening, generalized or systemic hypersensitivity reaction" [1].

Anaphylactic and anaphylactoid reactions represent life-threatening medical emergencies involving multiple organ systems. Activation of pathways leading to anaphylaxis and anaphylactoid reactions is from innumerable mediators. Regardless of the type of mediator, they cause basophil and mast cell activation leading to multiple physiologic alterations. These alterations can change vascular permeability and smooth muscle tone. Activation of inflammatory cells, via positive feedback cycles, leads to continued recruitment of inflammatory mediators and upregulation of the inflammatory cascade.

Anaphylaxis is a type I hypersensitivity, mediated by IgE bound to mast cells or basophils leading to release of cytokines such as histamine, leukotrienes, TNF, and others. *Anaphylactoid* reactions, however, are caused by direct mast cell activation without IgE as a mediator. There is, however, the same degranulation and cytokine release as with anaphylaxis. Thus, the clinical effects and subsequent treatments can be considered the same. The main difference is the fact that direct activation of mast cells in anaphylactoid reactions does not require prior exposure (and thus sensitization) to the allergen [2].

Onset of symptoms of anaphylactic-type reactions can be immediate to as much as an hour after exposure. Most commonly, dermatologic and gastrointestinal manifestations occur. These can include urticaria and angioedema, nausea, vomiting, and/or diarrhea. When manifestations are most severe, bronchospasm or upper airway angioedema may lead to respiratory failure. Shock may be present due to vasodilatation and capillary leak or direct myocardial suppression.

There is very little published on epidemiology of anaphylaxis, but expert consensus estimates the frequency to be approximately 50–2000 cases per 100,000 persons or a lifetime prevalence ranging from 0.05% to 2.0%, most frequently

J. Cohen
Boston MedFlight, Bedford, MA, USA

E. Marcolini (✉)
Departments of Emergency Medicine and Neurology, Divisions of Neurocritical Care and Emergency Neurology and Surgical Critical Care, SkyHealth Critical Care, Yale University School of Medicine, New Haven, CT, USA

© Springer Nature Switzerland AG 2020

J. R. Shiber, S. D. Weingart (eds.), *Emergency Department Critical Care*,
https://doi.org/10.1007/978-3-030-28794-8_27

affecting children and adolescents [3]. Rates of occurrence seem to be increasing, especially in this higher risk population. Accurate estimates of population incidence are very difficult due to underreporting, miscoding, and lack of a clear diagnostic standard. Approximately 1% of all emergency department visits in the United States are due to anaphylaxis and account for over 1500 deaths per year [4].

Thankfully, overall prognosis is good – with greater than 99% survival – though there is likely underreporting of fatalities due to nonspecific autopsy findings and potential lack of detailed peri-event details. Those at greatest risk for death are patients with previous history of reactive airway disease, particularly poorly controlled asthmatics [5]. Additional risk factors for severe disease include infancy, old age, and comorbid illness such as cardiovascular disease, mastocytosis, or severe atopy [6]. Based on published case series, it appears that when death occurs it develops early in the onset of illness, usually within 30 minutes, before reaching medical care [7].

Presentation

Patients presenting with anaphylaxis develop sudden (usually within minutes) symptom complex with potential rapid development of life-threatening respiratory or cardiovascular distress. These symptoms are usually accompanied by skin and/or mucosal changes, though upward of 20% of anaphylaxis occurs without "classic" allergic symptoms (i.e., urticaria). This is particularly true when the reaction is caused by ingested allergens [8].

Anaphylaxis and anaphylactoid reactions affect almost every organ system (See Table 27.1). Ultimately, it is cardiovascular and respiratory involvement that leads to the demise of patients if not recognized and treated urgently. A "foreign body" sensation in the throat can quickly progress to complete airway occlusion and respiratory collapse. Shock due to diminished venous return (vasodilation and volume contraction) may be preceded by a transient *increase in cardiac output* due to initial compensation. Subsequently, hemodynamic parameters will demonstrate decreased systemic vascular resistance, stroke volume, wedge pressure, and central venous pressure.

Table 27.1 Clinical effects of anaphylaxis and anaphylactoid reactions

Organ group	Presentation
Airway/breathing	Airway swelling/angioedema of airway Rhinorrhea/sneezing Hoarseness Stridor Dyspnea Wheezing Hypoxia Respiratory arrest Severe bronchospasm/status asthmaticus
Circulatory (45%)	Pale/clammy Tachycardia Hypotension Diminished level of consciousness Myocardial ischemia/ECG abnormality Cardiac arrest
Skin/mucosal change (80–90%)	May be just skin, just mucosa, or both Erythema Urticaria/hives Angioedema Pruritis Morbiliform rash
Gastrointestinal (45%)	Nausea Vomiting Diarrhea Cramping
Nervous system	Headache Dizziness Confusion Altered mental status

Approach

As with treatment of all acute life-threatening diseases, a systematic approach addressing each of the affected organ groups is appropriate. The ABCD approach utilized during cardiac arrest resuscitation addresses these and is familiar to most, if not all, healthcare practitioners. Treatment for all age groups is identical when suspicion for anaphylaxis is entertained. Basic cardiorespiratory monitoring should be in place including pulse-oximetry, noninvasive blood pressure monitoring, and 3-lead electrocardiographic tracings. If possible, remove the offending agent and decontaminate as appropriate (e.g., remove hymenoptera stinger, stop infusion, etc.). Further treatment will be dictated by clinical presentation.

Airway

For very mild upper respiratory distress, a trial of nebulized racemic epinephrine can be considered with close monitoring. It is important to recognize the potential for very rapid development of airway obstruction and possible need for advanced airway interventions. If airway swelling progresses beyond minimal complaints, endotracheal intubation should be seriously considered prior to complete obstruction. This should be performed by the most experienced provider utilizing adjuncts that improve first pass success in challenging airways (i.e., video laryngoscope, gum-elastic bougie, etc...) as minor irritation of an already inflamed glottis can rapidly progress to complete obstruction. Patients often attempt to compensate for airway narrowing via posture and accessory muscle usage. This compensation is abolished with typical rapid sequence intubation, potentially causing progression from airway narrowing to obstruction. Awake intubation utilizing sedation that maintains airway reflexes should be strongly considered (i.e., ketamine). Maintaining surgical airway equipment at bedside is also recommended with a low threshold for cricothyroidotomy.

Epinephrine

Epinephrine is considered the primary first-line, and most-important, treatment for anaphylaxis. Despite absence of randomized controlled trials (RCTs) proving benefit, its utility has physiologic plausibility with multiple reports of reversal of respiratory distress and anaphylactic shock.

Epinephrine affects both alpha and beta adrenergic receptors – addressing both respiratory and cardiovascular manifestations of anaphylaxis. Mediated via peripheral alpha adrenergic receptor agonism, reversal of vascular dilation occurs with apparent decrease in formation of perivascular edema. Direct beta-receptor agonism leads to bronchial relaxation, increased myocardial inotropy, and suppressed release of histamine and leukotrienes. Epinephrine seems to have its greatest effect on anaphylaxis the earlier it is given. This may be due to additional Beta-2 inhibitory receptors on MAST cells, allowing epinephrine to limit the severity of IgE-mediated reactions as well [9]. Adverse effects from epinephrine are extremely rare when given intra-muscularly; however, incidence of these effects increases when dosed intravenously.

Increased adverse effects from intravenous epinephrine, and varying unpredictable absorption from subcutaneous and inhaled delivery, makes intramuscular injection the preferred route; at least during the initial resuscitation. The recommended dosing of epinephrine is without the guidance of evidence. Recommendations are based on consensus standard as to what is safe and practical to draw up in an emergency (Table 27.2). This dosing should be repeated up to every 5 minutes as clinically indicated.

Continuous intravenous epinephrine following intramuscular dosing is a reasonable approach to manage ongoing anaphylactic reaction in patients who require repeated doses of IM epinephrine. Dosing ranges between 5 mcg/min and 15 mcg/min should be initiated and titrated to effect. Due to risks of harmful side effects, intravenous *bolus* dosing cannot be recommended for the routine management of patients who have a spontaneous perfusing cardiac rhythm. These side effects

Table 27.2 Volume dose of intramuscular epinephrine for anaphylaxis

Patient age	Volume of IM epinephrine at 1:1000 concentration
>12 years	0.5 ml
6–12 years	0.3 ml
>6 months–6 years	0.15 ml
<6 months	0.15 ml

include life-threatening hypertension, tachycardia, and myocardial ischemia. If the decision to use bolus dosing of intravenous epinephrine is made, repeated 50 mcg bolus (0.5 ml of 1:10,000) dosing should be utilized. The more dilute 1:10,000 concentration allows a little more of a safety margin as compared to the 1:1000 in intravenous dosing. While myocardial ischemia has been reported after using epinephrine, it should not be withheld for fear of increasing myocardial demand [6]. Intravenous bolus dosing in children is highly discouraged except when used by very experienced providers.

Bronchodilators

As acute asthma exacerbations can present very similarly to anaphylaxis, bronchodilators such as albuterol have a role in the management of both conditions. If clinically significant bronchospasm persists despite epinephrine and inhaled bronchodilators, an infusion of aminophyline can be considered. Intravenous magnesium sulfate may cause vasodilation and potentially exacerbate the shock state.

Intravenous Fluids

When coupled with vasodilation, capillary leak with intravascular fluid loss may lead to profound shock requiring large volume fluid resuscitation. There is no evidence supporting choice of one type of fluid over another – with the caveat that it is possible that some colloidal fluids may precipitate anaphylactic reactions. Intravenous or intraosseous access is appropriate to gain access to the intravascular space, but establishment of vascular access should not delay administration of intramuscular epinephrine.

Antihistamine

Evidence supporting use of antihistamines is weak, but also makes physiologic sense. A Cochrane review from 2007 was unable to recommend for or against the utility of antihistamines [10]. Antihistamines that antagonize H1 receptors theoretically can reduce histamine-mediated bronchospasm and vasodilation. Both H1 and H2 receptor antagonists may decrease skin manifestations of anaphylaxis; however they have NOT been clinically demonstrated to have any impact on life-threatening manifestations. Thus, they are of much lower priority when caring for these patients. It is recommended to administer 1 mg/kg (up to 50 mg) of diphenhydramine intravenously for patients with cutaneous manifestations. Ranitidine is an optional adjunct to the diphenhydramine [11].

Steroids

There is weak evidence supporting corticosteroids in preventing progression of, or shortening, anaphylactic reactions *following* initial resuscitation. Similar to antihistamines, a 2010 Cochrane review found no convincing benefit for glucocorticoids [12].The efficacy of early corticosteroids in treatment of asthmatic bronchoconstriction has been proven with some similar pathophysiology and many similar mediators to anaphylaxis. However, corticosteroids are not effective in the initial manifestations of anaphylactic reactions. Appropriate dosing ranges from 100 mg to250 mg of hydrocortisone equivalent every 6 hours. Intravenous dosing is recommended as enteral absorption cannot be guaranteed in shock or with potential mucosal edema [12].

Cardiac Drugs

Epinephrine is the first-line treatment for the treatment of anaphylaxis. Additionally, animal studies and case reports have demonstrated possible utility of other vasopressors and inotropes as rescue agents should epinephrine fail to have its desired effect. Glucagon is an option in patients refractory to epinephrine that are suspected of taking beta-blockers. Glucagon is thought to have receptors separate from the known/defined adrenergic receptors. Activation of this receptor appears to stimulate increased intracellular cAMP, promoting chronotropy and inotropy [13]. Glucagon is administered as a 1–5 mg bolus followed by a continuous infusion of 1–5 mg/hour.

Additional vasopressor infusions (including norepinephrine and dopamine) should be considered when vasodilation is refractory to epinephrine and glucagon therapy. Recently, vasopressin has also been added to the armamentarium to combat catecholamine-resistant vasodilation in anaphylaxis [14].

Diagnosis

While laboratory diagnosis of anaphylaxis is theoretically possible with serial-timed tryptase measurements, this is impractical and unavailable in the majority of emergency departments. This makes the diagnosis of anaphylaxis or anaphylactoid reactions a clinical one based on history and clinical findings. Tryptase is rapidly released from degranulating mast cells and quickly cleared. The peak of tryptase is approximately 1–2 hours after onset with a half-life of less than 2 hours. Sampling should occur after resuscitation has started and should not interfere with lifesaving therapy. Serum tryptase levels are not uniformly elevated in food-related anaphylaxis and thus should be interpreted with caution. Standard laboratory testing (i.e., blood count, metabolic panel) is not useful in the diagnosis of anaphylaxis [11].

Due to the need to make a clinical diagnosis at the bedside, and multisystem involvement of anaphylaxis and anaphylactoid reactions, it is necessary to keep a broad differential when evaluating these patients. While not always clear, an exposure history to an allergen of high risk may help make the diagnosis as well. The most commonly responsible agent is food, followed by medications, and insect bites [2, 8]. Disturbingly, there are increasing reports of reactions to medical treatments – including β-lactam antibiotics (40% medication-related reactions), latex, propofol, iodinated radiocontrast, nonsteroidal anti-inflammatory medication, and protamine (Moneret-Vautrin [15]). There is also a significant minority of cases without any identifiable trigger. So-called idiopathic reactions account for 6–27% of reported anaphylaxis/anaphylactoid reactions and may lead to diagnostic uncertainty on presentation [16, 17].

Follow-Up

Following resolution of anaphylaxis and its sequelae, consideration should be given to continued corticosteroid and antihistamine treatment for at least 3 days. Early recurrence of symptoms after complete resolution has been described (biphasic response) in 1–20% of patients with anaphylaxis. There is no reliable method to determine which patients are at risk for a biphasic response [18]. After all symptoms of anaphylaxis have resolved, it is reasonable to maintain the patient in a monitored setting for at least 24 hours.

On discharge from the hospital, all patients with anaphylaxis should be discharged with an epinephrine auto-injector along with education on when and how to use the device.

Heat-Related Injuries

The healthy human body varies its temperature daily by only +/−0.6 °C, this despite an average metabolic generation of over 1 °C/hour at rest or ten times that during strenuous activity [19]. The human thermoregulatory system attempts to control the transfer of this heat energy to the environment in order to maintain temperature within a homeostatic range. When this system fails or is overwhelmed, life-threatening injury can result.

Thermal energy (heat) is transferred to the environment in several ways—*radiation*, *evaporation*, *conduction*, and *convection*. Radiation is the primary method (60%) for heat transfer in the normal human while in conditions cooler than body temperature. This is due to the emission of infrared radiation from the skin [20]. Conduction accounts for another 15% of thermal energy loss. Conduction requires the presence of an object of lower temperature to be in contact with the body.

The energy transfer involves kinetic energy from molecules from a higher energy state (warmer) moving to a lower state (cooler). Finally, convection occurs when cool air replaces the warm layer of air that surrounds our skin – such as from wind. This process also occurs with blood flow just below the surface of the skin at the microvascular level. Evaporation, whereby water or sweat transforms from liquid phase to gaseous phase, accounts for another 20% of heat loss in temperate environments – primarily through insensible losses of breathing. As environmental temperatures increase above body temperature, evaporation becomes the primary method to dissipate heat energy. When these processes are unable to offload the thermal energy created by metabolism, hyperthermia results. As body temperature increases, symptoms as mild as "prickly heat" can progress to potentially fatal heat-related illness.

The hypothalamus is the body's thermostat – collecting input from sensors in the skin, muscles, and spinal cord. Integration of these signals triggers behavioral and physiologic changes to affect the amount and method of heat transfer to the environment. Blood flow to the skin can be increased (to over 8 liters/min), dilation of the peripheral venous system, and activation of sweat glands all influence this transfer. The success of these modalities in decreasing temperature depends on the condition of the person's skin and lungs along with ambient climate. Additionally, acclimatization can affect this transfer – as someone who has acclimated to hot environments for 7–10 days can produce 2–3 liters of sweat/hour releasing over 1700 kcals of heat per hour. In contrast, someone who has not acclimated may only produce 1 liter/hour. Acclimatization occurs as the hypothalamus develops a new, lower, threshold to start sweating along with increased amounts of sweat produced [21].

The most common heat-related injury presenting to the emergency department is heat exhaustion. Heat exhaustion presents as dehydration/volume depletion without significant aberration of hemodynamic or neurologic indices. Often, patients present with myalgias and flu-like complaints with mild hyperthermia (<39 °C). There is usually an aberrant sodium level – either hyponatremia (from volume replacement with plain water) or hypernatremia (from volume depletion from sweating). This condition only requires volume replacement and supportive care. When hemodynamic or neurologic impairment develops, the condition is defined as *heatstroke*.

Heatstroke is the most severe of heat-related illnesses and is defined as documented temperature greater than 41.1 °C or greater than 40.6 °C with neurologic impairment or anhidrosis [20]. The exact temperature at which an individual suffers neuro- or cardiovascular collapse varies based on comorbid conditions, medications, and other factors. Full recovery has been reported in temperatures as high as 46 °C, and death has been experienced at much lower temperatures. Heatstroke can be further classified into exertional and non-exertional (or classic) heatstroke. Exertional heatstroke (EHS) is typically found in young patients engaged in strenuous activity in a hot environment, while non-exertional heatstroke (NEHS) is typically in the extremes of age or with comorbid conditions that impair normal thermoregulatory response in environments of prolonged elevated temperatures – characteristic of heat waves. Cocaine-associated NEHS has also become an increasingly important contributor to heat wave lethality. Both EHS and NEHS are associated with high morbidity and are leading causes of mortality when there is a sustained, and uncharacteristic, elevation in climate temperatures. In the 2003 heat wave that affected Europe, there were over 14,800 victims of heatstroke in France alone [22, 23]. As climate change progresses, it can be assumed that visits to the emergency department for this condition will continue to increase.

Presentation

Heatstroke, on a subcellular level, appears very similar to other uncontrolled inflammatory states within the body. There is activation of inflammatory cytokines, interleukins, and heat shock protein. Translocation of lipopolysaccharides from the intestines occurs along with activation of coagulation cascades, potentially leading to regional, and later systemic microvascular malperfusion may cause or worsen shock and the inflammatory state. There appears to be a direct relationship between degree and duration of temperature elevation and the amount of injury that is produced [24].

The clinical history of exertional heatstroke is usually self-apparent; however the presentation of non-exertional heatstroke may be more challenging with nonspecific findings before onset of severe illness as the thermoregulatory system fails. Typically, there is irritability or alteration in mental status prior to onset of coma. Early recognition of those at increased risk for heatstroke is of important in order to change the trajectory of the illness. In addition to the extremes of age and comorbid conditions previously mentioned, those living without access to air conditioning (i.e., lower socioeconomic standing) or who are unable to compensate for increased heat due to occupation (fire-fighters, soldiers, industrial workers in protective gear) are also at increased risk.

Unchecked, heatstroke impacts a myriad of body systems. As previously noted, the neurologic system seems to be the first system affected in a clinically apparent manner. Hyperpyrexia can lead to direct cell death of neurons, primarily affecting the Purkinje cells within the cerebellum. Additionally, cerebral edema is common with small vessel hemorrhage. In addition to the acute decrease in mental status one would expect long-term effects on survivors due to these changes.

Hypotension is common, reflecting both volume depletion and peripheral vasodilation. Additionally, cardiac myocytes can be directly injured by elevated core temperatures leading to myocardial depression – a condition exacerbated by hypoperfusion. Most commonly, sinus tachycardia is present on electrocardiogram with QTc prolongation also noted (up to 60%) [25].

Acute Kidney Injury (AKI) is found in nearly all heatstroke patients, though acute renal failure requiring renal replacement therapy (RRT) is much less common. The need for RRT is 5–6 times more common with exertional heatstroke – likely due to increased muscle breakdown and rhabdomyolysis associated with strenuous exertion. This rhabdomyolysis may be severe, with associated profound hyperkalemia requiring emergent measures to prevent life-threatening arrhythmias [26]. Additionally, compartment syndromes may develop as muscles swell with exertion in conjunction with decreased arterial perfusion pressure.

On laboratory evaluation, dehydration is common (especially with exertional heatstroke) with laboratory values reflecting this; such as an elevated blood urea nitrogen and creatinine or hemo-concentration. In addition to the large volumes of fluid that are lost with sweating; sodium, potassium, and magnesium can also be depleted early on in the clinical course [26]. Significant muscle damage can ensue due to direct heat injury and lack of adequate perfusion. Rhabdomyolysis may occur and if significant can cause hyperkalemia as cells are lysed. Hypophosphatemia and hypocalcemia may also occur with the muscle injury [27]. Liver injury (as defined by elevation in liver enzymes) has been consistently described in heatstroke. Aspartate aminotransferase (AST) and alanine aminotransferase (ALT) often peak in the tens of thousands most commonly within the first 2–3 days but may be seen 2–3 weeks following insult. Jaundice may also occur. Creatinine kinase will be elevated with the presence of rhabdomyolysis with levels often in the 100,000's due to muscle necrosis. Urine myoglobin will be present as muscle cells lyse – this is detected with the presence of blood on urine dipstick with subsequent lack of red blood cells on microscopic evaluation. On arterial blood gas evaluation (ABG), a mixed metabolic acidosis and respiratory alkalosis is most commonly encountered. The acidosis would be expected from volume depletion and malperfusion while hyperthermia may lead to primary hyperventilation and alkalosis. It is important to correct the laboratory ABG values with correct temperature coefficients; as temperature impacts gas solubility. Both dissolved oxygen and carbon dioxide (PaO_2 and $PaCO_2$) will be higher than reflected on uncorrected samples. Evidence of Disseminated Intravascular Coagulation is occasionally found – ranging from asymptomatic to fulminant bleeding. The finding of DIC portends a very poor outcome with one study showing a 90% association with developing Acute Respiratory Distress Syndrome and subsequent mortality of 75% [28].

Approach

The primary goal in the treatment of heatstroke is to decrease the body temperature as quickly as possible while supporting the patient's cardiovascular system. Retrospective reviews of heat wave epidemics show that the majority of deaths occur shortly after the onset of hyperthermia – after the overwhelming of the body's compensatory mechanisms. Those that do not succumb to the cardiovascular collapse associated with the hyperthermia are at risk for developing multiorgan system failure and progressing to profound neurologic impairment and/or death [22, 29]. Survival has an inverse relationship with both duration and level of temperature elevation; the duration of hyperpyrexia has the greatest impact on outcome [30].

Removal of heat from the body should begin immediately once heatstroke is suspected, prior to initiation of transport if possible. There are multiple methods to attempt to cool the victim of heatstroke. The various modalities described take advantage of the thermal transfer principles previously described – *radiation*, *evaporation*, *conduction*, and *convection*. Throughout treatment, it is recommended to monitor continuous core temperature with a target 38.5–39 °C. We recommend a temperature decrement target of 0.2 °C/min. Once the measured temperature is at target, cooling measures should cease as the body will usually continue to cool another 1°–2 °C. Core temperature should be monitored via rectal, bladder, or esophageal probe as less invasive means are not reliable during active cooling.

The most rapid type of cooling is via conduction through immersion in ice water bath coupled with continuous massage of the skin and soft tissues of the extremities to promote local blood flow by inhibiting local vascoconstriction. This method has been shown to be the most efficient in terms of time to target temperature – and is recommended primarily for exertional heatstroke, when the patient is otherwise healthy, cooperative, and concerns for close hemodynamic monitoring are not necessary. Immersion of patients suffering from classic NEHS obtained rapid cooling, but the process was poorly tolerated and was associated with increased complications and death [24]. There have also been case reports of commercial external-cooling devices developed for post-cardiac arrest temperature management being used for treatment of heatstroke successfully [31].

Much more practical and familiar, utilization of evaporation and convection via wetting the patient and application of fans is very common. This method produces temperature control almost as fast as the immersion method, with the benefit of ability for standard hemodynamic monitoring. It is necessary to remove all of the patients clothing and intermittently spray the body with warm water while a fan continuously blows air across the person to encourage evaporation. It is not unreasonable to place ice-packs in the axilla and groin during this procedure to augment heat removal. Even helicopter rotor-wash has been used to facilitate this form of evaporative cooling in large groups suffering with this condition [32].

Other described cooling techniques include lavage of various body cavities with cooled fluids (gastric, peritoneal, thoracic, and rectal), though none have proven equal to the previously described evaporative or immersion techniques. Finally, ECMO and or cardiopulmonary bypass have been suggested as possible salvage therapy for the most severe cases.

Medication Management

Typical anti-pyretics (acetaminophen, ibuprofen, etc...) act via blockade of pyrogen activity on the hypothalamic set-point. As patients with heatstroke are hyperthermic due to inability to rid the body of excess heat, rather than alteration in the hypothalamic response, these medications have no role. They may, however, cause harm to already stressed or injured kidneys, livers, or coagulation systems.

Dantrolene has been found efficacious to treat anesthesia-induced malignant hyperthermia; however, it has been shown to be not helpful in animal models of heatstroke [33]. Neuroleptic medications – specifically chlorpromazine (10–50 mg IV every 6 hours) – historically had been used to treat shivering and resultant thermogenesis. As these medications carry multiple potential deleterious side effects including lowering of the seizure threshold and anticholinergic effects, we do not recommend their use. Benzodiazepines are a preferred agent to control shivering and treatment of any associated seizures. If shivering is refractory to benzodiazepines, neuromuscular blockade (with mechanical ventilation if not already started) should strongly be considered.

Rehydration and intravascular volume repletion should be individualized. Dehydration might not be as profound in non-exertional heatstroke but is usually profound in exertional heatstroke. Concomitant hypotension may be due to volume depletion, vasodilation, or primary cardiac dysfunction. While all patients with heatstroke should receive some intravenous fluid therapy, it is important to customize based on physiologic conditions. Patients who do not have hemodynamic improvement from initial cooling may benefit from more invasive monitoring. While there are multiple methods to assess hemodynamic status, measurement and trending of these hemodynamic values can serve to individualize therapy based on the underlying etiology. In general strictly alpha-adrenergic medications should be avoided due to their peripheral vasoconstriction that may interfere with heat energy transfer.

As previously described, rhabdomyolysis is a common complication of heatstroke – especially exertional heatstroke. When rhabomyolysis causes kidney injury, it becomes a major cause of patient morbidity. Prevention includes replacement of appropriate intravascular volume and reestablishment of adequate perfusion. Monitoring and correction of concomitant metabolic disturbances is crucial along with maintenance of adequate urinary output (1–3 ml/kg/hr). A small dose of mannitol (200–500 mg/kg) may be helpful to patients developing rhabdomyolysis with early oliguria after ensuring adequate intravascular volume. Mannitol may increase urinary blood flow and thus glomerular filtration rate. It is also hypothesized to be a free-radical scavenger thus decreasing damage to the renal tubules. If renal failure does occur, renal replacement therapy (e.g., hemodialysis) is usually necessary to control metabolic derangements, particularly the acidemia and hyperkalemia that go along with rhabdomyolysis. Utilization of sodium bicarbonate infusions with targeted alkalinization of the urine to a pH of 7.5–8.0 is also anecdotally reported to prevent the onset of acute kidney injury. However, this has been shown to be **not** helpful, and has **not** been shown to decrease need for renal replacement [34]. Thus we recommend reserving sodium bicarbonate infusions for correction of metabolic derangements, rather than for rhabdomyolysis without metabolic complication.

Following cooling and normalization of metabolic and hemodynamic indexes, these patients should be monitored for several days. As previously mentioned, cooling efforts should be discontinued when core temperature reaches 38.5–39.0 °C to avoid overshooting. Invasive temperature monitoring should continue for several days, as rebound hyperthermia may occur hours later and patients may be thermally unstable for days.

Accidental Hypothermia

Cold injury runs the gamut from nonfreezing injury to accidental hypothermia. The cases that present in the critical care setting will most likely be those of accidental hypothermia. These patients, even in the most severe circumstances, can survive with meticulous attention to clinical details. Hypothermia has been recognized as far back as 492 BC when the Persian general, Mardonios, describes men who died "by reason of cold" [35]. The diagnosis would not be described until the clinical mercury thermometer was developed in 1714 by Dr. Farenheit [36]. Even so, it took until 1866 to develop a thermometer that could take a clinical temperature in less than 5 minutes [37].

Accidental hypothermia can be acute or subacute, and can be associated with multiple other complicating factors, including trauma, toxins, and extremes of age. In the modern world, most accidental hypothermia occurs in urban settings, averaging 600 deaths annually in the United States. Half of these fatalities occur in patients over 65 years old. Mortality estimates can reach over 50 percent, depending on associated comorbidities and situational events [38]. The most common etiology of accidental hypothermia in a young healthy person is alcohol intoxication. Accidental hypothermia, by definition, includes those with core body temperatures less than 35 °C and can be further differentiated by severity into mild (32–35 °C), moderate (28–32 °C), and severe (less than 28 °C) [39].

The effects of hypothermia manifest in multiple organ systems, including cardiovascular, nervous, respiratory, hematologic, and renal. While an understanding of the cardiovascular effects is the most likely factor that can affect outcome; a focus on the optimization of the nervous system, helps determine quality of life upon recovery.

In the initial stage of hypothermia, cold stress, myocardial oxygen consumption is increased due to increased heart rate and afterload due to peripheral vasoconstriction. As core temperature continues to drop, pacemaker cells develop much slower depolarization; and the PR, QRS and QTc intervals become prolonged. This leads to a relative bradycardia and subsequent decreased cardiac output. Since it is the temperature affecting the pacer cells, atropine has no therapeutic effect. Cardiac slowing results in conduction time potentially outliving absolute refractory time, causing a reentrant rhythm and ultimately ventricular fibrillation. The classic ECG finding of J wave or Osborn wave, described in 1938, is found in roughly 80% of hypothermic patients, and best seen in leads II and V_6; but eventually develops in the precordial leads with further temperature drop [40].

Cardiac arrhythmia typically starts occurring at 29 °C, with degeneration into ventricular fibrillation and asystole at 20 °C [41]. The life-threatening arrhythmias can result from the decreased temperature itself, although other complicating factors can increase the propensity toward arrhythmia, including electrolyte abnormalities, hypovolemia, acid-base problems, mechanical manipulation (movement), sudden vertical positioning, and/or flooding of the myocardium with cold blood upon rewarming.

Afterdrop describes the situation where the patient's core temperature drops despite aggressive rewarming. This is primarily attributed to return of cold blood from the periphery to the core as vasodilation occurs with rewarming. Hypovolemia can worsen afterdrop, as evidenced by profound decreases in mean arterial pressure and peripheral vascular resistance during rewarming [42]. Contributing to the hypovolemic state of the hypothermic patient is a peripheral vasoconstriction resulting in compensatory diuresis.

Cerebral metabolism decreases by 6–10% per degree Celsius below 35 °C, and the brain takes a proportionately larger percentage of blood flow as the body's systems slow down. Cerebrovascular autoregulation remains intact, until core temperature drops below 25 °C, although it may be disrupted by other complicating factors such as trauma. Electroencephalogram (EEG) may not be diagnostic of cerebral dysfunction, as it becomes abnormal below 33 °C, and the abnormalities noted may also be due to other system issues, such as toxins or metabolic [43].

Multiple factors affect the respiratory system in accidental hypothermia. As the core temperature drops, the respiratory rate as well as carbon dioxide production drop, and ultimately the brainstem fails to control ventilation adequately. With lower temperature, the oxyhemoglobin dissociation curve shifts left with associated impaired oxygen release. Balancing this is a reduced oxygen consumption which causes a rightward shift.

Even in therapeutic hypothermia, the most significant infectious risk is pulmonary. This can be seen in accidental hypothermia, as well, as ciliary motility from cold is depressed, secretions can become significant, thoracic compliance is decreased, and respiratory muscles lose strength. These factors can contribute to the development of ARDS in the resuscitation phase and deserve meticulous attention.

Hypothermia results in significant coagulopathy that contributes to morbidity and mortality, as well. Cold temperatures depress clotting factor enzyme function and can cause thrombocytopenia by sequestration and reversible platelet dysfunction. Lab determination of clotting function can be difficult because enzymes deactivated by cold can be reactivated when samples are rewarmed in the lab. Fibrinolysis is also accelerated in hypothermia contributing further to coagulopathy. These mechanisms become significant at core temperatures below 34 °C. The aforementioned cold diuresis can also lead to increased viscosity and decreased rheology of red blood cells [44].

Presentation

Patients who succumb to accidental hypothermia may have comorbid factors that decrease inherent protective mechanisms, such as extremes of age, ethanol or other central nervous system depressants, preexisting infection, or trauma. Even though therapeutic hypothermia has been shown to improve outcome in post-cardiac arrest patients and possibly protective in significant intracranial injury, it is not found to be helpful in patients in shock [45, 46]. Induced hypothermia, by decreasing metabolism, reduces utilization of ATP protecting against its depletion. Uncontrolled accidental hypothermia, however, has been shown to increase mortality in trauma patients and others in hypovolemic shock because of the multiple system effects described above.

While the patient's history and predisposing factors lead to diagnosing hypothermia, certain physical exam findings will substantiate the diagnosis. Altered mental status is common, owing to central nervous system depression, and must be differentiated from other factors such as toxins. Heart sounds may be difficult to auscultate and pulses may be subtle, owing to bradycardia and hypotension. Hyperreflexia may dominate below 35 °C, but hyporeflexia ensues when core temperature drops below 32 °C [47]. Care must be taken to appreciate mechanism and the possibility of other injury, masked by hypothermia. Alcohol is a frequent complicating factor. The hypothermic patient may feel a warming sensation with ingestion of alcohol, but in reality, the alcohol causes cutaneous vasodilation resulting in heat loss through radiation and diminished shivering response. Severely hypothermic patients may exhibit paradoxical undressing due to altered decision-making, which may confound the picture.

Acid-base presentation will be a combination of respiratory acidosis from respiratory depression and metabolic acidosis from a drop in tissue perfusion, increased lactate production, and decreased hepatic metabolism. Cold blood also loses its ability to buffer; and the relative pH drop with increased carbon dioxide levels will double below core temperature of 28 °C [43].

The body's intrinsic protective mechanisms tend to maintain relative stability during the hypothermic phase of accidental hypothermia; during rewarming, however, the risk of instability greatly increases. Electrolytes must be fastidiously monitored and attended to, as they can fluctuate unpredictably during rewarming. Contributing factors include duration of hypothermia, speed of rewarming, and extent of hypothermic diuresis.

Hypokalemia is common, reflecting intracellular shift rather than frank loss. This is more common in chronically hypothermic patients, or those who have had a long duration of hypothermia. Hyperkalemia is not typical, and if observed, should raise index of suspicion for alternate etiologies such as rhabdomyolysis, renal failure, or other causes. Classic electrocardiographic (ECG) indications of hyperkalemia may be masked by hypothermia. As the myocardium is more sensitive to hyperkalemic changes, ventricular fibrillation occurs at levels lower than typical. Sodium, magnesium, and phosphate levels are unpredictably affected by hypothermia. Glucose levels initially may be elevated, due to insulin resistance, but eventually fall as glycogen is depleted. Aggressive surveillance for and treatment of hypoglycemia is critical due to the clear negative effect of hypoglycemia on neuronal cells. Blood urea nitrogen and creatinine are poor markers of volume during severe hypothermia, due to significant fluid shifts during the process of cooling and rewarming [48]. Hematocrit tends to rise with hypothermia because of intravascular fluid shifts and diuresis. Leukocytes may be artificially low due to bone marrow suppression and sequestration in the liver, spleen, and gut.

Approach

Resuscitation and rewarming of severely hypothermic patient ideally starts in the field. The decision to resuscitate should take into consideration evidence of lethal injuries such as severe trauma or asphyxia. Recognizing that pulses may be difficult to palpate due to bradycardia, hypotension, and cold environment, it is best to determine viability with more dependable markers of mortality, such as temperature below 12 °C or potassium above 12. The lowest temperature that a patient has successfully been resuscitated from is 20 °C [49]. ECG may be helpful, but if not available, chest compressions need careful consideration as rough handling can precipitate ventricular fibrillation and subsequent asystole. Defibrillation is rarely useful below 30 °C [49]. If a hypothermic patient is rescued from submersion, care must be taken to keep the patient supine until adequate resuscitation and rewarming has occurred, to reduce the risk of hypotension from relative vasodilation as the hydrostatic pressure from submersion is lost. Rewarming in the field is not typically a feasible option; best practice is to facilitate proper packaging with heated ventilation or external heat packs within a vapor barrier layer in order to insulate the patient from further heat loss.

In the emergency department, close attention to vital signs, including accurate core temperature monitoring is paramount. Esophageal temperature probes are the most accurate, although may not be practical, if the patient is not intubated. Rectal probes are the next best option, although with limitations of a time lag behind the rewarming trend in the brain and core, as well as the possibility of inaccuracy due to the presence of cold feces. Bladder temperatures will be unreliable and influenced by temperature of possible lavage fluids.

If central venous access is required, best location is femoral, to prevent myocardial irritation. Near-infrared spectroscopy may be helpful to increase the accuracy of pulse oximetry, which may be limited by vasoconstriction. Blood work is obtained, with consideration for the limitations described above and basic imaging to assess for significant traumatic injuries is completed.

Fluid administration is most likely necessary during resuscitation of the hypothermic patient. Ringer's lactate should be avoided since hepatic function is compromised and will not be able to metabolize lactate. As volume resuscitation progresses, biologic markers should include clinical signs such as pulmonary rales and S3 cardiac gallop, as laboratory values will be skewed for many of the reasons described above. Compartment syndrome is possible especially when frostbite is part of the clinical picture.

Rewarming

Depending on the core temperature, there are three options for rewarming: passive external, active external, and active core. Healthy patients with mild hypothermia can be passively rewarmed. This consists of drying the patient, blocking the body from further heat loss, and allowing the body to effect rewarming.

Active external rewarming can be considered for mild to moderate hypothermia and can be performed in various ways (Table 27.3). Decisions on method are based primarily on physiologic stability and resources available. Internal rewarming is recommended for moderate to severe hypothermia or when the patient demonstrates any hemodynamic instability. We typically will institute several internal rewarming mechanisms concurrently with external methods in severe hypothermia.

Table 27.3 Passive rewarming methods for accidental hypothermia

External warming method	Advantages	Disadvantages
Forced-air surface (e.g., Bair Hugger™)	Practical in emergency department Available in most hospitals Shivering and afterdrop minimized Low overall cost	Slow method especially with vasoconstriction
Forced-water energy transfer (e.g., Arctic Sun™)	Practical in emergency department Easy temperature titration Shivering and afterdrop minimized Available in many hospitals for targeted temperature management protocols	Expensive expendable components Restricts access to some parts of the body
Immersion (e.g., 40 °C water bath)	Low cost Widely available equipment (outside healthcare setting)	Not usually available in emergency department Difficult to monitor Difficult to control airway Susceptible to afterdrop Requires cooperative patient
Arteriovenous anastomosis rewarming [50] (e.g., distal extremities submerged in 44 °C water)	Low cost Readily available Minimize afterdrop Can also be used with localized negative pressure to induce vasodilation	Slow Labor-intensive Requires cooperative patient

Airway Rewarming

Airway rewarming is safe and relatively noninvasive. It is more effective when used with endotracheal intubation and coupled with humidification. The heat exchange works by gradient, so is more efficient when core temperatures are lower.

Warmed Infusion

Fluid resuscitation can be a significant source of heat and rewarming. A single liter of fluid at 42 °C can provide 14 kcal to a 70-kg patient at 28 °C and bring the core temperature up by nearly 0.33 °C. There are many commercial fluid warmers available. High-volume rapid infusers (e.g., Level-1, Belmont) can have flow rates of up to 500 ml/min. If these are not available, polyvinyl chloride bags packaging IV fluid is stable to be microwaved for about 2 minutes on high.

Warmed Internal Lavage

When using lavage for rewarming, it should not be the sole technique nor should fluids be heated beyond 45 °C. Fluid input and output should be carefully monitored and small aliquots utilized to avoid significant electrolyte disturbances and fluid shifts. The disadvantage of lavage is the relatively small surface area afforded for the rewarming process and for gastric lavage fluid escaping into the duodenum. In order to perform gastric lavage safely, the patient should be intubated for the concern for aspiration.

Peritoneal lavage has the advantage of a large surface area, the ability to detoxify drug overdoses and rhabdomyolysis, and the ability to directly rewarm the liver in the setting of possible toxicity or coagulopathy. Vigilance should be maintained for electrolyte shifts, especially for hypokalemia.

Closed thoracic lavage can be accomplished via two thoracentesis tubes placed in one or both thoracic cavities: antero-superior placement for infusion and postero-axillary for drainage. This method allows for the possibility of chest compressions. Alternatively, mediastinal irrigation can be accomplished through a lateral or median sternotomy, and allows for direct rewarming with 1–2 liters of warm fluid at a time. These methods should be considered a bridge to cardiopulmonary bypass.

Extracorporeal

Standard hemodialysis gives the advantage of rewarming while adjusting electrolyte and managing some toxic ingestions concurrently. Single vessel cannulation affords flow volumes of up to 250 ml/min, while two separate vessel catheters can achieve twice that flow rate. If an adequate blood pressure of 60 mm Hg is not attainable, then continuous venovenous or arteriovenous rewarming is an option. These methods can achieve flow rates of 375 ml/min (arteriovenous) and 400 ml/min (venovenous).

Cardiopulmonary bypass is an option for severe hypothermia in the unstable patient. Consideration is limited by criteria including potassium <10 mmol/L, combined with core temperature below 30 °C [51]. One significant advantage of cardiopulmonary bypass is that flow can be continuously maintained, even if spontaneous cardiac activity fails during the rewarming process. It is the fastest rewarming technique and has the ability to correct electrolyte abnormalities. Mean temperature increase can be up to 9.5 °C per hour [52]. Some advocate for the use of nitroglycerin to facilitate perfusion [53].

It is assumed that rapid rewarming is clinically beneficial; however, there is no published outcome data demonstrating this effect. The complications possible with rapid rewarming include DIC, pulmonary edema, hemolysis, and acute tubular necrosis.

Other Considerations

During rewarming from moderate or severe hypothermia, careful consideration should be given to the treatment of lethal rhythms such as pulseless electrical activity, ventricular fibrillation, and asystole. Contributors to these rhythms must include acid-base abnormalities, fluid shifts, and increased blood viscosity in addition to and in the setting of hypothermia. Strong data is lacking as to specific guidance for chest compressions in such a setting. Endotracheal intubation is advantageous, if not required during the process of rewarming. Oxygen consumption increases threefold for every rise of 1 °C. The risk of aspiration and the increased production of sputum along with ciliary blunting warrant intubation for airway protection alone. Rapid sequence intubation medications should be carefully chosen and judiciously used. Paralytics may not offer advantages in a patient with cold-induced trismus, and can have unpredictable efficacy in hypothermia. Decreased temperature contributes to increased protein binding, altered hepatic circulation and renal excretion, and prolonged metabolism.

Effects of vasoactive medications may vary. Dopamine is unique in that it can reverse cardiovascular depression in the setting of hypothermia [54]. It can be used in combination with labetalol and nitroglycerin to optimize both flow and pressure [55]. It is important to recognize the increased risk of limb ischemia from vasopressors in the presence of frostbite [53].

Summary

Environmental emergencies are a broad subject with somewhat indistinct diagnostic criteria due to the variety of presentations. Often encountered in conjunction with other diagnoses, they contribute greatly to the severity of other presentations. A common theme is that rapid identification and treatment greatly impacts outcome – even when the diagnosis may be uncertain. Keeping a high index of suspicion and maintaining attention to detail during the initial resuscitation is essential for a positive outcome.

References

1. Johansson SG, Bieber T, Dahl R, Friedman PS, Lanier BQ, Lockey RF, et al. Revised nomenclature for allergy for global use: report of the Nomenclature Review Committee of the World Allergy Organization, October 2003. J Allergy Clin Immunol. 2004;113:832–6.
2. Simons F. Anaphylaxis. J Allergy Clin Immunol. 2008;121:S402–7.
3. Lieberman P, Camargo CA, Bohlke K, Jick H, Miller RL, Sheikh A, Simons FE. Epidemiology of anaphylaxis: findings of the American College of Allergy, Asthma, and Immunology –Epidemiology

of Anaphylaxis Working Group. Ann Allergy Asthma Immunol. 2006;97:596–602.
4. Gaeta TJ, Clark S, Pelletier AJ, Camargo CA. National Study of US emergency department visits for acute allergic reactions,1993 to 2004. Ann Allergy Asthma Immunol. 2007;98:360–5.
5. Gonzalez-Perez A, Aponte Z, Vidaurre CF, Rodriguez LA. Anaphylaxis epidemiology in patients with and patients without asthma: a United Kingdom database review. J Allergy Clin Immunol. 2010;125:1098–104.
6. Simons FE, Adrusso LR, Biló MB, El-Gamal YM, Ledford DK, Ring J, et al. World allergy organization guidelines for the assessment and management of anaphylaxis. World Allergy Organ J. 2011;4:13–37.
7. Capps JA, Sharma V, Akwright PD. Prevalence, outcome, and pre-hospital management of anaphylaxis by first-aiders and paramedical ambulance staff in Manchester, UK. Resuscitation. 2010;81:653–7.
8. Keet CA, Wood RA. Food allergy and anaphylaxis. Immunol Allergy Clin N Am. 2007;27:193–212.
9. Bautista E, Simons FE, Simons KJ, Becker AB, Duke K, Tillet M, et al. Epinpehrine fails to hasten hemodynamic recovery in fully developed canine anaphylacitc shock. Int Arch Allergy Immunol. 2002;128:151–64.
10. Sheikh A, ten Broek V, Brown SG, Simmons FE. H1-antihistamines for the treatment of anaphylaxis: cochrane systematic review. Allergy. 2007;62:830–7.
11. Sampson HA, Muñoz-Furlong A, Campbell RL, Adkinson NF Jr, Bock SA, Branum A, et al. Second symposium on the definition and management of anaphylaxis: summary report—Second National Institute of Allergy and Infectious Disease/Food Allergy and Anaphylaxis Network symposium. J Allergy Clin Immunol. 2006;117:391–7.
12. Choo KJ, Simons E, Sheikh A. Glucocorticoids for the treatment of anaphylaxis: cochrane systematic review. Allergy. 2010;65:1205–11.
13. Pollack C. Utility of glucagon in the emergency department. J Emerg Med. 1993;11:195–205.
14. Schummer W, Schummer C, Wippermann J, Fuchs J. Anaphylactic shock: is vasopressin the drug of choice? Anesthesiology. 2004;101:1025–7.
15. Moneret-Vautrin DA, Morisset M, Flabbee J, Beaudouin E, Kanny G. Epidemiology of life-threatening and lethal anaphylaxis: a review. Allergy. 2005;60:443–51.
16. Lin RY, Schwartz LB, Curry A, Pesola GR, Knight RJ, Lee HS, et al. Histamine and tryptase levels in patients with acute allergic reactions: an emergency department-based study. J Allergy Clin Immunol. 2000;106:65–71.
17. Brown AF, McKinnon D, Chu K. Emergency department anaphylaxis: a review of 142 patients in a single year. J Allergy Clin Immunol. 2001;108:861–6.
18. Lieberman P. Biphasic anaphylactic reactions. Ann Allergy Asthma Immunol. 2002;95:341–8.
19. Keel CA. Regulation of body temperature in man. In: Wright S, editor. Sampson Wright's applied physiology., 13th ed. New York: Oxford University Press; 1982. p. 345–7.
20. Khosla R, Guntupalli K. Heat related illnesses. Crit Care Clin. 1999;15:251–63.
21. Armstrong LE, Stoppani J. Central nervous system control of heat acclimation adaptations: an emerging paradigm. Rev Neurosci. 2002;12:271–85.
22. Hernon D, Jougla E. The heat wave in France in August 2003. Rev Epidemiol Sante Publique. 2004;52:3–5. French.
23. Patz JA, Campbell-Lendrum D, Holloway T, Foley JA. Impact of regional climate change on human health. Nature. 2005;439:310–7.
24. Bouchama A, Dehbi M, Chaves-Carballo E. Cooling and hemodynamic management in heatstroke: practical recommendations. Crit Care. 2007;11:R54.
25. Akhtar MJ, al-Nozha M, al-Harthi S, Nouh MS. Electrocardiographic abnormalities in patients with heat stroke. Chest. 1993;104:411–4.
26. Farmer JC. Temperature-related injuries. In: Civetta JM, editor. Critical care. 3rd ed. Philadelphia: Lippincott-Ravens Publishers; 1997. p. 1451–63.
27. Tucker LE, Stanford J, Graves B, Swetnam J, Hamburger S, Anwar A. Classical heatstroke: clinical and laboratory assessment. South Med J. 1985;78:20–5.
28. Jiménez-Mejías ME, Montaño Díaz M, Villalonga J, Bollain Tienda E, López Pardo F, Pineda JA, et al. Classical heatstroke in Spain: analysis of 78 cases. Medicina Clin. 1990;94:481–9. Spanish.
29. Dematte JE, O'Mara K, Buescher J, Whitney CG, Forsythe S, McNamee T, et al. Near fatal heat stroke during the 1995 heat wave in Chicago. Ann Intern Med. 1998;129:173–81.
30. Tom PA, Garmel GM, Auerbach PS. Environment-dependent sports emergencies. Med Clin North Am. 1994;78:305–12.
31. Lee BC, Kim JY, Choi SH, Yoon YH. Use of an external-cooling device for the treatment of heat-stroke. Clin Exp Emerg Med. 2014;1:62–4.
32. Poulton TJ, Walker RA. Helicopter cooling of heatstroke victims. Aviat Space Environ Med. 1987;58:358–61.
33. Bouchama A, Cafege A, Devol EB, Labdi O, el-Assil K, Seraj M. Ineffectiveness of dantrolene sodium in the treatment of heatstroke. Crit Care Med. 1991;19:176–80.
34. Scharman EJ, Troutman WG. Prevention of kidney injury following rhabdomyolysis: a systematic review. Ann Pharmacother. 2013;47:90–105.
35. Herodotus. The History of Herodotus – vol. 2 [Macaulay GC, Trans.]. London: Macmillan & Co.; 1904. p. 78–9.
36. Haller JS. Medical thermometry—a short history. West J Med. 1985;142:108–16.
37. Kempainen RR, Brunette DD. The evaluation and management of accidental hypothermia. Respir Care. 2004;49(2):192–205.
38. Miller JW, Danzl DF, Thomas DM. Urban accidental hypothermia: 135 cases. Ann Emerg Med. 1980;9:456.

39. Petrone P, Asensio JA, Marini CP. Management of accidental hypothermia and cold injury. Curr Probl Surg. 2014;51:417–31.
40. Krantz MJ, Lowery CM. Giant Osborn waves in hypothermia. N Engl J Med. 2005;352:184.
41. Heimbach D, Jurkovich GJ, Gentilello LM. Accidental hypothermia. In: Shoemaker WC, Ayres SM, Grenvik A, Holbrook PR, editors. Textbook of critical care. 4th ed. Philadelphia: W.B. Saunders Co; 2000. p. 377–83.
42. Hayward JS, Eckerson JD, Kemna D. Thermal and cardiovascular changes during three methods of resuscitation from mild hypothermia. Resuscitation. 1984;11:21–3.
43. Danzl DF. Accidental hypothermia. In: Wilderness medicine. 6th ed. Philadelphia: Mosby, Auerbach; 2012. p. 116–42.
44. Poulos ND, Mollitt DL. The nature and reversibility of hypothermia-induced alterations of blood viscosity. J Trauma. 1991;31:996–8.
45. Bernard SA, Gray TW, Buist MD, Jones BM, Silvester W, Gutteridge G, et al. Treatment of comatose survivors of out-of- hospital cardiac arrest with induced hypothermia. N Engl J Med. 2002;346:557–63.
46. The Hypothermia after Cardiac Arrest Study Group. Mild therapeutic hypothermia to improve the neurologic outcome after cardiac arrest. N Engl J Med. 2002;346:549–56. [Erratum, N Engl J Med 2002; 346:1756.]
47. Maclean D, Emslie-Smith D. Accidental hypothermia. Philadelphia: JB Lippincott; 1977.
48. Giesbrecht GG. Cold stress, near drowning and accidental hypothermia: a review. Aviat Space Environ Med. 2000;71:733–52.
49. DaVee TS, Reineberg EJ. Extreme hypothermia and ventricular fibrillation. Ann Emerg Med. 1980;9:100–2.
50. Soreide E, Grahn DA, Brock-Utne JG, Rosen L. A non-invasive means to effectively restore normothermia in cold stressed individuals: a preliminary report. J Emerg Med. 1999;17:725–30.
51. Fischer A. Cardiopulmonary bypass. Presented at Immersion hypothermia task force, World Congress on Drowning. Amsterdam, June 26–28, 2002.
52. Splittgerber FH, Talbert JG, Sweezer WP, Wilson RF. Partial cardiopulmonary bypass for core rewarming in profound accidental hypothermia. Am Surg. 1986;52:407–12.
53. Long WB. Cardiopulmonary bypass for rewarming profound hypothermia patients: critical decisions in hypothermia. Annual International Forum, Portland, Ore, Feb 28, 1992.
54. Schroder T, Hering JP, Heidelmeyer CF, Pahl R, Sipinková I, Hellige G. Dopamine dependent diastolic dysfunction in moderate hypothermia. J Cardiovasc Pharmacol. 1994;23:689–702.
55. Zandstra D: Extracorporeal rewarming. Immersion hypothermia task force, World Congress on Drowning, Amsterdam, June 26–28, 2002.

Toxicology and OD

28

Mark Hincapie, Emily Fontane,
and Joseph R. Shiber

Critical Points

- Avoid pure beta blockers in cocaine or amphetamine toxicity, but labetalol or carvedilol is safe.
- Nalaxone can be given IV (start 0.2 mg), IM (0.4 mg), SQ (0.8 mg), or Intranasally (2 mg).
- Methadone, propoxyphene, and tramadol have a longer half-life and, there fore, will likely require repeated doses or a continuous infusion of naloxone.
- TCA overdose should be treated with IV fluids and IV sodium bicarbonate.
- Examine altered patients closely for transdermal drug patches (fentanyl, nicotine, nitroglycerin, lidocaine, scopolamine).
- Alcohol ingestion can cause hypoglycemia in young children.
- Consider giving NAC early for acetaminophen OD, but it can still be helpful even late with fulminant hepatic failure.

Introduction

After an exposure to any potential poison, the basic principles of assessment and stabilization of ABCD (Airway, Breathing, Circulation, Disability) still apply with the addition of an extra D for Decontamination. This includes removing any ongoing exposure or absorption by removing clothes that may be saturated with a toxin, irrigating the skin or manually brushing off cutaneous substances, and preventing further enteral absorption by using activated charcoal to bind the substance or to flush it out of the body using whole bowel irrigation. For some substances, certain patterns of toxicity known as toxidromes exist (See Fig. 28.1), and for some toxins, specific antidotes may be indicated in addition to supportive care (see Box 28.1) [1, 2].

Over 50,000 children younger than 5 years present to the emergency department each year for ingestion. Forty-eight percent of poison

M. Hincapie
Division of Pediatric Critical Care to Paediatric Emergency medicine, Jacksonville, FL, USA

E. Fontane
Department of Emergency Medicine, Division of Pediatric Emergency Medicine, University of Florida, College of Medicine, Jacksonville, FL, USA

J. R. Shiber (✉)
College of Medicine, University of Florida Health Science Center, Jacksonville, FL, USA
e-mail: Joseph.Shiber@jax.ufl.edu

© Springer Nature Switzerland AG 2020
J. R. Shiber, S. D. Weingart (eds.), *Emergency Department Critical Care*,
https://doi.org/10.1007/978-3-030-28794-8_28

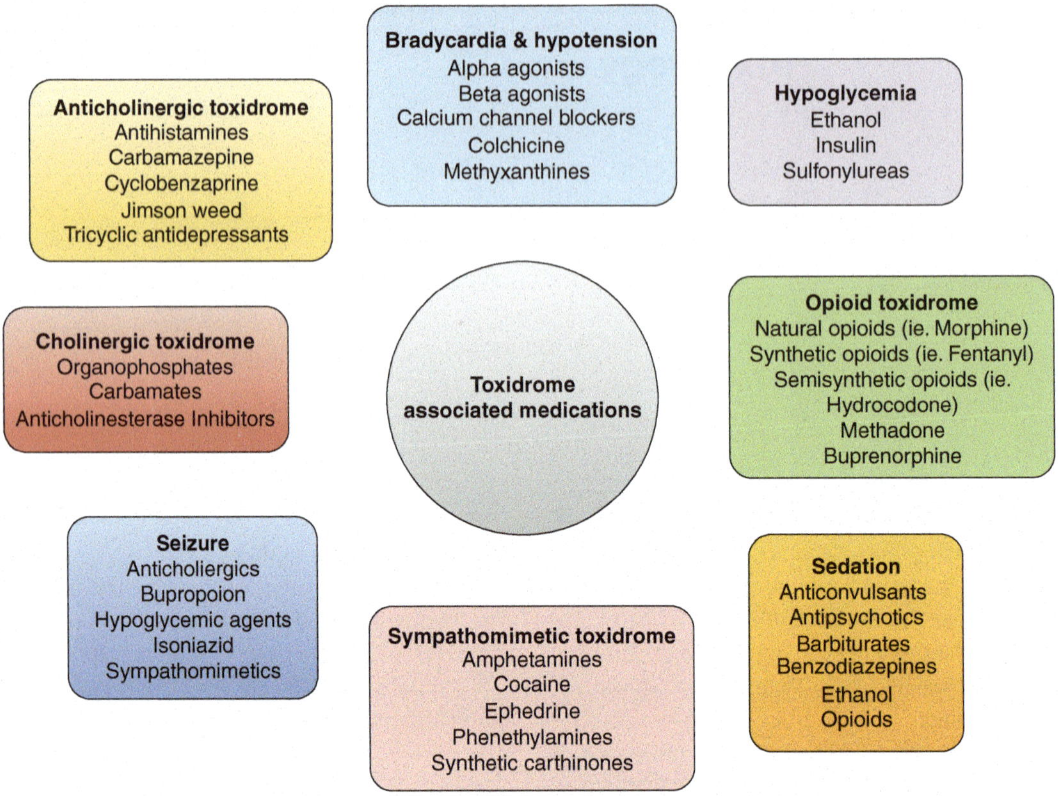

Fig. 28.1 Toxidromes and Common Poisoning Presentations. (Erickson [1], p. 5)

Box 28.1 Antidotes for common toxidromes (Erickson [1], p. 11)

Treatment-specific ingestions

Acetaminophen overdose: N-acetylcysteine (NAC)

Methanol or ethylene glycol overdose: Fomepizole

Anticholinergic overdose: Supportive and physostigmine

Beta blocker overdose: IVF, vasopressors, supportive, glucagon

Calcium channel blockers overdose: IVF, vasopressors, calcium, glucagon, insulin-euglycemia, intralipids

Cholinergic overdose: Decontamination, atropine, pralidoxirne, benzodiazepines

Digoxin overdose: Digoxin immune Fab, atropine, cardiac pacing

Iron overdose: Supportive, whole bowel irrigation, deferoxamine, exchange transfusion

Opioid overdose: Naloxone

Salicylate overdose: Activated charcoal, whole body irrigation, urinary alkalization

Sedative and hypnotics overdose: Flurnazenil

Sulfonylurea overdose: Observation, dextrose

center calls involve children less than 6 years of age (see Box 28.2). Poison control centers refer patients to the nearest emergency department and instruct parents to bring any prescription containers or fragments involved in any ingestion (see Box 28.3) [3–5].

Box 28.2 Mowry et al. [3]

2015 American Association of Poison Control Centers	% of pediatric exposures
Cosmetics and personal care products	13.6%
Household cleaning products	11.1%
Analgesics	9.1%
Foreign bodies	6.5%
Topical preparations	5.3%
Vitamins	4.6%
Antihistamines	4.4%
Pesticides	3.3%
Dietary supplements and homeopathic agents	3%
Plants	2.7%
GI preparations	2.6%
Antimicrobials	2.4%
Cold and cough preparations	2.1%
Cardiovascular drugs	2%

Box 28.3 Tarango and Liu [4]

Resources

American Association of Poison Control Centers

http://www.aapcc.org

1800 222 1222

Battery Ingestion Hotline

http://www.poison.org/battery

202 625 3333

Pill Identification

http://pillbox.nlm.nih.gov/pillimage/search.php

WHO Directory of Poison Centers

http://www.who.int/gho/phe/chemical_safety/poisons_centres/en/

A retrospective study found that contacting the poison control center decreased time to arrival by 12 min. A large study from 2007 to 2011 implicated 12 prescription medication ingestions in nearly half of all pediatric hospitalizations. Opioids (17.6%) and benzodiazepines (10.1%) were the most commonly implicated medication classes, and buprenorphine (7.7%) and clonidine (7.4%) were the most commonly implicated active ingredients. The top 12 ingestions included opioid-analgesics, benzodiazepines, sulfonylureas, beta blockers, centrally acting anti-adrenergics, calcium channel blocker, atypical antipsychotics, selective serotonin reuptake inhibitors, anticonvulsants, ACE inhibitors, skeletal muscle relaxants, and amphetamine simulants [5, 6].

Adult data shows that adverse drug events account for 5–20% of hospital admissions and 12% of ED visions, of which 50–70% are preventable. However, there is a significant gap in our understanding of the magnitude and impact of medication-related ED visits in pediatrics. In 2015, a large prospective observational study of pediatric patients presenting to the ED over 12 month period was conducted. This concluded that 65% of medication-related visits in pediatrics were deemed preventable; the probability of hospitalization was 6.5 times higher among patients with a medication-related visit compared to those without; the median hospital stay was twice as long; and medication-related causes account for 8% of pediatric ED visits accounting for 1 in 12 ED visits by pediatric patients [7–9].

In one study that spanned from 2001 to 2008, there was a 22% increase in poison control center calls, including those not referred to emergency departments, due to pharmaceutical-related medicines, such as opioid analgesics, sedatives, and hypnotics, and cardiovascular medications. Certain medications and household products have higher risks of death, and fatal ingestion in pediatrics is a rare event that typically occurs from opioid, sedatives, and cardiovascular prescription medications (see Box 28.4). Maintenance of airway, oxygenation, ventilation, and perfusion of organs is central to stabilizing any patient, child, or adult [4, 6, 10]

Box 28.4 Tarango and Liu [4]

High risk fatality-related medications

Antiarrythmics

Antimalarials

Antipsychotics

Beta blockers
Calcium channel blockers
Camphor
Clonidine
Opioids
Methyl salicylate
Sulfonylureas
Tricyclic antidepressants

Beta Blockers

Pathophysiology

Beta receptor blockade leads to reduced amounts of cyclic adenosine monophosphate, which causes bradycardia, hypotension, conduction blocks, heart failure, and hypoglycemia. Propranolol is meant to stabilize the membrane by inhibiting sodium channels. Toxic levels of propranolol cause QRS complex prolongation, negative inotropy, seizures, and coma. Sotalol inhibits potassium efflux causing QTc interval prolongation [11].

Patient Presentation

Beta blockers typically cause hypotension, bradycardia, and central nervous system depression.

Initial Stabilization

Early repletion of glycemic status and at least a 6 h observation is necessary as several beta blockers have delayed onset. Early use of glucagon activates the adenylate cyclase and is useful in the management of toxicity but may cause emesis, hyperglycemia, and tachyphylaxis. Transcutaneous or transvenous pacing may be needed for heart block or bradycardia not responding to glucagon [4, 11].

Calcium Channel Blockers

Pathophysiology

Calcium channel blockers (CCBs) act on the L-type calcium channels that mediate vasodilation, decrease inotropy, decrease dromotropy (AV node conduction), and decrease chronotropy. The blockade of calcium channels in the pancreas prevents insulin release and may cause hyperglycemia [4, 11].

Patient Presentation

Amlodipine, verapamil, nifedipine, and diltiazem toxicity cause bradycardia, hypotension, heart block diagnosed by ECG, and hyperglycemia.

Initial Stabilization

Measures that support blood pressure, stabilize calcium, and maintain euglycemia are central to calcium channel blocker toxicity treatment. These include vasopressors, intravenous fluids, calcium supplementation, and glucagon. Intralipid infusion should be considered as a potential treatment as it may act as a "lipid sink" and as a substrate for the myocardium. Cardiac pacing should also be considered to bradycardia or heart block [1, 4].

Camphor (*Vicks, Tiger Balm*)

Pathophysiology

Camphor was originally distilled from the camphor tree but is synthetically produced from turpentine oil. Upon absorption, camphor is rapidly oxidized to camphorol, which is metabolized by the liver to the glucuronide. Active metabolites get stored in fats and cleared over a prolonged period of time.

Its use in medicine spans as an anesthetic, antipruritic, antiseptic, and expectorant and is present as a topical or vaporized formulation. Most vaporized cold medications, topical anesthetics, and topical cold sore applications comprises camphor as the most common ingredient. Although the Federal Drug Administration banned products that contained more than 11% of camphor, there remain risks from oral toxicity. Tiger Balm contains 11% camphor, Vick's VapoRub contains 4.8% camphor, BenGay Ultrastrength contains 4% camphor, and *Orajel* contains 3% camphor [11].

Patient Presentation

Toddlers typically ingest or inhale camphor products causing nausea, vomiting, and burning of the mouth. Severe toxicity manifests with generalized pallor, dusky lips, irritability, hyperreflexia, myoclonic jerks, confusion, apnea, and coma. Seizures may be the initial presentation and may persist for up to 24 h. Respiratory failure or status epilepticus may lead to mortality.

Toxicity develops within 5–90 min from ingestion and can be identified from its odor, which is often a combination of camphor, eucalyptus, and menthol. Clinical toxicity resolves in 1 day and when symptoms subside, there are no documented long-term consequences [2, 11].

Diagnostics

Toxic toddler exposure to camphor occurs with approximately 500–1000 mg; however, levels are an impractical way to evaluate for toxicity.

Opioids

There are rapid increasing rates of pediatric opioid-related hospitalizations. Mortality has decreased from 2.8% to 1.3%; however, the rates of admission to the pediatric intensive care have doubled since 2004. Natural opioids (morphine, codeine), semisynthetic opioids (oxycodone, hydrocodone), and synthetic opioids (methadone, meperidine) are commonly used medications that are efficacious for analgesia and cough suppression but has been found to be problematic as they continue to be a health risk due to dependency, addiction, and toxicity [12].

From 1983 to 2000, the poison control centers documented 75,000 exposures to opioids and opioid-analgesic combinations in children less than the age of 6. Of note, nearly 54,000 of these events were due to opioid-analgesic combinations and half of these were due to acetaminophen-opioid combination [13].

Pathophysiology

Opioids target the mu, kappa, and delta receptors of the central nervous system while tramadol acts as a central acting analgesic that has both opioid and non-opioid properties. It has mu-specific receptor binding properties. Equi-analgesic doses of different opioids elicit the same respiratory depression [4, 13].

Patient Presentation

Mu receptor-targeted opioids cause analgesia, respiratory depression, gastrointestinal dysmotility, cough reflex inhibition, lethargy, nausea, tachycardia, agitation, seizures, confusion, and coma. Half-life depends on the specific opioid formulation with certain extended release preparations for morphine and oxycodone causing respiratory depression and symptoms for longer periods of time.

Tramadol overdose may sometimes lead to seizure activity, but there are no documented symptoms in children under 6 who ingested less than 10 mg/kg tramadol. Noncardiogenic pulmonary edema has long been associated with heroin use. Altered mental status effects include mild sedation, lethargy, and coma. High doses of opioids can lead to seizures but are most typical with meperidine and propoxyphene. There are minimal direct cardiovascular effects with most opiates; however, propoxyphene can widen the QRS complex and cause atrioventricular blockade. These medication-specific events require sodium bicarbonate, atropine, or isoproterenol [2, 13].

Documented cases of symptomatic children after codeine overdose showed that more than 5 mg/kg is typical and those who developed respiratory failure did so within 6 h of ingestion. Methadone, however, is the most toxic of opioid ingestion as case fatalities are documented with doses as little as 0.5 mg/kg. There is initial respiratory depression within 4–6 h. Therefore, it is imperative for close observation in the hospital. Fentanyl is found in parenteral, dermal, and oral formulations [13].

Methadone and buprenorphine – agents that counter addiction to heroine – and Loperamide – an antidiarrheal agent – are commonly the source for opioid toxicity. Victims often present with respiratory and central nervous system depression. Of the admissions from the emergency department to the intensive care unit, 37% required mechanical ventilation and 20% required vasopressors [4, 12].

Initial Stabilization

All patients with respiratory depression must have their airway properly managed according to ACLS & PALS guidelines. An extensive full body exam must be conducted as dermal opioid patches can be identified and have been culprits in pediatric case fatalities. Death from opioid overdose occurs from respiratory failure as there is markedly reduced responsiveness to hypercarbia, hypoxia, and eventually apnea [1].

Naloxone is an opioid receptor antagonist used to counter toxicity, and this must be administered in a timely fashion. Naloxone is given intravenously at 0.1 mg/kg with a maximum dose of 2 mg. Doses may be repeated every 2–3 min to a maximum combined dose of 10 mg. Naloxone's half-life is 30–100 min, so continuous infusion that is often titrated may be required for reversal of long-acting opioids. It can be given IM if no venous access but a higher dose should be given. Methadone, propoxyphene, and tramadol have a longer half-life and, therefore, will likely require continuous infusion of naloxone [4, 13].

Children must be admitted to the intensive care unit in the event of respiratory depression given the high risk for respiratory failure, coma, and seizures.

Salicylates

Salicylates are utilized as analgesics, anti-inflammatories, antipyretics, and inhibitors of platelet aggregation. Security measures over the last four decades included reducing dose strength per pill to 81 mg, minimizing packages to 36 tablets, and stronger tablets are not sweetened or flavored.

Non-aspirin salicylates include methyl salicylate, which is found in many over the counter creams, ointments, lotions, and medicated oils for use as an anti-inflammatory directly to muscles.

Pathophysiology

Methyl salicylates are readily metabolized to salicylic acid, but its severity is dependent on dosage, age, formulation, and the acuity to ingestion. The majority of non-aspirin salicylates occur from oral ingestion of oil of wintergreen or Asian herbal oils. Toxic levels of aspirin occur with 150 mg/kg with serious toxicity with 300–500 mg/kg [4, 10].

Salicylates uncouple oxidative phosphorylation, decrease adenosine triphosphate (ATP), and increase body temperature. The respiratory center of the CNS is the brain stem is directly stimulated causing hyperventilation and respiratory alkalosis, and eventually also an increased anion gap metabolic acidosis from mitochondrial poisoning.

It is important to determine the aspirin equivalent ingested dose with any salicylate ingestion. For instance, in the event of 5 mL BenGay (18.3% methyl salicylate) ingestion, this equates to 183 mg/mL; therefore, 5 mL is approximately 914 mg of methyl salicylate. The conversion factor is 1.4; therefore, this amount is equivalent to 1281 mg aspirin, which is an 85 mg/kg. Oil of wintergreen contains 98% methyl salicylate. As a potent liquid, 1 mL is equivalent to 1400 mg aspirin and 1 teaspoon (5 mL) is equivalent to 1400 mg of aspirin or approximately 22 adult aspirin tablets. Icy Hot Extra Strength, Bayer Muscle Joint Relief, Ben-Gay, and Tiger Balm ointments contain 30% methyl salicylate.

Additionally, certain Asian herbal remedies are composed of methyl salicylate, such as Red Flower Oil (67%), White Flower Oil (40%), and Tiger Oil (38%).

Volume of distribution amplifies the toxicity given the lipophilic nature of the drug, ultimately allowing for penetration to the brain, lung, and heart. Brain death, dysrhythmias from hypokalemia, and hypoxemia from pulmonary edema are the common causes of death. Patients who progressed to life-threatening toxicity nearly all had emesis within minutes to hours and then altered mental status, lethargy, or seizures. For this reason, a 6 h observation period is required for all potential serious salicylate ingestions [10, 14].

Patient Presentation

Direct stimulation of the CNS chemoreceptors triggers nausea and vomiting. Uncoupling of oxidative phosphorylation causes increased anaerobic metabolism and leads to fever. Fluid losses from emesis, dyspnea, and increased urinary output lead to dehydration and metabolic abnormalities. Vasoconstriction of the auditory vasculature leads to tinnitus. Effects on platelet aggregation and liver function occur as well.

Early onset symptoms are tinnitus, fever, tachypnea, diaphoresis, and abdominal distress. As the toxicity progresses, hyperpyrexia, lactic acidosis, respiratory alkalosis, and hypoglycemia are commonly seen and lead to multisystem organ dysfunction. Seizures, coma, hemodynamic instability, and noncardiogenic pulmonary edema are often severe cases. Severe toxicity mimics sepsis in that it causes tachypnea, hyperthermia, and altered mental status [4, 10, 11].

Diagnostics

Serum salicylate levels are a controversial topic as patients are typically symptomatic; however, some recommend salicylate levels if an anion gap or altered mental status is seen. Quantitative serum salicylate concentrations are attained at baseline and at 2 h intervals until there is a downtrend. Serum salicylate concentrations may downtrend, but the longer-lasting cellular events continue to target organs despite reassuring laboratory results. Unlike acetaminophen, where serum concentration is the only initial factor to evaluate, one must evaluate the patient as a whole.

The rapid ferric chloride test, if available, may be completed bedside and is a positive result when urine turns purple-brown when ferric chloride solution is added, but false positive can occur. The previous Done nomogram is out-dated and no longer used as it fails to predict toxicity based upon the serum concentration alone.

Serum concentration may peak after 24 h of the overdose, particularly with enteric-coated formulations. Bezoars may form which can affect absorption and serum levels. The tachypnea typically seen can be masked by opioids [4, 10, 11].

Initial Stabilization

Diminishing brain distribution is key to management. Acidemia increases the salicylate volume of distribution, which may lead to a falsely reassuring decrease in serum concentrations, despite an increasing toxicity. Therefore, respiratory alkalemia must be maintained.

Intubation may be required due to severe acidosis. Management is largely based on the victim's clinical status as serum salicylate levels are not always accurate, largely because of variable gastrointestinal absorption due to bezoar formation, long-acting formulations, and pylorospasm. Early gastrointestinal decontamination with several rounds of activated charcoal and aggressive fluid resuscitation can help to prevent central nervous system involvement, maintain tissue perfusion, and stabilize renal function [1, 2].

Urinary alkalization with sodium bicarbonate also has shown to increase elimination of salicylates by correcting acidemia, decreasing tissue distribution, and increasing urinary elimination. 150 mEq sodium bicarbonate is mixed in 1 L 5% dextrose and water, and 40 mEq potassium chloride to be given at a rate of 2–3 mL/kg/h and a goal urine pH greater than 7.5. To maintain normokalemia with urine alkalinization, potassium supplementation is very important.

Urine alkalinization is the first-line treatment for moderate-severe salicylate toxicity in patients not eligible for extracorporeal elimination. Severe toxicity involving hypotension, end-organ failure, severe acidosis, refractory medical management, and neurologic dysfunction are indications for hemodialysis, hemoperfusion, and peritoneal dialysis.

Hemodialysis preparation, if implemented, should be initiated in refractory cases in the emergency department, where coma, seizures, pulmonary edema, and severe metabolic disturbances develop. Hemodialysis has the benefit of correcting electrolyte abnormalities and improving serum salicylates. Additionally, exchange transfusion has been reported as an alternative in severe cases [4, 10, 14].

Tricyclic Antidepressants (TCA)

The tricyclic antidepressant (TCA) class includes imipramine, desipramine, amitriptyline, nortriptyline, doxepin, trimipramine, protriptyline, clomipramine, maprotiline, and amoxapine. The last 5 years has yielded a 200% growth in its usage in children less than 6. Children constitute 13% of TCA use and although they are second- or third-line therapies for depression, they are alternative therapies for obsessive-compulsive disorder, attention- deficit hyperactivity disorder, school phobias, and separation anxiety.

Pathophysiology

With the exception of maprotiline and amoxapine, all TCAs have the same side effect profile. Maproline has severe cardiac toxicity and amoxapine toxicity causes seizure activity. TCAs are the second most commonly prescribed psychotropic in children. Peak gastrointestinal absorption occurs between hour 2 and 8.

TCAs affect autonomic, central nervous, and cardiovascular systems. There are both central and peripheral anticholinergic effects. Inhibition of norepinephrine, serotonin, and dopamine into the presynaptic nerve terminals causes central sympathetic inhibition. Additionally, fast sodium channels are inhibited in the myocardium, which leads to conduction delays and dysrhythmias. Phase 0 of the action potential leads to slowed ventricular depolarization, thus prolonging QRS complexes, and phase 4 has slowed repolarization leading to prolonged QT intervals. The competitive inhibition of muscarinic acetylcholine receptors and histamine H1 receptors exert anticholinergic effects [15].

Patient Presentation

The history is integral to treatment as well. If the child is asymptomatic and the ingested dose is less than 5 mg/kg, home observation has been recommended. However, in cases of unknown ingestion or toxicity, the child must immediately be evaluated by a physician. Doses less than 6.67 mg/kg typically have not shown side effects beyond sedation. The large majority of case fatalities occur with doses greater than 30 mg/kg; therefore, a 10 kg toddler only would require 150 mg of a TCA to reach toxicity.

It is important to understand the name of the medication, its dose, and approximating how much of the bottle was ingested. TCAs typically come in 10 mg, 25 mg, 50 mg, 75 mg, 100 mg, and 150 mg tablets.

Clinical toxicity occurs by hour 6–8 of overdose and typically peaks within 24 h. For this reason, any symptomatic patient with abnormal vital signs, clinical exam findings, and/or EKG findings warrants admission.

Anticholinergic effects include dry mouth, dilated pupils, ileus, urinary retention, and tachycardia. Central nervous system effects typically cause delirium, agitation, hallucinations, convulsions, and coma. Seizure activity typically occurs within 2 h. The most dangerous life-threatening toxicity, however, remains cardiac dysrhythmias.

The most common dysrhythmia is sinus tachycardia from peripheral anticholinergic effects. Nevertheless, wide complex tachycardia, secondary to supraventricular tachycardia with aberrancy or ventricular tachycardia, is characteristic of TCA overdose. Additionally, there is a drug-induced Brugada syndrome that causes ST changes in leads V1, V2, and V3 [11, 14, 15].

Diagnostics

The amount of TCA determines toxicity. TCA serum levels are not helpful in the acute management of TCA toxicities as there is no correlation between serum level and clinical toxicity largely due to volume of distribution, drug half-life, genetic differences, pH-dependent protein binding, and tolerance.

Electrocardiogram changes occur in both children and adults. QRS prolongation and QTc prolongation are associated with seizure activity. Studies of acute TCA overdose-related seizures and dysrhythmias showed specific EKG findings including a QRS interval greater than 100 ms and an R wave amplitude greater than 3 mm in aVR.

Initial Stabilization

In the event of TCA-induced fast sodium channel blockade, sodium bicarbonate provides additional sodium, thus decreasing the QRS widening and suppressing dysrhythmias and alkalinization is a proven intervention in children.

Gastrointestinal decontamination is important for acute ingestions because there is rapid absorption initially and the anticholinergic aspect to TCAs leads to delayed emptying [2, 14, 15].

Stimulants

Cocaine and amphetamines represent the typical stimulant (also known as adrenergic) toxidrome. Cocaine use had been in decline in the previous decade in North America but has experienced a sudden resurgence with use by 1% of the population. The common presentation for stimulant toxicity is tachydysrhythmias, hypertension, acute coronary syndromes (ACS), stroke (ischemic and hemorrhagic), seizure, hyperthermia, acute renal failure, and behavioral agitation including hallucinations and psychosis. Usual physical exam findings include pupillary dilation, warm, flushed skin, diaphoresis, tachycardia, and psychomotor agitation. The potential differential diagnosis of someone with the constellation of symptoms and findings in addition to stimulant use would be withdrawal syndromes, pheochromocytoma, thyrotoxicosis, anticholinergic syndrome, and serotonin or neuroleptic malignant syndrome [16–18].

Cocaine and amphetamines are mono-amine (epinephrine, norepinephrine, dopamine, serotonin) agonists in the CNS and peripheral tissues. One particular issue with stimulant use is severe hyperthermia via multiple mechanisms that both increase heat generation (increased metabolic rate, increased motor activity) and heat retention while reducing heat dissipation (vasoconstriction, inhibiting appropriate behavioral adaptation) [18, 19].

The treatment strategy is to safely reduce the adrenergic overactivity (hypertension, tachycardia) safely while addressing any other potential adverse effects such as ACS, heart failure, stroke, or seizure. Calcium channel blockers and alpha-1 blockers may address hypertension and coronary vasospasm but not tachycardia. Beta blockers with alpha-blocking activity such as labetalol and carvedilol are safe and effective in treating hypertension and tachycardia; central alpha-2 agonists, such as clonidine or dexmedetomidine, also appear to work well. Agitation, anxiety, or seizures are best treated by benzodiazepines [20–22].

Hyperthermia may need to be treated by both external cooling (cooling blanket, ice packs, box fan) as well as internal cooling (chilled IV crystalloid infusion, esophageal cooling device, intravascular cooling catheter) if severe and the benefits are more than risks. The author's suggested manner for treating severe hyperthermia is as follows: cooling blanket under the patient to utilize conductive heat loss on the posterior body surface, infusion of 2 L of cold balanced salt solution (if not already chilled, place the IV solution bags in a emesis basin filled with ice water for 5–10 min prior to bolus), clothes removed to facilitate heat radiation, box fan at end of bed to promote convective heat loss, and wipe the patient down with tepid wet rags to increase evaporative heat exchange. Note, we do not typically use ice packs, unless no other options available, since it often induces shivering which increase heat generation and the chances of rhabdomyolysis. If shivering does occur, attempt to halt it with additional benzodiazepines, low-dose meperidine, or intravenous magnesium. In our experience, we can lower the core temperature by at least 2°C in 20–30 min and 4°C in 1 h which takes the patient out of dangerous zone for CNS damage and multi-organ failure [23–25].

Anticholinergics

Anticholinergic drugs should more accurately be called antimuscarinic agents as they do not block the nicotinic receptors but only the muscarinic. There are five muscarinic receptor subtypes, with the M1 receptors primarily in the CNS; delirium occurs when these M1 receptors, which function for cognition and attention, are blocked. The antagonism of peripheral muscarinic receptors (M2-5) cause the other features of the typical anticholinergic toxidrome: dry mouth, dilated pupils, blurry vision, tachycardia, dry, flushed skin, hyperthermia, and reduced bowel and bladder function (see Table 28.1). The delirium is commonly hyperactive with perceptual abnormalities including auditory and visual hallucinations [26–28].

The substances potentially causing this syndrome include multiple classes of medication (antihistamines, muscle relaxants, tricyclic antidepressants, antipsychotics) such as: scopolamine, atropine (including systemic effects from eye drops), diphenhydramine, chlorpheniramine, benztropine, dicyclomine, hydroxyzine, cyclobenzaprine, amitriptyline, olanzapine, and quetiapine, as well as the plants *jimson weed, angels trumpet, and belladonna* [28, 29].

Anticholinesterase (AChE) inhibitors, such a neostigmine or physostigmine, block the breakdown of acetylcholine increasing its level in the neuronal synapse to reverse the effects of anticholinergic drugs. The overload of acetylcholine can cause the cholinergic toxidrome consisting of bradycardia, salivation, bronchorrhea, vomiting, diarrhea, diaphoresis, and seizures, which is due to stimulation of nicotinic receptors in the hippocampus. The judicious use of physostigmine at an initial intravenous dose of 0.5–1 mg in adults, and 0.01–0.02 mg/kg in children has been found to be safe and effective. A second dose should not be given for at least 10–15 min with the maximum of 2 mg total in the first hour. The clear reversal of a delirious patient with suspected anticholinergic toxicity provides not only therapeutic effect, but confirms the diagnosis thereby avoiding unnecessary and possibly harmful procedures such as lumbar puncture or prolonged physical restraints. AChE inhibitors should potentially be avoided for patients at high risk of seizures or with potential cardiac toxicity from sodium channel blockers demonstrated by QRS prolongation on EKG [30–34].

Table 28.1 Signs of the anticholinergic toxidrome

Peripheral	Central
Dry warm skin	Altered mental status
Dry mucous membranes	Incoherent speech
Flushing	Carphologia[a]
Hyperthermia	Agitation
Mydriasis	Delirium
Decreased visual acuity	Hallucinations (auditory, visual, or tactile)
Photophobia	Seizures
Tachycardia	Coma

Adapted from Boroughf [26]

[a]Involuntary picking at imaginary objects, bedding, and clothing

Toxic Alcohols

Although ethanol obviously causes a well-known syndrome of intoxication, toxic alcohols refer to methanol, ethylene glycol, and isopropyl alcohol. The first two toxins will be discussed together since their mechanism of poisoning, metabolic derangements, and treatments are very similar. These substances may be found in cleaning agents or automotive fluids such as anti-freeze/coolants, wiper fluid, or brake fluid, while isopropyl alcohol is commonly found as rubbing alcohol or in hand sanitizers. All three toxins can cause exposure via ingestion, inhalation, or cutaneous absorption [35, 36].

Neither methanol nor ethylene glycol is directly toxic but is metabolized by alcohol dehydrogenase (ADH) to the toxins formaldehyde (and then formic acid) and glycolic acid (and then oxalic acid), respectively. All three toxins cause an increased osmolar gap, as also does ethanol, but methanol and ethylene glycol also cause a significant increased anion gap metabolic acidosis while isopropyl alcohol causes ketosis without acidosis. All three toxic alcohols can induce an intoxication syndrome as does ethanol inebriation but with potentially smaller volumes ingested [35–37].

Common complaints after methanol exposure are abdominal pain, nausea and vomiting, headache, dyspnea, blurry vision, and gait disturbance; these last two symptoms being due to the accentuated damage that occurs to the retina and brain. Ethylene glycol exposures may also present with abdominal pain, nausea and vomiting, and headache and also renal failure, seizures and cardiac dysrhythmias due to the accumulation of calcium oxalate crystals in the renal tubules and the resultant hypocalcemia. Isopropyl alcohol intoxication also has GI complaints and may cause hemorrhagic gastritis; in malnourished patients, hypoglycemia may occur [37–39].

The diagnosis can be challenging as no absolute laboratory test is rapidly available so that the clinician must use the surrogate assays of osmolar and anion gaps when they have suspicion based on a history of possible accidental exposure or intentional suicidality (See Fig. 28.2). The time period from exposure to symptoms is approximately 6–12 h for ethylene glycol and 12–24 h for methanol. At this time, a wide anion gap metabolic acidosis (WAGMA) should be present. Prior to that, the patient may have an increased osmolar gap, but as the metabolism of the primary substance is occurring, the osmolar gap decreases while the toxicity from the metabolites causes the acidosis and subsequent end organ toxicity. Using a Wood's lamp to identify fluorescence of the urine is not a reliable diagnostic test for ethylene glycol poisoning (even when fluorescein is present in the antifreeze added to assist mechanics in finding a leaking coolant system) [37, 40].

The primary therapeutic strategy for both methanol and ethylene glycol poisoning is to inhibit ADH thereby preventing the production of their toxic metabolites. Both ethanol and fomepizole have a much higher affinity for ADH than does the toxic alcohols. If ethanol is used (either intravenous or enteral) the target blood level is 100 mg/dL. This therapy requires ongoing administration of ethanol to maintain the therapeutic level and may induce hypoglycemia in children or

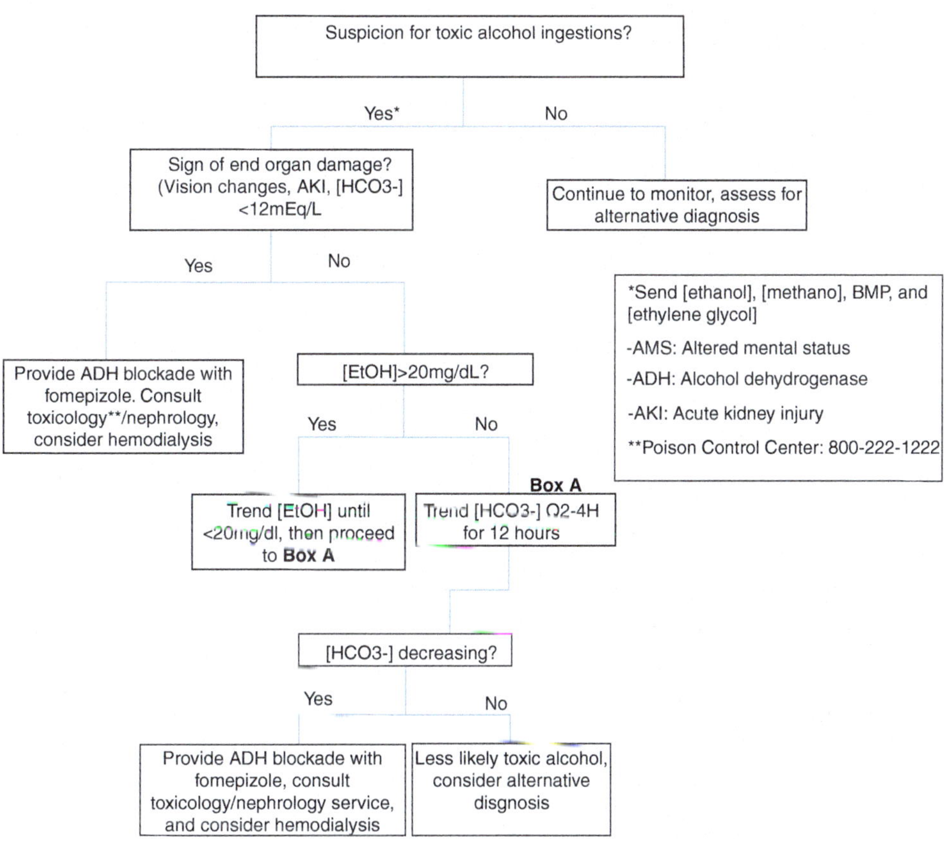

Fig. 28.2 An approach to the management of a possible toxic alcohol exposure. (Ng et al. [35])

malnourished adults. Fomepizole is effective and safe with the initial dose of 15 mg/kg over 30 min followed by 10 mg/kg every 12 h until the levels fall at least below 30 mg/dL. Hemodialysis can be used as a primary therapy or in addition to ethanol or fomepizole to hasten the clearance of the primary substance, which is actually increased with ADH inhibition [41, 42].

Acetaminophen

The leading over-the-counter analgesic in the world, acetaminophen (APAP), is unfortunately also responsible for most cases of acute liver failure (ALF) in the United States and Europe. Unintentional and chronic APAP overdose accounts for >50% of ALF. The maximum recommended daily dose of APAP in healthy adults is 650 mg orally every 4–6 h for a total of 4 g/day; this maximum is reduced to 2 g/day in adults with increased risk of hepatotoxicity. For children, the recommended dose is 10–15 mg/kg orally every 4–6 h for a total of 50–75 mg/kg in 24 h [43, 44].

It is not the APAP itself that is toxic but one of the active metabolites from the cytochrome p450 system *N*-acetyl-*p*-benzo-quinone imine (NAPQI). Normally the small amount of NAPQI produced (since ~90% of APAP is metabolized by glucuronidation or sulfation and excreted in the urine) is rapidly metabolized to a non-toxic product by glutathione (GSH). But in certain situations when GSH is depleted such as overdose, alcoholism, or malnutrition, then the NAPQI remains causing hepatocyte damage [45–49].

Activated charcoal decreases absorption of APAP if given with 4 h of ingestion. It should not be given if any concern over GI tract injury or airway maintenance as aspiration can be catastrophic. *N*-acetylcysteine (NAC) prevents hepatic damage by restoring GSH levels; it has also been found to improve cerebral edema, hemodynamic parameters, and hepatic function when ALF has already occurred from APAP toxicity. Using the Rumack-Mathew nomogram, an APAP level >100–200 ug/ml at 4 h should be considered for treatment with NAC (See Fig. 28.3). It can be given enterally (140 mg/kg load then 70 mg/kg

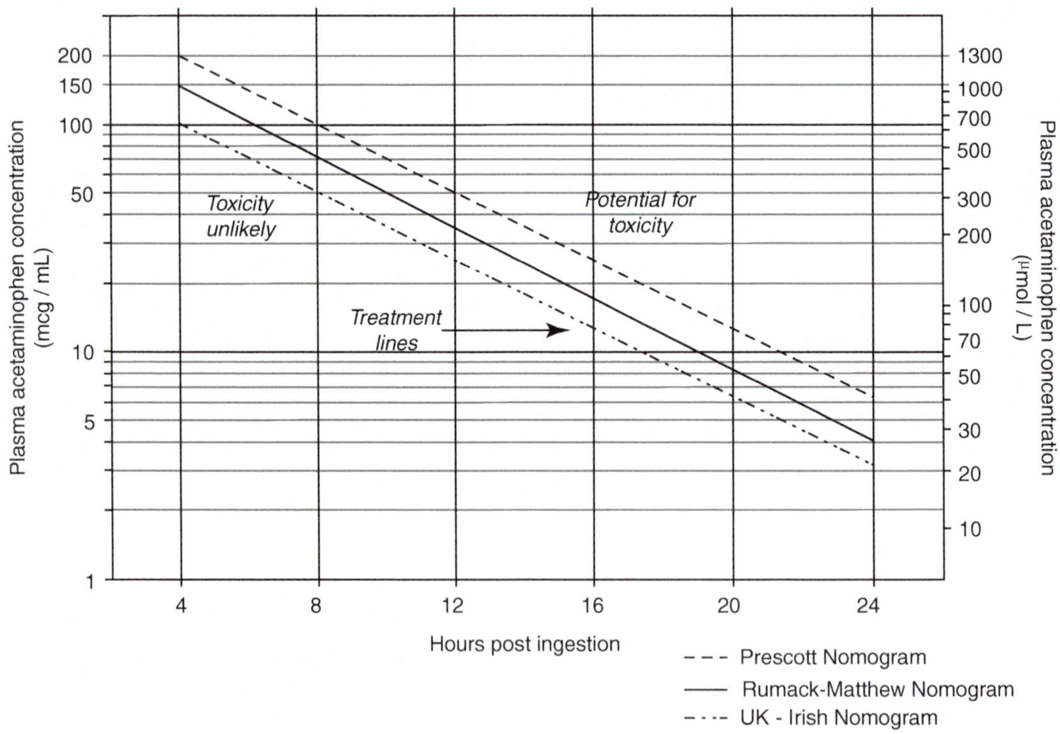

Fig. 28.3 Acetaminophen treatment nomograms. Treatment is recommended if the plasma acetaminophen concentration is above the *solid* (150 mg/L at 4 h) *line* in North America and Australia. In the UK and Ireland, the *dotted-dashed line* (100 mg/L at 4 h) is used to determine therapy with acetylcysteine. (Bateman [53])

Table 28.2 Acetylcysteine regimens

Regimen	Loading dose	Followed by	Total dose
21 h IV	150 mg/kg over 1 h	50 mg/kg over 4 h	300 mg/kg
		100 mg/kg over 16 h	
72 h PO	140 mg/kg	70 mg/kg every 4 h for 17 doses	1330 mg/kg

Table 28.3 Indications for ICU admission in acetaminophen poisoning

Significant acidosis
Any grade of encephalopathy
Coagulopathy requiring treatment
Significant renal failure

every 4 h for 18 doses) or intravenously (150 mg/kg over 1 h then 50 mg/kg over the next 4 h and then 150 mg/kg over the next 16 h) depending of the mental status and GI tract function of the patient (see Table 28.2). For indications for ICU admission, see Table 28.3. Liver transplant is the definitive therapy for ALF when continuing to decline, so urgent referral to a transplant center is indicated; but there has been some evidence that these patients may be supported by artificial or bioartificial extracorporeal liver support systems improving mortality [50–53].

Conclusion

Be vigilant for the possibility of poisoning and be aware of the potential toxidrome presentations. After initial evaluation and stabilization of the ABCDs, consider if decontamination is indicated and if a specific antidote may be available. Utilize the resources of the local Poison Control Center and consult specialists (Pharmacy, Toxicology, Nephrology, Hepatology) early for their assistance in tailoring treatment strategies such as hemodialysis.

References

1. Erickson TB. Toxicology (Chapter 18). In: APLS the pediatric emergency medicine resource. Jones & Bartlett Learning; Burlington, MA. 5th ed; 2012.
2. Olson KR, editor. Poisoning & drug overdose. 6th ed. New York: McGraw-Hill Companies Inc; 2007.
3. Mowry JB, Spyker DA, Brooks DE, et al. 2015 annual report of the American Association of poison Control Centers' National Poison Data System (NPDS): 33rd annual report. Clin Toxicol. 2016;54(10):943.
4. Tarango SM, Liu DR. Pediatric ingestions: emergency department management. EB Med. 2016;13(4):1–24.
5. Armenian P, Fleurat M, Mittendorf G, Olson KR. Unintentional pediatric cocaine exposures result in worse outcomes than other unintentional pediatric poisonings. J Emerg Med. 2017;52(6):825–32.
6. Bond GR, Woodward RW, Ho M. The growing impact of pediatric pharmaceutical poisoning. J Pediatr. 2012;160:265–70.
7. Lovegrove MC, Mathew J, Hampp C, et al. Emergency hospitalizations for unsupervised prescription medication ingestions by young children. Pediatrics. 2014;134(4):1009–15.
8. Zed PJ, Black KJ, Fitzpatrick EA, Ackroyd-Stolarz S, Murphy NG, Curran JA, MacKinnon NJ, Sinclair D. Medication-related emergency department visits in pediatrics: a prospective observational study. Pediatrics. 2015;135:435–43.
9. Zed PJ, Haughn C, Black KJ, Fitzpatrick EA, Ackroyed-Stolarz S, Murphy NG, MacKinnon NJ, Curran JA, Sinclair D. Medication-related emergency department visits and hospital admissions in pediatric patients: a qualitative systematic review. J Pediatr. 2013;163(2):477–83. https://doi.org/10.1016/j.jpeds.2013.01.042.
10. Davis JE. Are one or two dangerous? Methyl salicylate exposure in toddlers. J Emerg Med. 2007;32(1):63–9.
11. Brooks DE, Levine M, O'Connor AD, French RN, Curry SC. Toxicology in the ICU part 2: specific toxins. Chest. 2011;140:1072–85.
12. Kane JM, Colvin JD, Bartlett AH, Hall M. Opioid-related critical care resource use in US Children's Hospitals. Pediatrics. 2018;141(4):1–9.
13. Sachdeva DK, Stadnyk JM. Are one or two dangerous? Opioid exposure in toddlers. J Emerg Med. 2005;29(1):77–84.
14. Levine M, Brooks DE, Truitt CA, Wolk BJ, Boyer EW, Ruha AM. Toxicology in the ICU Part 1: general overview and approach to treatment. Chest. 2011;140:705–806.
15. Rosenbaum TG, Kou M. Are one or two dangerous? Tricyclic antidepressant exposure in toddlers. J Emerg Med. 2005;28(2):169–74.
16. United Nations Office on Drugs and Crime (UNODC). World drug report 2014; [Cited 2015 Nov 1]. www.unodc.org.
17. Substance Abuse and Mental Health Services Administration. 2011 National estimates of drug-related emergency department visits. [Cited 2015 Nov 1]. www.samhsa.gov.
18. Zimmerman JL. Cocaine intoxication. Crit Care Clin. 2012;28:517–26.
19. Matsumoto RR, Seminerio MJ, Turner RC. Methamphetamine-induced toxicity: an updated review on issues related to hyperthermia. Pharmacol Ther. 2014;144:28–40.

20. Richards JR, et al. Treatment of cocaine cardiovascular toxicity: a systematic review. Clin Toxicol. 2016;54:345–64.
21. Gordon CJ. Thermophysiological responses to hyperthermia drugs: extrapolating from rodent to human. Prog Brain Res. 2007;162:63–79.
22. Brody SL, Slovis CM, Wrenn KD. Cocaine-related medical problems. Am J Med. 1990;88:325–31.
23. Albertson TE, Derlet RW, Van Hoozen BE. Methamphetamine and the expanding complications of amphetamines. West J Med. 1999;170:214–9.
24. Krasnova IN, Cadet JL. Methamphetamine toxicity and messengers of death. Brain Res Rev. 2009;60:379–407.
25. West PL, McKeown NJ, Hendrickson RG. Methamphetamine body stuffers: an observational case series. Ann Emerg Med. 2010;55:190–7.
26. Boroughf WJ. Anticholinergic syndrome. In: Ciritical care toxicology. 2nd ed. Cham: Springer; 2017.
27. Dawson AH, Buckley NA. Pharmacological management of anticholinergic delirium – theory, evidence and practice. Br J Clin Pharmacol. 2016;81(3):516–24.
28. Hshieh TT, Fong TG, Marcantonio ER, Inouye SK. Cholinergic deficiency hypothesis in delirium: a synthesis of current evidence. J Gerontol A Biol Sci Med Sci. 2008;63:764–72.
29. Brann MR, Jørgensen HB, Burstein ES, Spalding TA, Ellis J, JonsS SVP, Hill-Eubanks D. Studies of the pharmacology, localization, and structure of muscarinic acetylcholine receptors. Ann N Y Acad Sci. 1993;707:225–36.
30. Triggle DJ, Filler R. The pharmacology of physostigmine. CNS Drug Rev. 1998;4:87–136.
31. Esterlis I, Hannestad J, Bois F, Seibyl J, Laruelle M, Carson R, Cosgrove K. Imaging acetylcholine effects on [123I] 5IA-85380 binding to beta2-nicotinic acetylcholine receptors: Physostigmine studies in human subjects. J Nucl Med. 2012;53:411.
32. Schneir AB, Offerman SR, Ly BT, Davis JM, Baldwin RT, Williams SR, Clark RF. Complications of diagnostic physostigmine administration to emergency department patients. Ann Emerg Med. 2003;42:14.
33. Arens AM, Shah K, Al-Abri S, Olson KR, Kearney T. Safety and effectiveness of physostigmine: a 10-year retrospective review. Clin Toxicol (Phila). 2018;56(2):101–7.
34. Betten DP, Vohra RB, Cook MD, et al. Antidote use in the critically ill poisoned patient. J Intensive Care Med. 2006;21:255–77.
35. Ng PCY, Long BJ, Davis WT, Sessions DJ, Koyfman A. Toxic alcohol diagnosis and management: an emergency medicine review. Intern Emerg Med. 2018;13(3):375–83.
36. Wiener SW. Toxic alcohols. In: Hoffman RS, Howland M, Lewin NA, et al., editors. Goldfrank's toxicologic emergencies. 10th ed. New York: McGraw-Hill; 2015.
37. Liesivuori J, Savolainen H. Methanol and formic acid toxicity: biochemical mechanisms. Pharmacol Toxicol. 1991;69:157–63.
38. Hodgman M, Marraffa JM, Wojcik S, et al. Serum calcium concentration in ethylene glycol poisoning. J Med Toxicol. 2017;13(2):153–7.
39. Dyer S, Mycyk MB, Ahrens WR, et al. Hemorrhagic gastritis from topical isopropanol exposure. Ann Pharmacother. 2002;36(11):1733–5.
40. Casavant MJ, Shan MN, Battels R. Does fluorescent urine indicate antifreeze ingestion by children? Pediatrics. 2001;107(1):113–4.
41. McMartin K, Jacobsen D, Hovda KE. Antidotes for poisoning by alcohols that form toxic metabolites. Br J Clin Pharmacol. 2016;81(3):505–15.
42. Jacobsen D, McMartin KE. Antidotes for methanol and ethylene glycol poisoning. Clin Toxicol. 1997;35:127–43.
43. Blieden M, Paramore LC, Shah D, Ben-Joseph R. A perspective on the epidemiology of acetaminophen exposure and toxicity in the United States. Expert Rev Clin Pharmacol. 2014;7:341–8.
44. Schilling A, Corey R, Leonard M, Eghtesad B. Acetaminophen: old drug, new warnings. Cleve Clin J Med. 2010;77:19–27.
45. Chiew AL, Gluud C, Brok J, Buckley NA. Interventions for paracetamol (acetaminophen) overdose. Cochrane Database Syst Rev. 2018;2:CD003328.
46. Dordoni B, Willson RA, Thompson RPH, Williams R. Reduction of absorption of paracetamol by activated charcoal and cholestyramine. BMJ (Clinical Research Ed). 1973;3:86–7.
47. Lancaster EM, Hiatt JR, Zarrinpar A. Acetaminophen hepatotoxicity: an updated review. Arch Toxicol. 2015;89(2):193–9.
48. Bunchorntavakul C, Reddy KR. Acetaminophen-related hepatotoxicity. Clin Liver Dis. 2013;17:587–607.
49. Suzuki A, Yuen N, Walsh J, et al. Co-medications that modulate liver injury and repair influence clinical outcome of acetaminophen-associated liver injury. Clin Gastroenterol Hepatol. 2009;7:882–8.
50. Heard KJ. Acetylcysteine for acetaminophen poisoning. N Engl J Med. 2008;359:285–92.
51. Bateman DN, Dear JW, Thanacoody HK, Thomas SH, Eddleston M, Sandilands EA, et al. Reduction of adverse effects from intravenous acetylcysteine treatment for paracetamol poisoning: a randomised controlled trial. Lancet. 2014;383(9918):607–704.
52. Craig DG, Lee A, Hayes PC, Simpson KJ. Review article: the current management of acute liver failure. Aliment Pharmacol Ther. 2010;31:345–58.
53. Bateman DN. Acetaminophen (Paracetamol). In: Brent J, Burkhart K, Dargan P, Hatten B, Megarbane B, Palmer R, editors. Critical care toxicology. Cham: Springer; 2016.

Oncologic Emergencies

29

David A. Wacker and Michael T. McCurdy

Introduction

With the overall incidence of cancer rising worldwide, management of a diverse set of emergencies stemming from underlying malignancy is increasingly common in emergency departments and intensive care units. Diagnosis of these conditions is complicated by their often nonspecific presenting symptoms, particularly in the setting of a known malignancy that may also cause a similar clinical picture. Nonetheless, vigilance must be maintained as these emergencies can threaten life and limb, and may respond to specific therapies. Malignant pericardial disease, hypercalcemia of malignancy, tumor lysis syndrome, metastatic spinal cord compression, superior vena cava syndrome, and leukostasis are reviewed in this chapter. For each section, a corresponding box briefly summarizes presentation and management.

D. A. Wacker
Department of Medicine, University of Minnesota Medical School, Minneapolis, MN, USA

M. T. McCurdy (✉)
Departments of Medicine and Emergency Medicine, University of Maryland School of Medicine, Baltimore, MD, USA

Malignant Pericardial Disease

Epidemiology and Pathophysiology

Though relatively rare in the general population, pericardial disease has been noted on autopsy in upward of 10% of cancer patients [1, 2]. Pericardial manifestations of disease include inflammation (pericarditis), pericardial neoplasm (often metastatic), effusion, and effusion-causing hemodynamic impairment (cardiac tamponade). Fortunately, approximately 70% of malignant pericardial disease is discovered incidentally and has no immediate clinical significance [2]. Clinically significant malignant effusion, however, tends to recur after drainage [3], and historically has a high likelihood of contributing to death [1].

The proportion of pericardial disease caused by malignancy largely corresponds to the geographic incidence of other diseases [2]. In most parts of the developed world, neoplasm is the underlying cause of approximately 7% of pericardial disease [4] and about a quarter of effusive pericardial disease [5]. In the developing world, however, malignancy is a less common cause of pericardial disease compared to tuberculosis and other diseases involving the pericardium [2].

Primary cardiac or pericardial neoplasms are rarely implicated in malignant pericardial disease, likely because of the extremely low incidence of these primary malignancies [1, 4]. The most common metastatic offenders are supradiaphragmatic

© Springer Nature Switzerland AG 2020

J. R. Shiber, S. D. Weingart (eds.), *Emergency Department Critical Care*,
https://doi.org/10.1007/978-3-030-28794-8_29

solid tumors, particularly lung and breast, hematologic malignancies, and melanoma [1, 4, 5].

Malignant pericardial effusion may occur through several mechanisms. Classically, pericardial metastasis is believed to occur by retrograde lymphatic flow from malignant lymph nodes into the pericardium [1]. The resulting pericardial metastatic lesions then interfere with the normal lymphatic and venous drainage of pericardial fluid, stimulating further fluid production from serosal surfaces [1]. Cancer patients may also develop "non-malignant" effusions due to impairment of pericardial lymphatic drainage by non-pericardial malignant disease, as a result of hypoalbuminemia, or as an adverse effect of treatment with radiation or chemotherapy [1, 2].

Cardiac tamponade is a life-threatening medical emergency that occurs when a pericardial effusion grows to a volume exceeding pericardial capacity. When this occurs, the increased intrapericardial pressure sequentially causes atrial and ventricular compression, severely limiting preload [6]. The manifestation of tamponade depends on the overall size of pericardial effusion, its rate of accumulation, and the patient's underlying hemodynamic state. The poorly distensible pericardium can adaptively stretch with gradual fluid accumulation on the order of even *a few* liters without significant cardiovascular effects, however, rapidly developing effusions of even a few hundred milliliters can cause hemodynamic collapse [6].

Clinical Presentation and Workup

The clinical manifestations of pericardial disease are varied and nonspecific. Classically, patients present with exertional dyspnea and chest pain [7, 8]. For patients with large, slowly accumulating effusions, as is often the case with malignant effusions, initial symptoms may result from mass effect on nearby structures, and may include nausea, early satiety, dysphagia, hoarseness, cough, and hiccups [3, 7]. Other systemic symptoms of pericardial disease, such as fatigue, malaise, or weakness, are often attributed to the known underlying malignancy [7].

Cardiac tamponade presents with shock, but concomitant signs may not be present. Pulsus paradoxus, a variation of systolic blood pressure of greater than 10 mmHg between inspiration and expiration, is the most sensitive sign but is only seen in approximately 80% of cases [9, 10]. Kussmaul's sign, increased jugular venous pressure with inspiration, is seen in only a quarter of cases [10, 11]. Beck's triad, which includes hypotension, elevated jugular venous pressure, and muffled heart sounds, is similarly rare [12]. Hypotension may not be present with tamponade, particularly if the patient is hypertensive at baseline [10, 13]. In some cases of gradual-onset tamponade, the presenting symptoms may be related to end-organ dysfunction, such as renal failure [6].

In addition to history and physical, workup for suspected pericardial disease should include a 12-lead electrocardiogram (EKG), chest X-ray, and transthoracic echocardiogram (TTE) [7, 14]. EKG will often demonstrate nonspecific ST-T changes or diminished QRS voltage; the classic finding of electrical alternans (alternating high and low QRS amplitude peaks, each representing beat-to-beat swinging of the heart within the pericardial sac) is present in less than 10% of cases of tamponade [1, 3]. Echocardiography secures the diagnosis by directly visualizing the pericardial effusion [7]. Adjunctive TTE findings, such as cardiac chamber collapse, can also assist in establishing a diagnosis of tamponade (see Fig. 29.1) [6].

Diagnostic pericardial drainage permits biochemical and cytological evaluation of suspected malignant effusions [7, 14]. In addition to cytological analysis, such fluid specimens should be tested for tumor markers, which include carcinoembryonic antigen (CEA), alpha-fetoprotein (AFP), and carbohydrate antigens (e.g., CA 125, CA 19-9), though no single tumor marker is highly sensitive for diagnosing malignancy [7, 15].

Clinical Management

Malignant pericardial effusion is a manifestation of advanced, and oftentimes end-stage, cancer [4]. Therefore, therapies and interventions should

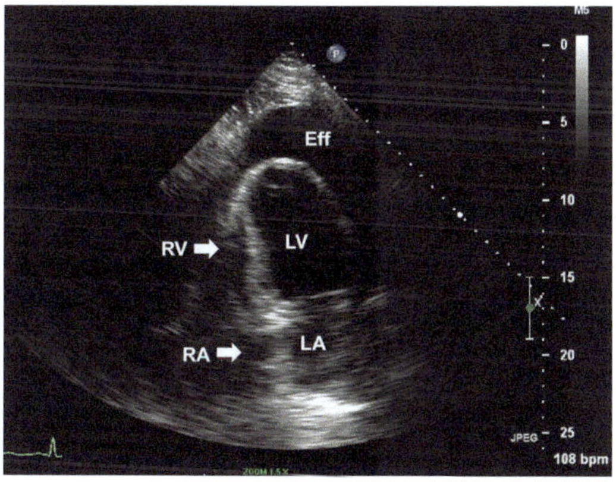

Fig. 29.1 Four-chamber apical echocardiogram demonstrating large pericardial effusion (Eff) with end-diastolic collapse of the right atrium (RA) and right ventricle (RV) consistent with tamponade physiology. Left atrium (LA) and left ventricle (LV) as marked. (Image courtesy of Dr. Matthew Peters, University of Maryland Medical Center)

be tailored to each individual patient's condition and goals of care [7, 16], which may range from aggressive drainage with curative intent to comfort measures only.

Tamponade-induced organ malperfusion is a life-threatening medical emergency requiring immediate therapeutic pericardiocentesis for definitive treatment, if compatible with goals of care. Pericardiocentesis performed under real-time echocardiogram guidance yields higher success and fewer complications compared to drainage using landmarks [17, 18]. Ultrasound may allow for identification of large, superficial fluid pockets accessible via an intercostal approach. In the absence of ultrasound, a subxyphoid approach is recommended. The needle should be inserted between the xyphoid process and left costal margin at a 15° vertical angle until the tip is deep to the rib cage, at which point the needle should be leveled and advanced toward the left shoulder until fluid is aspirated [6]. Reverse Trendelenberg patient positioning can facilitate drainage by promoting collection of fluid in the dependent portions of the pericardium.

Medical management of tamponade is controversial. Studies suggest that intravenous (IV) fluid administration and inotropes improve perfusion in anesthetized lab animals [19, 20], but these beneficial results were not reproducible and, in some cases, harmful in unanesthetized, euvolemic animals [6]. Patients believed to be hypovolemic should receive intravenous fluids and potentially empiric inotropes once euvolemic to temporize the clinical instability in preparation for a definitive pericardiocentesis. Positive pressure ventilation should be avoided whenever possible because intrathoracic pressure increases can worsen tamponade [6].

Treatment of malignant pericardial effusion without tamponade is nonemergent. Asymptomatic patients may be observed, as long as a diagnostic pericardiocentesis is unnecessary. When drainage is required, a modality should be chosen which is compatible with the patient's goals of care. Pericardiocentesis is minimally invasive and allows for short-term placement of a drainage catheter that can reduce the speed and frequency of fluid recurrence [1]. Additionally, pericardial infusion of sclerosing agents with or without chemotherapeutic effects (e.g., bleomycin, thiotepa) can decrease effusion recurrence [2, 3, 7]. Balloon pericardiotomy can be performed by guidewire insertion of a balloon catheter into the pericardial space via subxyphoid approach. The balloon is then inflated and withdrawn to dilate the pericardial opening, thus facilitating drainage [3]. Surgical intervention, which may include either a pericardial window to drain to the peritoneal or pleural spaces or a pericardiectomy [3, 14], effectively drains the effusion and facilitates access to diagnostic pericardial tissue specimens but at the expense of invasiveness. If procedural intervention is undesired or inappropriate, systemic chemotherapy or targeted radiation may provide some benefit, particularly for leukemias and lymphomas [3, 7].

Most studies comparing outcomes among the various therapies are observational in nature and inherently complicated by the study population [21–23], making it difficult to draw conclusive guidance. Therefore, management decisions, tailored to each particular patient's circumstances, remain at the practitioner's discretion. These decisions, however, should ideally include the patient, family, and potentially specialists in oncology, cardiology, and cardiac surgery (Table 29.3).

Hypercalcemia

Epidemiology and Pathophysiology

Malignancy has been shown to cause >40% of cases of hypercalcemia in the emergency department [24], and up to 30% of cancer patients may develop hypercalcemia during their course [25, 26]. Furthermore, malignancy-associated hypercalcemia is often a marker of advanced disease. Median survival of those afflicted is less than 2 months, and, even in the subgroup of patients with malignancies responsive to disease-specific therapy, survival only increases to 5 months [27, 28].

Under normal physiologic conditions, parathyroid hormone (PTH) and calcitriol primarily mediate calcium metabolism, with calcitonin playing a modest role [29]. PTH increases the serum calcium by promoting bone resorption, increasing renal calcium reuptake and phosphate elimination, and upregulating enzymatic conversion of vitamin D to calcitriol [29, 30]. Upon activation, calcitriol increases gastrointestinal uptake of calcium and phosphate and works in parallel with PTH to further promote bone resorption [31] (see Fig. 29.2).

Malignancy-associated hypercalcemia (MAH) occurs by four major mechanisms: (1) PTH-related protein (PTHrP) synthesis; (2) excess PTH secretion; (3) activated vitamin D overproduction; and (4) and direct bone osteolysis [26, 32]. In addition to PTHrP, human T-cell leukemia/lymphoma virus type 1 (HTLV-I)-related adult T-cell leukemia (ATL) cells have recently been demonstrated to express RANK ligand (RANKL) and Wnt-5a, both signaling molecules involved in activation of osteolysis [33].

Parathyroid hormone-related protein synthesis, or "humoral hypercalcemia," accounts for about 80% of cases of MAH [26]. Due to its structural homology to PTH [34], PTHrP activates pathways of calcium metabolism normally restricted to PTH. PTHrP secretion most commonly occurs in primary squamous cell cancers, particularly lung, esophagus, head and neck, cervical, ovarian, and endometrial cancer [25]. Less commonly, adenocarcinomas such as renal cell cancer may also generate PTHrP [25]. Very rarely, non-malignancy-associated PTHrP expression occurs [35].

Calcitriol, or activated vitamin D, overproduction, and local osteolysis from diffuse metastasis make up the vast majority of the remaining 20% of cases [25, 26]. Calcitriol overproduction is mostly seen in lymphomas (both Hodgkin and non-Hodgkin) [25, 31]. Macrophages expressing 1α-hydroxylase in malignant lymphatic tissue are thought to convert inactive vitamin D (25-OHD) to calcitriol (1,25-$(OH)_2D$) in an unregulated fashion [31, 36, 37]. This deregulation results from the ability of cytokines secreted

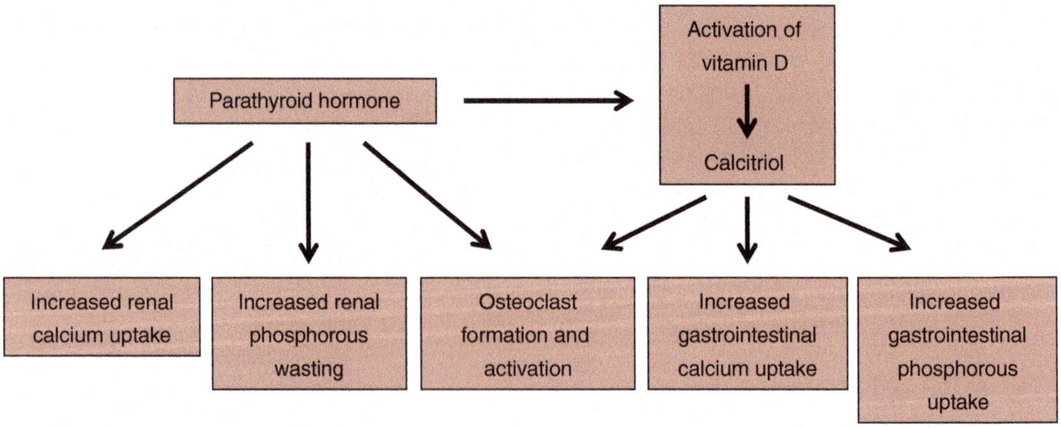

Fig. 29.2 Physiologic effects of parathyroid hormone (PTH) and activated vitamin D (calcitriol) on normal calcium metabolism

from malignant tissue to bypass feedback mechanisms normally regulated by PTH and other signals related to calcium metabolism [31]. Hypercalcemia from bony metastasis occurs only with diffuse disease and is believed to be caused by cytokine-mediated local osteolysis [16]. Despite its avidity for bone, prostate cancer interestingly does not manifest such findings as frequently as breast cancer, multiple myeloma, and lymphoma do, which further suggests a cytokine-mediated mechanism beyond simply bony destruction [16, 25].

Ectopic parathyroid hormone production is extremely rare in tumors external to the parathyroid and mainly limited to case reports [38–40]. Primary hyperparathyroidism occurring coincidentally with malignancy is thought to cause more than 10% of cases of MAH [41].

Excess PTH or PTHrP induces inappropriate renal tubular calcium reuptake, phosphaturia, and bone resorption [42]; however, only PTH stimulates production of calcitriol [43]. Even with PTH overproduction, most of the rise in serum calcium results from hormonal effects on the kidney and bone, while intestinal calcium uptake plays a lesser role [32]. Conversely, upregulated intestinal calcium absorption significantly, though not entirely, contributes to calcitriol-mediated hypercalcemia. Despite increased intestinal absorption, patients with elevated calcitriol levels can still develop hypercalcemia despite taking nothing by mouth [31].

Regardless of the underlying mechanism, hypercalcemia can precipitate significant hypovolemia by impairing renal water and sodium reabsorption [32]. The ensuing hypovolemia-induced renal injury can further impair calcium excretion [25, 32], creating a positive feedback loop in which hypercalcemia is maintained and augmented.

Clinical Presentation and Workup

Symptoms of hypercalcemia tend to be vague and nonspecific. Common findings include constipation, abdominal pain, nausea and vomiting, anorexia, polyuria, polydipsia, and neurological manifestations such as weakness, lethargy, and confusion [29] (Table 29.4). Further confounding the clinical picture, the rate of increase of serum calcium concentration may more profoundly affect symptom severity than its absolute value [25, 26]. The patient's age and comorbidities and the duration of hypercalcemia may also influence the presenting symptoms [32].

Renal and neurological abnormalities are the prevailing manifestations of MAH-induced organ injury. Acute kidney injury (AKI) is the most common renal manifestation of MAH. Nephrolithiasis and nephrocalcinosis, which are associated with chronic hypercalcemia, are seldom seen in MAH [29]. Severe hypercalcemia is associated with altered mental status leading to coma [27, 29], and development of associated posterior reversible encephalopathy syndrome (PRES) has been described [44]. If left untreated, severe hypercalcemia will ultimately lead to death [24, 25, 32].

Physical exam findings are usually nonspecific and are rarely helpful in reaching the diagnosis. On EKG, initial signs of hypercalcemia include QT interval shortening, while more severe hypercalcemia can cause bradydysrhythmias and heart block [25].

The most important step in the workup of hypercalcemia is an accurate measurement of the serum calcium concentration. Although the majority of serum calcium is rendered physiologically inert by binding to albumin and other proteins, this bound fraction of calcium is still included in total serum calcium measurements, obscuring the amount of physiologically active ionized (or "free") calcium [45]. Measurements of total serum calcium and serum albumin can approximate the ionized calcium fraction, but these are often inaccurate and do not account for the presence of other serum proteins or factors that influence protein avidity for calcium (e.g., medications, serum pH) [46]. Therefore, a serum ionized calcium level should be obtained when initially assessing for and managing hypercalcemia [45, 46].

Because initial therapy is the same regardless of the underlying cause of the hypercalcemia, initial measurement of PTH and PTHrP levels will not change the acute management. However, a serum PTH level is useful to rule out a concomitant primary hyperparathyroidism, especially in patients without widespread metastatic cancer or with cancers not usually associated with hypercalcemia [25, 47]. In one observational study, one in seven hypercalcemic cancer patients had coincidental primary hyperparathyroidism [41]. Because PTHrP suppresses PTH release, an elevated PTH level may suggest that PTHrP expression is not a significant factor in a particular patient's hypercalcemia [29]. In fact, a PTH level greater than 26 ng/L in the setting of hypercalcemia is 100% specific for predicting a negative PTHrP level [47]. A pretreatment PTHrP level may help predict response to bisphosphonate therapy. In one study, responders to bisphosphonate therapy had a median pretreatment PTHrP level of ~30 pg/mL, whereas the nonresponder median pretreatment PTHrP level was ~70 pg/mL [48].

An activated vitamin D (1,25-$(OH)_2D$) level should be obtained in patients with confirmed or suspected lymphoma (Hodgkin or non-Hodgkin), sarcoidosis, or other granulomatous disease. Imaging to assess skeletal tumor burden may similarly be helpful in cases suspicious for massive osteolysis due to direct bony metastasis. Assessing renal function (e.g., creatinine, blood urea nitrogen) and electrolyte levels (e.g., potassium, chloride, phosphorus, magnesium) helps to identify accompanying derangements frequently associated with hypercalcemia [24, 49]. Other factors may also contribute to the development of hypercalcemia, such as thiazide diuretics, exogenous calcium supplementation, hyperthyroidism, or granulomatous disease [26, 50]. All hypercalcemic patients benefit from medication management to minimize the pharmacologic impact on calcium intake and retention. Further testing for other contributing pathologies such as thyroid testing may be undertaken in patients whose malignancy does not seem concordant with degree of hypercalcemia, such as those who have malignancies not usually associated with hypercalcemia, or those without disseminated disease or elevation of PTH, PTHrP, or calcitriol.

Clinical Management

Severe (>14.0 mg/dL) or symptomatic hypercalcemia warrants immediate treatment [29], but any degree of hypercalcemia should be addressed [32]. To break the cycle of hypercalcemia-induced volume depletion, aggressive (e.g., 200–500 mL/hr or more) intravenous crystalloid should be promptly initiated [25, 26]. Patients with oliguria, either because of renal or heart failure, should also initially receive aggressive volume resuscitation, but management plans for hypervolemia, including diuresis, dialysis, or positive pressure ventilation, should be in place should this become necessary.

Historically, loop diuretics, which inhibit calcium reabsorption in the ascending limb of the loop of Henle, have been employed alongside fluid administration [32]. However, this calciuretic effect is insufficient to restore normocalcemia, and this therapy is associated with high complication rates [29, 51]. Loop diuretics should, therefore, be used to manage volume overload rather than force calciuresis. Thiazide diuretics should be avoided not only because of their potential to exacerbate volume depletion but also because they enhance distal tubule calcium reabsorption [25, 32].

Bisphosphonates, which are analogs of the bone catabolism by-product pyrophosphate, are the mainstay of hypercalcemia management [32, 52]. They reduce osteoclast function and viability and stabilize hydroxyapatite crystals, thus inhibiting bone catabolism [32]. Though bisphosphonates inhibit bone breakdown, they only minimally affect the accelerated renal calcium reabsorption generated by PTHrP and PTH [29, 42].

Though zoledronate has a faster onset and longer duration of effect than the less costly pamidronate, both MAH treatments are widely used because neither has demonstrated a superior longer-term outcome over the other [53, 54]. Response to pamidronate is dose-dependent, with nearly all patients showing response at the recommended dose of 90 mg given intravenously over 2–4 hours [29, 55]. The recommended dose of zoledronate is 4 mg intravenously over 5 minutes for initial treatment, and 8 mg for refractory hypercalcemia [53, 54]. Both agents reduce average peak serum calcium by 3–4 mg/dL usually within 7–10 days [53]. Bisphosphonates should be administered intravenously because oral bioavailability is unreliable [29].

Though generally safe, bisphosphonates can be associated with renal dysfunction or, in 10–30% of cases, with an acute phase reaction within 36 hours of administration [56]. The symptoms of fever, myalgia, arthralgia, and headache can be preempted by antihistamines and antipyretics administration [29]. Additionally, hypocalcemia, hypomagnesemia, and hypophosphatemia may occur in up to half of patients receiving bisphosphonate therapy [29].

Bisphosphonates are effective but require days to take effect [53], whereas calcitonin has a quicker onset (i.e., 12–24 hours) [25, 32]. Due to tachyphylaxis, calcitonin is most effectively used for situations requiring immediate reductions in serum calcium, such as seizures or dysrhythmia [32], and should be given concomitantly with longer-acting bisphosphonate therapy [25]. The recommended dose of calcitonin is 4–8 units/kg subcutaneously or intramuscularly every 6 hours [57]. This dose on average reduced serum calcium level by 1–3 mg/dL [57]. Side effects of calcitonin include abdominal cramping, nausea, and vomiting [57].

Denosumab is a human monoclonal antibody that inhibits the signaling protein RANK ligand (RANKL), which promotes bone resorption. Though not as well studied as bisphosphonates and with only case series to support its use, denosumab has successfully lowered calcium levels in patients recalcitrant to bisphosphonate therapy [58–60]. Similar to bisphosphonate therapy, it has been reported to induce hypocalcemia in some patients [61].

Gallium nitrate and plicamycin (mithramycin) have historically been used for treatment of MAH. Gallium nitrate is an osteoclast inhibitor rivaling pamidronate in terms of effectiveness [62]. Its use is limited, however, by both a prolonged 5-day intravenous administration time and renal toxicity. Typical dosing is 200 mg/m^2 per day administered as a continuous infusion over 5 days [63]. Another antihypercalcemic agent, plicamycin, inhibits nuclear transcription in osteoclasts, but its relatively robust side effect profile that includes hepatotoxicity, bone marrow suppression, platelet dysfunction, and clotting irregularities, limits its widespread use [29]. Although bisphosphonates have superseded these agents, they remain viable second-line therapies.

In cases where hypercalcemia is believed due to excessive vitamin D, administration of glucocorticoids can lower serum calcium levels by counteracting the effect of vitamin D [32]. The exact mechanism by which this occurs, however, remains debated [64]. Usual doses are 200–300 mg per day of intravenous hydrocortisone [29].

In severe hypercalcemia, hemodialysis can quickly and effectively reduce serum calcium concentration [65]. This treatment should be reserved for those patients who are recalcitrant to other means of calcium management, are dialysis-dependent, or have life-threatening manifestations of hypercalcemia, such as cardiac dysrhythmias or central neurological manifestations.

Antihypercalcemic agents lower serum calcium level in the short term but do not reduce tumor burden or PTH or PTHrP levels. Cancer therapy, if appropriate, should not be delayed in the hypercalcemic patient [26]. In general, chemotherapy in hypercalcemic patients has been associated with no further elevation of serum calcium concentration and, for some types of cancer, lowers it [66]. Chemotherapy should be chosen with careful attention to its effects on calcium metabolism, as some agents may actually induce hypercalcemia [67].

Tumor Lysis Syndrome

Epidemiology and Pathophysiology

Tumor lysis syndrome (TLS) is a constellation of metabolic derangements resulting from large-scale destruction of tumor cells, often following initiation of chemotherapy. Usually this consists of hyperuricemia, hyperkalemia, and hyperphosphatemia with subsequent hypocalcemia. In acute TLS, the breakdown of malignant cells occurs with sufficient speed that the body's usual mechanisms of homeostasis are overrun by the rapid release of these intracellular components. These homeostatic mechanisms are further impaired by the acute kidney injury (AKI) resulting from precipitation of calcium phosphate, uric acid, or both in the renal tubules [68]. Additionally, in patients with high tumor burden, serum levels of metabolites and minerals, especially phosphorus, are held in check due to rapid metabolic uptake by the tumor, but chemotherapy eliminates this mechanism, further contributing to their toxic accumulation [69].

Acute kidney injury frequently also accompanies TLS. This can be due to damage from uric acid or calcium phosphate crystal deposits in the tubules [70] or due to crystal-independent mechanisms of uric acid-mediated kidney damage [71, 72]. Furthermore, a clear etiology is often difficult due to comorbidities such as sepsis, hypovolemia, acute tubular necrosis, administration of nephrotoxic agents, and direct effect of the tumor (parenchymal infiltration or obstruction) [68, 73]. AKI accompanying TLS should be viewed as a sign of high morbidity; in one observational study, in-hospital mortality increased from 7% in patients with only TLS to 51% in patients with TLS and AKI [74].

Tumor lysis syndrome most commonly occurs with rapidly growing tumors such as Burkitt's lymphoma or acute lymphoblastic leukemia (ALL) [68], which exhibit treatment-induced TLS in up to 17% of cases [75]. Though much less common, TLS can also occur with proliferative solid tumors such as breast, testicular, and small cell lung cancer [68]. The overall incidence and diversity of TLS is increasing [76, 77]. The patients most at risk are those with tumors that are high burden, rapidly growing, and highly chemosensitive. Preexisting renal failure, hypovolemia, or hyperuricemia at the initiation of chemotherapy are also risk factors [68].

Clinical Presentation and Workup

Patients presenting with acute TLS may have a variety of symptoms, including nausea, vomiting, lethargy, confusion, edema, cardiac dysrhythmia, seizure, muscle cramps or myalgias, tetany, or cardiac arrest (Table 29.5). Most of these are a direct result of metabolite imbalance or resulting renal failure [68, 78]. Due to the nonspecific symptomatology, a high clinical suspicion is necessary, particularly in those with recent cytotoxic therapy for known malignancy with high tumor burden, but spontaneous TLS can also occur [79]. Electrocardiographic findings may include those related to hyperkalemia (P-wave flattening, PR and QRS interval prolongation, T-wave peaking) or hypocalcemia (QT interval prolongation) [80]. Workup should include measurement of serum potassium, ionized calcium, phosphate, urea nitrogen, creatinine, uric acid, and lactate dehydrogenase (LDH).

Because numerous pathologies can cause the signs and symptoms noted above, several formal definitions of tumor lysis syndrome have been proposed, of which the most widely employed is the Cairo–Bishop definition [68]. In this system, TLS is classified into laboratory TLS (LTLS) (see Table 29.1) and clinical TLS (CTLS), defined as AKI, dysrhythmia, or seizure in the presence of LTLS.

In addition to other metabolic components, tumor lysis can release large amounts of immunologic signaling proteins, such as cytokines, resulting in systemic inflammatory response syndrome (SIRS) [81]. If the diagnosis of sepsis is being entertained, cultures should be drawn and antibiotics should be started immediately while evaluating for possible TLS.

Table 29.1 Cairo–Bishop criteria for laboratory tumor lysis syndrome (LTLS). Two or more of the criteria listed must be met to establish the diagnosis of LTLS 68

Laboratory value	Criteria for LTLS
Uric acid	>8 mg/dL, or 25% increase from baseline
Potassium	>5 mEq/L, or 25% increase from baseline
Phosphorus	>4.5 mg/dL, or 25% increase from baseline
Calcium	<7 mg/dL, or 25% decrease from baseline

If AKI is present, renal imaging (e.g., ultrasound) can assess for obstruction. Urinalysis should be performed, and in oliguric, diuretic-naive patients, calculation of fractional excretion of sodium (Fe_{Na}) can differentiate between intrinsic and extrinsic renal etiologies. Though a urine uric acid-to-creatinine ratio greater than 1.0 was thought to identify a uric acid nephropathy [82], this finding has since been determined to be non-specific and is no longer recommended [83]. A symptom-specific workup such as brain imaging for neurological manifestations or abdominal imaging for gastrointestinal symptoms may also be necessary to rule out alternative causes.

Clinical Management

Aggressive intravenous fluid administration is the mainstay of therapy for patients with TLS. For patients with good urine output, initial volumes of 3 L/m^2/day are recommended [68]. Diuresis may be employed to manage hypervolemia, but this therapy may be deleterious in the hypovolemic or obstructed patient [78]. Once touted as enhancing uric acid clearance, guidelines no longer recommend urine alkalinization because alkaline urine promotes metabolic derangements [84], phosphate nephropathy [70], and xanthine crystal formation and resultant nephropathy [78, 81]. Patients with oliguria or anuria can be managed with similarly aggressive crystalloid administration and trials of diuresis, however plans should be in place for renal replacement therapy if urine output fails to improve with these interventions. In one observational study, half of all patients with newly diagnosed high-grade malignancy and AKI required renal replacement therapy [73].

Intravascular volume repletion is the primary means of reversing hyperphosphatemia [68]. Although the main source of serum phosphorus remains tumor lysis rather than enteric uptake, a low phosphate diet and administration of oral phosphate binders can still help. Avoidance of inadvertent exogenous phosphorus by oral supplement or in intravenous fluids is recommended [78].

Hypocalcemia results from ionized calcium and phosphorus precipitating into calcium phosphate, a compound with low solubility in blood and a proclivity for causing nephropathy. Asymptomatic hypocalcemia should not be repleted, as serum calcium levels will recover upon cessation of tumor lysis and resolution of hyperphosphatemia [68]. Hypocalcemia causing cardiac (e.g., heart block, dysrhythmia) or neurological (e.g., seizure, coma) symptoms should be immediately repleted using either intravenous calcium chloride if central access is available or calcium gluconate if administered peripherally.

Hyperkalemia should be managed just as from any other etiology. For those with an existing or impending dysrhythmia (e.g., QRS widening), an intravenous calcium bolus will stabilize cardiac myocytes for a brief period (less than 1 hour) [85], providing an opportunity to shift potassium intracellularly via intravenous insulin, bicarbonate, and inhaled beta-agonists. Total body potassium must then be removed, either by the patient's own kidney (augmented by loop diuresis if volume status permits) or renal replacement therapy [68, 78]. The patient's enteric tract may also be employed via potassium binders such as polystyrene sulfonate, but this should be used with caution due to the risk of associated colonic necrosis with this therapy [86]. Avoid giving exogenous potassium orally or in intravenous fluids.

Hyperuricemia results in urate crystal formation, which then leads to AKI. Aggressive hydration mitigates this outcome by reducing overall uric acid concentration and promoting renal clearance. Allopurinol, a xanthine analog which inhibits the breakdown of nucleic acids to uric acid, can be used to prevent further uric acid buildup, and is frequently used as a prophylactic measure or as active therapy in patients being treated for tumor lysis syndrome [78]. Allopurinol, however, can lead to serum xanthine buildup, which has limited solubility in blood and may ultimately cause xanthine nephropathy. Furthermore, allopurinol interferes with metabolism of nucleic acid analogs used as antimalignancy agents, such as 6 mercaptopurine and azathioprine, often necessitating dose reductions of these agents [68, 78]. Allopurinol should also be renally dosed [78].

Although allopurinol prevents uric acid production, no further enzymatic breakdown of existing serum urate exists in humans. In contrast, many mammalian species express urate oxidase, which converts uric acid into the more urine-soluble allantoin [68]. A recombinant form of urate oxidase, rasburicase, can effectively reduce elevated uric acid levels in as little as 4 hours [87, 88]. Those with glucose-6-phosphate dehydrogenase (G6PD) deficiency should not receive rasburicase because its by-product, hydrogen peroxide, may trigger a hemolytic crisis [68]. Methemoglobinemia may also occur as a result of rasburicase administration [89].

Initial studies with rasburicase demonstrated effective dosing with 0.2 mg/kg given intravenously every day for up to 7 days [87, 88]. However, weight-based dosing of 0.05 mg/kg as a single dose with repeat dosing only as needed is clinically effective [90, 91], as is single, fixed doses of 3–6 mg [92–94].

Whenever possible, appropriate pre-chemotherapy prophylaxis should be given to patients at elevated risk for TLS. A grading scale has been designed for this purpose which assigns patients to low (<1%), moderate (1–5%), or high (>5%) risk of TLS incidence based on (1) pretreatment renal function; (2) pretreatment serum phosphorus, uric acid, and potassium concentrations; and (3) disease type and burden [75]. For patients with acute myeloid leukemia (AML), elevated pretreatment white blood cell count and LDH level were determined to be independent risk factors for development of TLS [95]. Intermediate- and high-risk patients warrant aggressive hydration (>3 L/m^2/day), allopurinol therapy, and frequent laboratory monitoring. High-risk patients should be considered for prophylactic rasburicase [75].

Metastatic Spinal Cord Compression

Epidemiology and Pathophysiology

The vertebral column is the most common site of skeletal metastasis in the body [96]. Of patients with metastatic cancer, 40% develop spinal metastasis [96] and 5% experience spinal cord compression [97]. The majority of cases of cord compression occur following hematogenous metastasis to the marrow space of a vertebral body; only about 10–15% result from direct paravertebral malignancy extension through a neural foramen [98]. Animal data suggest that most spinal metastases travel from the marrow via the vertebral vein foramina to the anterior area of the spinal canal, where they expand extradurally until cord compression occurs. Rarely, infiltrative tumors migrate posterior to the cord before expanding [99]. Due to the usual spinal canal extension prior to cortical bone invasion of spinal metastases, plain radiographs may remain normal (i.e., low sensitivity) despite local tumor growth or cord involvement [99].

Metastatic spinal cord compression (MSCC) can also result from an intradural lesion, due either to an intramedullary tumor (e.g., glial cell tumor, neuroma) or to an extramedullary tumor extending or metastasizing to the intradural space [100]. Intradural compression lesions occur infrequently (<5% of cases of malignancy-related spinal cord compression) [100].

The primary mechanism by which neuronal injury occurs is vascular compromise. Occlusion or stenosis of the epidural venous plexus ultimately leads to breakdown of the blood–cord barrier and vasogenic edema [101]. At this stage, corticosteroids may temporarily stabilize against worsening compression and progression to permanent neural damage [101]. Without definitive management of the offending mass, however, arterial flow will eventually diminish, leading to cord ischemia and frank infarct [101]. The less common cause of neurologic injury is direct pressure of the tumor on the cord over time, leading to demyelination and axonal injury [101].

The majority of cases of MSCC result from prostate, breast, or lung cancer, each making up approximately 15–20% of total cases [97, 102]. Renal cell cancer, non-Hodgkin's lymphoma, and multiple myeloma each make up an additional 5–10% of total cases [97, 102]. Bone mass and blood flow distribution dictate the frequency of compressive metastatic lesions in each section of the spinal cord. Approximately 15% of cases involve the cervical spine, 60% the thoracic spine, and 25% the lumbosacral spine [102]. Importantly, 20–40% of patients with cord compression in one location will have at least one other locus of spinal metastasis [103–105].

Clinical Presentation and Workup

Back pain, usually caused by periosteal stretching and soft tissue invasion, is the most common and often the earliest symptom associated with MSCC. It is the initial symptom in 83–95% of cases of symptomatic MSCC, and up to 95% have back pain at the time of diagnosis [106, 107]. Because back pain is poorly specific for MSCC, the first onset of back pain usually precedes the ultimate diagnosis of MSCC by around 2 months [108, 109].

Weakness, usually of the lower extremities, is the next most common presenting symptom, with an incidence of 35–75%. Sensory loss is noted at presentation in 50–70% of MSCC cases, though this finding is often described as occurring later in the disease process than weakness. Sensory changes often start distally and move proximally toward the trunk. Autonomic dysfunction occurs late in the course, and bowel or bladder dysfunction rarely presents in isolation. Overall incidence of bowel or bladder dysfunction at presentation is 50–60% [106, 107].

Workup of MSCC begins with the history and physical. This diagnosis should at least be considered in any patient presenting with back pain, neurological deficit of the extremity, or bowel or bladder incontinence. A known history of cancer, especially with known spinal cord metastasis, provides a diagnosis with almost 100% specificity [110], but back pain is the first presenting manifestation of cancer in 20% of cases of MSCC [111]. A thorough neurological exam should be performed, including strength and sensation testing, deep tendon reflexes, and rectal tone. The full length of the spinal cord should be palpated for tenderness. The absence of any single symptom, including back pain or tenderness, does not rule out MSCC. By using magnetic resonance imaging (MRI), one observational study of asymptomatic patients with metastatic prostate cancer confirmed that 22 of 68 subjects (32%) had stenosis of the subarachnoid space or frank cord compression. Vertebral metastases were present in 65 of 68 subjects (96%) [112].

The gold standard test for MSCC is MRI (sensitivity 93%, specificity 97%) (see Fig. 29.3) [113, 114]. MRI is usually indicated even if the diagnosis has already been established either clinically or with other imaging modalities because up to 25% of patients have a lesion three

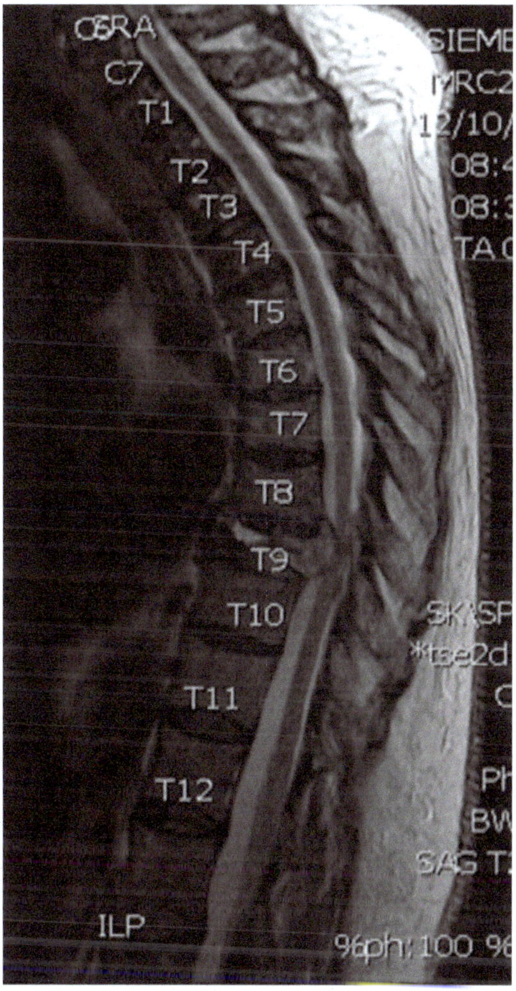

Fig. 29.3 T2-weighted MRI image demonstrating metastatic disease to thoracic vertebra number 9 (T9) with fracture of the vertebral body and impingement on the thecal sac and cord. (Image courtesy of Dr. Georgia Thomas, University of Maryland Medical Center)

or more vertebral levels away from the clinically determined level [104], 25–40% have multiple areas of compression [102–105], and up to 50% will have treatment changed based on MRI imaging [104, 115]. Due to the high morbidity associated with multiple lesions, both the thoracic and lumbar spine should be imaged in all patients suspected of MSCC. Whenever possible, the cervical spine should be included as well, but the 1% incidence of a secondary metastasis in the cervical spine lowers its priority for immediate imaging [116].

Prior to the widespread availability of MRI, plain radiographs, radionuclide scanning, and CT myelography were used to diagnose MSCC. The delayed appearance of abnormal plain radiographs in MSCC limits the utility of plain films [99], with observational studies demonstrating a 11–75% false negative rate for spinal metastasis [117–119]. Plain films showing evidence of vertebral destruction such as bony erosions or frank vertebral body collapse can only correctly predict the level of spinal cord involvement in 20% of cases [108].

Radionuclide scanning utilizes a radioactive tracer (usually ^{99m}Tc-labeled phosphates) to identify metastatic sites of increased bone turnover [120]. Though more sensitive than plain radiographs, radionuclide scans may overlook some metastatic sites seen on MRI, particularly prostate cancer and lumbar metastases [120]. Unlike MRI, radionuclide scanning provides no information about the spinal cord itself.

In situations where MRI is unavailable or contraindicated, spinal CT is considered the most informative study. If noncontrast scans suggest spinal metastasis, CT myelography can assess cord impingement by contrast injection into the subarachnoid space [118]. Sensitivity of this technique for detecting cord compression rivals that of MRI [121, 122].

While cerebrospinal fluid (CSF) protein levels may be elevated with MSCC, CSF cell counts and other laboratory values are generally unchanged [96], and such a workup is typically not indicated for MSCC. Despite historic concerns for spinal coning, a phenomenon in which pressure gradients created by spinal fluid drainage on one side of a complete subarachnoid obstruction results in paralysis below the level of the obstruction, lumbar puncture for CT myelography is now generally considered safe [96].

Clinical Management

The overall prognosis of patients with MSCC is relatively poor as this is a manifestation of disseminated cancer; however, proper and timely management can help to preserve ambulatory function and has been associated with increased median survival time [123]. Treatment includes immediate corticosteroid administration to control vasogenic edema, followed by correction of cord compression either by surgical decompression, radiation therapy, or by both (Table 29.6).

Corticosteroids provide the most immediate treatment for MSCC, as exact anatomic knowledge of the offending lesion is unnecessary and, unlike surgery or radiation, no significant logistical planning is required for their administration. In cases of high clinical suspicion, corticosteroids can be given empirically to reduce ischemia-induced vasogenic cord edema while awaiting further imaging and specialist consultation [101]. Randomized [124] and observational [125] trials of corticosteroids for MSCC have shown that subjects given an immediate bolus of intravenous dexamethasone followed by daily oral dexamethasone in combination with radiation therapy had both improved ambulation rates at 3- and 6-month intervals and improved pain scores compared to subjects receiving only immediate radiotherapy. These trials employed high-dose dexamethasone, approaching 100 mg for the bolus and daily doses, and 11% of subjects experienced adverse effects of steroid treatment [124]. However, a comparison of this high-dose therapy with a lower-dose regimen of 10 mg of intravenous dexamethasone followed by 16 mg orally daily in divided doses showed similar benefit [126]. Current guidelines suggest corticosteroids for any patient with neurological deficits believed to be secondary to MSCC [127]. A 10 mg IV bolus dose of dexamethasone followed by 16 mg orally per day is recommended for most patients [127].

Patients with significant neurological dysfunction, such as new paraplegia, may benefit from higher doses, usually 100 mg of dexamethasone as a bolus followed by 96 mg orally per day [127]. Patients with radiological spinal metastasis but without neurological deficits may be managed without steroids [127, 128].

Although corticosteroids may temporize vasogenic edema, spinal decompression must occur by surgery or radiation to prevent permanent neurological damage. Historically, surgical decompression was performed by posterior laminectomy. However, because cord compression usually results from an anterior mass effect, posterior laminectomy may not provide meaningful decompression [129]. Additionally, posterior laminectomy can destabilize the spinal column, leading to new neurological deficits in up to 25% [129]. Studies comparing radiotherapy alone with laminectomy or a combination of laminectomy and radiotherapy suggest that the addition of laminectomy does not improve outcomes and increases complications [107, 130–132].

More recently, surgical techniques for anterior decompression have been developed to replace diseased vertebral bodies with either a metal or cement spacer [129]. Surgical outcomes have improved, and most studies now suggest that cord decompression is optimally achieved by surgical intervention combined with radiation therapy. In one randomized, multicenter trial, those receiving surgery followed by radiation had higher median rates of regaining and maintaining ambulation, remaining continent, and surviving, than those receiving radiotherapy alone [133]. Several observational studies have noted improved outcomes with surgical intervention preceding radiation therapy [102, 134, 135] but one meta-analysis [136] and one observational study showed equivalence between combined therapy and radiation alone [137].

Current guidelines recommend surgery for any patient with MSCC who can tolerate it [127, 129]. Surgical decompression should particularly be considered in the following circumstances: Direct cord compression by bony fragments, spinal column instability, sphincter dysfunction, known radiation-insensitive tumor histology, and compression in an area that has already received a maximum allowable radiation dose [129]. Careful consideration should be given prior to pursuing this course, however, because 30-day postoperative mortality rates are as high as 13% and complication rates are as high as 54% [138]. Whenever possible, immediate surgery should be followed by radiation. Immediate radiation followed by delayed surgery has a significantly increased rate of wound complications and reduced 30-day continence and ambulation [139].

When surgery is not an option, radiation alone should be pursued. While radiation duration and dose will be determined by a radiation oncologist, a general knowledge of standard therapy is useful for the treating physician [140]. Randomized and observational trials comparing several-week courses of fractionated 30–100 Gy with a single 8 Gy fraction showed similar pain control, toxicity, survival, and ambulation between the two groups [141–145]. However, longer courses were associated with improved local tumor control and reduced rates of local recurrence [143, 146, 147]. Current guidelines therefore suggest a single fraction of 8 Gy for patients with poor overall prognosis, and a longer fractionated course for patients with good prognosis [127].

The recurrence rate of MSCC is about 20%, with a median interval to recurrence of 7 months [148]. In about half of these cases, repeat compression occurs at the same spinal level [148]. For these patients, current guidelines favor surgical intervention whenever possible [127, 140]. A second course of radiation is safe as long as doses are limited [149, 150], but posttreatment ambulation highly depends on pretreatment functional status [149]. In patients nearing spinal-toxic radiation doses, new radiotherapy techniques which deliver radiation with tighter focus, such as radiosurgery and stereotactic body radiation therapy, may provide viable options with little collateral exposure [151, 152].

Overall prognosis is generally poor for patients with MSCC, and median survival even with treatment is generally less than 1 year [153]. Factors indicating a poorer prognosis, both in terms of survival and functional outcome, include inability to walk before and after treatment [134, 153–155], metastatic lung or colorectal cancer [102, 156], interval from cancer diagnosis to MSCC of <15 months [157], visceral metastasis [157], and rapid progression of motor deficits (i.e., developing over ≤14 days) [158, 159]. Primary myeloma and breast and prostate cancer tend to be more radiosensitive and may, therefore, portend a better prognosis [154]. Prognostic factors derived from tumor-type-specific studies are listed in Table 29.2.

Superior Vena Cava Syndrome

Epidemiology and Pathophysiology

The superior vena cava (SVC) constitutes the final segment of venous return from the upper body to the heart. Because of its innately thin walls, relatively low venous pressure, and passage through a nondistensible area of the mediastinum, the SVC is susceptible to external compression [160]. External mass effect elevates central venous

Table 29.2 Review of factors prognosticating survival and positive functional outcome (retained or regained ambulatory, bowel, and bladder function) following therapy for MSCC by tumor type

Tumor type	Study	Factors associated with improved survival or functional status
Multiple myeloma	Douglas 2012 [200]	ECOG-PS score of 1–2 Ambulatory prior to therapy Absence of other bony metastases
Breast	Rades 2006 [201]	Ambulatory prior to therapy Absence of visceral metastases Motor deficits developed over greater than 7 days
Non-small cell lung	Rades 2012 [202]	ECOG-PS score of 1–2 Ambulatory prior to therapy Absence of visceral metastases No more than 1–2 vertebrae involved Motor deficits developed over greater than 7 days
Renal cell	Rades 2006 [144]	Motor deficits developed over greater than 14 days
Unknown primary	Douglas 2012 [203]; Rades 2007 [145]	Ambulatory prior to therapy Absence of visceral metastases Motor deficits developed over greater than 7 days

ECOG-PS score Eastern Cooperative Oncology Group – Performance Status score

Table 29.3 Critical action points: malignant pericardial disease

Presentation:
- *Pericardial effusion*:
  - *Symptoms*: Chest pain, dyspnea, nausea, dysphagia, cough
  - *Diagnostics*: large cardiac silhouette on X-ray, effusion on echo
- *Cardiac tamponade*:
  - Same as for effusion, but also shock
  - Elevated lactate, evidence of organ malperfusion
  - Cardiac chamber collapse on echo

Management:
- Should be determined based on patient prognosis and goals of care
- Immediate therapy: IV fluids and inotropes can be attempted
- Definitive therapy: Drainage of effusion as soon as possible for cardiac tamponade

Table 29.4 Critical action points: Hypercalcemia of malignancy

Presentation:
Symptoms: Constipation, abdominal pain, nausea, vomiting, anorexia, polyuria, polydipsia, neurological abnormality
Diagnostics: Shortened QT interval on EKG, elevation of serum *ionized* calcium

Management:
- Immediate therapy: Aggressive IV hydration: up to 500 mL/hr initially
- Definitive therapy:
  1. Pharmacotherapy
     - Calcitonin 4–8 u/kg subcut or IM q6hr
     - Zoledronate 4 mg IV once, OR
     - Pamidronate 90 mg IV once
  2. Initiation of antineoplastic therapy

Table 29.5 Critical action points: Tumor lysis syndrome

Presentation:
Symptoms: Nausea, vomiting, lethargy, confusion, edema, cardiac arrhythmia, seizure, myalgia
Diagnostics: Hyperuricemia, hyperkalemia, hyperphosphatemia, hypocalcemia, AKI. Peaked T waves and pan-interval prolongation on EKG
Management:
Immediate therapy: Aggressive IV hydration: 200 mL/kg/day. Diuresis or dialysis as needed
Standard management of hyperkalemia
Avoid repletion of calcium if the patient is asymptomatic
Rasburicase 3–6 mg IV once for hyperuricemia

pressures as high as 20–40 mmHg (normal 2–8 mmHg) [161]. Compression which compromises venous flow to point of symptomatic congestion or cardiac compromise constitutes superior vena cava syndrome (SVC syndrome).

Malignancy accounts for greater than 60% of SVC syndrome [160, 162], and over 90% of malignant SVC syndrome is due to primary lung cancer or lymphoma [163]. Intrathoracic infection (e.g., tuberculosis, syphilis, or histoplasmosis), goiter, benign idiopathic mediastinal fibrosis, intracaval thrombus, and foreign material in the SVC (e.g., venous catheter, pacemaker wires) are responsible for most of the nonmalignant cases [160].

SVC syndrome can also develop from flow restriction due to a large intraluminal clot, rather than an extraluminal mass, and the incidence of this etiology is increasing. While this can occur spontaneously, it is more likely to occur in a patient with an underlying hypercoagulable state [164] or with a foreign body (e.g., pacer wires, venous catheter) in the SVC [165, 166].

Clinical Presentation and Workup

Slowly developing SVC compression is often clinically silent, as development of collateral vessels ameliorates flow obstruction [167]. Patients with rapidly developing obstruction commonly present with symptoms of dyspnea and swelling of the upper extremities, face, and chest [162, 163]. Cough, chest pain, and dysphagia may also be present [162, 163]. Physical exam findings

Table 29.6 Critical action points: Metastatic spinal cord compression

Presentation:
Symptoms: Back pain, lower extremity weakness or numbness, bowel or bladder dysfunction
Diagnostics: Evidence of cord compression on whole spine MRI. Plain films or noncontrast CT scan may not have sufficient sensitivity
Management:
Immediate therapy: Dexamethasone: initial dose 10 mg intravenous
Definitive therapy: surgical decompression and/or radiation therapy

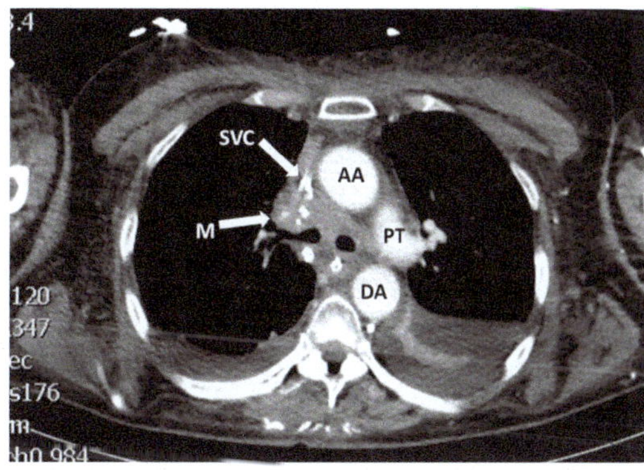

Fig. 29.4 CT scan of the thorax with intravenous contrast demonstrating a right mediastinal mass (M) compressing the SVC. Ascending aorta (AA), pulmonary artery trunk (PT), and descending aorta (DA) as marked

include facial, chest, and arm hyperemia, congestion, plethora, and edema. Jugular venous distention, cyanosis, vocal cord paralysis, blurred vision, and Horner's syndrome can also be present [160]. Chylous or exudative pleural effusions often accompany SVC compression [168].

Appropriate thoracic imaging is central to proper diagnosis and management of SVC syndrome. Plain films of the chest often demonstrate a superior mediastinal or right hilar mass [163]; though this does not confirm the diagnosis, it often prompts further imaging. Contrast-enhanced computed tomography (CT) of the chest has become a mainstay for the diagnosis and assessment of intrathoracic masses, and this modality adequately diagnoses SVC syndrome (see Fig. 29.4) [161]. Magnetic resonance imaging (MRI) of the chest may be useful when intravenous contrast is contraindicated or radiation needs to be minimized [160]. Other imaging modalities such as conventional venography and radionuclide scanning may be useful but are limited by invasiveness or availability [160].

Once diagnosed, an etiological workup is needed to ensure proper therapy. In cases of malignant etiology, a tissue diagnosis enables optimal selection of chemotherapeutics. Depending on the type of cancer, a suitable tissue sample can frequently be obtained by sputum cytology [163], but bronchoscopy, lymph node biopsy, mediastinoscopy, or even thoracotomy may be needed [163, 169, 170]. Although concern exists for delivering general anesthesia to those with SVC syndrome, little evidence exists to support this [162, 170–172]. In fact, the minimal or lack of increased risk from general anesthesia for patients with SVC syndrome should not obstruct the necessary tissue diagnosis. However, tracheal compromise, which more commonly occurs in children due to their smaller thoracic space [173], is an airway emergency and mandates its own particular precautions, for example, consideration of awake intubation to avoid sedation-induced complications [173].

Table 29.7 Critical action points: Superior vena cava syndrome

Presentation:
Symptoms: Dyspnea, edema of upper body, cough, chest pain, dysphagia
Diagnostics: Thoracic imaging – restriction of SVC flow due to either external compressive mass or internal clot
Management:
Immediate therapy: Elevate head of bed, provide supplemental oxygen if needed
Unless unstable, delay treatment to allow for diagnosis of mass, including tissue biopsy
Definitive therapy: Etiology-specific. Chemo and/or radiation for malignant SVC obstruction.

Clinical Management

Symptom management of SVC syndrome should begin with simple measures, such as head elevation and supplemental oxygen [160, 161] (Table 29.7). Steroids have historically been administered, but studies of this practice have never demonstrated benefit outside of case reports [160, 161]. Similarly, diuretics have historically been administered, but have no proven benefit in euvolemic patients and should be avoided since the patient has merely a regional increase in volume, and diuresis may induce hypotension by further reducing venous return to the heart [161, 174].

The need for a pretreatment tissue diagnosis and the rate and severity of progression of symptoms warrant urgent management of SVC patients. Despite its associated discomfort, SVC syndrome is only life-threatening when cerebral edema and airway or hemodynamic compromise exist [161, 175]. Though rare, severe SVC syndrome can also lead to right-to-left shunting of blood via systemic-to-pulmonary venous collateralization [176, 177], which can cause persistent hypoxemia. In stable patients, briefly delaying treatment for an imaging and a tissue diagnosis is safe and allows for etiology-specific management [160, 161, 174].

Definitive management depends on the etiology. A massive obstructing SVC thrombus should be treated with anticoagulation with or without thrombolysis [160, 166]. Whenever possible, foreign bodies (e.g., venous catheters) associated with thrombus should be removed [161].

Malignant SVC syndrome is managed with chemotherapeutics, radiotherapy, or both. In addition to reduction of tumor burden, the patient's own ongoing process of collateralization may also decrease SVC pressure, leading to symptomatic improvement [161]. Even with this management, though, the median survival of patients with malignant SVC syndrome is less than 1 year [160, 161, 178, 179].

SVC stenting may be beneficial when conventional treatment fails or is predicted to fail, as with poorly radio- and chemosensitive tumors [180, 181]. This intervention also immediately relieves obstruction in patients with hemodynamic or respiratory compromise [180]. Open bypass or surgical replacement of the SVC may be necessary, though this aggressive therapy is reserved for the most recalcitrant cases [182].

Leukostasis

Epidemiology and Pathophysiology

Hyperleukocytosis is defined as a white blood cell (WBC) count >100,000 cells/μL [183]. Though higher presenting WBC counts portend worse outcomes, this cutoff is arbitrary; patients with chronic lymphocytic leukemia (CLL) may tolerate counts greater than 500,000 cells/μL without complication, while certain forms of acute myeloid leukemia (AML) may cause complications with counts <100,000 cells/μL [183].

Among the known complications of hyperleukocytosis, leukostasis occurs when high WBC counts directly or indirectly induce vascular congestion, frequently in the lungs or central nervous system (CNS) [183]. Because the incidence of leukostasis does not correlate with cell count alone, leukostasis is believed to occur through two alternative mechanisms. First, the numerous large and nondeformable serum blast cells increase blood viscosity [183]. Second, certain leukemic subtypes and genetic translocations may trigger excessive cytokine-induced endothelial adhesion and vessel wall damage [183–185].

Because the gold standard tissue diagnosis is rarely initially available, the exact incidence of leukostasis is difficult to judge. Incidence seems dependent on the type and subtype of leukemia, with myeloid leukemia generally more prone and lymphocytic leukemia relatively spared [184]. Interestingly, the opposite is true of hyperleukocytosis, with incidence of 5–13% in AML and 10–30% in ALL [184]. Hypergammaglobulinemias due to multiple myeloma or Waldenström's macroglobulinemia may similarly cause hyperviscosity syndromes. The concentration of pathologic immunoglobin necessary to cause symptoms varies by type: approximately 3 g/dL for immunoglobulin M (IgM), 4 g/dL for immunoglobulin G (IgG), and 6 g/dL for immunoglobulin A (IgA) [186].

Clinical Presentation and Workup

Pulmonary leukostasis manifests as dyspnea, tachypnea, and hypoxemia [183]. Crackles may be heard on physical examination and bilateral opacities are frequently seen on chest imaging [183]. Symptoms of CNS leukostasis may include fever, confusion, dizziness, visual and auditory disturbances, headache, ataxia, delirium, and impaired level of consciousness [183] (Table 29.8). Head imaging may reveal intracranial hemorrhage [187–189] or may be grossly normal [183]. Other reported leukostatic complications include retinal hemorrhages, myocardial infarction, acute limb ischemia, priapism, renal vein thrombosis, and renal infarction [184, 190, 191].

The initial workup for leukostasis may be extensive. Blood work should include a cell count with peripheral smear, cytology, and immune staining. Imaging of afflicted systems may include an X-ray or chest CT for respiratory symptoms or a brain CT or MRI for CNS symptoms. Radiographic infiltrates and ground-glass opacities suggest pulmonary leukostasis, but normal imaging does not exclude the diagnosis [190]. CNS leukostasis may have brain imaging findings ranging from normal to intra-

Table 29.8 Critical action points: Leukostasis

Presentation:
Symptoms:
Pulmonary: Dyspnea, tachypnea, hypoxemia
Neurological: Altered level of consciousness, dizziness, headache, ataxia, visual disturbance
Labs/Imaging: Leukocytosis. Infiltrates or ground-glass opacities on chest imaging. Intracranial hemorrhage possible on head imaging
Management:
Immediate therapy: Initiate IV fluids. Avoid pRBC transfusions unless hemodynamically unstable
Definitive therapy: Leukoreduction with leukapheresis, hydroxyurea, and induction chemotherapy

cranial hemorrhage [183]. Blood gas studies in patients with hyperleukocytosis should be processed immediately to avoid the confounding "leukocyte larceny" or "leukocyte steal," which is the presence of falsely low measurements of oxygen saturation and partial pressure of oxygen (PaO_2) due to the highly abundant and metabolically active leukocytes' continued oxygen consumption in the phlebotomized sample [183].

Clinical Management

Because of overlapping symptoms and signs found in acute leukemia, leukostasis is a challenging diagnosis [192]. Most clinicians empirically treat leukostasis in patients with respiratory or CNS symptoms [183, 190]. However, simultaneous treatment of alternative etiologies, such as antibiotics for possible acute pneumonia in a patient with respiratory symptoms and lung infiltrates, may be warranted.

To reduce blood viscosity, patients with suspected leukostasis should receive intravenous fluids and [190] packed red blood cell (pRBC) transfusion should ideally be avoided [190]. Because of their much smaller contribution to blood viscosity, platelets and plasma may be given if needed to control bleeding [193].

To further manage this oncologic emergency, leukocyte reduction can be instituted with induction chemotherapy, administration of hydroxyurea, or leukapheresis. Leukapheresis entails continuous extraction of the patient's blood, selective removal of leukocytes, and return of the remaining fraction [183]. Leukapheresis rapidly reduces leukocyte counts by 20–50% in just a few hours but requires insertion of a large-bore central venous catheter or two large-bore peripheral IV lines in addition to special equipment and expertise not always readily available [183, 190]. Furthermore, existing studies on the effects of leukapheresis are nonrandomized, and their results generally demonstrate improvements in symptoms or short-term mortality [194, 195] without benefit on long-term outcomes [183, 196–198].

Hydroxyurea, a long-known antineoplastic agent which inhibits deoxyribonucleotide synthesis [199], can similarly reduce the leukemic burden by 50–80%, however its effects can take 24–48 hours to achieve maximal effect [184]. Regardless of the adjunctive therapy, induction chemotherapy, the definitive treatment, should be initiated as soon as possible [184].

Conclusion

The recognition and treatment of oncological emergencies pose unique challenges due to their diverse manifestations, often nonspecific presenting symptoms, and the often poor baseline functional status of such patients. Clinical vigilance and suspicion must be exerted when evaluating problems in cancer patients.

References

1. Press OW, Livingston R. Management of malignant pericardial effusion and tamponade. JAMA. 1987;257:1088–92.
2. Lestuzzi C. Neoplastic pericardial disease: old and current strategies for diagnosis and management. World J Cardiol. 2010;2:270–9.
3. Karam N, Patel P, deFilippi C. Diagnosis and management of chronic pericardial effusions. Am J Med Sci. 2001;322:79–87.
4. Imazio M, Demichelis B, Parrini I, et al. Relation of acute pericardial disease to malignancy. Am J Cardiol. 2005;95:1393–4.
5. Dragoescu EA, Liu L. Pericardial fluid cytology: an analysis of 128 specimens over a 6-year period. Cancer Cytopathol. 2013;121:242–51.
6. Spodick DH. Acute cardiac tamponade. N Engl J Med. 2003;349:684–90.
7. Imazio M, Adler Y. Management of pericardial effusion. Eur Heart J. 2013;34:1186–97.
8. Wilkes JD, Fidias P, Vaickus L, Perez RP. Malignancy-related pericardial effusion. 127 cases from the Roswell Park Cancer Institute. Cancer. 1995;76:1377–87.
9. Roy CL, Minor MA, Brookhart MA, Choudhry NK. Does this patient with a pericardial effusion have cardiac tamponade? JAMA. 2007;297:1810–8.
10. Argulian E, Messerli F. Misconceptions and facts about pericardial effusion and tamponade. Am J Med. 2013;126:858–61.
11. Cooper JP, Oliver RM, Currie P, Walker JM, Swanton RH. How do the clinical findings in patients with

pericardial effusions influence the success of aspiration? Br Heart J. 1995;73:351–4.
12. Guberman BA, Fowler NO, Engel PJ, Gueron M, Allen JM. Cardiac tamponade in medical patients. Circulation. 1981;64:633–40.
13. Argulian E, Herzog E, Halpern DG, Messerli FH. Paradoxical hypertension with cardiac tamponade. Am J Cardiol. 2012;110:1066–9.
14. Imazio M, Spodick DH, Brucato A, Trinchero R, Adler Y. Controversial issues in the management of pericardial diseases. Circulation. 2010;121:916–28.
15. Karatolios K, Pankuweit S, Maisch B. Diagnostic value of biochemical biomarkers in malignant and non-malignant pericardial effusion. Heart Fail Rev. 2013;18:337–44.
16. McCurdy MT, Shanholtz CB. Oncologic emergencies. Crit Care Med. 2012;40:2212–22.
17. Tsang TS, Enriquez-Sarano M, Freeman WK, et al. Consecutive 1127 therapeutic echocardiographically guided pericardiocenteses: clinical profile, practice patterns, and outcomes spanning 21 years. Mayo Clin Proc. 2002;77:429–36.
18. Maggiolini S, Bozzano A, Russo P, et al. Echocardiography-guided pericardiocentesis with probe-mounted needle: report of 53 cases. J Am Soc Echocardiogr. 2001;14:821–4.
19. Gascho JA, Martins JB, Marcus ML, Kerber RE. Effects of volume expansion and vasodilators in acute pericardial tamponade. Am J Physiol. 1981;240:H49–53.
20. Martins JB, Manuel WJ, Marcus ML, Kerber RE. Comparative effects of catecholamines in cardiac tamponade: experimental and clinical studies. Am J Cardiol. 1980;46:59–66.
21. Celik S, Lestuzzi C, Cervesato E, et al. Systemic chemotherapy in combination with pericardial window has better outcomes in malignant pericardial effusions. J Thorac Cardiovasc Surg. 2014;148:2288–93.
22. Lestuzzi C, Bearz A, Lafaras C, et al. Neoplastic pericardial disease in lung cancer: impact on outcomes of different treatment strategies. A multicenter study. Lung Cancer. 2011;72:340–7.
23. Saltzman AJ, Paz YE, Rene AG, et al. Comparison of surgical pericardial drainage with percutaneous catheter drainage for pericardial effusion. J Invasive Cardiol. 2012;24:590–3.
24. Lindner G, Felber R, Schwarz C, et al. Hypercalcemia in the ED: prevalence, etiology, and outcome. Am J Emerg Med. 2013;31:657–60.
25. Behl D, Hendrickson AW, Moynihan TJ. Oncologic emergencies. Crit Care Clin. 2010;26:181–205.
26. Stewart AF. Clinical practice. Hypercalcemia associated with cancer. N Engl J Med. 2005;352:373–9.
27. Ralston SH, Gallacher SJ, Patel U, Campbell J, Boyle IT. Cancer-associated hypercalcemia: morbidity and mortality. Clinical experience in 126 treated patients. Ann Intern Med. 1990;112:499–504.
28. Zhang SJ, Hu Y, Cao J, et al. Analysis on survival and prognostic factors for cancer patients with malignancy-associated hypercalcemia. Asian Pac J Cancer Prev. 2013;14:6715–9.
29. Sargent JT, Smith OP. Haematological emergencies managing hypercalcaemia in adults and children with haematological disorders. Br J Haematol. 2010;149:465–77.
30. Reagan P, Pani A, Rosner MH. Approach to diagnosis and treatment of hypercalcemia in a patient with malignancy. Am J Kidney Dis. 2014;63:141–7.
31. Seymour JF, Gagel RF. Calcitriol: the major humoral mediator of hypercalcemia in Hodgkin's disease and non-Hodgkin's lymphomas. Blood. 1993;82:1383–94.
32. Bilezikian JP. Management of acute hypercalcemia. N Engl J Med. 1992;326:1196–203.
33. Bellon M, Ko NL, Lee MJ, et al. Adult T-cell leukemia cells overexpress Wnt5a and promote osteoclast differentiation. Blood. 2013;121:5045–54.
34. Moseley JM, Kubota M, Diefenbach-Jagger H, et al. Parathyroid hormone-related protein purified from a human lung cancer cell line. Proc Natl Acad Sci U S A. 1987;84:5048–52.
35. Jacobs TP, Bilezikian JP. Clinical review: rare causes of hypercalcemia. J Clin Endocrinol Metab. 2005;90:6316–22.
36. Davies M, Hayes ME, Yin JA, Berry JL, Mawer EB. Abnormal synthesis of 1,25-dihydroxyvitamin D in patients with malignant lymphoma. J Clin Endocrinol Metab. 1994;78:1202–7.
37. Mudde AH, van den Berg H, Boshuis PG, et al. Ectopic production of 1,25-dihydroxyvitamin D by B-cell lymphoma as a cause of hypercalcemia. Cancer. 1987;59:1543–6.
38. Yoshimoto K, Yamasaki R, Sakai H, et al. Ectopic production of parathyroid hormone by small cell lung cancer in a patient with hypercalcemia. J Clin Endocrinol Metab. 1989;68:976–81.
39. Nussbaum SR, Gaz RD, Arnold A. Hypercalcemia and ectopic secretion of parathyroid hormone by an ovarian carcinoma with rearrangement of the gene for parathyroid hormone. N Engl J Med. 1990;323:1324–8.
40. Doyle MA, Malcolm JC. An unusual case of malignancy-related hypercalcemia. Int J Gen Med. 2013;7:21–7.
41. Ratcliffe WA, Hutchesson AC, Bundred NJ, Ratcliffe JG. Role of assays for parathyroid-hormone-related protein in investigation of hypercalcaemia. Lancet. 1992;339:164–7.
42. Rizzoli R, Thiebaud D, Bundred N, et al. Serum parathyroid hormone-related protein levels and response to bisphosphonate treatment in hypercalcemia of malignancy. J Clin Endocrinol Metab. 1999;84:3545–50.
43. Horwitz MJ, Tedesco MB, Sereika SM, Hollis BW, Garcia-Ocana A, Stewart AF. Direct comparison of sustained infusion of human parathyroid hormone-related protein-(1-36) [hPTHrP-(1-36)] versus hPTH-(1-34) on serum calcium, plasma 1,25-dihydroxyvitamin D concentrations, and frac-

tional calcium excretion in healthy human volunteers. J Clin Endocrinol Metab. 2003;88:1603–9.
44. Nakajima N, Ueda M, Nagayama H, Yamazaki M, Katayama Y. Posterior reversible encephalopathy syndrome due to hypercalcemia associated with parathyroid hormone-related peptide: a case report and review of the literature. Intern Med. 2013;52:2465–8.
45. Ladenson JH, Lewis JW, Boyd JC. Failure of total calcium corrected for protein, albumin, and pH to correctly assess free calcium status. J Clin Endocrinol Metab. 1978;46:986–93.
46. Slomp J, van der Voort PH, Gerritsen RT, Berk JA, Bakker AJ. Albumin-adjusted calcium is not suitable for diagnosis of hyper- and hypocalcemia in the critically ill. Crit Care Med. 2003;31:1389–93.
47. Fritchie K, Zedek D, Grenache DG. The clinical utility of parathyroid hormone-related peptide in the assessment of hypercalcemia. Clin Chim Acta. 2009;402:146–9.
48. Wimalawansa SJ. Significance of plasma PTH-rp in patients with hypercalcemia of malignancy treated with bisphosphonate. Cancer. 1994;73:2223–30.
49. Milionis HJ, Rizos E, Liamis G, Nikas S, Siamopoulos KC, Elisaf MS. Acid-base and electrolyte disturbances in patients with hypercalcemia. South Med J. 2002;95:1280–7.
50. Soyfoo MS, Brenner K, Paesmans M, Body JJ. Non-malignant causes of hypercalcemia in cancer patients: a frequent and neglected occurrence. Support Care Cancer. 2013;21:1415–9.
51. LeGrand SB, Leskuski D, Zama I. Narrative review: furosemide for hypercalcemia: an unproven yet common practice. Ann Intern Med. 2008;149:259–63.
52. Layman R, Olson K, Van Poznak C. Bisphosphonates for breast cancer: questions answered, questions remaining. Hematol Oncol Clin North Am. 2007;21:341–67.
53. Major P, Lortholary A, Hon J, et al. Zoledronic acid is superior to pamidronate in the treatment of hypercalcemia of malignancy: a pooled analysis of two randomized, controlled clinical trials. J Clin Oncol. 2001;19:558–67.
54. Major PP, Coleman RE. Zoledronic acid in the treatment of hypercalcemia of malignancy: results of the international clinical development program. Semin Oncol. 2001;28:17–24.
55. Nussbaum SR, Younger J, Vandepol CJ, et al. Single-dose intravenous therapy with pamidronate for the treatment of hypercalcemia of malignancy: comparison of 30-, 60-, and 90-mg dosages. Am J Med. 1993;95:297–304.
56. Drake MT, Clarke BL, Khosla S. Bisphosphonates: mechanism of action and role in clinical practice. Mayo Clin Proc. 2008;83:1032–45.
57. Silva OL, Becker KL. Salmon calcitonin in the treatment of hypercalcemia. Arch Intern Med. 1973;132:337–9.
58. Hu MI, Glezerman IG, Leboulleux S, et al. Denosumab for treatment of hypercalcemia of malignancy. J Clin Endocrinol Metab. 2014;99:3144–52. https://doi.org/10.1210/jc.2014-1001.
59. Hu MI, Glezerman I, Leboulleux S, et al. Denosumab for patients with persistent or relapsed hypercalcemia of malignancy despite recent bisphosphonate treatment. J Natl Cancer Inst. 2013;105:1417–20.
60. Boikos SA, Hammers HJ. Denosumab for the treatment of bisphosphonate-refractory hypercalcemia. J Clin Oncol. 2012;30:e299.
61. Teng J, Abell S, Hicks RJ, et al. Protracted hypocalcaemia following a single dose of denosumab in humoral hypercalcaemia of malignancy due to PTHrP-secreting neuroendocrine tumour. Clin Endocrinol (Oxf). 2014;81:940.
62. Cvitkovic F, Armand JP, Tubiana-Hulin M, Rossi JF, Warrell RP Jr. Randomized, double-blind, phase II trial of gallium nitrate compared with pamidronate for acute control of cancer-related hypercalcemia. Cancer J. 2006;12:47–53.
63. Chisholm MA, Mulloy AL, Taylor AT. Acute management of cancer-related hypercalcemia. Ann Pharmacother. 1996;30:507–13.
64. Lukert BP, Raisz LG. Glucocorticoid-induced osteoporosis: pathogenesis and management. Ann Intern Med. 1990;112:352–64.
65. Koo WS, Jeon DS, Ahn SJ, Kim YS, Yoon YS, Bang BK. Calcium-free hemodialysis for the management of hypercalcemia. Nephron. 1996;72:424–8.
66. Hassan BA, Yusoff ZB, Hassali MA, Othman SB, Weiderpass E. Impact of chemotherapy on hypercalcemia in breast and lung cancer patients. Asian Pac J Cancer Prev. 2012;13:4373–8.
67. Ipekci SH, Baldane S, Ozturk E, et al. Letrozole induced hypercalcemia in a patient with breast cancer. Case Rep Oncol Med. 2014;2014:608585.
68. Cairo MS, Bishop M. Tumour lysis syndrome: new therapeutic strategies and classification. Br J Haematol. 2004;127:3–11.
69. Koduri PR. Hyperphosphatemia and tumor lysis syndrome. Ann Hematol. 2005;84:696.
70. Desmeules S, Bergeron MJ, Isenring P. Acute phosphate nephropathy and renal failure. N Engl J Med. 2003;349:1006–7.
71. Shimada M, Johnson RJ, May WS Jr, et al. A novel role for uric acid in acute kidney injury associated with tumour lysis syndrome. Nephrol Dial Transplant. 2009;24:2960–4.
72. Wilson FP, Berns JS. Tumor lysis syndrome: new challenges and recent advances. Adv Chronic Kidney Dis. 2014;21:18–26.
73. Canet E, Zafrani L, Lambert J, et al. Acute kidney injury in patients with newly diagnosed high-grade hematological malignancies: impact on remission and survival. PLoS One. 2013;8:e55870.
74. Darmon M, Guichard I, Vincent F, Schlemmer B, Azoulay E. Prognostic significance of acute renal injury in acute tumor lysis syndrome. Leuk Lymphoma. 2010;51:221–7.
75. Cairo MS, Coiffier B, Reiter A, Younes A, TLS Expert Panel. Recommendations for the evalu-

ation of risk and prophylaxis of tumour lysis syndrome (TLS) in adults and children with malignant diseases: an expert TLS panel consensus. Br J Haematol. 2010;149:578–86.
76. McBride A, Westervelt P. Recognizing and managing the expanded risk of tumor lysis syndrome in hematologic and solid malignancies. J Hematol Oncol. 2012;5:75.
77. Duff DJ, Haddadin S, Freter C, Papageorgiou C. Gemcitabine and cisplatin-induced tumor lysis syndrome in a patient with gallbladder carcinoma: a case report. Oncol Lett. 2013;5:1237–9.
78. Coiffier B, Altman A, Pui CH, Younes A, Cairo MS. Guidelines for the management of pediatric and adult tumor lysis syndrome: an evidence-based review. J Clin Oncol. 2008;26:2767–78.
79. Hsu HH, Huang CC. Acute spontaneous tumor lysis in anaplastic large T-cell lymphoma presenting with hyperuricemic acute renal failure. Int J Hematol. 2004;79:48–51.
80. Van Mieghem C, Sabbe M, Knockaert D. The clinical value of the ECG in noncardiac conditions. Chest. 2004;125:1561–76.
81. Howard SC, Jones DP, Pui CH. The tumor lysis syndrome. N Engl J Med. 2011;364:1844–54.
82. Kelton J, Kelley WN, Holmes EW. A rapid method for the diagnosis of acute uric acid nephropathy. Arch Intern Med. 1978;138:612–5.
83. Tungsanga K, Boonwichit D, Lekhakula A, Sitprija V. Urine uric acid and urine creatine ratio in acute renal failure. Arch Intern Med. 1984;144:934–7.
84. Ten Harkel AD, Kist-Van Holthe JE, Van Weel M, Van der Vorst MM. Alkalinization and the tumor lysis syndrome. Med Pediatr Oncol. 1998;31: 27–8.
85. Weisberg LS. Management of severe hyperkalemia. Crit Care Med. 2008;36:3246–51.
86. Rogers FB, Li SC. Acute colonic necrosis associated with sodium polystyrene sulfonate (Kayexalate) enemas in a critically ill patient: case report and review of the literature. J Trauma. 2001;51:395–7.
87. Coiffier B, Mounier N, Bologna S, et al. Efficacy and safety of rasburicase (recombinant urate oxidase) for the prevention and treatment of hyperuricemia during induction chemotherapy of aggressive non-Hodgkin's lymphoma: results of the GRAAL1 (Groupe d'Etude des Lymphomes de l'Adulte Trial on Rasburicase Activity in Adult Lymphoma) study. J Clin Oncol. 2003;21:4402–6.
88. Bosly A, Sonet A, Pinkerton CR, et al. Rasburicase (recombinant urate oxidase) for the management of hyperuricemia in patients with cancer: report of an international compassionate use study. Cancer. 2003;98:1048–54.
89. Bucklin MH, Groth CM. Mortality following rasburicase-induced methemoglobinemia. Ann Pharmacother. 2013;47:1353–8.
90. Hummel M, Reiter S, Adam K, Hehlmann R, Buchheidt D. Effective treatment and prophylaxis of hyperuricemia and impaired renal function in tumor lysis syndrome with low doses of rasburicase. Eur J Haematol. 2008;80:331–6.
91. Knoebel RW, Lo M, Crank CW. Evaluation of a low, weight-based dose of rasburicase in adult patients for the treatment or prophylaxis of tumor lysis syndrome. J Oncol Pharm Pract. 2011;17:147–54.
92. Vines AN, Shanholtz CB, Thompson JL. Fixed-dose rasburicase 6 mg for hyperuricemia and tumor lysis syndrome in high-risk cancer patients. Ann Pharmacother. 2010;44:1529–37.
93. Trifilio S, Gordon L, Singhal S, et al. Reduced-dose rasburicase (recombinant xanthine oxidase) in adult cancer patients with hyperuricemia. Bone Marrow Transplant. 2006;37:997–1001.
94. McDonnell AM, Lenz KL, Frei-Lahr DA, Hayslip J, Hall PD. Single-dose rasburicase 6 mg in the management of tumor lysis syndrome in adults. Pharmacotherapy. 2006;26:806–12.
95. Montesinos P, Lorenzo I, Martin G, et al. Tumor lysis syndrome in patients with acute myeloid leukemia: identification of risk factors and development of a predictive model. Haematologica. 2008;93:67–74.
96. Byrne TN. Spinal cord compression from epidural metastases. N Engl J Med. 1992;327:614–9.
97. Loblaw DA, Laperriere NJ, Mackillop WJ. A population-based study of malignant spinal cord compression in Ontario. Clin Oncol. 2003; 15:211–7.
98. Sansur CA, Pouratian N, Dumont AS, Schiff D, Shaffrey CI, Shaffrey ME. Part II: spinal-cord neoplasms--primary tumours of the bony spine and adjacent soft tissues. Lancet Oncol. 2007;8:137–47.
99. Arguello F, Baggs RB, Duerst RE, Johnstone L, McQueen K, Frantz CN. Pathogenesis of vertebral metastasis and epidural spinal cord compression. Cancer. 1990;65:98–106.
100. Traul DE, Shaffrey ME, Schiff D. Part I: spinal-cord neoplasms-intradural neoplasms. Lancet Oncol. 2007;8:35–45.
101. Cole JS, Patchell RA. Metastatic epidural spinal cord compression. Lancet Neurol. 2008;7:459–66.
102. Constans JP, de Divitiis E, Donzelli R, Spaziante R, Meder JF, Haye C. Spinal metastases with neurological manifestations. Review of 600 cases. J Neurosurg. 1983;59:111–8.
103. Helweg-Larsen S, Hansen SW, Sorensen PS. Second occurrence of symptomatic metastatic spinal cord compression and findings of multiple spinal epidural metastases. Int J Radiat Oncol Biol Phys. 1995;33:595–8.
104. Cook AM, Lau TN, Tomlinson MJ, Vaidya M, Wakeley CJ, Goddard P. Magnetic resonance imaging of the whole spine in suspected malignant spinal cord compression: impact on management. Clin Oncol. 1998;10:39–43.
105. van der Sande JJ, Kroger R, Boogerd W. Multiple spinal epidural metastases; an unexpectedly frequent finding. J Neurol Neurosurg Psychiatry. 1990;53:1001–3.

106. Helweg-Larsen S, Sorensen PS. Symptoms and signs in metastatic spinal cord compression: a study of progression from first symptom until diagnosis in 153 patients. Eur J Cancer. 1994;30A:396–8.
107. Gilbert RW, Kim JH, Posner JB. Epidural spinal cord compression from metastatic tumor: diagnosis and treatment. Ann Neurol. 1978;3:40–51.
108. Levack P, Graham J, Collie D, et al. Don't wait for a sensory level--listen to the symptoms: a prospective audit of the delays in diagnosis of malignant cord compression. Clin Oncol. 2002;14:472–80.
109. Husband DJ. Malignant spinal cord compression: prospective study of delays in referral and treatment. BMJ. 1998;317:18–21.
110. Deyo RA, Rainville J, Kent DL. What can the history and physical examination tell us about low back pain? JAMA. 1992;268:760–5.
111. Schiff D, O'Neill BP, Suman VJ. Spinal epidural metastasis as the initial manifestation of malignancy: clinical features and diagnostic approach. Neurology. 1997;49:452–6.
112. Bayley A, Milosevic M, Blend R, et al. A prospective study of factors predicting clinically occult spinal cord compression in patients with metastatic prostate carcinoma. Cancer. 2001;92:303–10.
113. Li KC, Poon PY. Sensitivity and specificity of MRI in detecting malignant spinal cord compression and in distinguishing malignant from benign compression fractures of vertebrae. Magn Reson Imaging. 1988;6:547–56.
114. Husband DJ, Grant KA, Romaniuk CS. MRI in the diagnosis and treatment of suspected malignant spinal cord compression. Br J Radiol. 2001;74:15–23.
115. Colletti PM, Siegel HJ, Woo MY, Young HY, Terk MR. The impact on treatment planning of MRI of the spine in patients suspected of vertebral metastasis: an efficacy study. Comput Med Imaging Graph. 1996;20:159–62.
116. Schiff D, O'Neill BP, Wang CH, O'Fallon JR. Neuroimaging and treatment implications of patients with multiple epidural spinal metastases. Cancer. 1998;83:1593–601.
117. Portenoy RK, Galer BS, Salamon O, et al. Identification of epidural neoplasm. Radiography and bone scintigraphy in the symptomatic and asymptomatic spine. Cancer. 1989;64:2207–13.
118. O'Rourke T, George CB, Redmond J 3rd, et al. Spinal computed tomography and computed tomographic metrizamide myelography in the early diagnosis of metastatic disease. J Clin Oncol. 1986;4:576–83.
119. Rodichok LD, Harper GR, Ruckdeschel JC, et al. Early diagnosis of spinal epidural metastases. Am J Med. 1981;70:1181–8.
120. Gosfield E 3rd, Alavi A, Kneeland B. Comparison of radionuclide bone scans and magnetic resonance imaging in detecting spinal metastases. J Nucl Med. 1993;34:2191–8.
121. Hagenau C, Grosh W, Currie M, Wiley RG. Comparison of spinal magnetic resonance imaging and myelography in cancer patients. J Clin Oncol. 1987;5:1663–9.
122. Carmody RF, Yang PJ, Seeley GW, Seeger JF, Unger EC, Johnson JE. Spinal cord compression due to metastatic disease: diagnosis with MR imaging versus myelography. Radiology. 1989;173:225–9.
123. Helweg-Larsen S. Clinical outcome in metastatic spinal cord compression. A prospective study of 153 patients. Acta Neurol Scand. 1996;94:269–75.
124. Sorensen S, Helweg-Larsen S, Mouridsen H, Hansen HH. Effect of high-dose dexamethasone in carcinomatous metastatic spinal cord compression treated with radiotherapy: a randomised trial. Eur J Cancer. 1994;30A:22–7.
125. Greenberg HS, Kim JH, Posner JB. Epidural spinal cord compression from metastatic tumor: results with a new treatment protocol. Ann Neurol. 1980;8:361–6.
126. Vecht CJ, Haaxma-Reiche H, van Putten WL, de Visser M, Vries EP, Twijnstra A. Initial bolus of conventional versus high-dose dexamethasone in metastatic spinal cord compression. Neurology. 1989;39:1255–7.
127. Loblaw DA, Mitera G, Ford M, Laperriere NJ. A 2011 updated systematic review and clinical practice guideline for the management of malignant extradural spinal cord compression. Int J Radiat Oncol Biol Phys. 2012;84:312–7.
128. Maranzano E, Latini P, Beneventi S, et al. Radiotherapy without steroids in selected metastatic spinal cord compression patients. A phase II trial. Am J Clin Oncol. 1996;19:179–83.
129. Prasad D, Schiff D. Malignant spinal-cord compression. Lancet Oncol. 2005;6:15–24.
130. Young RF, Post EM, King GA. Treatment of spinal epidural metastases. Randomized prospective comparison of laminectomy and radiotherapy. J Neurosurg. 1980;53:741–8.
131. Sorensen S, Borgesen SE, Rohde K, et al. Metastatic epidural spinal cord compression. Results of treatment and survival. Cancer. 1990;65:1502–8.
132. Findlay GF. Adverse effects of the management of malignant spinal cord compression. J Neurol Neurosurg Psychiatry. 1984;47:761–8.
133. Patchell RA, Tibbs PA, Regine WF, et al. Direct decompressive surgical resection in the treatment of spinal cord compression caused by metastatic cancer: a randomised trial. Lancet. 2005;366:643–8.
134. Bach F, Agerlin N, Sorensen JB, et al. Metastatic spinal cord compression secondary to lung cancer. J Clin Oncol. 1992;10:1781–7.
135. Rades D, Huttenlocher S, Bajrovic A, et al. Surgery followed by radiotherapy versus radiotherapy alone for metastatic spinal cord compression from unfavorable tumors. Int J Radiat Oncol Biol Phys. 2011;81:e861–8.
136. Klimo P Jr, Thompson CJ, Kestle JR, Schmidt MH. A meta-analysis of surgery versus conventional radiotherapy for the treatment of metastatic spinal epidural disease. Neuro Oncol. 2005;7:64–76.

137. Rades D, Huttenlocher S, Dunst J, et al. Matched pair analysis comparing surgery followed by radiotherapy and radiotherapy alone for metastatic spinal cord compression. J Clin Oncol. 2010;28:3597–604.
138. Loblaw DA, Perry J, Chambers A, Laperriere NJ. Systematic review of the diagnosis and management of malignant extradural spinal cord compression: the Cancer Care Ontario Practice Guidelines Initiative's Neuro-Oncology Disease Site Group. J Clin Oncol. 2005;23:2028–37.
139. Ghogawala Z, Mansfield FL, Borges LF. Spinal radiation before surgical decompression adversely affects outcomes of surgery for symptomatic metastatic spinal cord compression. Spine. 2001;26:818–24.
140. Holt T, Hoskin P, Maranzano E, et al. Malignant epidural spinal cord compression: the role of external beam radiotherapy. Curr Opin Support Palliat Care. 2012;6:103–8.
141. Maranzano E, Trippa F, Casale M, et al. 8Gy single-dose radiotherapy is effective in metastatic spinal cord compression: results of a phase III randomized multicentre Italian trial. Radiother Oncol. 2009;93:174–9.
142. Maranzano E, Bellavita R, Rossi R, et al. Short-course versus split-course radiotherapy in metastatic spinal cord compression: results of a phase III, randomized, multicenter trial. J Clin Oncol. 2005;23:3358–65.
143. Rades D, Stalpers LJ, Veninga T, et al. Evaluation of five radiation schedules and prognostic factors for metastatic spinal cord compression. J Clin Oncol. 2005;23:3366–75.
144. Rades D, Walz J, Stalpers LJ, et al. Short-course radiotherapy (RT) for metastatic spinal cord compression (MSCC) due to renal cell carcinoma: results of a retrospective multi-center study. Eur Urol. 2006;49:846–52; discussion 52.
145. Rades D, Fehlauer F, Veninga T, et al. Functional outcome and survival after radiotherapy of metastatic spinal cord compression in patients with cancer of unknown primary. Int J Radiat Oncol Biol Phys. 2007;67:532–7.
146. Rades D, Lange M, Veninga T, et al. Final results of a prospective study comparing the local control of short-course and long-course radiotherapy for metastatic spinal cord compression. Int J Radiat Oncol Biol Phys. 2011;79:524–30.
147. Rades D, Fehlauer F, Schulte R, et al. Prognostic factors for local control and survival after radiotherapy of metastatic spinal cord compression. J Clin Oncol. 2006;24:3388–93.
148. van der Sande JJ, Boogerd W, Kroger R, Kappelle AC. Recurrent spinal epidural metastases: a prospective study with a complete follow up. J Neurol Neurosurg Psychiatry. 1999;66:623–7.
149. Maranzano E, Trippa F, Casale M, Anselmo P, Rossi R. Reirradiation of metastatic spinal cord compression: definitive results of two randomized trials. Radiother Oncol. 2011;98:234–7.
150. Nieder C, Grosu AL, Andratschke NH, Molls M. Update of human spinal cord reirradiation tolerance based on additional data from 38 patients. Int J Radiat Oncol Biol Phys. 2006;66:1446–9.
151. Wang XS, Rhines LD, Shiu AS, et al. Stereotactic body radiation therapy for management of spinal metastases in patients without spinal cord compression: a phase 1–2 trial. Lancet Oncol. 2012;13:395–402.
152. Ryu S, Rock J, Jain R, et al. Radiosurgical decompression of metastatic epidural compression. Cancer. 2010;116:2250–7.
153. Maranzano E, Latini P, Checcaglini F, et al. Radiation therapy in metastatic spinal cord compression. A prospective analysis of 105 consecutive patients. Cancer. 1991;67:1311–7.
154. Maranzano E, Latini P. Effectiveness of radiation therapy without surgery in metastatic spinal cord compression: final results from a prospective trial. Int J Radiat Oncol Biol Phys. 1995;32:959–67.
155. Helweg-Larsen S, Sorensen PS, Kreiner S. Prognostic factors in metastatic spinal cord compression: a prospective study using multivariate analysis of variables influencing survival and gait function in 153 patients. Int J Radiat Oncol Biol Phys. 2000;46:1163–9.
156. Sioutos PJ, Arbit E, Meshulam CF, Galicich JH. Spinal metastases from solid tumors. Analysis of factors affecting survival. Cancer. 1995;76:1453–9.
157. Rades D, Douglas S, Huttenlocher S, et al. Validation of a score predicting post-treatment ambulatory status after radiotherapy for metastatic spinal cord compression. Int J Radiat Oncol Biol Phys. 2011;79:1503–6.
158. Rades D, Blach M, Bremer M, Wildfang I, Karstens JH, Heidenreich F. Prognostic significance of the time of developing motor deficits before radiation therapy in metastatic spinal cord compression: one-year results of a prospective trial. Int J Radiat Oncol Biol Phys. 2000;48:1403–8.
159. Rades D, Heidenreich F, Karstens JH. Final results of a prospective study of the prognostic value of the time to develop motor deficits before irradiation in metastatic spinal cord compression. Int J Radiat Oncol Biol Phys. 2002;53:975–9.
160. Abner A. Approach to the patient who presents with superior vena cava obstruction. Chest. 1993;103:394S–7S.
161. Wilson LD, Detterbeck FC, Yahalom J. Clinical practice. Superior vena cava syndrome with malignant causes. N Engl J Med. 2007;356:1862–9.
162. Rice TW, Rodriguez RM, Light RW. The superior vena cava syndrome: clinical characteristics and evolving etiology. Medicine. 2006;85:37–42.
163. Armstrong BA, Perez CA, Simpson JR, Hederman MA. Role of irradiation in the management of superior vena cava syndrome. Int J Radiat Oncol Biol Phys. 1987;13:531–9.
164. de Jager CP, Rutten MJ, Lips DJ. "Benign" superior vena cava syndrome. Intensive Care Med. 2013;39:572–3.

165. Shaikh I, Berg K, Kman N. Thrombogenic catheter-associated superior vena cava syndrome. Case Rep Emerg Med. 2013;2013:793054.
166. Shaheen K, Alraies MC. Superior vena cava syndrome. Cleve Clin J Med. 2012;79:410–2.
167. Bechtold RE, Wolfman NT, Karstaedt N, Choplin RH. Superior vena caval obstruction: detection using CT. Radiology. 1985;157:485–7.
168. Rice TW. Pleural effusions in superior vena cava syndrome: prevalence, characteristics, and proposed pathophysiology. Curr Opin Pulm Med. 2007;13:324–7.
169. Jahangiri M, Goldstraw P. The role of mediastinoscopy in superior vena caval obstruction. Ann Thorac Surg. 1995;59:453–5.
170. Mineo TC, Ambrogi V, Nofroni I, Pistolese C. Mediastinoscopy in superior vena cava obstruction: analysis of 80 consecutive patients. Ann Thorac Surg. 1999;68:223–6.
171. Ahmann FR. A reassessment of the clinical implications of the superior vena caval syndrome. J Clin Oncol. 1984;2:961–9.
172. Ferrari LR, Bedford RF. General anesthesia prior to treatment of anterior mediastinal masses in pediatric cancer patients. Anesthesiology. 1990;72:991–5.
173. Jain R, Bansal D, Marwaha RK, Singhi S. Superior mediastinal syndrome: emergency management. Indian J Pediatr. 2013;80:55–9.
174. Schraufnagel DE, Hill R, Leech JA, Pare JA. Superior vena caval obstruction. Is it a medical emergency? Am J Med. 1981;70:1169–74.
175. Yu JB, Wilson LD, Detterbeck FC. Superior vena cava syndrome--a proposed classification system and algorithm for management. J Thorac Oncol. 2008;3:811–4.
176. Juan YH, Saboo SS, Anand V, Chatzizisis YS, Lin YC, Steigner ML. Superior vena cava syndrome associated with right-to-left shunt through systemic-to-pulmonary venous collaterals. Korean J Radiol. 2014;15:185–7.
177. Kim HC, Chung JW, Park SH, et al. Systemic-to-pulmonary venous shunt in superior vena cava obstruction: depiction on computed tomography venography. Acta Radiol. 2004;45:269–74.
178. Chan RH, Dar AR, Yu E, et al. Superior vena cava obstruction in small-cell lung cancer. Int J Radiat Oncol Biol Phys. 1997;38:513–20.
179. Chan RC, Chan YC, Cheng SW. Mid- and long-term follow-up experience in patients with malignant superior vena cava obstruction. Interact Cardiovasc Thorac Surg. 2013;16:455–8.
180. Sobrinho G, Aguiar P. Stent placement for the treatment of malignant superior vena cava syndrome – a single-center series of 56 patients. Arch Bronconeumol. 2014;50:135–40.
181. Marcy PY, Magne N, Bentolila F, Drouillard J, Bruneton JN, Descamps B. Superior vena cava obstruction: is stenting necessary? Support Care Cancer. 2001;9:103–7.
182. Li H, Jiang X, Sun T. Open surgery repair for superior vena cava syndrome after failed endovascular stenting. Ann Thorac Surg. 2014;97:1445–7.
183. Ganzel C, Becker J, Mintz PD, Lazarus HM, Rowe JM. Hyperleukocytosis, leukostasis and leukapheresis: practice management. Blood Rev. 2012;26:117–22.
184. Porcu P, Cripe LD, Ng EW, et al. Hyperleukocytic leukemias and leukostasis: a review of pathophysiology, clinical presentation and management. Leuk Lymphoma. 2000;39:1–18.
185. Stucki A, Rivier AS, Gikic M, Monai N, Schapira M, Spertini O. Endothelial cell activation by myeloblasts: molecular mechanisms of leukostasis and leukemic cell dissemination. Blood. 2001;97:2121–9.
186. Mehta J, Singhal S. Hyperviscosity syndrome in plasma cell dyscrasias. Semin Thromb Hemost. 2003;29:467–71.
187. Munoz J, Donthireddy V. CNS hyperleukocytosis. Blood. 2012;119:5953.
188. Naunheim MR, Nahed BV, Walcott BP, et al. Diagnosis of acute lymphoblastic leukemia from intracerebral hemorrhage and blast crisis. A case report and review of the literature. Clin Neurol Neurosurg. 2010;112:575–7.
189. Shiber JR, Fines RE. Cerebral hemorrhage due to hyperleukocytosis. J Emerg Med. 2011;40:674–7.
190. Majhail NS, Lichtin AE. Acute leukemia with a very high leukocyte count: confronting a medical emergency. Cleve Clin J Med. 2004;71:633–7.
191. Yen TH, Chang CT, Ng KK, Wu MS. Bilateral renal infarction in chronic myelomonocytic leukemia on blast crisis. Ren Fail. 2003;25:1029–35.
192. Wu YK, Huang YC, Huang SF, Huang CC, Tsai YH. Acute respiratory distress syndrome caused by leukemic infiltration of the lung. J Formos Med Assoc. 2008;107:419–23.
193. Jain R, Bansal D, Marwaha RK. Hyperleukocytosis: emergency management. Indian J Pediatr. 2013;80:144–8.
194. Novotny JR, Muller-Beissenhirtz H, Herget-Rosenthal S, Kribben A, Duhrsen U. Grading of symptoms in hyperleukocytic leukaemia: a clinical model for the role of different blast types and promyelocytes in the development of leukostasis syndrome. Eur J Haematol. 2005;74:501–10.
195. Bug G, Anargyrou K, Tonn T, et al. Impact of leukapheresis on early death rate in adult acute myeloid leukemia presenting with hyperleukocytosis. Transfusion. 2007;47:1843–50.
196. Oberoi S, Lehrnbecher T, Phillips B, et al. Leukapheresis and low-dose chemotherapy do not reduce early mortality in acute myeloid leukemia hyperleukocytosis: a systematic review and meta-analysis. Leuk Res. 2014;38:460–8.
197. De Santis GC, de Oliveira LC, Romano LG, et al. Therapeutic leukapheresis in patients with leukostasis secondary to acute myelogenous leukemia. J Clin Apher. 2011;26:181–5.

198. Pastore F, Pastore A, Wittmann G, Hiddemann W, Spiekermann K. The role of therapeutic leukapheresis in hyperleukocytotic AML. PLoS One. 2014;9:e95062.
199. Platt OS. Hydroxyurea for the treatment of sickle cell anemia. N Engl J Med. 2008;358:1362–9.
200. Douglas S, Schild SE, Rades D. A new score predicting the survival of patients with spinal cord compression from myeloma. BMC Cancer. 2012;12:425.
201. Rades D, Veninga T, Stalpers LJ, et al. Prognostic factors predicting functional outcomes, recurrence-free survival, and overall survival after radiotherapy for metastatic spinal cord compression in breast cancer patients. Int J Radiat Oncol Biol Phys. 2006;64:182–8.
202. Rades D, Douglas S, Veninga T, Schild SE. A validated survival score for patients with metastatic spinal cord compression from non-small cell lung cancer. BMC Cancer. 2012;12:302.
203. Douglas S, Huttenlocher S, Bajrovic A, Rudat V, Schild SE, Rades D. Prognostic factors for different outcomes in patients with metastatic spinal cord compression from cancer of unknown primary. BMC Cancer. 2012;12:261.

Obstetric Emergency Critical Care

30

Michael Buscher and Jennifer H. Edwards

Introduction

Management of critical illness in pregnancy can be intellectually challenging, emotionally devastating, and uniquely rewarding for the practitioner of adult emergency and critical care. Serious illness in pregnancy is rare; so, reliance on well-oiled patterns of recognition and management is often not possible. Yet, many pregnant women are resilient and can recover from critical illness without sequelae. The care these women receive may make an enormous difference in outcome. In this chapter, we cover the important aspects of the initial diagnosis and management of the most common critical illnesses that affect pregnant and peripartum patients in the United States. These include disease processes unique to the obstetric population; illnesses that are not limited to pregnancy but may strike with greater severity; and non-obstetric diseases for which there may be uncertainty about management because of the pregnancy, including cardiac arrest. In addition, we have provided tips on relevant pharmacology and diagnostic imaging in the pregnant patient.

[Disclaimer: Information provided on pharmacology and diagnostic imaging is not intended to be complete, replace good judgment or consultation with an obstetrician, pharmacist, or radiologist.]

General Principles of Management

An understanding of the altered physiology of pregnancy is essential (Tables 30.1, 30.2, 30.3, and 30.4). Many signs and symptoms of critical illness may at first be attributed to the normal experience of pregnancy, leading to delays in presentation and diagnosis.

Maternal positioning has broad clinical implications. The clinical effects of *supine hypotensive syndrome* become more pronounced as the gravid uterus enlarges greater than 20 weeks gestation and exerts increasing pressure on the IVC. Effects may be particularly significant in pathologic states in which there is increased dependence on preload/cardiac output to maintain blood pressure. Positioning the pregnant woman on her left side can prevent this, although a lateral tilt of at least 20 degrees or manual uterine displacement to the left is adequate to restore baseline hemodynamics.

Routine chest radiographs (CXR) should be avoided *if not necessary* to the evaluation, particularly in the first trimester; if done, the abdomen should be shielded. Thoracic ultrasonography may also be considered for the diagnosis of cardiopulmonary pathology. In general, women of

M. Buscher
Critical Care Medicine, Emergency Medicine, Yale New Haven Health, New Haven, CT, USA

J. H. Edwards (✉)
Intermountain Healthcare, Murray, UT, USA

© Springer Nature Switzerland AG 2020
J. R. Shiber, S. D. Weingart (eds.), *Emergency Department Critical Care*,
https://doi.org/10.1007/978-3-030-28794-8_30

Table 30.1 Cardiovascular adaptations in normal pregnancy

Physiologic parameter	Change	Time course	Clinical implications
Heart rate	↑ 15–20 bpm	Peaks 32–36 weeks	Mild tachycardia
Blood pressure	↓ 10–20%	Nadir 28 weeks	Mild (relative) hypotension
Stroke volume	↑	Throughout	–
Cardiac output	↑ 30–50% ↑ 60–80%	Peaks 25–32 weeks Within 15–20 minutes post partum	Blood pressure is increasingly supported by cardiac output in late pregnancy Third trimester and 4–6 hours after delivery are high risk times for patient with cardiac disease/risk factors
Ejection fraction (EF)	No change	–	Decreased EF on Echo signals pathology
ECG	Left-axis deviation	Late	–
CXR	Mild cardiomegaly	Late	–
Cardiac exam	Flow murmur	Throughout	Other murmurs can be pathological
CVP	No change	–	–

Refs. [115–117]

Table 30.2 Hematologic changes in normal pregnancy

Physiologic parameter	Change
Blood volume	↑ 30–50%
Hemodilution	Hgb ↓ about 1 gm
Platelets	No change
Procoagulants, including fibrinogen	↑↑
Colloid oncotic pressure	↓ about 15%

Ref. [25]

Table 30.3 Changes in common lab values during normal pregnancy

	Trend compared to nonpregnant adult female	Normal range in pregnancy
Hemoglobin (gm/dL)	↓	9.5–15 but generally >10
WBC (×10^3/mm^3)	↑	5.7–16.9 with left shift
Platelets (×10^9/L)	Slight ↓	Usually >150,000
HCO3- (mEq/L)	↓	18–22
BUN (mg/dL)	↓	3–12
Creatinine (mg/dL)	↓	0.4–0.8
Glomerular filtration rate	↑40–50%	–
Alkaline phosphatase (U/L)	↑ 2nd and 3rd trimesters	17–229
Serum albumin (g/dL)	↓	2.3–5.1
Bilirubin	No change to slight ↓	–
AST and ALT	Within normal reference range	–
LDH (U/L)	Usually within normal range, possible ↑	78–524
PT	Within normal reference range	–

Refs. [118, 119]

Table 30.4 Pulmonary adaptations in normal pregnancy

Physiologic parameter	Change	Time course	Clinical implications
Oxygen consumption	↑ 20–35%	Peaks at term	Decreased respiratory reserve
Minute ventilation	↑ 20–40%	Peaks at term	'Innocent hyperpnea'
Tidal volume	↑ 30–40%	Peaks at term	'Innocent hyperpnea'
Functional residual capacity	↓ 20%	–	Decreased respiratory reserve
Respiratory rate	No change	–	Significant or progressive dyspnea is not a normal finding in pregnancy

Refs. [117, 119]

reproductive age should be transfused with type-specific or O-negative blood. Central venous and arterial lines should be placed above the diaphragm due to increased pressure and poor venous return from the enlarged uterus.

In all cases, we recommend consulting an obstetrician (OB) or maternal–fetal medicine (MFM) specialist, checking fetal heart tones, and initiating continuous fetal monitoring at a gestational age sufficient for viability—this is often around 23–24 weeks but is institution-dependent. If preterm delivery is necessary prior to 34 weeks of gestation, there may be a role for administering steroids to aid in fetal lung maturation; this should be done in consultation with the obstetrician.

Many critically ill pregnant patients will require admission to an intensive care unit at a tertiary care hospital with MFM, transplant, or advanced cardiac services. Some catastrophic maternal pulmonary and cardiovascular illnesses can be very survivable. In these cases, our institution has had good outcomes with aggressive treatment including extra-corporeal membrane oxygenation (ECMO). Finally, perimortem cesarean section within 4 minutes of arrest may improve outcomes for both mother and fetus.

Epidemiology

Pregnancy-related deaths in the US have been increasing since 1987 and the current rate of 16 deaths per 100,000 live births is the highest in the developed world [1, 2]. This trend may be due in part to an increasing number of pregnant women with chronic medical conditions. Medical cardiovascular disease is now the single most common cause of pregnancy-related death in the US, accounting for 14.6% of maternal deaths. Infection and sepsis are the second leading causes of pregnancy-related death in the US and the leading causes in the UK [1, 3, 4]. Many women who suffer a pregnancy-related death do not make it to an intensive care unit—in one study, almost 60% of in-hospital maternal deaths occurred without admission to an ICU [2].

Fetal Physiology

Oxygen delivery to the fetus depends on uterine artery blood flow to the placenta and maternal oxygen content. The uterine artery is maximally dilated at baseline and unable to adapt to stress by local vascular adjustment. Conditions that lower maternal cardiac output or uterine artery blood flow (shock or vasoconstriction), as well as maternal hypoxia, will reduce oxygen delivery to the fetus. Maternal hypotension, exogenous or endogenous catecholamines, and alkalosis will cause uterine artery vasoconstriction. Factors that cause fetal acidosis may result in fetal hypoxia, as the fetal hemoglobin dissociation curve shifts to the right, limiting the ability of fetal hemoglobin to bind oxygen.

The fetus lives in a relatively hypoxic environment at baseline with an arterial PO_2 of 20–25 mmHg. Several compensatory mechanisms maintain oxygen delivery and protect the fetus from hypoxic insult. Fetal oxygenation is maintained until fetal oxygen content is reduced by more than 75%; irreversible brain damage begins only after 10 minutes without oxygen [5].

Hypoxia, hypercapnia, hypotension, shock, infection, acidosis, and alkalosis are harmful to both mother and fetus. However, the fetus may have a narrower window of tolerance than the mother for metabolic derangements. Continuous fetal heart rate monitoring after viable gestational age may provide early clues to maternal decompensation as well as fetal distress.

Cardiovascular Problems in Pregnancy

Cardiovascular disease is currently the leading cause of maternal mortality in the United States [1, 3]. The maternal cardiovascular system is significantly remodeled, usually reversibly, during pregnancy (Table 30.1). The third trimester, labor, and immediate postpartum period are the highest risk times for patients with cardiovascular disease. There are also hematologic changes that have broad clinical implications (Table 30.2). Cardiovascular medications routinely used and contraindicated in pregnancy are reviewed in Table 30.5.

Preexisting Heart Disease in Pregnancy

Maternal cardiac disease complicates 0.2–4% of pregnancies in industrialized Western countries, and in one study accounted for 14% of obstetric ICU admissions [6, 7].

Congenital Heart Disease and Pulmonary Arterial Hypertension

Residual disease almost always remains in women who have undergone catheter-based or surgical repair, and maternal response to physiologic changes in pregnancy can be unpredictable. Patients with prosthetic valves can often undergo a relatively normal pregnancy, and are usually managed with aspirin, twice-daily low-molecular weight heparin, or unfractionated heparin. Generally, regurgitant lesions are well tolerated, and obstructive lesions are poorly tolerated.

Eisenmenger syndrome and pulmonary arterial hypertension (PAH) are associated with a high (17–50%) mortality during pregnancy with the highest risk during the third trimester or the first few months after delivery [6, 8, 9].

Signs and Symptoms A physiologic S3 heart sound can often be auscultated in pregnancy, reflecting increased circulating volume. Symptoms that are *abnormal* during pregnancy include significant or progressive dyspnea, exertional chest pain, paroxysmal nocturnal dyspnea, orthopnea, sustained arrhythmias, pulmonary edema, dia-

Table 30.5 Cardiac drugs during pregnancy

Routinely used	
Anti-hypertensives	IV hydralazine, labetalol, nicardipine
	PO labetalol, nifedipine, hydralazine
	Nitroglycerin in myocardial ischemia
Heart failure	Furosemide, digoxin, beta blockers, milrinone, dobutamine, prostacyclin analogs, phosphodiesterase inhibitors
Vasopressors	All vasopressors have been used in pregnancy with the caveat that they may adversely affect uterine blood flow Norepinephrine, phenylephrine and vasopressin are routinely used in our institution
Anticoagulation and thrombolysis	Low molecular weight heparin is preferred over heparin for therapeutic and prophylactic anticoagulation in the stable patient. There are case reports of thrombolytics being safely given to pregnant women with life-threatening PE
ACLS	There are no changes to ACLS pharmacology during pregnancy and limited evidence suggests that no changes need to be made during maternal defibrillation or cardioversion [Nanson 2001]
Generally avoided	
ACE inhibitors, ARBs, amiodarone, warfarin, thiazide diuretics, spironolactone, statins, nitroprusside, calcium channel blockers	

Refs. [38, 120]

stolic murmurs, severe obstructive systolic murmurs, and an S4 gallop [8].

Differential diagnosis includes ischemic heart disease, peripartum cardiomyopathy, and pulmonary disease.

Initial evaluation and management should include a personal and family history, ECG, BNP, and transthoracic echocardiogram (TTE); consultation with a cardiologist, pulmonologist, or MFM specialist; hemodynamic monitoring and support as indicated. Women with PAH and those with CHD determined to be high risk by World Health Organization score or New York Heart Association grade should be managed by multidisciplinary critical care teams in specialized centers [10].

Acquired Ischemic Heart Disease

Acute coronary syndrome (ACS) is rare during pregnancy. Most acute myocardial infarctions (AMI) occur in multiparous women over the age of 30 during the third trimester, which is the period of greatest cardiovascular stress [11]. Pregnancy increases the risk of AMI two- to fourfold compared with age-matched nonpregnant women, with a sixfold risk immediately postpartum [12]. ACS in pregnant women may be caused by coronary spasm, in situ thrombosis and spontaneous coronary dissection, as well as acute plaque rupture or stenosis causing demand ischemia [12]. In addition to the usual ACS risk factors, pregnant women may face heightened risk from preeclampsia, gestational hypertension, thrombocytosis, and anemia.

Signs and symptoms include chest pain/pressure, exertional dyspnea, and diaphoresis. Some symptoms may overlap with common symptoms of normal pregnancy, which may delay diagnosis and treatment [12]. Clinical exam may reveal pulmonary edema.

Differential diagnosis includes peripartum cardiomyopathy, pulmonary embolism (PE), CHD, preeclampsia with pulmonary edema, pulmonary disease, and amniotic fluid embolism.

Initial evaluation includes ECG, basic labs, troponin, as well as CXR and BNP if indicated. CXR should be avoided if possible, especially during the first trimester.

Management Patients with STEMI should be taken for cardiac catheterization. The maternal abdomen should be shielded with lead, and fluoroscopy time should be limited. Because drug-eluting stents (DES) require a longer duration of antiplatelet therapy and their safety in pregnancy remains unstudied, PCI with a bare metal stent (BMS) is the current treatment of choice for pregnant women with STEMI [12]. Thrombolytic agents can be given if patients cannot undergo percutaneous coronary intervention (PCI) in the recommended time frame, although there is an approximately 8% risk of maternal hemorrhage [11–13].

Aspirin, nitrates, and beta-blockers are safe and effective for pregnant patients with ACS. Angiotensin-converting-enzyme (ACE) inhibitors and statins are contraindicated during pregnancy. There is a paucity of safety data regarding the use of thienopyridine derivatives (clopidogrel) and glycoprotein IIb/IIIa inhibitors in pregnant patients; most suggest using these for the shortest time possible. These agents may preclude regional anesthesia for labor and breastfeeding after delivery. It is recommended that patients taking GIIb/IIIa inhibitors undergo cesarean delivery to minimize the risk of fetal intracranial hemorrhage [11]. Patients without STEMI should undergo a workup similar to non-pregnant patients with symptoms of ACS. Most patients should be admitted to an ICU with MFM and cardiology consultation.

Hypertension in Pregnancy

Hypertension is one of the most common medical problems affecting the gravid patient, complicating 12% of all pregnancies [14]. The first important task is to determine whether it is due to preeclampsia because management and clinical sequelae of preeclampsia are different than for other causes of hypertension in pregnancy. In this section, we review the approach to severe hypertension in pregnancy.

Signs and Symptoms Hypertension in pregnancy is defined as a systolic blood pressure >140 mmHg or a diastolic pressure >90 mmHg

[15]. Evidence of end-organ damage and significant morbidity should be sought as in the non-pregnant population, as well as fetal distress. Note the signs and symptoms of preeclampsia (Table 30.6).

Differential Diagnosis Hypertension before 20 weeks of gestation suggests chronic essential hypertension, whereas hypertension that develops after 20 weeks indicates either gestational hypertension or preeclampsia. Gestational hypertension is an elevation in blood pressure during the second half of pregnancy or in the first 24 hours postpartum, without symptoms, proteinuria, or abnormal blood tests.

Initial evaluation is aimed at establishing the diagnosis and detecting morbidity, and should be broad including the following: complete blood count (CBC), comprehensive metabolic panel (CMP), serum uric acid, and lactic acid dehydrogenase (LDH), liver function tests (LFTs), UA (proteinuria), toxicology panel, and an ECG. CXR and brain imaging should be considered based on the patient's symptoms and presentation. Fetal heart tones should be checked.

Initial Management Patients with multiple blood pressures >160/100 should be started on parenteral antihypertensives. Antihypertensive medications that can be used safely in pregnancy include intravenous hydralazine or labetalol, or a titratable drip of labetalol or nicardipine. A nitroglycerin drip is a good option in cases of myocardial ischemia. Nitroprusside is not recommended if there are other options due to concern for fetal cyanide poisoning.

In the absence of significant morbidity, a reasonable ultimate goal is systolic pressures around 140 mmHg, and diastolic pressures around 90 mmHg, with care not to lower the MAP more than 25% in the initial phase of treatment. Lowering the blood pressure too rapidly can reduce cerebral, renal, myocardial, and uteroplacental perfusion.

Preeclampsia and Eclampsia

Preeclampsia is a disorder unique to pregnancy with serious adverse consequences for the mother and fetus. It is characterized by hypertension, proteinuria, and/or signs and symptoms listed in Table 30.6. In 2013, the American College of Obstetricians and Gynecologists removed proteinuria as a requirement for the diagnosis. Although hypertension is a defining feature of preeclampsia, the clinical presentation may be nonspecific and the disorder may involve every

Table 30.6 Preeclampsia—diagnostic criteria and severe features

Blood Pressure	≥140 systolic or ≥90 diastolic on 2 readings >4 hours apart after 20 weeks gestation in woman with previously normal BP **or** ≥160 systolic or ≥110 diastolic on 2 readings only minutes apart
	[a]≥160 systolic or ≥110 diastolic on 2 readings taken 4 hours apart while the patient is on bed rest unless antihypertensives initiated before this time
AND	
1. Proteinuria	>300 mg/24 hours (or extrapolated from a shorter collection)
OR	
2. New onset HTN with any of the following ([a]severe) features:	
Thrombocytopenia	[a]PLT <100,000/μL
Renal insufficiency	[a]sCr >1.1 mg/dL **or** 2× patient baseline
Impaired Liver Function	AST/ALT 2× normal [a](**and/or** severe, persistent RUQ/epigastric pain)
Pulmonary Edema	[a]clinical/radiographic
CNS or Visual symptoms	[a]Photopsia, scotomata, cortical blindness, retinal vasospasm, severe or persistent and progressive headache, altered mental status

Adapted from: Ref. [121]
[a]Designates severe features

system. Studies have suggested abnormal development of placental vasculature as a trigger. Preeclampsia affects approximately 3.4% of pregnancies in the United States, and the disease and its complications are among the most common reasons for obstetric ICU admission [16–19].

Eclampsia is the occurrence of new-onset seizures/coma in a patient with preeclampsia. The incidence of eclampsia in the United States is 0.04–0.1% [20, 21]. The maternal mortality rate is approximately 0.4–7.2% in developed nations, with a perinatal mortality rate of 11.8% in the US [21, 22]. The mechanism of eclamptic seizures is not clear. Most seizures are self-limited and last 1–2 minutes, with care during the event being supportive.

Signs and symptoms may be nonspecific and mistaken for a viral syndrome. The degree of hypertension and the presence of proteinuria, signs/symptoms, and laboratory abnormalities are highly variable [23]. Preeclampsia is divided into mild preeclampsia and preeclampsia with severe features (Table 30.6). Eclampsia presents with new onset generalized tonic–clonic seizures or coma, particularly in the third trimester. Preeclampsia/eclampsia may present as early as 20 weeks, but most cases are diagnosed after 34 weeks gestation through 1 month postpartum.

Clinical concerns include eclamptic seizures, posterior reversible encephalopathy, maternal intracranial hemorrhage, stroke, retinal detachment, pulmonary edema, ARDS, acute kidney injury, hepatic rupture or subcapsular hemorrage, hepatic infarction, HELLP syndrome, DIC, and placental abruption. Persistent thrombocytopenia, hemolysis, or organ dysfunction may indicate an alternative diagnosis of thrombotic thrombocytopenic purpura (TTP) or hemolytic uremic syndrome (HUS). Risk to the fetus from preeclampsia relates primarily to the condition of the mother as well as the gestational age at delivery.

Initial evaluation is broad and includes labs as listed above and in Table 30.6 for the pregnant patient with hypertension. Brain imaging is indicated after stabilization for patients with seizures or other neurologic symptoms.

Initial Management:

1. Blood pressure control is essential, but does not prevent progression of the disease.
2. In patients with preeclampsia, magnesium sulfate halves the risk of progression to eclampsia and likely reduces the risk of maternal death [24–26]. See Table 30.7 for dosing as well as treatment of magnesium toxicity.
3. In patients with eclampsia, magnesium sulfate is the anticonvulsive drug of choice (Table 30.7). Studies have shown that it is superior to benzodiazepines and antiepileptic drugs [27].
4. Supportive treatment of seizures as discussed in neurologic problems in pregnancy.
5. While it does not explain cases of postpartum eclampsia, most experts consider delivery of the placenta as the only curative treatment for antepartum preeclampsia and eclampsia. Women with mild preeclampsia at early gestational ages may be managed expectantly. Severe preeclampsia, eclampsia, HELLP syndrome, and fetal distress are indications for urgent delivery.

Peripartum Cardiomyopathy

Peripartum cardiomyopathy (PPCM) is a rare cause of heart failure that affects women in late pregnancy or early in the postpartum period.

Table 30.7 Magnesium for preeclampsia and eclampsia[a]

Loading dose	4–6 g IV over 15–30 minutes
Maintenance dose	2 g/hr IV Stop or reduce to 1 g/h for signs of toxicity[b]
Recurrent seizures (eclampsia)	2 g IV over 10–15 minutes
Treatment of magnesium toxicity[b]	*10 mL of 10% calcium gluconate over 10 minutes*

Ref. [20]

[a]Administration should be done in consultation with OB. Dosing reflects normal renal function. A loading dose of 5 g IM in each buttock for total of 10 g may be given in the absence of IV access

[b]Signs of magnesium toxicity include loss of patellar reflexes, somnolence, respiratory difficulty, cardiac dysrhythmias. Treatment of magnesium toxicity is administration of calcium, which competitively inhibits magnesium at the neuromuscular junction and decreases the toxic effects

PPCM is increasingly a cause of pregnancy-related death, now responsible for 11% of maternal deaths in the US [3]. The etiology remains unknown but is likely multifactorial [28]. Risk factors for PPCM include African descent, pregnancy with multiple fetuses, severe hypertension during pregnancy, obesity, cocaine abuse, or long-term (>4 weeks) oral tocolytic therapy with beta-adrenergic agonists such as terbutaline.

In more than half of patients diagnosed with PPCM, the left ventricular ejection fraction (LVEF) normalizes, usually within 6 months. LVEF >30% at presentation is a good prognostic sign but cannot be used to guide treatment. Those who do not improve by 6 months face 85% mortality at 5 years. These patients can be supported with mechanical assist devices and transplanted; however, they have higher rates of rejection and infection than other heart transplant recipients [29].

Signs and symptoms may be present at rest and include most commonly dyspnea, but also orthopnea, peripheral edema, fatigue, palpitations, chest pain, and cough. Most patients present in New York Heart Association (NYHA) class III or IV heart failure with a marked limitation of physical activity [29]. Nevertheless, the diagnosis can be challenging to make during late pregnancy when symptoms may overlap with the normal experience of pregnancy. PPCM is usually diagnosed within the first month after delivery, with 80% of cases diagnosed within the first 3 months [30]. When diagnosed before delivery, the average gestational age is approximately 37 weeks [31]. Patients with PPCM have a significantly heightened risk of thromboembolic disease and may present with this as well as decompensated heart failure.

PPCM is a diagnosis of exclusion. The 2011 European Society of Cardiology guidelines on the management of cardiovascular disease during pregnancy define PPCM as:

- An idiopathic cardiomyopathy
- Develops toward the end of pregnancy or within months of delivery
- With the absence of an identifiable cause
- With left ventricular (LV) systolic dysfunction, either dilated or nondilated, and an ejection fraction (EF) nearly always <45% [6]

The differential diagnosis includes CHD, diastolic heart failure secondary to hypertension, AMI, and pulmonary embolism.

Initial evaluation should include an ECG, BNP, cardiac enzymes and basic labs, TTE, CXR if there is concern for pulmonary edema, investigation for thromboembolism as indicated, and ultimately cardiac MRI and cardiac catheterization.

Initial management of acute presentations of PPCM with adequate perfusion begins with furosemide for preload reduction and relief of pulmonary edema, and vasodilators for afterload reduction. Evidence of poor perfusion (cool extremities, pallor, end organ damage) calls for inotropic support with dobutamine (pregnancy category B) or milrinone (pregnancy category C), and a low ejection fraction or evidence of thromboembolic disease may require anticoagulation. Beta blockade should be initiated early if the patient is not in a decompensated state. ACE inhibitors and aldosterone antagonists are contraindicated prior to delivery, although they are recommended postpartum. Cardiology should be urgently consulted for assistance in medical management and workup for additional therapies such as mechanical assist devices and transplantation. Most patients should initially be admitted to an ICU setting.

Pulmonary Embolism

Pregnancy and delivery are associated with an alteration in coagulation factors, stasis, and endothelial trauma—all three elements of Virchow's triad. Risk of thrombosis increases five- to tenfold during pregnancy, and by a factor of 9–22 in the 6 weeks following delivery with some heightened risk lasting for 12 weeks [25, 32]. Thromboembolic disease is a leading cause of maternal death in the US and UK, responsible for 9.6% of pregnancy-related deaths in the US between 2006 and 2010 [1, 2, 33].

Signs and symptoms may overlap with normal physiologic changes of pregnancy such as tachycardia, dyspnea, and leg swelling. DVT during pregnancy is more likely to be proximal, massive, and in the left lower extremity. Isolated iliac vein thrombosis may occur in pregnancy. Twenty percent of venous thromboembolic events during pregnancy and the postpartum period present as pulmonary embolism (PE) [34].

Initial evaluation is based on the 2011 American Thoracic Society (ATS) guideline, which was subsequently endorsed by the American College of Obstetricians and Gynecologists. The evidence supporting one imaging modality over the other is weak. In pregnant women with suspected PE and evidence of DVT, bilateral venous compression ultrasonography is the first-line test; anticoagulation should be started if positive for DVT, and further testing is indicated for negative scans. If there is suspicion for pelvic thrombosis, this should be followed with pelvis MRI or CT. If there is concern for PE, but no evidence of DVT, a chest radiograph should be obtained: a V/Q scan is recommended for patients with a normal CXR; a CT scan with pulmonary angiography is recommended for patients with an abnormal CXR. In a patient with a nondiagnostic V/Q scan, further imaging with a CTA is recommended rather than empiric treatment. In a patient for whom there is a reasonable suspicion of acute PE, bedside TTE showing an acutely dilated and hypocontractile right ventricle is enough evidence to begin empiric treatment.

The use of d-dimer as a screening test in pregnant women has not been validated. D-dimer levels are elevated in pregnancy, with particularly high levels in advanced gestational age, preeclampsia, and twin pregnancies. Nevertheless, it is possible that in the future, a negative test in conjunction with ultrasound may be useful for ruling out DVT/PE [35–37].

Initial management is anticoagulation with unfractionated heparin (UFH) or low molecular weight heparin (LMWH), with increasing preference to use LMWH in stable patients who are not at risk of bleeding from recent/imminent delivery or procedures [38]. For life-threatening PE, rescue therapies such as thrombolysis (systemic or catheter-directed), thrombectomy (surgical or catheter-assisted) and ECMO should be considered. While pregnancy is a relative contraindication, there are case reports of thrombolysis being used safely in pregnancy. Tissue plasminogen activator (tPA) is a large polypeptide that will not cross the placenta. Consultants may include a cardiothoracic surgeon, obstetrician, interventional radiologist, and intensivist.

Amniotic Fluid Embolism

Amniotic fluid embolism (AFE) is a catastrophic syndrome that classically occurs acutely during labor or in the immediate postpartum period. About 70% of cases occur before delivery. When it occurs postpartum, the time from delivery to the onset of symptoms is generally less than 45 minutes, although it can be delayed up to 48 hours. Most people who die do so within 7 hours [39]. AFE was once thought to be almost uniformly fatal; however, recent studies estimate that around one-fifth of women with this condition in the US will die [40]. Survivors frequently have long-term neurologic impairment.

The pathogenesis of AFE remains unclear. It appears to involve a breakdown in the barrier between maternal circulation and amniotic fluid and may be immune mediated [39]. It is no longer believed that amniotic fluid components cause an obstruction of the pulmonary vasculature.

Signs and symptoms may include premonitory symptoms; however, AFE usually presents abruptly and rapidly evolves to affect every system. The primary findings are sudden cardiovascular collapse with profound systemic hypotension, cardiac dysrhythmias, cyanosis, dyspnea or respiratory arrest, altered mental status and/or seizures, disseminated intravascular coagulation and hemorrhage, and pulmonary edema or ARDS [39, 40]. Most studies implicate a biphasic hemodynamic response to AFE, beginning with acute pulmonary artery hypertension and right heart failure followed quickly by left ventricular failure [40]. Profound hypoxemia may at first result from severe ventilation–perfusion mismatch, later from pulmonary edema. There have been rare cases associated with abortion, amniocentesis, and trauma.

Differential diagnosis includes the entities below:

Pulmonary embolism	Aortic dissection
Air embolism	Aspiration pneumonitis
Anesthetic complications	Transfusion reaction
Anaphylaxis to a medication	Sepsis
Myocardial infarction	Postpartum hemorrhage
Peripartum cardiomyopathy	Uterine rupture
	Placental abruption
	Eclampsia

Adapted from: Conde-Agudelo and Romero [40]

Initial evaluation should include echocardiography. Lab evaluation should be broad and include an ABG, lactate, and DIC studies.

Initial management is aimed at treating acute pulmonary hypertension with biventricular failure and supporting multisystem dysfunction. Immediate delivery of the fetus is paramount. A pulmonary artery catheter may help guide treatment. Treatment otherwise depends on the severity of illness and capabilities of the institution and involves support and rescue therapies including massive transfusion for hemorrhage and DIC; intubation and mechanical ventilation; pressors and inotropes; inhaled nitric oxide or prostacyclins; intraaortic balloon pump or ventricular assist devices; and ECMO/cardiopulmonary bypass.

Arrhythmias

Direct-current cardioversion and defibrillation are used to treat life-threatening arrhythmias in pregnancy. Other arrhythmias should be managed as they would be in a nonpregnant patient, with the avoidance of amiodarone. Vagal maneuvers, adenosine, beta-blockers, and digoxin have been safely used in pregnancy. There is a paucity of data regarding the safety of calcium channel blockers and some concern for maternal hypotension and fetal heart block; therefore, beta-blockers are preferred.

Cardiac Arrest

Cardiopulmonary arrest in pregnancy is uncommon. Major causes of cardiac arrest in pregnancy are listed in Table 30.8. Three major modifications to ACLS are suggested when treating pregnant patients in cardiac arrest: [41]

1. Secure the airway early with endotracheal intubation, preferably by an experienced provider, given inherent difficulty (See Table 30.9). A laryngeal device is not recommended due to increased risk of aspiration and altered airway physiology in pregnant patients.
2. Manual displacement of the uterus toward the left during chest compressions (chest compressions higher on the chest)
3. Consider perimortem cesarean delivery within 4 minutes of arrest

Aortocaval compression exerted by a uterus greater than 20 weeks gestation must be relieved to optimize the effectiveness of CPR. This is best achieved during CPR by manual displacement of

Table 30.8 Causes of cardiac arrest in pregnancy

Hemorrhage/hypovolemia
Placental abruption
Placenta previa
Hepatic hematoma
Ectopic pregnancy
Uterine rupture
Hypoxia
Hypermagnesemia/hyperkalemia
Acidosis
Hypoglycemia
Hypertension-related
Preeclampsia & eclampsia
Thrombosis/embolism
Pulmonary embolism
Myocardial infarction
Stroke
Amniotic fluid embolism
Tension pneumothorax
Tamponade (cardiac)
Trauma
Toxins
Sepsis
Anesthesia-related

Adapted from: Refs. [122, 123]

Table 30.9 Intubation in the pregnant patient

Risk	Response
Low oxygen reserve ➔	Preoxygenate
Airway hyperemia, friable mucosa ➔	Avoid nasotracheal intubation, suction readily available
Airway edema ➔	Use smaller endotracheal tube (6–7 mm)
Weight gain obscures anatomy ➔	Proper positioning ("sniffing" position)
Aspiration risk ➔	Cricoid pressure, rapid sequence induction, consider use of bicitrate if applicable,
Supine hypotensive syndrome ➔	Tilt patient or displace uterus to left after 20 weeks gestation

Adapted from Ref. [115]

the uterus to the left and not-left lateral positioning with a wedge, because the latter technique contributes to a reduction in chest compression force generation.

Perimortem cesarean section can be lifesaving for both mother and fetus. In addition to relieving aortocaval compression, it increases maternal blood volume and cardiac output. In healthy women who undergo cesarean delivery, cardiac output is increased by 30% and patients receive approximately 500 mL of autotransfusion [42]. Early cesarean delivery can have good outcomes for the fetus as well. It has been estimated that a fetus can survive for more than 10 minutes in conditions of asphyxia. In one review of surviving infants, 70% of the neonates had been delivered within 5 minutes of maternal death, and 93% within 15 minutes. Most had no neurologic sequelae [43]. If perimortem cesarean section is to be performed within 4 minutes of arrest, planning for the procedure must begin simultaneously with other maternal resuscitation efforts.

Respiratory Problems in Pregnancy

Shortness of breath is a common complaint during normal pregnancy because of physiologic changes (Table 30.4). It is vital to differentiate between dyspnea of pregnancy and pathologic causes of dyspnea that may result from pulmonary or cardiovascular disease. During evaluation, one must keep in mind several points: (1) pregnant women have decreased respiratory reserve and may quickly become hypoxic; (2) baseline arterial blood gas values differ from the nonpregnant patient (Table 30.10) and a PCO_2 of ≥40 portends respiratory failure; (3) some metabolic derangements driven by maternal respiratory insufficiency may be poorly tolerated by the fetus; and (4) intubation is likely to be difficult and high risk (Table 30.9).

Table 30.10 Changes in arterial blood gas values during pregnancy

	Pregnant	Nonpregnant adult
pH	7.40–7.47	7.35–7.45
PCO_2 (mmHg)	26–32	35–45
PO_2 (mmHg)	100–110	80–100
HCO_3^- (mEq/L)	18–21	22–26
$P(A\text{-}a)O_2$ (mmHg)	20	14

Asthma

Asthma is one of the most common chronic illnesses seen in pregnant women. In general, one-third of women with asthma get worse during pregnancy [44]. Improved asthma control may improve pregnancy outcomes. Exacerbations occur most frequently from 17 to 24 weeks, with decreased severity during the last 4 weeks of pregnancy. Exacerbations generally do not occur during labor, but may be incited by medications used in the peripartum period such as ergots and prostaglandin F2α (used for postpartum hemorrhage), indomethacin, morphine, and meperidine [45].

Differential diagnosis for women with severe symptoms includes viral infection (notably influenza), pneumonia, pulmonary edema, cardiomyopathy, and pulmonary embolism.

Initial evaluation includes a history of asthma and exacerbating factors, physical exam, and CXR if indicated. Peak expiratory flow rate (PEFR) generally does not change during pregnancy, especially if done while seated; therefore, this remains a useful tool to assess severity. Fetal heart tones should be checked. Arterial blood gases may help guide management (Table 30.10).

Initial management of the patient with a moderate-to-severe exacerbation who does not require immediate intubation includes high-dose, short-acting inhaled beta-2 agonist, inhaled ipratropium bromide, parenteral steroids, and supplemental oxygen with a goal oxygen saturation >95%. Noninvasive positive pressure ventilation (NPPV) may be used as a temporizing measure and is further discussed below in Airway Management. The following guidelines are an adjunct to clinical judgment: [46, 47]

1. Factors indicating ICU admission with intensivist coverage:
   (a) $PaCO2 \geq 40$ or
   (b) PEFR <25% of predicted
2. Factors indicating a need for intubation:
   (a) Severe symptoms and poor response to therapy
   (b) Inability to maintain a PaO2 >60 mmHg with 90% saturation despite supplemental oxygen
   (c) Inability to maintain a PaCO2 <40 mmHg
   (d) Worsening acidosis despite bronchodilator therapy (pH 7.2–7.25)
   (e) Exhaustion
   (f) Altered consciousness (drowsiness, confusion)

Pneumonia in Pregnancy

Pneumonia is the most common cause of fatal non-obstetric infection during pregnancy [48]. Community-acquired pneumonia is the norm with prevalence equivalent to that in the nonpregnant population, and *Streptococcus pneumoniae* the most frequently isolated pathogen [49]. Pregnant women are also at increased risk for aspiration pneumonia due to changes in the gastrointestinal system. Additional risk factors include preexisting maternal disease (HIV, asthma, and cystic fibrosis), anemia, cocaine use, and alcohol abuse [50].

Pneumonia is less well tolerated in pregnancy due to maternal physiologic adaptations (Table 30.4). Pregnant women have higher rates of complications from community-acquired pneumonia, including the need for mechanical ventilation (10–20%), bacteremia, and empyema [50]. The neonatal mortality rate due to antepartum pneumonia ranges from 1.9% to 12% with most deaths attributable to complications of preterm birth [50].

Signs and symptoms of bacterial pneumonia in pregnancy are the same as in nonpregnant women. Physical examination has limited sensitivity and specificity.

Initial evaluation should include CXR, assessment of oxygenation, and blood and sputum cultures. Bronchoscopy can be safely performed in pregnant patients.

Initial management for healthy pregnant women with no recent antibiotic or hospital exposure requiring hospitalization for pneumonia is shown in Table 30.11. The remainder of therapy is supportive with careful attention to maternal oxygenation and acid–base status, fetal monitoring when appropriate, and early preparation for intubation. American Thoracic Society and British Thoracic Society guidelines for severity assessment in pneumonia have been applied retrospectively to a limited series of pregnant patients and these may be useful in predicting the need for admission, ICU admission, and antibiotic choice [50].

Influenza in Pregnancy

Pregnant and postpartum women are at increased risk for severe pulmonary disease from H1N1 influenza. In the US, 5% of all deaths from the 2009 H1N1 Influenza pandemic were among pregnant women, although pregnant women represent only about 1% of the US population [51]. Most severe infections occurred in the second and third trimesters [52]. Comorbid asthma and obesity increase risk for complications [53]. Physiology responsible for the increased risk of severe disease may include suppression of cell-mediated immunity and pregnancy-related cardiac and respiratory changes. However, there remain two important modifiable factors: immunization, timely diagnosis, and treatment.

Maternal immunization during pregnancy is safe and protective for mother, fetus, and neonate [54–56]. Nevertheless, in the 2010–2011 flu sea-

Table 30.11 Antibiotics in pregnancy

Generally safe	Penicillins Cephalosporins Azithromycin Erythromycin (non-estolate) Clindamycin Gentamicin Nitrofurantoin Vancomycin Aztreonam
Broad spectrum empiric IV antibiotics for sepsis [1]	1. Vancomycin 15–20 mg/kg IV loading dose + Piperacillin/Tazobactam 4.5 gr IV every 6 hours 2. Gentamicin 1.5 mg/kg IV loading dose + Clindamycin 900 mg IV every 8 hours + Penicillin 3 m units IV every 4 hours
Empiric IV antibiotics for severe community acquired pneumonia	1. Azithromycin + [ceftriaxone/cefotaxime/ampicillin-sulbactam] 2. Aztreonam + gentamicin + azithromycin
Empiric IV antibiotics for postpartum endometritis [2, 3]	Clindamycin + gentamicin For patients with group B streptococcus ampicillin should be added or ampicillin–sulbactam can be considered for monotherapy
Empiric IV antibiotics for chorioamnionitis	Ampicillin + gentamicin. Add clindamycin for planned cesarean deliveries
Generally avoided or contraindicated in pregnancy	Tetracyclines (doxycycline, minocycline) Tigecycline Clarithromycin[a] Erythromycin estolate Fluoroquinolones[a] Chloramphenicol Kanamycin Streptomycin Sulfonamides[a]

Refs. [49, 70, 124–127]
[a]Safety information unclear, sometimes used

son, only 49% of pregnant women reported getting the vaccine [57].

Early diagnosis and treatment are key. Pregnant women who did not receive early antivirals were more likely to be admitted to the ICU or to die (relative risk 4.3) than were pregnant women who received antivirals within 48 hours [52]. Treatment is often delayed due to misattribution of symptoms to pregnancy, a high (up to 38%) false-negative rate of the rapid influenza test during flu season, and erroneous concerns that antivirals harm the fetus [52].

Signs and symptoms may be vague and systemic. There should be a high degree of suspicion for influenza in any pregnant patient presenting with respiratory and/or systemic complaints around flu season. *Differential diagnosis* includes preeclampsia, cardiopulmonary disease, bacterial pneumonia, HELLP syndrome, and acute fatty liver of pregnancy.

Initial evaluation should include CXR, rapid influenza screen, *and* a more reliable test such as viral culture or real time PCR.

Initial management involves early antivirals and supportive care. It is our practice to initiate treatment with oseltamivir at the time the test is sent and discontinue the drug when a reliable negative result becomes available. Some modifications to the use of oseltamivir may be beneficial for critically ill patients: (a) treatment may be initiated up to 4–5 days after illness onset; (b) doses of 150 mg BID appear to be well tolerated and may be beneficial in patients with normal renal function; (c) in patients with prolonged illness, it is reasonable to extend treatment beyond 5 days [58]. Other treatment is supportive with addition of antibiotics if bacterial superinfection is suspected; community-acquired, methicillin-resistant *Staphylococcus aureus* influenza-associated pneumonia carries a fatality rate of 25% [59].

Pregnant women critically ill with H1N1 influenza frequently require mechanical ventilation and treatment for ARDS. We have had some success using ECMO in these cases and therefore advocate early consideration of transfer to an ECMO center for patients with severe pulmonary disease. Fetal outcomes largely depend on severity of maternal illness. It is unclear whether early delivery improves maternal outcomes in these cases, but it may be wise in the setting of rapid decompensation when proning or initiation of ECMO is imminent.

ARDS and Noncardiogenic Pulmonary Edema

Incidence of ARDS in pregnant women is believed to be similar to that in the general population, but may be up to 10 times higher than incidence in nonpregnant women of similar (reproductive) age [60, 61]. The reasons for this probably lie in the altered physiology of pregnancy, and infections or diseases specific to pregnancy such as AFE that frequently involve ARDS (see Cardiovascular Problems in Pregnancy). Maternal mortality from ARDS in pregnancy is thought to be similar to that or slightly better than in the general population [60].

Etiologies for ARDS in the Obstetric Population Severe sepsis or septic shock is the most common cause of ARDS in both the obstetric and nonobstetric populations. The source of sepsis may not be immediately apparent. Acute pyelonephritis seems to be an especially important cause of obstetric sepsis-related ARDS. Up to 7% of pregnant women with acute pyelonephritis may develop respiratory failure [60, 62]. Other considerations relevant to the pregnant woman include influenza, bacterial/aspiration pneumonia, chorioamnionitis, endometritis, and retained products of conception.

Severe preeclampsia and eclampsia, as well as some tocolytic medications such as the beta-2 adrenoreceptor agonists terbutaline and ritodrine, can cause pulmonary edema with acute hypoxemic respiratory failure. The mechanism for both is unclear and may involve a combination of cardiogenic and noncardiogenic factors. Noncardiogenic factors include the decreased oncotic pressure normal to pregnancy along with increased permeability of the pulmonary capillary membranes and excessive resuscitation with IV fluids characteristic of the disease and treatment. These processes generally respond to cessation of the offending drug, delivery of the fetus, and gentle diuresis or fluid conservative therapy.

Initial Management

1. Identify and direct therapy at the underlying cause (above).
2. Supportive care including airway and ventilator management (below).
3. Closely monitor fetus if it is of viable gestational age.

Airway Management

The approach to airway management in the pregnant patient is unique in two ways. The first involves assessing the need for intubation. A pregnant woman has decreased respiratory reserve and increased oxygen consumption at baseline (Table 30.4). Evaluation should take into account alterations in normal arterial blood gas values during pregnancy (Table 30.10). A $PaCO_2$ of ≥40 represents woefully inadequate ventilation. Respiratory acidosis, alkalosis, and prolonged hypoxemia may be poorly tolerated by the fetus.

Noninvasive positive pressure ventilation (BiPAP, CPAP) is an acceptable temporizing measure, but carries a heightened risk of aspiration in pregnant women. It should be used cautiously and never in women with altered mental status or a condition that is not expected to improve quickly.

Second, a pregnant woman must be presumed to have a difficult and potentially high-risk airway. Difficulty of obtaining an airway, as indicated by Mallampati score, increases as pregnancy progresses [63]. A pregnant patient may become hypoxic quickly when apneic and is at increased risk for aspiration. Challenges and modifications to intubating the pregnant patient are outlined in Table 30.9.

Mechanical Ventilation

There are two general considerations when mechanically ventilating a pregnant patient. First, care should be taken with maternal positioning to avoid supine hypotensive syndrome. Second, the fetus may have a narrow window of tolerance for prolonged maternal hypoxia, hypercapnia, and acid–base abnormalities.

Tidal Volumes There is evidence that lung protective ventilation may be beneficial to all mechanically ventilated patients, not just those with ARDS [64]. It is reasonable to initiate mechanical ventilation on volume control with a tidal volume of 6 ml/kg *ideal body weight (IBW)*. This is calculated from the patient's height, and therefore will not change with pregnancy.

Respiratory Rate There is no evidence to guide whether settings should attempt to mimic the mild respiratory alkalosis that naturally occurs during pregnancy. In general, both maternal alkalosis and acidosis should be avoided if possible. In very sick women, permissive hypercapnia may be necessary. Limited data suggest that a maternal PCO_2 between 45 and 55 mmHg is tolerated by the fetus [60].

Oxygenation—FiO_2 and PEEP Adequate fetal oxygenation probably requires a maternal PO_2 of 70–90 mmHg [60]. This should be accomplished with the lowest possible FiO_2, and with positive end expiratory pressure (PEEP). Increasing PEEP up to a certain point will improve oxygenation and protect against lung injury, but can decrease cardiac preload causing cardiac output to fall. Pregnant women may be more vulnerable to this, as venous return may already be impaired due to pressure from the uterus on the IVC.

Sedatives and Paralytics There is good evidence supporting the short-term use of nondepolarizing neuromuscular blocking agents, such as cisatracurium, in ARDS with refractory hypoxemia [65]. Short-term use of these agents produces no adverse fetal effects. Sedation with benzodiazepines, propofol, and opiates is also believed to be safe during pregnancy with the following (albeit conflicting) caveats. Early in pregnancy, the lowest possible dose of benzodiazepines should be used, as there is a theoretical risk of cleft palate. Sedating medications used near the time of delivery may mean that the neonate requires immediate intubation. On the other hand, pregnant women may metabolize medications more effectively than other adult patients; therefore, higher doses and multiple synergistic medications are sometimes necessary to achieve adequate sedation.

Proning There is also good evidence that early proning improves survival in adults with severe ARDS [66]. Clearly this is logistically difficult in women at advanced gestational stages; moreover, continuous fetal monitoring becomes challenging. Our practice has been to consider delivery by cesarean section if it seems likely that a pregnant woman will require proning and the fetus is of viable age. Limited data support ECMO as a salvage intervention. At the time of proning, it may be prudent to contact an ECMO center if there is one in the area.

Infections in Pregnancy

Sepsis in Pregnancy

Sepsis is one of the five leading causes of pregnancy-related death around the world, with the highest rates in developing countries, and increasing rates in the United States and United Kingdom [1, 4]. Common sources of sepsis include pyelonephritis, retained products of conception, chorioamnionitis or endomyometritis, pneumonia, necrotizing fasciitis, and intraabdominal infections. The principal etiologic agents are endotoxin producing aerobic Gram-negative rods, Gram-positive bacteria, fungal infections, and polymicrobial infections. *Escherichia coli, enterococci,* and *beta-hemolytic streptococci* are the three most frequently recovered organisms.

Signs and symptoms of sepsis in pregnancy may initially overlap with normal physiologic changes of pregnancy. Similar to the general population, lactic acid levels correlate with risk of maternal morbidity and adverse outcomes from sepsis during pregnancy [67]. Scoring systems such as the Acute Physiology and Chronic Health Evaluation and Simplified Acute Physiology Score have not been validated in the pregnant population.

Initial evaluation and management should focus on early detection of sepsis and intervention. The physiologic adaptations that occur in normal pregnancy are broadly applicable here (Tables 30.1, 30.2, 30.3, and 30.4). Fetal compromise results mainly from maternal decompensation. Below are some considerations unique to the management of sepsis during pregnancy.

1. Early, appropriate antibiotics reduce mortality and morbidity in sepsis for all patients. Two commonly used broad-spectrum antibiotic regimens that are safe in pregnancy are shown in Table 30.11.
2. Maternal acid–base status deserves special attention because alkalosis can cause uteroplacental vasoconstriction and acidosis can cause fetal hypoxemia and distress.
3. Goal of 95% O2 saturation and PaO2 ≥70 mmHg due to fetal reliance on an O2 gradient for adequate oxygenation [60]
4. Frequent reevaluation of maternal respiratory status during resuscitation, as she is more likely to develop pulmonary edema.
5. CVP is not altered during pregnancy but is a poor indicator of fluid responsiveness in general [68].
6. SvO2 progressively decreases in the later stages of pregnancy; therefore, achieving goals of 70–75% may be neither feasible nor necessary [26].
7. Bedside TTE is an important early tool to evaluate fluid status/myocardial function.
8. Vasopressors can restrict uterine blood flow, but in general, maternal benefits outweigh this risk. Norepinephrine is a good first choice.
9. Relative adrenal insufficiency and the use of corticosteroids in septic pregnant patients have not been studied [69].

Pyelonephritis

Women are at greater risk for pyelonephritis during pregnancy because of a reduction in renal concentrating ability, smooth muscle relaxation causing ureteral dilatation, and bladder changes that lead to urinary stasis and vesicoureteral reflux. The most common organisms responsible for pyelonephritis are *Escherichia coli*, *group B streptococci*, and *Klebsiella* species. *Signs and symptoms* are similar to those in the nonpregnant patient with the possible exception of an increased susceptibility for respiratory insufficiency. *Initial evaluation* includes blood and urine cultures.

Initial management includes parenteral beta-lactam antibiotics with modifications according to local antibiograms, and hospitalizaton until afebrile for at least 24 hours. If patients fail to respond to initial antibiotic therapy, imaging with renal ultrasound or magnetic resonance imaging should be obtained to rule out hydronephrosis, nephrolithiasis, abscess, or obstruction.

Postpartum Endometritis

Infection of the endometrium occurs after 1–3% of vaginal births, and up to 20% of cesarean births [70, 71]. The infection is generally polymicrobial involving bacteria from the genital tract and may spread into the myometrium (endomyometritis) or parametrium (parametritis) [72, 73]. Risk factors include chorioamnionitis, prolonged labor, multiple cervical examinations, internal monitoring, manual removal of the placenta, maternal diabetes, or anemia, and HIV infection.

Signs and Symptoms Postpartum fever (>38 °C), tachycardia, midline lower abdominal pain and uterine tenderness, purulent lochia, malaise, anorexia, and uterine bleeding.

Initial Evaluation Thorough history, physical and exclusion of other etiologies for postpartum fever. Ultrasound has not been shown to assist with diagnosis, but may be useful in identifying retained products of conception [74]. Blood and endometrial cultures are not routinely obtained [75]. Blood cultures should, however, be obtained in immunosuppressed or septic patients.

Initial management should focus on maternal resuscitation, early parenteral antibiotics (Table 30.11), and hospital admission, although oral antibiotics have been used for outpatients with very mild symptoms.

Chorioamnionitis

Infection of the chorion and amnion can occur when organisms of the lower genital tract ascend into the lower uterine segment during labor or after rupture of membranes, or after invasive procedures, including pelvic exams in the last month of pregnancy. Patients with chorioamnionitis remain at increased risk for sepsis after delivery, especially cesarean delivery. Most infections are polymicrobial [76].

Signs and symptoms include fever, tachycardia, uterine tenderness, change in amniotic fluid color and purulent vaginal discharge.

Initial evaluation should focus on the following diagnostic criteria: Maternal fever >38 °C (the essential criterion) *and* the presence of one or two of the following: (1) maternal leukocytosis (>15,000 cells/mm3), (2) maternal tachycardia (>100 bpm), (3) fetal tachycardia (>160 bpm), (4) uterine tenderness, and (5) foul odor of amniotic fluid.

Initial management includes resuscitation, prompt initiation of intrapartum antibiotics (Table 30.11), and consultation with the obstetrics team for delivery [76].

Septic Pelvic Thrombophlebitis

This is an uncommon complication of childbirth and gynecologic procedures. It occurs more frequently after cesarean than vaginal delivery, and has also been reported after a variety of gynecologic procedures. Signs and symptoms include spiking fevers within a few days after delivery or surgery that often fails to respond to antibiotics. Often there is no abdominal tenderness. Initial evaluation for infection should include blood cultures, which are often negative. Diagnosis of septic pelvic thrombosis can be challenging, and requires a high degree of suspicion. Contrast-enhanced MRI or CT may aid in diagnosis, although no formal imaging recommendations exist. The gold standard is a surgical specimen. Initial management has traditionally been antibiotics and therapeutic anticoagulation.

Appendicitis in Pregnancy

Acute appendicitis is the most common general surgery emergency in pregnancy. The diagnosis may be challenging as evidenced by the increased rate of rupture and associated complications in pregnant women, especially in the third trimester [77]. The risk of fetal loss increases when the appendix perforates (36% fetal loss with perforation versus 1.5% without perforation) and when there is generalized peritonitis or a peritoneal abscess [78].

Signs and Symptoms Pregnant women are more likely to have an atypical presentation of appendicitis. While pain at or near McBurney's point occurs in the majority of cases, pain may localize to the mid- or upper right abdomen in the third trimester as the appendix is pushed cephalad. There may be less peritoneal irritation evident on exam, as the gravid uterus pushes the abdominal wall away from the inflamed appendix.

Initial Evaluation The initial imaging modality is often graded compression ultrasonography; however, there is a wide variation in the reported diagnostic performance of this test [79]. If the diagnosis remains in doubt, MRI, usually without gadolinium, is an excellent option. CT is usually avoided due to concerns about the radiation dose to the fetus during abdominal/pelvic imaging; however, modifications to the CT protocol can limit fetal radiation exposure.

Initial treatment should begin with preoperative antibiotics, although definitive treatment of acute appendicitis is appendectomy. Open laparotomy is associated with fewer complications than laparoscopy in pregnancy. Maternal and fetal outcomes are worse with conservative (antibiotics alone) management. A higher negative laparotomy rate in pregnant women is generally considered acceptable, although not without risk to the fetus [78].

HIV in Pregnancy

Pregnant women with HIV infection are at risk for the same complications as the nonpregnant HIV-infected population; however, some of these have special significance in pregnancy.

Pulmonary Arterial Hypertension While still rare, the prevalence of PAH is 6–12 times greater in HIV-infected patients than in those without HIV. Patients with PAH have a high risk of death during pregnancy [80].

Postpartum Hemorrhage Ergot alkaloid drugs such as methergine, commonly used to treat postpartum hemorrhage, should be avoided if at all possible in patients taking CYP3A4 enzyme inhibitors (protease inhibitors) due to an exaggerated vasoconstrictor response. In addition, HIV + patients should receive CMV-negative blood if possible.

Pneumocystis jiroveci pneumonia is the most common cause of AIDS-related death in pregnant women in the United States. Trimethoprim–sulfamethoxazole, although in other cases normally avoided near term in pregnancy, is the treatment of choice, with steroids added as for the nonpregnant patient [81].

Obstetric Hemorrhage

Hemorrhage is the fifth leading cause of pregnancy-related death in the United States, and is the leading cause of maternal mortality worldwide [1]. Postpartum hemorrhage (PPH) is one of the most common obstetric reasons for ICU admission with most hemorrhage occurring within 1 hour following delivery [26]. Women can also experience antepartum hemorrhage, as well as delayed postpartum hemorrhage up to 6 weeks following delivery.

Postpartum Hemorrhage

The most common cause of PPH is uterine atony (60–70%), followed by retained placental products (20–30%), obstetric trauma (<10%), and more rarely, uterine inversion [26]. Coagulation disorders may also result in hemorrhage. Delayed or secondary PPH usually occurs as a result of retained placental tissue, endometritis, genital tract tears, and rarely arteriovenous fistulas or pseudoaneurysms.

Major postpartum hemorrhage is an emergency and successful management requires an aggressive, coordinated, multidisciplinary approach. Institutional massive transfusion protocols should be activated early. In addition to the emergency medicine physician, care of the patient with PPH should involve multiple nurses, obstetricians, intensivists, anesthesiologists, the laboratory, blood bank, and possibly interventional radiology (IR). Evaluation and management should take place simultaneously. Poor outcomes may result from delayed recognition and underresuscitation.

Evaluation Detecting and appreciating the severity of PPH can at times be surprisingly difficult. Lack of overt bleeding does not rule out hemorrhage, as the uterus and pelvis can sequester liters of blood. Early hemodynamic changes may be subtle due to the increased blood volume of pregnancy and relative resilience of young women; this may only consist of mild (relative) tachycardia and tachypnea in the absence of hypotension. In addition, the hemoglobin can be falsely reassuring if labs are obtained before fluid resuscitation. In a setting of increased risk, hemorrhage should remain at the top of the differential diagnosis. In the case of visible bleeding, studies have shown that visual estimates of hemorrhage are commonly inaccurate, with frequent underestimation by at least 30–50% [82]. Systemic signs of hemorrhagic shock are not specific to etiology and include restlessness and anxiety, pallor, cool and clammy extremities, oliguria or anuria, sinus tachycardia, and hypotension.

Initial management begins with (a) addressing hypovolemia and anemia; (b) preventing dilutional coagulopathy, acidosis, and hypothermia; and (c) hemodynamic support if absolutely necessary, although vasopressors can mask signs of ongoing anemia and hypovolemia, thereby derailing the resuscitation. These principles do not differ significantly from response to massive hemorrhage in trauma, and indeed the terms "golden hour" and "lethal triad" have equal relevance here. Young women can survive the initial hemorrhage only to die hours later from the sequelae of inadequate or delayed resuscitation.

Simultaneously one should identify and control the source of hemorrhage. An obstetrician is key to this process.

1. Establish adequate IV access; transfuse with blood, plasma, platelets and cryo; resuscitate with crystalloid (warmed); warm the patient; and check ABGs to assess acid–base status.
2. Place a urinary catheter—a distended bladder can interfere with uterine contractility.
3. Bimanual massage for uterine atony.
4. Manual uterine exploration to remove retained products of conception
5. Uterotonics: Add 40 units *oxytocin* to 1 liter of NS or LR. Start the infusion at a rate of 10–40 milliunits per minute and titrate to maintain uterine contraction. If no IV access, give 10 units IM with expected response in 3–5 minutes. Additional agents are methylergonovine and prostaglandins (Carboprost, PGF2alpha, and Hemabate). These medications may have hemodynamic and respiratory side effects, especially when given quickly. If uterotonics do not reverse atony within 30 minutes, invasive intervention is indicated [83].
6. Tranexamic acid and recombinant factor VIIa (off label)—one must balance concerns about thrombotic complications with the latter [84].
7. Procedural interventions: balloon tamponade (OB), uterine artery embolization (IR), or operative intervention such as uterine artery ligation, B-Lynch suture, or cesarean hysterectomy.

Antepartum Hemorrhage

Antepartum hemorrhage occurs in 1 in 20 pregnant women and is rarely life threatening to the mother or fetus [26]. Causes include ectopic pregnancy, abortion, and trauma. Placental abruption and uterine rupture are two causes of antepartum hemorrhage that can lead to significant maternal and fetal morbidity and mortality.

Placental abruption is the most common etiology of antepartum hemorrhage, and involves premature separation of the placenta from the decidua basalis. This may result from trauma or vascular or placental abnormalities. Presentation is variable and may include vaginal bleeding, uterine tenderness, painful tetanic contractions, nonreassuring fetal heart rate patterns, or simply preterm labor. In major abruption, the uterus can feel "woody" as blood infiltrates the myometrium. Up to 5 liters of blood can extravasate into the uterus. This is a clinical diagnosis; ultrasonography is not sensitive, but if positive for abruption, it is diagnostic. Treatment depends on the clinical status of mother and fetus, and varies from close observation and monitoring to immediate delivery.

Uterine rupture is a rare life-threatening cause of antepartum hemorrhage. This may result from trauma, or it may occur at the site of prior gynecologic or obstetric surgery. It can occur antenatally or postpartum, but is usually first suspected postpartum in the setting of intractable hemorrhage. Clinical presentation can be variable, but may include abdominal pain, cramping, rigidity, guarding, and signs of hypovolemia/hemorrhage. An abnormal fetal lie, inability to discern the fundus, and easy palpation of fetal parts also signal possible uterine rupture. Maternal hemorrhage can be life threatening and fetal prognosis is poor. Treatment is maternal resuscitation and laparotomy, possibly with hysterectomy.

Neurologic Emergencies in Pregnancy

It is unknown if brain physiology is altered by pregnancy; however, metabolic, hematologic, and vascular changes can contribute to neurologic pathology. The differential diagnosis for a pregnant patient with headache, seizures, and/or altered consciousness should be the same as for the nonpregnant patient with special emphasis on eclampsia and the entities described below. Other neurologic diseases that may present in the peripartum period include brain tumors (pregnancy may worsen vasogenic edema) and ischemic stroke (risk is highest postpartum).

Seizures

Seizures are the most common neurologic complication of pregnancy with preexisting epilepsy being the most frequent cause [20]. However, *new onset* seizures, especially in the third trimester or postpartum period, should be considered eclampsia until proven otherwise. Eclampsia is discussed with preeclampsia in Cardiovascular Disorders of Pregnancy.

Although still debated, some historical evidence points to a worsening of seizures during pregnancy among those with a history of epilepsy [20, 85]. It is not clear whether this increase is related to an increased susceptibility or declining levels of antiepileptic drugs in the pregnant patient, the latter occurring due to poor compliance over fears of teratogenicity, decreased GI absorption, increased volume of distribution, or increased renal and hepatic clearance. Seizures result in a severe lactic acidosis, increased cardiac output, transient increase in blood pressure, increased intraabdominal pressure, and increased blood flow to the brain and muscles, notably with a corresponding decrease in blood flow to the viscera and uterus [20].

Initial Evaluation When a pregnant patient presents with a seizure, two questions need to be answered: (1) Does the patient have a history of seizures and if not, (2) could this represent eclampsia? If the answer to both questions is "no" the differential should be broadened to include the other disorders in this section as well as causes of seizure in the general population.

Initial management should focus on support and rapid seizure control.

1. Left lateral positioning to prevent venocaval compression and aspiration.
2. Supplemental oxygen as needed with careful attention to airway protection and the need for intubation.
3. Thiamine and glucose—empirically or if the blood glucose is less than 40–60 mg/dL
4. Magnesium sulfate if secondary to eclampsia, see section on Preeclampsia and Eclampsia, and Table 30.7.
5. If not secondary to eclampsia, treat with IV lorazepam, then if necessary load with fosphenytoin or levetiracetam.
   (a) There is no consensus on the antiepileptic drug of choice for status epilepticus in pregnancy. Valproic acid, phenytoin, phenobarbital, and carbamazepine are all FDA Pregnancy Category D. Levetiracetam is FDA Pregnancy Category C and may be a good first-line option (15–20 mg/kg over 15 minutes) if it works [86].
6. Labs: Electrolytes, glucose, liver, and renal function tests and levels of antiepileptic drugs the patient may have been taking.

Cerebral Venous Thrombosis

This is the presence of thrombosis in the dural venous sinuses, which drain blood from the brain. While an uncommon condition, pregnancy is an independent risk factor for the development of CVT and the condition can be devastating [87]. Most cases occur during the third trimester or puerperium [87]. Mortality for pregnancy-related cerebral venous sinus thrombosis is 25–30%, and those that survive often suffer long-term neurologic sequelae [20].

Signs and symptoms of CVT include headache, focal seizures, paresis, papilledema, altered mental status, and intracranial hypertension. Headache is the most common symptom and occurs in 95% of patients [88]. Headache can be gradual or abrupt in nature. The diagnosis requires a high degree of suspicion.

Initial evaluation should include MRI with venography. The MRI scans will often show bilateral hemorrhagic infarcts. CT with venography is an alternative if MRI is unavailable, although the sensitivity is not as high. Traditional cerebral angiography with particular attention to the venous phase can also diagnose CVT, with the benefit of being able to mechanically intervene during the procedure.

Initial management of CVT involves therapeutic anticoagulation with UFH or LMWH. Both treatment modalities are safe, and may improve outcomes even in patients with preexisting hemorrhagic infarcts. Directed thrombolysis is reserved for patients with profound neurologic symptoms, or those that worsen despite treatment with heparin [20]. Seizures should be controlled with antiepileptic drugs and basic maneuvers to reduce intracranial pressure. Neurology and possibly neurosurgery should be consulted on all patients with CVT.

Intracranial Hemorrhage

Intracranial hemorrhage is a rare but serious problem during pregnancy. Common causes include ruptured aneurysm, arteriovenous malformations (AVMs), hypertensive intraparenchymal bleed, eclampsia, bleeding disorders, malignancy, and cocaine abuse. Subarachnoid hemorrhage (SAH) carries a threefold increased risk during pregnancy, with >85% of hemorrhages occurring in the second or third trimester [89]. AVMs, although a rare cause of SAH in the general population, account for nearly half of SAH in gravid patients [90]. *Signs and symptoms*, *initial evaluation*, and *management* of intracranial hemorrhage in the pregnant patient do not differ significantly from the nonpregnant population.

Gastrointestinal Disease in Pregnancy

Gastrointestinal Physiology

Abdominal organs are displaced cephalad, posterior, and lateral by the growing uterus. Progesterone-associated relaxation of smooth muscles results in decreased lower esophageal sphincter tone and GI tract hypomotility, leading to an increased risk of aspiration pneumonitis and pneumonia. The two major gastrointestinal disorders specific to pregnancy involve the liver. While a slightly elevated alkaline phosphatase is normal in pregnancy, elevated transaminases or evidence of liver failure should prompt a search for pathology such as hepatitis, HELLP syndrome, or acute fatty liver of pregnancy (AFLP). AFLP and HELLP syndrome can be difficult to distinguish. See Table 30.3 for normal lab values.

HELLP Syndrome

The syndrome of *h*emolysis, *e*levated *l*iver enzymes, and *l*ow *p*latelets (HELLP) is a serious, potentially fatal complication of pregnancy that affects between 1 and 3 per 1000 pregnancies [26, 91]. The maternal mortality rate is estimated between 1% and 3%, and is usually attributed to DIC or hemorrhage. The perinatal mortality rate is approximately 30%, with many fetuses born prematurely or with intrauterine growth restriction [91]. More than 70% of cases occur antenatally, usually before 37 weeks [26, 92].

There is overlap between HELLP syndrome and preeclampsia, but the relationship remains unclear. For example, up to 20% of patients with HELLP syndrome do not have antecedent hypertension or proteinuria as would be seen in preeclampsia [26, 92].

Signs and symptoms are often nonspecific with a highly variable clinical presentation [93]. The most common symptom is abdominal pain with tenderness in the epigastrium or right upper quadrant. Other symptoms include nausea, vomiting, headache, and general malaise [94]. Because presentation is often nonspecific and may suggest a viral syndrome, the diagnosis can be missed by not checking basic labs.

Initial evaluation should include a complete set of labs, a liver panel (specifically AST, ALT, and bilirubin), serum LDH, haptoglobin, coagulation panel, and peripheral blood smear. Ultrasound or CT may be useful if there is concern for hepatic complications. There are two major classifications—the Mississippi Classification and Tennessee Classification. While all criteria must be met for a diagnosis of the complete form of HELLP, patients can be diagnosed with partial or incomplete HELLP. Complete HELLP can develop rapidly in patients with the incomplete form.

Tennessee Classification:

1. Hemolysis
    (a) Schistocytes on blood smear
    (b) Elevated indirect bilirubin
    (c) LDH >600 IU or bilirubin >1.2 mg/dL
    (d) Low serum haptoglobin (≤25 mg/dL)
2. Elevated liver enzymes
    (a) AST >70 U/L
3. Low platelets
    (a) <100,000/mm^3

Differential diagnosis includes TTP, HUS, cold agglutinins, and acute fatty liver of pregnancy (AFLP). Women with HELLP syndrome often have more severe liver dysfunction than in other conditions with the exception of AFLP. HELLP syndrome and AFLP can be difficult to differentiate—this is discussed in the section on AFLP below. Clinical concerns should also include the major life-threatening complications of HELLP syndrome—hepatic hemorrhage, and/or infarction, subcapsular hematoma, liver rupture, and multisystem organ failure [26].

Initial management should focus on stabilization of maternal blood pressure and coagulopathies. Definitive treatment for HELLP is expeditious delivery of the fetus [26]. Subcapsular hematomas and ruptures require surgical intervention. Patients with suspected or diagnosed HELLP should be cared for at a tertiary care center with consultants including obstetrics, particularly a maternal–fetal medicine team, and possibly general surgery and interventional radiology.

Acute Fatty Liver of Pregnancy

AFLP is an uncommon but potentially fatal complication of pregnancy [95]. This disease has a rising incidence and declining maternal and fetal mortality due to better recognition, identification of milder cases and aggressive early care [96, 97]. Maternal mortality rates have fallen from as high as 85% to 0–10% and fetal mortality is now 8–25% [25, 98]. Maternal death is most often related to severe coagulopathy.

AFLP is characterized by hepatic microvesicular steatosis related to fetal deficiency of long-chain 3-hydroxyacyl coenzymes dehydrogenase—a fatty acid beta-oxidation enzyme [26]. A fetus that is homozygous for the mitochondrial mutations is unable to metabolize long-chain fatty acids. The excess fatty acids overflow into maternal circulation, causing hepatotoxicity.

Signs and symptoms may be vague and usually develop in the late third trimester, with rare cases reported in the second trimester. AFLP is more common in women with multiple gestations and possibly in underweight mothers. History may reveal that the patient's other children have metabolic problems. Symptoms include vomiting, abdominal pain, malaise, anorexia, edema, and headache. Physical findings may include jaundice, right upper quadrant abdominal tenderness, tachycardia, asterixis, fever, altered mental status, evidence of ascites, oliguria, scleral icterus, and mucous membrane bleeding.

Initial evaluation: Characteristic laboratory findings may include:

1. Elevated PT.
2. Hyperbilirubinemia.
3. Alkaline phosphatase, which is mildly elevated in normal pregnancy, is usually elevated to a greater degree in AFLP.
4. A moderate transaminitis (250–500 U/mL). Levels >1000 U/mL should raise concern for other conditions such as a viral hepatitis.
5. Hypoglycemia with as many as 75% of patients requiring a 10% dextrose drip in one study [99].
6. Frequently elevated serum ammonia, uric acid and lipase, and evidence of renal insufficiency.

Differential Diagnosis The diagnosis of AFLP is usually made clinically and may be most efficiently reached by excluding other more common causes of liver dysfunction in pregnancy including HELLP syndrome, preeclampsia, viral hepatitis, and cholestasis of pregnancy. It may be difficult or impossible to differentiate AFLP and HELLP syndrome. Compared with

HELLP syndrome, AFLP is more strongly characterized by evidence of hepatic insufficiency such as encephalopathy, coagulopathy, and hypoglycemia, whereas HELLP syndrome is more strongly associated with thrombocytopenia and hypertension. Preeclampsia is not usually accompanied by jaundice, hypoglycemia, or significant coagulopathy. Viral hepatitis is rarely associated with high uric acid levels and will commonly have transaminases above 1000 U/L. Cholestasis of pregnancy is characterized by intense pruritus and an elevated alkaline phosphatase without the other symptoms and signs common to AFLP. Conclusive diagnosis of AFLP requires a liver biopsy, but this is rarely performed due to the underlying coagulopathy. While the sensitivity of radiography is poor for diagnosing AFLP, it is reasonable to obtain imaging to exclude biliary obstruction as the cause of symptoms.

Initial management should be aimed at the stabilization of maternal glucose levels and correction of coagulopathy. The definitive treatment is urgent delivery of the fetus. These patients are best cared for at a tertiary-care medical center with high-risk obstetric services. Delay in diagnosis and delivery can result in liver failure, death, or need for transplantation.

Renal/Urinary System Problems in Pregnancy

Renal Physiology in Normal Pregnancy A pregnant woman's kidneys must handle excretory load from the fetus as well as from her own increased metabolism. In patients with no preexisting kidney disease, glomerular filtration rate increases during pregnancy as evidenced in a fall in levels of serum creatinine (Table 30.3). A pregnant woman with normally functioning kidneys may need higher or more frequent dosing of renally cleared drugs.

Acute Kidney Injury There are no obstetric illnesses that cause isolated injury to the kidneys. Acute kidney injury frequently accompanies systemic diseases such as preeclampsia/eclampsia, HELLP syndrome, and other illnesses such as sepsis similar to the nonpregnant population. With lower normal values for serum BUN and creatinine, the threshold for diagnosing acute kidney injury is also lower. A previously healthy pregnant woman with a creatinine as low as 1.0 likely has acutely impaired renal function and may suffer toxicity from renally cleared drugs such as magnesium sulfate.

Chronic Kidney Disease In patients with preexisting kidney disease, renal function may decline during pregnancy. Hypertension and a serum creatinine above 1.5 mg/dL during pregnancy are risk factors for the permanent exacerbation of underlying kidney disease. Chronic kidney disease is associated with worse maternal and fetal outcomes [100].

Infections Ureteral stasis may contribute to an increased incidence of urinary tract infections and pyelonephritis.

Endocrine Problems in Pregnancy

Diabetic Ketoacidosis (DKA)

Pregnancy is a "diabetogenic" state and many factors make pregnant women more susceptible to DKA. DKA remains a major concern when diagnosed in pregnancy because of maternal morbidity, and fetal morbidity and mortality. DKA can lead to maternal dehydration, hypotension, metabolic acidosis, and electrolyte disturbances severe enough to cause arrhythmias. Maternal acidosis can impair fetal oxygenation and tissue perfusion. DKA carries a perinatal mortality rate of 9–35% [101].

Signs and symptoms of DKA are variable and similar to those in the nonpregnant population. In pregnancy, DKA can occur with serum glucose levels much lower than those seen in nongravid patients, and is not infrequently the initial presentation of a new diagnosis of diabetes [102].

Initial evaluation and management of DKA in pregnancy do not differ significantly from that in nonpregnant patients. History and exam should reveal an identifiable trigger for DKA, with insulin cessation and infection being the most common. While acidosis may be poorly tolerated by the fetus, there has been no benefit shown from more liberal use of bicarbonate in pregnant women with DKA. Continuous fetal heart rate monitoring should be started if the fetus is of viable gestation. Often, signs of fetal distress serve as an alert to the degree of maternal metabolic derangement. Delivery should be delayed until the mother is metabolically stabilized.

Thyroid Disease

Thyroid disorders are the second most common endocrine disorder in pregnancy. Thyroid tests must be interpreted in light of the normal physiologic changes of pregnancy. There is a 50% increase in thyroxine-binding globulin (TBG) by 20 weeks gestation; in order to keep free T4 levels normal, total T3 and T4 levels also increase until mid-gestation [103]. The increase in TBG is due to the effects of estrogen and decreased hepatic clearance. Serum thyroid-stimulating hormone (TSH) levels decrease in the first trimester due to human chorionic gonadotrophin (hCG) elevation, but increase in later pregnancy, albeit not to prepregnancy levels [103].

Thyroid Storm

Thyroid storm is estimated to occur in 1–2% of pregnancies already complicated by hyperthyroidism and receiving thioamide therapy [104]. The condition is rare and diagnosis can be difficult, but it is potentially fatal if not recognized and treated early.

Signs and symptoms of thyroid storm include cardiovascular compromise, hyperpyrexia, and central nervous system changes. Patients may be in shock or coma when presenting to the ED. The differential diagnosis is broad and includes heart failure and sepsis, which may present concomitantly [105].

Initial evaluation should include a comprehensive laboratory evaluation, including serum TSH, total T4/T3, and free T4/T3. Diagnosis of hyperthyroidism is based on a suppressed TSH with elevated *free* T4.

Initial Management Empiric treatment should be started in consultation with an endocrinologist and MFM specialist before laboratory results become available [103]. Radioactive iodine is contraindicated in all stages of pregnancy, and methimazole is recommended as the first-line antithyroid medication except during the first trimester [105, 106].

Initial ED treatment may consist of the following: [105, 106]

1. Methimazole 20–30 mg once to reduce production of thyroid hormones and block peripheral conversion of T4 to T3.
   (a) In the first trimester, use propylthiouracil (PTU) 300 mg PO/NG every 6 hours.
2. Iodide: 1 hour *after* the patient is given PTU (to block release of stored hormone)
   (a) Sodium iodide (1 g IV every 12 hours), or
   (b) SSKI (10 drops PO every 8 hours)
3. Steroids (hydrocortisone 50–80 mg every 8 hours; dexamethasone 2 mg every 6 hours; or prednisone 60 mg every day) to block release of stored hormone and the peripheral conversion of T4 to T3.
4. Propanolol (60–80 mg PO every 4 hours or 1 mg/min IV) or esmolol (250–500 μg/kg loading, then 50–100 μg/kg/min infusion) for tachycardia.

Trauma in Pregnancy

Epidemiology There are approximately 4.1 injury-related hospital admissions per 1000 deliveries [107]. The most common types of trauma during pregnancy include motor vehicle collisions (MVCs; 48%), falls (25%), and assaults (17%) [108]. Blunt trauma (91%) far exceeded the incidence of penetrating injury (9%) in a retrospective review [109].

Mechanisms of Injury In blunt trauma, the abdominal wall, uterine myometrium, and amniotic fluid act as buffers to direct fetal injury. The fetus may still be injured if the direct forces are significant or in cases of indirect injury such as compression, deceleration, coup–countercoup effects, or shearing. In patients involved in MVCs, the type of restraint system affects the frequency of uterine rupture and fetal death [110]. A lap belt alone can cause too much forward flexion and uterine compression, leading to uterine rupture and placental abruption. A lap belt worn too high can lead to uterine rupture. A lap and shoulder belt combination reduces the risk of fetal injury. Unrestrained occupants have a higher risk of premature delivery and fetal death. There does not appear to be an increase in pregnancy-specific risks associated with airbags.

In penetrating trauma, the risk of uterine injury increases as the gravid uterus enlarges. The dense myometrium and amniotic fluid serve to decrease the energy of the penetrating object and may actually protect maternal viscera; however, fetal morbidity and mortality can be as high as 73% [108, 109]

Obstetrical Injuries Placental abruption and uterine rupture are reviewed in more detail under Obstetric Hemorrhage (Antepartum).

1. *Placental abruption* is a common cause of fetal death after significant trauma. It can occur in 7–9% of minor traumas in late pregnancy, and in 13% of severe traumas [111]. Management depends on the degree of hemorrhage and clinical status of the woman and fetus, and may include close monitoring or immediate delivery.
2. *Uterine rupture*, while very rare, is estimated to occur 45 times more frequently in maternal assault than in pregnant women not exposed to trauma [112]. Maternal hemorrhage can be life threatening and fetal prognosis is poor. Laparotomy, possibly with hysterectomy, is indicated.

Initial Evaluation and Management The American College of Surgeons recommends first assessing and resuscitating the mother, then assessing the fetus before conducting the secondary survey [110]. Below are considerations unique to the pregnant patient.

Primary survey:

1. Airway: Presume it is difficult and high risk (Table 30.9).
2. Breathing: Chest tubes should be placed 1–2 rib interspaces higher given the elevated diaphragm in pregnancy.
3. Circulation:
   (a) Supine patients at greater than 20 weeks or unknown gestation should be tilted left side down at least 20–30 degrees, or the uterus manually displaced to relieve aortocaval pressure.
   (b) Pregnant women may lose a significant amount of blood before typical signs of hypovolemia occur. Transfuse with type specific or O negative blood.
   (c) Perimortem cesarean delivery should be considered, acknowledging that the limited data for this is derived from patients suffering nontraumatic cardiac arrest.
4. Fetal Assessment:
   (a) Fetal heart tones (normal range 120–160 beats/min)
   (b) Urgent obstetric consultation [ATLS]

Secondary Survey:

1. Early vaginal and rectal exam, noting dilation and effacement of the cervix, and the presence of blood and/or amniotic fluid. If there is vaginal bleeding in the second or third trimester, cervical exam should be deferred until placenta previa is excluded by ultrasound.
2. Focused abdominal sonography for trauma (FAST) exam is useful to identify major life threats. In experienced hands, the ultrasound can also be used to estimate gestational age, calculate fetal heart rate, amniotic fluid volume, and placental position.

Studies:

1. Kleihauer–Betke (KB) screen in addition to trauma labs.

2. Medically indicated radiographic studies, including CT scans, should not be delayed, although abdominal shielding should be used where possible.
3. Continuous fetal tocodynamic monitoring and a complete ultrasonographic evaluation should be obtained in consultation with OB.

Nonemergent management:

1. Consult a general/trauma surgeon and OB early.
2. Tocodynamic monitoring of all patients with a viable pregnancy.
   (a) Asymptomatic patients with normal findings can be monitored for 6 hours.
   (b) Patients with symptoms or abnormal fetal monitoring should continue to be monitored for at least 24 hours.
3. Rh immunoglobulin therapy should be given within 72 hours of injury to all Rh-negative patients.
   (a) The KB screen can miss minor degrees of feto-maternal hemorrhage that are still able to sensitize the Rh-negative mother.
4. Tetanus prophylaxis is safe in pregnancy.

Diagnostic Imaging During Pregnancy

There is often uncertainty and anxiety associated with the decision to expose pregnant women to ionizing radiation, primarily due to concern for embryonic/fetal risk and the paucity of data to support clinical decision-making. In most cases, if medically indicated, the risk to the mother of not doing the procedure is greater than is the risk of potential harm to the fetus [113].

Exposure to <5 Rad There is no evidence of an increased risk of fetal anomaly, growth restriction, or pregnancy loss. While controversial, with 1–2 rad there *may be* an increased risk of childhood cancer (~1 in 1000 children per rad) [114]. See Table 30.12 for doses involved in common radiologic tests.

Table 30.12 Fetal exposure in common radiologic tests[a]

Procedure	Fetal exposure
Chest X-ray (2 views)	0.00002–0.00007 rad
Abdominal X-ray (1 view)	0.1 rad
Hip X-ray (1 view)	0.2 rad
CT head	<1 rad
CT chest	<1 rad
Helical CT for PE	0.013 rad
V–Q scan for PE	0.037 rad
CT abdomen & lumbar spine	3.5 rad

Adapted from: Refs. [114, 128]
[a]*These are estimations of fetal exposure. Exact doses are difficult to determine and will depend on factors such as shielding, equipment, and scan protocols*

Exposure to 5–50 Rad The risk of fetal malformation appears to increase above 10 rad. Between 5 and 10 rad, the risk is less clear. In the first 14 days following conception, exposure to doses above 5 rad will lead to either undamaged survival or embryonic loss. After 14 days, the risk of loss is less, but the fetus remains at risk of malformations. The chance of causing CNS malformations is greatest between weeks 8 and 15, usually associated with doses of *20–40 rad*, with no proven risk beyond 25 weeks gestation [113, 114].

Most radiopaque agents for CT scanning have not been studied in pregnant humans, although animal studies suggest that they are not teratogenic. Because of case reports of neonatal hypothyroidism associated with iodinated contrast media, contrast should be avoided unless deemed necessary by the radiologist. Radiopaque agents used with CT should not interfere with lactation or the ability to breastfeed [114].

MRI and ultrasonography are not associated with known adverse effects on the fetus and should be considered as an alternative, when appropriate.

We recommend consultation with a radiologist for any questions regarding nonemergent imaging and for assistance using low-exposure techniques when available. When multiple studies need to be performed, it may be helpful to consult an expert in dosimetry calculation [114].

References

1. Pregnancy mortality surveillance system [Internet]. Atlanta: Centers for Centers for Disease Control and Prevention; 2014. [cited 2015 January 23]. Available from: http://www.cdc.gov/reproductivehealth/maternalinfanthealth/pmss.html.
2. Wanderer JP, Leffert LR, Mhyre JM, Kuklina EV, Callaghan WM, Bateman BT. Epidemiology of obstetric-related ICU admissions in Maryland: 1999–2008*. Crit Care Med. 2013;41(8):1844–52.
3. Berg CJ, Callaghan WM, Syverson C, Henderson Z. Pregnancy-related mortality in the United States, 1998 to 2005. Obstet Gynecol. 2010;116(6):1302–9.
4. Cantwell R, Clutton-brock T, Cooper G, et al. Saving mothers' lives: reviewing maternal deaths to make motherhood safer: 2006–2008. The eighth report of the confidential enquiries into maternal deaths in the United Kingdom. BJOG. 2011;118(Suppl 1):1–203.
5. Lapinsky SE, Kruczynski K, Slutsky AS. Critical care in the pregnant patient. Am J Respir Crit Care Med. 1995;152(2):427–55.
6. Regitz-Zagrosek V, Blomstrom Lundqvist C, Borghi C, et al. ESC guidelines on the management of cardiovascular diseases during pregnancy: the task force on the management of cardiovascular diseases during pregnancy of the European Society of Cardiology (ESC) Eur Heart J. 2011;32(24):3147–97.
7. Mahutte NG, Murphy-Kaulbeck L, Le Q, Solomon J, Benjamin A, Boyd ME. Obstetric admissions to the intensive care unit. Obstet Gynecol. 1999;94(2):263–6.
8. Naderi S, Raymond R. Pregnancy and heart disease [Internet]. Cleveland (OH): Center for Continuing Education, Cleveland Clinic; 2014 [cited 2015 Feb 23]. Available from: http://www.clevelandclinicmeded.com/medicalpubs/diseasemanagement/cardiology/pregnancy-and-heart-disease/.
9. Regitz-Zagrosek V, Seeland U, Geibel-Zehender A, Gohlke-Bärwolf C, Kruck I, Schaefer C. Cardiovascular diseases in pregnancy. Dtsch Arztebl Int. 2011;108(16):267–73.
10. Duarte AG, Thomas S, Safdar Z, et al. Management of pulmonary arterial hypertension during pregnancy: a retrospective, multicenter experience. Chest. 2013;143(5):1330–6.
11. Roth A, Elkayam U. Acute myocardial infarction associated with pregnancy. J Am Coll Cardiol. 2008;52(3):171–80.
12. Simpson LL. Maternal cardiac disease: update for the clinician. Obstet Gynecol. 2012;119(2 Pt 1):345–59.
13. Demchuk AM. Yes, intravenous thrombolysis should be administered in pregnancy when other clinical and imaging factors are favorable. Stroke. 2013;44(3):864–5.
14. Vidaeff AC, Carroll MA, Ramin SM. Acute hypertensive emergencies in pregnancy. Crit Care Med. 2005;33(10 Suppl):S307–12.
15. Report of the national high blood pressure education program working group on high blood pressure in pregnancy. Am J Obstet Gynecol. 2000;183(1):S1–22.
16. Abalos E, Cuesta C, Grosso AL, Chou D, Say L. Global and regional estimates of preeclampsia and eclampsia: a systematic review. Eur J Obstet Gynecol Reprod Biol. 2013;170(1):1–7.
17. Ananth CV, Keyes KM, Wapner RJ. Pre-eclampsia rates in the United States, 1980–2010: age-period-cohort analysis. BMJ. 2013;347:1–9.
18. Fujitani S, Baldisseri MR. Hemodynamic assessment in a pregnant and peripartum patient. Crit Care Med. 2005;33(10 Suppl):S354–61.
19. Steegers EA, von Dadelszen P, Duvekot JJ, Pijnenborg R. Pre-eclampsia. Lancet. 2010;376(9741):631–44.
20. Karnad DR, Guntupalli KK. Neurologic disorders in pregnancy. Crit Care Med. 2005;33(10 Suppl):S362–71.
21. Aagaard-tillery KM, Belfort MA. Eclampsia: morbidity, mortality, and management. Clin Obstet Gynecol. 2005;48(1):12–23.
22. Sibai BM. The HELLP syndrome (hemolysis, elevated liver enzymes, and low platelets): much ado about nothing? Am J Obstet Gynecol. 1990;162(2):311–6.
23. Sibai BM, Stella CL. Diagnosis and management of atypical preeclampsia-eclampsia. Am J Obstet Gynecol. 2009;200(5):481.e1–7.
24. Duley L, The Magpie Trial Collaborative Group. Do women with pre-eclampsia, and their babies, benefit from magnesium sulphate? The Magpie Trial: a randomised placebo-controlled trial. Lancet. 2002;359:1877–90.
25. Foley M, Strong JT, Garite T. Obstetric intensive care manual. 4th ed. New York: McGraw-Hill; 2010.
26. Neligan PJ, Laffey JG. Clinical review: special populations--critical illness and pregnancy. Crit Care. 2011;15(227):1–10.
27. Duley L, Henderson-Smart D. Magnesium sulphate versus diazepam for eclampsia. Cochrane Database Syst Rev. 2003;4(CD000127):1–21.
28. Sliwa K, Förster O, Libhaber E, et al. Peripartum cardiomyopathy: inflammatory markers as predictors of outcome in 100 prospectively studied patients. Eur Heart J. 2005;27(4):441–6.
29. Murali S, Baldisseri MR. Peripartum cardiomyopathy. Crit Care Med. 2005;33(10 Suppl):S340–6.
30. Baughman KL. Management of a case of peripartum cardiomyopathy. Nat Clin Pract Cardiovasc Med. 2006;3(9):514–8.
31. Elkayam U, Akhter MW, Singh H, et al. Pregnancy-associated cardiomyopathy: clinical characteristics and a comparison between early and late presentation. Circulation. 2005;111(16):2050–5.
32. Kamel H, Navi BB, Sriram N, Hovsepian DA, Devereux RB, Elkind MS. Risk of a thrombotic event after the 6-week postpartum period. N Engl J Med. 2014;370(14):1307–15.

33. Lapinsky SE. Cardiopulmonary complications of pregnancy. Crit Care Med. 2005;33(7):1616–22.
34. James AH. Pregnancy and thrombotic risk. Crit Care Med. 2010;38(2 Suppl):S57–63.
35. Chan WS, Chunilal S, Lee A, Crowther M, Rodger M, Ginsberg JS. A red blood cell agglutination D-dimer test to exclude deep venous thrombosis in pregnancy. Ann Intern Med. 2007;147(3):165–70.
36. Kovac M, Mikovic Z, Rakicevic L, et al. The use of D-dimer with new cutoff can be useful in diagnosis of venous thromboembolism in pregnancy. Eur J Obstet Gynecol Reprod Biol. 2010;148(1):27–30.
37. Tan M, Huisman MV. The diagnostic management of acute venous thromboembolism during pregnancy: recent advancements and unresolved issues. Thromb Res. 2011;127(Suppl 3):S13–6.
38. Bates SM, Greer IA, Middeldorp S, et al. VTE, thrombophilia, antithrombotic therapy, and pregnancy: antithrombotic therapy and prevention of thrombosis, 9th ed: American College of Chest Physicians Evidence-Based Clinical Practice Guidelines. Chest. 2012;141(2 Suppl):e691S–736S.
39. Moore J, Baldisseri MR. Amniotic fluid embolism. Crit Care Med. 2005;33(10 Suppl):S279–85.
40. Conde-Agudelo A, Romero R. Amniotic fluid embolism: an evidence-based review. Am J Obstet Gynecol. 2009;201(5):445.e1–13.
41. Vanden Hoek TL, Morrison LJ, Shuster M, et al. Part 12: cardiac arrest in special situations: 2010 American Heart Association guidelines for cardiopulmonary resuscitation and emergency cardiovascular care. Circulation. 2010;122(18 Suppl 3):S829–61.
42. Mallampalli A, Guy E. Cardiac arrest in pregnancy and somatic support after brain death. Crit Care Med. 2005;33(10 Suppl):S325–31.
43. Katz VL, Dotters DJ, Droegemueller W. Perimortem cesarean delivery. Obstet Gynecol. 1986;68(4):571–6.
44. Dombrowski MP, Schatz M, Wise R, et al. Asthma during pregnancy. Obstet Gynecol. 2004;103(1):5–12.
45. Kwon HL, Belanger K, Bracken MB. Effect of pregnancy and stage of pregnancy on asthma severity: a systematic review. Am J Obstet Gynecol. 2004;190(5):1201–10.
46. Dombrowski MP, Schatz M. ACOG practice bulletin #90: asthma in pregnancy. Obstet Gynecol. 2008;111(2 Pt 1):457–64.
47. Busse WW, et al. National Asthma Education and Prevention Program. Working group report on managing asthma during pregnancy: recommendations for pharmacologic treatment. Bethesda: National Institutes of Health; National Heart, Lung, and Blood Institute; 2004.
48. Brito V, Niederman MS. Pneumonia complicating pregnancy. Clin Chest Med. 2011;32(1):121–32.
49. Barton JR, Sibai BM. Severe sepsis and septic shock in pregnancy. Obstet Gynecol. 2012;120(3):689–706.
50. Goodnight WH, Soper DE. Pneumonia in pregnancy. Crit Care Med. 2005;33(10 Suppl):S390–7.
51. Kourtis AP, Read JS, Jamieson DJ. Pregnancy and infection. N Engl J Med. 2014;370(23):2211–8.
52. Louie JK, Acosta M, Jamieson DJ, Honein MA. Severe 2009 H1N1 influenza in pregnant and postpartum women in California. N Engl J Med. 2010;362(1):27–35.
53. Moreno R, Rhodes A. From the bedside to the bench: how to improve the care of critically ill pregnant patients with influenza. Crit Care Med. 2011;39(5):1199–200.
54. Zaman K, Roy E, Arifeen SE, et al. Effectiveness of maternal influenza immunization in mothers and infants. N Engl J Med. 2008;359(15):1555–64.
55. Madhi SA, Cutland CL, Kuwanda L, et al. Influenza vaccination of pregnant women and protection of their infants. N Engl J Med. 2014;371(10):918–31.
56. Håberg SE, Trogstad L, Gunnes N, et al. Risk of fetal death after pandemic influenza virus infection or vaccination. N Engl J Med. 2013;368(4):333–40.
57. Centers for Disease Control and Prevention. Influenza vaccination coverage among pregnant women – United States, 2010–2011 influenza season. MMWR. 2011;60:1078–82.
58. Influenza antiviral medications: summary for clinicians [Internet]. Atlanta: Centers for Disease Control and Prevention; 2015 [cited 2015 January 23]. Available from: http://www.cdc.gov/flu/professionals/antivirals/summary-clinicians.htm.
59. Sheffield JS. Methicillin-resistant Staphylococcus Aureus in obstetrics. Am J Perinatol. 2013;30(2):125–9.
60. Cole DE, Taylor TL, Mccullough DM, Shoff CT, Derdak S. Acute respiratory distress syndrome in pregnancy. Crit Care Med. 2005;33(10 Suppl):S269–78.
61. Lapinsky SE. Pregnancy joins the hit list. Crit Care Med. 2012;40(5):1679–80.
62. Hill JB, Sheffield JS, Mcintire DD, Wendel GD. Acute pyelonephritis in pregnancy. Obstet Gynecol. 2005;105(1):18–23.
63. Munnur U, de Boisblanc B, Suresh MS. Airway problems in pregnancy. Crit Care Med. 2005;33(10 Suppl):S259–68.
64. Neto AS, Cardoso SO, Manetta JA, et al. Association between use of lung-protective ventilation with lower tidal volumes and clinical outcomes among patients without acute respiratory distress syndrome: a meta-analysis. JAMA. 2012;308(16):1651–9.
65. Papazian L, Forel JM, Gacouin A, et al. Neuromuscular blockers in early acute respiratory distress syndrome. N Engl J Med. 2010;363(12):1107–16.
66. Guérin C, Reignier J, Richard JC, et al. Prone positioning in severe acute respiratory distress syndrome. N Engl J Med. 2013;368(23):2159–68.
67. Albright CM, Ali TN, Lopes V, Rouse DJ, Anderson BL. Lactic acid measurement to identify risk of morbidity from sepsis in pregnancy. Poster (# 571)

presented at: 34th Annual Meeting of the Society for Maternal Fetal Medicine; 2014 Feb 3–8; New Orleans, LA.
68. Marik PE, Baram M, Vahid B. Does central venous pressure predict fluid responsiveness? A systematic review of the literature and the tale of seven mares. Chest. 2008 July;134(1):172–8.
69. Fernández-Pérez ER, Salman S, Pendem S, Farmer JC. Sepsis during pregnancy. Crit Care Med. 2005;33(10 Suppl):S286–93.
70. Mackeen AD, Packard RE, Ota E, Speer L. Antibiotic regimens for postpartum endometritis. Cochrane Database Syst Rev. 2015;(2):CD001067.
71. Smaill FM, Grivell RM. Antibiotic prophylaxis versus no prophylaxis for preventing infection after cesarean section. Cochrane Database Syst Rev. 2014;(10):CD007482.
72. Rosene K, Eschenbach DA, Tompkins LS, Kenny GE, Watkins H. Polymicrobial early postpartum endometritis with facultative and anaerobic bacteria, genital mycoplasmas, and chlamydia trachomatis: treatment with piperacillin or cefoxitin. J Infect Dis. 1986;153(6):1028–37.
73. Giraldo-Isaza MA, Jaspan D, Cohen AW. Postpartum endometritis caused by herpes and cytomegaloviruses. Obstet Gynecol. 2011,117(2 Pt 2):466–7
74. Mulic-Lutvica A, Axelsson O. Postpartum ultrasound in women with postpartum endometritis, after cesarean section and after manual evacuation of the placenta. Acta Obstet Gynecol Scand. 2007;86(2):210–7.
75. Locksmith GJ, Duff P. Assessment of the value of routine blood cultures in the evaluation and treatment of patients with chorioamnionitis. Infect Dis Obstet Gynecol. 1994;2(3):111–4.
76. Tita AT, Andrews WW. Diagnosis and management of clinical chorioamnionitis. Clin Perinatol. 2010;37(2):339–54.
77. Abbasi N, Patenaude V, Abenhaim HA. Management and outcomes of acute appendicitis in pregnancy: population-based study of over 7000 cases. BJOG. 2014;121(12):1509–14.
78. McGory ML, Zingmond DS, Tillou A, Hiatt JR, Ko CY, Cryer HM. Negative appendectomy in pregnant women is associated with a substantial risk of fetal loss. J Am Coll Surg. 2007;205(4):534–40.
79. Williams R, Shaw J. Ultrasound scanning in the diagnosis of acute appendicitis in pregnancy. Emerg Med J. 2007;24(5):359–60.
80. Sitbon O, Lascoux-Combe C, Delfraissy JF, et al. Prevalence of HIV-related pulmonary arterial hypertension in the current antiretroviral therapy era. Am J Respir Crit Care Med. 2008;177(1):108–13.
81. Ahmad H, Mehta NJ, Manikal VM, et al. Pneumocystis carinii pneumonia in pregnancy. Chest. 2001;120(2):666–71.
82. Stafford I, Dildy GA, Clark SL, Belfort MA. Visually estimated and calculated blood loss in vaginal and cesarean delivery. Am J Obstet Gynecol. 2008;199(5):519.e1–7.
83. Herbert W, Zelop CM. ACOG practice bulletin #76: postpartum hemorrhage. Obstet Gynecol. 2006;108(4):1039–47.
84. Ducloy-Bouthors AS, Jude B, Duhamel A, et al. High-dose tranexamic acid reduces blood loss in postpartum haemorrhage. Crit Care. 2011;15(2):R117.
85. Harden CL, Hopp J, Ting TY, et al. Practice parameter update: management issues for women with epilepsy – focus on pregnancy (an evidence-based review). Quality Standards Subcommittee and Therapeutics and Technology Assessment Subcommittee of the American Academy of Neurology and American Epilepsy Society. Neurology. 2009;73(2):126–32.
86. Brophy GM, Bell R, Claassen J, et al. Guidelines for the evaluation and management of status epilepticus. Neurocrit Care. 2012;17(1):3–23.
87. Saposnik G, Barinagarrementeria F, Brown RD, et al. Diagnosis and management of cerebral venous thrombosis: a statement for healthcare professionals from the American Heart Association/American Stroke Association. Stroke. 2011;42(4):1158–92.
88. Kimber J. Cerebral venous sinus thrombosis. QJM. 2002;95(3):137–42.
89. Tate J, Bushnell C. Pregnancy and stroke risk in women. Womens Health (Lond Engl). 2011;7(3):363–74.
90. Carvalho CS, Resende F, Centeno MJ, Ribeiro I, Moreira J. Anesthetic approach of pregnant woman with cerebral arteriovenous malformation and subarachnoid hemorrhage during pregnancy: case report. Braz J Anesthesiol. 2013;63(2):223–6.
91. Guntupalli SR, Steingrub J. Hepatic disease and pregnancy: an overview of diagnosis and management. Crit Care Med. 2005;33(10 Suppl):S332–9.
92. Sibai BM, Ramadan MK, Usta I, Salama M, Mercer BM, Friedman SA. Maternal morbidity and mortality in 442 pregnancies with hemolysis, elevated liver enzymes, and low platelets (HELLP syndrome). Am J Obstet Gynecol. 1993;169(4):1000–6.
93. Martin JN, Perry KG, Miles JF, et al. The interrelationship of eclampsia, HELLP syndrome, and prematurity: cofactors for significant maternal and perinatal risk. Br J Obstet Gynaecol. 1993;100(12):1095–100.
94. Haram K, Svendsen E, Abildgaard U. The HELLP syndrome: clinical issues and management. BMC Pregnancy Childbirth. 2009;9:8.
95. Sheehan HL. The pathology of acute yellow atrophy and delayed chloroform poisoning. BJOG. 1940;47:49–62.
96. Riely CA. Acute fatty liver of pregnancy. Semin Liver Dis. 1987;7(1):47–54.
97. Brooks RR, Feller CM, Maye JP. Acute fatty liver of pregnancy: a case report. AANA J. 2002e;70(3):215–7.
98. Kaplan MM. Acute fatty liver of pregnancy. N Engl J Med. 1985;313(6):367–70.
99. Castro MA, Fassett MJ, Reynolds TB, Shaw KJ, Goodwin TM. Reversible peripartum liver failure: a new perspective on the diagnosis, treatment,

and cause of acute fatty liver of pregnancy, based on 28 consecutive cases. Am J Obstet Gynecol. 1999;181(2):389–95.
100. Jungers P, Chauveau D. Pregnancy in renal disease. Kidney Int. 1997;52(4):871–85.
101. Carroll MA, Yeomans ER. Diabetic ketoacidosis in pregnancy. Crit Care Med. 2005;33(10 Suppl):S347–53.
102. Montoro MN, Myers VP, Mestman JH, Xu Y, Anderson BG, Golde SH. Outcome of pregnancy in diabetic ketoacidosis. Am J Perinatol. 1993;10(1):17–20.
103. Stagnaro-green A, Pearce E. Thyroid disorders in pregnancy. Nat Rev Endocrinol. 2012;8(11): 650–8.
104. Belfort MA. Grand rounds: critical care in OB: part 4, navigating a thyroid storm [Internet]. Ohio: Contemporary OB/GYN; 2006 [cited 2015 Jan 2]. Available from: http://contemporaryobgyn.modernmedicine.com/contemporary-obgyn/news/clinical/clinical-pharmacology/grand-rounds-critical-care-ob-part-4-navigati.
105. Mestman JH. Hyperthyroidism in pregnancy. Best Pract Res Clin Endocrinol Metab. 2004;18(2):267–88.
106. De Groot L, Abalovich M, Alexander EK, et al. Management of thyroid dysfunction during pregnancy and postpartum: an endocrine society clinical practice guideline. J Clin Endocrinol Metab. 2012;97(8):2543–65.
107. Kuo C, Jamieson DJ, McPheeters ML, Meikle SF, Posner SF. Injury hospitalizations of pregnant women in the United States, 2002. Am J Obstet Gynecol. 2007;196(2):161.e1–6.
108. El Kady D. Perinatal outcomes of traumatic injuries during pregnancy. Clin Obstet Gynecol. 2007;50(3):582–91.
109. Petrone P, Talving P, Browder T, et al. Abdominal injuries in pregnancy: a 155-month study at two level 1 trauma centers. Injury. 2011;42(1):47–9.
110. American College of Surgeons, Committee of Trauma. Advanced trauma life support, student course manual. 9th ed. Chicago: American College of Surgeons; 2012.
111. Schiff MA, Holt VL. Pregnancy outcomes following hospitalization for motor vehicle crashes in Washington state from 1989 to 2001. Am J Epidemiol. 2005;161(6):503–10.
112. El-Kady D, Gilbert WM, Anderson J, Danielsen B, Towner D, Smith LH. Trauma during pregnancy: an analysis of maternal and fetal outcomes in a large population. Am J Obstet Gynecol. 2004;190(6):1661–8.
113. Valentin J. Annals of the ICRP, Publication 84, Pregnancy and medical radiation. Elsevier Health Sciences; 2000.
114. American College of Obstetricians and Gynecologists. ACOG committee opinion No. 299: guidelines for diagnostic imaging during pregnancy. Washington (DC): American College of Obstetricians and Gynecologists. Obstet Gynecol. 2004;104:647–51.
115. Strek ME. Chap. 5, Pregnancy and critical illness. In: ACCP critical care medicine board review. 21st ed. Glenview: American College of Chest Physicians; 2009.
116. Norwitz ER, Robinson JN. Pregnancy-induced physiologic alterations. In: Belfort M, editor. Critical care obstetrics. 5th ed. Oxford: Wiley-Blackwell; 2010.
117. Yeomans ER, Gilstrap LC. Physiologic changes in pregnancy and their impact on critical care. Crit Care Med. 2005;33(10 Suppl):S256–8.
118. Abbassi-Ghanavati M, Greer LG, Cunningham FG. Pregnancy and laboratory studies: a reference table for clinicians. Obstet Gynecol. 2009;114(6):1326–31.
119. Belfort M, Saade GR, Foley MR, Phelan JP, Dildy GA. Critical care obstetrics. 5th ed. Oxford: Wiley-Blackwell; 2010.
120. Post T, editor. UpToDate [internet]. Waltham (MA): UpToDate; 2015. Accessed 23 Jan 2015.
121. American College of Obstetricians and Gynecologists, Task Force on Hypertension in Pregnancy. Hypertension in pregnancy: executive Summary. Report of the American College of Obstetricians and Gynecologists' Task Force on Hypertension in Pregnancy. Obstet Gynecol. 2013;122(5):1122–31.
122. Campbell TA, Sanson TG. Cardiac arrest and pregnancy. J Emerg Trauma Shock. 2009;2(1):34–45.
123. Neumar RW, Otto CW, Link MS, et al. Part 8: adult advanced cardiovascular life support: 2010 American Heart Association guidelines for cardiopulmonary resuscitation and emergency cardiovascular care. Circulation. 2010;122(18 Suppl 3):S729–67.
124. MMWR: Prevention of Perinatal Group B Streptococcal Disease. Atlanta: Centers for Disease Control and Prevention. 2010;59:10.
125. American College of Obstetricians and Gynecologists. ACOG Committee Opinion No. 494: sulfonamides, nitrofurantoin, and risk of birth defects. Obstet Gynecol. 2011;117:1484–5.
126. Norwitz ER, Greenberg JA. Antibiotics in pregnancy: are they safe? Rev Obstet Gynecol. 2009;2(3):135–6.
127. Nahum GG, Uhl K, Kennedy DL. Antibiotic use in pregnancy and lactation: what is and is not known about teratogenic and toxic risks. Obstet Gynecol. 2006;107(5):1120–38.
128. Winer-Muram HT, Boone JM, Brown HL, Jennings SG, Mabie WC, Lombardo GT. Pulmonary embolism in pregnant patients: fetal radiation dose with helical CT. Radiology. 2002;224(2):487–92.

Care of the Newborn

31

Morgen Bernius and Fernando Mena

Abbreviations

ACLS Advanced Cardiac Life Support
AHA American Heart Association
CHD Congenital Heart Disease
CPAP Continuous Positive Airway Pressure
ECMO Extracorporeal Membrane Oxygenation
ED Emergency Department
ELBW Extremely Low Birth Weight
$ETCO_2$ End-tidal Carbon Dioxide
ETI Endotracheal Intubation
ETT Endotracheal Tube
HIE Hypoxic Ischemic Encephalopathy
IO Intraosseous
IVC Inferior Vena Cava
LBW Low Birth Weight
LMA Laryngeal Mask Airway
MAS Meconium Aspiration Syndrome
MSAF Meconium Stained Amniotic Fluid
NICU Neonatal Intensive Care Unit
NRP Neonatal Resuscitation Program
PALS Pediatric Advanced Life Support
PaO_2 Partial Pressure of Oxygen
PEEP Positive End Expiratory Pressure
PIP Positive Inspiratory Pressure
Pox Pulse Oximetry
PPHN Persistent Pulmonary Hypertension of the Newborn
PPV Positive Pressure Ventilation
UV Umbilical Vein
VLBW Very Low Birth Weight

Introduction

Since the beginning of time, babies have been born without medical support or intervention. Current numbers show that the great preponderance of births proceed without any resuscitative support at all. Ten percent, however, will need some intervention to begin breathing and fewer than 1% will require more extensive resuscitation [1–4].

The Neonatal Resuscitation Program (NRP) is a comprehensive training curriculum that details the key interventions involved in resuscitation of both premature and term newborns. It describes in detail the problems that may arise in this population and how to combat them. While most Emergency Physicians are certified in ACLS and even PALS, few are NRP certified and, unfortunately, the ACLS and PALS algorithms and lessons cannot be applied to care of the neonatal population.

M. Bernius (✉)
Department of Emergency Medicine, Medstar Franklin Square Medical Center, Baltimore, MD, USA

F. Mena
Department of Pediatrics, MedStar Franklin Square Medical Center, Baltimore, MD, USA

© Springer Nature Switzerland AG 2020
J. R. Shiber, S. D. Weingart (eds.), *Emergency Department Critical Care*,
https://doi.org/10.1007/978-3-030-28794-8_31

Because most infants do not require any intervention at birth and most high-risk infants are delivered at tertiary care centers—in delivery rooms with highly trained personnel—our experience with these patients (and therefore our comfort level) is likely limited. But, as Emergency Physicians, we know that although only a small percentage of infants born will require extensive resuscitation, one may very well end up in our Emergency Department (ED).

This chapter will serve as your guide to the management of that patient.

Pathophysiology

Transition From Fetal Circulation *(Fig. 31.1)* In fetal circulation, the right and left sides of the heart function as parallel circuits, with only a small amount of blood passing through the pulmonary circulation. All oxygen and carbon dioxide exchange occurs across the placental membrane. Oxygenated blood flows from the placenta through the umbilical vein back to the fetus, where half then flows through the hepatic circulation and the other half through the ductus venosus to the inferior vena cava (IVC) (Table 31.1). Blood from the lower extremities and from the umbilical vein mixes in the IVC and returns to the right atrium, where it is shunted across the foramen ovale to the left atrium, then to the left ventricle (Table 31.1). Blood from the left ventricle is pumped into the ascending aorta, then to the coronary and cerebral arteries and the upper extremities. Deoxygenated blood from the superior vena cava also flows into the right atrium, but primarily then to the right ventricle through the tricuspid valve. The right ventricle pumps blood toward the pulmonary circulation, but because it is so vasoconstricted in utero, most of the blood from the right ventricle is shunted through the ductus arteriosus into the descending aorta (Table 31.1). This blood then travels through the descending aorta to both the umbilical arteries and the lower part of the fetal body. Very little blood from the left ventricle travels across the aortic isthmus to the descending aorta to mix with blood from the right ventricle via the ductus arteriosus. Therefore, the coronaries, cerebral arteries, and upper extremities receive blood with a higher partial pressure of oxygen (PaO_2) than the umbilical arteries and lower extremities. In utero, the low PaO_2 causes the pulmonary vessels to be vasoconstricted, while the lungs themselves are expanded with the alveoli filled with fluid rather than air [1].

Three major changes occur at birth to allow transition from fetal circulation to that of a newborn [1]. First, clamping of the umbilical cord removes the low resistance placental circuit from the system and results in an increase in systemic blood pressure. Second, the baby takes its first breaths, replacing the alveolar fluid with oxygenated air and forcing that fluid into the pulmonary lymphatic system. Surfactant present in the alveoli facilitates their expansion, then "splints" them open to provide enough surface area for gas exchange to occur [5]. Oxygen can then be absorbed into the pulmonary circulation, which quickly raises the PaO_2 of that circuit. Third, the increased PaO_2 in the pulmonary circulation causes the vascular resistance in that circuit to drop, decreasing resistance to blood flowing from the right ventricle. Because of that decreased pulmonary vascular resistance, combined with the increased systemic blood pressure, blood starts preferentially to flow through the pulmonary circulation rather than the ductus arteriosus, causing it to vascoconstrict. Constriction of the ductus arteriosus is also a function of increased PaO_2. When hypoxemia exists, it causes both the ductus to remain open and pulmonary vascular resistance to remain high, and a vicious cycle ensues forcing blood to continue to shunt through the ductus and bypass the pulmonary circulation.

The majority of these changes occur within seconds after birth, but the full transition from fetal to neonatal blood oxygen levels has been shown to be a slower and continual increase, extending over a period of 5–10 minutes before reaching an oxygen saturation of at least 90% [1, 6].

Transition of the Premature Infant A number of differences among premature infants may render the normal newborn transition more diffi-

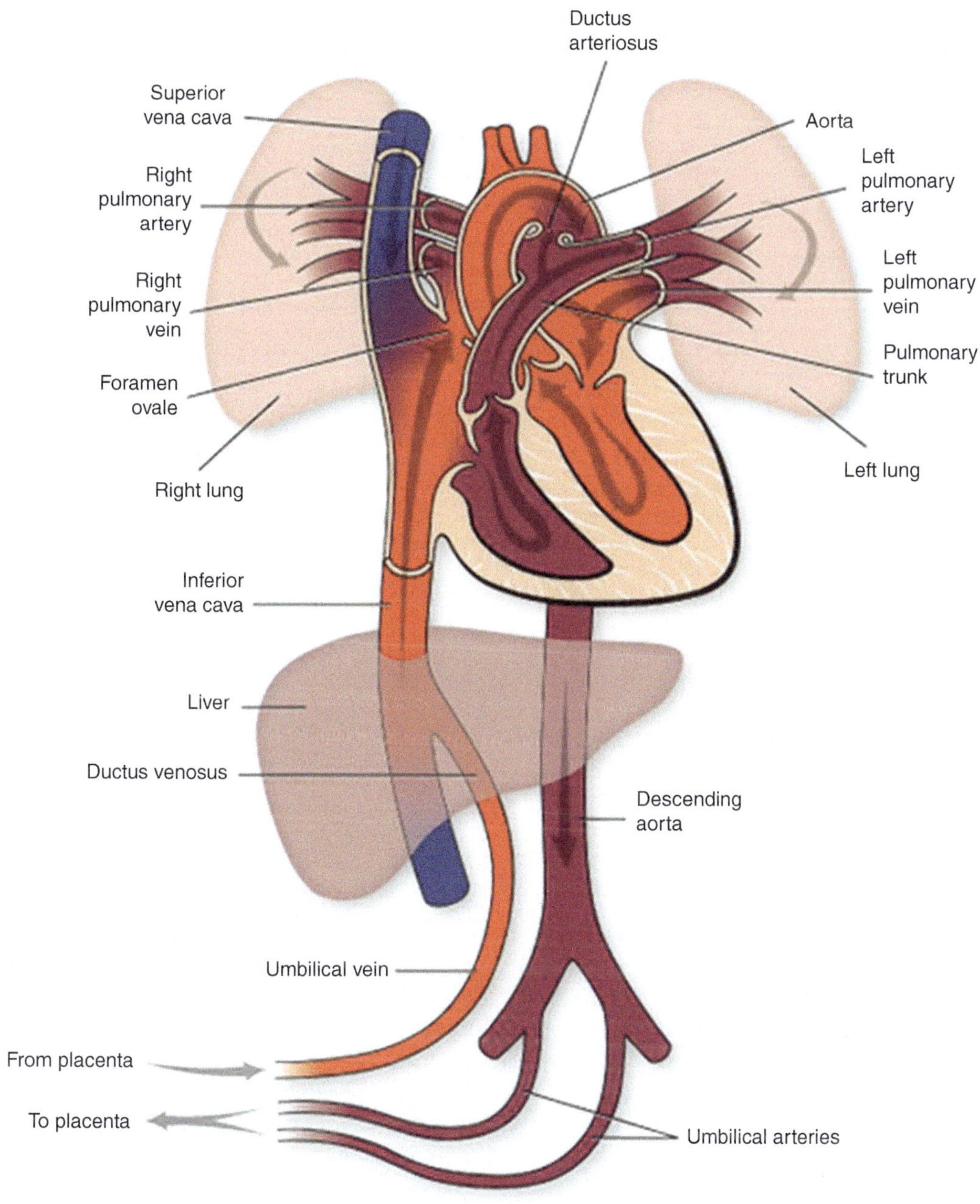

Fig. 31.1 Diagram of fetal circulation. (Reprinted with permission http://www.heart.org/en/health-topics/congenital-heart-defects/symptoms%2D%2Ddiagnosis-of-congenital-heart-defects/fetal-circulation. ©2015 American Heart Association, Inc.)

cult. Surfactant production only begins around 24–28 weeks' gestational age and infants born at fewer than 35 weeks may still be deficient. Without adequate surfactant, infants have more difficulty expanding their alveoli and preventing their collapse upon expiration [5]. The repeated expansion and collapse of alveoli also may trigger an inflammatory response, in which plasma proteins are exuded onto the epithelial surface of the alveoli, further inhibiting surfactant function

Table 31.1 Definitions (in the order they appear in the text)

Ductus venosus	In utero, shunt of oxygenated blood from the umbilical vein, bypassing the liver, to the IVC. This ductus closes upon clamping of the umbilical cord and eventually becomes the ligamentum venosus
Foramen ovale	A flap valve in the atrial septum that shunts more highly oxygenated blood from the IVC via the right atrium to the left atrium
Ductus arteriosus	In utero, shunt from the pulmonary artery to the descending aorta. This shunt remains open in utero because of low PaO_2 and the presence of circulating prostaglandins
Persistent pulmonary hypertension of the newborn (PPHN)	Pulmonary vasoconstriction that causes ventilation perfusion mismatch with hypoxemia and persistent intra- and extracardiac right to left shunting of blood, causing a failure of the normal transition of the fetal to newborn circulation
Acrocyanosis	A blue hue to the hands and feet seen at birth from decreased circulation to the extremities. This is not in itself an indication of decreased blood oxygen levels
Central cyanosis	Cyanosis present throughout the body, including the mucous membranes and tongue, indicative of decreased blood oxygen levels
"Vigorous" infant	An infant with strong respiratory efforts, good muscle tone, and a heart rate greater than 100 bpm
Preductal oxygen saturation	The pulse ox probe is placed on the *right wrist* to detect the saturation of the blood received from the aorta prior to the ductus arteriosus where mixing occurs with blood with lower oxygen levels from the pulmonary artery
Preterm	<37 weeks
Moderate to late preterm	34 to <37 weeks
Very preterm	28 to <32 weeks
Extremely preterm	<28 weeks
Low birth weight	<2500 g
Very low birth weight (VLBW)	<1500 g
Extremely low birth weight (ELBW)	<1000 g

and causing adhesions on those epithelial surfaces, and making re-expansion of the alveoli even more difficult [5].

Premature infants often lack the muscular strength to make the vigorous respiratory efforts required to generate adequate inspiratory pressures to expand the alveoli and replace the fetal fluid with air. A softer and more flexible chest wall also means increased work of breathing and often leads to paradoxical chest wall movement, thereby lowering achievable tidal volumes [5]. Additionally, immature brain development often means a decreased or even absent respiratory drive.

Thermoregulation is also more difficult in the premature infant because of decreased fat stores, thinner skin, and a large body surface area relative to body mass.

Premature babies are also more likely to be born with an infection, a common stimulus for premature labor; they have a smaller relative blood volume and are therefore more vulnerable to the effects of blood loss and hypovolemia; they are more susceptible to oxidative cell damage from increased oxygen exposure; and finally, they have extremely fragile vessels in their brains that may bleed easily [1, 7].

Potential Problems During Transition Many problems can occur in the transition process of a newborn. Some can begin in utero (such as infections or compromised placental or uterine blood flow), which may trigger early and unexpected labor. Most problems occur after birth however, and the algorithm for neonatal resuscitation addresses those potential issues in a stepwise fashion.

Respiratory problems are encountered most often. Because of a blocked airway from secretions or meconium, inadequate respiratory drive or strength of inspirations, or lung immaturity (as outlined above), the lungs may not fill with air and fluid may not be forced from the alveoli. Without adequate lung expansion and oxygen exposure, the PaO_2 of the pulmonary circuit remains low, and therefore pulmonary arterioles remain constricted. This vasoconstriction may occur even if the lungs expand, and can lead to persistent pulmonary hypertension (PPHN) of the newborn (Table 31.1). Inadequate lung inflation and pulmonary vasoconstriction also result in systemic hypoxemia.

Systemic hypotension may also occur in cases of extreme blood loss or may result from neonatal hypoxia causing decreased cardiac contractility or bradycardia with resulting low blood pressures [1].

Patient Presentation

Identifying Patients at Risk Before Birth Many risk factors help identify infants who may require resuscitation, although in the ED there often is no time to identify these historical factors and one must always be prepared for a potential resuscitation. However, when significant risk factors are recognized, and if appropriate resources in your own facility are absent, arrangements for transfer of the mother to a tertiary care center should be considered as soon as possible.

Antepartum risk factors pertinent in the ED setting include maternal issues such as diabetes, hypertension, preeclampsia, ongoing infection, substance abuse, lack of prenatal care, a history of previous fetal or neonatal death, and advanced maternal age (over 35 years). Other risk factors are pregnancy-related and include premature rupture of membranes, multiple gestations, fetal malformation or anomalies, diminished fetal activity, bleeding in the second or third trimester, post-term gestation, and diminished fetal activity [1]. Intrapartum risk factors that pertain to ED deliveries include breech or other abnormal presentations, prolapsed cord, premature or precipitous labor, prolonged (greater than 18 hours) rupture of membranes, prolonged (greater than 24 hours) labor, chorioamnionitis, meconium-stained amniotic fluid, abruptio placentae, placenta previa, or significant intrapartum bleeding [1].

The four most urgent questions to ask in a time-sensitive scenario are the gestational age, characteristics of the amniotic fluid if rupture of membranes has occurred, number of babies, and any additional risk factors [1].

Identifying Patients in Need of Resuscitation The NRP recommends a rapid assessment of three characteristics to determine which infants likely do *not* require resuscitation [1]:

Is it a term gestation?
Is there good muscle tone?
Is the infant crying or breathing?

If the answer to all three questions is yes, then the infant typically should not require resuscitation and may be allowed to remain in physical contact with the mother and routine care provided (dry, keep warm, position airway, and clear airway secretions if needed). If the answer to any question is no, then resuscitative efforts should be initiated.

In past teachings, skin color, and its transition from blue to pink, was considered an important component of the initial assessment because it was thought to be the quickest and most visible sign of the baby's state of oxygenation. Most babies display acrocyanosis (a blue hue to the hands and feet from decreased circulation to the extremities) at birth, which is not indicative of decreased blood oxygen levels. Central cyanosis (cyanosis present throughout the body, including the mucous membranes and tongue) on the other hand may indicate hypoxemia (Table 31.1). Studies have shown, however, that this clinical assessment is rather unreliable and depends on provider experience and skin pigmentation [1]. Therefore, it is no longer considered a component of the critical initial assessment to determine resuscitation needs.

Initial Stabilization

Overview In 2010, the American Heart Association (AHA) changed its recommendations for adult resuscitation of primary cardiac arrest patients from A-B-C (Airway-Breathing-

Circulation) to C-A-B, stressing the importance of initiating compressions over establishing ventilation. For pediatric patients, the order was changed as well. Ventilation is still of primary importance because most pediatric arrests are of a respiratory etiology, but compressions should not be delayed while ventilatory support is established. Neonatal resuscitation however remains A-B-C, focused primarily on establishment of an airway and ventilation, since nearly all of the problems encountered in a distressed neonate are solved with these interventions [1].

Once the rapid assessment of the newborn is performed and it is determined that the patient is either not at term, displays poor tone, or lacks adequate respiratory effort, the process of resuscitation begins. Neonatal resuscitation includes a sequence of four categories of intervention: initial steps of stabilization (including temperature regulation, clearing the airway, and stimulation); ventilation; chest compressions; and administration of epinephrine and/or volume expansion (Fig. 31.2) [7].

Initial Steps of Stabilization

Temperature Regulation Because newborn babies are wet and susceptible to significant heat loss at birth, the first step in resuscitation is to dry the infant and provide warmth. For most newborns, warmth is best provided via kangaroo care, consisting of skin-to-skin contact between mother and baby under her clothing or a towel or blanket. This position obviously does not allow for resuscitation, but for those vigorous term infants who are breathing spontaneously, it is a simple and effective method [8].

Infants who do require resuscitative efforts should be dried with towels (removing damp ones after use) and placed on a radiant warmer. The radiant warmer is prepared by setting it at 36.5 °C and attaching the temperature probe to a bag of normal saline placed on the warmer. The baby should remain uncovered for full visualization during resuscitative efforts. Hats are helpful to reduce heat loss.

Clearing the Airway Once dried, the infant should be placed in the supine position on the warmer with the neck in a neutral to slightly extended "sniffing" position. In cases where the infant has a large occiput due to molding, edema, or prematurity, it may help to place a rolled towel under the shoulders [1]. In the past, all infants had intrapartum oropharyngeal and nasopharyngeal bulb suctioning performed, but suctioning is no longer routinely recommended, even in infants at risk for difficult transitions, as it may induce a vagal response and further impair circulation [7, 9, 10]. Current recommendations are to suction infants only if it is deemed necessary to clear obvious airway secretions, if secretions are obstructing the airway, if there is meconium-stained fluid, or if they are thought to require positive pressure ventilation (PPV) [1, 7]. Airway suctioning can be performed with a bulb syringe or a suction catheter (Table 31.2). Be mindful of too vigorous deep suction as you may injure tissues and stimulation of the posterior pharynx may produce a vagal response leading to bradycardia and apnea [7].

Passage of meconium occurs most often in term or postterm infants and it may be the result of fetal distress or hypoxia in utero. The presence of meconium-stained amniotic fluid (MSAF) may be associated with fetal bradycardia, fetal acidosis, and low apgar scores [9]. Aspiration of meconium can cause physical airway obstruction leading to atelectasis, and potentially even air leak or pneumothorax; chemical irritation causing an inflammatory pneumonitis; and inactivation and decreased synthesis of surfactant [11]. Meconium-aspiration syndrome (MAS) should be suspected in infants born through MSAF who may be hypoxic and exhibit signs of respiratory distress immediately after birth [9]. Characteristic radiographic findings may not be distinguishable from transient tachypnea of the newborn initially but can evolve over days to a typical hyperinflated appearance with diffuse patchy densities [11].

Neonatal Resuscitation Algorithm—2015 Update

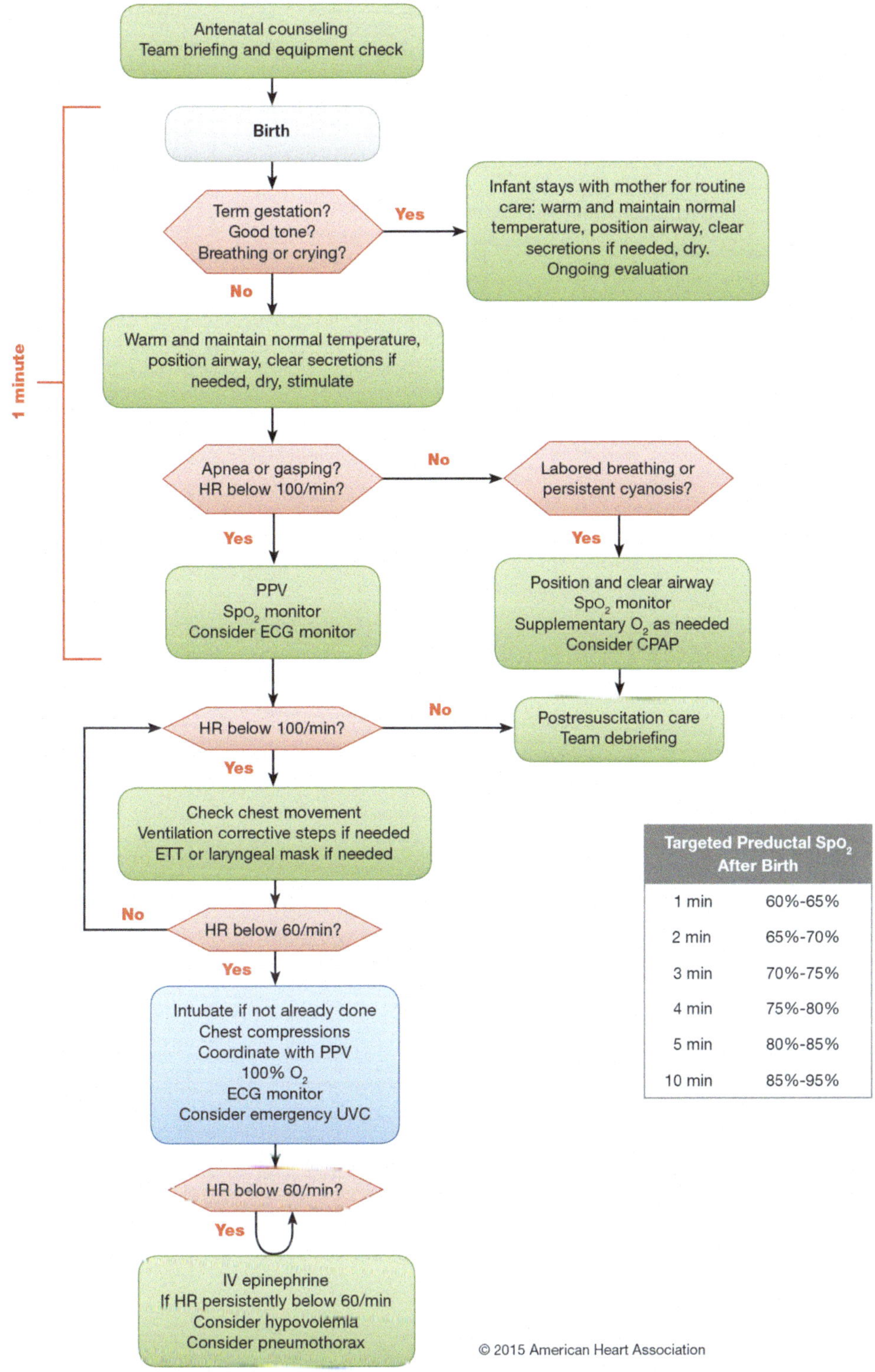

Targeted Preductal SpO_2 After Birth	
1 min	60%-65%
2 min	65%-70%
3 min	70%-75%
4 min	75%-80%
5 min	80%-85%
10 min	85%-95%

Fig. 31.2 Neonatal resuscitation algorithm. (**permission granted. ©2015 American Heart Association)

Table 31.2 Procedures in neonatal resuscitation

Procedure	Tools	Technique
Suctioning the airway	Bulb syringe 12 F or 14 F suction catheter (10 F for premature infants) Wall suction with negative pressure of apx 80–100 mmHg when the catheter is occluded	In the case of copious secretions, turn the infant's head to the side to allow pooling and facilitate suctioning. The mouth should be suctioned before the nose to prevent aspiration of intraoral contents if nasal suctioning results in a gasping breath. To avoid a vagal response, do not suction too deeply or aggressively [1, 8, 21, 22]
Deep tracheal suctioning for thick secretions or a plug preventing ventilation	Laryngoscope 12 F or 14 F suction catheter Endotracheal tube (ETT) Meconium aspirator device Wall suction with negative pressure of apx 80–100 mmHg when the catheter is occluded	First, prepare the meconium aspirator by attaching it to the suction source. Insert the appropriate size ETT for gestational age into the trachea. Now, attach the meconium aspirator to the ETT and occlude the port on the meconium aspirator to apply suction for approximately 3 seconds as you slowly pull the tube out. While monitoring for bradycardia with pulse checks, repeat the same process until no more meconium can be suctioned, or there is a drop in heart rate [1]
Endotracheal intubation	Straight blade laryngoscope (No. 0 for preterm and No. 1 for term infants) Appropriate sized uncuffed ETTs (2.5 mm, 3.0 mm, 3.5 mm, 4.0 mm) Stylet $ETCO_2$ detector or capnography Self-inflating bag, T-piece resuscitator, or flow-inflating bag 5 F to 8 F suction catheters for suctioning inside the ETT *see Table 31.7 for equipment sizes by age	Premedication is not indicated in neonatal resuscitation. Insert the laryngoscope and suction as needed until the vocal cords are visualized. Most ETTs for newborns have a black line near the tip of the tube called a "vocal cord guide" which should be placed at the level of the cords to guide depth of insertion. A rough estimate of the appropriate distance from the tip of the tube to the vermillion border is 6 cm plus the baby's weight in kg [1]. Confirm tube placement with $ETCO_2$, auscultation, and clinical response. Intubation attempts should last no longer than 20–30 seconds [18, 1]
Orogastric tube placement	8 F feeding tube (6 F in ELBW) 20 mL syringe	Use the tube to measure the distance from the bridge of the nose to the earlobe and down to the xiphoid. Insert the tube through the mouth the desired distance, then attach the syringe and gently suction for gastric contents. Remove the syringe and leave the end of the tube open to vent, then tape to the infant's cheek to secure [1]
Chest compressions	Second provider	Chest compressions should be performed using 2 thumbs on the sternum to compress while the hands encircle the ribs and the fingers support the spine. The 2-finger technique using the middle and index fingers is no longer preferred because there is less ability to control the depth of compressions. Pressure should be directed vertically, compressing the chest to a depth of approximately one-third the anterior-posterior diameter [1, 8]. Chest compressions and ventilations must always be coordinated in the newborn, even when they are intubated, with one ventilation after every three compressions, giving a total of 30 breaths and 90 compressions per minute. It is helpful for the person performing the compressions to count out loud: one, two, three, breath, one, two, three, breath

Umbilical line placement	3.5 F or 5 F Umbilical vein catheter Sterile gloves Antiseptic solution Umbilical tape 3 mL syringe filled with normal saline 3-way stopcock Scalpel	Attempts should be made to perform this procedure in a sterile fashion, though that may not be feasible in a resuscitation scenario and the line may be changed later. The umbilical stump should be cleaned with antiseptic solution and the umbilical tape tied loosely around the base so it may be tightened if there is significant bleeding. Use the syringe attached to a stopcock and then the catheter to prefill the umbilical catheter with normal saline, then close the stopcock off to the catheter. Cut the cord with the scalpel perpendicularly below the clamp (at least 1–2 cm from the skin). The umbilical vein is the larger single thin-walled hole contrasted with the two small thick-walled arteries. Insert the catheter guiding it caudally 2–4 cm (the shorter distance in premature infants) until there is blood return when the stopcock is opened and the syringe is drawn back
Intraosseous access	Smallest available IO needle Alternative: 18 gauge needle	Depending on the type of needle, shorten it prior to insertion to prevent likely penetration of the posterior wall of the bone. Using sterile technique, identify the flat portion of the tibia 1 cm below the tibial tuberosity. Support the leg on a firm surface without placing your hand behind the leg. Insert the needle using a gentle but firm twisting motion through the bony cortex perpendicular to the bone. Stop advancing when there is a sudden decrease in resistance. Remove the stylet if present and attempt to aspirate marrow. If you are unable to aspirate but feel the needle is likely in the appropriate position, then try to flush the needle and feel for extravasation of fluid into the anterior or posterior lower leg. Alternative locations for IO placement include the distal femurs
Surfactant administration	Surfactant (dose per kilogram depends on the brand) Sterile supplies: 5 ml syringe with 16 or 18 g needle 5 or 6 F feeding catheter Spare ETT (same size as used for intubating the newborn) Scissors Sterile gloves	Patient needs to be intubated. Prewarm the surfactant bottle by gently rolling between your hands without shaking. Sterilely draw the desired volume of surfactant into the syringe. Dispose of the needle and set the syringe containing the surfactant aside. Introduce the feeding tube all the way through the spare ETT. Trim the excess feeding tube right at the distal tip of the ETT so when it is introduced through the ETT into the newborn's trachea, the feeding tube will not go beyond the tip. Connect the syringe to the feeding tube hub and prime it with the surfactant. Place the newborn supine and ask an assistant to disconnect the ETT from the bag. Introduce the feeding tube into the ETT and administer the first aliquot of surfactant as a rapid bolus. Remove the feeding tube, reconnect the ETT to the bag, position the infant on his side, and provide PPV at a slightly increased PIP for 30 seconds. Place the infant back in the supine position and if stable, repeat the previous steps with the remaining aliquot with the infant positioned on the opposite side. The number of aliquots delivered [2–4] depends on the brand of surfactant. Some experts recommend giving the whole dose as a slower bolus through a side port in the ETT without interrupting ventilation

In the past, recommendations called for deep tracheal suctioning to be performed on any infants with meconium-stained amniotic fluid. Later this recommendation was amended and the focus was placed on the infant's appearance, and whether or not they are vigorous at birth (Table 31.1). This is no longer the case and routine intubation and suction for meconium-stained fluid is not recommended as there is insufficient evidence to support the practice and there is evidence that it may induce harm [7, 9]. Current recommendations focus on the infant's need for resuscitation. If the infant is not vigorous, with poor tone and depressed respirations, or the heart rate remains below 100 bpm despite initial steps of stabilization, then you should establish ventilation and proceed with PPV [1, 7]. It is important to note, however, that the presence of meconium in amniotic fluid may indicate fetal distress and increases the risk that the infant will require resuscitation and potentially tracheal intubation [7].

Stimulation Primary apnea (defined as true apnea or gasping respiratory efforts) may occur in a stressed newborn after an initial period of rapid breathing. During primary apnea, tactile stimulation (including the process of drying and suctioning, as well as slapping or flicking the soles of the feet or gently rubbing the back, trunk, or extremities) will provoke the baby to initiate breathing [1].

The much more dangerous secondary apnea may occur when cardiorespiratory depression persists during primary apnea, causing the infant to attempt a brief period of gasping breaths before entering this phase. When the infant is in secondary apnea, no amount of stimulation will result in a resumption of spontaneous respiratory activity [1]; if a couple of back rubs or flicks of the feet have not prompted spontaneous respiratory effort, then it is time to initiate PPV.

Assessing Respirations and Heart Rate During the initial seconds of stabilization, respiratory rate and depth should quickly increase with tactile stimulation. Rate can be counted by observing for good chest rise or by auscultation. Heart rate can be best determined by physical examination using a stethoscope to auscultate along the left side of the chest. If a baby is breathing effectively, the heart rate should be at least 100 bpm. Heart rate can also be determined by feeling for a pulse at the base of the umbilical cord where it attaches to the abdomen. Most ED physicians lack experience in detecting an umbilical pulse, and it may be more difficult if the vessels are constricted, so our recommendation is always to use the stethoscope to auscultate a precordial pulse. If you still have difficulty, a pulse oximetry (Pox) probe or cardiac leads should be quickly placed. Typically, providers tap out the heart rate on the bed so other members of the team can follow the rate. You may count the number of beats in a 6 second period and multiply by 10 for a quick estimate that will not cause any delay in the resuscitation algorithm sequence [1].

Continuing to the Next Step: Ventilation These first steps of drying, suctioning, and stimulating the infant are often occurring simultaneously as heart rate and respiratory rate are also being evaluated. The entire initial process should only take approximately 30 seconds to complete [1]. If the infant is apneic or gasping, or the heart rate is less than 100 bpm, then immediately proceed to provide PPV and apply the Pox monitor (Table 31.3) [1].

If the baby is breathing spontaneously but has labored breathing or remains cyanotic, repeat efforts should be made to clear the airway, a Pox monitor should be applied, and continuous positive airway pressure (CPAP) should be considered (Table 31.3) [1]. For infants with persistent cyanosis and hypoxia confirmed by Pox monitoring, but without a low heart rate or increased work of breathing, blow-by oxygen may be administered using a face mask or an open oxygen tube held close to the baby's mouth and nose and with the provider's hand cupped toward the baby's face, but without making physical contact (Table 31.3) [1]. Flow-inflating bags and masks and T-piece resuscitators may also be used to provide free-flow oxygen, but those are seldom available in the ED setting. Self-inflating bags are the most common device used in the ED but cannot provide free-flow oxygen. See the discussion

Table 31.3 Indications for Interventions

Intervention	Indication
Free-flow supplemental oxygen	Persistent cyanosis (and confirmed hypoxia) in an infant with a normal heart rate and no increased respiratory effort
Positive pressure ventilation	Apneic or gasping infant Heart rate below 100 bpm despite stimulation Hypoxia despite supplemental oxygen increased to 100%
CPAP	Heart rate greater than 100 bpm with persistent cyanosis or increased work of breathing
Endotracheal intubation	Inability to ventilate with bag-valve-mask ventilation despite corrective efforts Persistent requirement for PPV Initiation of chest compressions Special situations (e.g., surfactant administration and diaphragmatic hernia)
Chest compressions	Heart rate below 60 bpm despite adequate ventilation for 30 seconds
Epinephrine administration	Heart rate remains below 60 bpm despite 60 seconds of coordinated chest compressions and effective ventilations

below regarding oxygen concentrations for resuscitations to determine how much oxygen should be applied with free-flow support.

Ventilation

Ventilation of the newborn is the most critical intervention performed in neonatal resuscitation, and most compromised newborns will quickly respond with improved heart rates [1, 7]. At the time ventilatory support is initiated, Pox monitoring should also be started. The use of Pox as a required early intervention in neonatal resuscitation is rather recent and is critical for titrating oxygen administration. Because the ductus arteriosus may remain open for a period of time after birth, allowing blood with lower oxygen levels to cross from the pulmonary artery and mix into the descending aorta, the Pox probe should be placed on the *right wrist*, which receives blood from the aorta prior to the ductus arteriosus to detect a preductal saturation (Table 31.1) [1]. Pox monitoring allows for a continuous pulse assessment without requiring interruption of resuscitation efforts, but the reality is that it may not provide accurate readings in low flow states and it may take 1–2 minutes to apply correctly and obtain a reading [7].

Oxygen Administration In the past, the recommendations for resuscitation of any newborn with persistent cyanosis or respiratory distress included the administration of 100% oxygen. Studies have conclusively shown, however, that asphyxiated term infants exposed to 100% oxygen during resuscitation (as compared to ambient air) have increased mortality, increased myocardial and kidney injury, reduced cerebral circulation, delayed recovery (as demonstrated by lower 5-minute apgar scores and heart rates), increased resuscitation time requirements, and signs of increased oxidative stress for up to 4 weeks after birth [12, 13]. Excess oxygen exposure, especially in preterm infants and infants who have experienced hypoxic events, is thought to lead to increased free oxygen radical generation which can result in cellular damage [12].

Initiation of resuscitation with 21% oxygen (room air), on the other hand, has been shown to result in earlier initiation and maintenance of spontaneous respiratory efforts without any increase in neurodevelopmental disabilities [6]. Meta-analyses of several randomized controlled trials comparing use of 21% oxygen versus 100% oxygen in initiation of resuscitation in term newborns showed increased survival in patients given room air [7, 14, 15].

Most delivery rooms use blended oxygen during neonatal resuscitation, guided by preductal saturations. Normal preductal saturations rise slowly from the in utero value of 60% in uncompromised term infants over the first 10 minutes of life to the neonatal value of over 90% [1, 7]. Current recommendations are that resuscitation of term newborns be initiated with room air and oxygen concentrations gradually increased with the use of a blender to target typical preductal saturations for the age in minutes (Table 31.4) [7, 16].

Most delivery rooms utilize T-piece resuscitators attached to blenders to control both the per-

Table 31.4 Normal preductal oxygen saturations [1, 7]

Minutes after birth	Target saturation (%)
1 minute	60–65
2 minutes	65–70
3 minutes	70–75
4 minutes	75–80
5 minutes	80–85
10 minutes	85–95

Table 31.5 Delivering various oxygen concentrations using self-inflating bags and a gas source of 100% oxygen [17]

% oxygen delivered	Oxygen flow rate	PIP
<40%	0.25 L/min	Noncontributory
≤40%	0.5 L/min	35–40 cmH_2O
>40%	0.5 L/min	20–25 cmH_2O
40–60%	1 L/min	35–40 cmH_2O
>60%	1 L/min	20–25 cmH_2O
Apx 100%	5 L/min	Noncontributory

centage of oxygen being delivered and ventilatory pressures. This is the device that provides the most reliable and controlled peak inspiratory pressure (PIP) and positive end expiratory pressure (PEEP) for neonatal resuscitation. Most EDs, however, are stocked with only self-inflating bags. A study by Thio et al. evaluated oxygen delivery of four common self-inflating bags (Laerdal, Ambu, Parker Healthcare, and Mayo Healthcare) at different oxygen flow rates and PIPs [17]. While there were differences among the brands, the study found in general that self-inflating bags with a reservoir can deliver varying oxygen concentrations when a blender is unavailable (Table 31.5). The use of self-inflating bags with varied oxygen flow rates and PIPs may be a useful method in the ED, where obtaining a blender and T-piece resuscitator for the unlikely event of a neonatal resuscitation may be unrealistic. However, if feasible, we recommend purchasing a T-piece resuscitator for use in the ED.

After 30 seconds of resuscitation with effective PPV that expands the lung with visible chest rise, if the heart rate remains below 60 bpm, the oxygen concentration should be increased to 100% and chest compressions should be initiated [1, 7, 11].

If the newborn improves to the point that preductal saturations remain above 85–90%, oxygen concentration may be titrated back down to room air. If respiratory effort is adequate and heart rate is greater than 100 bpm, but central cyanosis or low oxygen saturations persist despite CPAP and oxygen, a trial of PPV should be considered [1]. For infants who are effectively ventilated but for whom cyanosis and hypoxia persist, problems such as congenital heart disease (CHD) or PPHN need to be considered [1].

Positive Pressure Ventilation Indications for PPV include an apneic or gasping infant, a heart rate below 100 bpm despite stimulation, or hypoxia despite provision of supplemental oxygen where the concentration has been increased to 100% (Table 31.3) [1]. If an infant has a heart rate below 100 bpm despite a brief period of stimulation or remains cyanotic despite administration of free-flow oxygen, continuing to attempt these measures is futile and there should be no delay in initiating PPV. In a retrospective review of neonatal resuscitations, ineffective PPV was identified as the most frequent cause of severe neonatal depression and the need for intensive resuscitation [18]. ED physicians are well versed in the art of bag-valve-mask ventilation, but without experience, performing this task on the much smaller scale of the neonate can still be challenging.

The equipment needed includes appropriate size masks and bags, a manometer to gauge pressures delivered and, in case they are necessary, appropriate sized endotracheal tubes (ETTs), laryngoscope blades, and laryngeal mask airways (LMAs). Cushioned-rimmed face masks in newborn and premature sizes should be available. As with an older child or adult patient, the appropriate size mask should cover the chin, mouth, and nose (but not the eyes) of the infant in order to provide an airtight seal. PPV may be administered using a flow-inflating (or anesthesia) bag, a T-piece resuscitator, or the neonatal self-inflating bag most commonly found in EDs. Self-inflating bags should have an oxygen reservoir attached to provide a more constant concentration of oxygen. The appropriate size bag should have a minimum volume of 200 mL and a maximum of 750 mL

[1]. The tidal volume required for a term newborn is only 4–6 mL/kg, or 10–25 mL, which would be a very difficult volume to deliver in a controlled manner using a larger bag [1].

Adequacy of ventilation can be assessed by evaluating for good chest rise as well as the response of the infant's heart rate and oxygen saturations. Without experience, it is easy to ventilate too aggressively and, even with adequate ventilation, chest rise may not always be visible, or stomach inflation may be mistaken for chest rise [1, 19, 20]. To accompany the clinical assessment in guiding ventilatory efforts, all self-inflating bags should be equipped with an integral pressure gauge or an attached pressure manometer to monitor inspiratory pressures. Initial PPV should be performed at a rate of 40–60 breaths per minute, with initial inspiratory pressures of approximately 20 cmH_2O [1, 7, 21]. In some term babies without spontaneous ventilation, in order to clear the alveoli of their fluid, high pressures (up to 30–40 cmH_2O) may be necessary for the first several breaths [7, 21–24]. Once functional residual capacity has been established, inspiratory pressures may be decreased while continuing to assess for adequate chest movement and monitoring heart rate and Pox.

Use of an end-tidal Carbon Dioxide ($ETCO_2$) detector placed between the self-inflating bag and the face mask may be considered to facilitate early recognition of an obstructed airway during bag-valve-mask ventilation. Leone et al. found that use of the PediCap allowed providers more quickly to recognize an obstructed airway by visualizing the lack of color signal change as opposed to trying to appreciate an inadequate degree of chest rise and auscultating for absent or unequal breath sounds [19]. When no color change was visible, providers knew to adjust their ventilation technique to correct the error, while infants with color change and poor clinical response to ventilation required other interventions.

Once PPV is initiated, the provider should observe for a rapid increase in heart rate and Pox readings, typically within the first 5–10 breaths [1]. Whether or not an $ETCO_2$ detector is used, the provider should be observing for adequate chest rise, and a second provider should auscultate for adequate breath sounds. If there is no color change, poor chest rise, or lack of bilateral breath sounds, then the ventilation corrective sequence should be performed.

Table 31.6 Ventilation corrective sequence: MR SOPA [1]

Mask adjustment	Reapply the mask to ensure an adequate seal, slight increase in pressure on the mandible to pull it into mask
Reposition airway	Place infant in sniffing position, towel roll under shoulders as needed.
Suction	Check for excess secretions, suction as necessary
Open mouth	Ventilate through an open mouth to bypass potentially obstructed nares
Pressure increase	Gradually increase airway pressures to 30–40 cmH_2O until good chest rise and equal breath sounds are present
Airway alternative	Consider ETI or LMA to improve ventilation efforts

The mnemonic for this sequence is "MR SOPA": *M*ask adjustment, *R*eposition airway, *S*uction mouth and nose, *O*pen mouth, *P*ressure increase, and *A*irway alternative (Table 31.6) [1, 25].

To adjust the mask, simply reapply with enhanced but gentle pressure to pull the jaw into the mask cushion and ensure a good seal. Repositioning the airway includes checking that the infant is in the appropriate sniffing position and adding a towel roll under the shoulders if necessary. The mouth and nose should be suctioned if necessary for excess secretions. Because of their small nares and potential for secretions, attempts should be made to ventilate with the mouth open, especially in premature infants. Pressure may be slowly increased every few breaths to 30 cmH_2O until the infant has visible chest rise and equal bilateral breath sounds. If the other components of the corrective sequence have been addressed and there is still inadequate chest rise, the pressure may cautiously be increased to 40 cmH_2O [1]. Finally, if all of these adjustments have not corrected the inability to ventilate, an alternate airway, such as an ETT or LMA should be considered (Table 31.7).

Attempts to wean and discontinue PPV can be made once the heart rate is greater than 100 bpm and stable [1]. The rate and pressure of ventila-

Table 31.7 Equipment sizes by weight and gestational age [1]

Weight (g)	Gestational age (weeks)	Tube size (mm)	ETT suction catheter size (Fr)	Laryngoscope blade size
Below 1000	Below 28	2.5	5 F or 6 F	00
1000–2000	28–34	3.0	6 F or 8 F	0
>2000	>34	3.5	8 F	1

tion may be gradually reduced while observing for spontaneous respiratory efforts. If the infant can sustain respiratory efforts and maintain a heart rate over 100 bpm, then PPV may be discontinued. If preductal oxygen saturations remain in the target range, supplemental oxygen can also be weaned as tolerated [1].

Continuous Positive Airway Pressure CPAP allows oxygen delivery under lower pressures of about 4–6 cmH_2O to improve work of breathing, distend the alveoli and prevent their collapse during expiration, and improve gas exchange [5]. It has also been shown to improve ventilation-perfusion matching, decrease pulmonary vascular resistance, reduce incidences of apnea, and enhance surfactant release which further stabilizes the alveoli [5].

Many delivery rooms utilize CPAP for infants with heart rates in the normal range (above 100) and spontaneous respirations, but with increased respiratory effort (grunting or retractions) or persistent hypoxia and cyanosis [1]. If after several minutes of CPAP support the infant still has an increased work of breathing, PPV is indicated.

In the delivery room, CPAP is typically delivered using a face mask connected to a flow-inflating bag or to a T-piece resuscitator and adjusting the flow-control valve or PEEP. Unfortunately, CPAP cannot be delivered using the self-inflating bags present in most EDs. The NRP suggests that CPAP may be deliverable using some mechanical ventilators, but this method is quite cumbersome, as it requires a relatively long preparation time and is not suitable for resuscitation scenarios. The T-piece resuscitator is now the standard of care in delivery rooms and would be the ideal tool for use in the ED as well. If one is not available, then a flow-inflating bag with a manometer would be the next best option. If neither is available to deliver CPAP and the infant remains hypoxic or distressed, then PPV using a bag-valve-mask or endotracheal intubation (ETI) and full ventilator support would be the only other option.

Endotracheal Intubation Indications for ETI in neonatal resuscitation include inability to ventilate with bag-valve-mask ventilation despite corrective efforts, a persistent requirement for PPV, the initiation of chest compressions, and special situations such as surfactant administration or diaphragmatic hernia (Table 31.3) [1, 7].

While ED physicians have plenty of experience in ETI of adult and often pediatric patients, ETI of the newborn tends to be a unique skill that may be difficult to acquire and, like other skills, only improves with experience (Table 31.2) [26]. The NRP recommends providers spend no more than 30 seconds trying to intubate, with PPV by mask in between intubation attempts, and close monitoring for deterioration during those attempts [1, 26].

Laryngeal Mask Airway Because ETI of the neonate is a potentially difficult skill when not practiced, and practice opportunities may be hard to come by, ED neonatal resuscitation equipment should include an LMA as a rescue device. Only the size 1 LMA is appropriate for newborns. As a rescue device, the LMA requires less training and practice than ETI, may be placed rapidly, and has a high rate of successful first-time placement. Among its disadvantages is the existence of air leaks, which may lead to gastric distension and an inability to deliver adequate ventilatory pressures; in addition, suctioning cannot be performed through the LMA [1, 18].

Continuing to the Next Step in Resuscitation: Chest Compressions If after 30 seconds of effective ventilation the infant is improving and the heart rate is greater than 60, but still less than 100, continue to administer PPV. Respiratory effort, Pox, and heart rate should be reassessed at least every 30 seconds while other complications such as hypovolemia and pneumothorax are considered [1]. An orogastric tube should also be considered at this time (Table 31.2).

If after 30 seconds of adequate ventilation with supplemental oxygen, CPAP, or PPV, the infant's heart rate is still below 60 bpm, then the ED provider should continue to the next step in the resuscitation algorithm: chest compressions (Table 31.3) [1, 7]. Most often, effective ventilation will result in an increase in heart rate. However, if the compromising event was substantial enough, myocardial function may have been affected.

Chest Compressions

When chest compressions are initiated, ETI is strongly recommended if it has not been done prior to this point, and the oxygen concentration should be increased to 100%. Sixty seconds of well-coordinated chest compressions and ventilation should be performed before stopping to reassess heart rate. Chest compressions and ventilations must be coordinated in the newborn, even when intubated, with one ventilation given after every three compressions for a total of 30 breaths and 90 compressions per minute (Table 31.2).

If the heart rate has improved to over 60 bpm, then compressions are discontinued and the ventilatory rate should be increased back to 40–60 breaths per minute from the coordinated rate of 30 breaths per minute, and oxygen administration can be titrated back down as guided by preductal saturations [1].

If the heart rate remains below 60 bpm despite 60 seconds of coordinated chest compressions and effective ventilations, preparations should be made to proceed to the next step in the algorithm: medication administration (Table 31.3) [1, 7]. While preparing for this next intervention and obtaining vascular access, continue coordinated chest compressions and ventilation with brief periodic checks of the heart rate. Use of a cardiac monitor is the preferred method for assessing heart rate during chest compressions. You may also assess the heart rate using a stethoscope or a Pox but there are limitations to these methods [1]. There should also be constant reassessment of the quality of ventilation by observing adequate chest rise and auscultating for good breath sounds, confirming ETT placement, administering appropriate supplemental oxygen, and delivering quality and coordinated chest compressions [1].

Medication Administration

Epinephrine is the drug of choice in neonatal resuscitation. As long as the heart rate remains below 60 bpm, chest compressions and PPV are continued and repeat doses of epinephrine are given until the heart rate rises above 60 bpm [1]. Once the heart rate improves to over 60 bpm, compressions and epinephrine administration are discontinued, and PPV continues until it is over 100 bpm and the infant has spontaneous respiratory effort.

Intravenous Access The most easily manageable intravenous access in the newborn is the umbilical vein (UV), but many ED physicians may not be comfortable with this procedure if they have never performed it in the past (Table 31.2). In reality, umbilical line placement, though intimidating, is a technically simple procedure to perform. An alternative is placement of an intraosseous (IO) needle, which most ED physicians have been trained to perform (Table 31.2). Studies comparing UV catheter placement versus IO placement by inexperienced providers found the IO to be easier and faster [16]. In newborns, IOs are placed preferentially in the proximal tibia, then distal femur, medial or lateral malleoli, and iliac crests [16].

In the past, the endotracheal route of medication administration was considered an equally viable option. Like ACLS and PALS recommendations, however, the endotracheal route is now typically only used to give a single dose of epinephrine while intravenous access is being secured [1, 27]. With the use of the IO in the ED setting, there likely would not be enough of a delay to warrant use of the endotracheal route at all.

Epinephrine The recommended dose of epinephrine in neonatal resuscitation is 0.1–0.3 mL per kg of the 1:10,000 concentration [1]. Since this concentration contains 0.1 mg of epinephrine per mL, this dose is the equivalent of 0.01–0.03 mg per kg. Dosing of the epinephrine should be followed with a 0.5–1 mL flush of normal saline [1, 7, 27].

If the epinephrine must be given via the endotracheal route while efforts are being made to establish intravenous access, a higher dose of 0.5–1 mL per kg of the 1:10,000 solution (or 0.05–0.1 mg per kg) should be used [1, 7].

Chest compressions should be continued for 1 minute after epinephrine administration via the intravenous route, slightly longer if it is given endotracheally, before a pulse check is performed. Repeat doses may be given every 3–5 minutes until the heart rate improves to over 60 bpm. If the baby has had evidence of blood loss, appears pale, or is still responding poorly to resuscitative efforts suggesting the possibility of hypovolemia, volume administration may be considered [1].

Volume Administration Volume expansion is not routinely used during neonatal resuscitation unless there is evidence of acute blood loss or clinical factors suggest that possibility. Blood loss may occur via the umbilical cord, in cases of placenta previa or, occasionally, into the maternal circulation without external evidence of hemorrhage. Clinically, hypovolemic infants may display pallor, sluggish capillary refill time, weak pulses, persistent bradycardia, and a poor response to resuscitative efforts.

Volume expansion is given as a 10 mL per kg dose of normal saline or, in cases of suspected or proven severe anemia, type O Rh-negative packed red blood cells. Ringer's lactate is no longer recommended in neonatal resuscitation [1, 7]. The fluids should be given slowly over 5–10 minutes rather than as a rapid bolus, especially in premature infants, because a potential risk of intracranial hemorrhage exists with rapid volume expansion. If there is no significant improvement after the first dose, a second 10 mL per kg dose may be considered.

Other Medications Naloxone administration is not recommended for newborns during initial resuscitative efforts, even for those with respiratory depression. Instead, ventilatory support as outlined above is the mainstay of management [1, 7]. The use of sodium bicarbonate during resuscitation to correct metabolic acidosis is controversial and not without risk. In the acidotic infant, emphasis again should be on adequate ventilation. Consultation with a neonatologist should be considered before administering sodium bicarbonate.

Resuscitation of the Premature Infant

Prematurity is defined as a gestational age of less than 37 weeks at birth (Table 31.1) [28]. This category is further broken down by the WHO into very preterm (less than 32 weeks) and extremely preterm (less than 28 weeks). In 2007, the American Academy of Pediatrics endorsed a nomenclature proposed by an expert panel in 2005 that recommended that babies born between 34 weeks and 36 6/7 weeks gestation be referred to as late preterm infants to reflect the fact that these infants have a greater risk of morbidity and mortality than term infants [29]. Premature infants are also categorized by birth weight, that is, as low birth weight (LBW) which is less than 2500 grams; very low birth weight (VLBW) which is less than 1500 grams; and extremely low birth weight (ELBW) which is less than 1000 grams [30].

Resuscitation of the preterm infant follows the same algorithm as that of the term infant. There are, however, certain factors unique to this population that deserve discussion. Premature babies are in fact as fragile as they appear, from the delicate network of germinal matrix capillaries in their brains to their immature surfactant-deficient lungs. Attention must focus on avoiding cold stress, excessive ventilation pressures, trendelenburg positioning, and rapid changes in CO_2 levels, blood pressure, and volume [1]. They must be handled gently as they are dried and stimulated and bagged, despite the nervous energy any ED provider undoubtedly will have when resuscitating a premature infant.

Temperature Regulation When the delivery of a premature infant is anticipated, recommendations are to increase the ambient temperature of the resuscitation area to 74–77 °F, preheat the radiant warmer, and place a warming pad under the towels on the resuscitation table [1]. ED personnel rarely have the luxury of advance notice (beyond the estimated time of arrival given by prehospital providers calling with a consult) but should implement these preparations when possible. The recommendation for heat conservation unique to VLBW infants, or those delivered at less than 29 weeks gestation, is use of a polyethylene plastic bag (e.g., a sheet of plastic food wrap or a food-grade one gallon plastic bag) to wrap the infant in up to the neck immediately after birth [1, 7, 31]. This is done instead of drying the infant with towels, and the infant should remain in this plastic throughout the resuscitation process. There is a small risk that this may produce hyperthermia, so the baby's temperature should be monitored as resuscitation efforts allow, with a goal axillary temperature of approximately 36.5 °C [1, 8]. Chemical heat mattresses are also quite effective at maintaining body temperature and are easy to use. Because the large surface area of a newborn's head results in significant evaporative heat loss, a head cap should be placed to prevent hypothermia [32].

Ventilation

Oxygen There is no defined optimal oxygen concentration for resuscitation of premature infants, though to reach target saturations somewhat higher concentrations may be required for premature infants than for term infants [6, 25]. Target preductal saturations are the same for premature infants as term infants (Table 31.3) though they may be slightly slower to reach those goals [1, 25, 33].

Current recommendations are to initiate resuscitation with an oxygen concentration of 30% for premature infants and titrate according to anticipated preductal saturations for the age in minutes [1, 6]. Most studies on oxygen administration in this population are done using blenders and titrating accordingly. In the ED, if a blender is not available and the only options include room air or 100% oxygen administration, based on the literature it is not possible for us to make a recommendation as to which you should use to initiate resuscitation. Using room air has a high treatment failure rate, and using 100% oxygen has the potential for early and possibly long-term toxic effects in premature infants who have yet to develop their natural antioxidant defenses [6, 33]. If you need to resuscitate a preterm infant, a T-piece resuscitator and oxygen blender would be the ideal equipment to use. If only a self-inflating bag is available, then it might be best to adjust the concentration of oxygen delivered to the infant by varying the flow rates and PIP as reviewed in Table 31.4, though this has not been studied for resuscitation of preterm infants.

Positive Pressure Ventilation The same criteria are used for assisting ventilations in the premature infant as in the term infant, but the ED provider must be aware of the increased susceptibility to injury in these babies with immature lungs. Initial inflation pressures in the premature infant should be around 20–25 cmH_2O [1]. The best indicator of effective ventilation will be a prompt increase in the heart rate. If this does not occur, then assess for chest rise and bilateral breath sounds. Keep in mind that adequate chest rise in the premature infant may be barely perceptible, or may not be visible at all in the VLBW infant covered in plastic [1, 19]. Premature infants may also be more difficult to ventilate with a mask because of their relatively large tongues and small mandibles, causing them to be more prone to obstruction [34]. Proper positioning of the airway and a good mask fit are of the utmost importance. While bagging the overweight adult with a big tongue, short neck, and facial hair requires the full strength of both hands and forearms, bagging of the premature infant requires a delicate touch, precision, and fingertip finesse. Keep this in mind even as you may feel your own palpitations and your mind races to recall your neonatal resuscitation algorithm, and you will "first do no harm."

Positive End Expiratory Pressure While there is insufficient information about the value of PEEP during the initial resuscitation, NRP recommends that it be utilized in the premature infant if ongoing ventilation is necessary. If the baby is intubated, use a PEEP of 5 cmH_2O for premature infants [1].

Continuous Positive Airway Pressure CPAP may be especially useful in the preterm infant whose surfactant-deficient lungs are more susceptible to collapse with expiration, and to damage from repeated collapse and reinflation [1]. Its use in premature infants has been associated with decreased need for intubation, decreased oxygen requirement, fewer days on mechanical ventilation, and less use of postnatal steroids [5]. CPAP should be considered for premature infants who, like term infants, are breathing spontaneously and have a heart rate above 100, but have persistent cyanosis, low Pox, or increased work of breathing. In the delivery room, CPAP is provided via a mask or CPAP nasal prongs attached to a T-piece resuscitator or flow-inflating bag. If this equipment is not available and prolonged support is anticipated (especially in a preterm infant), intubation and mechanical ventilation might be a better option until the infant can be transported to a neonatal intensive care unit (NICU) [7, 35].

Medications Infants born at less than 30 weeks gestation benefit from early surfactant administration after resuscitation, though the guidelines for timing of administration and indications for its use are not precisely defined. Surfactant is relatively expensive and has an approximate 36-month shelf life, so it may not be available in the ED. It is acceptable to await the NICU transport team and allow them to administer surfactant if the receiving physician deems it to be necessary [1]. However, in ELBW infants it is often not until surfactant is administered that an increase in heart rate is seen and resuscitation efforts become effective, so we would strongly recommend having a dose available (Table 31.2).

Noninitiation and Termination of Resuscitation

Noninitiation of Resuscitation Conditions in which it is considered acceptable not to initiate resuscitation efforts include a confirmed gestational age of less than 23 weeks or birth weight less than 400 grams, anencephaly, a confirmed lethal genetic disorder (such as trisomy 13) or malformation, or when an otherwise unacceptably high likelihood of death or severe disability exists [1, 7]. Parents may request that resuscitation efforts not be initiated for patients in the "gray zone" where survival rates are still low and morbidity rates are high, such as infants in the 23–24 week gestational age range [1, 7, 36]. These recommendations, however, are made for NICU staff who have the benefit of prenatal consultations with families and complete access to prenatal records. In the ED it is best not to make irreversible decisions prior to the birth of the infant, and even when the gestational age is expected to be less than 23 weeks, the ED physician must keep in mind that except in cases of in vitro fertilization where exact dates are known, due dates are estimates and may be off by several weeks depending on how they were calculated and the recall of the mother.

Termination of Resuscitation Resuscitation efforts may be terminated if there has been no detectable heart rate for a period of at least 10 minutes [1, 7]. At this point, the infant's chance of survival is extremely low, and any who does survive will suffer severe disabilities. At this point, attention should turn to the family members. When death is considered inevitable and resuscitation efforts are discontinued, the parents should be offered an opportunity to hold the infant before and after its death. Consider allowing the family to choose a name, obtain a weight and length and photograph, or even a footprint or lock of hair if so desired [37].

Definitive Treatment Infants who require resuscitation are at significant risk of deterioration after initial stabilization. Once effective ventilation and circulation have been established, newborns should be transferred to an environment where close monitoring and anticipatory care can be provided.

Temperature Regulation Thermoregulation is an important part of post-resuscitative care. This may be achieved using kangaroo care for the infant no longer requiring intervention or temperature monitoring on the radiant warmer. Unintentional hyperthermia should be avoided, defined as a body temperature above 37.5 °C [38].

Therapeutic hypothermia has been shown in several randomized controlled studies of infants 36 weeks of age and older with hypoxic-ischemic encephalopathy (HIE) to result in significantly lower mortality and neurodevelopmental disability at 18 months, but it must be initiated within 6 hours after birth and requires a very well-defined protocol to perform [1, 39–41]. Arrangements should be made for transfer to a facility that can perform this service as soon as possible, so it can be initiated within the required window of time for infants who are candidates. If a newborn is deemed eligible for hypothermia, all heat sources should be turned off until arrival of the transport team.

Respiratory Support Infants who require continued respiratory support after initial resuscitation should receive heated and humidified oxygen to prevent heat loss and drying of the mucosa [1]. Infants who need continued support are also at risk for further complications from their difficult transition and require close monitoring until they are transferred to a NICU [1].

Laboratory Studies All infants, especially those who are premature, have relatively low glycogen stores, and the stress of a difficult transition will rapidly deplete those supplies. Infants who have required resuscitation should have glucose levels checked immediately after stabilization, then every 30–60 minutes until levels are stable or they are transferred to definitive care [1, 7]. You may treat as instructed by your NICU consultant, but if levels are over 25 and less than 40 and the infant is able to take oral fluids, consider feeding. If they are unable to feed, or if levels are less than 25, you may give dextrose as 2 mL/kg bolus of $D_{10}W$ and start an intravenous glucose infusion [42]. Healthy term infants should not require routine glucose testing unless they are symptomatic. Symptoms may include lethargy, jitteriness, tremors, or tachypnea.

Other laboratory studies that may be considered as appropriate for each individual case include blood gas analysis and hemoglobin measurements.

Post-Resuscitation Complications

Persistent Pulmonary Hypertension of the Newborn PPHN is the persistent vasoconstriction of the pulmonary circuit in those infants who were hypoxemic or acidemic at the time of birth. It usually occurs in infants 34 weeks and older, and is most often managed with mechanical ventilation and supplemental oxygen to help vasodilate the pulmonary vasculature. More severe cases may require therapies such as inhaled nitric oxide or extracorporeal membrane oxygenation (ECMO) [1]. Supportive care in the ED prior to transport includes likely intubation with mechanical ventilation, sedation, and avoidance of hypoxemic episodes.

Pneumothorax The possibility of pneumothorax should be considered in any infant who is not responding to resuscitation efforts or with an acute deterioration, especially those who are intubated. As with any adult patient with acute deterioration while being artificially ventilated, the "DOPE" mnemonic—dislodged tube, obstructed tube, pneumothorax, or equipment failure—will help a diagnosis.

Seizures Infants with HIE from a period of perinatal asphyxiation may have seizures after a period of several hours after birth. Any seizing infant should have a glucose value checked first and treated accordingly, after which anticonvulsant treatment with Phenobarbital may be necessary [1].

Apnea Infants with HIE or premature infants may have episodes of apnea or hypoventilation in the immediate postnatal period. Again, close monitoring is necessary until the time of transfer to definitive care [1].

Premature Infants

Postresuscitation preterm infants require close monitoring of glucose values, as well as cardiorespiratory monitoring for apnea and bradycardia episodes typical in the extremely premature infants. Hypothermia should be avoided and oxygen saturations should be closely monitored for lows and highs with attempts to maintain them in the normal range for their age. Prompt initiation of antibiotics should also be considered since infection is a potential cause of premature delivery and can have a significant impact on outcomes [1].

Critical Points

To determine which infants likely do not require resuscitation, the NRP recommends a rapid assessment of three characteristics:

Is it a term gestation?
Is there good muscle tone?
Is the infant crying or breathing?

Neonatal resuscitation includes a sequence of four categories of intervention: initial steps of stabilization (including temperature regulation, clearing the airway, and stimulation); ventilation; chest compressions; and administration of epinephrine and/or volume expansion.

Routine suctioning is no longer recommended for all infants. Infants should be suctioned only if it is deemed necessary to clear obvious airway secretions or if they will require PPV.

Routine intubation and tracheal suctioning of the newborn delivered through MSAF is no longer recommended. Intubation should only be performed if it is deemed necessary during resuscitation to provide PPV.

Ventilation of the newborn is the most critical intervention performed in neonatal resuscitation, and most compromised newborns will quickly respond with improved heart rates.

The use of Pox to monitor preductal saturations is a required early intervention in neonatal resuscitation to titrate administered oxygen.

The use of 3 lead ECG monitoring is recommended for the rapid and accurate measurement of a newborn's heart rate.

Current recommendations are that resuscitation of term infants be initiated with room air and oxygen concentrations gradually increased with the use of a blender to target typical preductal saturations.

Current recommendations are that resuscitation of premature infants be initiated with 30% oxygen and titrate with use of a blender to target typical preductal saturations.

Indications for PPV include an apneic or gasping infant, a heart rate below 100 bpm despite stimulation, or hypoxia despite provision of supplemental oxygen where the concentration has been increased to 100%.

Ventilation corrective sequence (MR SOPA): mask adjustment, reposition airway, suction mouth and nose, open mouth, pressure increase, and airway alternative.

Indications for ETI include inability to ventilate with bag-valve-mask ventilation despite corrective efforts, a persistent requirement for PPV, the initiation of chest compressions, and special situations such as surfactant administration or diaphragmatic hernia.

Chest compressions are indicated for patients who have a heart rate below 60 bpm despite 30 seconds of adequate ventilation. Chest compressions in the newborn must be given in coordination with ventilations, even when the infant is intubated.

Debriefing and simulation are excellent ways of improving knowledge and practice skills.

References

1. American Academy of Pediatrics and American Heart Association. Textbook of neonatal resuscitation. 7th ed. Elk Grove Village: American Academy of Pediatrics; 2016.
2. Thio M, Bhatia R, Dawson JA, Davis PG. Oxygen delivery using neonatal self-inflating resuscitation bags without a reservoir. Arch Dis Child Fetal Neonatal Ed. 2010;95:F315–9.
3. Perlman JM, Risser R. Cardiopulmonary resuscitation in the delivery room: associated clinical events. Arch Pediatr Adolesc Med. 1995;149:20–5.
4. Barber CA, Wyckoff MH. Use and efficacy of endotracheal versus intravenous epinephrine during neonatal cardiopulmonary resuscitation in the delivery room. Pediatrics. 2006;118:1028–34.
5. Halamek LP, Morley C. Continuous positive airway pressure during neonatal resuscitation. Clin Perinatol. 2006;33:83–98.
6. Finer N, Saugstad O, Vento M, Barrington K, Davis P, Duara S, et al. Use of oxygen for resuscitation of the extremely low birth weight infant. Pediatrics. 2010;125:389–91.
7. Wyckoff MH, Aziz K, Escobedo MB, Kapadia VS, Kattwinkel J, Perlman JM, Simon WM, Weiner GM, Zaichkin JG. Part 13: Neonatal resuscitation: 2015 American Heart Association guidelines update for cardiopulmonary resuscitation and emergency cardiovascular care. Pediatrics. 2015;136:S196.
8. Watkinson M. Temperature control of premature infants in the delivery room. Clin Perinatol. 2006;33:43–53.
9. Velaphi S, Vidyasagar D. Intrapartum and post delivery management of infants born to mothers with meconium-stained amniotic fluid: evidence-based recommendations. Clin Perinatol. 2006;33:29–42.
10. Vain NE, Szyld EG, Prudent LM, Wiswell TE, Aguilar AM, Vivas NI. Oropharyngeal and nasopharyngeal suctioning of meconium-stained neonates before delivery of their shoulders: multicentre, randomized controlled trial. Lancet. 2004;364:597–602.
11. Garcia-Prats JA. Clinical features and diagnosis of meconium aspiration syndrome. UTD [Internet]. 2013 [cited 2014 Oct 12]. Available from: http://www.uptodate.com/contents/clinical-features-and-diagnosis-of-meconium-aspiration-syndrome.
12. Saugstad OD, Ramji S, Vento M. Oxygen for newborn resuscitation: how much is enough? Pediatrics. 2006;118:789–92.
13. Richmond S, Goldsmith JP. Air or 100% oxygen in neonatal resuscitation? Clin Perinatol. 2006;33:11–27.
14. Davis PG, Tan A, O'Donnell CP, Schulze A. Resuscitation of newborn infants with 100% oxygen or air: a systematic review and meta-analysis. Lancet. 2004;364:1329–33.
15. Rabi Y, Rabi D, Yee W. Room air resuscitation of the depressed newborn: a systematic review and meta-analysis. Resuscitation. 2007;72:353–63.
16. Engle W. Intraosseous access for administration of medications in neonates. Clin Perinatol. 2006;33:161–8.
17. Thio M, Van Kempen L, Rafferty AR, Bhatia R, Dawson JA, Davis PG. Neonatal resuscitation in resource-limited settings: titrating oxygen delivery without an oxygen blender. J Pediatr. 2014;165:256–60.
18. Mora EU, Weiner GM. Alternative ventilation strategies: laryngeal masks. Clin Perinatol. 2006;33:99–110.
19. Leone TA, Lange A, Rich W, Filner NN. Disposable colorimetric carbon dioxide detector use as an indicator of a patent airway during noninvasive mask ventilation. Pediatrics. 2006;118(1):e202–4.
20. Tracy M, Downe L, Holberton J. How safe is intermittent positive pressure ventilation in preterm babies ventilated from delivery to newborn intensive care unit? Arch Dis Child Fetal Neonatal Ed. 2004;89:F84–7.
21. Stenson BJ, Boyle DW, Szyld EG. Initial ventilation strategies during newborn resuscitation. Clin Perinatol. 2006;33:65–82.
22. Vyas H, Milner AD, Hopkin IE, Boon AW. Physiologic responses to prolonged and slow-rise inflation in the resuscitation of the asphyxiated newborn infant. J Pediatr. 1981;99:635–9.
23. Boon AW, Milner AD, Hopkin IE. Lung expansion, tidal exchange, and formation of the functional residual capacity during resuscitation of asphyxiated neonates. J Pediatr. 1979;95:1031–6.
24. Lindner W, Vossbeck S, Hummler H, Phlandt F. Delivery room management of extremely low birth weight infants: spontaneous breathing or intubation? Pediatrics. 1999;103(5 Pt 1):961–7.
25. Zaichkin J, Weiner G. Neonatal resuscitation program (NRP) 2011: new science, new strategies. Neonatal Netw. 2011;30(1):5–13.
26. O'Donnell CP, Kamlin OF, Davis PG, Morley CJ. Endotracheal intubation attempts during neonatal resuscitation: success rates, duration, and adverse effects. Pediatrics. 2006;117:e16–21.
27. Wyckoff MH, Wyllie J. Endotracheal delivery of medications during neonatal resuscitation. Clin Perinatol. 2006;33:153–60.
28. World health organization, prevention of perinatal morbidity and mortality. Public health papers. Geneva: WHO; 1969. p. 42.
29. Engle WA, Tomashek KM, Wallman C, Committee on Fetus and Newborn, American Academy of Pediatrics. "Late-preterm" infants: a population at risk. Pediatrics. 2007;120:1390–401.
30. Fanaroff A, Fanaroff J. Klaus and Fanaroff's care of the high-risk neonate. 6th ed. Philadelphia: Elsevier Saunders; 2013. p. 105.

31. Cramer K, Wiebe N, Hartling L, Crumley E, Vohra S. Heat loss prevention: a systematic review of occlusive skin wrap for premature neonates. J Perinatol. 2005;25:763–9.
32. Trevisanuto D, et al. Heat loss prevention in very preterm infants in delivery rooms: a prospective, randomized, controlled trial of polyethylene caps. J Pediatr. 2010;156(6):914–7, 917 e1.
33. Rabi Y, Singhal N, Nettel-Aguirre A. Room-air versus oxygen administration for resuscitation of preterm infants: the ROAR study. Pediatrics. 2011;128:e374–81.
34. Finer N, Rich W, Wang C, Leone T. Airway obstruction during mask ventilation of very low birth weight infants during neonatal resuscitation. Pediatrics. 2009;123:865–9.
35. Morley CJ, Davis PG, Doyle LW, Brion LP, Hascoet JM, Carlin JB. Nasal CPAP or intubation at birth for very preterm infants. N Engl J Med. 2008;358:700–8.
36. Batton D. Antenatal counseling regarding resuscitation at an extremely low gestational age. Pediatrics. 2009;124:422–7.
37. MacDonald H. American Academy of Pediatrics, Committee on Fetus and Newborn. Perinatal care at the threshold of viability. Pediatrics. 2002;110(5):1024–7.
38. Wariki WMV, Mori R. Interventions to prevent hypothermia at birth in preterm and/or low-birth-weight infants: RHL commentary (last revised: 1 June 2010). [cited 2014 Nov 30]. The WHO Reproductive Health Library; Geneva: World Health Organization. Available from: http://apps.who.int/rhl/newborn/cd004210_Warikiwmv_com/en/.
39. Gluckman PD, Wyatt JS, Azzopardi D, Ballard R, Edwards AD, Ferriero DM, Polin RA, Robertson CM, Thoresen M, Whitelaw A, Gunn AJ. Selective head cooling with mild systemic hypothermia after neonatal encephalopathy: multicentre randomized trial. Lancet. 2005;365:663–70.
40. Shankaran S, Laptook AR, Ehrenkranz RA, Tyson JE, McDonald SA, Donovan EF, Fanaroff AA, Poole WK, Wright LL, Higgins RD, Finer NN, Carlo WA, Duara S, Oh W, Cotton CM, Stevenson DK, Stoll BJ, Lemons JA, Guillet R, Jobe AH. Whole-body hypothermia for neonates with hypoxic-ischemic encephalopathy. N Engl J Med. 2005;353:1574–84.
41. Azzopardi DV, Strohm B, Edwards AD, Dyet L, Halliday HL, Juszczak E, Kapellou O, Levene M, Marlow N, Porter E, Thoresen M, Whitelaw A, Brocklehurst P. Moderate hypothermia to treat perinatal asphyxia encephalopathy. N Engl J Med. 2009;361:1349–58.
42. From the American Academy of Pediatrics. Clinical report: postnatal glucose homeostasis in late-preterm and term infants. Committee on Fetus and Newborn. Pediatrics. 2011;127(3):575–9.

32

Pediatrics 1: Intro, Airway, Respiratory, Cardiac, Neuro

Emily Fontane, Mark Hincapie, and Nico Chiriboga

Introduction

Care of the critically ill child in the emergency room is often challenging. Fortunately, the majority of children who visit the ED are not suffering from life-threatening diseases, and those presentations are not the intent of this chapter. We will provide brief overviews of the presentation, diagnosis, and treatment of the most common life-threatening diseases in children and focus on providing tools that will help the emergency department team recognize children who are critically ill and in impending organic failure. We will highlight the importance of teamwork, including not only the ED team but also consulting pediatric specialists when caring for the critically ill child.

E. Fontane (✉)
Department of Emergency Medicine, Division of Pediatric Emergency Medicine, University of Florida, College of Medicine, Jacksonville, FL, USA

M. Hincapie
Division of Pediatric Critical Care to Paediatric Emergency medicine, Jacksonville, FL, USA

N. Chiriboga
Division of Pediatric Critical Care, University of Florida, Department of Pediatrics in the College of Medicine, Jacksonville, FL, USA

Anatomical and Physiological Differences

Children are not simply small adults as there are several differences in anatomy and physiology that differentiate them from adults. The care of pediatric patients ranges from newborns to fully grown adolescents, and recognizing these anatomical and physiological differences is vital. Certain congenital and acute diseases present anatomical and physiologic differences of their own. One of the most challenging sources of anatomical differences is the pediatric airway. Table 32.1 highlights some of these differences. The most common congenital disease in children, trisomy 21, further exacerbates some of these differences like the larger tongue and the shorter neck.

Children have a much more intense vagal response potentially causing bradycardia when inserting an endotracheal tube or airway adjunct. Another important difference is the smaller lungs, especially in infants and newborns, making it critical to use an appropriately sized bag-valve-mask when providing assisted ventilation and using only the volumes necessary to expand the chest.

Children's chests, especially in some congenital conditions, are less compliant. They are dependent on the movement of their diaphragm for breathing and have a reduced functional residual capacity. Some disease processes like chronic lung disease of prematurity, cystic fibrosis, and asthma further complicate these differences. Finally, the cardio-

© Springer Nature Switzerland AG 2020

J. R. Shiber, S. D. Weingart (eds.), *Emergency Department Critical Care*,
https://doi.org/10.1007/978-3-030-28794-8_32

Table 32.1 Anatomical differences of the pediatric airway

Head	Prominent Occiput
Neck	Shorter
Tongue	Larger and occupies more relative space in mounth
Larynx	Higher than adult (above C2-C3)
Epiglottis	Friable, Ω shape
Vocal Cords	Short and concave. Diameted smaller
Tracheal Cartilage	Softer, less calcified

vascular system of children has several differences including a smaller circulating blood volume but more physiologic reserve, especially by increasing heart rate and vascular tone, than that of adults. This presents a challenge in the diagnosis of shock as *blood pressure change is a late finding and usually signals impending cardiovascular collapse.*

Table 32.2 Vital sign differences

Age (years)	Respiratory rate (/min)	Heart rate (/min)	Systolic blood pressure (mmHg)
<1	30–40	110–160	70–90
1–2	25–35	100–150	80–95
2–5	25–30	95–140	80–100
5–12	20–25	80–120	90–110
>12	15–20	60–100	100–120

Initial Assessment of the Critically Ill Child

The evaluation of children in the ED requires a rapid recognition of the critically ill as they can quickly deteriorate without immediate intervention. The provider must maintain a high index of suspicion to be able to recognize the signs of impending deterioration. The focus of critical care support in the ED (and in any other setting) should be recognizing impending organ failure to prevent cardiopulmonary collapse. Vital signs differ across age groups, and recognition of abnormalities is an important first step and can help monitor response to therapy (Table 32.2).

DIRECT

Society of Critical Care Medicine developed a methodology for the approach to critically ill child using the acronym DIRECT: D for detection, meaning to form a fast impression of the child's status; I for intervention – so after detecting a physiologic abnormality, quickly intervene to avoid further deterioration; after each intervention, the child should be reassessed (hence the R) to evaluate the effect of the interventions; throughout these steps, healthcare providers should maintain effective communication and teamwork (EC and T in DIRECT) as they should contact the referral pediatric institution and specialists early on and maintain effective communication with them throughout the ED resuscitation up to the moment of transfer.

Initial Impression

As you walk into the patient's room, quickly form an impression by the assessment of three principal systems: behavior, respiratory, and cardiovascular. These three, in combination with vital signs, form the Pediatric Early Warning Score which we will discuss later.

Behavior

Quickly observe how the child is acting; it is important to know the child's age and developmental stage and if the child suffers from developmental delay. *In general, a child that is active, playful, and feeding appropriately is not critically ill.* One of the most important tools is asking the parent/caregiver if the child's current behavior is his usual. Table 32.3 highlights some behavioral characteristics of an ill child.

A change in behavior alone, with no respiratory or cardiovascular abnormalities, is usually a sign of isolated neurologic dysfunction, so consider etiologies such as CNS infection, trauma, metabolic derangements, and ingestions. When neurologic dysfunction combines with respiratory or cardiovascular compromise, this can be a sign of respiratory failure or impending cardiopulmonary failure.

Table 32.3 Behavioral characteristics of the sick child

Lethargy
Confusion
Not Moving
Sleeping more than usual and not waking up for feeds
Irritable and not consolable by parent
Not latching on to breast or not taking bottles
Not reactive to stimulation
No reaction to painful stimuli

Respiratory

Respiratory emergencies are common, and most cardiac arrests in children are of respiratory etiology, and as such, rapid intervention to prevent respiratory failure is of paramount importance to prevent cardiac arrest and death. Children's use of compensatory mechanisms to support ventilation and oxygenation are excellent indicators of respiratory dysfunction. Start with assessment of age-appropriate respiratory rate (see Table 32.2). In general, respiratory rate > 10 breaths/min higher than the age average can point toward respiratory difficulty. Fever can cause tachypnea, and young infants can have normal periods of rapid breathing, followed by pauses and then normalization of the respiratory rate called periodic breathing, which is a normal variant. Next, assess the child's respiratory effort: First, the child's position. Older children tend to favor a position which expands their chest's capacity and allows better use of their accessory muscles – bending forward and laying their hands on their legs or knees known as *tripoding*. Second, use of accessory muscles – intercostal, subcostal (abdominal), and supracostal (neck) muscles – to assist in ventilation is a sign of respiratory distress. *Nasal flaring and head bobbing are more ominous signs of impending respiratory failure, as is grunting*. This usually consists of a low-pitched, repetitive mewing sound used to generate higher end expiratory pressures to maintain oxygenation (especially in infants). Desaturation might only be a late finding when respiratory distress overwhelms the compensatory mechanisms mentioned above causing hypercapnia, hypoxia/hypoxemia, or both leading to neurologic dysfunction as the metabolic needs of the brain and other organs are not met. If not rapidly corrected, it can quickly evolve into cardiopulmonary failure and arrest.

Cardiovascular

Quickly assess the patient's skin for signs of peripheral vasoconstriction: pallor, duskiness, cyanosis, or mottling (a more ominous sign). Measure capillary refill in both upper and lower extremities as there are conditions (like ductal-dependent heart disease) where these may be different. Heart rate more than 30 above the average for age (see table) is a sensitive indicator of cardiovascular dysfunction. It is important to separate fever as a factor for tachycardia and skin pallor, but if a child is febrile, a low threshold should be maintained for septic shock. With compensated *warm* shock, the child's compensatory mechanisms are sufficient to maintain end-organ perfusion with blood pressure usually normal at this stage (a reason why the use of blood pressure to assess a child's cardiovascular status can be misleading!). As these compensatory mechanisms are overwhelmed (see section on shock), perfusion to end organs decreases, and blood pressure drops. Decreased perfusion to the brain will lead to changes in behavior. This is known as uncompensated *cold* shock which, if not quickly corrected, may result in cardiopulmonary failure.

Conditions worsening respiratory conditions
Prematurity
Chronic lung disease of prematurity
Asthma
Congenital heart disease
Chronic kidney disease
Neuromuscular conditions

Respiratory Failure

Introduction

Respiratory failure can be of ventilation (with hypercapnia), oxygenation (with hypoxia), or mixed with both failing. As respiratory failure progresses, the child will become more obtunded and eventually lethargic due to respiratory acidosis or low cerebral oxygenation. If allowed to progress, respiratory failure will eventually lead to respiratory arrest and/or cardiopulmonary arrest.

Etiology

The main entities that lead to respiratory failure are viral infections like croup and bronchiolitis as well as bacterial infections like tracheitis, epiglottitis (now rare due to routine HIB vaccination), pneumonia, and asthma.

Diagnosis

The diagnosis of respiratory failure can be made on clinical grounds usually by a combination of tachypnea (RR more than 10 above average for age), use of accessory muscles, and, as it progresses, with abnormalities in behavior (ranging from irritability to obtundation and lethargy). *Chest radiography or lab tests are not needed to diagnose respiratory failure although are useful for its etiology.* Blood gasses should be arterial or capillary as venous are not as accurate for respiratory acidosis and hypercarbia.

Management

The goal of immediate treatment for respiratory failure consists of supporting ventilation and oxygenation, but some therapies are tailored for the underlying etiology.

Bronchiolitis

Acute bronchiolitis is one of the most common presentations to outpatient clinics, EDs, and inpatient pediatric services and consists of upper respiratory symptoms combined with viral invasion and inflammation of the lower airways (bronchi) which leads to air trapping and increased mucus production with plugging. It almost exclusively presents in children 0–2 years of age. After that age, other diagnoses like asthma exacerbations are more likely.

Etiology

Most cases of bronchiolitis are caused by respiratory syncytial virus (RSV), but human metapneumovirus, parainfluenza, rhinovirus, and influenza viruses can also be implicated. The incidence of bronchiolitis waxes and wanes seasonally.

Risk Factors

Most children with bronchiolitis have a mild course, but some have a higher risk of severe disease: infants <12 weeks of age and premature infants (especially born <31 weeks or who developed chronic lung disease of prematurity, congenital heart disease, neuromuscular disorders, and chronic health conditions). When evaluating children with any of these risk factors, the clinician should have a lower threshold for admission and more aggressive interventions.

Presentation and Diagnosis

Bronchiolitis is diagnosed exclusively on history and physical examination: a combination of nasal congestion, cough, audible wheezing, tachypnea, and retractions. Auscultation will reveal a combination of transmitted upper airway sounds, crackles, and wheezing. Younger infants and premature infants can present with episodes of apnea. Nasal flaring, grunting, and head bobbing usually point toward more severe respiratory distress. Desaturation, cyanosis, and pallor are also late and ominous signs; lethargy and altered mental status are usually late findings but reveal severe respiratory disease. Chest X-ray abnormalities are common, and atelectasis may correlate more severe disease. Viral panels are not necessary for the diagnosis of bronchiolitis, and negative results do not rule out bronchiolitis.

Management

The management of bronchiolitis is mainly supportive with nasal suctioning decreasing the work of breathing and need for ventilatory support, and saline can be used to liquify secretions to assist suctioning. The decision to start ventilatory support should not be based solely on the presence of tachypnea and retractions, as these are present in some degree in all children with bronchiolitis; the criteria should include severe respiratory distress, respiratory failure, hypoxia (SaO2 < 90%), and hypercarbia. In the last decade, use of noninvasive forms of ventilation has decreased the need for intubation and mechanical ventilation. High-flow nasal cannula (HFNC) humidifies and warms air to make higher liter flow more tolerable, provides PEEP at higher flows (we recommend to start at least at 6 L for smaller infants and 10 L for older children), and improves ventilation. CPAP and BIPAP are other important noninvasive forms of ventilation that can be used when HFNC has failed or is not available. PEEP and inspiratory pressures should be individualized to the needs of the child. Smaller infants may benefit from noninvasive mechanical ventilation using a RAM cannula programmed for PIP, PEEP, rate, and pressure support. Blood gasses should be obtained to demonstrate hypercarbia and respiratory acidosis as a baseline before initiating supportive measures. The decision to intubate a child with bronchiolitis should be after the use of noninvasive support has failed. The use of sedation and paralysis, plus the presence of an endotracheal tube, makes clearing of secretions more difficult and can prolong the disease, as well as causes secondary complications. Consultation with the pediatric critical care specialist in the facility which will be receiving the patient should occur when starting any ventilator support. Some facilities can receive patients on HFNC on their general pediatric wards, and it is important for emergency physician to know floor and ICU admission criteria for their local pediatric hospitals.

Bronchodilators have not decreased rates of admission but were actually associated with an increased length of stay as their side effects usually negate beneficial effects in studies of children with mild disease. Although with severe disease and respiratory failure, a rescue dose of bronchodilator (we recommend racemic epinephrine) can be used. Nebulized hypertonic saline did not decrease the rate of admissions but did reduce LOS by 1 day in children staying for more than 72 hours (the average is 2.4 days). Finally, the supportive treatment of bronchiolitis should also include adequate hydration which can be provided through a nasogastric tube or through an IV if a child is not tolerating PO or is requiring ventilatory support.

Status Asthmaticus

Asthma consists of inflammation, bronchial edema, bronchial smooth muscle spasm, and increased secretions from a hyperactive response to stimuli or antigens. Most cases are not severe and respond well to bronchodilator therapy and steroids, but cases resistant to bronchodilator therapy (status asthmaticus) can be life-threatening.

Etiology

The classical tetrad is airway inflammation, bronchoconstriction, increased mucus production, and remodeling of the airway architecture. Most patients have concomitant atopy and a family history of atopy or asthma. Asthma exacerbations are usually brought around by triggers including viral or bacterial infections, cold temperatures, pollen, dust, smoke, or chemicals.

Presentation/Diagnosis

The diagnosis usually can be made on the basis of history and physical examination as many patients have already received a diagnosis of asthma and reactive airway disease, have a history of prior wheezing, or have family history of asthma. During viral peak seasons, it is often challenging to distinguish younger patients with an asthma/reactive airway disease from those with bronchiolitis. *Children who have had previous ICU admissions or intubations tend to have more severe exacerbations and should be more closely monitored.* An exacerbation which does not initially respond to beta-agonist therapy and steroids is considered *status asthmaticus* (SA), and it is a common cause of pediatric respiratory failure. *Children (especially toddlers) with unilateral wheezing and respiratory distress (especially if first episode) should be evaluated for foreign body aspiration.* In SA, because of the obstructive nature of the disease, respiratory failure is usually hypercarbic. Altered mental status and lethargy in combination with signs of respiratory distress should prompt an evaluation for respiratory failure, including obtaining blood gasses. Hypoxia may initially worsen with beta-agonist therapy as it opens the airways a V/Q mismatch ensues. A chest X-ray is not necessary in patients presenting with asthma, but high fever and focal findings on physical exam (crackles, dullness to palpation, fremitus) will require evaluation for secondary pneumonia.

Assessing disease severity is important, but obtaining peak flow values can be challenging in smaller children. Several clinical scores like the pediatric asthma score have been developed and validated. Higher scores on the PAS are predictive of more severe exacerbations and the need for more support.

Management

Most patients presenting with asthma exacerbations have a mild clinical course, but those with SA will require frequently inhaled beta-agonists and continued steroid treatment. Prevention of respiratory failure in these patients is key, and aggressive management will prevent it in most cases.

Airway

Airway interventions are not usually necessary, but airway patency should be assessed, maintained, and reevaluated constantly throughout the patient's ED course.

Breathing

Support of breathing, especially ventilation, is the mainstay of treatment in respiratory failure due to asthma. Hypoxia usually ensues after initial bronchodilator therapy due to V/Q mismatching and can be treated with oxygen delivery devices like nasal cannula or face mask. The mainstay of treatment for the underlying bronchoconstriction is inhaled beta-agonists. For SA timed doses of beta-agonists are usually insufficient, and continuous treatment (10–20 mg/h) is usually necessary. Anticholinergic agents like ipratropium can be useful in severe cases, as these have a modest synergistic bronchodilator effect. The bronchi might be so constricted that they do not allow passage of inhaled agents to lower airways so that parenteral treatments like magnesium sulfate, terbutaline, albuterol, or epinephrine may be needed. Magnesium sulfate has traditionally been given as a bolus dose of 50 mg/kg, but a continuous infusion (50 mg/kg/h over 4 hours) may be more effective. In SA with respiratory failure, IV steroid therapy should be initiated rapidly – methylprednisolone bolus dose of 2 mg/kg with a maximum of 60 mg and 1 mg/kg doses every 6 hours. Other corticosteroids like hydrocortisone are used in some institutions. Any of these measures should be done in consultation with the receiving facility. Other bronchodilators like theophylline are usually limited to the ICU setting as they require close monitoring.

Support of ventilation tends to be more challenging, and noninvasive methods should be attempted as children tend to tolerate BIPAP well; initiate it slowly and individualize settings to suit the child and presentation. Sedation should be used sparingly and by trained providers as it can decrease respiratory drive, further worsening the patient's hypercarbia. *Intubation should be left as a last resort as sedation and paralysis make clearance of secretions very difficult and often worsen air trapping.* Ketamine can be useful for intubation as it has a modest bronchodilator effect but can also increase airway secretions. Intubation should be performed by the most experienced provider in pediatric airways. *Selection of ventilator mode and settings should include a long expiratory time (usually a low-rate and low-moderate tidal volume) allowing for permissive hypercapnia.* Therapies like *Heliox* can be helpful in decreasing turbulent airflow but may be limited to the ICU setting. Management should be done in close communication with the receiving PICU facility. Blood gasses should be obtained early and frequently as elevated PCO2 (or even a normal value when tachypneic) is predictive of impending respiratory failure as most children with SA are initially hypocarbic due to intact compensatory mechanisms.

Circulation

Children with SA tend to present with some degree of dehydration due to increased insensible losses and decreased oral intake. Many of the treatments for SA will increase heart rate, decrease diastolic filling and stroke volume, and cause vasodilation. Inhaled beta-agonists have a strong ß2 activity but also bind to ß1 receptors causing tachycardia. This tachycardia is usually well tolerated by children but when hypovolemic or with smooth muscle relaxants like magnesium sulfate can cause a decreased cardiac output and organ perfusion. Thus, it is important to assess the patient's baseline circulatory status and perform frequent reassessments especially when on continuous albuterol. Early determination of the need for IV access and parenteral fluids should be made. For children with underlying arrhythmias or heart disease, the L isomer of albuterol (levalbuterol) has been marketed as a safer option, but so far no difference in its effectiveness or side effect profile has been found.

Upper Airway Obstruction

Etiology

Upper airway obstruction can be caused by infectious and noninfectious causes. The most common noninfectious cause is foreign bodies, more prevalent in toddlers, as they are learning to crawl and walk, and in young children. Common foreign bodies are peanuts, round fruits, sausages, and small toys.

Croup, or laryngotracheitis, is an inflammatory process of the glottis and subglottis. It is the most common infectious cause of infectious upper airway obstruction in children. It is caused by viruses, most commonly parainfluenza but also RSV, influenza virus, and HMPV. Epiglottitis remains an important cause of infectious upper airway obstruction in children and can be deadly when not diagnosed and treated in a timely manner. It is classically caused by HIB, but the incidence of this infection has decreased due to vaccination. Finally, bacterial tracheitis is a less common but potentially deadly cause of infectious upper airway obstruction. It is usually preceded by a viral infection (croup). Although it can be difficult to isolate a causative organism, *S. aureus* has been found to be the most likely etiology for bacterial tracheitis.

Clinical Presentation

The hallmark presentation of upper airway obstruction is stridor which, depending on the affected site, can be inspiratory, expiratory, or biphasic. Respiratory distress, dysphonia, and generalized distress are also common. Hypoxia may occur due to severe obstruction, but as obstruction worsens, a mixed respiratory failure develops. Fever is common with infectious causes. Croup is usually benign but severe cases can be deadly if not treated rapidly. It usually presents with biphasic stridor only during exertion (mild) or at rest (moderate-severe) and often with nasal congestion and a barking cough. Patients with epiglottitis and tracheitis usually have high-grade fevers and are toxic-appearing. They will also have more severe respiratory distress and will commonly be assuming a tripod position. Epiglottitis tends to cause severe throat pain in older children, but younger patients might present with rapid-onset respiratory distress, muffled voice, and drooling. Patients with tracheitis tend to have cough with grossly purulent secretions. If not treated quickly, upper airway obstruction can rapidly degenerate to hypoxic cardiopulmonary arrest.

Management

Patients with upper airway obstruction require rapid interventions to relieve the obstruction and improve respirations. ABCDEs should be rapidly assessed, intervened upon, and reassessed.

Airway

Upper airway obstruction requires immediate evaluation of airway patency and interventions to relieve obstruction. Patients will commonly arrive in severe respiratory failure or in cardiac arrest. Direct laryngoscopy should be attempted to visualize the airway and look for the foreign body. It can be difficult to remove the foreign body and instrument the airway. Needle cricothyrotomy can be lifesaving until a laryngoscope and bronchoscope can be inserted by an experienced provider to remove the obstruction. For croup, relief of upper airway obstruction usually consists of rapid initiation of steroids (PO dexamethasone is a good choice given its long half-life) and an inhaled agent with vasoconstricting and respiratory smooth muscle dilating properties, most commonly racemic epinephrine. Humidified oxygen delivered through devices that can deliver PEEP (HFNC, CPAP, BIPAP) can also be helpful. In severe cases, *Heliox* can increase laminar flow through the airway and improve oxygenation. Every effort should be made to decrease stimulation of the child as airflow through the airway tends to become more turbulent with agitation. Only about 1% of cases of croup require intubation, but when required an uncuffed tube 0.5 cm less than the age-appropriate diameter should be used. If possible, muscle paralysis should be avoided given possible collapse of the airway causing difficulty providing bag-valve-mask (BVM) ventilation. For epiglottitis, rapid assessment and intervention of the airway should be performed in the most controlled setting; if possible the child (especially under 5 years old) should be immediately taken to the OR to be intubated by an anesthesiologist or ENT. With decreasing rates of HIB, some studies have found that in selected children older than 5 years of age, observation in a PICU without intubating does not increase mortality. The role of steroids in epiglottitis is contentious, and given that they might depress the immune system, they are generally not indicated. Airway management in tracheitis follows similar principles of those in epiglottitis.

Breathing

Close evaluation of respiratory status should be undertaken on all patients with upper airway obstruction. Hypoxia is usually ominous and should be rapidly corrected. Most of the interventions mentioned in the airway section will correct hypoxia in upper airway obstruction. If a patient is intubated for upper airway obstruction, ventilator settings should attempt to minimize volutrauma and barotrauma given that patients with upper airway obstruction may rapidly develop auto-peep. Ventilator management principles are similar to those mentioned in the asthma section.

Circulation

Patients with upper airway obstruction, especially those with foreign bodies, frequently present in cardiac arrest. PALS algorithms should be followed until establishment of an airway or final removal of the foreign body restores oxygenation and ventilation. While patients with croup rarely require interventions to restore circulation, racemic epinephrine causes tachycardia, and patients receiving more than one dose should be under telemetry monitoring. Patients with epiglottitis and tracheitis frequently present with concomitant septic shock, and the principles stated in the shock section of this chapter should be followed.

Cardiac Emergencies

Cardiac emergencies in the pediatric population can be categorized by age. Please refer to the neonatal chapter for a review of cardiac emergencies in the neonatal period. After the neonatal period (1–2 months), cardiac emergencies in the pediatric population are most likely to be due to postoperative congenital heart disease, arrhythmias, and acquired heart disease.

Congenital heart diseases that may present emergently after the strict neonatal period include hypoplastic left heart syndrome (HLHS) and coarctation of the aorta (CoA) . These congenital heart lesions are dependent on a patent ductus arteriosus for adequate circulatory function. The infant with undiagnosed HLHS or CoA in distress is brought to the pediatric emergency department for color change, poor weight gain, difficulty breathing, sweating during feeding, fussiness, or excessive crying. Cardiogenic instability or shock in a 2-month-old infant due to closure of the ductus arteriosus is treated by administering prostacyclin as for the neonate.

Congestive heart failure in children is most commonly due to congenital heart anomalies and precedes cardiogenic shock. Myocarditis should be considered in all children with new-onset congestive heart failure. Usual symptoms are poor feeding and crying in infants and fatigue, abdominal pain, and difficulty breathing in the older child. Findings on exam include jugular venous distension, diaphoresis, hepatic congestion, a cardiac gallop (S3 hear sound), and respiratory distress with rales.

Supraventricular Tachycardia (SVT)

Supraventricular tachycardia (SVT) is the most common sustained arrhythmia in children. SVT is the most common symptomatic tachyarrhythmia that requires medical therapy in children and occurs in 1 of 250 to 1000 children. Infants with SVT and ventricular preexcitation (Wolff-Parkinson-White syndrome – WPW) are known to have up to 30% prevalence of congenital heart disease (CHD). Infants without ventricular preexcitation who present with SVT at <1 year of age have a similar prevalence of CHD.

In a large population of pediatric patients with SVT who were referred for radiofrequency catheter ablation, they found that accessory pathways (APs) as with WPW allowing for AVRT (A-V Re-entry Tachycardia) are more prevalent than AVNRT (A-V Nodal Re-entry Tachycardia) at all ages (see Fig. 32.1) while AVNRT occurs with greater relative frequency in older pediatric patients. Males are more likely to have APs than females, and females older than 12 years of age are more likely to have AVNRT than males. SVT generally exceeds 180 beats per minute in children/adolescents and 220 beats per minute in infants.

The management strategy for children with SVT is based on the physiological status of the patient. Stable patients with adequate perfusion (normal capillary refill time, mental status, and blood pressure) are managed with vagal maneuvers (ice pack to face for young children, or carotid massage, or Valsalva maneuvers – the authors' favorite is having the child take a deep breath and either forcefully exhale through a straw or inflate an exam glove "balloon") or adenosine: initial dose (0.1 mg/kg IV rapid push) and subsequent doses (increase by 0.1 mg/kg to a maximum of 12 mg/dose). Other treatment options are listed in Table 32.4. Those who have evidence of poor perfusion or hypotension receive synchronized DC cardioversion. The initial energy dose is 0.5–1 J/kg. For subsequent doses, double the energy dose to a maximum of 2 J/kg if initial dose is ineffective. Consider analgesia and sedation when possible, but do not delay cardioversion when the child is in extremis. A continuous ECG should be obtained before and during interventions to capture changes in the rhythm. If time and the clinical status allow, it is extremely valuable to obtain a full 12-lead ECG during the tachycardia, in addition to repeating it once sinus rhythm has been restored to determine if pre-excitation is present (since this can only be detected when in sinus rhythm) (see Fig. 32.2).

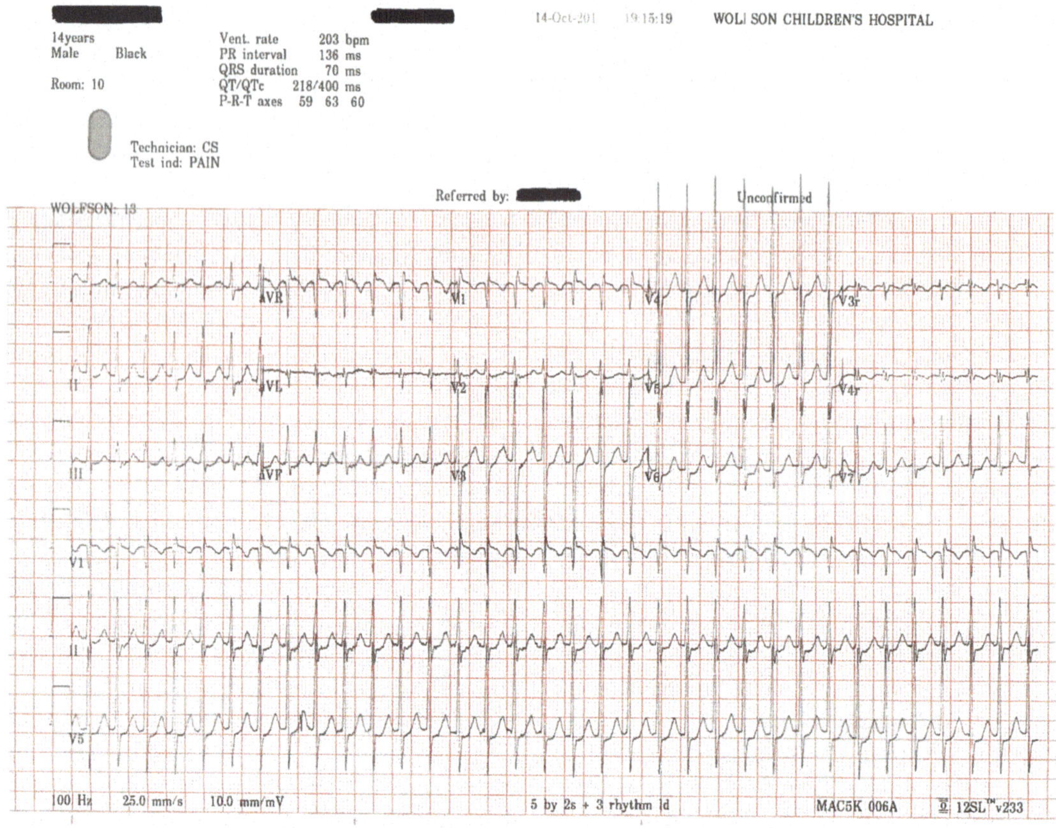

Fig. 32.1 EKG 1

Table 32.4 Pharmacological therapy for acute episodes of SVT

Medication	Pharmacological effect	Bolus injection	Adverse effects
Adenosine	Slows sinus rate	0.1–0.4 mg/kg	Chest pain, asystole/bradycardia
	Slows AV conduction velocity		Arrhythmias, bronchospasm
Amiodarone	Depresses sinus node	5 mg/kg	Arrhythmias
	Increases AVN refractoriness		Increases the defibrillation threshold
	Increases refractory period of Aps		Makes cardioversion more difficult
Esmolol	Prolongs AVN refractory time	100–500 mg/kg 1 min	Hypotension; short half-life
Procainamide	Increases atrial & ventricular	3–6 mg/kg over 5 min	Hypotension
	refractory period (including in APs)	max 100 mg	
Verapamil	Slows AV nodal conduction	0.1 mg/kg over 2 min	Hypotension, sinus bradycardia, heart block*

*do NOT give if <1 yr

Cardiogenic Shock

Mortality due to shock of all types has decreased in the last two decades due to implementation of evidence-based guidelines emphasizing prompt diagnosis and rapid goal-directed interventions to reverse shock and restore normal respiratory and cardiac function. In 2003, researchers were able

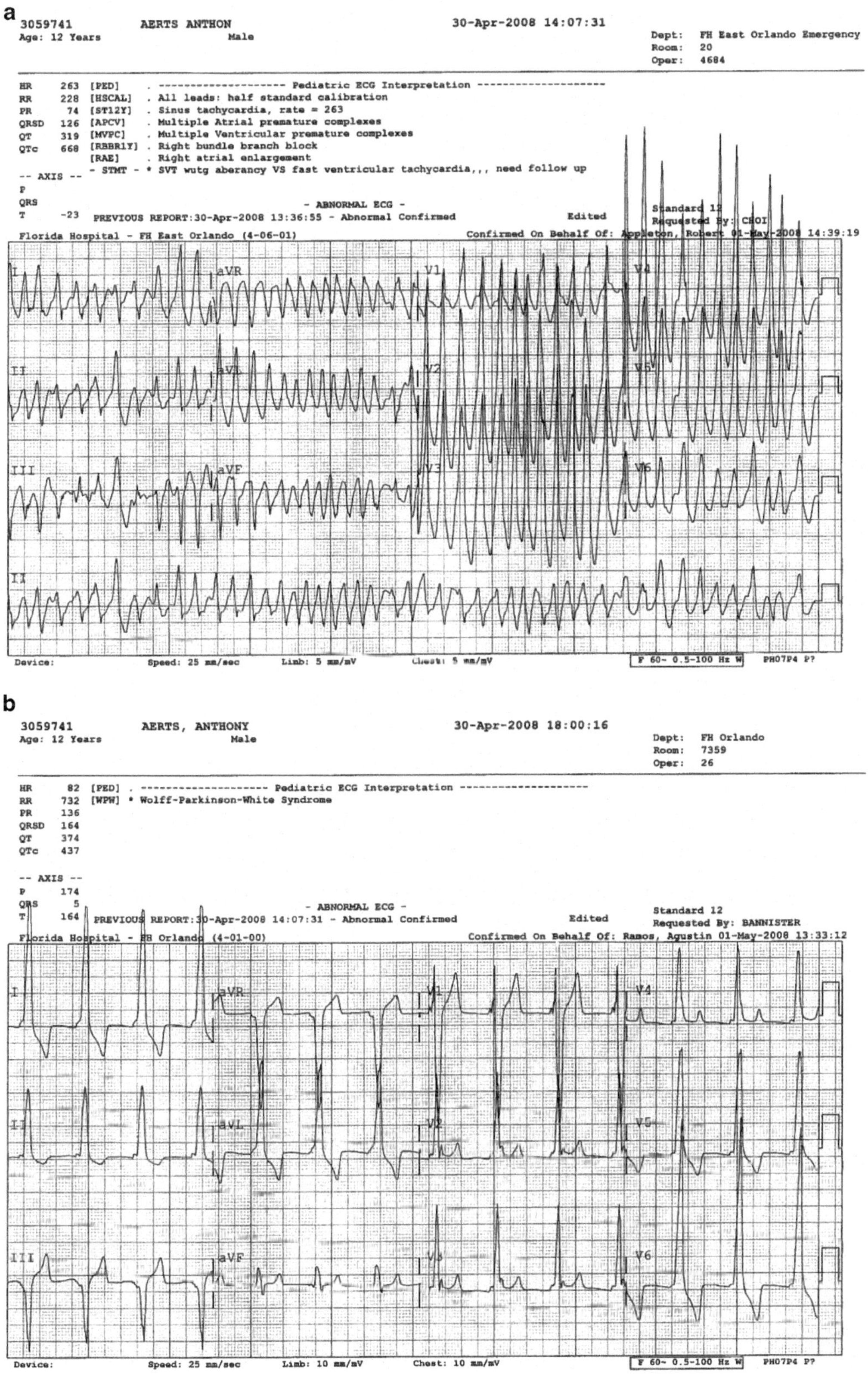

Fig. 32.2 EKG 2A & B

to show that reversal of shock within the first hour of presenting to a community hospital was associated with improved functional outcome. Older children and adolescents like adults will have an increase in cardiac rate and contractility when acutely ill. Infants and young children on the other hand have a relatively fixed stroke volume (bradycardia critically lowers cardiac output) and higher baseline heart rates limiting improvement in cardiac output by increasing heart rate.

The increase in SVR common in acutely ill infants and young children will maintain their blood pressure in a reassuring range during compensated shock. The abrupt decompensation to uncompensated shock may seem like it occurred without warning if a healthcare provider relies on the blood pressure as reassurance of adequate perfusion. Avoid the pitfall of reliance on normal blood pressures as a sign of adequate perfusion. Instead, tachycardia and tachypnea are harbingers of early shock until proven otherwise. Although increased SVR is a physiologic response to illness, it will compromise cardiac output in a child with hypovolemia or decreased myocardial function. Optimally, compensated shock should be detected within the first 5 minutes of presentation in order to reverse course within the first hour and protect major organ function.

Cardiogenic shock is the least common of the four categories of shock (also hypovolemic, obstructive, and distributive) in children but the one potentially requiring the most specialized therapies, labs, equipment, and teamwork. It is due to cardiac dysfunction and decreased cardiac output. The most common etiologies of cardiogenic shock from primarily cardiac causes after the neonatal period and not due to pre- or postoperative congenital heart disease include myocarditis, cardiomyopathies, arrhythmias, and trauma. End-organ damage may be already present in the emergency department. Warner and Stevenson describe acute decompensated heart failure by noting whether hypoperfusion or congestion is present: neither (warm/dry); congestion only (warm/wet); hypoperfusion only (cold/dry); both (cold/wet) (see Fig. 32.3). Children with acute

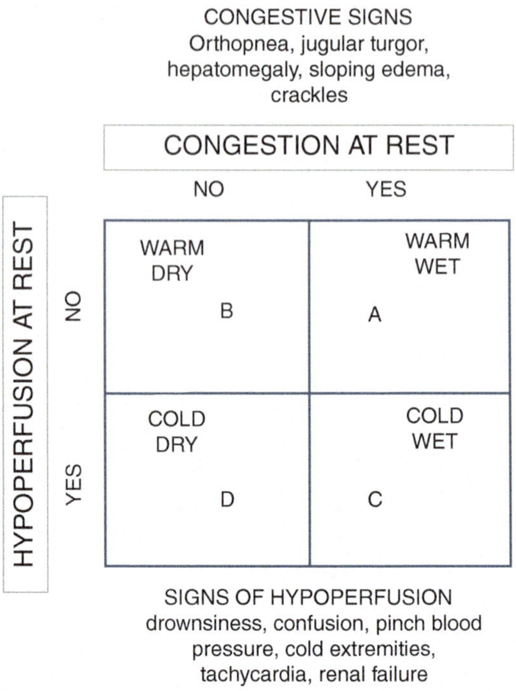

Fig. 32.3 Possible signs and symptoms of cardiogenic shock (Brissaud et al. [32])

decompensated heart failure can present with tachycardia, tachypnea, normal or low blood pressure, irritability or depressed cognition, enlarged liver, cool or mottled extremities, difficulty breathing, sweating during feeding, fussiness, and excessive crying. Extremity edema and jugular venous distention may be seen in adolescents. The successful stabilization of cardiogenic shock in the pediatric emergency department is dependent on rapid detection, intervention, and transfer to the intensive care unit to forestall multiorgan failure and ensure best functional outcome. Following the tenets of emergency medicine resuscitation using the primary survey to both evaluate and intervene is paramount. Bedside serial cardiac ultrasonography, 12-lead electrocardiography, portable chest X-ray, NT pro-BNP (see Figs. 32.4 and 32.5), and communication with an intensivist and cardiologist as soon as cardiogenic shock is recognized ensure fluid teamwork and specialist involvement in decision-making. A formal echocardiogram if not readily available in the PED setting is obtained in the PICU. The goal

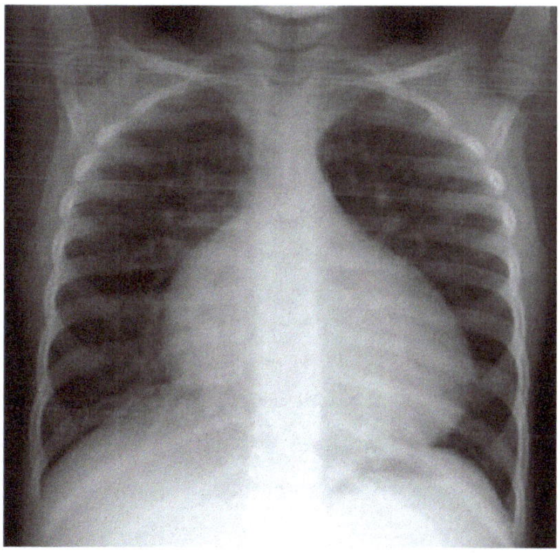

Fig. 32.4 Chest X-ray of child with cardiomegaly and pulmonary congestion (Tissot et al. [39])

of initial treatment is to restore adequate perfusion to tissues and optimize gas exchange with a goal of >95% oxygen saturations. The aim of initial patient management is to restore adequate oxygen delivery to peripheral tissues. This relies on emergency support (early recognition, monitoring, access), optimizing ventilation/gas exchange (oxygen therapy ± noninvasive or invasive ventilation with a saturation objective of >95% except in cyanotic heart disease patients), optimizing the preload and afterload (volume expansion or diuretics and fluid restriction, inotropes, discontinuation of deleterious medication), and treating curable causes (fluid and electrolyte balance, rhythm, or thromboembolic disorders; pneumothorax, tamponade, infection) (see Table 32.5).

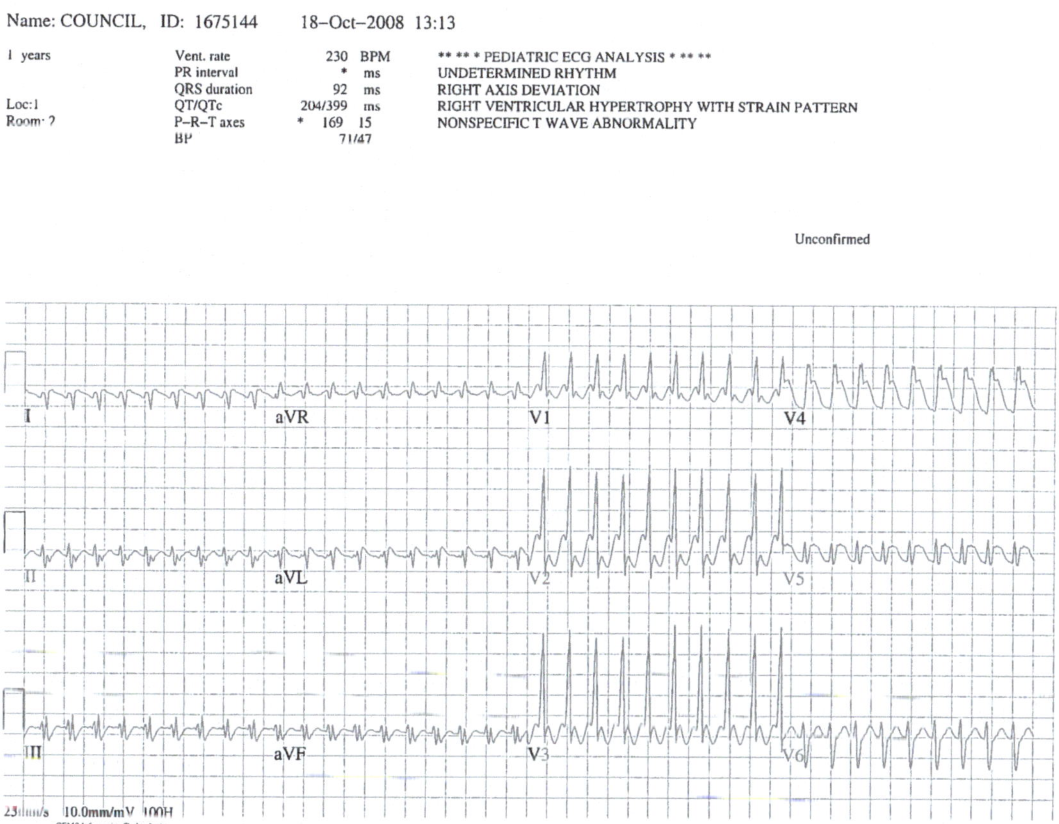

Fig. 32.5 CXR and EKG 3

Table 32.5 Medications for cardiogenic shock

Medication	Dose	Physiologic effect
Epinephrine	0.1–1 mcg/kg/min IV/IO	Inotrope, chronotrope, vasodilator in low doses, pressor in high doses
Dobutamine	2–20 mcg/kg/min IV/IO	Inotrope, chronotrope, vasodilator
Dopamine	2–20 mcg/kg/min IV/IO	Inotrope, chronotrope, renal and splanchnic vasodilator in low doses, pressor in high doses
Norepinephrine	0.1–0.2 mcg/kg/min IV/IO	Vasopressor (slight chronotrope & inotrope)
Milrinone	0.375–0.750 mcg/kg/min IV/IO	Inotrope, chronotrope, vasodilator

Seizures and Status Epilepticus

A seizure is defined as the physical manifestation of abnormal and excessive synchronized discharges of neurons associated with disturbance of consciousness, while epilepsy is a condition in which a person is prone to recurrent unprovoked seizures. An aura is that portion of the seizure experienced before loss of consciousness occurs and for which memory is retained. Todd's phenomenon is a transient focal neurologic deficit following a focal or secondarily generalized seizure.

Simple Febrile Seizure

Simple febrile seizure is a seizure that is associated with fever (= or > 100.4 °C), is brief (although most resources quote <15 minutes, a more clinically useful time limit is <5 minutes), is generalized (convulsive tonic-clonic), and does not recur within 24 hours. The post-ictal period is usually brief (<30–45 minutes). Alternatively, complex febrile seizure is a seizure associated with fever that is prolonged, focal, or recurrent within a 24-hour period.

Simple febrile seizure is the most common neurologic event in children less than 5 years old. Most children who experience simple febrile seizure with cessation at home are brought to the emergency department because the condition is universally frightening to caregivers. The typical patient is a febrile child 6–36 months old who presents to the emergency department after seizure activity has terminated usually during the post-ictal period and has a family history of febrile seizures. Occurrence of simple febrile seizures in children peaks at 18 months of age. Only 6–15% of simple febrile seizures occur after 4 years of age. To satisfy the criteria for simple febrile seizure, the patient must be 6–60 months old, have a fever, have no known neurologic or developmental deficits or seizure disorder, and have a short post-ictal period that spontaneously resolves in the emergency department with the patient returning to normal baseline neurologic status.

The AAP published clinician guidelines in 1996 emphasizing the benign nature of simple febrile seizures with recommendations to limit the work up to a search for the cause of the fever. The AAP Subcommittee on Febrile Seizures published a revision to the 1996 guidelines in 2011 essentially corroborating the recommendations of the first practice guidelines, "a simple febrile seizure does not usually require further evaluation, specifically electroencephalography, blood studies, or neuroimaging." Clinicians are advised to consider meningitis and perform a lumbar puncture in all children 6–12 months presenting with febrile seizure and other clinical concerns worrisome for a more serious systemic or neurologic process. Lumbar puncture is advocated as an option in infants who are otherwise well but whose immunization status is unknown, incomplete, or lacking and in infants pretreated with antibiotics.

Since the guidelines were published, several studies have shown little benefit from aggressive neurodiagnostic testing in the patient with spontaneous and complete recovery from a simple febrile seizure (see Fig. 32.6).

Patients with simple febrile seizures have a 50% chance of recurrence if their first simple febrile seizure occurs before 12 months of age and a 30%

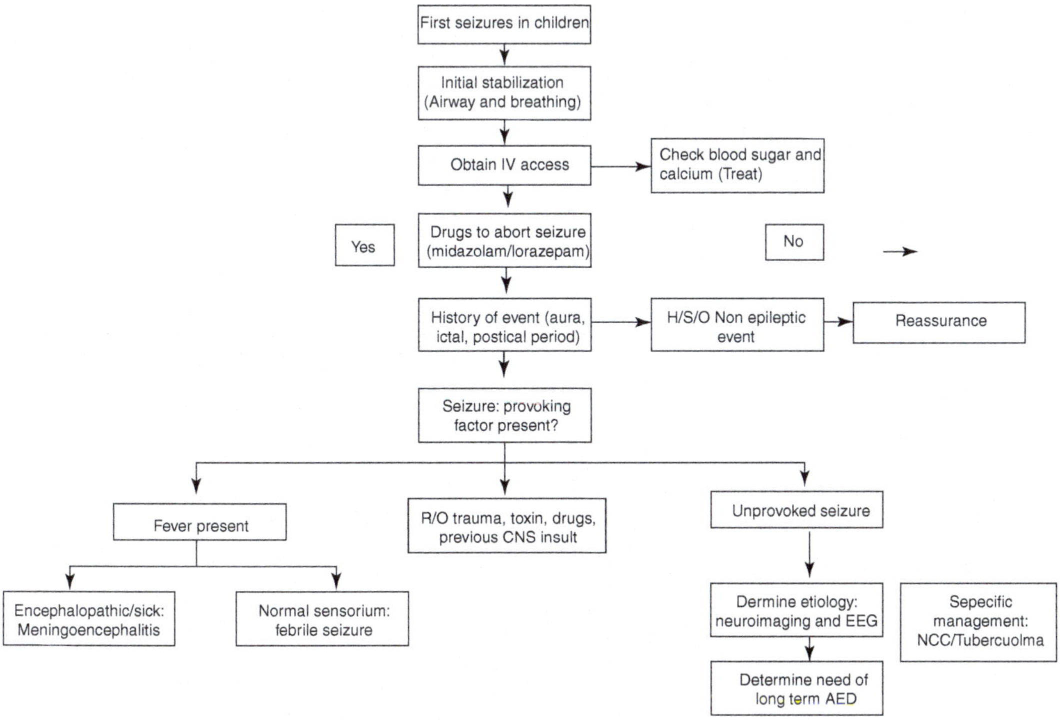

Fig. 32.6 Evaluation of first seizure

chance of recurrence if their first SFS occurs after 12 months. They have only a slightly higher risk of developing epilepsy than the general pediatric population. Caregiver education is important. Caregivers should be informed that a febrile seizure may recur even when scheduled antipyretic dosing is administered in the hopes of preventing fevers. Prior to discharge, caregivers should receive education on basic life support (basic first aid) in case of seizure recurrence. They should be reassured of the normally benign nature of simple febrile seizures and informed of the excellent prognosis associated with a simple febrile seizure. Although a simple febrile seizure is benign, complex febrile seizures can progress to status epilepticus. Caregivers should be instructed to provide BLS and activate EMS as soon seizure activity is recognized.

Status Epilepticus

Status epilepticus is defined by professional specialty organizations as a seizure that is so prolonged or frequently repeated as to create a fixed and lasting condition. A seizure lasting >30 minutes or recurrent seizures lasting >30 minutes from which the patient does not regain consciousness are the functional definition of SE. The brain suffers irreversible excitotoxicity after 30 minutes of seizure activity without recovery of consciousness (PCNA). A more clinically practical definition with therapeutic and outcome implications is any seizure lasting ≥5 minutes; a vast majority of self-limiting generalized convulsive seizures stop within 5 minutes of onset.

SE is a common pediatric neurologic emergency affecting about 20 per 100,000 children per year. 40% of SE occurs in children younger than 2 years of age. Common causes of SE are fever in children with and without epilepsy, low antiseizure medication level in children with known epilepsy, and acute or remote symptomatic. It occurs in 10–20% of children with epilepsy and may be the presenting manifestation. Prognosis is linked to etiology and patient age. Outcome may be affected by duration of

SE. Refractory SE carries a high morbidity and mortality.

The findings of a study of cultured neurons subjected to prolonged burst activity helped explain the loss of efficacy of antiepileptic drugs that act at the GABA receptor during SE. The study showed that prolonged neuronal activity (seizure activity) caused GABA receptors to be internalized by the neuron. The clinical implication is that the longer seizure activity persists untreated, the less likely it is for antiseizure medications with action at GABA receptors to have a therapeutic effect. Most antiseizure medications in the SE armamentarium act at the GABA receptor. A goal of The Established Status Epilepticus Treatment Trial currently in progress is to investigate medication choices in benzodiazepine refractory SE. Until more information is available, early and timely recognition and treatment of SE are critical to obtain the best patient outcomes and avoid complications requiring invasive airway management and prolonged ICU care. A recent study and editorial highlight the lack of improvement in mortality over the last 30 years for SE in the pediatric population. Studies that looked at patient management in the emergency setting reveal that clinician adherence to consensus guidelines is often suboptimal.

In an attempt to improve adherence to guidelines, several recommendations have been proposed including SE code teams (as with trauma or stroke code teams); EMR SE order sets with medication dose per weight; changing nomenclature from first-, second-, and third-line treatment to emergent, urgent, and refractory treatment; wall posters with delineated SE treatment algorithms; training all emergency team members including prehospital personnel to administer emergent treatment followed by urgent treatment within 10 minutes; better education of caregivers on rectal dosing of antiseizure medication and on the importance of routine follow-up; and identifying patients with hyperutilization of emergency services for targeted caregiver seizure and SE education (see Table 32.6).

In order to ensure the best patient outcomes, the management of SE requires strict adherence to current neurocritical care consensus treatment guidelines while implementing the initial steps of resuscitation medicine including protection and monitoring of neurologic function, protection and optimization of airway and breathing, securing vascular access, monitoring of cardiorespiratory status, initiating investigation of etiology or trigger, and initial planning for safe transfer to definitive care. These tasks are performed in tandem in

Table 32.6 Stepwise treatment for pediatric seizures and status

Status Epilepticus Algorithm

Pre-Arrival
Prepare equipment:
- Non-rebreather, BVM
- Suction, oral/nasal airway, pulse ox
- IV, mucosal atomizer, IO, iStat and Dstix
- Medications

Ongoing seizure > 5 minutes
Recurrent seizure without return to baseline mental status

Seizure	Status Epilepticus (5 min)	Early Refractory SE (10 min)	Refractory SE (20 min)	Established SE (30 min)
Anti-epileptics Lorazepam (Ativan) OR 0.1 mg/kg IV/IM (max 4mg) Midazolam (Versed) OR 0.1 mg/kg IV (max 4mg) 0.2 mg/kg IN 13-40kg:5mg IM, >40kg:10mg Diazepam (Valium) 2-5yo 0.5 mg/kg PR 6-11yo 0.3 mg/kg PR ≥12yo 0.2 mg/kg PR (max 20) **Diagnostics / Therapeutics** Airway, oxygen, pulse ox Glucose, iStat (Na, Ca) Tx hypertension, fever IV access (or IO)	**Anti-epileptics** Repeat benzodiazepine q 5min up to 2 more doses Fosphenytoin OR 20-30 mg/kg PE (max 1gm) IV (150mg/min) Phenytoin 20-30mg/kg (max 1 gm) IV (50mg/min) **Diagnostics / Therapeutics** Consider ingestions (INH, TCA, ETOH) Chem panel incl Mg, PO4 Anti-epileptic drug levels CBC, LFTs, coags, Utox, ICON Consider neurology consult	**Anti-epileptics** Levetiracetam (Keppra) 20-40 mg/kg (max 3gm) IV at 5mg/kg/min Valproate 20-40 mg/kg IV at 5mg/kg/min (avoid in patients with liver disease, thrombocytopenia, metabolic disorder) **Diagnostics / Therapeutics** Consider head CT Consider lumbar puncture EKG Neurology consult	**Anti-epileptics** Phenobarbital 20-40 mg/kg IV at 2mg/kg/min Consider empiric pyridoxine If < 2yo, 100mg IV Consider empiric thiamine & glucose If suspect ETOH abuse, thiamine 100mg IV **Diagnostics / Therapeutics** Prepare to intubate Admit PICU Consider central line Arrange continuous EEG	**Coma induction** Midazolam 0.2 mg/kg (max 10mg) IV then infusion 0.1 mg/kg/hr Pentobarbital 5 mg/kg IV then infusion 0.5mg/kg/hr **Add-on options** Ketamine 1.5 mg/kg IV, then infusion at 1 mg/kg/hr Propofol 2 mg/kg IV, then infusion *in adults only* 1 mg/kg/hr, titrate up to effect* General anesthesia

Abend NS et al. Semin Pediatr Neurol 2014;21(4):263-274

*Risk of propofol infusion syndrome in children

order to prevent secondary injury due to hypoxia, hypotension, acidosis, and hyperpyrexia.

The most important role of the emergency clinician team is to adequately treat SE in a timely manner in order to prevent inadequate dosing and delays in dosing of antiseizure medications. Because nearly one-half of patients who no longer have clinical (convulsive) seizures remain in nonconvulsive SE, EEG monitoring in the ED is essential for assessment of treatment effect.

Neuroimaging is delayed until patient is stable for transfer to another area or outside the emergency care unit. MRI is preferred, but trauma patients and patients suspected to have an intracranial lesion should have emergent CT neuroimaging. Communication with the neuroradiologist prior to imaging to share patient history and clinical exam findings optimizes study interpretation.

Consultation with pediatric neurology, pediatric critical care, trauma surgery, neurosurgery for complicated cases, refractory SE, trauma patients, or patients with signs of elevated intracranial pressure should be done as soon as possible.

References

Introduction

1. Advanced Life Support Group (ALSG). Advanced paediatric life support: the practical approach. 5th ed. ISBN: 978-1-444-34020-4. BMJ Books; 2011.
2. Akre M, Finkelstein M, Erickson M, Liu M, Vanderbilt L, Billman G. Sensitivity of the pediatric early warning score to identify patient deterioration. Pediatrics. 2010;125(4) https://doi.org/10.1542/peds.2009-0338. Murray J, Williams LA. An integrative review of pediatric early warning system scores. Pediatr Nurs. 2015;41(4):165–174.
3. Fontane E, Savage R, Eldridge D, Perkin R. Pediatric emergency medicine manual. Greenville: ECU Printing; 2007.
4. Gill C, Kissoon N. Pediatric life support update: 2015 American Heart Association highlights. Pediatr Emerg Care. 2017;33(8):585–93.
5. Gold DL, Mihalov LK, Cohen DM. Evaluating the Pediatric Early Warning Score (PEWS) system for admitted patients in the pediatric emergency department. Acad Emerg Med. 2014;21(11):1249–56. https://doi.org/10.1111/acem.12514
6. Jayashree M, Singhi SC. Initial assessment and triage in ER. Indian J Pediatr. 2011;78:1100.
7. Mehra B, Gupta S. Common pediatric medical emergencies. Indian J Pediatr. 2018;85(1):35–43.
8. Pierre L, Pringle E, editors. Pediatric fundamental critical care support. 3rd ed: Society of Critical Care Medicine. Mount Prospect, IL; 2018.
9. Shaffner DH, Nichols DG. Rogers textbook of pediatric intensive care. Philadelphia: Lippincott Williams & Wilkins; 2016.

Airway

10. Fuchs S. Pediatric office emergencies. Pediatr Clin North Am. 2013;60(5):1153–61.
11. Langley EW, Gigante J. Anaphylaxis, urticaria and angioedema. Pediatr Rev. 2013;34(6):247–57.
12. Mandal A, Kabra SK, Lodha R. Upper airway obstruction in children. Indian J Pediatr. 2015;82(8):737–44.
13. McDougall RJ. Paediatric emergencies. Anaesthesia. 2013;68(Suppl 1):61–71.
14. Rafei K, Lichenstein R. Airway infectious disease emergencies. Pediatr Clin North Am. 2006;53(2):215–42.
15. Smith KA, Flori HR. Critical care in the pediatric emergency department. Pediatr Clin North Am. 2018;65(6):1119–34.
16. Virbalas J, Smith L. Upper airway obstruction. Pediatr Rev. 2015;36(2):62–73.

Respiratory

17. Beers SL, Abramo TJ, Bracken A, Wiebe RA. Bilevel positive airway pressure in the treatment of status asthmaticus in pediatrics. Am J Emerg Med. 2007;25(1):6–9.
18. Carroll CL, Sala KA. Pediatric status asthmaticus. Crit Care Clin. 2013;29(2):153–66. https://doi.org/10.1016/j.ccc.2012.12.001.
19. Choi J, Lee GL. Common pediatric respiratory emergencies. Emerg Med Clin North Am. 2012;30(2):529–63.
20. Cundiff KM, Gerard JM, Flood RG. Critical care interventions for asthmatic patients admitted from the emergency department to the pediatric intensive care unit. Pediatr Emerg Care. 2018;34(6):385–9. https://doi.org/10.1097/pec.0000000000001163.
21. Hardasmalani MD, DeBari V, Bithoney WG, Gold N. Levalbuterol versus racemic albuterol in the treatment of acute exacerbation of asthma in children. Pediatr Emerg Care. 2005;21(7):415–9.
22. Irazuzta JE, Chiriboga N. Magnesium sulfate infusion for acute asthma in the emergency department. Jornal De Pediatria. 2017;93:19–25. https://doi.org/10.1016/j.jped.2017.06.002.
23. Jat KR, Khairwa A. Levalbuterol versus albuterol for acute asthma: a systematic review and meta-analysis. Pulm Pharmacol Ther. 2013;26(2):239–48.

24. Messinger AI. Management of pediatric community-acquired bacterial pneumonia. Pediatr Rev. 2017;38(9):394–409.
25. Pardue Jones B, Fleming GM, Otillio JK, Asokan I, Arnold DH. Pediatric acute asthma exacerbations: evaluation and management from emergency department to intensive care unit. J Asthma. 2016;53(6):607–17.
26. Ralston SL. Clinical practice guideline: the diagnosis, management, and prevention of bronchiolitis. Pediatrics. 2014;134(5):e1474–502. https://doi.org/10.1542/peds.2015-2862.
27. Ramratnam SK, Bacharier LB, Guilbert TW. Severe asthma in children. J Allergy Clin Immunol Pract. 2017;5(4):889–98.
28. Rehder KJ. Adjunct therapies for refractory status asthmaticus in children. Respir Care. 2017;62(6):849–65.
29. Richards AM. Pediatric respiratory emergencies. Emerg Med Clin North Am. 2016;34(1):77–96.
30. Vo P, Karasch VS. Respiratory failure. Pediatr Rev. 2013;35(2):476–86.

Cardiac

31. Abdulla R, Luxenberg DM. Cardiac interpretation of pediatric chest x-ray. In: Abdulla R, editor. Heart diseases in children. Boston: Springer; 2011.
32. Brissaud O, et al. Experts' recommendations for the management of cardiogenic shock in children. Ann Intensive Care. 2016;6:14.
33. De Caen AR, et al. Part 12: pediatric advanced life support. Circulation. 2015;132:S526–42.
34. Diaz-Parra S, et al. Use of adenosine in the treatment of SVT in the pediatric emergency department. Pediatr Emerg Care. 2014;30:388–93.
35. Hitz MP, Bertram H, Köditz H, et al. Levosimendan for bridging in a pediatric patient with Alström syndrome awaiting heart-lung transplantation. Clin Res Cardiol. 2008;97:846.
36. Lerman BB, et al. SVT: mechanistic insights deduced from adenosine. Circ Arrhythm Electrophysiol. 2018;11:e006953.
37. Lewis J, et al. Acute management of refractory and unstable pediatric SVT. J Pediatrics. 2017;181:177–82.
38. Manole MD, Saladino RA. Emergency department management of the pediatric patient with SVT. Pediatr Emerg Care. 2007;23:176–89.
39. Tissot C, da Cruz EM, Miyamoto S. Cardiac failure. In: Munoz R, Morell V, Cruz E, Vetterly C, editors. Critical care of children with heart disease. London: Springer; 2009.
40. Pacheco GS, LeetchA. Pediatric cardiopulmonary arrest and post-arrest care. Critical concepts in pediatric emergency medicine. Relias Media, Morrisville, NC; 2015. Online.
41. Quattrocelli A, et al. Age makes a difference: symptoms in pediatric SVT. J Arrhythm. 2018;34:565–71.
42. Rohit M, Shrivastava S. Acyanotic and cyanotic congenital heart diseases. Indian J Pediatr. 2018;85:454.
43. Smith AH. Arrhythmias in cardiac critical care. Ped Crit Care Med. 2016;17:S146–54.
44. Wackel P, Cannon B. Hear rate and rhythm disorders. Pediatr Rev. 2017;38:243–53.
45. Woods WA, McCulloch MA. Cardiovascular emergencies in the pediatric patient. Emerg Med Clin N Am. 2005;23:1233–49.

Neuro

46. Abend NS, Loddenkemper T. Management of pediatric status epilepticus. Curr Treat Options Neurol. 2014;16:301.
47. Abend NS, Loddenkemper T. Pediatric status epilepticus management. Curr Opin Pediatr. 2014;26:668–74.
48. Abend NS, et al. Anticonvulsant medications in the pediatric emergency room and ICU. Pediatr Emerg Care. 2008;24:705–21.
49. Abend NS, et al. Status epilepticus and refractory status epilepticus management. Semin Pediatr Neurol. 2014;21:263–74.
50. Guterman EL, Betjemann JP. Status epilepticus mortality – improving or status quo? JAMA Neurol. 2019;76(8):885–6.
51. Mittal R. Recent advances in febrile seizures. Indian J Pediatr. 2014;81:909.
52. Stredny CM, et al. Towards acute pediatric status epilepticus intervention teams: do we need "seizure codes"? Seizure. 2018;58:133–40.

33 Pediatrics 2: Trauma, Abuse, Drowning, Burns

Emily Fontane, Mark Hincapie, and Nico Chiriboga

Polytrauma

Introduction

Unintentional and intentional injuries remain the leading cause of death in the United States for children 1–18 years of age and account for more years of life lost than sudden infant death, cancer, and infectious disease combined. Trauma, in general, is the leading cause of childhood death around the world, including developed countries. Specifically, injuries associated with motor vehicles are the most common cause of death in children regardless of age and include pedestrians and occupants (Figs. 33.1 and 33.2).

Fifty percent of pediatric trauma deaths occur in the prehospital setting. Restoration of spontaneous circulation prior to arrival to the trauma center by cardiopulmonary resuscitation (CPR) leads to a 50% survival without neurological deficits. However, CPR lasting more than 15 minutes with or without fixed pupils on arrival is typically an indicator of high mortality. Seriously injured children have better outcomes at a children's hospital or trauma center that integrates both pediatric and adult trauma services. A pediatric trauma score (PTS) was adapted in the 1980s, and it continues to be utilized today as a means to identify polytrauma in a timely fashion (Fig. 33.3).

A PTS has a minimum score of −6 and a maximum score of +12. A PTS score less than 0 was indicative of 100% mortality, and a PTS score greater than 8 had a mortality of 0%. Scores between 0 and 8 had mortalities that increased with lower scores.

Having a variety of sizes for vascular access (IV, IO, CVL), airway equipment, and vital signs is important in the emergency department. A pediatric-specific airway cart should always be available with a checklist of items, which may be sized according to the Broselow color system. The Broselow tape on initial evaluation may be the only way to rapidly determine dosing for medications, boluses, and products. It is important to note that not all hospitals employ the Broselow tape, but alternative standardized methods must be clearly available and labeled to provide expedient care, especially in the event of polytrauma (Fig. 33.4).

Common sites of polytrauma include the head, chest, abdomen and genitourinary and musculoskeletal systems. Between 3 and 27% of children die from polytrauma, most commonly from severe traumatic brain injury. As a result, apnea,

E. Fontane (✉)
Department of Emergency Medicine, Division of Pediatric Emergency Medicine, University of Florida, College of Medicine, Jacksonville, FL, USA

M. Hincapie
Division of Pediatric Critical Care to Paediatric Emergency medicine, Jacksonville, FL, USA

N. Chiriboga
Division of Pediatric Critical Care, University of Florida, Department of Pediatrics in the College of Medicine, Jacksonville, FL, USA

© Springer Nature Switzerland AG 2020
J. R. Shiber, S. D. Weingart (eds.), *Emergency Department Critical Care*,
https://doi.org/10.1007/978-3-030-28794-8_33

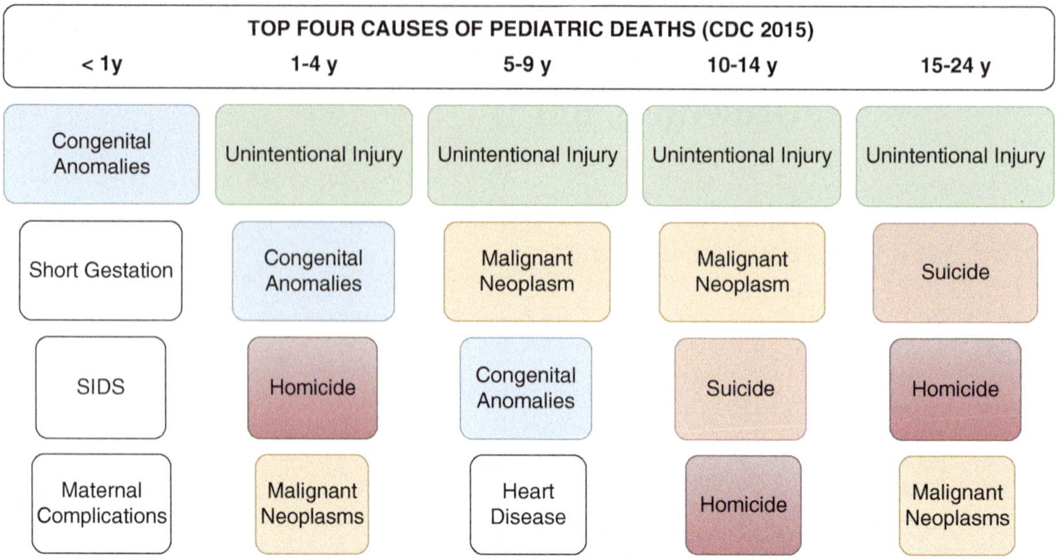

Fig. 33.1 Top four causes of pediatric deaths (CDC 2015)

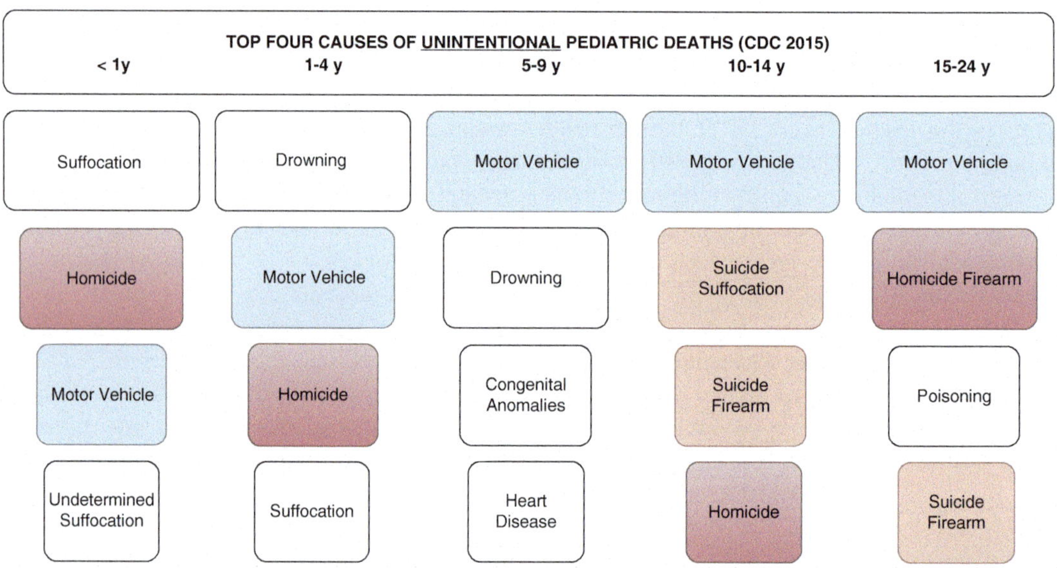

Fig. 33.2 Top four causes of unintentional pediatric deaths (CDC 2015)

hypoventilation, and hypoxia are markedly more common than hypovolemic shock in these circumstances, hence the emphasis on establishing an airway and maintaining breathing. Any trauma can lead to increased metabolism and heat loss; therefore, preservation of thermoregulation throughout interventions should be maintained. Airway, breathing, and circulation must be monitored closely as combination of acidosis, hypothermia, and coagulopathy is a very poor determinant of prognosis.

Airway

Pathophysiology

There are several unique aspects to the pediatric airway: the oropharynx is largely occupied by the

	-1	+1	+2
Weight	<10 kg <22 lb	10-20 kg 22-44 lb	>20 kg >44 lb
Airway	Intubated Cricothyroidotomy Tracheostomy	Oral Airway Nasal Airway Oxygen	Normal
Systolic BP	<50 mm Hg weak or absent pulses	50-90 mm Hg Palpable Carotid Pulse Palpable Femoral Pulse	>90 mm Hg Good peripheral pulses
Consciousness	Coma Unresponsive	Obtunded Loss of Consciousness	Awake
Fracture	Open Multiple	Single Closed	None Seen None Suspected
Skin	Tissue Loss Gunshot Wound Stab Wound through Fascia	Contusion Abrasion Laceration &1t;7 cm through Fascia	None Visible

PTS Score < 0: 100% mortality ←→ PTS Score > 8: 0% mortality

Fig. 33.3 Pediatric trauma score

tongue and tonsils, the larynx and the vocal cords are more anterocephalad than in older individual, and secretions can often accumulate in the retropharyngeal space. The trachea is 5 cm long in the infant and extends to 7 cm by 18 months of age. *Typically, an appropriate calculation of endotracheal tube (ETT) depth (centimeter) is "three multiplied by the appropriate tube size."*

Patient Presentation

As always, airway patency is a priority and oftentimes requires a definitive airway for oxygenation and ventilation.

Length-based resuscitation tapes should be utilized given the diversity in child size, and standard practice should be to obtain ETT one size larger and one size smaller than predicted (ATLS Peds).

Initial Stabilization

Smaller children have a larger discrepancy with the occiput and the midface, often requiring a 1 inch padding beneath the torso to ensure cervical spine stabilization. Optimal neutral positioning is obtained when the midfacial plane is parallel to the spinal board.

The jaw-thrust maneuver may help keep the airway patent until a definitive airway is established. If unconscious, an oral airway can be placed; however, placement is different than in adults as backwards insertion with 180° rotation leads to soft tissue oropharyngeal injury. Preoxygenation is necessary before attempting placement of a definitive airway.

Diagnostics

Auscultation is necessary alongside a secondary confirmation (including airways placed in the field) such as waveform capnography, end-tidal CO_2 detection, or chest radiograph. However, given the increased risk for endotracheal tube dislodgement due to the shorter trachea, reevaluation of the airway is important.

Premature 3kg	0-6 months 3.5kg	6-12 months 7 kg	1-3 years 10-12kg	4-7 years 16-18kg	8-10 years 24-30 kg
Mask premie, newborn Oral Airway infant Bag-Valve infant Laryngoscope 0 Miller (Straight) ETT 2.5-3.0 uncuffed Stylet 6 Fr Suction 6-8 Fr	Mask newborn Oral Airway infant, small Bag-Valve infant Laryngoscope 1 Miller (Straight) ETT 3.0-3.5 uncuffed Stylet 6 Fr Suction 8 Fr	Mask pediatric Oral Airway small Bag-Valve pediatric Laryngoscope 1 Miller (Straight) ETT 3.5-4.0 cuffed or uncuffed Stylet 6 Fr Suction 8-10 Fr	Mask pediatric Oral Airway small Bag-Valve pediatric Laryngoscope 1 Miller (Straight) ETT 4.0-4.5 cuffed or uncuffed Stylet 6 Fr Suction 10 Fr	Mask pediatric Oral Airway medium Bag-Valve pediatric Laryngoscope 2 Miller (Straight) or Macintosh (Curved) ETT 5.0-5.5 uncuffed Stylet 14 Fr Suction 14 Fr	Mask adult Oral Airway medium, large Bag-Valve pediatric, adult Laryngoscope 2-3 Miller (Straight) or Macintosh (Curved) ETT 5.5-6.0 cuffed Stylet 14 Fr Suction 14 Fr
IV catheter 22-24 gauge BP cuff premie, newborn	IV catheter 22 gauge BP cuff newborn, infant	IV catheter 22 gauge BP cuff infant, child	IV catheter 20-22 gauge BP cuff child	IV catheter 20 gauge BP cuff child	IV catheter 18-20 gauge BP cuff child, adult
OG/NG 8 Fr Chest Tube 10-14 Fr Urinary Catheter 5 Fr Feeding Cervical Collar N/A	OG/NG 10 Fr Chest Tube 12-18 Fr Urinary Catheter 5-8 Fr Feeding Cervical Collar N/A	OG/NG 12 Fr Chest Tube 14-20 Fr Urinary Catheter 8 Fr Cervical Collar Small	OG/NG 12 Fr Chest Tube 14-20 Fr Urinary Catheter 10 Fr Cervical Collar Small	OG/NG 12 Fr Chest Tube 20-28 Fr Urinary Catheter 10-12 Fr Cervical Collar Small	OG/NG 14 Fr Chest Tube 28-32 Fr Urinary Catheter 12 Fr Cervical Collar Medium

Fig. 33.4 Broselow tape

Definitive Treatment

Orotracheal intubation is the "most reliable means of establishing an airway and administering ventilation" and is warranted in severe traumatic brain injury, airway instability, ventilatory failure, severe hypovolemia in the setting of altered mental status, or need of surgical intervention.

The cricoid ring of a small child forms a seal around an uncuffed endotracheal tube; however, if age-appropriate, cuffed endotracheal tubes are known to improve ventilatory exchange and cerebral blood flow.

Given advances, there are no longer concerns of tracheal necrosis with cuffed endotracheal tubes with cuffed pressures < 30 mm Hg as safe.

Atropine sulfate of 0.1–0.5 mg should be considered in infants requiring rapid sequence intubation to block bradycardia from laryngeal manipulation. Note, however, that PALS recommends 0.02 mg/kg with no minimum dose and reports that there is conflicting evidence. It is not required but can certainly be considered in the setting of bradycardia.

Unlike adults, nasotracheal intubation is not recommended due to the sharp angle created from the glottis, risk of penetrating the brain, and damage to the adenoids.

Temporizing measures such as the laryngeal mask airway may be needed, but note that cricothyroidotomy in emergencies is not recommended in children less than 12 years of age.

Breathing

Pathophysiology

"Hypoxia is the most common cause of pediatric cardiac arrest" ATLS.

Normal spontaneous tidal volumes of 4–6 mL/kg are common in infants and children, but clear titration to as high as 10 mL/kg may be required in assisted ventilation. However, barotrauma is always a concern in pediatrics; therefore, an adult bag-valve-mask device should never be utilized in those less than 30 kilograms.

Patient Presentation

Re-establishing ventilation and perfusion is a priority as early introduction of sodium bicarbonate infusion may exacerbate metabolic acidosis and lead to worsening hypercarbia.

Definitive Treatment

In the event of hemothorax, pneumothorax, or hemopneumothorax, the site of chest tube insertion remains the same as in adults – the fifth intercostal space and anterior to the midaxillary line. Tunneling a chest tube above a rib superior-posteriorly is important due to their thinner chest wall.

Circulation

Pathophysiology

A child's physiologic reserve may allow for preservation of a systolic blood pressure with greater volume loss so that early assessment of heart rate and skin perfusion are more important indicators of hypovolemia and shock. Please refer to the table (adapted from ATLS) for further details of circulatory compensation in children.

Patient Presentation (Fig. 33.5)

Initial Stabilization

Appropriate estimation of volume resuscitation can be calculated with the use of Broselow tape. Two peripheral IVs (antecubital fossa if possible) should be started in any critically ill or injured child. Intraosseous placement can be a temporizing access for up to 24 hours in the anteromedial tibia, antero-distal femur, distal tibia above the medial malleolus, or the anterior superior iliac spine. A 5–10 mL normal saline flush should be used after administration of medications. A bolus or infusion may be necessary to overcome some baseline resistance but understanding that tissue necrosis and compartment syndrome must be avoided.

Avoid intraosseous placement with cellulitis, osteomyelitis, areas of previous attempts, or fracture.

MILD BLOOD VOLUME LOSS <30%	MODERATE BLOOD VOLUME LOSS 30% to 45%	SEVERE BLOOD VOLUME LOSS 45%
CARDIOVASCULAR increased heart rate weak, thread *peripheral* pulse normal SBP 80 to 90 + 2 x age (years) normal pulse pressure	**CARDIOVASCULAR** markedly increased heart rate weak, thread *central* pulses normal SBP 80 to 90 + 2 x age (years) normal pulse pressure	**CARDIOVASCULAR** tachycardia then bradycardia weak, thread central pulses hypotension with SBP <70 + 2 x age (years) narrowed pulse pressure undetectable DBP
CENTRAL NERVOUS SYSTEM Anxious Irritable Confused	**CENTRAL NERVOUS SYSTEM** Lethargy Dulled Response to Pain	**CENTRAL NERVOUS SYSTEM** Comatose
SKIN Cool Mottled Prolonged Capillary Refill	**SKIN** Cyanotic Markedly Prolonged Capillary Refill	**SKIN** Pale Cold
URINARY OUTPUT low to very low	**URINARY OUTPUT** minimal	**URINARY OUTPUT** none

Fig. 33.5 Classifaction of hemorrhagic shock

Definitive Treatment

If there are concerns of ongoing bleeding, after the second or third crystalloid bolus of 20 cc/kg (so 40–60 cc/kg total), it is appropriate to consider a 10–20 ml per kilogram of packed red blood cells, a concept accepted as the "damage control resuscitation" in ATLS. The balanced administration of fluids with packed red blood cells, fresh frozen plasma, and platelets may avoid worsening acidosis, hypothermia, and coagulopathy. Following a hospital site-based mass transfusion protocol may simplify and improve the resuscitation. At any facilities in which there are delays in blood product administration, crystalloid fluids are the acceptable alternative until transfer to another facility.

Chest/Thoracic Trauma

Pathophysiology

The pediatric skeleton is not completely ossified and therefore pliable, which increases risk for visceral organ damage without fracture. When rib fractures are seen in children, significant force should always be assumed. Thoracic injury is less common than abdominal or cranial injuries; however isolated thoracic injury has a 4–12% mortality that increases to 25–40% with concomitant injuries. However, significant injuries to the thorax rarely are singular in children, and polytrauma should always be considered.

Tension pneumothorax is the most common life-threatening injury in pediatric chest injuries, largely due to the mobility of the mediastinum.

Patient Presentation

Nearly four out of five thoracic injuries are due to blunt force from motor vehicles, pedestrian accidents, falls, and recreational injuries. However, penetrating wounds are more common in adolescents. Pulmonary contusion is one of the most common thoracic injuries and may lead to pulmonary hemorrhage, edema, and consolidation. The reduced lung compliance ultimately causes ventilation-perfusion mismatch and shunting, thus worsening hypercarbia, and hypoxia. If the area affected is large, then ARDS and acute respiratory failure may develop.

Initial Stabilization

Rapid management for pneumothorax is always necessary, whether it is a simple pneumothorax or a tension pneumothorax, as chest tube placement may be necessary. Note that patients may be asymptomatic with simple pneumothorax. French tube sizing is the diameter in millimeters multiplied by three.

Diagnostics

Pulmonary contusions remain the most common pediatric thoracic trauma however may not immediately show on chest radiograph until 4–6 hours later. Many pediatric centers utilize CT angiogram in the event of first rib injury due to the proximity to the great vessels, although pediatric studies do not readily yield the same association as adults. Tension pneumothorax is a clinical diagnosis so that chest radiograph is not utilized to diagnose as it delays management. Hemothorax occur in 7–29% of chest injuries and are seen on chest radiograph as opacification, blunting of the costodiaphragmatic angle, and/or an air-fluid level.

In ARDS, chest radiography may indicate pulmonary infiltrates within several hours of the injury, but many children are initially stable as hypoxemia develops over time and may lead to a change in mental status. Careful monitoring of interval blood gases and chest radiographs should be ongoing.

Definitive Treatment

Most injuries to the chest are treated similarly to adults and can be managed with supportive care and/or tube thoracostomy. Tracheal deviation, hypotension, unequal breath sounds, and jugular venous distention are indicative of tension pneumothorax and warrant immediate needle decompression followed by a tube thoracostomy (Leeper). Proper management of hemothorax is imperative due to the risk of atelectasis, poor lung expansion, shunting, and fibrosis leading to a trapped lung.

Surgical intervention is warranted if the initial chest tube drainage is greater than 15 mL/kg or has subsequent drainage of greater than 2 mL/kg/hour.

Cardiac and great vessel injuries although rare (0.03% incidence) occur from high-energy trauma, and patients may rapidly deteriorate. In the event of cardiac tamponade, hypotension, jugular venous distension, muffled heart sounds, and an abnormal subxiphoid, focused assessment with sonography for trauma (FAST) is elicited. If this were to occur, pericardiocentesis, pericardial window, and thoracotomy are options for immediate therapy. *Therefore, prompt contact with the surgery or cardiothoracic team is necessary before deterioration.*

ED thoracotomy is only indicated in pediatric patients with penetrating wounds that have active deterioration of vital signs en route or in the trauma bay.

Severe Traumatic Brain Injury

Introduction

Traumatic brain injury (TBI) is the leading cause of death and disability in those greater than 1 year of age. Seventeen percent of polytrauma have closed head injuries and often lead to long-term disability. Mechanisms of pediatric TBI are primarily a result of motor vehicle crashes, bicycle crashes, falls, assaults, and child abuse. Eighteen percent have severe TBI defined by a Glasgow Coma Scale (GCS) between 3 and 8. *A modified GCS verbal score is utilized for children less than four years of age.*

Pathophysiology

TBI can be subdivided into primary injury, the immediate damage at the time of trauma, and secondary injury, the cellular changes that occur due to neurological deterioration. The goal of severe TBI management relates to limiting and/or preventing secondary injury due to hypotension, hypoxia, hyperglycemia, seizures, and hyperthermia while optimizing cerebral blood flow. There is a loss of cerebral autoregulation in severe TBI that can compromise cerebral blood flow, perfusion pressure, and metabolism. Pediatric populations differ from adult brain injuries in that they have lower circulating blood volume, less cerebrospinal fluid volume, and open cranial sutures and fontanelles. Infants may hemorrhage significantly into the subgaleal, subdural, or intraventricular spaces, which is masked by these pediatric anatomic differences. Overt bulging fontanelles or cranial suture diastases indicate serious injury, and urgent neurosurgical involvement is necessary

Altered mental status, focal neurologic findings, neck pain, torticollis, substantial torso

injury, diving, and high-risk motor vehicle crash are highly associated with cervical spine injury.

Initial Stabilization

Persistent vomiting requires gastric decompression to prevent aspiration and may indicate elevated intracranial pressure. Systolic blood pressure less than the 75 percentile for age is associated with worse neurological outcomes.

Diagnostics

The Eastern Association for the Surgery of Trauma (EAST) guidelines on blunt cerebrovascular injury state that all pediatric trauma patients should be evaluated with the same adult criteria.

Early neuroimaging is imperative in the event of severe TBI upon the completion of primary and secondary surveys and once hemodynamic stability is ensured. Computed tomography (CT) of the head without contrast is preferred for the assessment of intracranial hemorrhage or skull fracture and detects 62–75% of pediatric head injuries. In the event of polytrauma, it would be appropriate to obtain combined imaging of the chest, abdomen, or pelvis. MRI is not an accepted practice in the event of severe pediatric TBI due to timing, inability to closely evaluate the patient, and consequences of sedation. *New studies have identified routine follow-up CT imaging more than 24 hours after admission as unnecessary unless there is neurological deterioration, increased intracranial pressures, or the need for postoperative evaluation of hematoma.*

If unable to admit to a pediatric intensive care unit, then arrange for immediate transfer to a tertiary or quaternary center.

Definitive Treatment (Fig. 33.6)

Spinal Trauma

Pathophysiology

One in five children with cervical damage has injuries at multiple levels.

Thirty-five percent of pediatric trauma is a result of motor vehicle accidents, and the most common area of injury is the head and neck (Fig. 33.7).

Vertebral and pelvic fractures are most worrisome not only due to high impact injury but that they each have five other concomitant injuries on average and a nearly 1% mortality rate.

Spinal injury without radiographic abnormalities (SCIWORA) is a unique feature to pediatric spinal trauma given the anatomical differences. Its incidence ranges from 5% to 67% but is most common in children less than 8 years.

Patient Presentation

SCIWORA presents with transient paresthesia or even subjective paralysis and occurs in 30–40% of children with traumatic myelopathy.

Initial Stabilization

A large-scale study found that a patient that is alert, with no cervical tenderness, no focal neurologic deficit, no intoxication, and no painful distracting injury does not warrant cervical spine imaging. All other children must have their cervical spine immobilized with an appropriately fitted cervical collar and evaluated by a three-view plain film or CT.

SCIWORA patients must be immediately immobilized to prevent progression of neurologic dysfunction and evaluated by MRI if CT scan is negative for injuries.

Diagnostics

Screening lateral cervical spine radiographs have a sensitivity of 75%; however, additional imaging may be necessary. *Unlike adults, lateral cervical radiographs that show prevertebral soft tissue swelling may be a result of crying.* There is increased sensitivity with CT and less likelihood for repeat plain films.

Definitive Treatment

History and index of suspicion of spinal trauma should not preclude further management, even with a normal cervical spine series. Consult pediatric orthopedic and spinal colleagues early. Pediatric fractures adapt to more stress, remodel more than adults, and heal in shorter time.

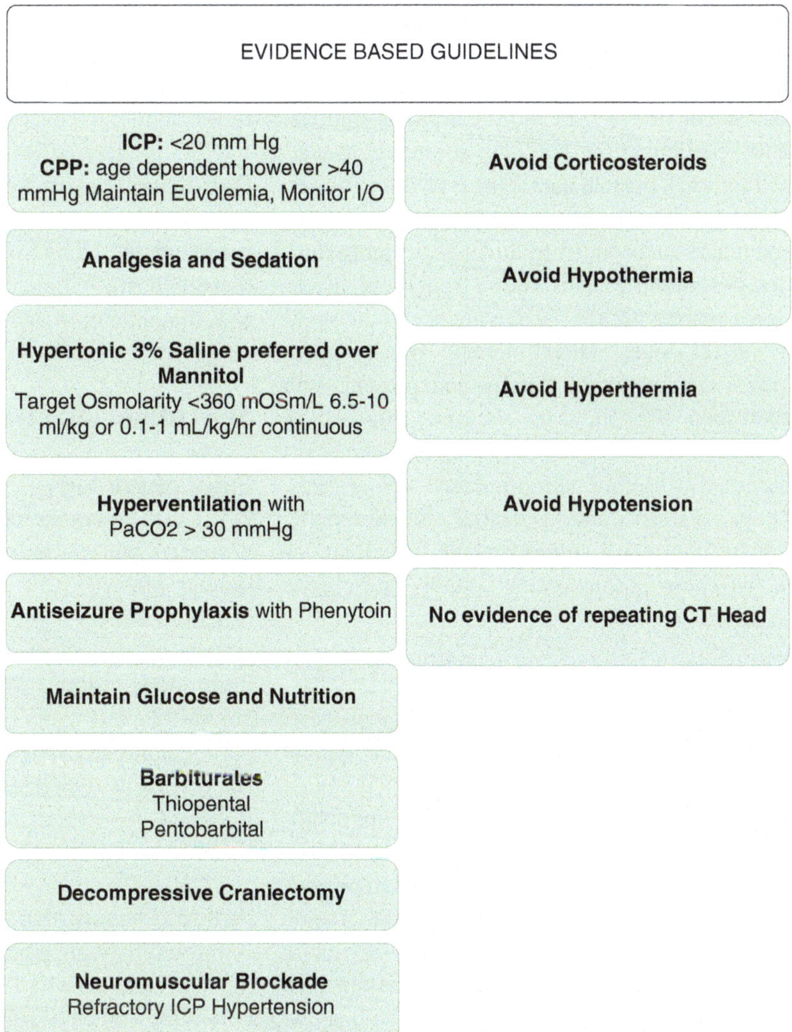

Fig. 33.6 Evidence-based guidelines

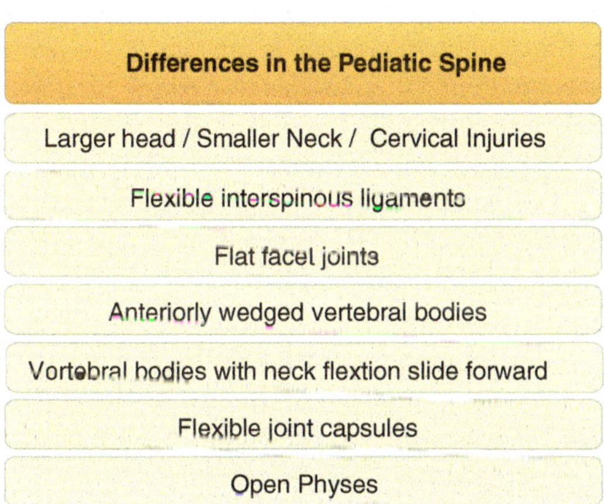

Fig. 33.7 Differences in the pediatric spine

Abdominal Trauma

Introduction

Most polytrauma injuries result from blunt trauma where internal bleeding may be undetected.

Overall, abdominal injuries occur in 8–27% of pediatric polytrauma most commonly from MVC and falls.

Patient Presentation

Children, unlike adults, may be stable initially but deteriorate rapidly due to physiologic reserve, difficulty to evaluate abdominal visceral injuries with ultrasound, and the absence of abdominal wall ecchymosis in children. Unlike hepatic and splenic injuries, duodenal and pancreatic injuries only occur in 3–5% of intra-abdominal injuries. These particular injuries occur secondary to seat-belt injuries, bicycle handlebars, or direct blows. Major hollow viscus injuries like in the stomach and intestines occur from direct penetrating injuries, crush injuries, perforation from rapid distension, shearing injuries, and avulsions of the small bowel mesentery. Diaphragmatic injuries occur in 4% of abdominal trauma and present with chest pain radiating to the shoulder, shortness of breath, and abdominal pain. Upon persistent crying, gastric distention accumulates causing respiratory distress and potential diaphragmatic rupture. Possible findings include bowel sounds in the chest, absent breath sounds, and classic scaphoid abdomen.

Initial Stabilization

Keep in mind that orogastric tube decompression is preferred in infants, rather than the typical nasogastric tube. The emergency physician must always be mindful of the need for prompt operative intervention in the event of hemorrhagic shock, especially given the pediatric high physiologic reserve. There is extreme high importance of continued re-evaluation, particularly of volume and hemodynamic status, by the trauma team. In the event of hepatic or splenic injury with active extravasation seen on CT, it is important to obtain serial hematocrit, serial clinical evaluations, and serial radiographic examinations.

Diagnostics

"Diagnostic adjuncts for assessing abdominal trauma include CT, FAST, and diagnostic peritoneal lavage (DPL)."

In centers without surgeons, CT evaluation should not preclude transport for definitive care.

CT of the abdomen is indicated in possible intraperitoneal and retroperitoneal abdominal injuries but still may miss up to 13% of hollow viscus injuries (mostly small bowel). FAST may not identify up to one-third of solid organ injuries in children given the intraparenchymal injuries that are more difficult to detect and does not detect retroperitoneal injuries. Although DPL is listed in ATLS, it must only be performed by the acting surgeon as the procedure interferes with future abdominal evaluations and imaging.

Definitive Treatment

Emergency surgical laparotomy is indicated if hemodynamics remain uncontrolled and one of the diagnostic adjuncts are indicative of intra-abdominal hemorrhage.

Musculoskeletal Trauma

Pathophysiology

Any crush injury to the physis leads to a worst prognosis but can be very difficult to detect on radiograph.

Compartment syndrome is a clear consequence of musculoskeletal injuries, intravenous infiltration, clotting disorders, septicemia, and animal bites. It results when a myofascial compartment has an increase in pressure affecting tissue perfusion, which leads to muscular and nerve ischemia. Concomitant rhabdomyolysis, hyperkalemia, and renal failure may also occur.

Patient Presentation

A thorough orthopedic evaluation of the spine, pelvis, and extremities is very important. Oftentimes, ecchymosis, swelling, and crepitus are key findings in an unresponsive patient.

An isolated closed femur fracture may lead to a drop in hematocrit by 4%, which may not lead to shock; therefore, shock in the face of this fracture should involve detailed evaluation for other sources of blood loss.

Initial Stabilization

Surgical fixation is common in polytrauma; therefore, orthopedics must be contacted early during initial stabilization.

Compartment syndrome can be identified by the "five Ps," pain, paresthesia, paralysis, pallor, and pulselessness, but these findings are less reliable in pediatrics. Pain occurs early and is typically out of proportion both at rest and during passive motion, while pallor and pulselessness are late findings. Any limb evaluated for compartment syndrome must have any splint or dressing removed, and the orthopedic team must be immediately contacted as a pressure > 30–45 mmHg warrants fasciotomy. Neurovascular evaluation of all limbs, particularly distal perfusion, is part of any orthopedic inspection.

Diagnostics

Plain radiographs are integral to the polytraumatic patient. If abnormal plain films are found, immediate consultation of the orthopedic team is necessary.

Definitive Treatment

Fractured extremities are splinted not only to help facilitate transport in the facility and minimize pain but mainly to enhance thorough trauma evaluation. Although there is no optimal time for definitive fracture fixation in polytraumatic children, it is suggested within 24–72 hours after stabilization.

Child Abuse

Introduction

More than 2 million Child Protective Service (CPS) reports are made for suspected child maltreatment. Approximately one in five of those reports are due to concerns of physical abuse. Each year, 650,000 of these reports are substantiated, and approximately 1500 childhood deaths occur due to child abuse or neglect. Seventy-one percent of fatalities from maltreatment occur in those less than 3 years of age with nearly 76% of suspected child abuse involved children under 1 year of age.

Severe TBI from child abuse occurred at 12 months on average, while severe TBI from accidental injuries occurred at 8 years on average.

Child abuse patients are more likely to sustain severe head injuries in comparison with other pediatric trauma patients and as a result suffer higher mortality rates and higher rates of neurological dysfunction, such as impairment of eyesight and hearing, cerebral palsy, developmental delay, and cognitive delay.

The rate of abuse in those less than 1 year of age has risen since 2010, while rates in other groups remain the same.

Pathophysiology

Abusive head trauma has higher incidence of hypoxic ischemic insult rather than diffuse axonal injury. Avulsion of the bridging veins between the brain and dura causes subdural hematomas from shaking or direct impact. Accidental subdural hematoma is not common as it requires an acceleration and deceleration high-energy mechanism of injury that is typically greater than a fall from a height of 4 ft. There are several theories to retinal hemorrhage in child abuse. For one, the abrupt increased intracranial pressure causes venous obstruction, which is further exacerbated by increased intrathoracic pressure due to thoracic compression. Causes of retinal hemorrhage also include traumatic birth, cardiopulmonary resuscitation, hematological disease, and ruptured vascular malformation. Therefore, they must be interpreted in the context of clinical presentation. However, *retinal hemorrhage and rib fractures are rare events in infants and children from accidental trauma*.

Rib fractures are thought to be a result of violent shaking with anterior and posterior compressive movements. Sixty to eighty percent of femoral fractures in those less than 1 year of age are due to child abuse. However, studies indicate that lower extremity fractures in those older than two are rarely due to child abuse trauma. Additionally, abdominal injuries most commonly occur as a result of mid epigastric injury due to compression of abdominal viscera against the spine causing hematoma, perforation, or laceration. Interestingly, no fall has ever been reported as a cause of intestinal perforation.

Patient Presentation

It is important for the practitioner to understand the unique associations to trauma from child abuse in order to protect the child from further harm. It is imperative to document the interaction with family or caregivers during the initial evaluation. It is not uncommon for discrepant details to be offered, but one must catalog the changing history thoroughly.

A landmark study in 2010 documented the differences between accidental and abusive bruising injuries in children less than 4 years of age. In it, the "T (torso) E (ear) N (neck)-4" mnemonic was derived to assist the practitioner in identifying higher likelihood for abuse. Within the accident group, bruising within the torso, ear, and neck was absent or rare regardless of the cause and identified as common bruising sites for the abused in children less than 4 years of age. Bruises in pre-cruising infants are rare and when present occur as small bruises over the bony prominences (Fig. 33.8).

Fifty to seventy percent of abusive head trauma is caused by the patient's father or father figure, but in general, perpetrators are more likely to be a mother 41% of the time, father 21% of the time, and both parents 21% of the time. The highest rate is not in young adults or teenage parents but those aged 25–34 years.

Low GCS score on initial evaluation, retinal hemorrhages, intracranial hemorrhage, and cerebral edema were all found to be independent factors for mortality in abusive head trauma. It was found that those with abusive head trauma and moderate traumatic brain injury had a similar mortality rate to those with severe traumatic brain injury due to accidental injuries.

Unexplained Loss of Consciousness or Shock

Infants with abusive head trauma often present with sudden infant death syndrome (SIDS), seizures, coma, or apnea.

Retinal Hemorrhage

Retinal hemorrhage does not occur in mild or moderate TBI and rarely occurs (6%) in severe TBI but elicits 74% sensitivity and 94% specificity for abusive head trauma. It is seen as more sensitive than retinal folds, traumatic retinoschisis, and optic nerve sheath hemorrhages.

Abdominal Injury

Abdominal injury in traumatic child abuse is less common than head trauma, musculoskeletal injury, or burns. *It represents less than 1% of all pediatric trauma admissions.* As with blunt abdominal injury, hemoperitoneum is the primary concern.

Fractures

Patterns of bruising or burns as well as fractures can be elicited through careful soft tissue evaluation. The identification of an identifiable fracture places the patient at risk for multiple fractures, and 80% of occult fractures found by skeletal survey occur in children under the age of two.

Fractures can be elucidated by direct physical exam and symptoms or incidental findings of fracture callus on specific radiographs or skeletal survey. Correlating fracture with developmental milestones is important to assist with diagnosis of child abuse. Stairway or low-level falls more commonly cause head, neck, and distal extremity injury in 70–90% of cases, while truncal injuries and femoral fractures are rare events. Although

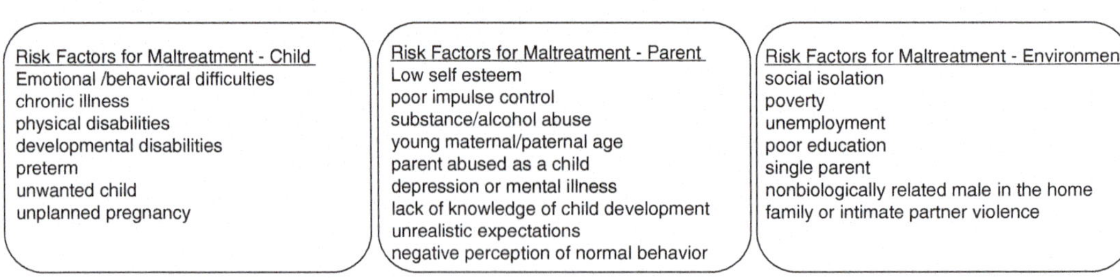

Fig. 33.8 Risk factors for maltreatment

spiral fractures are pathognomonic of abuse in nonambulating children, transverse fractures were found in the majority of fractures in a study. Additionally, midshaft and metaphyseal humeral fractures are more likely due to child abuse, while supracondylar fractures are typically accidental. Rib fractures, the most commonly detected occult fracture in child abuse, require a high-energy mechanism in children and occur in 85–100% of child abuse. Fractures typically occur in the posterior rib, although studies have also shown that the anterior and lateral ribs are affected as well.

External and Soft Tissue Trauma

Sources of injuries can often be obvious such as branding injuries; however, bruising can be difficult at times. For this reason, patterns of bruises are important to recognize. Bruises of the buttocks, perineum, and abdomen, or bruises of different ages, or immersion burns which create a stocking distribution of the buttocks and lower extremities are highly suspicious for abuse.

Diagnostics (Figs. 33.9 and 33.10)

There is a low threshold for head CT/MRI, especially when history is inconclusive or suspicious for abuse, as the need to rule out intracranial injuries is imperative when there is altered mental status, vomiting, scalp injury, facial injury, and neck injury.

The skeletal survey is mandatory in all suspected physical abuse in those under the age of 2. As high-quality skeletal surveys may not be available in the emergency department in the evening,

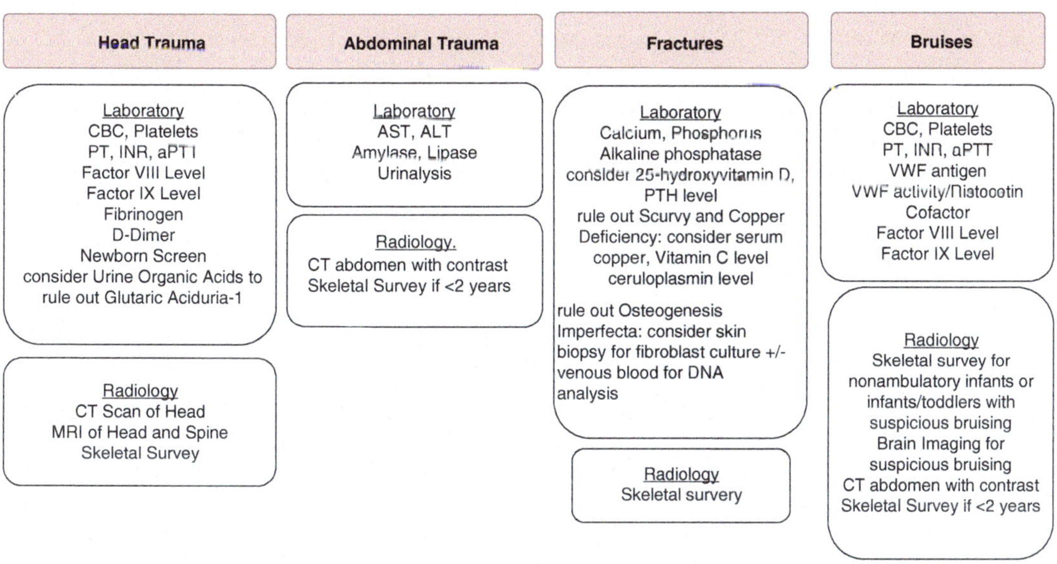

Fig. 33.9 Radiographic and laboratory testing for suspected non-accidental trauma

Indications for Skeletal Survey (sometimes referred to as "**Kempe**" Series)
- less than 2 years with obvious abusive injuries
- less than 2 years with any suspicious injury
  Nonambulatory infants with bruises, skin injuries, oral injuries
  Injuries not consistent with the history provided
- infants with unexplained, unexpected sudden death
- unexplained intracranial injuries, including hemorrhage and hypoxic-ischemic injury household contacts of an abused child less than 2 years
- twins of abused infants and toddlers

Fig. 33.10 Indications for skeletal survey (sometimes referred to as "Kempe" series)

the American Academy of Pediatrics recommends hospitalization. *Although skeletal surveys are difficult to conduct on stabilized children on life support, efforts should be made to obtain the study in a timely fashion as results have a direct effect on any investigation.* Due to the development of fracture calluses, repeat imaging in 1–2 weeks is necessary as injuries may not have been seen on initial radiologic exam.

Submersion Injury

Introduction

Although there has been significant decline in the rate of submersion hospitalizations, *drowning is the second leading cause of unintentional injury death in children aged 1–19* with 91% unintentional and not related to boating accidents. *Female submersion rates peak at 1–2 years of age, while male submersion rates are bimodal in toddlers and adolescents.*

The World Health Organization estimates 400,000 drowning deaths each year worldwide. Seven percent of all human injury-related deaths are attributed to drowning. The First World Congress on Drowning defined drowning as a process of pulmonary impairment as a result of submersion in fluid and may be fatal or nonfatal.

Children less than 4 years of age have the highest mortality rate from drowning, most commonly in swimming pools or open water. Adolescents likely drown due to swimming or boating accidents and are unlikely to receive bystander resuscitation because they are often dead at the scene.

For every death, there are approximately two nonfatal drowning victims that are admitted to the hospital, and 20% of the survivors have severe sustained neurological disability.

Compared to non-epileptic children, epileptic pediatric patients are 4–14 times at risk of submersion. Recent evidence has associated swimming lessons with an 88% reduction in the drowning events for children less than 4 years of age. However, some suggest that increased swimming proficiency increases exposure risk to water and submersion accidents. Pre-existing medical conditions, the initial ECG rhythm, the duration of suspension of cerebral flow, and the quality of life support are important factors that influence outcome. Immersion times greater than 25 minutes are associated with the highest mortality rates.

Pathophysiology

Primary hypoxic ischemic injury to the brain is irreversible due to inadequate metabolic substrate reserves, and the central tenet of resuscitation is the prevention of secondary neuronal injury. The exact mechanism of human drownings remains unclear. However, there is a consensus belief that prolonged apnea and laryngospasm occur initially resulting in hypoxemia and hypercapnia. With progressive hypoxemia, laryngospasm subsides predisposing the patient to aspiration of fluid causing acute lung injury and acute respiratory distress syndrome (ARDS).

Appropriate ventilator protective strategies can be implemented, such as tidal volumes of 6 mL/kg or less with adequate positive end expiratory pressure for alveolar recruitment, as large TV have been found to decrease cerebral venous flow and decrease cardiac output and mean arterial pressure which would worsen CPP. Permissive hypercapnia is not encouraged without proper intracranial monitoring.

Submersion injuries can be differentiated from other cardiac arrests in that hypothermia decelerates neural tissue death and cerebral blood flow continues for a brief interval. Rapid cold water submersions, particularly less than 5 °C, have shown potential protective effects to cerebral organ function before hypoxia occurs due to decreased oxygen demand. Submersion duration has been found to be a direct measure of cerebral anoxia with duration over 5–10 minutes worsening prognosis. In the retrospective study by Suominen et al., the median submersion time for deaths was 16 minutes, and survival with minimal neurological dysfunction was 5 minutes.

Patient Presentation

Drowning victims are often covered in wet clothing that will be removed by the rescue team. Cyanosis, tachypnea, and persistent tachycardia in combination with abnormal pulse oximetry are key indicators of respiratory distress. Severe signs and symptoms of submersion victims include abnormal lung auscultation, severe cough, frothy sputum, altered mentation, hypotension, and tachycardia.

According to several retrospective submersion studies, unreactive pupils and a GCS score of 5 or less in the PICU were two strong independent factors that predicted poor neurological outcome.

There is no need to hospitalize submersion victims if there are no signs or symptoms of aspiration (normal pulmonary examination and need for oxygen) after a 4–6 hour observation period.

Diagnostics

The initial chest radiograph should be obtained however may not reflect acute lung injury until hours later. Normal initial head computed tomography scan has no prognostic benefit in submersion victims. If the patient is awake, alert, and oriented, head imaging is not recommended, unless there is known trauma or a change to clinical status (Schmidt). Neurologic monitoring, including EEG and neuroimaging, and somatosensory evoked potentials, after submersion resuscitation, are helpful for prognostication but not required.

Initial Stabilization

Prehospital management is to re-establish oxygenation and ventilation before the development of cardiac arrest. In the event of cardiac arrest, cardiopulmonary resuscitation (CPR) enacted by bystanders while awaiting EMS arrival *has shown to increase the likelihood of neurological recovery.*

Removal of wet clothing and warming with thick blankets are advised. Shivering has been found to be a positive prognostic sign. Core temperature body temperature should be obtained upon initial resuscitation.

Immediate neurologic function is not a dependable predictor of outcome. If the child is spontaneously breathing, victims should be placed in the right lateral decubitus position with head down to prevent aspiration. If bag-valve-mask resuscitation is necessary, cricoid pressure is recommended as it may limit gastric aspiration. Continuous or bi-level positive airway pressure is required for treatment of hypoxia at times. Intubation may be required as supraglottic airway devices are not very effective.

Associated injuries such as fracture or dislocation of the cervical spine and thoracic and intra-abdominal injuries in shallow water must be considered. Spinal stabilization with a cervical collar should be prioritized in the event of significant mechanism for cervical spine injury, altered mental status, focal neural deficits, or a significant injury. However, spinal immobilization should not be prioritized over resuscitation and preservation of the airway.

The Heimlich maneuver or abdominal compressions have not been shown to be beneficial in drowning as they delay CPR and may lead to vomiting and aspiration. Electrocardiographic monitoring is recommended early on; however, defibrillation is often rendered ineffective with a hypothermic myocardium, particularly less than 28 °C. In these circumstances, chest compressions support circulation until core temperature can be raised.

The neurological admission on admission in the emergency department is not predictive of outcome. For this reason, serial examinations of consciousness, pupil size and reactivity, brain stem reflexes, and motor strength are integral to admission. *Hemodynamic status in the emergency department and neurologic status in the ICU are highly predictive of outcome. pH less than 7 is associated with poorer prognosis.*

Pulmonary edema typically presents within 4 hours. Clinical symptoms of hemoptysis, rales, abnormal radiography, and hypoxia are indicative of aspiration and must be carefully monitored. Continuous pulse oximetry and blood gases should be obtained with the intention of preventing hypoxia and secondary neurological injury.

Hypoxemia and respiratory and metabolic acidosis must be aggressively treated with ventilatory support and hemodynamic support with isotonic crystalloids.

Target post-cardiac arrest patient's core temperature of 32–34 °C for 12–72 hours with slow rewarming at a rate of 0.5 °C per hour has shown higher rates of neurologic outcomes. Additionally, immediate treatment of hyperthermia is imperative. Prophylactic antibiotics and corticosteroids are not beneficial, unless there is evidence of infection or sepsis. Seizures are common in hypoxic brain injuries, but unlike TBI, prophylactic anticonvulsant medications and intracranial monitoring are not always necessary. Better outcomes result from the avoidance of hypoglycemia, hyperglycemia, and large or rapid fluctuations of glucose, so the goal should be to maintain it at 80–110 mg/dL.

Severe Burns

Introduction

The incidence of burns is higher in children than in adults with scald burns and then contact burns the most common etiologies. Advancements in burn management have reduced overall mortality.

Pathophysiology

Burns are characterized as superficial (previously first degree), superficial partial, deep partial (previously second degree), and full thickness (previously third degree). Superficial burns are blanching and dry, have no blisters, and heal within 3–6 days without scarring. Superficial partial-thickness burns involve blanching, weeping, and blisters and heal within 7–20 days without scarring. Deep partial-thickness burns are non-blanching, weeping sites that require more than 21 days to heal and lead to scars and contracture. Finally, full-thickness burns are typically dry, non-painful, and non-blanching which require prolonged duration of healing. Children tend to have thinner skin, which leads to deeper injuries.

Heat spreads rapidly in the oropharynx, and inhalational thermal injuries are commonly seen above the carina. Lower airway thermal injuries are typically secondary to steam exposure and only occur in 5% of patients. Thermal injuries release inflammatory mediators by the endothelial and nerve cells such as complement, kinins, histamine, serotonin, prostaglandins, neuropeptides, and oxygen free radicals. Mediators allow for third spacing and increase capillary permeability leading to pronounced volume deficits and additional tissue damage in large burns.

Chemical inhalation injuries occur due to combustion by-products that affect both the upper and lower respiratory tracts. Chemical inhalation injuries cause bronchoconstriction, increased vascular permeability, and ventilatory dysfunction. Protein leakage and alveolar collapse evolve and cause significant airway compromise up to 48 hours after injury.

Carbon monoxide and cyanide are common toxicities in house fires and must be addressed immediately. Carbon monoxide (CO) is 200 times more potent than oxygen in binding to hemoglobin, which displaces oxygen and increases carboxyhemoglobin. Additionally, CO and cyanide inhibit aerobic respiration through the mitochondrial electron transport chain. These agents not only are commonly present in fire exposure but also act synergistically, thus only requiring smaller concentrations. If one is expected, both should be treated. Hypermetabolic responses lead to glycogen depletion and to eventual hypoglycemia, hence the importance of dextrose in resuscitative fluids for younger burn victims.

Patient Presentation

Frequent re-evaluation over the course of 72 hours is important as inflammation evolves and partial-thickness burns can easily become full-thickness burns.

Initial Stabilization

Emergency physicians should recognize criteria for referral to a burn center. These factors include any full-thickness burns; partial-thickness burns greater than 10% TBSA; burns to the face, hands, feet, genitourinary area, or major joints; electrical or chemical burns; suspected inhalational injuries; burns with inhalational injury; comorbid conditions that can affect resuscitation and treatment; significant associated traumatic injuries; injuries that exceed the hospital parameters; and cases requiring comprehensive social or rehabilitative needs.

Burn estimates at the scene or non-specialty centers overestimate the TBSA; therefore, initial hydration at 1.5 maintenance lactated Ringer is appropriate when transport time is short. Upon immediate stabilization, it is important to simultaneously contact the regional burn center to coordinate immediate transport and care.

Signs of airway compromise include facial burns, singed nasal hairs, carbon-laden sputum, stridor, work of breathing, and tachypnea. Direct evaluation of the supraglottic and oropharyngeal areas for burns or edema is required by a specialist via direct laryngoscopy. Severe full-thickness burns to the neck are a high risk for airway compromise up to 36 hours later when edema is most severe. Routine bronchoscopy with lavage has been associated with decreased mortality due to prevention of atelectasis and reducing inflammation.

Primary survey requires supplemental oxygen, and early intubation with the appropriately sized cuffed endotracheal tube must always be considered because of airway narrowing as children have rapid decreases in cross-sectional areas to their airway. Tracheostomy is rarely indicated unless it is difficult to establish the airway and there are extensive burns. Poor chest wall compliance from edema and eschars and the systemic inflammatory response syndrome (SIRS) directly contribute to impending respiratory failure, which requires up to 72 hours of close hospital observation.

Carbon monoxide exposure must be treated with 100% oxygen because it decreases the half-life of carboxyhemoglobin, while hydroxycobalamin binds cyanide and excretes it in the urine.

The delicate balance between providing adequate perfusion, decreasing crystalloid fluids, and avoiding organ dysfunction from hypoperfusion is imperative in burn victims.

Burn injuries in children that are less than 10% TBSA should be repleted with oral rehydration therapy. However, enteral tube and oral rehydration are not rapid methods in maintaining circulation for larger burns. For this reason, the Parkland formula was devised to provide adequate oral, enteral, or intravenous hydration based on patient size and burn injury. The Parkland formula estimates 4 mL/kg/% TBSA resuscitation; however, the Shriners Burns Hospital-Galveston is more accurate in victims less than 23 kg. The Galveston formula provides maintenance and resuscitation requirements of 5000 mL/m2 TBSA and 2000 mL/m2 TBSA. There are no randomized controlled trials between the two formulas to date; however, *these formulas underestimate volume in smaller burns and overestimate volume in larger burns*. These formulas provide estimates for resuscitation over the first 24 hours of injury. Half of the volume should be administered within the first 8 hours of the burn injury with the second half volume administered over the subsequent 16 hours.

Lactated Ringer is the initial resuscitative fluid. Dextrose is added for children less than 30 kg and less than 5 years of age. The use of colloids (5% albumin) within 8–12 hours after injury decreases crystalloid volume requirements, decreases third spacing, and decreases length of stay. Frequent re-evaluation of end-organ perfusion is imperative therefore hourly urine output goals of 1 mL/kg/h via indwelling urinary catheter. Overall, proper management of circulation in burn victims prevents acute renal failure, multiple organ abnormalities, and mortality.

Urine output has been extensively studied and found to be the most cost-effective and least invasive manner of evaluating burn resuscitation victims.

However, over-resuscitation has been documented to have caused abdominal compartment syndrome, need for extremity escharotomies, pericardial effusion, prolonged intubation from acute respiratory distress syndrome, multiple organ dysfunction, and death.

After airway, breathing, and circulation are addressed, the wound itself must be evaluated closely. Depth and size of the burn injury determine resuscitative efforts and determine transfer to a regional trauma burn center.

Many burn centers have adopted laser Doppler imaging (LDI) on the initial assessment of burn injuries to measure tissue perfusion in the dermal vasculature, as it increases the accuracy of burn depth assessment.

The surface of the victim's palm and fingers is approximately 1% of total body surface area (TBSA) and is a technique utilized to quickly estimate affected burn areas. Additionally, the "rule of nines" has been a practical method in estimating TBSA affected in adults but is less dependable in children; and the Lund and Browder chart provides age-appropriate TBSA estimates.

Standard care involves daily dressing changes, debridement, and topical antimicrobials. Long-acting silver dressings as well as biosynthetic dressings may improve re-epithelialization and decrease the amount of painful dressing changes.

Circumferential full-thickness injuries compromise both arterial and venous blood flow causing ischemic tissue loss; therefore, these injuries require immediate surgery consultation. When they occur to the chest, restrictive chest expansion will lead to hypoxia, hypercapnia, and impending respiratory failure. For this reason, escharotomy as deep as the hypodermis is promptly required, often by a surgeon. Linear incisions are typically made on opposite sides of the injury.

The standard of care for deep partial-thickness and full-thickness burns involves early excision and coverage using autologous or non-autologous skin grafts. The excision of necrotic or devitalized tissue reduces inflammatory mediators, decreases infection, preserves the dermis, and decreases scar formation. Split-thickness skin grafts are harvested to the superficial dermis and require 7–10 days.

Pain management cannot be understated and often requires potent, short-acting medications. Intranasal or IV fentanyl can often be used in the emergency department; however, extensive injuries may require ketamine often in combination with a benzodiazepine or longer-acting opiates. Low doses of ketamine are analgesic, and higher doses provide anesthesia. Benefits occur from prevention of narcotic use and the possibility of central respiratory depression. Additionally, nitrous oxide has been increasingly documented as safe and effective for children in the emergency department.

The tetanus vaccine should be administered to children with burns deeper than superficial-thickness, who have not received booster immunizations in more than 5 years. Additionally, those who have not received the immunization to date should also receive the tetanus immune globulin.

Definitive Treatment (Fig. 33.11)

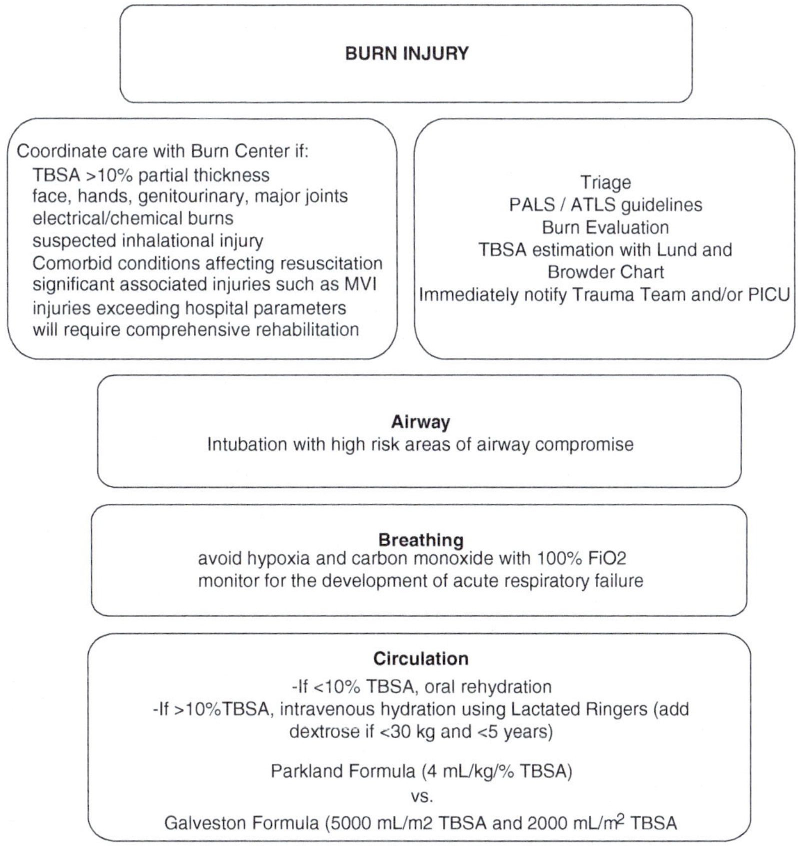

Fig. 33.11 Burn injury

References

Polytrauma

1. Kay RM, Skaggs DL. Pediatric polytrauma management. J Pediatr Orthop. 2016;26(2):268–77.
2. Tuggle DW, Snow SK, AAP Committee On Pediatric Emergency Medicine, Council On Injury, Violence, And Poison Prevention, Section On Critical Care, Section On Orthopaedics, Section On Surgery, Section On Transport Medicine, Pediatric Trauma Society, Society Of Trauma Nurses, Pediatric Committee. Management of pediatric trauma. Pediatrics. 2016;138(2):1–9. https://doi.org/10.1542/peds.2016-1569.
3. Tepas JJ, Ramenofsky ML, Mollitt DL, et al. The Pediatric Trauma Score as a predictor of injury severity: an objective assessment. J Trauma. 1988;28(4):425–9.
4. Falcone RA, Haas L. Organizing the hospital for pediatric trauma care. In: Pediatric trauma: CRC Press; 2017.
5. Robertson JO, Vogel AM. Pediatric ICU management. In: Pediatric trauma: CRC Press; 2017.
6. Leeper CM, Gaines BA. Pediatric thoracic trauma. Pediatric trauma. https://doi.org/10.4324/9781315113746.
7. Gillory L, Naik-Mathuria B. Pediatric abdominal trauma. https://doi.org/10.4324/9781315113746.
8. Au J, Janzen N. Pediatric genitourinary trauma. Pediatric trauma. https://doi.org/10.4324/9781315113746.
9. Hill JF, Robertson AK. Pediatric orthopedic trauma: spine and pelvis trauma. Pediatric trauma. https://doi.org/10.4324/9781315113746.
10. Schroeder K, Rosenfeld S. Pediatric orthopedic trauma: an overview of pediatric musculoskeletal trauma. Pediatric trauma. https://doi.org/10.4324/9781315113746.
11. May MM, Shenava VR. Lower extremity fractures. Pediatric trauma. https://doi.org/10.4324/9781315113746.
12. McFadyen JG, Ramaiah R, Bhananker SM. Initial assessment and management of pediatric trauma patients. J Crit Illn Inj Sci. 2012;2(3):121–7.
13. Henry S, editor. ATLS. 10th ed: Pediatrics. Chicago. American College of Surgeons (ACS); 2018.

14. Anderson V, Godfrey C, Rosenfeld JV, Catroppa C. Predictors of cognitive function and recovery 10 years after traumatic brain injury in young children. Pediatrics. 2012;129:e254–61. https://doi.org/10.1542/peds.2011-0311.
15. Vedantam A, Whitehead WE. Treatment of severe pediatric head injury: evidence-based practice. Pediatric trauma. https://doi.org/10.4324/9781315113746.
16. O'Lynnger TM, Shannon CN, Le TM, Greeno A, Chung D, Lamb FS, Wellons JC. Standardizing ICU management of pediatric traumatic brain injury is associated with improved outcomes at discharge. J Neurosurg Pediatr. 2016;17(1):19–26.
17. Leonard JC, Kuppermann N, Olsen C, Babcock-Cimpello L, Brown K, Mahajan P, Adelgais KM, Anders J, Borgialli D, Donoghue A, Hoyle JD, Kim E, Leonard JR, Lillis KA, Nigrovic LE, Powell EC, Rebella G, Reeves SD, Rogers AJ, Stankovic C, Teshome G, Jaffe D. Factors associated with cervical spine injury in children after blunt trauma. Ann Emerg Med. 2011;58:145–55.
18. Stocchetti N, Maas AIR, Chieregato A, van der Plas AA. Hyperventilation in head injury. Chest J. 2005;127(5):1812–27.
19. Bromberg WJ, Collier BC, Diebel LN, Dwyer KM, Holevar MR, Jacobs DG, Kurek SJ, Schreiber MA, Shapiro ML, Vogel TR. Blunt Cerebrovascular Injury. J Trauma. 2010;68(2):471–7.
20. Kochanek PM, Carney N, Adelson PD, Ashwal S, Bell MJ, Bratton S, Carson S, Chesnut RM, Ghajar J, Goldstein B, Grant GA, Kissoon N, Peterson K, Selden NR, Tasker RC, Tong KA, Vavilala MS, Wainwright MS, Warden CR. Guidelines for the acute medical management of severe traumatic brain injury in infants, children, and adolescents-second edition. Pediatr Crit Care Med. 2012;13(1):1–82.
21. Sahuquillo J. Decompressive craniectomy for the treatment of refractory high intracranial pressure in traumatic brain injury. Cochrane Database Syst Rev. 2006;25(1):1–41.

Child Abuse

22. Christian CW, Committee on Child Abuse and Neglect. The evaluation of suspected child abuse. Pediatrics. 2015;1337–54.
23. Cox CS, Jackson ML, Aertker BM. Trauma from child abuse. In: Pediatric trauma: CRC Press; 2017.
24. Davis FC, Coats TJ, Fischer R, Lawrence T, Lecky FE. A profiled of suspected child abuse as a subgroup of major trauma patients. Emerg Med J. 2015;32:921–5. https://doi.org/10.1136/emermed-2015-205285.
25. Shein SL, Bell MJ, Kochanek PM, Tyler-Kabara EC, Wisniewski SR, Feldman K, Makoroff K, Scribano PV, Berger RP. Risk factors for mortality in children with abusive head trauma. J Pediatr. 2012;161(4):716–22.
26. Pierce MC, Kaczor K, Aldridge S, O'Flynn J, Lorenz DJ. Bruising characteristics discriminating physical child abuse from accidental trauma. Pediatrics. 2010;125(1):67–74.
27. DiPietro MA, Brody AS, Cassady CI, Kleinman PK, Wyly JB, Applegate KE, Wood BP, Zerin JM, Mercado-Deane MG, Seibert JJ. Diagnostic imaging of child abuse. Pediatrics. 2009;123:1430–5.
28. Belfer RA, Klein BL, Orr L. Use of the skeletal survey in the evaluation of child maltreatment. Am J Emerg Med. 2001;19(2):122–4.

Submersion Injuries

29. Bowman SM, Aitken ME, Robbins JM, Baker SP. Trends in US pediatric drowning hospitalizations, 1993–2008. Pediatrics. 2012;129:275–81. https://doi.org/10.1542/peds.2011-2491.
30. Moler FW, Hutchison JS, Nadkarni VM, Silverstein FS, Meert KL, Holubkov R, Page K, Slomine BS, Christensen JR, Dean M. Targeted temperature management after pediatric cardiac arrest due to drowning: outcomes and complications. Pediatr Crit Care Med. 2016;18(8):712–20. https://doi.org/10.1097/PCC.0000000000000763.
31. Brenner RA, Bull MJ, Agran P, Dowd MD, Garcia V, Gardner HG, Smith G, Tenenbein M, Weiss JC, Wright J. Prevention of drowning in infants, children, and adolescents. Pediatrics. 2003;112(2):440–5.
32. Habib DM, Fecklenburg FW, Webb SA, Anas NG, Perkin RM. Prediction of childhood drowning and near-drowning morbidity and mortality. Pediatr Emerg Care. 1996;12(4):255–8.
33. Quan L, Kinder D. Pediatric submersions: prehospital predictors of outcome. Pediatrics. 1992;90(6):909–13.
34. Suominen P, Baillie C, Korpela R, Rautanen S, Ranta S, Olkkola KT. Impact of age, submersion time and water temperature on outcome in near-drowning. Resuscitation. 2002;52:247–54.
35. Suominen P, Kyriacou DN, Arcinue EL, Peek C, Kraus JF. Effect of immediate resuscitation on children with submersion injury. Pediatrics. 1984;94(2):137–42.
36. Romlin BS, Winberg H, Janson M, Nilsson B, Bjork K, Jeppsson A, Drake G, Claesson A. Excellent outcome with extracorporeal membrane oxygenation after accidental profound hypothermia (13.8 °C) and drowning. Crit Care Med. 2015:521–5. https://doi.org/10.1097/CCM.0000000000001283.
37. Orlowski JP. Drowning, near-drowning, and ice-water drowning. J Am Med Assoc. 1988;260(3):390–1.
38. Salomez F, Vincent JL. Drowning: a review of epidemiology, pathophysiology, treatment, and prevention. Resuscitation. 2004;63:261–8. https://doi.org/10.1016/j.resuscitation.2004.06.007.
39. Quan L, Cummings P. Characteristics of drowning by different age groups. Inj Prev. 2003;9:163–8.

40. Topjian AA, Berg RA, Bierens J, Branche CM, Clark RS, Friberg H, Hoedemaekers CW, Holzer M, Katz LM, Knape JT, Kochanek PM, Nadkarni V, van der Hoeven JG, Warner DS. Brain resuscitation in the drowning victim. Neurocrit Care. 2012;17(3):441–67. https://doi.org/10.1007/s12028-012-9747-4.
41. Hirshberg E, Larsen G, Van Duker H. Alterations in glucose homeostasis in the pediatric intensive care unit: hyperglycemia and glucose variability are associated with increased mortality and morbidity. Pediatr Crit Care. 2008;9(4):361–6. https://doi.org/10.1097/PCC.0b013e318172d401.
42. Schmidt AC, Sempsrott JR, Hawkins SC, Arastu AS, Cushing TA, Auerbach PS. Wilderness medical society practice guidelines for the prevention and treatment of drowning. Wilderness Environ Med. 2016;27:236–51.
43. Harries M. ABC of resuscitation near drowning. Br Med J. 2003;327:1336–8.

Severe Burns

44. Webman RB, Shupp JW, Burd RS. General principles of resuscitation and supportive care: burns. In: Pediatric trauma: CRC Press; 2017.
45. Centers for Disease Control and Prevention (CDC). Updated recommendations for use of tetanus toxoid, reduced diphtheria toxoid and acellular pertussis (Tdap) vaccine from the Advisory Committee on Immunization Practices, 2010. MMWR Morb Mortal Wkly Rep. 2011;60:13.
46. Hettiaratchy S, Papini R. ABC of burns Initial management of a major burn: II assessment and resuscitation. BMJ. 2004;329:101–3.

Fluids and Vasoactive Agents

34

James Dargin

Introduction

Fluids and vasoactive agents are the principal means of restoring tissue perfusion and oxygen delivery in patients with circulatory shock. A basic knowledge of the physiologic determinants of arterial pressure is helpful in understanding the role of fluid resuscitation and vasoactive agents in the treatment of shock. Mean arterial pressure (MAP), the primary determinant of organ blood flow, is the product of cardiac output (CO) and systemic vascular resistance (SVR):

$$\text{MAP} = \text{CO} \times \text{SVR}$$

CO is generated by both heart rate (HR) and stroke volume (SV). SV is determined by three factors: preload, afterload, and cardiac contractility.

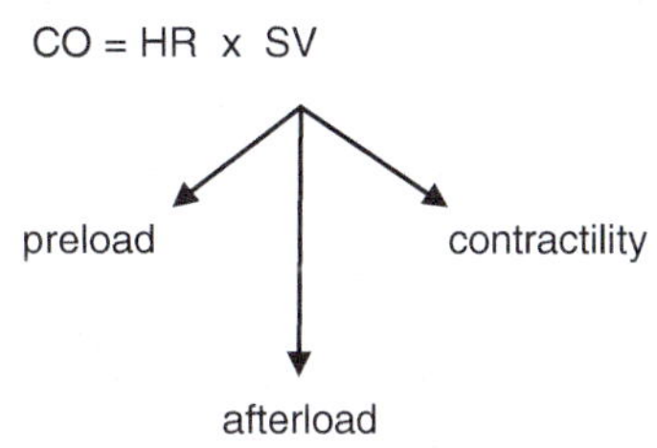

In simplistic terms, the hypotensive patient can be thought of as having either insufficient SV or insufficient SVR. Low SV could be related to inadequate preload (hypovolemic shock) or a reduction in cardiac contractility (cardiogenic shock). At the bedside, SV can be estimated by measuring the pulse pressure:

$$\text{Pulse pressure} = \text{Systolic blood pressure} - \text{Diastolic blood pressure}$$

Thus, a patient with hypotension and a narrow pulse pressure (e.g., 80/60 mmHg) likely has a reduced SV. Patients with a reduced SV typically have cool extremities and delayed capillary refill. Clinical evaluation of the patient can help to differentiate the causes of reduced SV (Fig. 34.1). Patients with low SVR (distributive shock) typically have warm extremities with

J. Dargin (✉)
Tufts University School of Medicine, Medical Intensive Care Unit, Boston, MA, USA

Pulmonary and Critical Care Medicine, Lahey Hospital & Medical Center, Burlington, MA, USA
e-mail: James.M.Dargin@Lahey.org

© Springer Nature Switzerland AG 2020

J. R. Shiber, S. D. Weingart (eds.), *Emergency Department Critical Care*,
https://doi.org/10.1007/978-3-030-28794-8_34

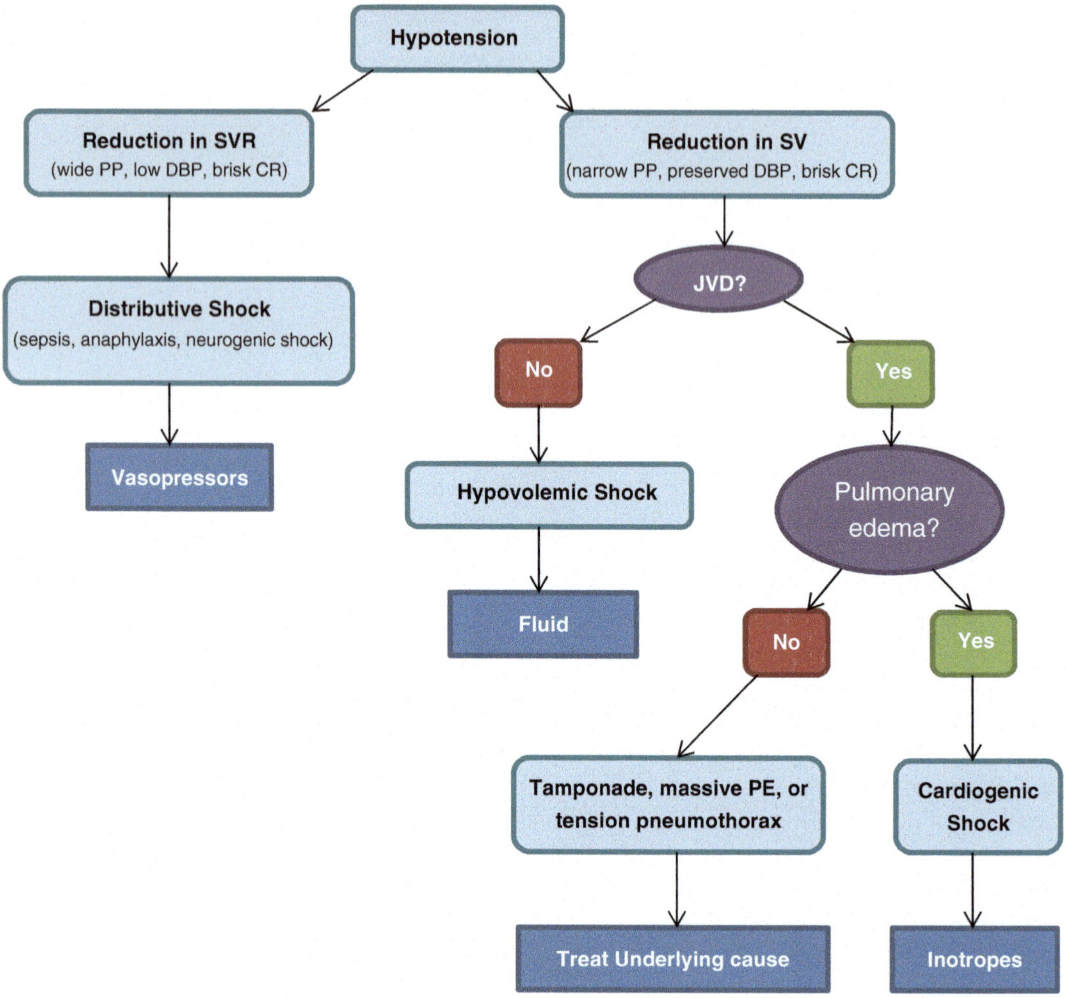

Fig. 34.1 Diagnostic approach to the patient with hypotension to guide the use of fluids and vasoactive agents. The algorithm provides an illustrative framework for the use of fluids and vasoactives. Causes of shock may be multifactorial and require additional treatments (e.g., distributive shock may also require fluids). Abbreviations: JVD jugular vein distention, SV stoke volume, DBP diastolic blood pressure, PP pulse pressure, SVR systemic vascular resistance, CR capillary refill, PE pulmonary embolus

brisk capillary refill. Distributive shock is also characterized by a preserved or elevated SV but low resistance, resulting in a drop in diastolic blood pressure and a wide pulse pressure (e.g., 85/25 mmHg). Determining the underlying pathophysiology of the patient's shock state is fundamental to providing the proper treatment with either fluids or vasoactives (Fig. 34.1). For example, the patient with a reduction in preload (hypovolemic shock) will require aggressive fluid resuscitation, whereas the patient with a reduction in contractility may require inotropic support. The patient with a reduced SVR often requires vasoconstricting agents in addition to fluid resuscitation to achieve adequate perfusion pressure.

Fluids

The primary determinant of cardiac output is preload and, as Starling's Law of the Heart demonstrates, increasing preload with an intravenous fluid bolus will increase cardiac output (Fig. 34.2)

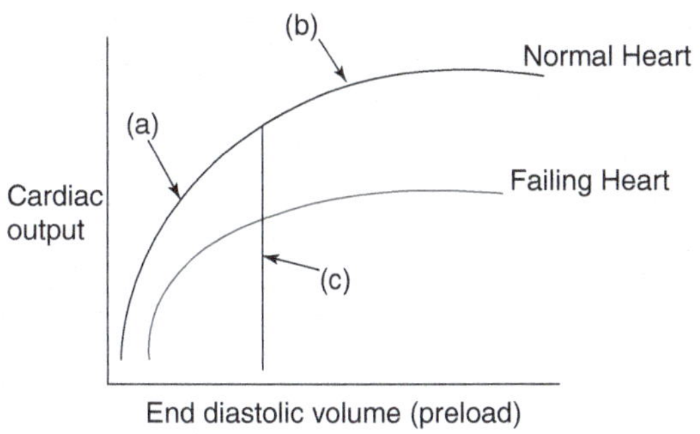

Fig. 34.2 Relationship between preload and cardiac output (Starling's Law of the Heart).[1] On the steep portion of the Starling curve, volume expansion will increase cardiac output (**a**). Once the heart is operating on the flat part of the curve, further fluid resuscitation will not improve cardiac output (**b**). Note that the slope of the curve (preload vs. cardiac output) depends on the systolic function. Thus, a given value of preload may result an in increase in cardiac output for the normal heart, or no improvement in cardiac output for the failing heart (**c**)

[1]. Thus, the fundamental reason for giving a patient a fluid bolus is to increase cardiac output, which will help to raise the blood pressure and improve tissue perfusion and oxygen delivery. An intravenous fluid bolus will not only improve cardiac output in patients with hypovolemic shock, but often with other causes of shock as well (distributive, obstructive, and neurogenic) because the healthy, euvolemic heart operates on the ascending limb of the Starling curve. Moreover, certain kinds of distributive shock may have a component of hypovolemia, as is the case of sepsis where capillary leak causes effective hypovolemia. Thus, in a patient presenting to ED with undifferentiated shock, augmenting preload with a fluid bolus will tend to improve cardiac output in most cases, except for the patient with a failing heart. As such, the vast majority of patients in the ED with shock tend to be fluid responsive at initial presentation, and a fluid challenge makes good sense as an early resuscitation effort.

Multiple studies have shown that *early*, aggressive fluid resuscitation improves outcomes in patients with shock, particularly in sepsis [2, 3]. However, repeated fluid boluses in a patient who is no longer fluid responsive may simply precipitate pulmonary edema and hypoxemia, worsen cardiac output as the heart is pushed onto the descending portion of the Starling curve (Fig. 34.2), and cause tissue edema, all of which *impair* oxygen delivery to tissues. As critically ill patients are increasingly remaining in the ED for prolonged periods of time, the difficulty comes in predicting which patients are still fluid responsive after the third, fourth, or fifth liter of fluid. In fact, only about half of ICU patients will increase their cardiac output when given an intravenous fluid bolus [4]. Furthermore, excessive fluid resuscitation has been associated with worse outcomes in the critically ill [4–6]. Continuing to attempt fluid resuscitation in a hypotensive patient who is no longer fluid responsive is not only counterproductive, but simply delays the appropriate therapy, which is typically a vasoactive agent. Thus, haphazardly fluid resuscitating patients in shock is not without risk, and careful consideration should be undertaken to determine if the patient is fluid responsive (i.e., will respond with an increase in CO when given additional preload).

Determining Fluid Responsiveness

For many years, clinicians have relied upon the measurement of central venous pressure (CVP) to guide fluid resuscitation. The traditional teaching was that CVP can serve a surrogate measure of end diastolic volume (preload). It was assumed that if CVP was low, then the patient was on the ascending part of Starling's curve and would respond to a fluid bolus with an increase in CO. Conversely, if the CVP was high, then the patient was no longer fluid responsive. However, multiple studies have shown CVP to be a poor predictor of fluid responsiveness [7]. In fact, CVP has been shown to be as accurate as a coin toss in determining if a patient is fluid responsive or not [8]. The poor predictive value of CVP may be due to a number of factors, including the fact that CVP is a poor surrogate measure of preload and that CVP is affected by other variables, such as positive end expiratory pressure (PEEP), left ventricular (LV) compliance, and cardiac contractility. Given the convincing evidence that CVP does not accurately predict fluid responsiveness, CVP should *not* be used to guide

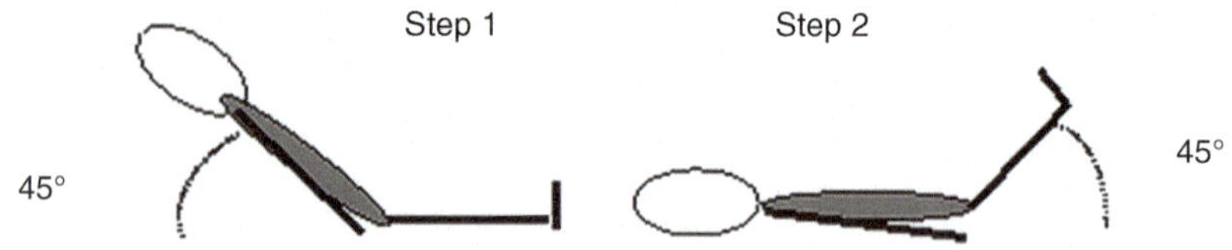

Fig. 34.3 The passive leg raise maneuver. Step 1. The patient is placed in the supine position and the blood pressure and pulse pressure (systolic minus diastolic blood pressure) are measured. Step 2. The legs are then lifted to 45 degrees for approximately 30 seconds and the blood pressure is measured again. An increase in pulse pressure or systolic pressure with passive leg raise indicates that the patient is fluid responsive

fluid resuscitation. In the ICU setting, more invasive and complicated methods of measuring fluid responsiveness can be utilized, including pulse pressure variation (the reader is referred to reference [9] for a concise review of the topic). In the ED, a passive leg raise maneuver can be used as a quick and inexpensive technique to accurately determine fluid responsiveness. The maneuver involves laying the patient supine and then measuring the blood pressure. The legs are then lifted to 45 degrees for approximately 30 seconds and the blood pressure is measured again (Fig. 34.3). This maneuver equates to a "reversible fluid challenge" using venous blood from the legs. An increase in pulse pressure or systolic pressure indicates that the patient is fluid responsive. Passive leg raise has been shown to be highly accurate in predicting fluid responsiveness [10].

Crystalloids Versus Colloids

Clinicians have a broad range of products to choose from when fluid resuscitating patients (Table 34.1). Fluids are typically categorized as crystalloid (normal saline, Ringer's lactate) and colloid (hetastarch, albumin) solutions. The colloid solutions contain large molecules that tend not to cross a healthy, intact capillary membrane. Colloid solutions can be hypooncotic (e.g., 5% albumin) or hyperoncotic (e.g., 25% albumin, dextrans, and hydroxyethyl starches). The oncotic pressure helps to retain the fluid in the intravascular space. Although the osmotic pressure of crystalloid solutions can likewise help to expand the intravascular space, the ions in crystalloid solutions are able to freely cross the capillary membrane. In fact, only 25% of a normal saline bolus will remain in the intravascular space, and 75% will distribute into the extravascular space [13]. Because colloids are thought to more effectively maintain fluid in the intravascular space than crystalloids, less colloid fluid is required for the same degree of intravascular expansion as a crystalloid solution. There is no accepted standard volume that should be given for a fluid bolus. Most clinical studies use 500 cc of crystalloid (or slightly less if colloid is used) given rapidly over 15–30 minutes to assess whether or not a patient's cardiac output increases with volume expansion [4].

Controversy has raged for decades regarding the choice of crystalloid versus colloid solutions for resuscitating patients with shock [14]. A number of large, high quality trials in recent years have shed light on the debate over crystalloids versus colloids. In general, there is little convincing evidence to the clinical benefit of colloids over crystalloids. Furthermore, there is potential for harm in some cases with use of colloid solutions. In one of the largest trials examining crystalloids versus colloids for resuscitation from hypovolemic shock, there was no benefit to using one solution over the other in terms of mortality. However, the colloid group received less fluid, had more days without vasopressors, and fewer days without mechanical ventilation [15]. It bears mentioning that colloids are also significantly more expensive than crystalloid solutions (Table 34.1).

Balanced Versus Unbalanced Crystalloid Solutions

The two most commonly used crystalloid solutions for resuscitating the critically ill are isotonic saline and Ringer's lactate. Ringer's lactate is

Table 34.1 Properties of commonly used intravenous fluids

	Plasma	Normal saline	Ringer's lactate	5% Albumin	Hetastarch 6%
Osmolality (mOsm/L)	290	308	273	309	310
Na (mEq/L)	140	154	130	130–160	154
Cl	100	154	109	130–160	154
K	4	0	4	0	0
Ca	2	0	3	0	0
Lactate	2	0	28	0	0
Potential side effects	–	Acidosis	–	Infection Anaphylaxis	Pruritis Hypersensitivity Kidney injury Coagulopathy
Cost	–	$1.46/L	$1.48/L	$91.54/250 mL [11]	$29.69/500 mL [12]

considered a "balanced" solution with an electrolyte composition that closely resembles plasma (Table 34.1). In contrast, normal saline is not considered to be a balanced solution owing to its relatively high chloride content compared to plasma. The use of normal saline for fluid resuscitation first appeared in the medical literature in the late 1800s and has become the most commonly used crystalloid solution in the United States [16].

Normal saline has a sodium concentration that is similar to that of plasma, but the solution is not truly "normal" in that the chloride concentration is approximately 1.5 times that of plasma. High chloride concentration in the renal tubules during saline resuscitation causes afferent vasoconstriction and reduced renal blood flow, a phenomenon that appears to be more pronounced during hypovolemia [17]. The high chloride levels resulting from resuscitation with normal saline also lead to a reduction in serum bicarbonate levels and a nonanion gap metabolic acidosis. In patients with renal failure, the acidosis may result in an increase in the serum potassium levels due to shifting of potassium out of the intracellular space. Other balanced solutions such as Plasmalyte and Ringer's lactate may avoid the untoward biochemical effects of normal saline. In fact, the use of balanced solutions has been associated with a lower postoperative mortality in surgical patients and lower rates of acute kidney injury and renal replacement therapy in ICU patients [18, 19]. There is also some evidence that resuscitation of critically ill patients with sepsis using balanced solutions may be associated with a lower mortality [20].

Albumin

Albumin-containing solutions were first used as a resuscitation fluid on the battlefield in World War II [21]. Human albumin in saline is expensive to produce, and the solution can theoretically transmit infection, although it is heat-treated to kill viruses. In the Saline versus Albumin Fluid Evaluation (SAFE) trial, almost 7000 ICU patients were randomized for resuscitation with normal saline or albumin [22]. The SAFE trial showed no difference in mortality or other outcomes with albumin versus normal saline even in patients with hypoalbuminemia [22]. Albumin is associated with a higher rate of mortality in traumatic brain injury patients and should probably be avoided in this population [23]. Given the cost of albumin compared to crystalloid solutions and the paucity of data showing clear benefit in patient outcomes, it is difficult to support the routine use of albumin for resuscitating patients with shock. However, several studies have shown potential mortality benefit specifically in patients with sepsis resuscitated with albumin [24, 25]. Current consensus guidelines recommend using crystalloids as the initial fluid of choice for patients with sepsis and to consider the use of albumin in patients who require "substantial amounts of crystalloids [26]."

Hydroxyethyl Starches

Hydroxyethyl starches (HES), the most commonly used and best studied semisynthetic colloid solutions, are derived from hydroxyethyl substitution of plant starches. The hydroxyethyl substitution prevents these molecules from being broken down by amylases in the blood, thus prolonging their oncotic effect in the blood and maintaining intravascular volume. However, this resistance to breakdown also tends to promote the accumulation of HES in the skin and kidney, causing pruritus and kidney injury, respectively. HES may also impair coagulation and can cause hypersensitivity reactions [27, 28]. The colloids are dissolved in a carrier solution, which is commonly isotonic saline. Most solutions used in the United States now contain 6% HES as higher concentrations have been associated with adverse effects. Four HES products are FDA approved for treatment of hypovolemia: HESPAN (6% HES 450/0.7 in 0.9% sodium chloride; Braun Medical Inc), Hetastarch (6% in 0.9% sodium chloride, generic equivalent to Hespan; Teva Pharmaceuticals USA), HEXTEND (6% HES 450/0.7 in physiologic solution; BioTime Inc), and Voluven (6% HES 130/0.40 in normal saline Fresenius Kabi USA, LLC). Multiple trials comparing hydroxyethyl starches to crystalloid solutions in patients with sepsis showed that starches were associated with a higher rate of acute kidney injury, renal replacement therapy, and possibly mortality [27, 29, 30]. After a review of multiple randomized trials and meta-analyses, the FDA released a "black box warning" in 2013 against the use of HES solutions in critically ill adult patients, including those with sepsis and in patients with preexisting renal dysfunction [31].

Vasoactives

Vasoactive agents help to restore tissue perfusion in shock states by increasing cardiac contractility (inotropes) or by increasing vasomotor tone (vasopressors). Most vasoactive agents exert their hemodynamic effects by acting on adrenergic receptors located within the heart and vascular smooth muscle (Table 34.2). Stimulation of alpha-1 subtype receptors located in vascular smooth muscle cells increases the production of

Table 34.2 Pharmacologic properties of commonly used vasoactive agents

Agent	Receptor activity			Indications	IV dosing	Side effects
	β1	α	Other			
Dopamine[c]	++	++	dopamine	Shock with bradycardia	1–20 mcg/kg/min	Tachyarrhythmias
Norepinephrine	+	+++	________	First line for septic shock Cardiogenic shock with hypotension	1–40 mcg/min	Tachyarrhythmias
Phenylephrine	0	++	________	Shock with tachyarrhymias	20–200 mcg/min	Bradycardia
Epinephrine	+++	+++	________	Anaphylactic shock Septic shock with low cardiac output	1–20 mcg/min	Tachyarrhythmias Mesenteric and myocardial ischemia Lactic acidosis
Dobutamine	+++	0	*β2*	Cardiogenic shock Septic shock with low cardiac output	2–20 mcg/kg/min	Tachyarrhythmias Hypotension
Milrinone[a]	0	0	PDE inhibitor	Cardiogenic shock RV failure	0.25–0.75 mcg/kg/min	Tachyarrhythmias Hypotension
Vasopressin	0	0	V1	Use with norepinephrine for septic shock	0.03 or 0.04 U/min	Limb ischemia[b] Mesenteric ischemia[b] Bradycardia

+ Minimal stimulation, ++ moderate stimulation, +++ potent stimulation
Abbreviations: *PDE* phosphodiesterase, *RV* right ventricular, *min* minute
[a]Side effects may be more pronounced in patients with renal failure
[b]More common at doses higher than 0.04 units/minute
[c]Dopamine binds dopamine, alpha, β1 receptors in a dose-dependent fashion

diacylglycerol and inositol triphosphate, resulting in an increase in intracellular calcium and vasoconstriction of both arteries and veins. The beta-1 receptor subtype is primarily located in the heart. Stimulation of this receptor increases intracellular cAMP, resulting in an influx of calcium into cardiac myocytes, leading to enhanced cardiac contractility. Although adrenergic agonists are primarily used for their vasoactive properties, some agents have beneficial effects outside of the cardiovascular system. For example, the beta-2 receptor subtype is not only located in vascular smooth muscle where it causes vasodilation, but also in bronchioles where stimulation causes bronchodilation. The clinical effects of different vasoactive agents depend on the relative affinity for different receptors and the dose of the agent used.

Vasoactive agents are generally short-acting and delivered as a continuous infusion, allowing for rapid titration based on the patient's hemodynamic response. Vasoactive medications should be administered through a central venous catheter as infiltration of the medications into the subcutaneous tissue during peripheral intravenous administration can cause soft tissue necrosis. In the case of life-threatening hypotension, vasoactive agents can be given temporarily through peripheral intravenous catheters or intraosseous access until central access is established. In the event that an adrenergic agent infiltrates subcutaneously, the adrenergic antagonist phentolamine can be administered subcutaneously directly into the site of extravasation to help prevent soft tissue necrosis.

Phenylephrine

Phenylephrine is a synthetic adrenergic agent with pure alpha-1 activity and causes vasoconstriction. Phenylephrine does not act directly on the heart, but the pure vasoconstricting effects can cause reflex bradycardia. Phenylephrine does not appear to be as potent a vasoconstrictor as other agents (e.g., norepinephrine), but may be a useful agent when tachyarrhythmias are of concern. One must be careful using this agent in patients with impaired left ventricular function (cardiogenic shock or sepsis induced left ventricular dysfunction), as the pure increase in afterload and lack of beta-1 activity may adversely affect myocardial function [32].

Norepinephrine

Norepinephrine is an endogenous neurotransmitter released from postganglionic sympathetic nerves and has potent alpha-1 effects, resulting in vasoconstriction. Norepinephrine possesses beta-1 affinity as well and modestly increases heart rate and cardiac contractility. This agent can precipitate tachyarrhythmias, although less so than more potent beta-1 agonists, such as dopamine or epinephrine. Clinical trials have shown norepinephrine to be a more potent vasopressor than dopamine with fewer tachyarrhythmias [33]. Although the potent vasoconstricting effects of norepinephrine could theoretically impair blood flow to vital organs, animal models of sepsis have demonstrated *improved* renal blood flow as MAP increases with norepinephrine titration [34].

Dopamine

Dopamine is an endogenous catecholamine precursor of norepinephrine and epinephrine. Dopamine binds dopamine, beta, and alpha receptors in a dose-dependent fashion. At low doses of <5 mcg/kg/minute, dopamine receptor activity results in dilation of renal, mesenteric, cerebral, and coronary vessels. Activation of dopamine receptors in the kidney also increases urinary sodium excretion. At moderate doses of 5–10 mcg/kg/minute, beta-1 agonism predominates, resulting in an increase in heart rate and stroke volume. The inotropic effects of dopamine are fairly modest compared to other agents, such as dobutamine and epinephrine. At higher doses, above 10 mcg/kg/minute, alpha effects cause peripheral vasoconstriction. Although dopamine demonstrates dose dependent receptor activity, the precise dosages at which particular clinical effects occur are less predictable in individual patients and dopamine should be titrated based on the clinical response rather than theoretical dosing. The chronotropic effects make dopamine useful in patients with hypotension and relative bradycardia. Dopamine was once used at low doses (<5 mcg/kg/min) in an attempt to increase renal blood flow and urine output to prevent acute kidney injury. Large trials have shown no benefit to this practice in terms of renal outcomes and dopamine should not be used for this indication [35]. Although dopamine has the potential for vasodilating mesenteric vessels through dopaminergic activity, most studies show impaired gut mucosal perfusion with dopamine [36].

Epinephrine

Epinephrine is a naturally occurring catecholamine released from the adrenal medulla. Epinephrine has strong affinity for alpha and beta receptors, has both inotropic and chronotropic effects, and is the most potent vasoconstrictor used in clinical practice. The potent beta-1 effects can precipitate tachyarrhythmias, which may limit its use in some patients. Although epinephrine can increase cardiac oxygen demand and should be used cautiously in patients with coronary artery disease, this agent has not been associated with adverse cardiac effects when used to treat septic shock [37]. Epinephrine causes glycogenolysis in the liver, increased glucagon, and decreased insulin, resulting in hyperglycemia. Epinephrine causes increased serum lactate levels, which occurs as a result of increased glycolysis and glycogenolysis in skeletal muscle rather than a result of global tissue hypoperfusion [38].

Dobutamine

Dobutamine is synthetic catecholamine with potent beta-1 activity, resulting in an increase in heart rate and cardiac contractility. Dobutamine also possesses modest beta-2 activity, which causes peripheral vasodilation. In patients with decompensated heart failure and a preserved blood pressure, the beta-1 effect improves cardiac output and the vasodilatory effect reduces afterload, thus "unloading" the failing heart. In patients without baseline hypotension, the blood pressure tends to remain normal despite the vasodilatory effects of dobutamine. The inotropic effects of dobutamine can increase myocardial work and oxygen consumption and should be used with caution in patients with cardiac ischemia. This agent can also cause tachyarrhythmias, which limits its use in some patients.

Milrinone

Milrinone is a phosphodiesterase inhibitor that increases cyclic AMP. The effect on the heart is to increase heart rate and SV. Milrinone also acts in in vascular smooth muscle to cause vasodilation, which may result in hypotension, particularly in hypovolemic patients. Milrinone can cause tachyarrhythmias, but may cause less tachycardia than catecholamines, such as dobutamine and epinephrine [39].

Milrinone has a relatively long half-life of approximately 2 hours compared to minutes for most other vasoactive agents. This agent is renally cleared and can cause hypotension and tachyarrhythmias in patients with renal failure. Although a loading dose can be used when starting milrinone, most clinicians avoid this practice in the critically ill, as hypotension often occurs. Milrinone causes pulmonary vasodilation and can be particularly useful when treating right ventricular failure by reducing afterload for the failing right heart [40].

Vasopressin

Vasopressin is an endogenous hormone released into the circulation from the pituitary in the setting of hypotension. Vasopressin acts on V_1 receptors in smooth muscles cells to cause vasoconstriction via phosphatidyl-inositol-calcium signaling pathway, as well as an increased sensitivity to catecholamines. There is some evidence that vasopressin may cause more peripheral and mesenteric ischemia than other vasoactive agents, particularly in the setting of hypovolemia, underscoring the importance of adequate fluid resuscitation prior to starting this medication [41]. The pure increase in afterload with vasopressin may be deleterious in patients with depressed left ventricular function. Vasopressin can also cause bradycardia via a baroreceptor mechanism. The adverse effects of vasopressin appear to be dose-dependent, and doses higher than 0.03–0.04 units/minute are often avoided for this reason.

Septic Shock

For many years, dopamine and norepinephrine were used interchangeably as first-line agents for the treatment of septic shock. However, multiple randomized trials have shed light on the use of these agents in the management of septic shock. Clinical trials suggest that dopamine may be associated with an increased mortality when compared to norepinephrine [42]. Furthermore, dopamine appears to be less effective at restoring blood pressure and more arrhythmogenic than norepinephrine [33]. As such, norepinephrine is currently recommended as the first-line vasoactive agent for septic shock [26]. Dopamine should be considered in patients with relative bradycardia, owing to its chronotropic effects. There are relatively few clinical trials examining the role of phenylephrine in the treatment of septic shock [43]. Phenylephrine may be less potent than norepinephrine and therefore less effective at maintaining blood pressure. For these reasons, this agent is not routinely used in septic shock. However, the pure alpha effects make this agent a useful alternative to norepinephrine, dopamine, and epinephrine in patients with tachyarrhythmias.

Although sepsis is traditionally thought of as a "high cardiac output" shock state, sepsis-induced left ventricular dysfunction is not uncommon [44]. In patients with septic shock and evidence of a low cardiac output state (low central venous oxygen saturation despite adequate fluid resuscitation, cool extremities, and delayed capillary refill) agents with inotropic properties may be of utility [3]. For example, dobutamine is often used to augment cardiac output in patients with sepsis-related left ventricular dysfunction. When used in patients with septic shock, dobutamine is generally used in combination with norepinephrine to prevent hypotension from the vasodilatory effects of dobutamine. Epinephrine can also be used as a single agent for patients with septic shock and evidence of low cardiac output, owing to its combination of inotropic and vasoconstricting properties. Studies examining epinephrine versus combination dobutamine–norepinephrine for sepsis have shown no difference in mortality between these agents [45]. Epinephrine was not associated with an increased risk of severe arrhythmias or myocardial or limb ischemia in these studies. However, epinephrine reduces gut mucosal perfusion in sepsis when compared to norepinephrine or combination norepinephrine–dobutamine [46, 47]. Epinephrine increases lactate levels, precluding the use of this laboratory study as an endpoint of resuscitation when using epinephrine infusions. Epinephrine can also be added to high-dose norepinephrine in patients with refractory septic shock.

Vasopressin levels initially increase manifold to supraphysiologic levels early in the setting of sepsis, and then decrease dramatically to inappropriately low levels [48]. Combination treatment with vasopressin and norepinephrine in patients with septic shock results in lower norepinephrine requirements without an increase in adverse events. Patients with less severe septic shock (those requiring 5–15 mcg/min of norepineprhine) have a reduction in mortality when treated with combination vasopressin–norepinephrine [49]. Vasopressin has been associated with a reduction in heart rate in septic shock and may be of use in patients experiencing to tachyarrhythmias from norepinephrine. Although vasopressin is a potent vasoconstrictor, it does not appear particularly efficacious for septic shock when used as a single agent and is associated with increase complications and mortality compared to norepinephrine [50]. In clinical practice, intravenous vasopressin is typically added at a low dose, fixed rate of 0.03 or 0.04 units/hour to moderate doses of norepinephrine (5–15 mcg/kg) in patients with septic shock.

Decompensated Heart Failure and Cardiogenic Shock

In patients with a low cardiac output state and evidence of inadequate tissue perfusion (oliguria, low central venous oxygen saturation, lactic acidosis, etc.), inotropes are often used to augment cardiac contractility. Dobutamine and milrinone are commonly used in patients with preserved blood pressure. These medications augment cardiac contractility and their vasodilating effects help to reduce afterload for the failing heart. Milrinone tends to cause more pulmonary vasodilation than dobutamine and can be useful in patients with right ventricular failure, especially in the setting of pulmonary hypertension [40]. Milrinone also tends to cause less tachycardia than dobutamine. In patients with hypotension and a low output state, dobutamine or milrinone can still be used despite their vasodilatory effects. However, in the setting of hypotension these inotropes must be administered in conjunction with a vasoconstricting agent, such as norepinephrine, in order to maintain blood pressure and coronary perfusion. It should be noted that milrinone has a relatively long half-life of hours, and unlike dobutamine, cannot be rapidly titrated down if the patient develops hypotension.

Dopamine is often used as a single agent for patients with cardiogenic shock and hypotension owing to its dual inotropic and vasoconstricting effects. However, in a large randomized trial comparing dopamine to norepinephrine for the treatment of shock, a subgroup analysis showed that patients with cardiogenic shock had a higher mortality and increased arrhythmias with the use of dopamine [42]. For this reason, norepinephrine may be a better first-line agent than dopamine for cardiogenic shock and hypotension. Epinephrine has been compared to combination dobutamine–norepinephrine in patients with cardiogenic shock and epinephrine was associated with a higher rate of tachyarrhythmias, lactic acidosis, and impaired gastric mucosal perfusion [51]. Phenylephrine is generally avoided in cardiogenic shock, as it adversely affects cardiac performance by increasing afterload without any favorable effects on cardiac contractility.

Neurogenic Shock

Patients with neurogenic shock have lost sympathetic input to the heart and vasculature as a result of a cervical spine injury. Vagal tone predominates, characteristically resulting in hypotension and bradycardia. For this reason, dopamine has been used as a first-line agent in light of its chronotropic and vasoconstricting properties [52]. There is some evidence that titrating vasopressors to achieve a supraphysiologic MAP of 85–90 mmHg may augment spinal cord perfusion and improve neurologic outcome in neurogenic shock [53].

Anaphylaxis

Epinephrine not only helps to restore hemodynamic stability, but also reduces mucosal edema in the upper airway and causes bronchodilation in patients with anaphylaxis. Therefore, epinephrine remains the first-line agent for this condition, given that it can counteract all of the life-threatening effects of an allergic reaction, including shock, airway edema, and bronchospasm. Epinephrine should be administered *intramuscularly* in the lateral thigh at a dose of 0.3–0.5 mg of **1:1000 (1 mg/mL)** solution for initial treatment of anaphylaxis [54]. The intramuscular dose can be repeated one to two times every 5 minutes as necessary based on the clinical response. In cases of impending circulatory collapse or conditions refractory to intramuscular therapy, epinephrine should be administered with the **1:10,000 (0.1 mg/mL)** solution intravenously at a rate of 1–20 mcg/minute and titrated to achieve a normal blood pressure.

Postintubation Hypotension

Hypotension occurs in up to a quarter of tracheal intubations performed in the ED [55]. Although hypotension can occur for a number of reasons, this complication frequently occurs as a result of vasodilation and sympatholysis from induction agents. The vasodilating effects of induction agents can be counteracted with the use of a bolus dose of phenylephrine, a technique that has been described in the anesthesia literature for reversing hypotension related to spinal anesthesia [56]. Bolus-dose phenylephrine can be prepared by mixing 2 mL of 10 mg/mL phenylephrine solution into a 250 mL bag of sterile D5W. Then 10 cc of this solution (80 mcg/mL) can be drawn up into a sterile syringe and administered in aliquots of 1–2 mL (80–160 mcg) as an intravenous bolus every few minutes as a need to stabilize the blood pressure. This technique is a good temporizing measuring following intubation until induction-related hypotension resolves or until a vasopressor infusion can be prepared and administered continuously.

Titration of Vasoactive Agents

Blood pressure is the most commonly used endpoint for titration of vasopressor agents. Providing an exact blood pressure to target for all patients is difficult, and in reality, the proper target for blood pressure likely varies from patient to patient. For example, a patient with baseline poorly controlled hypertension may have signs of inadequate organ perfusion despite a "normal blood pressure." The target blood pressure also may vary with the underlying shock state. For example, a higher endpoint blood pressure may improve neurologic outcome for neurogenic shock [53]. Clinical signs of global tissue perfusion, such as urine output and mental status, can be helpful to determine if a target blood pressure is adequate for individual patients. Nevertheless, clinicians need some minimum blood pressure to target while titrating vasopressors. MAP, rather than systolic blood pressure, is the driving pressure for peripheral blood flow, and there is some evidence that MAP may be a more accurate measure of end-organ perfusion than systolic blood pressure [57, 58]. Autoregulation maintains blood flow to vital organs at a constant level despite changes in perfusion pressure. However, below a MAP of 60 mmHg, organ perfusion becomes pressure-dependent. Thus, a MAP >65 mmHg is often cited as a minimum blood pressure target for titrating vasopressors in patients with shock [3, 59].

References

1. Katz AM. Ernest Henry Starling, his predecessors, and the "law of the heart". Circulation. 2002;106(23):2986–92.
2. Lee SJ, Ramar K, Park JG, Gajic O, Li G, Kashyap R. Increased fluid administration in the first three hours of sepsis resuscitation is associated with reduced mortality: a retrospective cohort study. Chest. 2014;146(4):908–15.
3. Rivers E, Nguyen B, Havstad S, Ressler J, Muzzin A, Knoblich B, et al. Early goal-directed therapy in the treatment of severe sepsis and septic shock. N Engl J Med. 2001;345(19):1368–77.
4. Michard F, Teboul JL. Predicting fluid responsiveness in the ICU patients: a critical analysis of the evidence. Chest. 2002;121(6):2000–8.
5. Vincent JL, Sakr Y, Sprung CL, Ranieri VM, Reinhart K, Gerlach H, et al. Sepsis in European intensive care units: results of the Soap study. Crit Care Med. 2006;34(2):344–53.
6. Wiedemann HP, Wheeler AP, Bernard GR, Thompson BT, Hayden D, deBoisblanc B, et al. Comparison of two fluid-management strategies in acute lung injury. N Engl J Med. 2006;354(24):2564–75.
7. Marik PE, Cavallazzi R. Does the central venous pressure predict fluid responsiveness? An updated meta-analysis and a plea for some common sense. Crit Care Med. 2013 Jul;41(7):1774–81.
8. Marik PE, Baram M, Vahid B. Does central venous pressure predict fluid responsiveness? A systematic review of the literature and the tale of seven mares. Chest. 2008;134(1):172–8.
9. Marik PE, Monnet X, Teboul JL. Hemodynamic parameters to guide fluid therapy. Ann Intensive Care. 2011;21(1):1.
10. Monnet X, Rienzo M, Osman D, Anquel N, Richard C, Pinsky MR, et al. Passive leg raising predicts fluid responsiveness in the critically ill. Crit Care Med. 2006;34:1402–7.
11. Lexicomp® Online. [Internet]. c1978–2014. Hetastarch (Lexi-Drugs). [Updated Nov 12, 2014; cited Nov 15, 2014]. Available from: https://online.lexi.com/.
12. Lexicomp Online. [Internet]. c1978–2014. Albumin (Lexi-Drugs). [Updated Sept 19, 2014, cited Nov 15, 2014]. Available from: https://online.lexi.com/.
13. Moore FD, Dagher FJ, Boyden CM, Lee CJ, Lyons JH. Hemorrhage in normal man. I. Distribution and dispersal of saline infusions following acute blood loss: clinical kinetics of blood volume support. Ann Surg. 1966;163:483–504.
14. Falk JL, Rackow EC, Weil MH. Colloid and crystalloid fluid resuscitation. Acute Care. 1983–84;10(2):59–94.

15. Annane D, Siami S, Jaber S, Martin C, Elatrous S, Declere AD, et al. Effects of fluid resuscitation with colloids vs crystalloids on mortality in critically ill patients presenting with hypovolemic shock: the CRISTAL randomized trial. JAMA. 2013;310(17):1809–17.
16. Churton E. Leed general infirmary: a case of scirrhus of the pylorus, with excessive vomiting; repeated intravenous injections of saline solution; remarks. Lancet. 1888;132:620–1.
17. Wilcox CS. Regulation of renal blood flow by plasma chloride. J Clin Invest. 1983;71(3):726–35.
18. McCluskey SA, Karkouti K, Wijeysundera D. Hyperchloremia after noncardiac surgery is independently associated with increased morbidity and mortality: a propensity-matched cohort study. Anesth Analg. 2013;117(2):412–21.
19. Yunos NM, Bellomo R, Hegarty C, Story D, Ho L, Bailey M. Association between a chloride-liberal vs chloride-restrictive intravenous fluid administration strategy and kidney injury in critically ill adults. JAMA. 2012;308:1566–72.
20. Raghunathan K, Shaw A, Nathanson B, Sturmer T, Brookhart A, Stefan MS, et al. Association between the choice of IV crystalloid and in-hospital mortality among critically ill adults with sepsis. Crit Care Med. 2014;42(7):1585–91.
21. McDermid RC, Raghunathan K, Romanovsky A, Shaw AD, Bagshaw SM. Controversies in fluid therapy: type, dose and toxicity. World J Crit Care Med. 2014;3(1):24–33.
22. Finfer S, Bellomo R, Boyce N, French J, Myburgh J, Norton R, et al. A comparison of albumin and saline for fluid resuscitation in the intensive care unit. N Engl J Med. 2004;350:2247–56.
23. Myburgh J, Cooper DJ, Finfer S, Bellomo R, Norton R, Bishop N, et al. Saline or albumin for fluid resuscitation in patients with traumatic brain injury. N Engl J Med. 2007;357(9):874–84.
24. Delaney AP, Dan A, McCaffrey J, Finfer S. The role of albumin as a resuscitation fluid for patients with sepsis: a systematic review and meta-analysis. Crit Care Med. 2011;39:386–91.
25. Finfer S, McEvoy S, Bellomo R, McArthur C, Myburgh J, Norton R, et al. Impact of albumin compared to saline on organ function and mortality of patients with severe sepsis. Intensive Care Med. 2011;37(1):86–96.
26. Dellinger RP, Levy MM, Rhodes A, Annane D, Gerlach H, Opal SM, et al. Surviving sepsis campaign: international guidelines for management of severe sepsis and septic shock: 2012. Crit Care Med. 2013;41(2):580–637.
27. Myburgh JA, Finfer S, Bellomo R, Billot CA, Gattas D, et al. Hydroxyethyl starch or saline for fluid resuscitation in intensive care. N Engl J Med. 2012;367(20):1901–11.
28. Treib J, Haass A, Pindur G. Coagulation disorders caused by hydroxyethyl starch. Thromb Haemost. 1997;78(3):974–83.
29. Brunkhorst FM, Engel C, Bloos F, Meier-Hellmann A, Ragaller M, Weiler N, et al. Intensive insulin therapy and pentastarch resuscitation in severe sepsis. N Engl J Med. 2008;358(2):125–39.
30. Perner A, Haase N, Guttormsen AB, Tenhunen J, Klemenzson G, Aneman A, et al. Hydroxyethyl starch 130/0.42 versus Ringer's acetate in severe sepsis. N Engl J Med. 2012;367(2):124–34.
31. FDA Safety Communication: Boxed Warning on increased mortality and severe renal injury, and additional warning on risk of bleeding, for use of hydroxyethyl starch solutions in some settings. [Internet]. [Revised Nov 15, 2013; cited Nov 15, 2014]. Available from: http://www.fda.gov/biologicsbloodvaccines/safetyavailability/ucm358271.htm.
32. Ducrocq N, Kimmoun A, Furmaniuk A, Hekalo Z, Maskali F, Poussier S, et al. Comparison of equipressor doses of norepinephrine, epinephrine, and phenylephrine on septic myocardial dysfunction. Anesthesiology. 2012;116(5):1083–91.
33. DeBacker D, Biston P, Devriendt J, Madl C, Chochrad D, Aldecoa C, et al. Comparison of dopamine and norepinephrine in the treatment of shock. N Engl J Med. 2010;362(9):779–89.
34. Bellomo R, Kellum JA, Wisniewski SR, Pinsky MR. Effects of norepinephrine on the renal vasculature in normal and endotoxemic dogs. Am J Respir Crit Care Med. 1999;159(4 Pt 1):1186–92.
35. Kellum JA, Decker JM. Use of dopamine in acute renal failure: a meta-analysis. Crit Care Med. 2001;29(8):1526–31.
36. Marik PE, Mohedin M. The contrasting effects of dopamine and norepinephrine on systemic and splanchinic oxygen utilization in hyperdynamic sepsis. JAMA. 1994;272(17):1354–7.
37. Levy B. Bench-to-bedside review: is there a place for epinephrine in septic shock? Crit Care. 2005;9(6):561–5.
38. Levy B, Gibot S, Franck P, Cravoisy A, Bollaert PE. Relation between muscle N+K+ ATPase activity and raised lactate concentrations in septic shock: a prospective study. Lancet. 2005; 365(9462):871–5.
39. Tisdale JE, Patel R, Web CR, Borzak S, Zarowitz BJ. Electrophysiologic and proarrhythmic effects of intravenous inotropic agents. Prog Cardiovasc Dis. 1995;38(2):167–80.
40. Price LC, Wort SJ, Finney SJ, Marino PS, Brett SJ. Pulmonary vascular and right ventricular dysfunction in adult critical care: current and emergency options for management: a systematic literature review. Crit Care. 2010;14(5):R169.
41. Barrett LK, Orie NN, Taylor V, Stidwell RP, Clapp LH, Singer M. Differential effects of vasopressin and norepinephrine on vascular reactivity in a long-term rodent model of sepsis. Crit Care Med. 2007;35(10):2337–43.
42. DeBacker D, Aldecoa C, Njimi H, Vincent JL. Dopamine versus norepinephrine in the treat-

ment of septic shock: a meta-analysis. Crit Care Med. 2012;40(3):725–30.
43. Morelli A, Ertmer C, Rehber S, Lange M, Orecchioni A, Laderchi A, et al. Phenylephrine versus norepinephrine for initial hemodynamic support of patients with septic shock: a randomized, controlled trial. Crit Care. 2008;12(6):R143.
44. Court O, Kumar A, Parrillo JE, Kumar A. Myocardial depression in sepsis and septic shock. Crit Care. 2002;6(6):500–8.
45. Annane D, Vignon P, Renault A, Bollaert PE, Charpentier C, Martin C, et al. Norepinephrine plus dobutamine versus epinephrine alone for management of septic shock : a randomised trial. Lancet. 2007;370:676–84.
46. Meier-Hellmann A, Reinhart K, Bredle DL, Specht M, Spies CD, Hanneman L. Epinephrine impairs splanchnic perfusion in septic shock. Crit Care Med. 1997;25(3):399–404.
47. Duranteau J, Sitbon P, Teboul JL, Vicaut E, Anguel N, Richard C, et al. Effects of epinephrine, norepinephrine, or the combination of norepinephrine and dobutamine on gastric mucosa in septic shock. Crit Care Med. 1999;27(5):893–900.
48. Russell JA. Bench to bedside review: vasopressin in the management of septic shock. Crit Care. 2011;15(4):226.
49. Russell JA, Walley KR, Singer J, Gordon AC, Hebert PC, Cooper DJ, et al. Vasopressin versus norepinephrine infusion in patients with septic shock. N Engl J Med. 2008;358(9):877–87.
50. Lauzier F, Levy B, Lamarre P, Lesur O. Vasopressin or norepinephrine in early hyperdynamic septic shock: a randomized clinical trial. Intensive Care Med. 2006;32(11):1782–9.
51. Levy B, Perez P, Perny J, Thivilier C, Gerard A. Comparison of norepineprhine-dobutamine to epineprhine for hemodynamics, lactate metabolism, and organ function variables in cardiogenic shock: a prospective, randomized pilot study. Crit Care Med. 2011;39(3):450–5.
52. Blood pressure management after acute spinal cord injury. Neurosurgery. 2002;50(3):S58–62.
53. Vale FL, Burns J, Jackson AB, Hadley MN. Combined medical and surgical treatment after acute spinal cord injury: results of a prospective pilot study to assess the merits of aggressive medical resuscitation and blood pressure management. J Neurosurg. 1997;87(2):239–46.
54. Simons FE, Gu X, Simons KJ. Epineprhine absorption in adults: intramuscular versus subcutaneous injection. J Allergy Clin Immunol. 2001;108(5):871–3.
55. Heffner AC, Swords D, Kline JA, Jone AE. The frequency and significance of postintubation hypotension during emergency airway management. J Crit Care. 2012;27(4):417.
56. Doherty A, Ohashi Y, Downey K, Carvalho JC. Phenylephrine infusion versus bolus regimens during cesarean delivery under spinal anesthesia: a double-blind randomized clinical trial to assess hemodynamic changes. Anesth Analg. 2012;115(6):1343–50.
57. Pinsky MR, Payen D. Functional hemodynamic monitoring. Crit Care. 2005;9(6):566–72.
58. Lehman LW, Saeed M, Talmor D, Mark R, Malhotra A. Methods of blood pressure measurement in the ICU. Crit Care Med. 2013;41(1):34–40.
59. LeDoux D, Astiz ME, Carpati CM, Rackow EC. Effects of perfusion pressure on tissue perfusion in septic shock. Crit Care Med. 2000;28(8):2729–32.

Blood Products

35

Joseph R. Shiber

Critical Points

- The initial Hgb and Hct in acute blood loss do not reflect the actual extent of hemorrhage.
- Clinical evaluation is required to judge the degree of acute blood loss by vital signs and physical examination: tachycardia, orthostasis, narrowed pulse pressure, pallor, cool extremities, and delayed capillary refill.
- Even critically ill patients with chronic anemia can tolerate Hgb level of 7 g/dL, except those with preexisting coronary, pulmonary, or cerebrovascular disease.
- A 70-kg man has a circulating blood volume of ~5 L (70 cc/kg so 70 × 70 = 4900), so 10u of whole blood.
- Transfusion of 10 or more units of RBC in 24 h meets criteria for mass transfusion.
- Risk factors that predict the need for massive transfusion include abnormal vital signs on presentation with tachycardia (HR >120) and hypotension (SBP <90), pH below 7.25, initial Hct less than 32%, a penetrating mechanism of trauma, and a positive FAST.
- The platelet count should be kept higher than 50,000/μL in a patient who is actively bleeding and even higher (>100,000/μL) for microvascular bleeding involving the central nervous system.
- If signs or symptoms of a transfusion reaction emerge, the blood product should be halted immediately, while the patient is assessed and the blood bank is notified.

Introduction

A total of 1.4 million units of red blood cell (RBC) concentrates, also known as packed RBCs, and 1.6 million units of platelets are transfused in the United States each year [1]. The number of transfusions in ICUs declined slightly, as physicians adopted more conservative transfusion policies despite the fact that the total number of transfusions increased by 6% during the past decade [2–4]. In this chapter, the indications for blood product administration – whole blood, packed RBCs, platelets, fresh frozen plasma (FFP), cryoprecipitate, and albumin – are reviewed and the procedures for safe and expedi-

J. R. Shiber (✉)
College of Medicine, University of Florida Health Science Center, Jacksonville, FL, USA
e-mail: Joseph.Shiber@jax.ufl.edu

© Springer Nature Switzerland AG 2020
J. R. Shiber, S. D. Weingart (eds.), *Emergency Department Critical Care*,
https://doi.org/10.1007/978-3-030-28794-8_35

ent transfusion are described, along with the potential adverse effects associated with blood product administration and the recommended treatment of these complications.

Transfusion of blood products are intended to prevent and treat shock, hypovolemia, and coagulopathy; to maintain oxygen-carrying capacity; and to maintain vascular oncotic pressure without causing adverse effects [5–8]. In the original era of transfusion medicine, whole blood was commonly given, with a preference for "fresh" whole blood (stored for less than 24 h at 22 °C). A unit of whole blood (450 mL at collection, with 60 mL of anticoagulant added, for a total volume of 510 mL) has a shelf life of 35 days, but the platelet function and coagulant factor quickly degrade. Modern blood-banking practices, including the separation of whole blood into distinct components, increase the viability of blood products. For example, packed RBCs have a shelf life of 42 days, and frozen RBC concentrates, typically reserved for autologous donation or rare antibody cross-matched blood, can be kept for 10 years, but must be used within 24 h of thawing [7]. Previously, whole blood transfusion was rarely given outside combat hospital situations, but it is now being used at some civilian trauma centers [7, 9].

A single unit of packed RBCs will raise the hemoglobin (Hgb) level by approximately 1 g/dL and the hematocrit (Hct) by 3% in a 70-kg patient without ongoing blood loss [3, 7]. The average half-life of a transfused RBC is 57.7 days as compared to 120 days of a "native host" RBC. Patients with pure RBC aplasia typically require a two-unit transfusion approximately every 2 weeks [7].

For a critically ill or injured patient, "emergency release" blood is type O, the universal RBC donor; O Rh-negative blood is a precious resource and is reserved for girls and women with childbearing potential in order to prevent Rh (D) antibody complications [1]. Type-specific blood, which can be given if necessary, for ongoing hemorrhage or uncorrected shock after the emergency release blood, is usually available 15 minutes after the specimen is received in the blood bank. Cross-matching will take 45–60 minutes if no antibodies are detected [1, 3]. Platelets, plasma, and cryoprecipitate must be ABO compatible but do not require cross-matching. AB plasma is the universal plasma donor since it does not contain anti-A or anti-B antibodies. Platelets are usually available in 5–15 minutes, and plasma and cryoprecipitate in 5–30 minutes, respectively, due to their thawing of different volumes of frozen blood product [1, 9].

Red Blood Cell Transfusion

Indications for RBC transfusion are listed in Table 35.1. RBC transfusion can increase oxygen delivery, expand blood volume, alleviate symptoms of acute blood loss anemia, and relieve cardiac ischemia [10, 11]. A clear distinction needs to be made between chronic anemia, which can be well tolerated by otherwise healthy individuals, and acute hemorrhage, which represents loss of red cell mass and intravascular volume. The initial Hgb and Hct in acute blood loss do not reflect the actual extent of hemorrhage since the recruitment of interstitial and intracellular fluid into the intravascular space is not immediate. Unless crystalloid or colloid is given to replace the blood volume lost, Hgb and Hct will significantly underestimate the hemorrhage [7, 12]. Clinical evaluation is required to judge the degree of acute blood loss by vital signs and physical examination findings such as tachycardia, orthostasis, narrowed pulse pressure (decreased systolic pressure due to reduced cardiac filling and output but increased diastolic

Table 35.1 Indications for red blood cell transfusion

Evidence of class 3–4 hemorrhagic shock
Acute blood loss of >15–20% estimated blood volume
Symptomatic anemia in a euvolemic patient
Hgb <7 g/dL in a critically ill patient
Hgb <8 g/dL in a patient with an acute coronary syndrome or ischemic stroke
Hgb <9 g/dL preoperatively with expected blood loss of >500 mL
Hgb <10 g/dL in a possibly euvolemic patient with evidence of tissue hypoxemia
Sickle cell acute chest syndrome if Hgb <10 g/dL or Hgb-SS >30%

pressure due to intense vasoconstriction), pallor, cool extremities, and delayed capillary refill. Frank arterial hypotension is a late finding in acute blood loss [3].

At rest, oxygen delivery is four times greater than tissue utilization in a healthy person. Even with an isolated decrease in Hgb to 10 g/dL, oxygen delivery will still be twice that needed for resting consumption [13]. Signs and symptoms of anemia are unlikely to be evident at Hgb values above 7 or 8 g/dL in healthy patients. Even critically ill patients with chronic anemia can tolerate an Hgb level of 7 g/dL, except those with preexisting coronary, pulmonary, or cerebrovascular disease [5, 7, 11]. The anemic patient has a diminished arterial oxygen content but is able to increase oxygen delivery by increasing cardiac output and increasing coronary blood flow through vasodilation. Myocardial oxygen extraction increases from 25% at baseline up to approximately 50% where the anaerobic threshold is reached and myocardial lactate levels increase [7]. Therefore, the current recommendations for packed RBC transfusions are more liberal in patients with coronary artery disease, particularly those with acute myocardial ischemia [1, 6, 13, 14]. Clinical judgment and data such as lactate levels and/or central venous oxygen saturation should be used to assess each case individually for the benefits and risks of transfusion versus the risks of ongoing anemia [1, 12, 14].

In a previously healthy patient with blood loss of less than 20–25% of blood volume without ongoing blood loss, only volume restoration with crystalloid or colloid is needed [3, 6]. If the total blood volume loss exceeds 20–25% (with a normal blood volume of 70 mL/kg), regardless of the presenting blood indices, RBC transfusion may be indicated. Transfusion can be indicated at even lower percentages of blood volume loss if there is a high risk of ongoing hemorrhage such as in a trauma patient, a woman with postpartum hemorrhage, or a patient with high-risk gastrointestinal bleeding, such as in end-stage liver disease. Patients with sickle cell anemia can require RBC transfusion to begin in the emergency department such as in acute chest syndrome where an Hct goal of 30% and an Hgb-sickle of less than 30% should be targeted [8].

Massive Transfusion

The term massive transfusion describes the administration of more than 10 units of blood, or an amount equal to the patient's total blood volume (TBV), within 24 h [3]. Updated dynamic definitions also include replacement of >50% of TBV within 3 h, and transfusion of >4 RBC units within 1 h with anticipated need for ongoing blood products [15–17]. Massive transfusion is needed by 1–3% of civilian trauma patients as well as with gastrointestinal bleeding, ruptured abdominal aortic aneurysm, ruptured ectopic pregnancy, and obstetric or postpartum hemorrhage [9, 18]. Risk factors that predict the need for massive transfusion include any of the following: abnormal vital signs on presentation (tachycardia and hypotension), pH below 7.25, Hct less than 32%, a penetrating mechanism of trauma, and evidence of hemoperitoneum on bedside ultrasonography (FAST) [18]. Critically ill or injured patients who have sustained significant blood loss are likely to present with coagulopathy resulting from platelet and clotting factor consumption as well as tissue hypoperfusion, acidosis, and hypothermia, all causing dysfunction of the remaining coagulation factors and platelets [3, 9, 18]. Resuscitation with crystalloid, colloid, or packed RBCs alone can cause further dilutional coagulopathy. Early trauma-induced coagulopathy (ETIC) develops in up to 56% of severely injured patients within 30 minutes of injury, even prior to PRBC and fluid resuscitation. The mechanism of coagulopathy involves not only the factors mentioned above but also increased thrombomodulin expression on endothelial cells due to hypoperfusion, which leads to protein C activation and inhibition of factors V and VIII. Fibrinolysis is also enhanced by accelerated plasmin formation and depletion of plasminogen activator inhibitor- 1 (PAI-1) leading to hyperfibrinolysis and subsequent fibrinogen depletion. Development of ETIC is an independent predictor of mortality separate from the injury severity [15, 19–21].

Hemostatic resuscitation (Table 35.2) describes the early use of all blood components in order to give the equivalent of whole blood in an effort to prevent or treat the coagulopathy associated with massive transfusions [15]. Using an equal ratio of packed RBC units, FFP, and platelet units (so-called 1:1:1 resuscitation) is the nearest substitute for whole blood and has been associated with decreased mortality in trauma patients receiving massive transfusion [3, 9, 18]. A transfusion made up of this 1:1:1 (one unit each of PRBC, FFP, and platelets) would be 645 ml and have a Hct of 29–30%, a platelet count of 80–90 × 10^9/L, and approximately 60–65% of coagulation factor activity, which is clearly not equal to whole blood [9]. For this reason, crystalloid and colloid infusion should be limited in patients requiring massive transfusion to prevent further dilutional coagulopathy and thrombocytopenia, while allowing permissive hypotension without shock (lower than "normal" BP target but enough to support end-organ function) until definitive control of hemorrhage has been achieved. The strategy of hemostatic resuscitation includes giving plasma and platelets early to limit ongoing hemorrhage requiring more blood products [9, 18].

Point-of-care testing of hemostasis using thromboelastography (TEG) may be helpful at identifying coagulopathy and guiding the blood products used during MTP [15, 16, 22]. Conventional coagulation assays, such as PT and aPTT, are not very useful in the prediction of the need for MTP nor for directing blood component therapy during the ongoing resuscitation due to their slow turnaround times. TEG can be available more rapidly and provide quantitative measurements of the individual components involved in hemostasis. Unlike PT and aPTT which only measure secondary hemostasis, TEG is able to measure all of the phases necessary for adequate clot formation such as platelet function in primary hemostasis, coagulation factor activity (VII, VIII, and X), and cross-linking of the fibrin to strengthen the clot. TEG also detects hyperfibrinolysis, a main contributor to ETIC which is not detected by conventional coagulation assays. A critical usage for TEG is to help determine "medical" from "surgical" bleeding in a postoperative patient since if it is found that a bleeding patient has abnormalities on TEG (Figs. 35.1 and 35.2), then the appropriate component will be given and then a repeat TEG will be checked to verify correction; if the patient is still bleeding when all aspects of hemostasis are normal by TEG, then the bleeding is not due to coagulopathy, but instead a vascular source that requires a surgical/mechanical intervention. Use of TEG can be considered part of goal-directed hemostatic resuscitation, similar to serum lactate in a shock patient, since it is checked initially and then repeated after interventions until it normalizes and the patient has had clinical improvement. Using TEG to guide blood product administration has been shown to reduce the transfusion requirements and need for MTP activation but has not been found thus far to conclusively reduce mortality in these patients [15, 16, 21, 23, 24].

Table 35.2 Hemostatic resuscitation guidelines

Expedite control of hemorrhage to reduce the need for blood products and prevent consumptive coagulopathy and thrombocytopenia
Limit crystalloid infusion to prevent dilutional coagulopathy
Goal systolic blood pressure of 80–100 mm Hg until definitive hemorrhage control is achieved
Transfuse at 1:1:1 ratio of packed RBCs/FFP/platelets (1 apheresis unit = 5 platelet units)
Frequently monitor potassium, ionized calcium, lactate, and blood gas values

Common Initial MTP "Package": 6 PRBC units (O- for women and O+ for men), 4–6 Plasma units (AB initially but A can be given safely), 1 Platelet apheresis with Cryoprecipitate given on an individual basis. Implementing a MTP is generally believed to improve the speed by which blood products are available by optimal coordination between the blood bank, laboratory services, and clinical team [25].

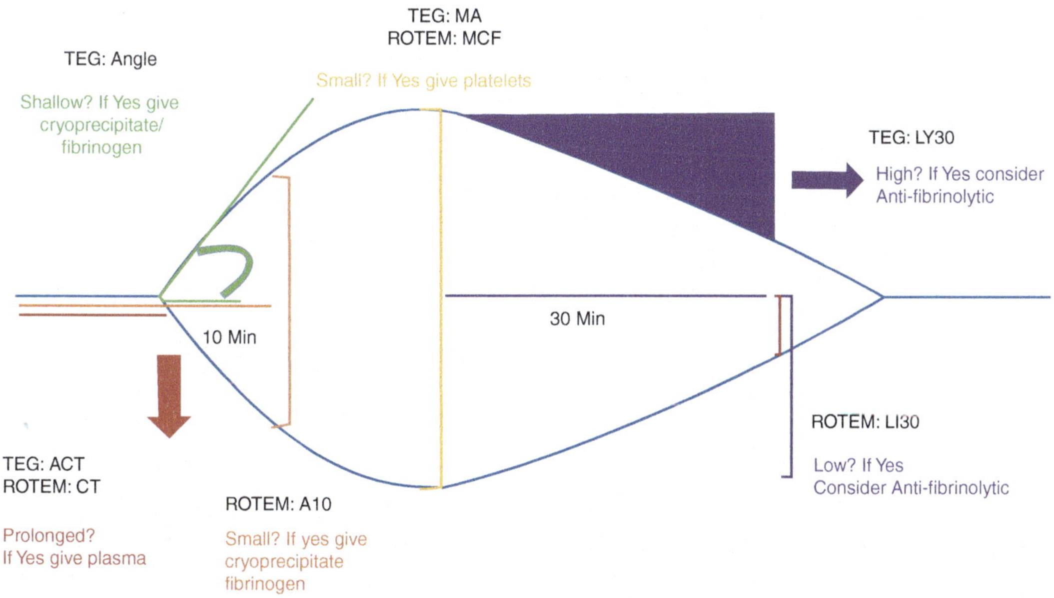

Fig. 35.1 Representative thromboelastogram tracing (Moore et al. [39])

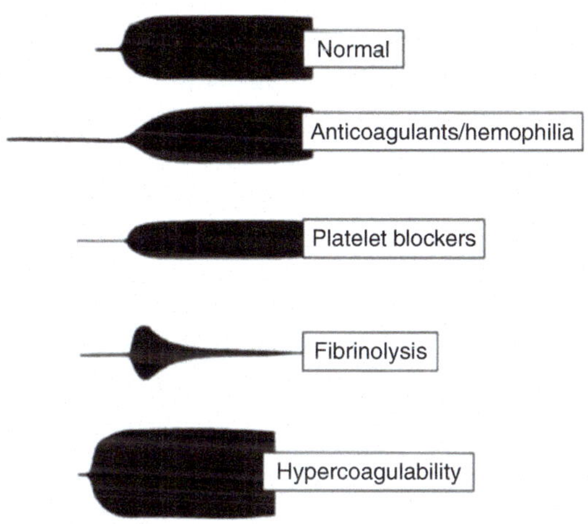

Fig. 35.2 Examples of normal compared to abnormal TEG tracings (da Luz et al. [40])

Platelet Transfusion

Platelet units are obtained by separating them from single-donor units of whole blood or, more commonly, by apheresis. An apheresis platelet unit, which contains 4.2 × 10^{11} platelets, is equivalent to four to six individual platelet units, each containing 8 × 10^{10} platelets [2, 12]. Each unit also contains approximately 50 mL of plasma [7]. Platelets are stored at room temperature (22 °C) for up to 5 days. Each platelet unit can be expected to increase the platelet count of a 75-kg patient by 5000–10,000/μL, and an apheresis unit will raise the count by 20,000–40,000/μL [8, 16]. Approximately one-third of all circulating platelets, whether transfused or native ones released from the marrow, are pooled in the spleen; this number is larger in patients with splenomegaly. The in vivo lifespan of a platelet is 9–10 days [26].

The indications for platelet transfusion in nonbleeding critically ill patient are different from the intent of transfusions to control bleeding. To maintain the integrity of the vascular endothelium by filling the gaps in the junctions between endothelial cells requires 7000 platelets per microliter. When the number of circulating platelets falls below 7000, mucosal surfaces start to bleed and measured blood in the stool increases [7, 26]. The platelet count should be kept higher than 50,000/μL in a patient who is actively bleeding and even higher (>100,000/μL) if the patient has microvascular bleeding, particularly if it involves the central nervous system

Table 35.3 Guidelines for platelet transfusions in various clinical scenarios

Stable patient without increased bleeding risk: <10,000/μL
Patient with increased bleeding risk: <20,000/μL
For bedside procedure: <20,000–30,000/μL
For most surgery: <40,000–50,000/μL (except neurologic/ ophthalmologic surgery: <100,000/μL)
For bleeding: <50,000/μL (except central nervous system or retinal bleeding: <100,000/μL)

or retina [6, 7]. To decrease the chance of hemorrhage in a patient without recognized risk factors for bleeding, platelets should be transfused when the count is below 10,000/μL. Platelet transfusion thresholds for other clinical scenarios are listed in Table 35.3.

Platelet transfusion is contraindicated in certain groups of patients with thrombocytopenia such as thrombotic thrombocytopenic purpura, hemolytic uremic syndrome, or heparin-induced thrombocytopenia, as it will "add fuel to the fire" and worsen the microvascular thrombosis. Platelet transfusion may not be deleterious but is unlikely to be effective in patients with thrombocytopenia caused by immune-mediated platelet destruction [6, 8, 26].

Plasma Transfusion

One unit of plasma contains between 200 and 280 mL of fluid volume. After separation from whole blood, it can be frozen for up to 1 year but must be used within 24 h after thawing [7]. Each milliliter of FFP contains approximately 1 unit of each coagulation factor and 2 mg of fibrinogen. One unit of FFP contains about 500 mg of fibrinogen, twice as much as is in a unit of cryoprecipitate but in a much larger volume, and should increase clotting factors by 5% [27]. A critically ill hemorrhaging patient should initially receive AB plasma, which is usually immediately available but in limited supply so that subsequent units can be group A if type type-specific plasma is not available and is well tolerated without complications [7, 8]. Since it takes 25–30 minutes to thaw frozen plasma, it is necessary to keep some already thawed immediately available for critical patients [15, 17].

There is a difference between the use of plasma transfusion to prevent bleeding and to treat bleeding. Spontaneous bleeding does not usually occur until the prothrombin time (PT), partial thromboplastin time (PTT), or international normalized ratio (INR) is more than 1.5 times higher than normal; therefore, there is little benefit from plasma transfusion in a nonbleeding patient with coagulation function tests below these levels. The exception is patients in need of neurosurgical or ophthalmologic procedures, who may be at increased risk for devastating results of hemorrhage; in these situations, a value of 1.3 times higher than normal is the threshold for plasma transfusion [8]. The dose that will commonly achieve hemostasis is 10–20 mL/kg which would raise clotting factor levels by 15–30%, but 30 mL/kg should be given if the patient is critically ill and bleeding [7, 8, 27]. This dose may be repeated in 4–6 h to maintain adequate factor levels, or a constant infusion may be given until hemostasis is achieved. Prothrombin complex concentrate (PCC) has been used for congenital bleeding disorders and for reversal of warfarin induced coagulopathy but has not been fully evaluated in critically hemorrhaging patients. It contains factors II, VII, IX, and X in varying amounts between different products. PCC provides similar effects as FFP but in a smaller volume that can be infused quickly and does not need to be thawed [15, 28].

The common clinical indications for plasma transfusion are listed in Table 35.4. It can take

Table 35.4 Indications for plasma transfusion

Massive transfusion protocol
Hemorrhage in liver disease
Disseminated intravascular coagulation
Multiple coagulation factor deficiency
Thrombotic thrombocytopenic purpura
Rapid reversal of warfarin effect
Prevention of bleeding if PT/PTT/INR >1.5 × normal (except for central nervous system or retinal bleeding, then >1.3 × normal)
Acute angioedema caused by C1 esterase inhibitor deficiency

12–18 h for vitamin K to correct the factor deficiency (II, VII, IX, and X) induced by warfarin, so in a symptomatic or high-risk patient, plasma transfusion is indicated for more rapid reversal. Vitamin K should still be given in order for the liver to make new host clotting factors as the transfused factors have a short half-life and although the PT/INR will drop initially it will rise again if Vitamin K is not given. If a single factor deficiency is known to be present, it is preferable to use specific replacement factors that are purified, that are standardized in activity, and that carry an extremely low risk of infectious disease transmission (or no risk if they are made by a recombinant process) [7, 8]. Plasma transfusion is also indicated for treatment of thrombotic thrombocytopenic purpura, hemolytic uremic syndrome, and the syndrome of hemolysis, elevated liver enzymes, and low platelets. Plasmapheresis can also be required, but there can be a delay in obtaining vascular access and the staffing necessary for plasmapheresis, so early administration of plasma in the emergency department can be lifesaving [7, 8]. Acute angioedema, particularly if caused by C1 esterase inhibitor deficiency, is also an indication for plasma administration. Plasma transfusion may be necessary for disseminated intravascular coagulation if bleeding is the clinical feature causing the most concern.

A newly recognized but important benefit of plasma transfusion is the impact on endothelial cell function. By effects on the endothelial cells and the extracellular matrix, plasma reduces endothelial permeability, improves thrombin generation, and vascular vasomotor stability. These favorable effects decrease vascular space loss into the interstitial tissue, help maintain arterial blood pressure, and support hemostasis [27].

Cryoprecipitate Transfusion

Cryoprecipitate is obtained when a unit of frozen plasma is thawed at 4 °C. The 10–15 mL of plasma that precipitates out of this thawing contains fibrinogen, factor VIII, von Willebrand factor, and factor XIII. Each unit of cryoprecipitate contains 80–100 units of factor VIII activity and 150–200 mg of fibrinogen [6, 8, 14]. This is a smaller amount of fibrinogen than is contained in plasma but it is more concentrated, so cryoprecipitate can be a better choice when volume overload is a concern. As with FFP, cryoprecipitate requires ABO compatibility but not cross-matching.

A dose of 2–4 units/kg can be expected to increase the fibrinogen level by 60–100 mg/dL [7]. A fibrinogen level above 150–200 mg/ dL is the goal of cryoprecipitate transfusion for any bleeding patient; below this level, PT and PTT values will be elevated despite sufficient clotting factors. Below 150–200 mg/dL level, perioperative and postoperative bleeding increases [28]. Cryoprecipitate transfusion is indicated for any deficient fibrinogen state such as with massive transfusion, disseminated intravascular coagulation, congenital hypofibrinogenemia, or reversal of thrombolytic therapy; it is also indicated for factor XIII deficiency [7, 8, 15]. Transfusion of cryoprecipitate is an option for factor VIII deficiency and von Willebrand disease if the respective factor concentrates are unavailable. It has also been given for bleeding abnormalities associated with uremia, but desmopressin is the preferred treatment for this disorder [7, 8].

Albumin Transfusion

Albumin provides 80% of intravascular oncotic pressure so that patients with disease states associated with low albumin levels such as cirrhosis and nephrotic syndrome can require albumin transfusion to aid in maintaining intravascular volume. Albumin is derived from human sources but is heat treated so that it is unable to transmit viruses. It is available as a 5% solution, which is oncotically equivalent to normal plasma, and a 25% solution, which is hyperoncotic and able to pull three to four times the volume administered from the interstitial space into the vascular space [8]. The typical dose is 50–100 mL, but if the patient does not have adequate extravascular

Table 35.5 Indications for albumin transfusion

Nephrotic syndrome resistant to diuretics
Volume replacement with plasmapheresis
Fluid resuscitation for sepsis or burns associated with interstitial edema
Prevention of vascular collapse after large-volume paracentesis

hydration, then additional isotonic fluids should also be given. After 4 h, 50% of infused albumin is lost to the extravascular space. Indications for albumin transfusion are listed in Table 35.5.

Adverse Effects of Transfusions

Complications from blood component therapy include acute immunologic transfusion reactions, allergic reactions, volume overload, viral or bacterial transmission, acute lung injury, and immunomodulating effects associated with an increased risk of nosocomial infection and multiorgan failure (Table 35.6) [11, 14, 26, 29, 30]. The risk of a transfusion-related adverse event is 10%, and the risk of it being a serious event is 0.5% [1]. ABO incompatibility reactions, previously the leading cause of transfusion-related morbidity and mortality, have decreased with improved clerical and nursing documentation and verification policies. Unfortunately, they have been replaced by transfusion-related acute lung injury (TRALI) [31]. The third most common cause of serious transfusion-related complications, including death, is bacterial contamination of blood products [1].

Hemolytic transfusion reactions occur when preformed IgM against ABO antigens causes complement activation and intravascular hemolysis. Patients experience fever, chills, dyspnea, hypotension, tachycardia, and diffuse myalgias along with hemoglobinemia and hemoglobinuria. The haptoglobin level will fall and bilirubin will be elevated. The main causes of hemolytic transfusion reactions are patient misidentification and clerical blood-banking errors.

Nonhemolytic transfusion reactions are caused by an amnestic response against non-ABO erythrocyte antigens that were not identified by the cross-match testing. Complement is not activated, but RBCs are cleared by the reticuloendothelial system 2–10 days later. The clinical picture is less severe than with hemolytic transfusion reactions, and there is modest elevation of bilirubin without hemoglobinemia and hemoglobinuria [1, 8]. Allergic reactions are common, occurring in about 1% of all transfusions. Most are mild, consisting of pruritus and hives; frank anaphylaxis is rare.

Table 35.6 Clinical presentation of the transfusion reaction types

Acute hemolytic	Fever, chills, dyspnea, tachycardia, hypotension, back/flank pain
Febrile	Fever, chills (patient not ill appearing)
Mild allergic	Urticaria, pruritus
Anaphylactic	Bronchospasm, dyspnea, angioedema, tachycardia, hypotension
TRALI	Dyspnea, decreased arterial oxygen saturation, fever, hypotension, normal/low central venous pressure
Hypervolemic	Dyspnea, headache, tachycardia, hypertension, elevated central venous pressure
Septic	Fever, chills, hypotension, tachycardia, vomiting

The risk of disease transmission per unit of blood transfused is 1:2 million for HIV, 1:500,000 for hepatitis B, and 1:2 million for hepatitis C [8, 26]. The risk for bacterial infection transmission (which is highest for platelets, since they are stored at room temperature to keep their activity) is 1:2000–3000 platelet units. Fortunately, only 1 in 5000 contaminated units causes sepsis [16, 32]. Bacteria can be transferred if the skin preparation at the phlebotomy site was unsterile, if the donor had transient bacteremia, if a blood-banking procedure was not sterile, or if the integrity of the bag or tubing was breeched. Gram-negative rods (*Serratia*, *Pseudomonas*, *Yersinia*, *Enterobacter*, and *Salmonella*) and gram-positive cocci (*Staphylococcus* and *Streptococcus*) are the most common organisms [7].

TRALI occurs after 1 in 1000–5000 units of blood products are transfused, the highest risk being associated with plasma-containing transfusions [7, 33, 34]. It is caused by the transfusion recipient's having neutrophils that are already "primed" by a prior stimulus (e.g., trauma, infection, and malignancy) and adherent to the pulmonary endothelium, which are then stimulated by donor antileukocyte antibodies in the blood product [35]. The activated neutrophils cause diffuse pulmonary capillary leak, leading to noncardiogenic pulmonary edema. Dyspnea, decreased oxygen saturation, and bilateral fluffy pulmonary infiltrates, with a normal left ventricular end-diastolic pressure, occur within 6 h after transfusion. TRALI typically resolves within 72 h but has a mortality rate of up to 20% [36, 37].

Prevention of adverse effects is crucial and begins with scrupulous adherence to blood-bank policies to prevent incompatibility reactions. Irradiation of blood products, which prevents donor leukocytes from replicating, should be ordered for patients at risk for graft-versus-host disease as follows: severe cellular immunodeficiency (but not AIDS), currently on potent chemotherapeutic regimens, after bone marrow transplant, and those receiving transfusions from biologic relatives. Graft-versus-host disease has no effective treatment and a 90% mortality rate [6–8]. All blood products should be given with an isotonic non-calcium-containing solution such as normal saline to prevent hemolysis and clotting [8]. Unless the patient is in hemorrhagic shock, the transfusion should be started at a slow rate for the first 15 minutes while the patient is monitored closely for signs of a transfusion reaction since the main determinant of the severity of such a reaction is the volume of blood transfused [7].

If any signs or symptoms suggesting a transfusion reaction emerge, the blood product should be halted immediately while the patient is assessed, and the blood bank is notified. If the allergic reaction is mild, the patient should be treated with acetaminophen and diphenhydramine, and the transfusion can be continued safely. An anaphylactic reaction should be treated appropriately, and the patient should not be rechallenged by continuing the transfusion. Treatment for hemolytic transfusion reactions includes intravenous volume expansion and diuretics to maintain urine output at more than 100 mL/h and bicarbonate to raise the urinary pH above 7.0. The treatment of TRALI is supportive: Oxygen and positive-pressure ventilation are effective, but there is no role for diuretics or steroids [36, 37].

Each blood product should be given over a maximum of 4 h to decrease bacterial contamination [7, 8]. If the patient's volume status is labile or if there is concern about congestive heart failure, each unit can be split by the blood bank so it can be given even more slowly and diuretics may be administered [24]. Rapid transfusion, as in a massive transfusion protocol, can be associated with hypothermia if more than 100 mL/min of volume is given for more than 30 minutes without using a blood-warming device. Other complications of rapid transfusion include hypocalcemia due to citrate toxicity, alkalosis due to citrate conversion, and hyperkalemia due to potassium release from stored erythrocytes [6–8]. Each 1 mL of blood contains 1 mg of iron, so there are about 250 mg in a unit of packed RBCs [7]. This iron load can be helpful in a patient with iron deficiency, but it could be deleterious to a patient who requires frequent transfusions.

Transfusions activate an inflammatory cascade and have immunomodulating effects that are associated with immunosuppression, increased risk of nosocomial infections, acute lung injury, and increased mortality [2, 14, 29]. An example of the importance of considering the risk versus the benefit of the transfusion is demonstrated by one study that found that patients hospitalized for acute coronary syndrome had improved outcome if they received an RBC transfusion for an Hgb of less than 8 g/dL, particularly if they were elderly, but they had a worse outcome if they were transfused when their Hgb was above 8 g/dL [13].

Adjunctive Therapies

Several nonblood products may be considered to augment or replace a transfusion strategy in specific situations. Recombinant activated factor VII (rFVIIa) initiates the extrinsic coagulation pathway when complexed with tissue factor at sites of injury. Currently, rFVIIa is approved by the U.S. Food and Drug Administration (FDA) only for the treatment of hemophilia and factor VII deficiency; however, it has been used with some success in coagulopathic trauma patients, decreasing the need for massive transfusion, the amount of total blood products transfused, and the incidence of organ failure. An increase in vascular thromboembolic events in treated patients has been documented and overall has not been shown to improve outcomes in trauma or surgical patients [9, 18]. Desmopressin increases endothelial cell release of von Willebrand factor molecules. Desmopressin is FDA approved for the treatment of hemophilia A and von Willebrand disease type 1, but it is also used clinically for uremic bleeding at a dose of 0.3 ug/kg administered intravenously [27]. Aminocaproic acid inhibits plasmin, and is approved by the FDA for the enhancement of hemostasis in any hyperfibrinolytic state such as certain acute leukemias or after fibrinolytic therapy [9, 18]. Tranexamic acid (TXA), another antifibrinolytic, has been shown to reduce mortality in military and civilian trauma patients, particularly if given early (<3 h from injury but preferably within the first hour) [38]. If ETIC is confirmed by hyperfibrinolysis on TEG, then TXA should be administered even if later than 3 h from injury since it will still have benefits and appears to have minimal risk. Additionally, it should be given whenever an MTP is initiated; the dose is 1 g load and then 1 g infusion over 8 h [15, 38].

Conclusion

The transfusion of blood products is common practice in the management of critically ill patients. Critically ill patients often remain in the emergency department for exceedingly long periods awaiting an ICU bed; it is imperative that emergency physicians know the indications for transfusion of blood products as well as have the ability to recognize and manage complications of blood product transfusion, namely allergic reactions, hemolytic reactions, anaphylaxis, and TRALI. Blood and blood products can be lifesaving but can also have adverse effects, so that the benefit of transfusion should be clearly indicated and outweigh the potential risks before being given.

References

1. Despotis GJ, Zhang L, Lublin DM. Transfusion risks and transfusion-related pro-inflammatory responses. Hematol Oncol Clin North Am. 2007;21:147–61.
2. Brandt MM, Rubinfeld I, Jordan J, et al. Transfusion insurgency: practice change through education and evidence-based recommendations. Am J Surg. 2009;197:279–83.
3. Peterson SR, Weinberg JA. Transfusions, autotransfusions, and blood substitutes. In: Feliciano DV, Mattox KL, Moore EE, editors. Trauma. 6th ed. New York: McGraw-Hill; 2008. p. 235–42.
4. American Association of Blood Banks. National Blood Bank Data Resource Center. Available at: www.aabb.org. Accessed on 6 July 2010.
5. Hebert PC, Tinmouth A. Anemia and red blood cell transfusion in critically ill patients. In: Fink MP, editor. Textbook of critical care. 5th ed. Philadelphia: Elsevier Saunders; 2005. p. 1421–6.
6. Isbister JP. Blood component therapy. In: Fink MP, editor. Textbook of critical care. 5th ed. Philadelphia: Elsevier Saunders; 2005. p. 1427–35.
7. Cushing MM, Ness PM. Blood cell components. In: Hoffman R, editor. Hematology: basic principles and practice. 5th ed. Philadelphia: Churchill Livingstone; 2008. p. 146–54.
8. McPherson M, Pincus P. Transfusion administration. In: Henry S, editor. Clinical diagnosis and management by laboratory methods. 21st ed. Philadelphia: W.B. Saunders; 2006. p. 486–99.
9. Perkins JG, Cap AP, Weiss BM, et al. Massive transfusion and nonsurgical hemostatic agents. Crit Care Med. 2008;36:S325–39.
10. Napolitano LM, Corwin HL. Efficacy of red blood cell transfusion in the critically ill. Crit Care Clin. 2004;20:255–68.
11. Napolitano LM, Kurek S, Luchette FA, et al. Clinical practice guideline: red blood cell transfusion in adult trauma and critical care. Crit Care Med. 2009;37:3124–39.
12. Isbister JP. Decision making in perioperative transfusion. Transfus Apher Sci. 2002;27:19–28.
13. Aronson D, Dann EJ, Bonstein L, et al. Impact of red blood cell transfusion on clinical outcomes in patients with acute myocardial infarction. Am J Cardiol. 2008;102:115–9.
14. Marik PE, Corwin HL. Efficacy of red blood cell transfusion in the critically ill: a systematic review of the literature. Crit Care Med. 2008;36:1654–67.
15. Pham HP, Shaz BH. Update on massive transfusion. Br J Anaesth. 2013;111(S1):71–82.

16. Johansson PI, Sorenson AM, Larsen CF, et al. Low hemorrhage-related mortality in trauma patients in a Level I trauma center employing transfusion packages and early thromboelastography-directed hemostatic resuscitation with plasma and platelets. Transfusion. 2013;53:3088–99.
17. Sorenson B, Fries D. Emerging treatment strategies for trauma-induced coagulopathy. Br J Surg. 2012;99(S1):40–50.
18. Sihler KC, Napolitano LM. Massive transfusion: new insights. Chest. 2009;136:1654–67.
19. Kashuk JL, Moore EE, Sawyer M, et al. Primary fibrinolysis is integral in the pathogenesis of the acute coagulopathy of trauma. Ann Surg. 2010;252:434–42.
20. Ives C, Inaba K, Branco BC, et al. Hyperfibrinolysis elicited via thromboelastography predicts mortality in trauma. J Am Coll Surgeons. 2012;215:496–502.
21. Rugeri L, Levrat A, David JS, et al. Diagnosis of early coagulation abnormalities in trauma patients by rotation thrombelastography. J Thromb Haemost. 2007;5:289–95.
22. Cotton BA, Faz G, Hatch QM, et al. Rapid thromboelastography delivers real-time results that predict transfusion within 1 hour of admission. J Trauma. 2011;2:407–14.
23. Teodoro de Luz L, Nascimento B, Rizoli S. Thromboelastography (TEG): practical considerations on its clinical use in trauma resuscitation. Scan J Trauma Resusc Emerg Med. 2013;21:29–37.
24. Bollinger D, Seeberger MD, Tanaka KA. Principles and practice of thromboelastography in clinical coagulation management and transfusion practice. Transfusion Med Rev. 2012;26:1–13.
25. del Junco DJ, Holcomb JB, Fox EE, et al. Resuscitate early with plasma and platelets or balance blood products gradually: PROMMTT study. J Trauma Acute Care Surg. 2013;75:S24–30.
26. Slichter SJ. Platelet transfusion therapy. Hematol Oncol Clin North Am. 2007;21:697–729.
27. Seghatchian J, Samama MM. Massive transfusion: an overview of the main characteristics and potential risks associated with substances used for correction of a coagulopathy. Transfus Aphe Sci. 2012;47:235–43.
28. Fries D. The early use of fibrinogen, prothrombin complex concentrate, and recombinant-activates factor VIIa in massive bleeding. Transfusion. 2013;53:91S–5S.
29. Wahl WL, Hemmila MR, Maggio PM, Arbabi S. Restrictive red blood cell transfusion: not just for the stable intensive care unit patient. Am J Surg. 2008;195:803–6.
30. Beale E, Zhu J, Chan L, et al. Blood transfusion in critically injured patients: a prospective study. Injury. 2006;37:455–65.
31. Chaiwat O, Lang JD, Vavilala M, et al. Early packed red blood cell transfusion and acute respiratory distress syndrome after trauma. Anesthesiology. 2009;110:351–60.
32. MacLennan S, Williamson LM. Risks of fresh frozen plasma and platelets. J Trauma. 2006;60:S46–50.
33. Marik PE, Corwin HC. Acute lung injury following blood transfusion: expanding the definition. Crit Care Med. 2008;36:3080–4.
34. Benson AB, Moss M. Trauma and acute respiratory distress syndrome: weighing the risks and benefits of blood transfusions. Anesthesiology. 2009;110(2):216–7.
35. Silliman CC. The two-event model of transfusion-related acute lung injury. Crit Care Med. 2006;34:S124–31.
36. Skeate RC, Eastlund T. Distinguishing between transfusion related acute lung injury and transfusion associated circulatory overload. Curr Opin Hematol. 2007;14:682–7.
37. Triulzi DJ. Transfusion-related acute lung injury: current concepts for the clinician. Anesth Analg. 2009;108:770–6.
38. The CRASH-2 collaborators. The effects of tranexamic acid on death, vascular occlusive events, and blood transfusion in trauma patients with significant haemorrhage: a randomized placebo-controlled trial. Lancet. 2010;376:23–32.
39. Moore HB, Gonzalez E, Moore EE. TEG/ROTEM-driven resuscitation in trauma. In: Martin M, Beekley A, Eckert M, editors. Front line surgery. Cham: Springer; 2017.
40. da Luz LT, Nascimento B, Rizoli S. Scand J Trauma Resusc Emerg Med. 2013;21:29. https://doi.org/10.1186/1757-7241-21-29.

36 Inter-hospital Transfer of the Critically Ill

Adam B. Schlichting, Azeemuddin Ahmed, Joshua D. Stilley, and Nicholas M. Mohr

Introduction

Although the initial resuscitation of a critically ill patient should be similar regardless of a hospital's capabilities, unavailability of specialty resources may dictate that critically ill emergency department (ED) patients be transferred to other hospitals for definitive care. As recently as 2012, only 27% of US hospitals were capable of providing one of four defined specialized services: cardiac catheterization for percutaneous coronary intervention (PCI), stroke care, trauma care, or pediatric critical care [1]. Furthermore, only 53% of hospitals in the US have critical care units [2]. Critically ill patients frequently present to other hospitals, and inter-hospital transfer is a crucial part of their care. The 1986 Emergency Medical Treatment and Active Labor Act (EMTALA) defines globally how transfers occur and the requirements for a federally compliant transfer.

Resuscitation should not be delayed for transfer, and the need for definitive therapy after transfer should be balanced carefully with the priorities of resuscitation. Transitioning a critically ill patient from the relative safety of an ED to the transport environment can be daunting. In this context, transferring a critically ill patient from one medical facility to another is perhaps one of the most common and risky procedures a physician performs. This chapter will present a history of inter-hospital transfer, discuss the evolving regionalization of tertiary care services, outline the legalities and requirements for transferring patients, and provide a framework for safely facilitating inter-hospital transfer of the critically ill.

Regionalization

The Institute of Medicine (IOM) has described regionalization as the coordination of resources to optimize condition-specific care for patients across a geographic area [3, 4]. Citing multiple examples of improved outcomes, the 2006 IOM report on the *Future of Emergency Care in the United States Health System* recommended that the US further develop a "coordinated,

A. B. Schlichting (✉)
Department of Emergency Medicine, Department of Internal Medicine, University of Iowa Healthcare, Iowa City, IA, USA
e-mail: adam-schlichting@uiowa.edu

A. Ahmed
Department of Emergency Medicine, University of Iowa Carver College of Medicine, Iowa City, IA, USA

J. D. Stilley
Department of Emergency Medicine, University of Iowa, Iowa City, IA, USA

N. M. Mohr
Department of Emergency Medicine, Department of Anesthesia, University of Iowa Carver College of Medicine, Iowa City, IA, USA

© Springer Nature Switzerland AG 2020
J. R. Shiber, S. D. Weingart (eds.), *Emergency Department Critical Care*,
https://doi.org/10.1007/978-3-030-28794-8_36

regionalized, accountable system" for emergency medical care [4]. The evidence cited by the IOM focused on explicit, formalized networks for transferring patients with conditions including trauma, ST-elevation myocardial infarction (STEMI), postcardiac arrest care, and acute ischemic stroke. Although not included in the IOM report, explicit transfer would also apply to referral to a regional burn center.

Regionalization of trauma care in the US was first introduced after the 1973 Emergency Medical Systems Services Act. Since implementation, regionalized trauma care has improved mortality, functional outcomes, and cost-effective care [5–10]. Similarly, outcomes of patients with STEMI transferred to regional referral centers have decreased 30-day mortality, reinfarction, and stroke [11, 12]. Even patients with acute ischemic stroke who are treated at a regional stroke center have 11–38% decreased 1 year mortality [13–15].

Survival to hospital discharge for patients with nontraumatic out-of-hospital cardiac arrest of any rhythm is 10.4 % (95% CI, 9.7–11.2%) [16]. Regionalized systems of care for patients resuscitated from nontraumatic cardiac arrest have reported that neurologically intact survival approaches 43%, with no difference in outcome regardless of where the patient initially presented [17]. In 2010, the American Heart Association published a policy statement advocating for regionalized care of patients resuscitated from out-of-hospital cardiac arrest [18].

Please refer to chapters 8, 11, 21, 23, and 24 of this text for more detailed management of critically ill ED patients with acute coronary syndrome, cardiac arrest, stroke, and trauma, respectively. In many diseases with specific, specialized rescue treatments, however, hospital volume is associated with improved outcomes, and transferring patients to specialty care and decreasing practice variability improves outcome.

Less formalized, implicit regionalized transfer networks have also evolved for specialized care of nonspecific critically ill patients, neurosurgical emergencies, toxicologic emergencies, and hand trauma [19]. These networks have largely developed as a result of inadequate distribution of specialists. For example, if a hand surgeon operates at only a single hospital in a region, that center may become the de facto hand center, despite having no specific designation as such. Similarly, as only half of US hospitals have inpatient critical care units [2], centers with critical care units often become critical care specialty centers within that region.

Knowing the Capabilities of Your Hospital

As a clinician, knowing the technical capabilities and human resources of your hospital is an essential component of the daily practice of medicine. Admitting a critically ill patient to a hospital that lacks the ability to treat him can place a patient at risk. Conversely, transferring a patient who could have been treated locally can jeopardize patient safety and stretch health care resources. It is the clinician's duty to understand local and regional resources to find the hospital most appropriate for a patient's health care. There are five main areas that must be assessed as part of understanding the hospital environment in which one practices (Table 36.1).

First, the clinician should understand the physician and nursing care that a facility can offer. This includes the specialty affiliations, training, number of physicians, advanced practice providers, nurses, and support staff. The availability and willingness of these clinicians to provide critical care and perform life-saving procedures must also be considered. Included in this assessment is a review of prehospital provider staffing, skills, and comfort in caring for critically ill patients. Second, a review of physical resources is needed to include beds in the emergency department, hospital floors, step-down units, and the intensive care unit. In addition, it is important to assess the number and readiness of the operating rooms and availability of special procedural suites for cardiac catheterization and interventional radiology. Third, evaluating the availability of specialized equipment (i.e., advanced airway equipment, ventilators, advanced monitoring devices, and transvenous pacemakers) needed for the provi-

Table 36.1 Five areas of assessment for understanding local hospital environment capabilities

Category	Description	Examples
Personnel	Number of physicians, advanced practice providers, nurses, support staff with specialty training	Intensivists, neurosurgeons, interventional radiologists, interventional cardiologists, hand surgeons, gastroenterologists, clinical pharmacists, respiratory therapists
Physical resources	Number of ED beds, inpatient floor beds, ICU beds, operating rooms, procedural suites	Cardiac catheterization lab, interventional radiology suite, endoscopy suite
Specialized life sustaining equipment	Advanced equipment necessary for managing specific critical illnesses	Advanced airway equipment, ventilators, transvenous pacemakers, renal replacement therapies, intra-aortic balloon pump, extracorporeal membrane oxygenation
Specialized diagnostic equipment	Advanced radiologic and laboratory testing modalities	Magnetic resonance imaging, ventilation/perfusion scanning, blood gas analyzer, mass spectrometry
Specialized therapeutics	Rapid availability of medications and products necessary for management of critically ill patients	Antibiotics, vasoactive medications, factor replacement therapies, anti-dysrhythmic agents, blood products

sion of critical care must be assessed. Fourth, the breadth and availability of laboratory and radiographic testing modalities should be noted as this can affect the intensity of care provided. Finally, clinicians should review the drug formulary specific for critical care, including antibiotics, vasoactive agents, anti-dysrhythmic agents, drug antidotes and anticoagulant reversal medications, as well as capabilities of transfusion and blood bank services. Understanding the local hospital environment is an important component of providing critical care, as inefficient processes or unavailable equipment can overshadow excellent clinical care and lead to crisis.

The Emergency Medical Treatment and Active Labor Act (EMTALA)

The inter-hospital transfer of critically ill patients is largely defined by the 1986 Emergency Medical Treatment and Active Labor Act (EMTALA). This legislative mandate became known as the "anti-dumping" law, as it prohibited refusal of service to any patient presenting to an emergency department who receives federal payment through the Medicare program, regardless of a patient's ability to pay for services. This legislation explicitly applies to patients without Medicare, making EMTALA nearly universally applicable. All patients are legally entitled to a screening examination for emergency medical conditions and, should an emergency medical condition be identified, to appropriate stabilizing therapy. Furthermore, if a patient requires interventions or therapies not available, it is the responsibility of the physician to transfer the patient to a facility capable of appropriately managing his condition [20–22]. With passage of EMTALA, referral centers were also required to accept transfers of patients with life-threatening conditions without considering the patient's ability to pay for services.

EMTALA involves several very specific definitions that influence the way clinicians interpret the law. Emergency physicians are trained to recognize an "emergency medical condition," but EMTALA specifically defines this term (Table 36.2). EMTALA also defines an appropriate, medically indicated transfer as a transfer to a facility that can provide a level of care necessary to treat a medical condition that is unavailable at the transferring facility (Table 36.3). The transferring facility is required to provide appropriate stabilization and resuscitation prior to transfer. "To stabilize" is defined as providing "medical treatment of the condition as may be necessary to assure, within reasonable medical probability that no material deterioration of the condition is likely to result from or occur during the transfer

Table 36.2 EMTALA-defined emergency medical condition [20]

"A medical condition manifesting itself by acute symptoms of sufficient severity (including severe pain) such that the absence of immediate medical attention could reasonably be expected to result in: (i) placing the health of the individual (or, with respect to a pregnant woman, the health of the woman or her unborn child) in serious jeopardy, (ii) serious impairment to bodily functions, or (iii) serious dysfunction of any bodily organ or part."
"With respect to a pregnant woman who is having contractions: (i) that there is inadequate time to effect a safe transfer to another hospital before delivery, or (ii) that transfer may pose a threat to the health or safety of the woman or the unborn child." [20]

Table 36.3 EMTALA-defined appropriate transfer [20]

Transferring hospital provides stabilization of the patient and treatment, within the capacity of the sending facility to minimize morbidity and mortality
Receiving hospital must have capacity and qualified personnel to manage the patient and must agree to accept the patient in transfer
Transferring hospital must send all available, appropriate records and test results pertaining to the emergency medical condition; it is understood documentation may not be complete at the time of transfer
Transferring facility must select qualified personnel and appropriate equipment, capable of responding to foreseeable deterioration during transport

of the individual from a facility." [20] This mandate does not preclude transferring unstable patients, provided that (a) benefits of transfer outweigh risks or (b) a patient or family requests transfer. For facilities that do not have a physician present, transfer of unstable patients to a more appropriate medical center can also be arranged after a qualified provider has discussed the case with the supervising physician at the sending facility. The sending clinician must arrange for the receiving hospital to accept the patient in transfer and provide appropriate medical data and records. Furthermore, the transferring clinician must certify that the benefits to the patient outweigh the risks of the transfer, informed consent of the patient or their family has been obtained, if possible, and an appropriately trained, qualified provider accompanies the patient en-route [20].

Some authors continue to oppose EMTALA as it is an unfunded mandate, but penalties for violation are severe. Hospitals violating EMTALA may be fined up to $50,000 per occurrence. In addition, physicians who either knowingly misrepresent the condition of the patient or who transfer a patient inappropriately accounting for risks and benefits can be subject to fines up to $50,000. Legally, the transferring physician is responsible for the well-being of the patient until arrival of the patient at the receiving facility, again reiterating the importance of following the EMTALA-delineated protocol. Inter-hospital transfer should be conducted in accordance with a well-defined institutional protocol that is defined well before an EMTALA-compliant transfer is requested.

Timing in the Transfer Process

The timing of appropriate transfer is often a source of debate. In general, a patient who clearly will require tertiary transfer should be transferred early. An intubated patient in a hospital without an ICU does not derive any further value by continuing a workup in the referring hospital. Trauma patients who meet criteria for trauma center transfer, for instance, should have a basic evaluation, specifically identifying life threats for which emergent ED intervention would be required prior to transfer. A comprehensive diagnostic workup should be deferred to the receiving hospital. Patients who are more complicated or for whom the disposition is unclear should undergo more extensive ED workup, but in all cases, once the treating clinician has collected enough data to determine the appropriate disposition (e.g., transfer decision and destination), inter-facility transfer should be initiated, knowing that arranging transfer may take a considerable amount of time. Delays in initiating transfer can render safe transport unattainable, as clinical decompensation can occur while transfer is arranged.

Additional factors that need to be considered in making the transfer timing decision include the clinical condition of the patient, distance and time to the receiving facility, mode of transportation, the skill set of the transporting providers, and whether the transferring facility has the clinical and provider assets to continue adequately caring for the patient. The balance that the clinician must maintain is stabilizing the patient adequately without wasting time, while transferring patients who have been optimized for transfer.

Transfer Procedures

Transferring emergent patients can be a complicated procedure, but transfer itself should not be an emergency. Inter-hospital transfer requires coordination of two health-care systems, several health-care providers, and a transporting agency. The transfer should be conducted in accordance with guidance specified through federal regulation and local custom. Most of the transfer negotiation should be conducted prior to a transfer event through transfer agreements and standardized transfer procedures.

Identify Patient Appropriate for Transfer

The first step in initiating transfer of a critically ill patient is identifying a patient who would benefit from care at another institution. The ideal transfer patient is one for whom the transferring institution is incapable of offering a specific procedure, consultant, or other capability that is necessary for expeditious standard care, especially as it relates to improved survival free from disability. Often this decision is obvious, but occasionally patients fall into a "gray area" where the capability of your inpatient facility to care for a critically ill patient is in question. In these scenarios, early consultation with local inpatient physicians can help to guide appropriate disposition. It is also critically important when new clinicians begin working in an ED that the available inpatient services and capabilities of local inpatient centers are elucidated, as described in "Knowing the capabilities of your hospital" above. Especially in rural areas, these transfer arrangements are often clear. Absent guidance from these two sources, experienced emergency department nursing staff can be a useful resource in guiding selection of a transfer destination.

In selecting patients appropriate for an EMTALA-compliant transfer, one must be explicit about the indication for transfer. For instance, a hospital without access to an intensive care unit must transfer patients requiring mechanical ventilation. Hospitals without interventional cardiology services must transfer patients who require emergent cardiac catheterization. In addition, patients or families may request inter-hospital transfer at any time, regardless of the capabilities of the transferring center—these transfers are permissible outside of EMTALA mandates. Transferring a patient for a service available at the local hospital without this patient request, however, would be a violation of federal law.

Obtain Consent for Transfer

The next step in the transfer process is obtaining the consent of the patient or family. As with any medical procedure, transfer offers a patient benefits, but it also places them at unique risks. These risks may be higher in critically ill patients, and can include risks of clinical deterioration, a lack of adequate transfer medical resources, delays in time-sensitive care, risks of transport itself, inadequate handoff communication, and neglected patient preferences. Patients who are unable to make their own medical decisions (e.g., unconscious patients, intubated patients receiving chemical sedation, patients with illness that prevents them from having the capacity to make their own decisions) rely on the experience and knowledge of their medical providers to advocate on their behalf. Such advocacy may require the independent practitioner to initiate transfer without patient or family consent.

Most hospitals have a packet of forms that must be completed for a patient who will be transferred to another hospital. That documentation is mostly required by federal regulation, and includes a transfer consent document. Although this document is used to illustrate a patient's informed consent, the document alone is insufficient – this is only the documentation of a conversation between a provider and a patient that the risks and benefits of transfer have been discussed and the patient agrees with transfer. A portion of the form typically allows the provider to indicate when patients are unable to consent for themselves.

Identify Receiving Facility and Discuss Case with Accepting Physician

Once a consenting patient has been identified for transfer, the next step is identifying a receiving clinician. This is one scenario where an experienced colleague can be a useful consultant, because local transfer patterns and transfer agreements often dictate the recipient of a critically ill transfer patient. Some centers accept transfers directly for admission to an ICU (preferable for a patient with a clear diagnosis and treatment plan), while others request transfer to the emergency department for further evaluation and ultimate inpatient disposition. Your local transfer center will have a protocol that it uses to guide the ultimate transfer recipient.

Most tertiary referral centers have a central telephone number that connect referring physicians to tertiary accepting physicians. In some systems, ED nursing staff or unit clerks can initiate the early steps of inter-hospital transfer (e.g., faxing patient information, requesting a specialty clinician, evaluating tertiary center bed availability). The goal of the initial contact with the accepting hospital is to (1) screen for the capacity to care for your patient (e.g., available ICU beds) and (2) request consultation with the accepting clinician. In some centers, this accepting clinician is an intensivist or other specialty physician, and in other centers, this clinician is an emergency physician.

Once the capacity and capability of a center to care for your patient is established, you will be connected with an accepting clinician. That clinician is talking with you to screen for (1) the ability of his institution to care for your patient's problem and (2) your compliance with EMTALA mandates. Preparing well for the telephone interaction is one successful strategy for simplifying the transfer process. Using a checklist to guide your oral presentation may provide additional structure and help to ease the acceptance of your transfer patient (Table 36.4). Some centers that participate in telemedicine networks conduct transfer through a telemedicine connection, which may allow for more comprehensive sharing of patient data.

While it is always important to share information that will aid the accepting clinician in providing ongoing care, it is prudent to avoid discussing your patient's insurance status or ability to pay for care. Focusing on medical care alone avoids the impression that your patient's transfer is noncompliant with EMTALA mandates.

Identify Appropriate Transfer Crew

The next step in safely transporting a critically ill patient to a receiving facility is identifying the appropriate level of training for the crew to accompany the patient, which is often closely associated with the mode of transport. The crew training component of the inter-facility transfer cannot be underestimated. A retrospective cohort of more than 5000 urgent ground transports revealed that a critical event associated with mechanical ventilation, hemodynamic instability, or transport duration occurred in nearly 1 in 15 transports [23]. An important factor in predicting decompensation was the level of training of the transport crew, with significantly higher odds of decompensation among patients transferred by paramedics as compared to critical care paramedics (OR 1.6, 95% CI 1.1 to 2.2) [23].

The transferring clinician bears the obligation to select the team appropriate for the transfer. In order to properly evaluate the options available, it is very important that one understands the capabilities and scope of practice of the various out-of-hospital medical professionals. There is a wide degree of variation in title and capabilities of providers between countries, so practitioners should familiarize themselves with local conven-

Table 36.4 Structured oral presentation for transfer consultation

Checklist	Example Presentation
1. Introduce yourself, your location, and your role in your medical center	1. *Good afternoon, I'm Dr. McGillicutty, an emergency physician at St. Mary's Hospital in Springfield*
2. Introduce your patient, with relevant identifiers	2. *I'm calling you about Bart Michaels. Would you like a birth date?*
3. Explicitly state your request	3. *I would like to transfer him to your facility for ongoing ICU care . . .*
4. List the most important diagnosis and the reason for transfer, along with the service you are unable to provide	4. *. . . because he has pneumonia and I have intubated him. I don't have an ICU that can care for an intubated patient*
5. Present a brief synopsis of the case, including relevant vital signs and laboratory data. Detail interventions you have performed and the patient's current status	5. *He is a 74-year-old patient from a local nursing home with a history of diabetes mellitus who came in with a 5-day history of progressive cough and progressive altered mental status. On arrival, he was febrile to 39.1° and hypoxic to 78%. I tried oxygen by facemask, but he continued to have a respiratory rate into the 40s and was altered, so I just finished intubating him. His laboratory tests are remarkable for a white blood cell count of 18,000 and a creatinine of 3.1, but his lactate is normal at 1.4 and the remainder of his labs are unremarkable. He has a right lower lobe infiltrate on his chest X-ray, and he is doing well on the ventilator with an FiO2 of 60%. I've given him 2 liters of normal saline and a dose of cefepime and vancomycin. After intubation, his vital signs have normalized, and he is stable for transfer.*
6. Summarize the proposed method of transport and any additional information that will be sent with your patient.	6. *I will plan to send his laboratory studies, his EKG, and a summary of his ED care with him, and I will burn his two chest X-rays to a CD for you, too. He'll be coming by ground ambulance, and I think he is ready for admission to the ICU*
7. Invite questions or clarifications	7. *Is there any additional information that I can get for you?*
8. Thank the accepting clinician	8. *Thank you for your time, and let me know if there is anything else I can do!*
9. Record the name of the accepting physician (for the transfer document)	9. *Can I get your name please as the accepting clinician?*

tions. Within the United States, the clinician may refer to the National EMS Scope of Practice Model, which is a component of the National Highway Traffic Safety Administration's EMS Agenda for the Future [24]. The National EMS Scope of Practice model defines four levels of EMS licensure for out-of-hospital providers.

The *Emergency Medical Responder (EMR)* is the first level of trained care above the average layperson, and EMR is tasked with initiating immediate lifesaving care to critically ill patients. These first responders are not meant to be the sole provider during field care and transport, but rather function to allow faster access to the sick and injured. Many law enforcement officers and most firefighters will be trained to the level of the EMR. Their scope of practice includes the use of automated external defibrillators, limited airway devices such as bag valve masks, the use of auto injectors for peer or self-care, and basic trauma care. EMRs spend 48–60 hours in initial training and must participate in continuing education. Very rarely will an EMR participate in the inter-hospital transport of a critically ill patient as part of the core team, but depending on location and circumstances, may serve an adjunctive role.

The *Emergency Medical Technician (EMT)* is the next level of trained provider and is capable of providing basic emergency care and transportation of critically ill patients. The EMT can provide care independently or may work alongside providers with more advanced training and certification. The EMT has built upon the skills of the EMR with added qualifications in the use of airway devices such as oral and nasal airways as well as assisting the patient with a limited number of a patient's medications (i.e., albuterol and nitroglycerin). The EMT may also administer certain over-the-counter medications as approved by the EMS medical director. There is also a higher level of trauma training including the use of spinal immobilization devices, traction devices, and advanced hemorrhage control. The EMT will spend 150–190 hours in training and must participate in continuing education. An EMT can provide a basic level of care which may be appropriate to transfer a psychiatric patient or a patient with an isolated extremity fracture that needs monitoring alone, but these types of situations are not usually applicable to critically ill patients.

The *Advanced Emergency Medical Technician (AEMT)* is the next higher level of trained provider, capable of providing basic and some advanced level of patient care and transportation. The AEMT is able to use esophageal/tracheal devices including the King LT® and LMA® as well as the ability to monitor blood glucose levels. The number and range of medications available also increase. The AEMT can start IVs, deliver medications via the intramuscular, subcutaneous, and sublingual routes, as well as by aerosol. They can administer narcotic antagonists, nitroglycerin, epinephrine, glucagon, and albuterol. Intravenous fluids and D50 are available to the AEMT but all other IV medications are reserved for providers with additional training and certification. Training for the AEMT requires 150–250 hours beyond EMT, and AEMTs must participate in continuing education. An AEMT may participate in the transport of a critically ill or injured patient mainly as a secondary care provider based on location and circumstances.

The *Paramedic* provides the most advanced level of EMS care and is heavily involved in the transport of critically ill patients. They may employ a wide range of life-saving skills (based on their respective protocols) including needle cricothyrotomy, needle decompression of a pneumothorax, rapid sequence intubation (RSI), advanced cardiac life support, and administration of a variety of medications as determined by the EMS medical director. Paramedic training can require 1000–2000 hours beyond that required for the EMT, and some paramedic programs allow students to complete an associate's or bachelor's degree with their paramedic training.

Some paramedics will obtain additional education to become certified as *Critical Care Paramedics*, which better prepares them to provide advanced critical care transport mainly in the inter-hospital environment. Critical Care Paramedics have enhanced training in noninvasive ventilation, advanced airway and ventilation management including surgical airways and ventilators, chest tube maintenance, central venous line maintenance, expanded pharmacologic formulary usage, interpretation of laboratory data, 12-lead ECG interpretation, monitoring and maintaining intra-aortic balloon counterpulsation pumps, and invasive hemodynamic monitoring. Critical Care Paramedics also have specific education in flight physiology and transfer considerations such as safety, patient packaging, and practice in a closely confined space.

Critical Care Transport Nurses are not defined in National EMS Scope of Practice Model but are essential to the critical care transport team, especially in the air medical environment. These nurses often come from an emergency medicine and/or critical care background and have focused their careers on out-of-hospital care. They are experienced and knowledgeable in the realm of advanced life support to include airway, ventilation, and hemodynamic management as well as the delivery of basic and advanced pharmaceuticals. In addition, critical care transport nurses may be able to provide RSI as well as surgical airways as part of their scope of practice as defined by their medical director. Some nurses may possess EMT or paramedic training as well, and may also have undertaken out-of-hospital transport training similar to the Critical Care Paramedic.

In some cases, a specialty team may be employed to conduct the transport. Examples of specialty transport teams include neonatal or pediatric transport teams, extracorporeal membrane oxygenation (ECMO) teams, and high-risk OB teams who maintain advanced levels of skill and experience with their specific patient population. Often these teams must be dispatched from a referral center, which will likely delay arrival of the team to the patient. A transferring clinician must balance the time factors with training factors for a specialty transport team.

Identify Appropriate Transfer Mode

Multiple factors must be taken into consideration when deciding how to transfer a critically ill patient between hospitals. Selecting the most appropriate mode of transport requires consideration of the acuity of illness, expected clinical course and interventions that will be required en route, local EMS resources, the desired speed and distance of transit (time out of a hospital), and the prevailing weather conditions. While patients may be transported by aircraft (rotor wing or fixed wing), ambulance (advanced life support or basic life support crew), or by private vehicle, this chapter will only focus on the former two in our treatment of transferring critically ill patients.

Intimately related to mode of transfer is the level of training of the crew. Some ground ambulance systems operate with paramedics at all times while others adjust the crew makeup based on the patient's condition and transfer request. It therefore behooves the physician transferring a critically ill patient to understand local practice. Paramedic ground services are highly capable of transporting the majority of patients, but there are important limitations to understand.

Traditionally, ground ambulance services (even with advanced training and protocols) may not possess the level of clinical experience and/or scope of practice that air ambulance can provide. This difference is a reflection of the very narrow practice niche for air ambulances, which were created to transport the most critical patients with time sensitive conditions. Air ambulances are almost universally staffed with a combination of *Critical Care Paramedics*, *Critical Care Transport Nurses*, and occasionally physicians. These crew members can therefore provide a higher level of critical care intervention during transit and prior to departure than most ground-based crew, although the specifics of training and crew resources vary for each transport service.

The most common modality for air-medical transport is rotor wing aircraft (e.g., helicopters), which allow for easy access to hospitals and can be deployed quickly and efficiently. Helicopters range from single engine, single pilot helicopters to multi-engine, two pilot aircraft with the capability to fly in poor weather conditions. Fixed wing aircraft are also used for transfers, especially in remote areas far from referral centers as this allows for a rapid transfer over long distances. Because of the necessity of a runway, ground ambulances are used to transport patients to and from airports/airstrips.

Another limitation of ground ambulances is speed, which equates to time out of the hospital. Ground ambulances are slower than air ambulances, but they often are stationed near the point of departure, so out-of-hospital time is only minimized on longer transfers. Air ambulances can travel more quickly than ground ambulances, and their ability to access remote locations where road access is difficult can be a significant advantage.

The largest limitation of either ground or air transportation is weather. Ground ambulances are susceptible to road conditions such as icy roads or floods while air ambulance transport can be cancelled by fog or high winds. If poor weather conditions preclude air transportation, a coherent backup plan must be available to activate ground-based backup transportation.

Other limitations on helicopter transport include large patient size, as helicopter capabilities may limit the weight of patients that can be safely transported. Patients who are physically and/or emotionally volatile can place the helicopter and crew at risk. Should a potentially volatile patient require helicopter transport, sedation, and possible endotracheal intubation should be strongly considered versus transporting by ground with a critical care transport team. In addition, women in active labor most likely will not be able to be transported by air safely, as patient and provider position in the aircraft may be suboptimal; there may be inadequate lighting and the inability to turn the patient most certainly exists. Also, patients exposed to hazardous chemicals may not be able to be transported safely as they risk contaminating the cabin space, which can potentially incapacitate the pilot and/or the medical crew. Patients who have been properly decontaminated may be safely transported by air ambulance. Finally, patients with a small pneumothorax can safely be transported by air at nonmountainous altitudes, as tube thoracostomy may not be routinely necessary [25].

Finally, the rate of fatal crashes for rotor wing air ambulances is higher than in all sectors of aviation, and 1993–2002 saw an increase in the number of accidents [26]. This risk is sobering, and should be considered when deciding on whether air medical transport is necessary.

Despite seemingly significant advantages, the list of conditions for which air-based transport has demonstrated improved patient outcome is very short. Some suggest that air ambulances are overutilized, especially in patients who do not require specific time-sensitive interventions [27]. For many conditions (even for critically ill and injured patients), ground transport offers a level of care and time-to-destination that equals that of air transport [28–30].

Moving critically ill patients is not without risk, but dangers can be minimized through carefully matching patient characteristics with an appropriate transport mode and optimally trained crew [31]. Familiarity with out-of-hospital systems of care is essential for caring for critically ill patients.

"Package" Patient and Documentation for Transfer

Once a patient has been accepted for transfer and a mode of transport has been defined, the astute clinician should prepare or "package" the patient for transit. This includes both clinical stabilization and preparation of transfer documentation. EMTALA and good medical practice dictate that patients being transferred are stabilized within the transferring center's capabilities. This may require endotracheal intubation, initiation of vasopressor therapy, volume resuscitation, blood transfusion, initiation of transcutaneous pacing, or other life-saving procedures tailored to a patient's medical condition. One challenge for a transferring clinician can be anticipating the interventions that might be required prior to arrival in the accepting center, but one should avoid delaying stabilizing interventions solely for transfer.

In general, ED-based interventions are safer than interventions during transit. For a patient not protecting his airway, for instance, a controlled intubation in the ED is usually safer than intubation during flight or in an ambulance. Patients who have been hypotensive will be much safer in transit if vasopressor therapy is initiated prior to departure. Patients with tension pneumothorax should have tube thoracostomy performed prior to transport, balancing the risks and benefits of additional procedures to maximize a patient's safety. A transferring clinician's objective is to make transit itself as safe as possible by anticipating clinical decompensation and emergencies prior to departure. An experienced and knowledgeable transfer crew can also help anticipate potential decompensation and recommend predeparture interventions.

Adequate vascular access should also be assured prior to the initiation of a transfer. For most patients, high quality peripheral intravenous catheters will be adequate, but if the patient requires significant resuscitation or vasopressors, central access should be considered. If venous access is difficult, intraosseous access for transport is acceptable for patients in extremis.

Preparing documentation for transfer requires completing the EMTALA-compliant transfer form, the patient's consent for transfer, any certifications for ambulance transfer required by your institution, and providing records to accepting clinicians. Figure 36.1 shows an example of an EMTALA-compliant transfer form.

Compiling records to accompany a patient is often completed in concert with nursing and clerical staff. The transferring clinician should carefully consider the data that will be required to continue caring for a patient. Often, the chart

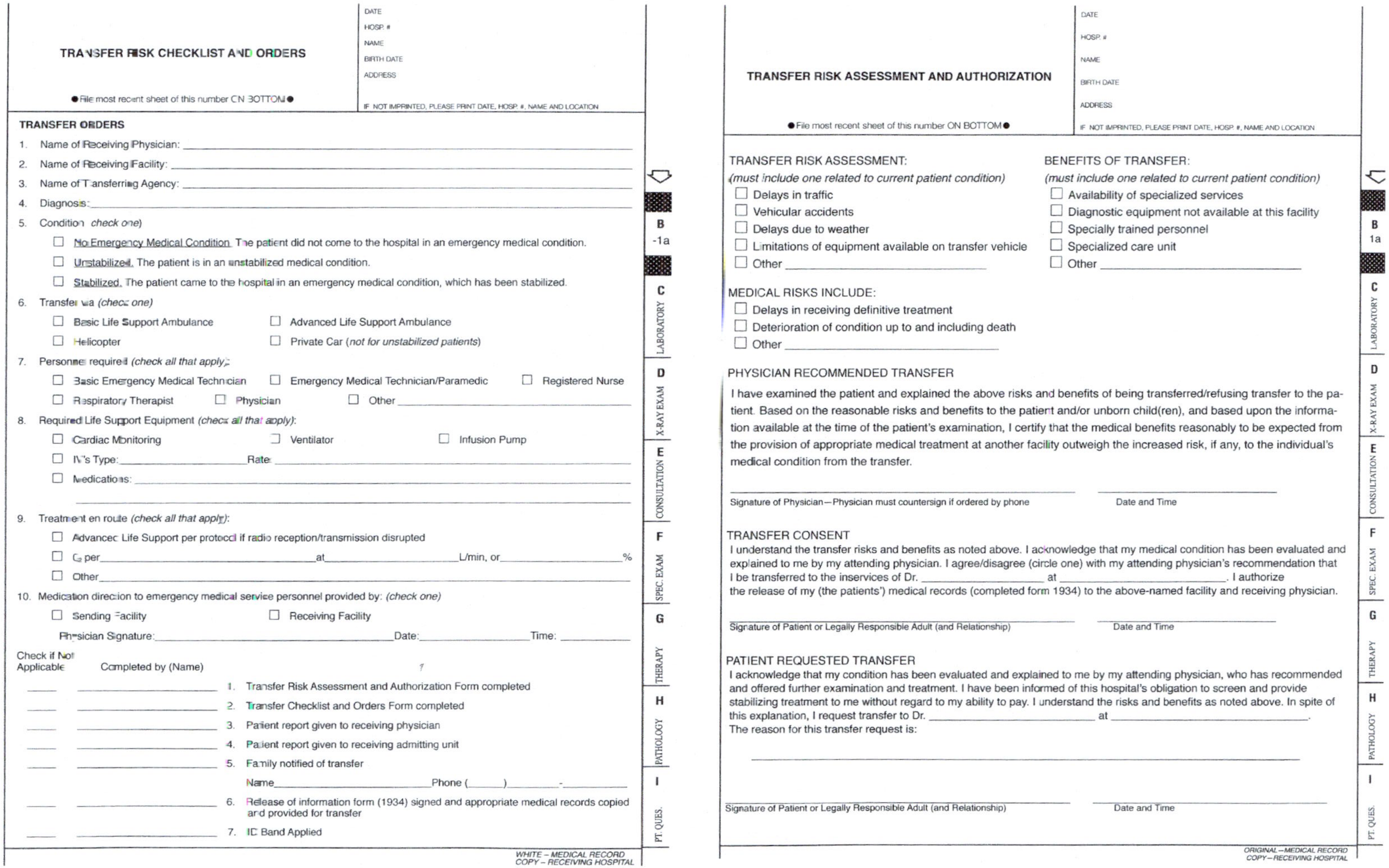

TRANSFER RISK CHECKLIST AND ORDERS

DATE
HOSP. #
NAME
BIRTH DATE
ADDRESS
IF NOT IMPRINTED, PLEASE PRINT DATE, HOSP. #, NAME AND LOCATION

● File most recent sheet of this number ON BOTTOM ●

TRANSFER ORDERS

1. Name of Receiving Physician: ______
2. Name of Receiving Facility: ______
3. Name of Transferring Agency: ______
4. Diagnosis: ______
5. Condition (*check one*)
   - ☐ No Emergency Medical Condition. The patient did not come to the hospital in an emergency medical condition.
   - ☐ Unstabilized. The patient is in an unstabilized medical condition.
   - ☐ Stabilized. The patient came to the hospital in an emergency medical condition, which has been stabilized.
6. Transfer via (*check one*)
   - ☐ Basic Life Support Ambulance ☐ Advanced Life Support Ambulance
   - ☐ Helicopter ☐ Private Car (*not for unstabilized patients*)
7. Personnel required (*check all that apply*):
   - ☐ Basic Emergency Medical Technician ☐ Emergency Medical Technician/Paramedic ☐ Registered Nurse
   - ☐ Respiratory Therapist ☐ Physician ☐ Other ______
8. Required Life Support Equipment (*check all that apply*):
   - ☐ Cardiac Monitoring ☐ Ventilator ☐ Infusion Pump
   - ☐ IV's Type: ______ Rate: ______
   - ☐ Medications: ______
9. Treatment en route (*check all that apply*):
   - ☐ Advanced Life Support per protocol if radio reception/transmission disrupted
   - ☐ O_2 per ______ at ______ L/min, or ______ %
   - ☐ Other ______
10. Medication direction to emergency medical service personnel provided by: (*check one*)
   - ☐ Sending Facility ☐ Receiving Facility

Physician Signature: ______ Date: ______ Time: ______

Check if Not Applicable	Completed by (Name)	
___	______	1. Transfer Risk Assessment and Authorization Form completed
___	______	2. Transfer Checklist and Orders Form completed
___	______	3. Patient report given to receiving physician
___	______	4. Patient report given to receiving admitting unit
___	______	5. Family notified of transfer Name ______ Phone (___) ___-___
___	______	6. Release of information form (1934) signed and appropriate medical records copied and provided for transfer
___	______	7. ID Band Applied

WHITE – MEDICAL RECORD
COPY – RECEIVING HOSPITAL

B -1a C LABORATORY D X-RAY EXAM E CONSULTATION F SPEC. EXAM G THERAPY H PATHOLOGY I PT. QUES.

TRANSFER RISK ASSESSMENT AND AUTHORIZATION

DATE
HOSP. #
NAME
BIRTH DATE
ADDRESS
IF NOT IMPRINTED, PLEASE PRINT DATE, HOSP. #, NAME AND LOCATION

● File most recent sheet of this number ON BOTTOM ●

TRANSFER RISK ASSESSMENT:
(*must include one related to current patient condition*)
- ☐ Delays in traffic
- ☐ Vehicular accidents
- ☐ Delays due to weather
- ☐ Limitations of equipment available on transfer vehicle
- ☐ Other ______

BENEFITS OF TRANSFER:
(*must include one related to current patient condition*)
- ☐ Availability of specialized services
- ☐ Diagnostic equipment not available at this facility
- ☐ Specially trained personnel
- ☐ Specialized care unit
- ☐ Other ______

MEDICAL RISKS INCLUDE:
- ☐ Delays in receiving definitive treatment
- ☐ Deterioration of condition up to and including death
- ☐ Other ______

PHYSICIAN RECOMMENDED TRANSFER

I have examined the patient and explained the above risks and benefits of being transferred/refusing transfer to the patient. Based on the reasonable risks and benefits to the patient and/or unborn child(ren), and based upon the information available at the time of the patient's examination, I certify that the medical benefits reasonably to be expected from the provision of appropriate medical treatment at another facility outweigh the increased risk, if any, to the individual's medical condition from the transfer.

Signature of Physician—Physician must countersign if ordered by phone ______ Date and Time ______

TRANSFER CONSENT

I understand the transfer risks and benefits as noted above. I acknowledge that my medical condition has been evaluated and explained to me by my attending physician. I agree/disagree (circle one) with my attending physician's recommendation that I be transferred to the inservices of Dr. ______ at ______. I authorize the release of my (the patients') medical records (completed form 1934) to the above-named facility and receiving physician.

Signature of Patient or Legally Responsible Adult (and Relationship) ______ Date and Time ______

PATIENT REQUESTED TRANSFER

I acknowledge that my condition has been evaluated and explained to me by my attending physician, who has recommended and offered further examination and treatment. I have been informed of this hospital's obligation to screen and provide stabilizing treatment to me without regard to my ability to pay. I understand the risks and benefits as noted above. In spite of this explanation, I request transfer to Dr. ______ at ______.
The reason for this transfer request is: ______

Signature of Patient or Legally Responsible Adult (and Relationship) ______ Date and Time ______

ORIGINAL—MEDICAL RECORD
COPY—RECEIVING HOSPITAL

B 1a C LABORATORY D X-RAY EXAM E CONSULTATION F SPEC. EXAM G THERAPY H PATHOLOGY I PT. QUES.

Fig. 36.1 Sample EMTALA-compliant transfer document. (From courtesy of University of Iowa Hospitals and Clinics)

is not complete at the time of transfer, so one should carefully select the documents that will enhance the care that a patient will receive. In most locations, it is acceptable to fax or send electronic records to the receiving facility. For instance, awaiting final laboratory studies before initiation the transfer is not necessary. The patient can be transferred if a mechanism exists to transmit the data as it becomes available. In general, this documentation should include:

1. A narrative summary of the presentation, including events that occurred in the ED. This narrative summary could be satisfied by the ED chart, but if the chart is not complete, a separate short narration that includes the history and events should be included. This documentation is especially important for patients who are unable to provide their own history, or where additional history has been obtained from corroborating sources (e.g., care facility, EMS, family, etc.).
2. Documentation from previous encounters (primarily for patients transferred from a care facility, another hospital, or where EMS provided relevant historical data).
3. Medications administered in the emergency department prior to transfer.
4. Laboratory studies.
5. Radiology studies (including both the official narrative reading and the original digital images).
6. Relevant historical data from the transferring medical system – this may not always be relevant, but for patients being transferred to a new medical system, records pertaining to diagnostics or therapeutics could be useful (e.g., historical cardiac catheterization reports, surgical procedure notes).
7. Current medication and allergy list (if available).
8. Contact information for family or next of kin.
9. Name of transferring clinician with contact information for further contact.
10. Transfer form and informed consent document.

Handoff to Transfer Crew

The final aspect to the transfer is the information provided to the transport personnel. The conscientious provider will directly provide a verbal report to the crew assuming care of a critically ill patient prior to transfer. This task should not be delegated exclusively to nursing staff, especially for critically ill patients. Establish clearly who is providing medical control for the patient en route (e.g., transferring provider, accepting provider, EMS medical director), and your expectation for potential changes of condition during transit. Often medical providers can anticipate clinical decompensation, so discussing expectations and potential solutions with the transport personnel can provide some additional guidance. The experienced transfer crew can also raise their concerns for stability of the patient during the transport, and collaborative discussions regarding measures to improve stability, such as endotracheal intubation, which can be more safely performed in the ED prior to departure, may further prevent decompensation. Providing this comprehensive handoff is a respectful way to ensure continuity of care.

Timing of Departure

Ultimately, the exact time of departure from the sending facility to the receiving hospital is a nuanced decision that should be arrived at as a team, but it is the sending clinician who is responsible for the care and safety of the patient until arrival at the receiving hospital. Clear communication between hospital-based providers and out-of-hospital providers is essential to successful transfer, as mistiming or mismanaging the transfer of care can lead to disastrous consequences.

Transitions of Care

One significant risk of inter-hospital transfer is the discontinuity of care between providers. Patient handoff is a recognized opportunity for error, and inter-hospital transfer constitutes several critical patient handoffs. Often, a brief telephone conversation is unable to fully relay the details of care to the accepting clinician, and most providers feel that transfer handoff communication is inadequate [32, 33].

Transitions are a dangerous time for patients, too. Not only is it inconvenient for one's provider to feel uncomfortable with the details of transfer, but this represents a period of vulnerability during which medical error is common and the consequences of error are more significant [34, 35]. Critically ill patients have a large database of information that accompanies their transfer, and much of this information is vitally important for the receiving clinician. Providers on both sides of the transfer may be busy and distracted during the transfer telephone call, and critical details may be neglected for brevity.

It is imperative that transferring and receiving clinicians dedicate appropriate time and attention to the transfer handoff to minimize handoff risks for patients. Using a standardized communication tool may improve handoff communication [36–38] and a checklist can assure that appropriate written documentation accompanies the patient during transfer. This rigor is especially important for patients who are being transported to an intermediate location (e.g., emergency department) prior to an ultimate inpatient destination.

Establishing standing transfer agreements with local tertiary centers and standardized handoff communication are two strategies that transferring emergency providers can use to alleviate some of the barriers to effective transfer communication.

Quality Assurance and Quality Improvement

As part of clinical operations, facilities that transfer patients with critical illness should engage in mechanisms to evaluate transfer quality and safety. After transport occurs, most clinicians will be distracted by competing clinical demands. Contacting the accepting clinician 1–3 days after the transfer can be a constructive way to provide internal follow-up and share patient progress with the team who helped care for a critically ill patient. Establishing mechanisms with accepting centers to receive this information effectively can be one strategy to strengthen the transfer relationship between transferring EDs and tertiary referral centers.

Often, transports involving an unexpected decompensation or complication are peer-reviewed, but a system should exist where a representative sample of transports are examined on a routine basis. A transferring emergency department's clinical medical director often conducts these reviews, and multidisciplinary representation may provide additional insight into transfer procedures. Performance indicators must be specific, measurable, action-oriented, relevant, and timely in order for them to be impactful [39]. Particular attention should be focused on ensuring compliance with patient care protocols, transport times, patient turnaround times, patient deterioration, medical control utilization, and additional metrics that can be tailored to the needs of the involved hospitals. Having a clear mechanism for follow up regarding quality and safety practices is essential for an efficient, effective, and safe transfer network.

Futility Decisions

Some patients benefit little from inter-hospital transfer. These patients should be identified early in their course and resources should be sought to provide care locally, avoiding the cost and potential harm of inter-hospital transfer. In general, these patients should be treated locally through established policies and systems of care, either through protocol or through consultation with physicians at a local referral center.

Patients persistently in cardiopulmonary arrest, for instance, have very low survival. Data suggest that high quality cardiopulmonary resuscitation (CPR) and rapid reversal of underlying causes of cardiac arrest offer patients the greatest likelihood of survival. Patients who achieve return of spontaneous circulation may benefit from regionalized care in high volume cardiac arrest centers [17], but patients currently requiring CPR are unlikely to benefit from immediate transfer. The one exception to this premise may be for referral centers that offer emergency extracorporeal cardiopulmonary resuscitation (E-CPR) life support, although patient survival is likely enhanced primarily through detailed transfer protocols that include EMS transport directly to an E-CPR capable center.

Other patients unlikely to benefit from transfer are critically ill patients with rapidly progressive, life-limiting conditions who have expressed their intention to limit interventions for their comfort. These patients could present with a variety of conditions (e.g., septic shock, intracerebral hemorrhage, postcardiac arrest), but the expected clinical outcome is death regardless of transfer. Many patients prefer to die near their home and their family [40]. While these conditions may be managed locally, successfully caring for these patients requires coordination and prior planning. It may also require mechanisms for tertiary specialist consultation for discussion about prognosis and treatment options. Admitting these critically ill patients locally to a hospital unprepared to manage them should rarely occur; rather, it should be considered as part of a palliative care effort to provide services for patients close to their homes

Conclusions

Emergency physicians are capable of caring for a vast array of patients with medical and surgical emergencies, but when the severity of illness or injury exceeds the capabilities of a local hospital, transfer to a referral center is indicated. Complex critically ill or injured patients often require specialty services, and patients require transfer to other medical facilities for definitive care. The process guiding acute medical transfers is legislated by EMTALA, which dictates requirements that a transferring physician must meet. Interhospital transfer is a common but risky procedure, and only by understanding the resources, priorities, mechanisms, and prior planning of transfer networks can clinicians align with patients in achieving optimal regionalized medical treatment.

References

1. Wang HE, Yealy DM. Distribution of specialized care centers in the United States. Ann Emerg Med. 2012;60:632–7 e7.
2. Halpern NA, Pastores SM. Critical care medicine in the United States 2000-2005: an analysis of bed numbers, occupancy rates, payer mix, and costs. Crit Care Med. 2010;38:65–71.
3. National Academy of Sciences IoM, Committee on the Future of Emergency Care in the United States Health System. Hospital-based emergency care: at the breaking point: National Academies Press; 2007.
4. Regionalizing emergency care: workshop summary: The National Academies Press; 2010.
5. MacKenzie EJ, Rivara FP, Jurkovich GJ, et al. A national evaluation of the effect of trauma-center care on mortality. N Engl J Med. 2006;354:366–78.
6. Jurkovich GJ, Mock C. Systematic review of trauma system effectiveness based on registry comparisons. J Trauma. 1999;47:S46–55.
7. Mackenzie EJ, Rivara FP, Jurkovich GJ, et al. The impact of trauma-center care on functional outcomes following major lower-limb trauma. J Bone Joint Surg Am. 2008;90:101–9.
8. Mann NC, Mullins RJ, MacKenzie EJ, Jurkovich GJ, Mock CN. Systematic review of published evidence regarding trauma system effectiveness. J Trauma. 1999;47:S25–33.
9. Nathens AB, Jurkovich GJ, Cummings P, Rivara FP, Maier RV. The effect of organized systems of trauma care on motor vehicle crash mortality. JAMA. 2000;283:1990–4.
10. MacKenzie EJ, Weir S, Rivara FP, et al. The value of trauma center care. J Trauma. 2010;69:1–10.
11. Westfall JM, Kiefe CI, Weissman NW, et al. Does interhospital transfer improve outcome of acute myocardial infarction? A propensity score analysis from the cardiovascular cooperative project. BMC Cardiovasc Disord. 2008;8:22.
12. De Luca G, Biondi-Zoccai G, Marino P. Transferring patients with ST-segment elevation myocardial infarction for mechanical reperfusion: a meta-regression analysis of randomized trials. Ann Emerg Med. 2008;52:665–76.
13. Kim DH, Cha JK, Bae HJ, et al. Organized comprehensive stroke center is associated with reduced mortality: analysis of consecutive patients in a single hospital. J Stroke. 2013;15:57–63.
14. Meretoja A, Roine RO, Kaste M, et al. Effectiveness of primary and comprehensive stroke centers: PERFECT stroke: a nationwide observational study from Finland. Stroke. 2010;41:1102–7.
15. Xian Y, Holloway RG, Chan PS, et al. Association between stroke center hospitalization for acute ischemic stroke and mortality. JAMA. 2011;305:373–80.
16. Go AS, Mozaffarian D, Roger VL, et al. Heart disease and stroke statistics--2014 update: a report from the American Heart Association. Circulation. 2014;129:e28–e292.

17. Heffner AC, Pearson DA, Nussbaum ML, Jones AE. Regionalization of post-cardiac arrest care: implementation of a cardiac resuscitation center. Am Heart J. 2012;164:493–501.. e2
18. Nichol G, Aufderheide TP, Eigel B, et al. Regional systems of care for out-of-hospital cardiac arrest: a policy statement from the American Heart Association. Circulation. 2010;121:709–29.
19. Feazel L, Schlichting AB, Bell GR, et al. Achieving regionalization through rural inter-hospital transfer. Am J Emerg Med. 2015;33:1288.
20. Office UGP. 1395DD – THE PUBLIC HEALTH AND WELFARE. United States Code 2006; 2006 Edition, Supplement 4, Title 42.
21. Kindermann S, Mutter R, Pines J. Emergency Department Transfers to Acute Care Facilities, 2009. HCUP statistical brief #155. Rockville: Agency for Healthcare Research and Quality; 2013.
22. American College of Emergency P. EMTALA and on-call responsibility for emergency department patients. Policy statement. Ann Emerg Med. 2013;62:441–2.
23. Singh JM, MacDonald RD, Ahghari M. Critical events during land-based interfacility transport. Ann Emerg Med. 2014;64:9–15. e2.
24. Administration NHTS. The national EMS scope of practice model. DOT HS. 1007;810:657.
25. Braude D, Tutera D, Tawil I, Pirkl G. Air transport of patients with pneumothorax: is tube thoracostomy required before flight? Air Med J. 2014;33:152–6.
26. Plevin RE, Evans HL. Helicopter transport: help or hindrance? Curr Opin Crit Care. 2011;17:596–600.
27. Wormer BA, Fleming GP, Christmas AB, Sing RF, Thomason MH, Huynh T. Improving overtriage of aeromedical transport in trauma: a regional process improvement initiative. J Trauma Acute Care Surg. 2013;75:92–6; discussion 6.
28. Borst GM, Davies SW, Waibel BH, et al. When birds can't fly: an analysis of interfacility ground transport using advanced life support when helicopter emergency medical service is unavailable. J Trauma Acute Care Surg. 2014;77:331–6; discussion 6–7.
29. Munoz D, Roettig ML, Monk L, Al-Khalidi H, Jollis JG, Granger CB. Transport time and care processes for patients transferred with ST-segment-elevation myocardial infarction: the reperfusion in acute myocardial infarction in Carolina emergency rooms experience. Circ Cardiovasc Interv. 2012;5:555–62.
30. Hesselfeldt R, Gyllenborg J, Steinmetz J, Do HQ, Hejselbaek J, Rasmussen LS. Is air transport of stroke patients faster than ground transport? A prospective controlled observational study. Emerg Med J. 2014;31:268–72.
31. Warren J, Fromm RE Jr, Orr RA, Rotello LC, Horst HM, American College of Critical Care M. Guidelines for the inter- and intrahospital transport of critically ill patients. Crit Care Med. 2004;32:256–62.
32. Ammon AA, Fath JJ, Brautigan M, Mehta R, Matthews J. Transferring patients to a pediatric trauma center: the transferring hospital's perspective. Pediatr Emerg Care. 2000;16:332–4.
33. Ligtenberg JJ, Arnold LG, Stienstra Y, et al. Quality of interhospital transport of critically ill patients: a prospective audit. Crit Care. 2005;9:R446–51.
34. Jeffs L, Lyons RF, Merkley J, Bell CM. Clinicians' views on improving inter-organizational care transitions. BMC Health Serv Res. 2013;13:289.
35. Smith D, Burris JW, Mahmoud G, Guldner G. Residents' self-perceived errors in transitions of care in the emergency department. J Grad Med Educ. 2011;3:37–40.
36. Ilan R, LeBaron CD, Christianson MK, Heyland DK, Day A, Cohen MD. Handover patterns: an observational study of critical care physicians. BMC Health Serv Res. 2012;12:11.
37. Mullan PC, Macias CG, Hsu D, Alam S, Patel B. A novel briefing checklist at shift handoff in an emergency department improves situational awareness and safety event identification. Pediatr Emerg Care. 2015;31(4):231–8.
38. Starmer AJ, O'Toole JK, Rosenbluth G, et al. Development, implementation, and dissemination of the I-PASS handoff curriculum: a multisite educational intervention to improve patient handoffs. Acad Med. 2014;89:876–84.
39. El Sayed MJ. Measuring quality in emergency medical services: a review of clinical performance indicators. Emerg Med Int. 2012;2012:161630.
40. Fischer S, Min SJ, Cervantes L, Kutner J. Where do you want to spend your last days of life? Low concordance between preferred and actual site of death among hospitalized adults. J Hosp Med. 2013;8:178–83.

Ultrasound for Shock Evaluation, Resuscitation, and Critical Care Procedures

37

Daniel Haase and Rohit Patel

Introduction

Critical care ultrasonography is a new discipline with real-time adaptation to the critically ill patient. These patients' main adversary is time to diagnosis or treatment of condition causing morbidity and/or mortality. Speed of decision-making is very important in this population and the ability to perform serial bedside limited ultrasound examinations to answer specific emergent conditions can be lifesaving and help confirm correct treatment. The use of ultrasound in critical care settings has been shown to be safe, accurate, and repeatable and provides data that may not be found with other routine methods of physical examination [1]. Quality of care is also improved by the use of ultrasound in many emergency and intensive care unit applications. The use of real-time ultrasound guidance during central line insertion to prevent complications is one of the Agency for Healthcare Research and Quality's highly rated patient safety practices designed to decrease medical errors [2]. This has also been shown in many other procedures performed in the critically ill patient such as arterial line access, thoracentesis, pericardiocentesis, paracentesis, and even peripheral line access [3]. The healthcare provider must be able to acquire and interpret the images, make the bedside clinical decision, and use it in real-time to implement and monitor changes in management. When a brief echocardiographic examination is added to the physical exam, diagnostic accuracy can be increased [4, 5]. In the following sections, point of care ultrasound applications are discussed individually; then we will show how you can put the individual applications together to evaluate shock and hypoxia in the resuscitation of a critically ill patient.

Training

Healthcare providers who take care of critically ill patients manage conditions that relate to all anatomical regions. Management consists of evaluations of multisystem disease states and performing various high-risk procedures. Ultrasound training standards are required for developing clinical care providers and physicians with skills to perform ultrasound enhanced point of care applications that involve many regions of the body [6–8]. The American College of Chest Physicians has suggested that ultrasound competency for critical care includes modules in the following areas: pleural, vascular, thoracic, and cardiac. The purpose of their document was to describe the components of competence so that healthcare providers can

D. Haase
University of Maryland School of Medicine, Baltimore, MD, USA

R. Patel (✉)
University of Florida Health, Gainesville, FL, USA
e-mail: rohitpatel@ufl.edu

© Springer Nature Switzerland AG 2020
J. R. Shiber, S. D. Weingart (eds.), *Emergency Department Critical Care*,
https://doi.org/10.1007/978-3-030-28794-8_37

have specific goals of training while they develop their skills. Competence is distinguished from certification, which is defined as the process by which competence is recognized by an external agency [9]. As ultrasound grows in each specialty, we will begin to see more competence-based training during residency or fellowship training [10]. In fact, many medical schools are now incorporating ultrasound in the preclinical years in order to help students grasp anatomy through visualization of ultrasound, and as a result this training should become easier for the individual throughout their graduate training years in all different specialties that are incorporating ultrasound into their curriculum [11].

Simulation of point of care ultrasound applications is very straightforward. Many applications can be practiced on "phantom" models or even more sophisticated computer-based models used frequently in echocardiogram applications. There has been a shift in medical procedural training from experience based (where training experience is defined by number of procedures performed) to competency based (which involves development of models specifically designed to assess procedural skill). It is well known that individuals acquire skills at different rates and therefore require different durations of training to become competent [12, 13]. The societal views of physician or healthcare provider practice to provide objective evidence of acquired skill have changed to assure accountability to the general public to improve quality of care, and therefore many of the applications we will discuss have many studies to assess competence [14]. One must understand that these applications are meant to answer specific bedside questions, and many of these "limited" or "focused" exams are meant to be adjuncts to other clinical indicators for management (e.g., urine output, central venous pressure, etc.). More complex measurements or evaluations should be reserved for formal ultrasound examinations performed by trained ultrasound specialists and interpreted by radiologists or cardiologists. For this reason, in each application we describe below, we will clarify the limited or focused question to be answered by the critical care healthcare provider at the bedside who will subsequently make immediate and patient care changing decisions.

Cardiac

Background Critical care echocardiography (CCE) is a broad and dynamic topic. The focus of CCE should be goal oriented or problem focused. Specifically for emergency medicine (EM) CCE, questions might include: Is the patient volume responsive? Will the patient benefit from an inotrope? Does the patient have acute right heart strain or failure? In this section, we will address basic CCE, beginning with practical ultrasound skills, image acquisition and adequacy, and what measurements or functional questions can be obtained in each view. Then, we will address practical specific emergency medicine critical care scenarios.

We will focus on basic CCE and only mention advanced CCE applications. Though there is not an official flow through the basic CCE exam, the following progression is most common. The transducer of choice for CCE is the phased array transducer – it provides appropriate footprint, frequency, and resolution for cardiac imaging.

Probe Type Cardiac (phased array) transducer: 2–5 MhZ

Basic Echocardiography and Views

Probe Type Cardiac (phased array) transducer: 2–5 MhZ

Parasternal Long-Axis View (PSL)

While standing on the patient's left, with the phased array transducer in the sonographer's left hand, the transducer is placed in the left third, fourth, or fifth intercostal space, just lateral to the patient's sternum. The machine should be in cardiac presets and the index marker should be pointed towards the patient's right shoulder, such that the left ventricular (LV) cavity is on the left of the screen. Manipulations (angulation, tilting, and rotation) of the transducer will be made until the ideal parasternal long view is achieved. This includes bisection of the mitral valve (MV) and aortic valve (AV) and should include the LV chamber in its longest dimension. The apex of the LV will not be in view. Depth should be set such that the posterior pericardium and descending aorta are in the view (Figs. 37.1, 37.2, 37.3, and 37.4).

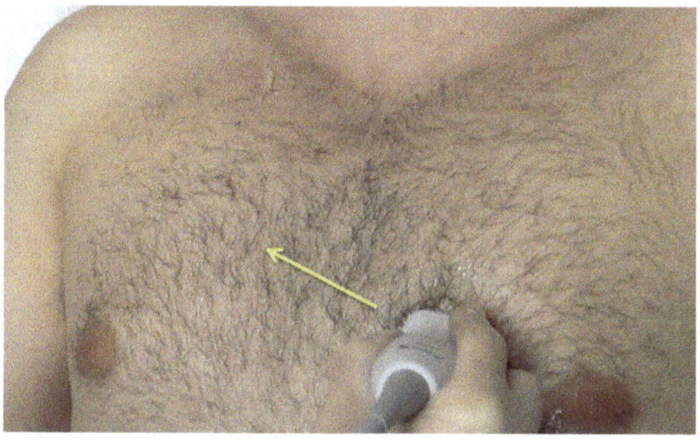

Fig. 37.1 Probe location and orientation for a parasternal long-axis view. Index marker is pointed towards the patient's right shoulder

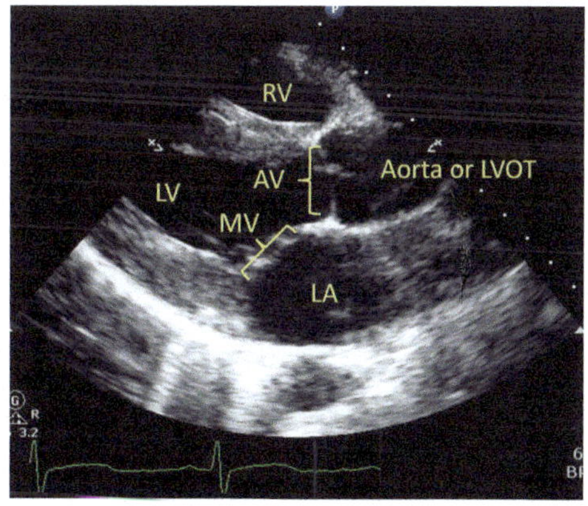

Fig. 37.3 PSL view at end systole. AV has just closed, and MV yet to open. Note the septum and LV free wall are thickened compared to diastole and the LV chamber size is decreased

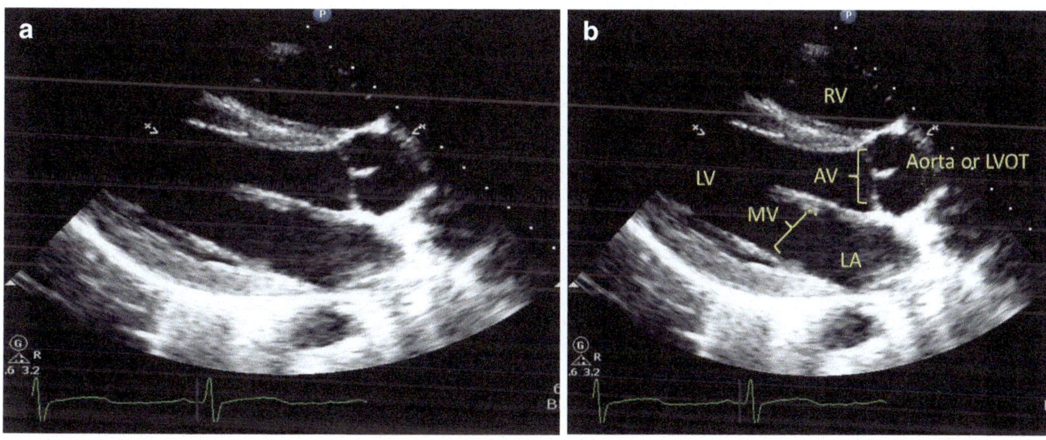

Fig. 37.2 (**a**, **b**) PSL view in diastole. Note that the MV is still open, while the AV is closed

Fig. 37.4 Assessments in parasternal long-axis view

Basic	Advanced
LV systolic function – visual, EPSS, FS	LVEF
LV size and preload	Aortic valve
Pericardial effusion	Mitral valve
Pleural effusion	LVOT diameter and aortic root
	LV/RV wall thickness

Parasternal Short-Axis (PSS) View

The PSS view is obtained after the PSL by rotating the transducer 90° clockwise (now towards the patient's left shoulder) – no further manipulation of the transducer should be necessary. Some sonographers find it easier to keep the transducer steady in the left hand and rotate the transducer with the right hand from the base of the transducer. This prevents unintended movements, other than the 90° rotation to the cross-sectional view of the LV.

There are three typical levels of the PSS: aortic valve, mitral valve, and mid-papillary. By angling towards the right shoulder, one can see the base of the heart, AV, and tricuspid valve (TV), and angling towards the left hip, one can see the apex of the LV. In the mid-papillary view, which most frequently used for assessing LV systolic function, the RV will still be seen at the top of the screen and is crescent-shaped in a normal exam (Figs. 37.5, 37.6, 37.7, and 37.8).

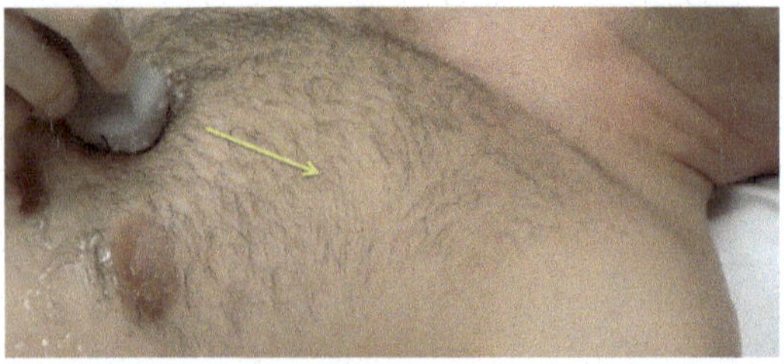

Fig. 37.5 The index marker has been rotated approximately 90° clockwise and is now pointed towards the patient's left shoulder

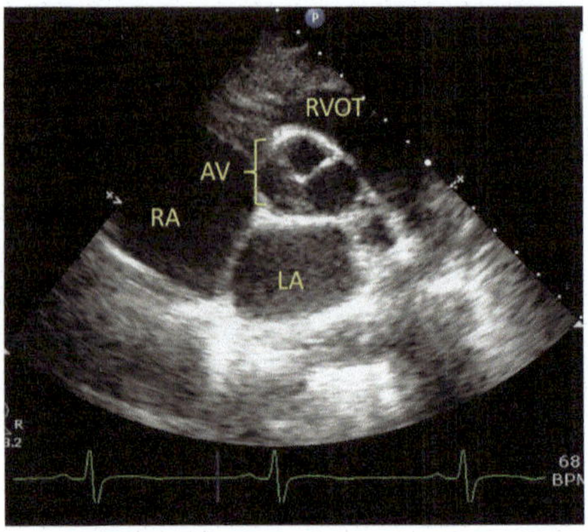

Fig. 37.7 PSS view at AV level. Note that all three valves can be visualized. TV not seen

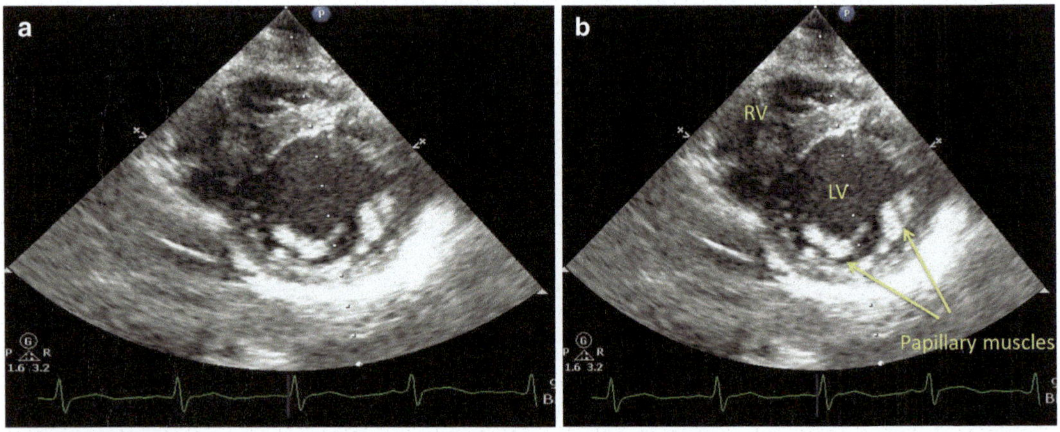

Fig. 37.6 (**a**, **b**) PSS view at the mid-papillary level. RV is normal sized and crescent shaped, and LV has normal filling volume and is round

Fig. 37.8 Assessments in parasternal short-axis view

Basic	Advanced
LV systolic function	LV wall thickness and segmental wall motion
RV size and septal flattening	Tricuspid valve
Pericardial effusion	Pulmonic valve
	Pulmonary arteries

Apical Four-Chamber (A4C) View

With the index marker continuing to point towards the 2–3 o'clock position, the transducer should be placed at the apex of the heart, which is best localized at the point of maximal impulse. This can be difficult to find. In older and larger patients with cardiomyopathy, the apex will be located quite laterally (anterior to midaxillary line) and LV oriented more horizontally. In young, slender patients, the apex will be more medial, and LV oriented more vertically. Although not always feasible, placing the patient, at least partially, in the left lateral decubitus position may help optimize the view by bringing the heart in direct contact with the chest wall. The depth must also be increased, especially if the apex is located laterally.

The ideal image for the A4C can be quite difficult, especially in the critically ill patient. In patients with hyperinflation from asthma and COPD or in patients with high PEEP or APRV, the heart may be pushing inferiorly or the apex may be obscured by lung tissue. However, this view is also frequently the most useful and provides nearly all the required information to adequately assess RV and LV function in the critically ill patient.

An ideal A4C view is comprised of three components:

1. The septum should be in the center of the screen and oriented vertically on the screen.
2. The apex, MV, and TV should all be bisected – this gives maximal cavity size to the LV.
3. The RV should be in maximal diameter, best achieved by transducer rotation (Figs. 37.9, 37.10, and 37.11).

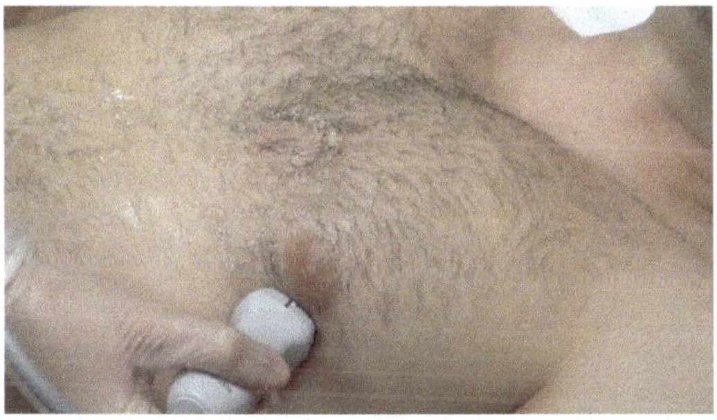

Fig. 37.9 Transducer location for A4C view, index marker remains pointed to the patient's left shoulder

Subcostal (Subxiphoid) View

The transducer should be placed just below the xiphoid process, pointed towards the left shoulder, with a fair amount of downward pressure and a flattened angle to the skin. Switching from a pencil to overhand grip may be necessary to achieve the appropriate angle. The probe marker should be directed towards the 3 o'clock position. The ideal image will be a four-chamber view, with the right side of the heart at the top of the screen, left heart at the bottom, and the apex on the right of the screen (Figs. 37.12, 37.13, and 37.14).

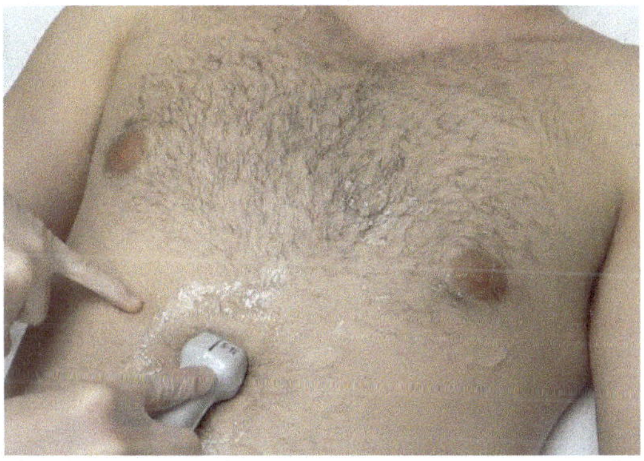

Fig. 37.12 Transducer moved to the epigastrium with the index marker to the patient's left. Note the overhand grip on the transducer and shallow angle with the abdomen

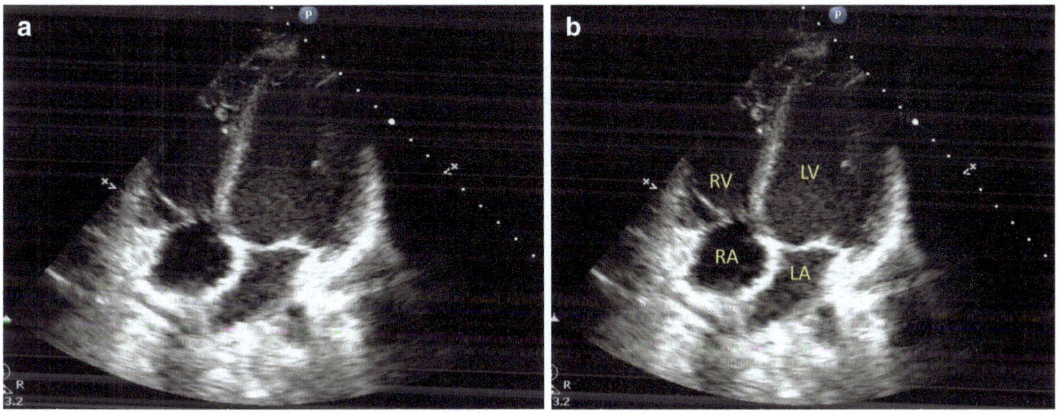

Fig. 37.10 (**a**, **b**) A4C view at end diastole. Note the size relationship between the RV and LV

Fig. 37.11 Assessments in apical four-chamber view

Basic	Advanced
LV size and systolic function	Aortic valve
RV size and function	Mitral valve
TAPSE	Tricuspid valve
Pericardial effusion	LV diastolic function
	Velocity-time integral

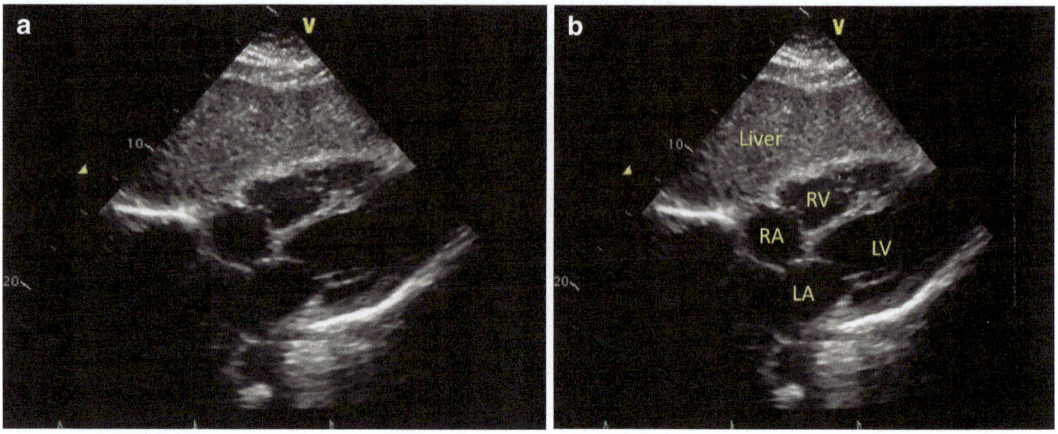

Fig. 37.13 (**a**, **b**) Subxiphoid view at end diastole. Note how the liver is used as an acoustic window

Fig. 37.14 Assessments in subxiphoid view

Basic	Advanced
LV size and systolic function	Aortic valve
RV size and function	Mitral valve
Pericardial effusion	Tricuspid valve

Chart 4
Assessments in SC:

- Basic ➔ LV systolic function, RV size and function, pericardial effusion
- Advanced ➔ Aortic valve, mitral valve, tricuspid valve

Inferior Vena Cava (IVC)

Coming from the subcostal view, and keeping focused on the cavoatrial junction, the IVC can be most easily imaged by rotating the transducer counterclockwise until the index mark is oriented towards the 12 o'clock position. Now, the IVC can be seen in its longitudinal orientation. The IVC can also be viewed from a lateral position at the midaxillary line with the index marker at the 12 o'clock position, giving a sagittal view, using the liver as an acoustic window.

By following the cavoatrial junction throughout the rotation from the subcostal view, one ensures that the structure in question is indeed the IVC and not the aorta. Recognizing the spatial relationship between the two structures is important, as are pulsatility, wall thickness, and color Doppler flow. Visualization of the IVC draining into the RA is 100% specific for identification of the IVC. IVC collapsibility index (IVC-CI) can be assessed in this view (Fig. 37.15).

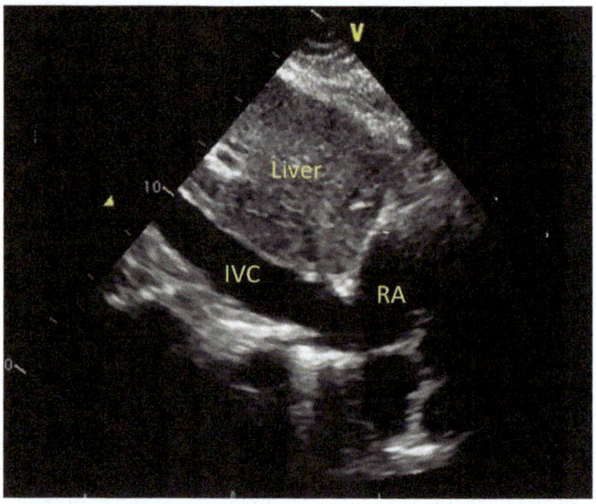

Fig. 37.15 IVC draining into the RA

LV Systolic Function

Emergency Question My patient is hypotensive or in a shock state, what is their left ventricular function? Would my patient benefit from an inotrope?

Probe Type Cardiac (phased array) transducer: 2–5 MhZ

Clinical Scenario Approximately 1/3 of critically ill patients have left ventricular systolic dysfunction during their ICU stay, whether it be preexisting, from acute ischemia or from a secondary cause such as sepsis. In patients with shock, LV systolic function must be assessed, because the treatment for LV systolic dysfunction is much different from other shock states.

Further, LV systolic function is relative to the clinical situation. Numerically quantifying LVEF is frequently unnecessary in the acute setting, as the clinical scenario may only query whether or not the patient would benefit from an inotrope. The ACCP suggests that basic competence of this skill should only distinguish between hyperdynamic function, normal function, mild-moderate dysfunction, and severe dysfunction [15]. Therefore, time-consuming quantitative and semiquantitative measures should not be routinely used for determining LV systolic function, but only used to support clinical decision-making or in unclear clinical scenarios.

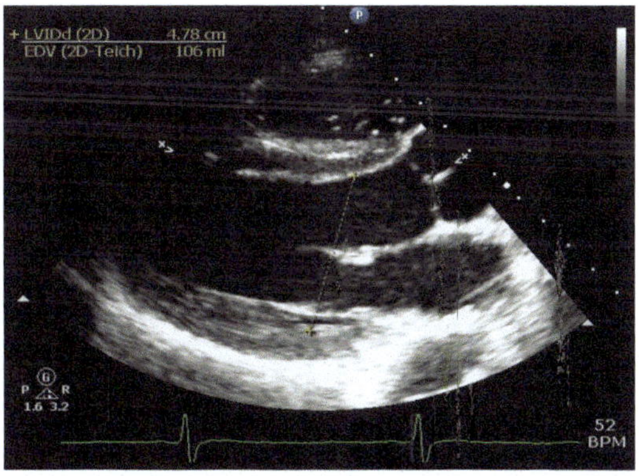

Fig. 37.16 PSL view at end diastole with a measurement of the LVIDd

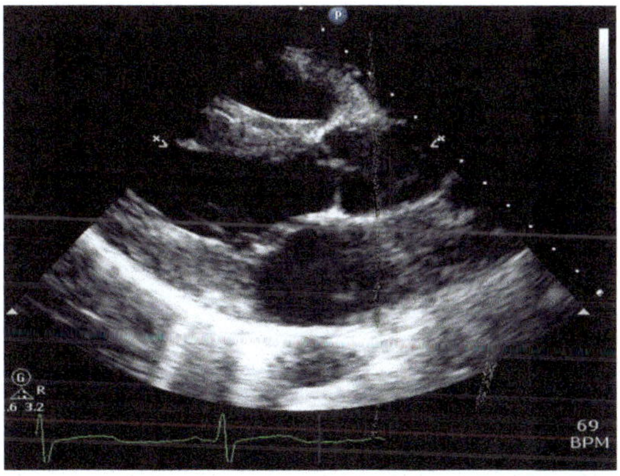

Fig. 37.17 PSL view at end systole. Note the difference in LV wall thickening and LV chamber size

Scanning Technique

Qualitative Assessment of LV Systolic Function

The left ventricle should contract symmetrically, and the LV cavity should reduce in size approximately 40% on bedside echocardiography – this is true for all four main cardiac views. Determinations of dysfunction or hyperdynamic function are relative to normal function.

Assessment of LV systolic function can be difficult to the novice sonographer, as there is no single objective measure that definitively quantifies function. Most experts agree that LV systolic function determination on echocardiography is multifactorial determination, using multiple views, modes, and measurements, and ultimately is a composite decision of the interpreting physician [16, 17] (Figs. 37.16 and 37.17).

When assessing for a hyperdynamic states, the interpreting physician must be careful to assess LV preload. LV systolic function may be artificially increased when the LV preload is decreased (Figs. 37.18 and 37.19).

The term "underfilled" most accurately describes LV preload and can be quantified using LV end-diastolic diameter (LVIDd). If the patient is severely hypovolemic, the LV does not have time to fill, or there is decreased LV preload from RV dysfunction, and then the LVIDd may be decreased. If there is decreased LV filling, the LVEF will be artificially increased, though the actual stroke volume and cardiac output may be normal or decreased. If LVIDd is normal or increased, this may be a marker of LV dilation cardiomyopathy, and its value must be used with caution. One must distinguish between a hyperdynamic LV that has normal and abnormal pre-

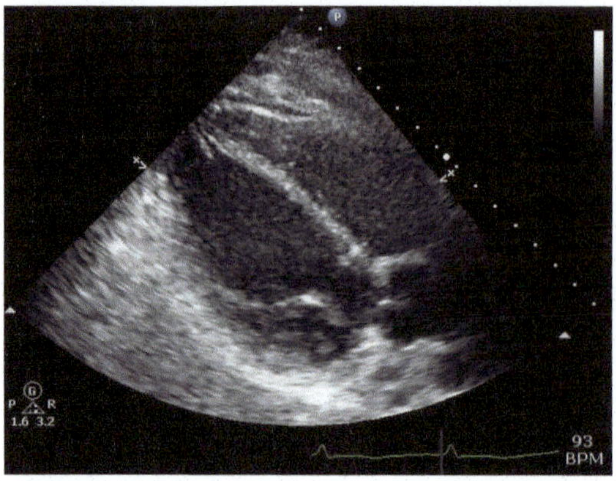

Fig. 37.18 PSL view at end diastole with normal LV preload

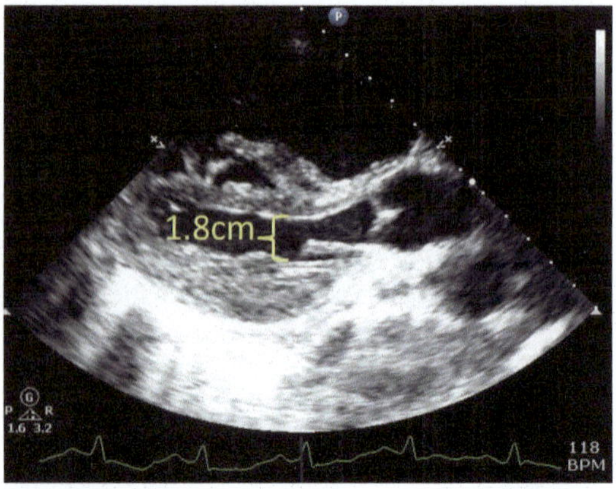

Fig. 37.20 PSL view with severe LV compression from RV dilation. Note the very small LVIDd

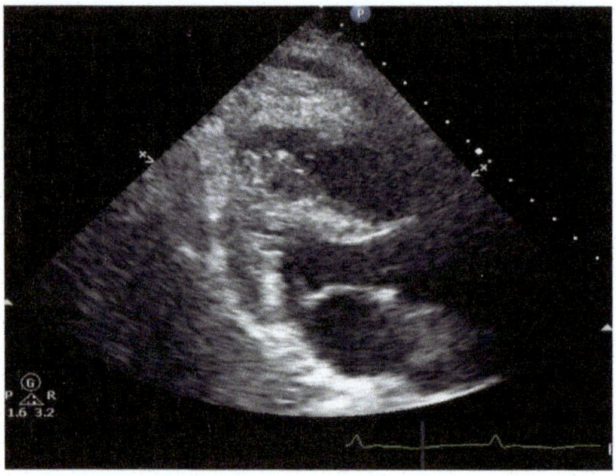

Fig. 37.19 PSL view at end systole with hyperdynamic function

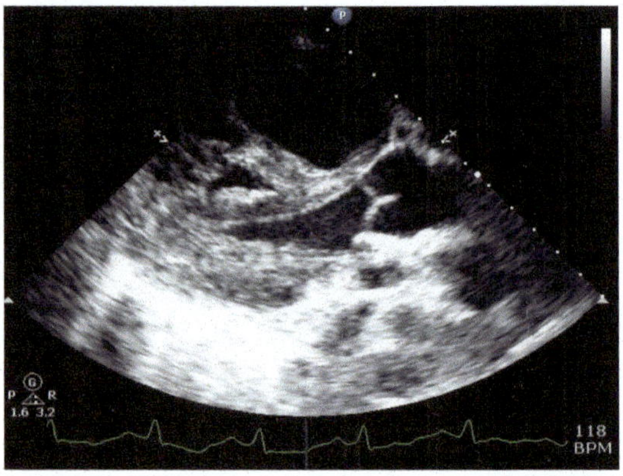

Fig. 37.21 PSL with "kissing" left ventricle. The LV ejects most of its volume, but the actual stroke volume is likely diminished

load because the treatments are different [18] (Figs. 37.20 and 37.21).

Quantitative and Semiquantitative Assessments

The American Society of Echocardiography recommends the modified Simpson's method to quantify the LVEF. Although this method may be accurate, it is complex, time-consuming, and not appropriate in point-of-care CCE [18].

Again, there is no single quantitative value that determines LVEF. These measures may help to assist the inexperienced sonographer in making an overall assessment, but their clinical utility is limited.

E-Point Septal Separation (EPSS)

EPSS is a quantitative measure of LV systolic function that is obtained in the parasternal long view. It is limited in scenarios of mitral stenosis and aortic regurgitation. During early diastole, mitral inflow is the greatest, and the anterior leaflet of the mitral valve swings open, coming in close proximity to the intraventricular septum in normal, healthy patients. When LV systolic function is decreased and very little of the blood in the LV is ejected, very little blood flows through the mitral valve during diastole. Thus, the anterior leaflet of the MV does not come as close to the septum, and the EPSS is reduced [19–21].

To measure EPSS, the M-mode cursor is placed through the tip of the anterior mitral leaflet, and the distance between the tip of the mitral leaflet and the intraventricular septum is measured. The closer the anterior mitral leaflet is to the septum, the greater the mitral inflow to the left ventricle and, thus, the better the LVEF (Figs. 37.22, 37.23, and 37.24).

EPSS can be performed successfully by emergency physicians and, with the low incidence of mitral stenosis, should be fairly reliable [20]. Because it looks at filling of the LV, it does not look at specific segments of LV contractility, but rather at global systolic function of left ventricle. However, if EPSS is not measured at the tip of the mitral leaflet, EPSS will be overestimated.

Fractional Shortening (FS) (Fig. 37.25)

$$\text{Fractional Shortening}: \frac{\left[(\text{LV end-diastolic diameter})-(\text{LV end-systolic diameter})\right]}{(\text{LV end-diastolic diameter})}$$

Fractional shortening assumes symmetric contractile function throughout the LV – i.e., the base and apex are contracting similarly and there are no focal segmental wall abnormalities. This is a key reason that FS measurements can often be misleading – it only assesses function at a single point.

Most sonographers who choose to use fractional shortening use M-mode for their measurements. It ensures the measurements are in the same axis, which can be helpful. Further, another view to assess function may be helpful in the overall assessment. Fractional shortening can be done in both the parasternal long- and

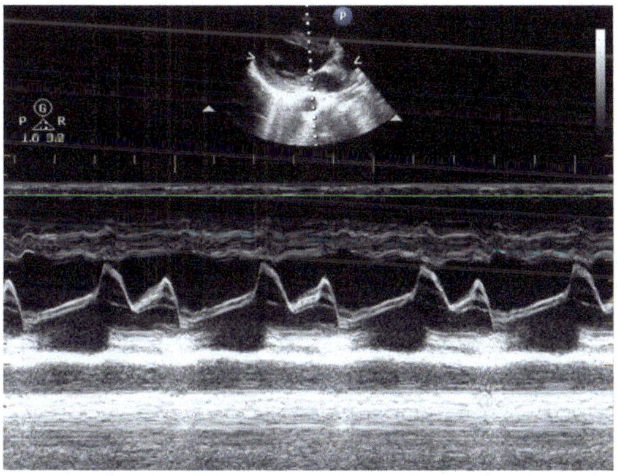

Fig. 37.22 EPSS of 0.3 cm, suggesting normal LV function

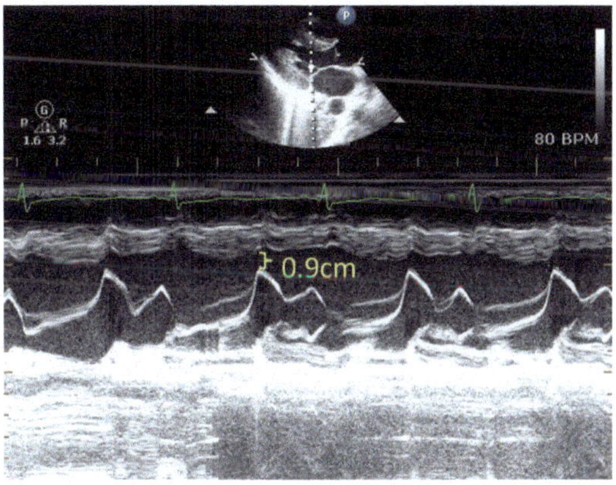

Fig. 37.23 EPSS of 0.9 cm in same patient when cursor not aligned properly. LV function would be underestimated with this image

Fig. 37.24 Suggested values for E-point septal separation (EPSS). Reference values for EPSS are not well validated and are variable throughout the literature

EPSS Value	LV function estimation
</= 0.7 cm	Normal LV function
0.8–1.6 cm	Mild-moderate LV dysfunction
>/= 1.7 cm	Severe LV dysfunction

Fig. 37.25 Suggested values for fractional shortening (FS)

Fractional Shortnening %	LV function estimation
>45%	Hyperdynamic LV function
30–45%	Normal LV function
15–30%	Mild-moderate LV dysfunction
<15%	Severe LV dysfunction

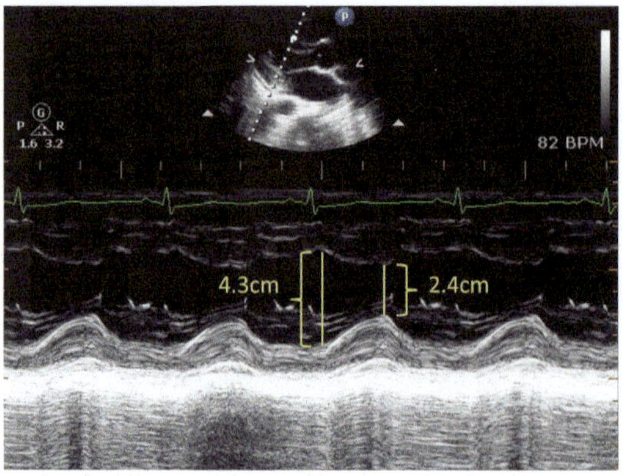

Fig. 37.26 PSL view with FS measurements. FS is 44%, suggesting normal LV function

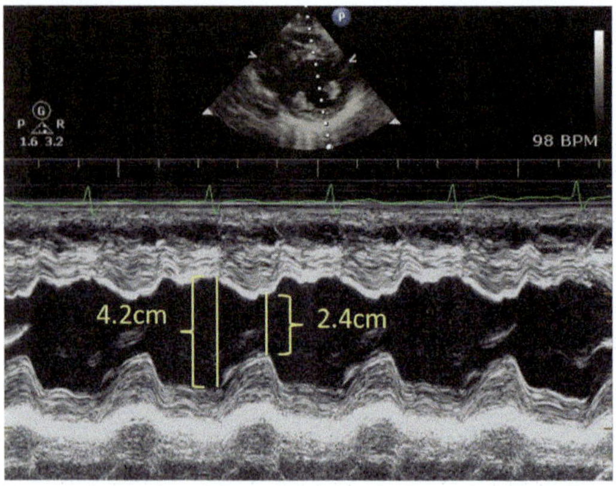

Fig. 37.27 PSS view with FS in same patient. FS is 43%, supporting normal LV function

parasternal short-axis views [22] (Figs. 37.26, 37.27, and 37.28).

RV Function

Emergency Question Does the patient have acute right heart strain or failure?

Probe Type Cardiac (phased array) transducer: 2–5 MhZ

Clinical Scenario RV dysfunction is a complex disease and has a wide variety of causes (e.g., massive pulmonary embolism, RV infarction, acute respiratory distress syndrome, sepsis, hypoxia, acidosis). In patients with shock, the RV

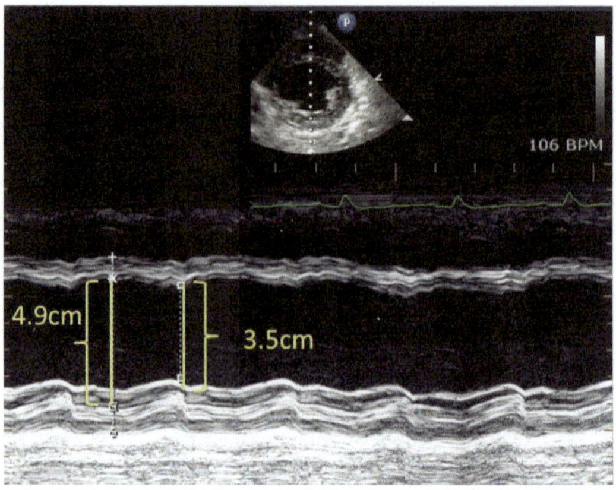

Fig. 37.28 PSS view with FS of 29%, suggesting mild-moderate LV dysfunction

should be routinely evaluated because it is an underdiagnosed contributor to shock.

Distinguishing between acute and chronic RV dysfunction using echocardiography can be challenging, but is important in clinical management of patients. While the general principles of acute and chronic right heart failure are similar (volume and pressure reduction), clinical management depends on the etiology of the RV dysfunction.

For instance, acute massive PE might get thrombolytics and inotropic support, acute RV ischemic might get reperfusion therapy and possibly mechanical support (e.g., RVAD), and ARDS or severe hypoxia-induced RV failure may get an inhaled vasodilator such as nitric oxide or epoprostenol. In patients with long-standing pulmonary hypertension, focus is more on pulmonary vasodilators and preload reduction, depending on the WHO classification of pulmonary hypertension.

RV anatomy and function is more complex than the LV and is more difficult to visualize with echocardiography than the LV. Whereas systolic and diastolic function of the LV are quite distinct, there are less so in the RV because the RV free wall is less muscular and more compliant; thus acute volume and pressure overload are intricately related.

Understanding RV physiology is critical to echocardiographic assessment of the RV. The RV does not have circumferential myocardial fibers causing symmetric contraction. Instead, the RV gains the majority of its systolic function from the longitudinal contraction of the RV cavity, resulting in a bellows-like action. RV free wall contraction and LV contraction contribute a smaller portion to RV systolic function [23–25].

Scanning Technique Assessment of RV function should be a routine part of echocardiography. The RV can be assessed in all views, though the apical four-chamber and subxiphoid views provide the most reliable and useful information. Though no measurements or true qualitative assessments of the RV are done in the parasternal long view, the sonographer may note an abnormally large RV in this view. In severe RV failure, LV compression may be noted in the parasternal long-axis view.

In the parasternal short-axis view, the RV is at the top of the screen and crescent-shaped and typically isn't significantly noticed by the sonographer. When failed, the RV is enlarged and the increased pressure causes intraventricular septal flattening towards the LV. This finding is frequently called the "D-sign" because the LV cavity in cross section has changes from its typical circular appearance to a "D-shaped" appearance (Fig. 37.29).

On the apical four-chamber view, the RV should be no greater than 1/2 to 2/3 the size of the LV and should be triangular in shape. In failure, the RV free wall dilates outward and the RV can appear equal in size or even larger than the LV. "McConnell's sign" is frequently used to describe RV dilation and hypokinesis with apical sparing. When observed, McConnell's sign suggests acute RV failure and is frequently seen with massive pulmonary embolism [26] (Figs. 37.30 and 37.31).

Tricuspid annular plane systolic excursion (TAPSE) is a reliable quantitative measure of RV function. After obtaining an adequate apical four-chamber view, the M-mode cursor is placed through the lateral tricuspid annulus, and the longitudinal movement of the annulus is measured. Measuring TAPSE does not require visualization of the RV free wall, which is often quite challenging.

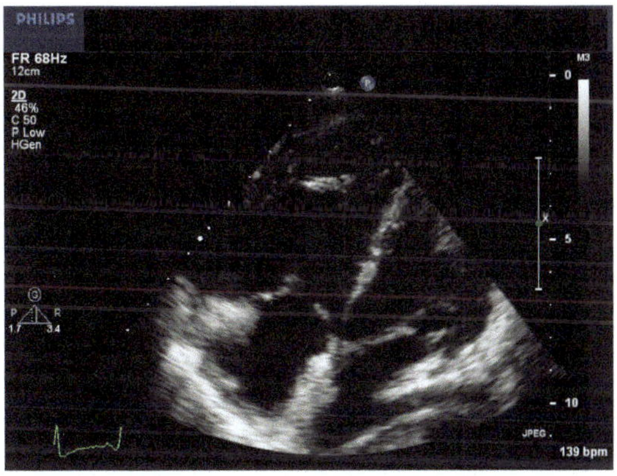

Fig. 37.30 A4C with severe RV dilation. RV is actually larger than the LV

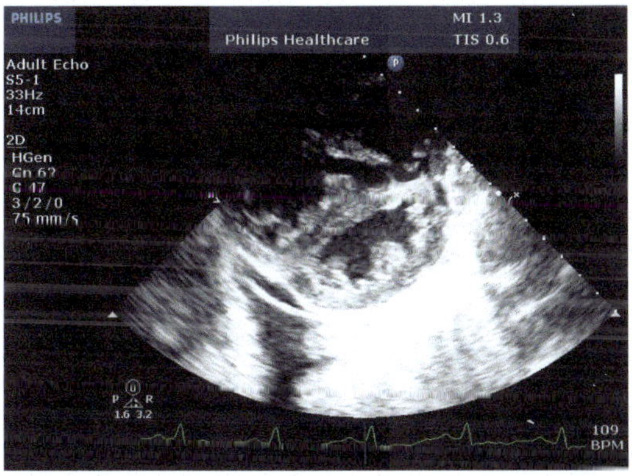

Fig. 37.29 PSS view with significant septal flattening from RV dilation

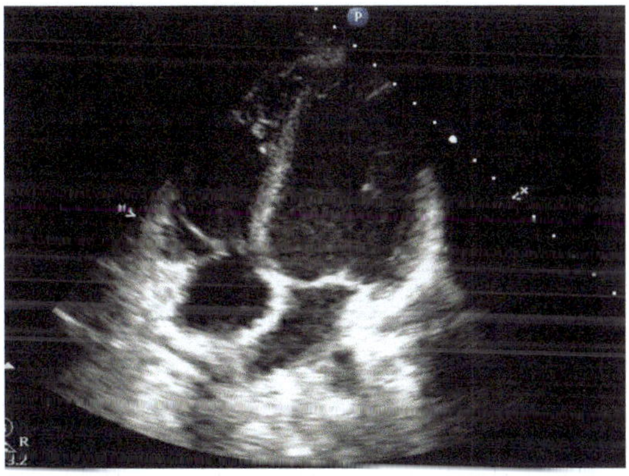

Fig. 37.31 A4C with normal LV/RV size ratio of approximately 0.6:1

The subxiphoid view also allows for side-by-side size assessment of the RV/LV ratio. The RV and LV cavities should be in the longest diameter, and the TV and MV should be in view to accurately assess the size ratio (Fig. 37.32).

Supporting Literature While a few semiquantitative measures of RV function do exist, the most well-validated, reproducible, and prognostic is tricuspid annular plane systolic excursion (TAPSE). After obtaining an adequate A4C view, the M-mode cursor is placed through the lateral tricuspid annulus, and the longitudinal movement of the annulus is measured. Measuring TAPSE does not require visualization of the RV free wall, which is often quite challenging [27, 28] (Figs. 37.33, 37.34, and 37.35).

A 2014 multicenter, observation cohort study of patients with symptomatic, but without hemodynamic, instability showed that patients with TAPSE <1.6 cm had greater all-cause mortality at 30 days. A decreased TAPSE was also associated with most other markers of RV failure (i.e., RV end-diastolic diameter, RV/LV end-diastolic diameter, systolic pulmonary artery pressures). TAPSE does have limitations, specifically in patients with LV systolic dysfunction, as reduced LV function has been shown to affect TAPSE [29].

Other quantitative measures of RV/LV size ratio and RV systolic function do exist and are accurate, but are more time-consuming and complex measurements outside the scope of the emergency department intensivist. And, as has been shown with many other assessment, experienced echocardiographer assessments are as reliable and accurate as quantitative measures [30–32].

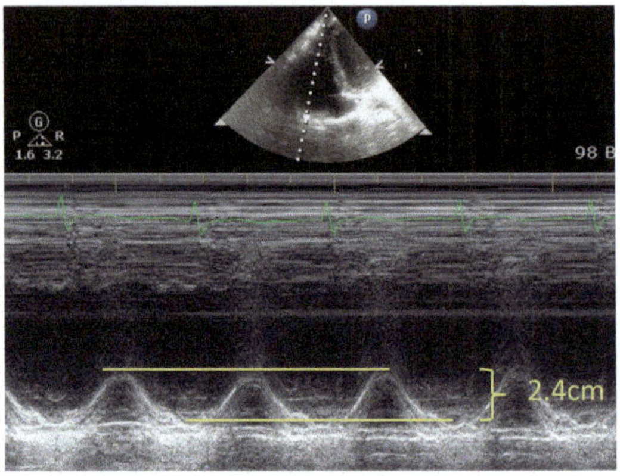

Fig. 37.34 M-mode cursor through lateral tricuspid annulus with normal function

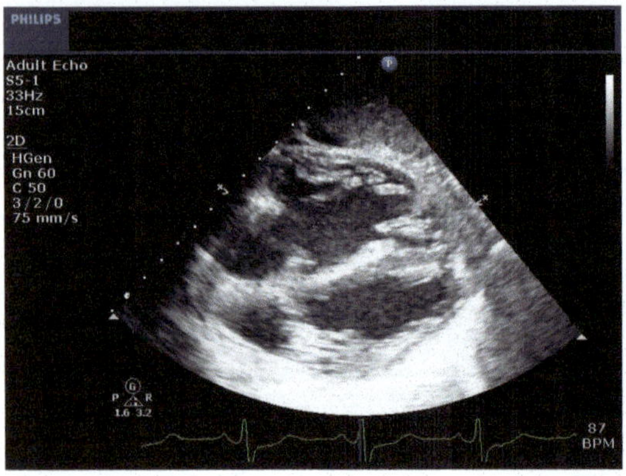

Fig. 37.32 Subxiphoid view with RV dilation and wall thickening

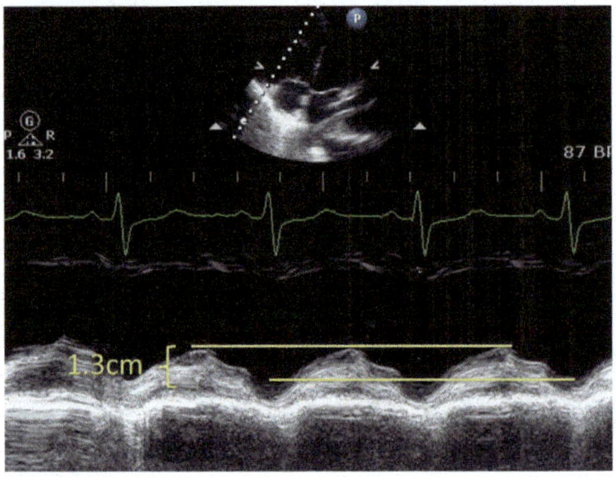

Fig. 37.35 TAPSE 1.3 cm, suggesting mild-moderate RV dysfunction

Fig. 37.33 TAPSE values and RV function

TAPSE measurement	RV function estimation
>1.6 cm	Normal RV function
1.0–1.6 cm	Mild-moderate RV dysfunction
<1.0 cm	Severe RV dysfunction

Pericardial Effusion and Cardiac Tamponade

Emergency Question Does the patient have a pericardial effusion? If so, is it causing cardiac tamponade?

Probe Type Cardiac (phased array) transducer: 2–5 MhZ

Clinical Scenario Patients can have pericardial effusion for a variety of reasons – trauma, post-cardiac surgery, malignancy, uremia, etc. The presence of a pericardial effusion can be easily assessed by bedside ultrasound by novice sonographers. However, the presence of cardiac tamponade is a bit more difficult to assess, and the sonographer must use clinical findings to make the diagnosis.

The most common symptom of pericardial tamponade is dyspnea. Physical exam findings may include Beck's triad of muffled heart tones, elevated jugular venous pressure, and hypotension, but are not required for diagnosis. Pulsus paradoxus (a drop in systolic blood pressure >10 mmHg during inspiration) is useful when present, as are low-voltage QRS complexes or electrical alternans on EKG. However, these subtle findings are rarely present and may not be identified in the emergent situation [33].

As pericardial fluid accumulates, the increased pressure overcomes the filling pressure of the right atrium. Decreased venous return and right heart filling may cause arterial hypotension and global hypoperfusion. The pericardial effusion may continue to increase pericardial pressure, eventually causing diastolic collapse of the right ventricle, which results in hemodynamic collapse [34].

In patients who have chronic pericardial effusions, the fibrous pericardium can stretch over time, allowing for a large volume of fluid to accumulate prior to hemodynamic compromise. Pericardial effusions from trauma, cardiac surgery, or even infection may accumulate more quickly, causing cardiac tamponade physiology from a relatively smaller volume of fluid [34, 35].

Bedside echosonography is the most useful tool in diagnosis pericardial tamponade. Early findings will include a pericardial effusion and diastolic collapse of the right atrium, as it is under the lowest pressure. As tamponade progresses, early diastolic collapse of the right ventricle occurs, followed by late diastolic collapse, which is a premorbid condition, requiring immediate intervention. Placing M-mode through the right ventricular free wall and correlating diastole with the EKG lead is most helpful in discerning right ventricular diastolic collapse [36–38].

Scanning Technique With the patient in the supine or semirecumbent position, the phased array transducer should be used to obtain a parasternal long view. In this view, pericardial fluid is most frequently seen posterior to the left ventricle and atrium. In large effusions, it may be seen anterior to the right ventricle, but this is often difficult to visualize, due to the smaller footprint of the phased array transducer. The effusion may also be visualized in parasternal short view, but provides less diagnostic information (Fig. 37.36)

The subxiphoid and apical four-chamber views allow for optimal visualization of the right atrium and ventricle – it is in these views that tamponade will be diagnosed. Because the right atrium is under the lowest pressure, its collapse during diastole is the most sensitive for diagnosing cardiac tamponade [34–36]. Diastolic collapse can be seen on 2D imaging by correlating

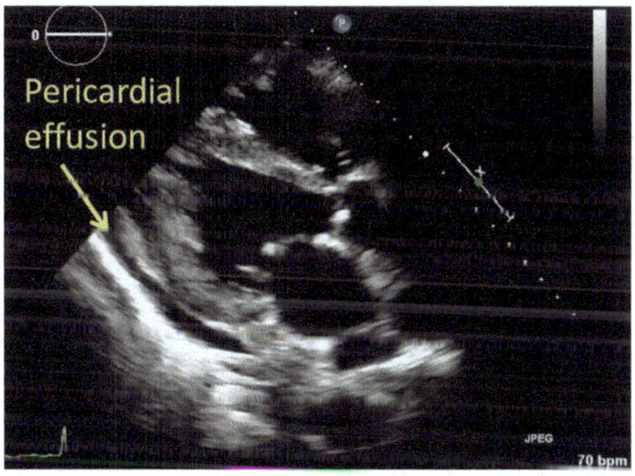

Fig. 37.36 PSL view demonstrating a posterior pericardial effusion

the image to the EKG and valve opening (recall that diastole occurs between the T wave and QRS complex on EKG, on echo, and the mitral and tricuspid valves will be open, but the aortic valve closed). Diastolic collapse of the right ventricular free wall may also be diagnosed using M-mode imaging. Again, correlation to the EKG tracing is crucial in diagnosing tamponade (Figs. 37.37, 37.38, 37.39, and 37.40)

In patients with large pericardial effusions or in those that have a "swinging heart," it may be difficult to assess diastolic collapse because the heart may move in and out of view.

Other echocardiographic findings of patients with tamponade physiology should include a dilated, non-collapsing IVC [38]. This is due to the decreased filling of the right atrium and ventricle from increased pericardial pressures. Left ventricular diastolic volumes may be decreased as well, causing the LV to appear hyperdynamic and underfilled [35, 37].

It is important to distinguish between a pericardial effusion and pleural effusion, as the management strategies are quite different. This is best done in the parasternal long view, where a pericardial effusion is visualized behind the left atrium, but anterior to the descending aorta. Pleural effusions are located posterior to the descending aorta (Figs. 37.41 and 37.42).

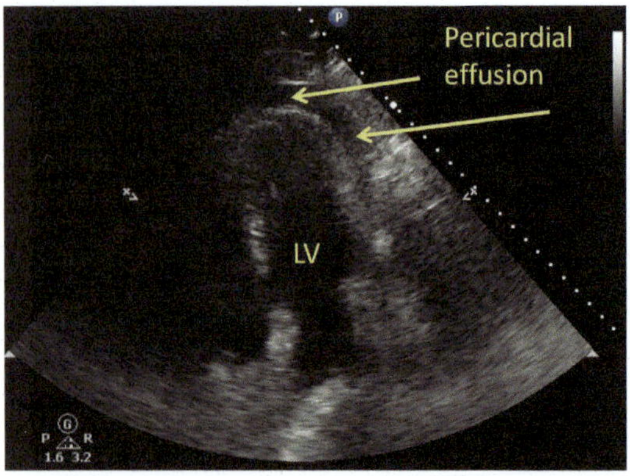

Fig. 37.37 A4C view demonstrating pericardial effusion. The RV/RA is difficult to visualize

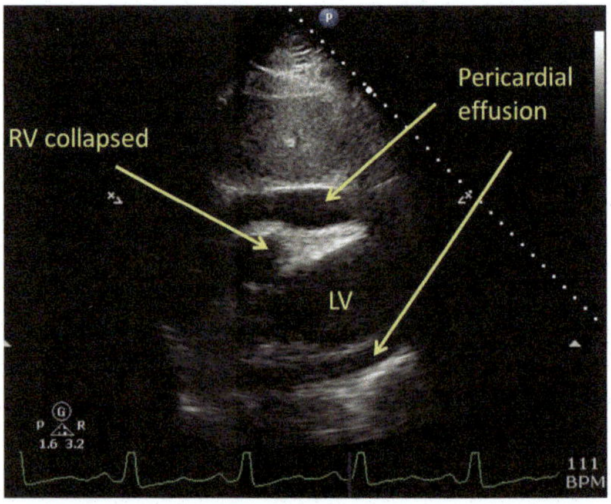

Fig. 37.39 Subxiphoid view with collapsed RV, demonstrating evidence of cardiac tamponade

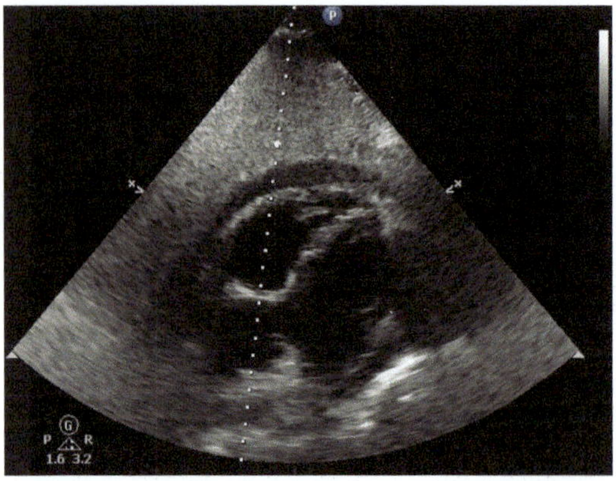

Fig. 37.38 Subxiphoid view with a pericardial effusion at end diastole. RV is full and does not demonstrate tamponade. Also demonstrates appropriate M-mode cursor alignment for tamponade assessment

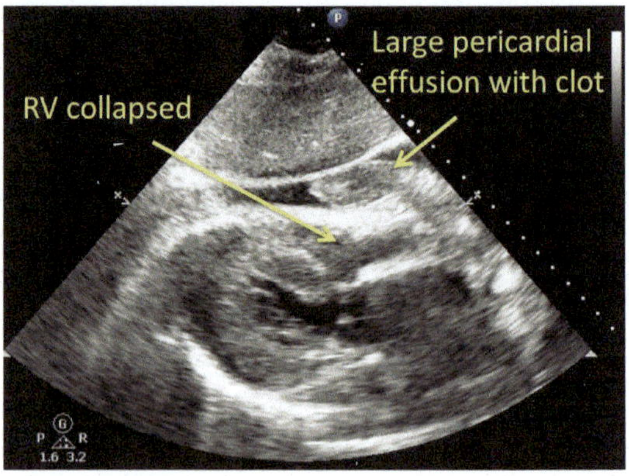

Fig. 37.40 PSL view with pericardial effusion and RV collapse. Note the large pericardial clot. Patient was a type A aortic dissection with retrograde dissection into the pericardium. Patient also has significant left ventricular hypertrophy

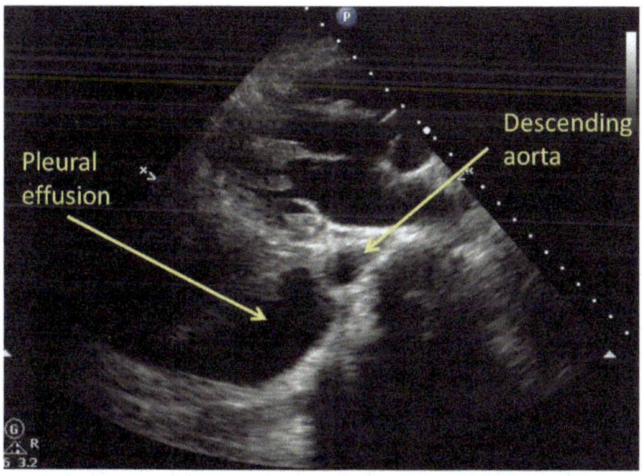

Fig. 37.41 PSL view with pleural effusion. Note that the effusion is posterior to the descending thoracic aorta

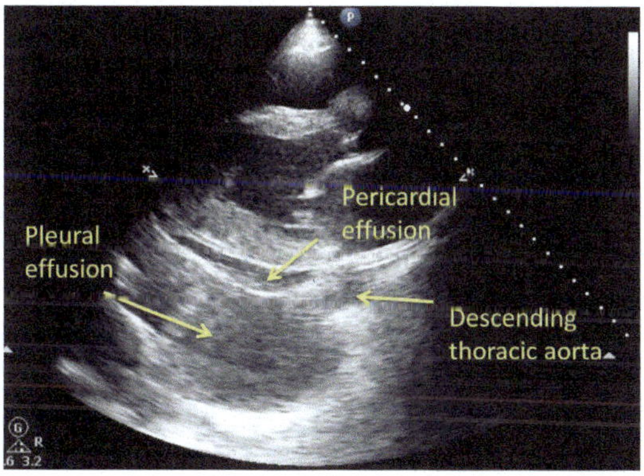

Fig. 37.42 PSL view with both a pericardial and pleural effusion. Again, note the relationships to the aorta

Supporting Literature After the diagnosis of cardiac tamponade has been established, volume resuscitation should be initiated immediately. Reversing any hypovolemia is critical, and increased right atrial and ventricular filling pressures with volume repletion may temporize the tamponade physiology, allowing for drainage of the effusion – either by pericardiocentesis or pericardiotomy by a surgeon [34, 35].

IVC Collapsibility and Echocardiographic Measures of Fluid Responsiveness

Emergent Question(s) Would my patient benefit from a fluid bolus or is their shock "volume responsive"? What echocardiographic measures predict fluid responsiveness?

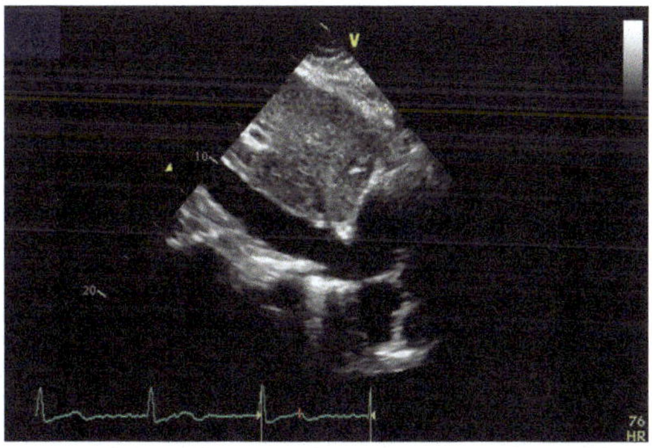

Fig. 37.43 Longitudinal view of the IVC draining into the RA

Probe Type Cardiac (phased array) or abdominal (curvilinear) probe: 2–5 MhZ

Clinical Scenario Many patients who are hypotensive or in a shock state will benefit from IV fluid administration. However, in those patients with volume overload or in those that have already received significant fluid resuscitation, additional IV fluids may be harmful.

Scanning Technique Recall that the IVC can be identified by starting in the subcostal cardiac view and rotating the transducer counterclockwise until the index marker is oriented towards the 12 o'clock position. Now, the IVC can be seen in its longitudinal orientation (see section "Basic Echocardiography and Views" for further details regarding general IVC scanning techniques and identification) (Fig. 37.43).

The IVC size is usually measured 1–2 cm distal to the hepatic vein, and collapsibility is visually measured (greater than or less than 50%) or actually measured by using the M-mode during inspiration. If an epigastric approach is difficult due to bowel gas, abdominal wounds, or surgical dressing, the IVC can also be viewed from a lateral position at the midaxillary line with the index marker at the 12 o'clock position, giving a sagittal view, using the liver as an acoustic window (Fig. 37.44).

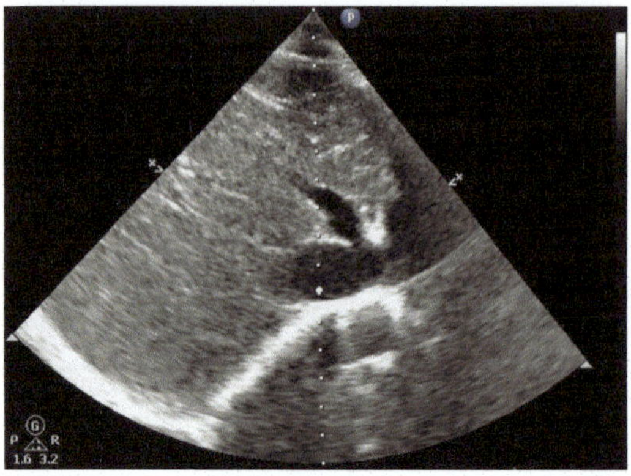

Fig. 37.44 IVC in longitudinal view. The M-mode cursor is place 1–2 cm left of the hepatic vein

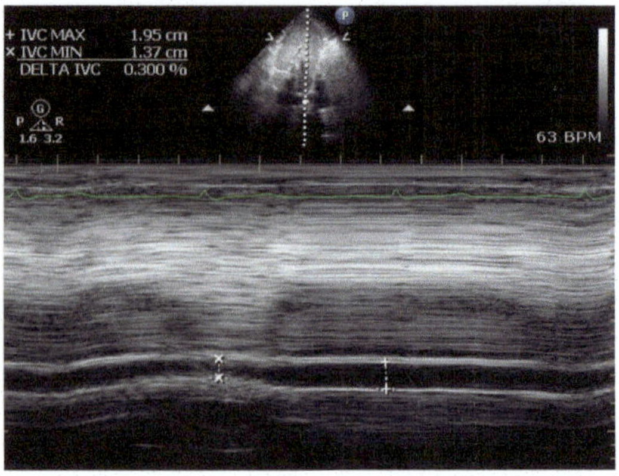

Fig. 37.46 IVC in M-mode with an IVC-CI of 30%

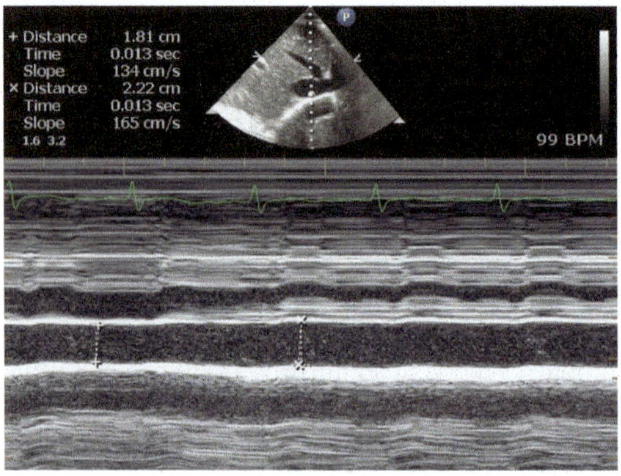

Fig. 37.45 IVC in M-mode with minimal collapsibility

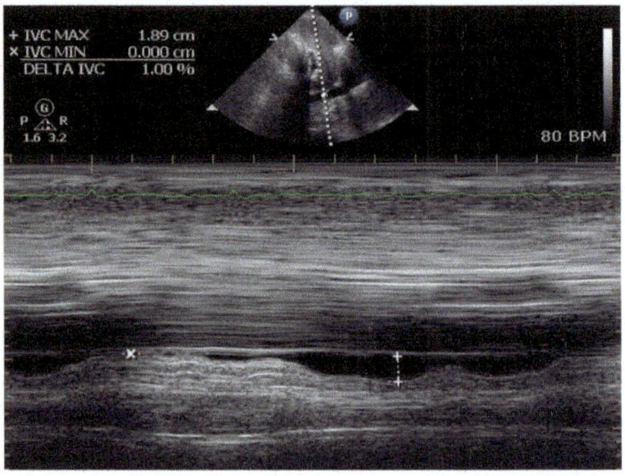

Fig.37.47 IVC in M-mode with an IVC-CI of 100%

Assessment of IVC collapsibility can be done in a variety of ways, but typically M-mode is used in the longitudinal view of the IVC. As the diaphragm moves inferiorly during inspiration, the IVC may move in and out of plane and can often be mistaken for complete collapsibility. The walls of the IVC must remain distinct throughout respirations to be an adequate exam. Also in longitudinal view, the plane may also be off-axis and not at its maximal diameter throughout the respiratory cycle [39]. Thus, it is recommended that a combination of transverse and longitudinal views and B-mode visual assessment and M-mode quantification be used to completely assess IVC collapsibility (Figs. 37.45, 37.46, and 37.47).

Supporting Literature Risk of organ failure and mortality is influenced by systemic perfusion, but positive fluid balance may worsen patient outcomes [40, 41]. Evaluation of the inferior vena cava size and collapsibility is a potential method of noninvasive adjunct to estimate central venous pressure. Bedside ultrasound evaluation of the inferior vena cava can estimate central venous pressure with acceptable predictive value and reliability between operators [42, 43]. The size and collapsibility of the inferior vena cava has been used in the non-acute settings for estimation of right atrial pressures. IVC diameters less than 2 cm in many studies have been shown as a great predictor of low CVP. IVC diameters greater than 2 cm are less predictive and in some studies have found that 25% of patients with IVC diameters greater than 2 cm have correlations with central venous pressure less than 10 mm HG [44–46]. However, IVC diameter may correlate well with CVP; CVP is unlikely an accurate predictor of volume responsiveness [47].

IVC-CI also correlates with CVP [48, 49], but more importantly has been shown to predict volume responsiveness, in both intubated and non-intubated patients [50–52]. PEEP and spontaneous breathing change intrathoracic pressure dynamics and greatly affect venous return and preload responsiveness. Assessment for preload responsiveness has only been studied in flow-limited, volume-cycled ventilation in patients who aren't spontaneously breathing above the set ventilator rate. Other caveats include presumption of normal sinus rhythm, normal intra-abdominal pressure, and absence of RV dysfunction. So, while IVC-CI is a good predictor of volume responsiveness, its generalizability to all critically ill patients is likely limited.

IVC-CI is the most heavily studied surrogate of volume responsiveness, but other measures include subclavian, internal jugular, and femoral collapsibility. These have yet to be completely validated and their usefulness is currently limited [53, 54].

Bedside echocardiography can also be used to assess stroke volume variation (SVV) by using pulsed wave Doppler measurements of flow through the aortic valve. Cardiac output (CO) can also be assessed through measurements of LVOT diameter and velocity time integral (VTI). These measurements are somewhat advanced, and single values of cardiac output may not be particularly helpful. However, when measured serially in response to interventions such as passive leg raise (PLR), they are quite accurate in predicting volume responsiveness [55]. While technically more advanced than IVC-CI, they are accurate and clinically useful to the experienced sonographer [56] (Figs. 37.48, 37.49, and 37.50)

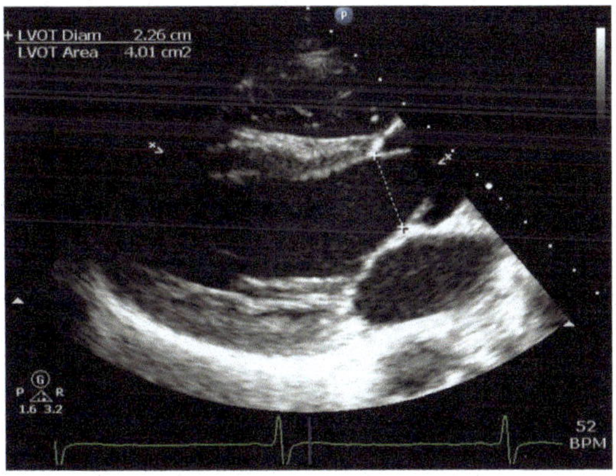

Fig. 37.48 PSL view during systole demonstrating how to measure LVOT

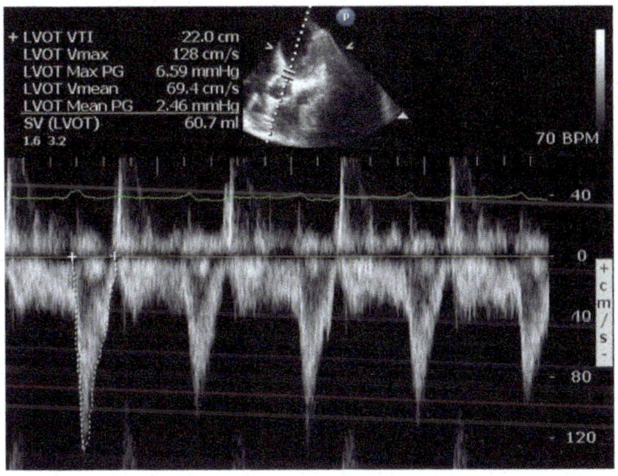

Fig. 37.49 A4C with pulsed-wave Doppler through the aortic valve demonstrating LVOT-VTI tracing

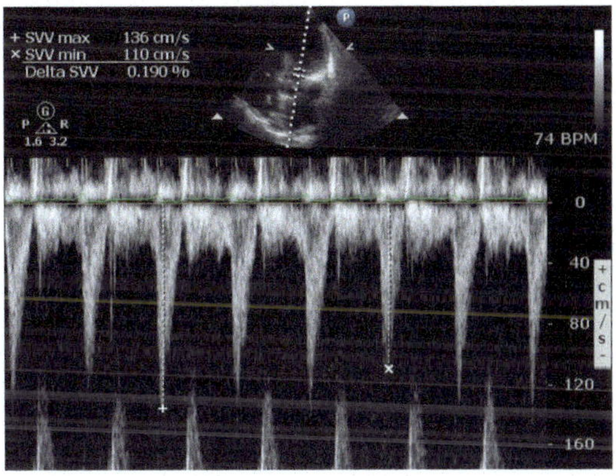

Fig. 37.50 SVV can be calculated using stroke volume assessments on echo

Vascular

Aorta

Emergent Question Is the aorta enlarged?

Probe Type Cardiac (phased array) or abdominal (curvilinear) probe: 2–5 MhZ

Critical Care Scenario Patients who are hypotensive should be evaluated for aortic aneurysm and possible dissection. If an abnormally high aorta size is found in a patient who is hypotensive, the clinician should consider aortic dissection as a possible cause of the hypotension. The ability for limited exam to detect aortic dissection is not accurate, and the limited exam must be used to help provide guidance for further definitive imaging or treatment in case the patient is unstable for transfer to radiological suite.

Scanning technique The patient should be in the supine position. The probe marker is towards the patient's right side for obtaining transverse views of the aorta and towards the patient's head for the longitudinal views. Gentle pressure is applied in the epigastric region to push bowel gas out of the way (Fig. 37.54). The aorta should be imaged from the proximal celiac trunk to the distal bifurcation. It's usually visualized as the circular vessel immediately anterior to the vertebral body (Fig. 37.51). Both transverse and longitudinal planes should be measured at its maximal diameter from outside wall to outside wall. A measurement should be made near the celiac trunk and another measurement distal to the iliac bifurcation. The transverse measurement is preferred due to "cylinder" effect and underestimation of aortic size in the longitudinal measurements (Fig. 37.52). Abdominal aorta size greater than 3 cm and iliac arteries size greater than 1.5 cm are an indication of abnormal size (Fig. 37.53). Another common challenge is ensuring the aorta is imaged and not the inferior vena cava. The inferior vena cava has both sides bordered by the liver, whereas the aorta does not. Other landmarks such as the spinal shadow and celiac takeoffs should be used to confirm appropriate vessel is evaluated (Fig. 37.54).

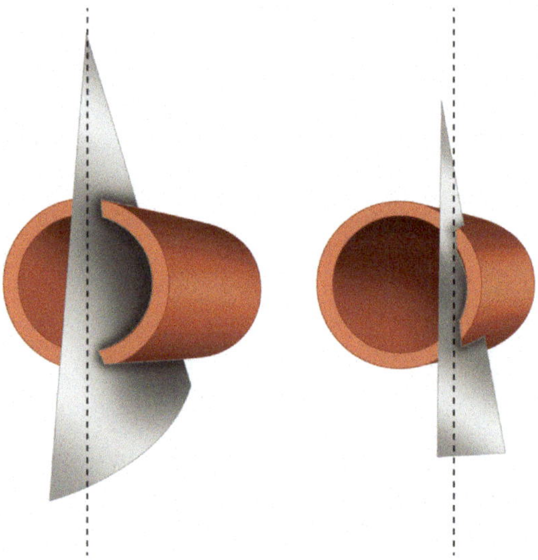

Fig. 37.52 Cylinder effect showing underestimation of size in longitudinal view. (Source: Ma OJ, Mateer JR, Reardon RF, Joing SA. *Ma and Mateer's emergency ultrasound, Third Edition*. www.accessemergencymedicine.com. Copyright © The McGraw-Hill Companies, Inc)

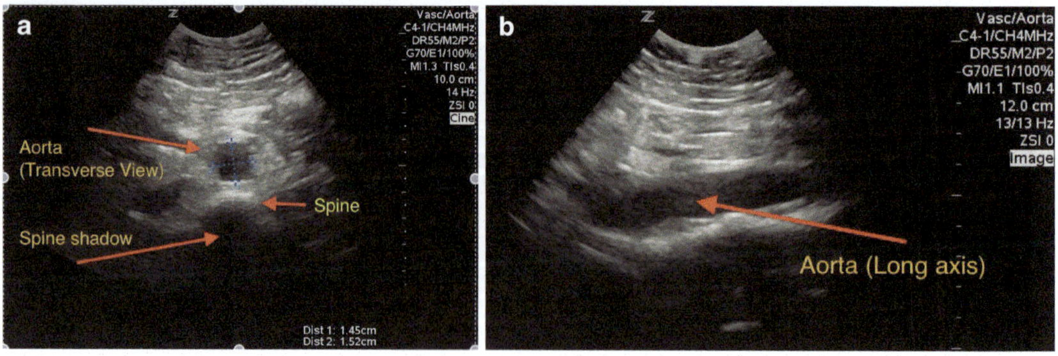

Fig. 37.51 (**a**) Aorta in transverse view. (**b**) Aorta in longitudinal view

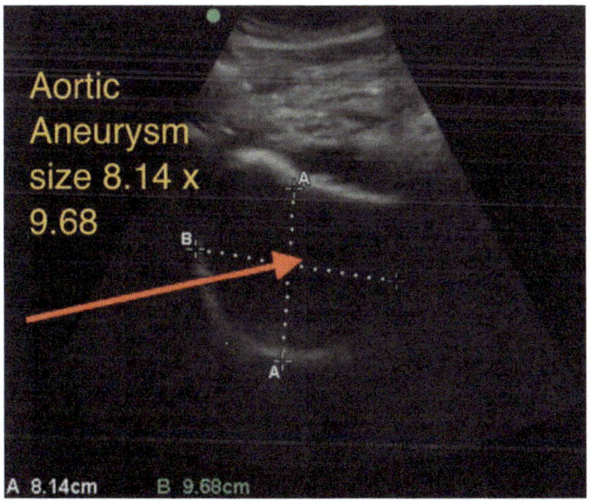

Fig. 37.53 Aortic aneurysm

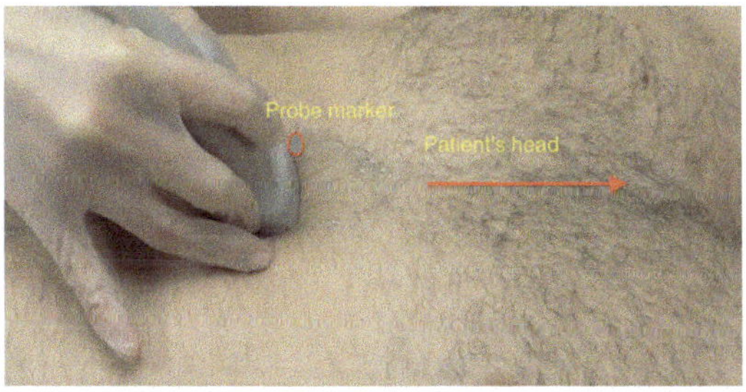

Fig. 37.54 Probe location-transverse view

Supporting Literature Imaging of the aorta is becoming applicable for many situations. A class B recommendation was given by the US Preventive Services Task Force for one time ultrasound screening for abdominal aortic aneurysms in men between ages of 65 and 75 who had ever smoked. This led to the addition of screening for abdominal aortic aneurysms into Medicare reimbursement [57, 58]. Also there have been many studies that have shown that emergency physicians are able to obtain these views comparable to computed tomography scans [59–61].

Deep Vein Evaluation (Deep Femoral Vein, Superficial Femoral Vein, Popliteal Vein)

Emergent Question Is the common femoral or popliteal vein fully compressible?

Probe Type Vascular probe (linear array, high frequency): 7.5–10 MhZ

Critical Care Scenario Patients who are unable to be transferred to radiological suites for evaluation of pulmonary embolism may benefit from evaluation of lower extremity deep veins. Also in patients who are in acute resuscitation, finding a deep vein thrombosis may provide the clinician with more confidence in making the decision for heparin or intra-arrest thrombolytic agents.

Scanning Technique Most patients in the emergent setting will be unable to sit in the best position to evaluate the lower extremity veins (with legs hanging off the bed). Most patients are supine and the visualization of the deep veins of the lower extremity can be improved by externally rotating the leg. The probe marker should be directed towards the patient's right side. If the veins are collapsible with pressure, the vein is patent and there is no clot present. If the veins do not collapse with pressure, there may be a clot within the lumen of the vessel preventing collapse. If the artery is seen in relationship to the vein (which is preferred), the amount of pressure applied should be even and just enough show some small deformity in the artery visualized. The strength and direction of compression is important since if not done strong enough, one might think there is a thrombus when there is not, and if done too aggressively one might miss early thrombi formation that is not clearly seen in the lumen of the vessel. Also, the pressure should be applied evenly and perpendicular to the skin, if pressure applied at angle, the vessel may appear not to collapse. The most common examinations are the "two-point" and the "three-point" studies, where two-point examination studies the common femoral vein and the popliteal vein and the three-point examination adds the superficial femoral vein. The two-point examination has been well validated in the outpatient population [62–64]. The three-point examination is recommended as there have been studies that show higher incidence of clots isolated to the superficial femoral vein in asymptomatic patients [65, 66]. In a study by Kory et al., they found their sensitivity would have decreased from 88% to 82% if the superficial femoral vein was not included; and as a result they recommend a three-point protocol [67]. The common femoral vein should compress fully and done at the greater saphenous takeoff (Fig. 37.55). Then you can move just a bit distal to image the deep/superficial femoral vein junction. The last location to evaluate is the popliteal vein behind the knee. In the supine patient, the operator can lift the leg and place the probe behind the knee. One must not mistake the lymph node for a clotted femoral vein and can be best prevented by scanning proximal and distal or turning your probe to the longitudinal axis, as a lymph node will not continue in either direction more than a few centimeters and appears as a circular structure in longitudinal views (Fig. 37.56).

Supporting Literature Venous thromboembolism has been shown to lead to significant morbidity and mortality when undiagnosed in the emergently ill patient [68–70]. It has also been shown that clinicians with focused training in ultrasound can perform accurate proximal lower extremity deep vein studies, with a study from Blaivas et al. showing that emergency medicine physicians with 5 hours of training achieved a 98% agreement with formal ultrasound [71–73]. Most studies done on this topic had examinations that were limited to the proximal veins secondary to the undefined clinical relevance of calf vein thrombosis in the intensive care units, the much lower sensitivity of ultrasound to diagnose calf deep vein thrombosis, and the increased time this would require [63, 74].

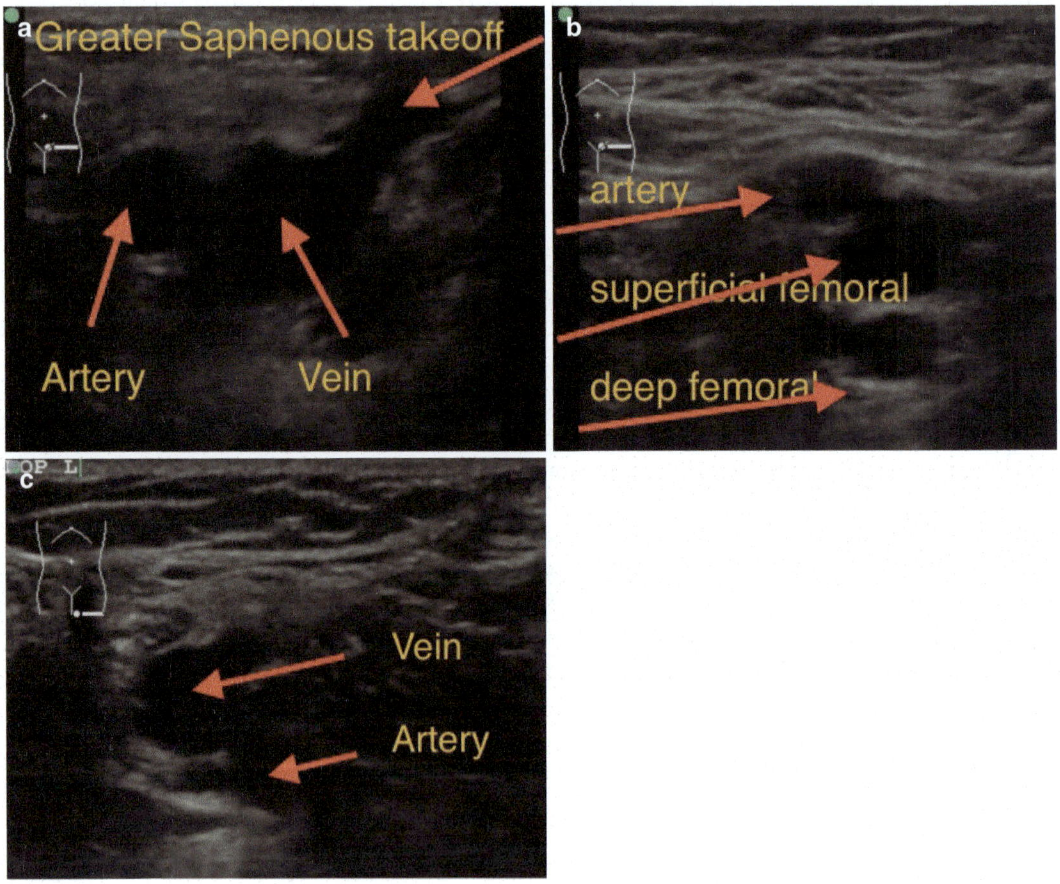

Fig. 37.55 Common femoral at greater saphenous (**a**), superficial femoral (**b**), popliteal (**c**)

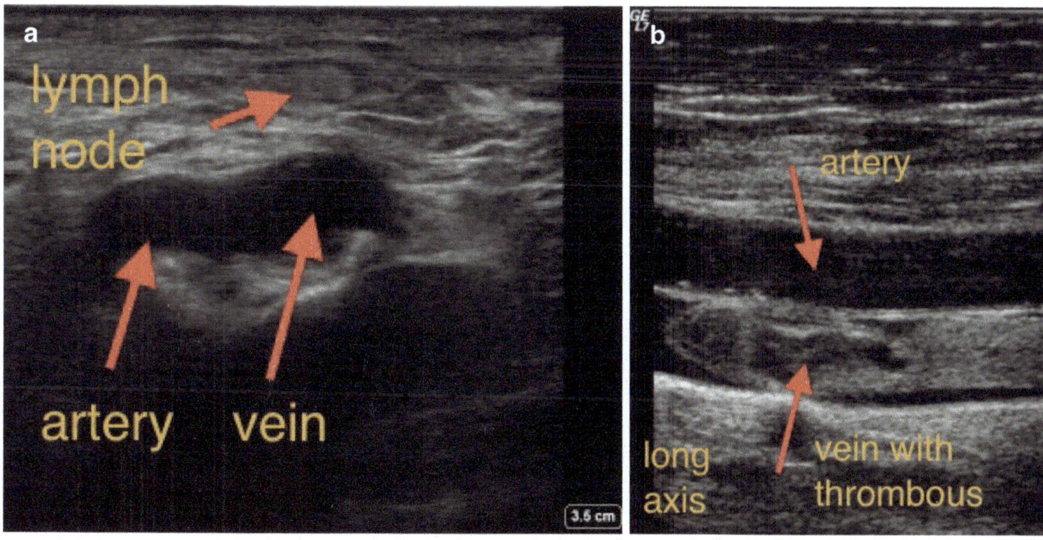

Fig. 37.56 Lymph node (**a**) and deep vein thrombosis (**b**) in comparison

Lung

General Information Many specialties are now incorporating lung ultrasound into specific scenarios faced by each one in routine basis. Several new studies over the past 10 years with growing terminologies with differences in evaluation, approach, nomenclature, and techniques of evaluation have led to international evidence-based recommendations for point of care lung ultrasound [75]. Many times transportation of emergently ill patients is impossible and the ability to evaluate the lung at bedside can be very helpful in decision-making for the treatment plan. Each of the individual applications below will be discussed and then combined to form the basis of evaluation of patients in shock from hypoxia or respiratory failure. The "BLUE" protocol and "ICU-sound" protocol both found that diagnostic accuracy of lung ultrasound to differentiate dyspneic patients is increased greatly [76, 77].

Pneumothorax

Emergent Question(s) Is a lung point present? Do I have absence of lung sliding? Do I have absence of B lines? Do I have absence of a lung pulse?

Probe Type Vascular (linear array) probe: 5–10 MhZ preferred for evaluation of pleural interface, but can use curvilinear (2–5 MhZ) probe in resuscitation/trauma-type situations where other lung abnormalities are being evaluated. The high-frequency linear array probe can be better when analyzing lung sliding or teaching a novice.

Clinical Scenario The patient who cannot be easily transported to radiological suite or arrest patient who has ongoing resuscitation efforts so that portable imaging cannot be performed. Also, acute trauma situations where patient is decompensating and concern for pneumothorax as a potential cause.

Scanning Technique The patient usually is in the supine position, so most of the studies performed have evaluated for pneumothorax in the supine position. The sonographer's hand must remain stabilized to prevent artifact, which may make it more difficult to evaluate the sonographic signs of pneumothorax. The probe marker is placed towards the patient's head. The probe is first placed on the sternum in which the operator will see an ultrasound image with large shadowing artifact from the sternum. First move laterally towards the right chest and identify the pleural

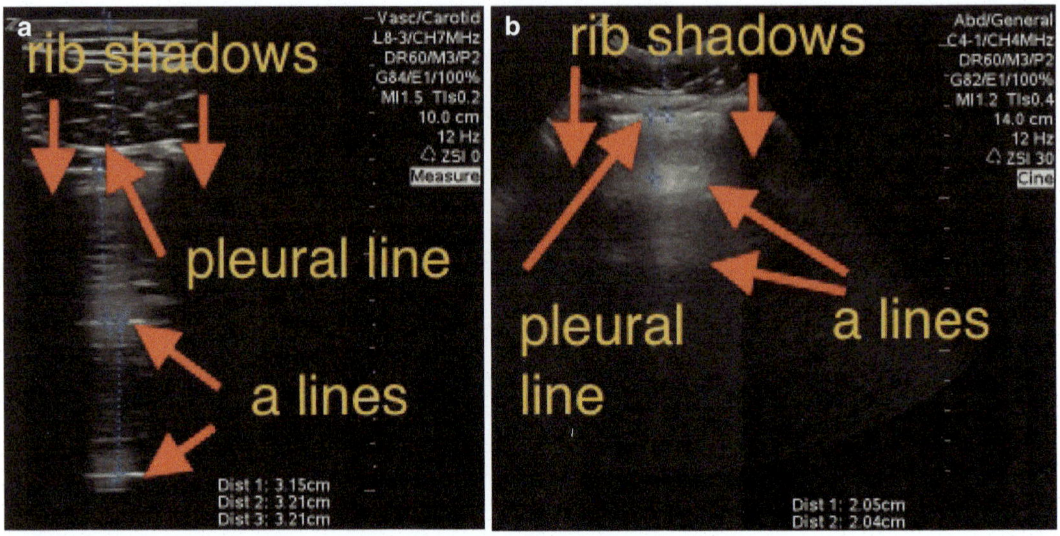

Fig. 37.57 (**a**) Rib shadows with pleural line (linear array probe); (**b**) rib shadows with pleural line and A lines (phased array probe)

line between two rib interfaces (Fig. 37.57). Evaluation consists of identifying "lung sliding" which is the side to side movement of the pleural line with breathing. Lung sliding is the regular rhythmic movements synchronized with respiration that occur between the parietal and visceral pleura that are in direct contact (without air between them). Once air is between the two layers, the movement seen is absent. If you see lung sliding, there is no pneumothorax in that part of the chest wall examined. The exam can continue laterally towards the mid axillary line. The same is repeated on the left side (may need to go more towards the head due to the cardiac chambers obscuring the lung views). The evaluation for pneumothorax entails the search for a lung point, which is the point where the visceral pleura and parietal pleura are against each other without air interposition and slides with respiration and corresponds to the lateral edge of the pneumothorax [78]. This can be seen between two ribs as part of the interface with sliding present (representing the parietal and visceral pleural without air between them) and the other part without sliding present (representing air between the parietal and visceral pleura). The more lateral on the chest wall this lung point manifests, the larger the pneumothorax in supine patients. This may be useful since size of the lung collapse usually determines treatment and establishes the prognosis for the pneumothorax [79, 80].

Other sonographic signs of pneumothorax besides absence of lung sliding described above include absence of B lines and absence of lung pulse. B lines are artifacts found that originate from the visceral pleura (B lines discussed further in section "Pulmonary Edema or Interstitial Syndrome"), and their presence proves that the visceral pleura is opposing the parietal and therefore excludes pneumothorax at that point in the chest wall (Fig. 37.58). B lines can be present in other processes such as pneumonia, pulmonary contusion, pulmonary fibrosis, or aspiration. Last, if a lung pulse is found, there is no pneumothorax. The lung pulse refers to the rhythmic movements of the visceral upon the parietal due to the cardiac oscillations [81]. One must be careful not to use only lung sliding as a determinant of pneumothorax, as this sign is also found in apneic patients, "mainstem intubations" where one lung is ventilated, acute lung injury (ALI), lung fibrosis, pneumonia, blebs, and various other lung disease processes. In the emergent setting, the absence of any movement of the pleural line, either horizontal (lung sliding) or vertical

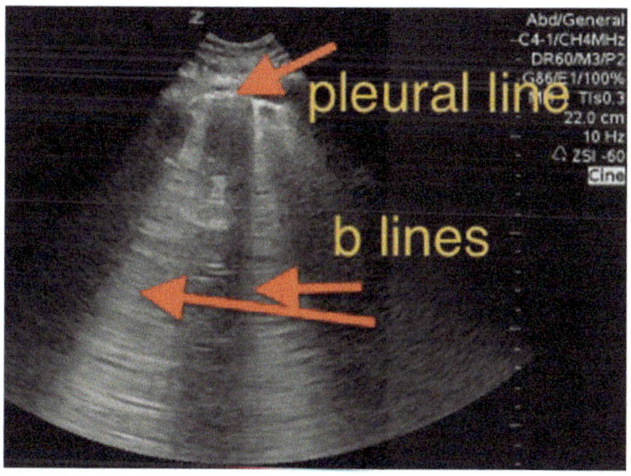

Fig. 37.58 B lines

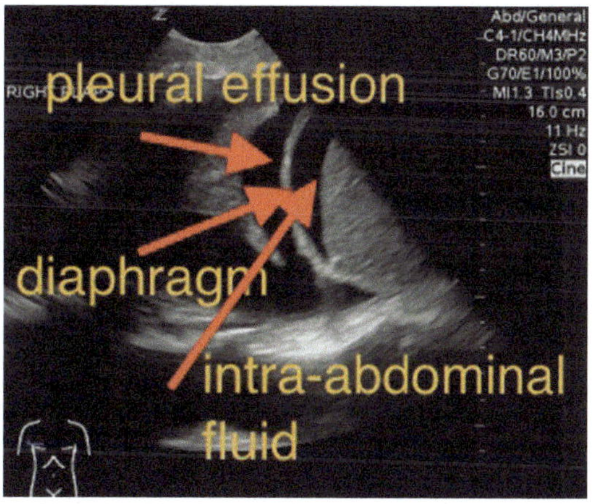

Fig. 37.59 Diaphragm with ascites and pleural fluid

(lung pulse), coupled with absence of B lines allows for diagnosis of pneumothorax without searching for the lung point [82].

Supporting Literature Supine chest radiography is not sensitive for diagnosis of pneumothorax [83, 84]. Lung ultrasound is more accurate than chest radiography in ruling out pneumothorax and can benefit evaluation in cardiac arrest or unstable patients [85–87]. According to the international recommendations, lung ultrasound more accurately rules out the diagnosis of pneumothorax than supine anterior chest radiography. Although mentioned that the lung point can be used to determine size of pneumothorax, the international point of care recommendations also state that due to controversy over the pathophysiology of expansion of pneumothorax, and lack of evidence in human studies, ultrasound is not a reliable method to assess the volume of pneumothorax as compared to computed tomography and concluded the need for additional evidence [88]. Also the treatment may depend on many other clinical factors that are out of the scope of this text.

Pleural Effusion

Emergent Question Do I have a moderate or large pleural effusion that the patient might benefit from acute drainage, either improving oxygenation, alleviating dyspnea, or improving ventilation?

Probe Type Cardiac (phased array) or abdominal (curvilinear) probe: 2–5 MhZ

Clinical Scenario Patients who have acute respiratory failure, hypoxia, or increased work of breathing on the ventilator may benefit from evacuation of pleural fluid. Patients in the acute trauma bay also can benefit from this by using as part of the extended FAST exam to identify hemothorax.

Scanning Technique Small effusions may be better visualized with patient sitting in the upright position, but of interest to us in the emergent setting are the moderate to large effusions. Most of these patients will be limited to the supine position. The probe marker is positioned towards the patient's right and placed in the midaxillary line. The diaphragm is a very important structure to identify and so the exam is best to start with identification of the renal and liver interface, since this is an easily identifiable structure in most patients. Once this location is identified, the probe is moved towards the patient's head along the midaxillary line and the liver/diaphragm interface should be noted and recorded. This is very important in that many patients with pleural effusions may also have ascites. The diaphragm must be visualized in relationship in order to correctly identify pleural fluid (Fig. 37.59). Once the area visualized is confirmed to be above the diaphragm, the probe can be angled slightly towards

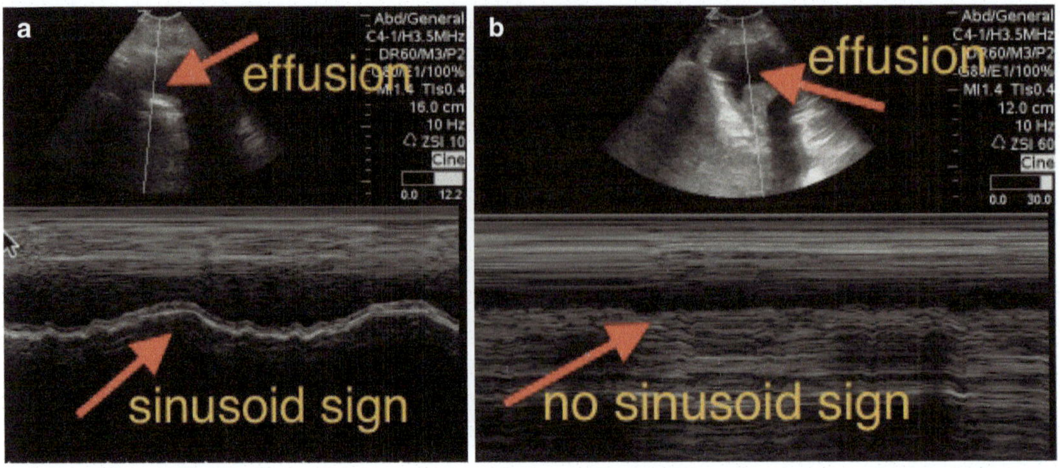

Fig. 37.60 (**a**) Moderate to large effusion, with split screen showing sine wave "sinusoid" sign; (**b**) moderate to large effusion with no sinusoid sign

the bed to better visualize the whole lung field. An anechoic space between the parietal and visceral pleura and respiratory movement of the lung within the effusion (sinusoid sign) is present in almost all free effusions (Fig. 37.60). This sign is a dynamic sign showing variation of interpleural distance during respiration. This can be visualized in M-mode as a sine wave when the M-mode line is positioned over the visceral pleura through the effusion [89, 90]. If the lung is not freely moving, the lung is sometimes referred to as "trapped." This might be an indicator that removal of fluid may "un-trap" the lung so that oxygenation can be improved. An effusion with internal echoes (mobile particles or septa) suggests an exudate or hemorrhage. While most transudates are anechoic, some exudates can also be anechoic and therefore thoracentesis may be needed to further classify [91, 92]. This technique can be done on the side of interest to the clinician or in part of an acute respiratory failure algorithm done on both sides.

Supporting Literature In the evaluation of pleural effusion, ultrasound is more accurate than supine radiography and is as accurate as computed tomography. Also, in opacifications seen on chest radiography, lung ultrasound should be used to distinguish between effusions and consolidations [93]. Balik et al. have shown that you can estimate the drainage that can be done with a formula, although it is not used frequently due to underestimation of volume [94, 95]. Also if one is attempting to reduce the work of breathing and increase respiratory muscle efficiency, the consideration of removal of pleural fluid should be made even though there have not been validated criteria for decision-making process [96]. Many times the decision to drain can be made on clinical parameters such as reduced chest wall compliance, difficulty weaning, refractory hypotension or when ultrasound suggests, and infectious effusion (homogenous echogenicity, septation, fibrin strands, nodular pleural changes) [97].

Pneumonia or Lung Consolidation

Emergent Question Do I see a lung consolidation with air bronchograms?

Probe Type Cardiac (phased array) or abdominal (curvilinear) probe: 2–5 MhZ

Clinical Scenario Patients who are in respiratory failure with unknown etiology and unstable for transfer to radiological suite might benefit from evaluation of the lung fields for large consolidations that might be the etiology. This examination can also be helpful in differentiating consolidation from pleural effusions in the acutely hypoxic patient.

Scanning Technique The acutely ill patient is usually in the supine position. The probe marker is towards the patient's head and the operator should start the exam with the probe on the sternum. The image obtained will be a shadow artifact from bony sternum. First move towards the right anterior chest and then move laterally towards the posterior thorax. Multiple areas can be studied and the various types of pneumonias produce abnormalities at many locations on the chest wall (Fig. 37.61). The sonographic sign we are looking for is a subpleural echo-poor region or one with a tissue-like echo texture ("tissue-like sign") (Fig. 37.62). Also, one of the most important criteria is a positive air bronchogram within the tissue-like sign and has been shown to be found in 70–97% of cases [98–100] (Fig. 37.63a). Atelectasis has to be differentiated from pneumonia. Atelectasis is normal due to large pleural effusion and moves within an effusion; it is moderately echoic and sharply demarcated. Air bronchograms indicating pneumonia can sometimes be seen as moving to and fro with respirations or ventilator breaths and are referred to as "dynamic" air bronchograms and mean bronchial patency and rule out obstructive atelectasis [101]. Pneumonia appears as a hypoechogenic area with poorly defined borders and presence of B lines with lung sliding reduced or absent. Multiple lenticular echoes, representing air trapped in the smaller airways, are also frequently observed (Fig. 37.63b).

Supporting Literature Lung ultrasound should be considered an accurate tool in ruling in lung consolidations when compared to chest radiography. In mechanically ventilated patients, lung ultrasound should be considered because it is more accurate than chest radiography in differential diagnosis of consolidation which includes

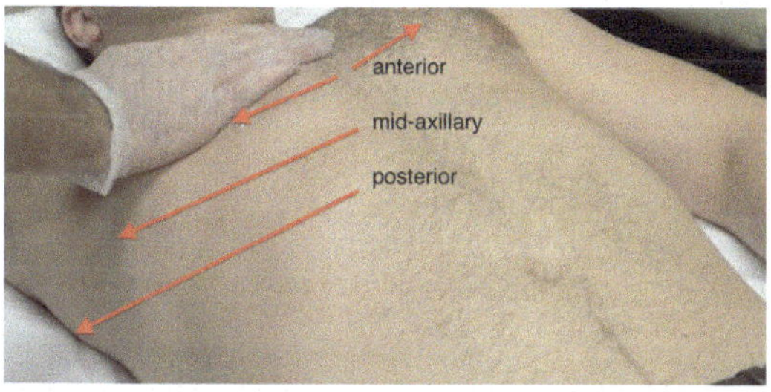

Fig. 37.61 Chest zones for evaluation of pneumonia

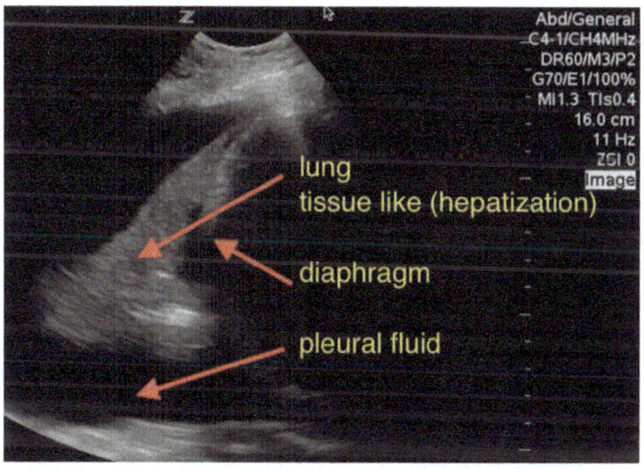

Fig. 37.62 Tissue-like sign

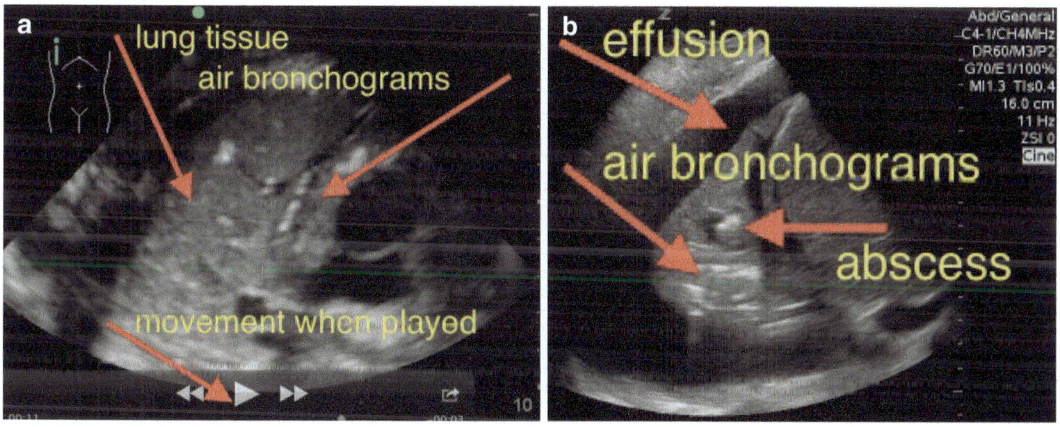

Fig. 37.63 (**a**) Air bronchogram; (**b**) lenticular echoes with abscess

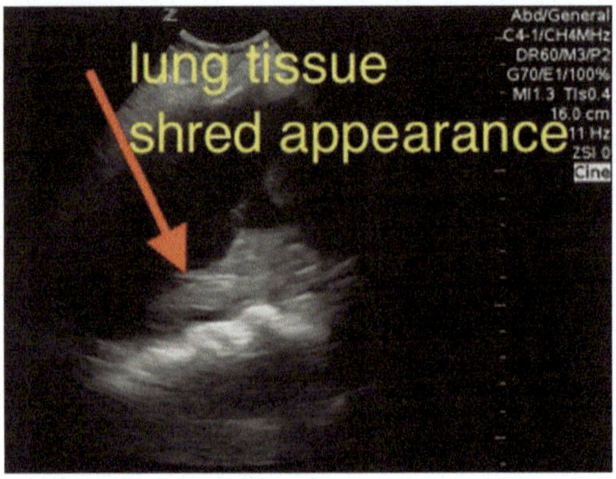

Fig. 37.64 Shredded lung sign

pneumonia, atelectasis, or pulmonary embolism [102]. In many recent studies it has been shown that lung ultrasound can be highly effective in evaluating pulmonary conditions such as pneumonia [103, 104]. High diagnostic accuracy was found in multiple studies where CT scan alone was the gold standard [105–107]. Bedetti et al. have shown that clinicians are able to detect presence of pulmonary interstitial syndrome after fewer than 10 examinations and total training time of 30 minutes [108] (Fig. 37.64).

Pulmonary Edema or Interstitial Syndrome

Emergent Question(s) Is my patient in a fluid overload state? Are B lines with lung sliding present?

Probe Type Cardiac (phased array) or abdominal (curvilinear) probe: 2–5 MhZ

Clinical Scenario In patients who present with severe dyspnea or acute respiratory failure requiring noninvasive ventilation or endotracheal intubation, evaluation for pulmonary edema can be performed. States such as hypertensive emergency, cardiogenic shock, or neurogenic pulmonary vasodilation can all cause similar lung patterns.

Scanning Technique The acutely ill patient is usually in the supine position. The probe marker is towards the patient's head and the operator should

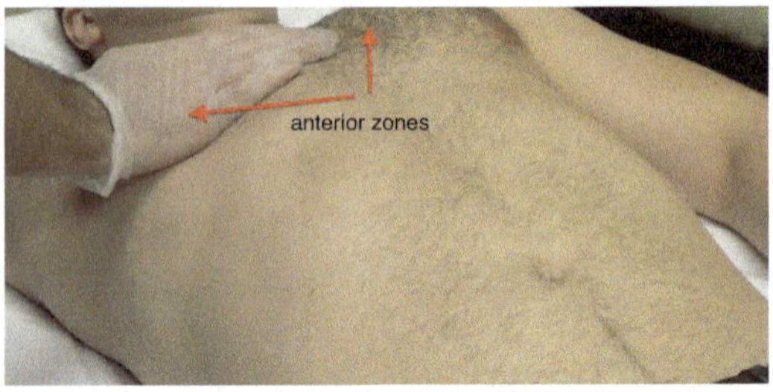

Fig. 37.65 Areas of chest to examine

start the exam with the probe on the sternum. The image obtained will be a shadow artifact from bony sternum. First move towards the right anterior chest and then move laterally towards the posterior thorax. Multiple areas can be studied and the various types of pneumonias produce abnormalities at many locations on the chest wall (Fig. 37.65). A more rapid two-region scan may be sufficient in some cases (anterior chest in the supine patient). B lines are vertical hyperechoic reverberation artifacts that arise from the pleural line and extend to the bottom of the ultrasound screen without fading. These lines can either be associated with lung sliding or not associated with lung sliding. The anatomic and physical basis of B lines is not clear at this time and could be related to alveolar wall thickening. Multiples of these lines are the sonographic sign of lung interstitial syndrome. A positive region is defined by the presence of more than 3 B lines in a longitudinal plane between the ribs (Fig. 37.66). Focal B lines can be present in normal lung. In cardiogenic pulmonary edema, these B lines are associated with lung sliding, with homogenous distribution in anterior bilateral chest exam, and "spared" areas are not observed, and the pleural line is rarely involved [109]. Pulmonary edema produces a transudate in this scenario, which is not supposed to generate inflammatory adherences (a factor that may affect lung sliding). In contrast, the findings in diffuse parenchymal lung disease include: pleural line abnormalities (irregular, fragmented pleural line), subpleural abnormalities (small echo-poor areas), and nonhomogenous distribution of B lines. In acute respiratory distress syndrome (ARDS), anterior subpleural consolidations, absence of lung sliding, "spared" areas of normal parenchyma, pleural line abnormalities (irregular fragmented pleural line),

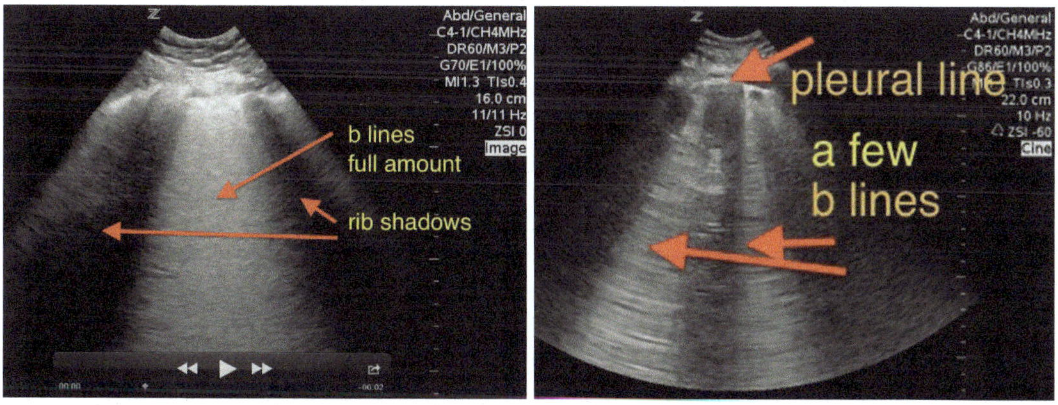

Fig. 37.66 B lines

and nonhomogenous distribution of B lines can be found [110]. Evaluation of B lines allows monitoring of response to therapy in cardiogenic pulmonary edema.

Supporting Literature Chest radiography can be used to diagnose pulmonary edema, but overall accuracy may be as low as 69% and findings of pulmonary edema can lag behind clinical changes [111, 112]. Many studies have now shown that lung ultrasound can be used to distinguish between cardiogenic and non-cardiogenic causes of dyspnea [113, 114]. Also B lines have been shown to correlate with more recognized methods of identifying pulmonary edema. Chest radiography [115], computed tomography [116], pulmonary capillary wedge pressure, quantitative measurements of extravascular lung water, and natriuretic peptide levels have all been correlated to B lines using lung ultrasound [117, 118]. The presence of B lines has also been shown to be dynamic, disappearing in patients undergoing hemodialysis [119].

Abdomen

Extended Focused Assessment with Sonography in Trauma (EFAST)

Background The focused assessment with sonography for trauma (FAST) was first described in Europe in the 1980s, with the first US studies in the 1990s, resulting in the subsequent replacement of diagnostic peritoneal lavage at most centers by the turn of the century [120–122].

The concept of ultrasonographic assessment of hemothorax was introduced in the late 1990s [123]. The extended FAST (EFAST) which first included ultrasonographic assessment of the pneumothorax was introduced in the 2000s [124–126]. The FAST is now the standard of care, endorsed by the American College of Surgeons in its Advanced Trauma Life Support (ATLS) course and by the American College of Emergency Physicians [127, 128].

Probe Type Abdominal (curvilinear) transducer (2–5 MhZ) is suggested for the abdominal portion of the EFAST and for assessment of hemothorax. It can also be used for xiphoid cardiac view, but we recommend switching to the cardiac (phased array) transducer (2–5 MhZ) if obtaining an adequate view is difficult. Finally, the vascular (linear array) transducer (5–10 MhZ) is best for evaluation of lung sliding, but this can also be done with the curvilinear transducer. The entire EFAST can be performed with the curvilinear transducer, but the sonographer should switch to the ideal transducer if time permits or if views are inadequate or indeterminate.

Scanning Technique The traditional FAST exam assesses four different areas – hepatorenal space, splenorenal space, pelvis, and pericardium. The extended FAST (EFAST) includes assessment of the thorax for pneumothorax and hemothorax.

Hepatorenal Space Morrison's pouch RUQ – In blunt trauma, most sonographers start their FAST assessment in the RUQ, as Morrison's pouch is the most sensitive location for the presence of peritoneal free fluid [120, 121]. Placing the patient in Trendelenburg position may help to increase that sensitivity even more [129].

With the index marker towards the patient's head, the sonographer should use the liver as an acoustic window, assessing the hepatorenal space. If positive, anechoic fluid will appear between the liver and kidney, frequently accumulating near the caudal tip of the liver. The sonographer should visualize the entire interface between the two organs, as small amounts of free fluid may not be visible in a single view (Figs. 37.67, 37.68, and 37.69).

Continuing to use the liver as a window, the transducer should now be directed upwards towards the right hemidiaphragm. The diaphragm appears as a thick, hyperechoic line at the top border of the liver on the left of the screen. When present, anechoic blood will denote a hemothorax on the other side of the diaphragm (see section "Pleural Effusion" for further details regarding scanning technique).

Splenorenal Space or LUQ With the index marker pointed towards the patient's head, the spleen should be used as an acoustic window to assess the splenorenal space. In comparison to the RUQ, the ideal acoustic window for the LUQ is typically somewhat higher and more posterior. Again, the entire interface between the spleen and kidney should be visualized. It is common that free fluid accumulates above the spleen, just below the diaphragm due to the ligamentous anatomy, so one must be sure to observe the interface between the left hemidiaphragm and spleen. The left hemothorax should also be assessed in this view, looking for hemothorax above the diaphragm (Figs. 37.70, 37.71, and 37.72).

Pelvis or Pouch of Douglass The pelvis should be assessed using a transverse view of the urinary bladder by placing the transducer just above the pubic symphysis with the index

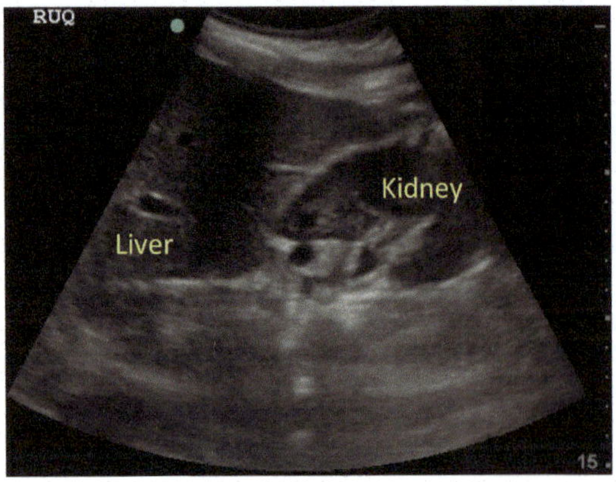

Fig. 37.67 Normal RUQ FAST. Note the hyperechoic fascial line between the liver and kidney

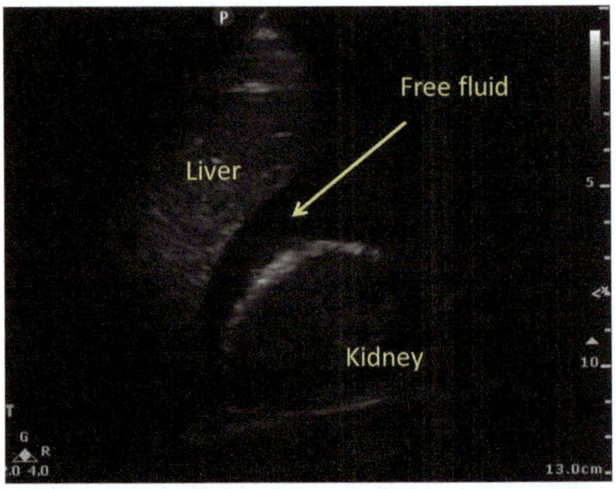

Fig. 37.68 RUQ FAST with a moderate amount of free fluid

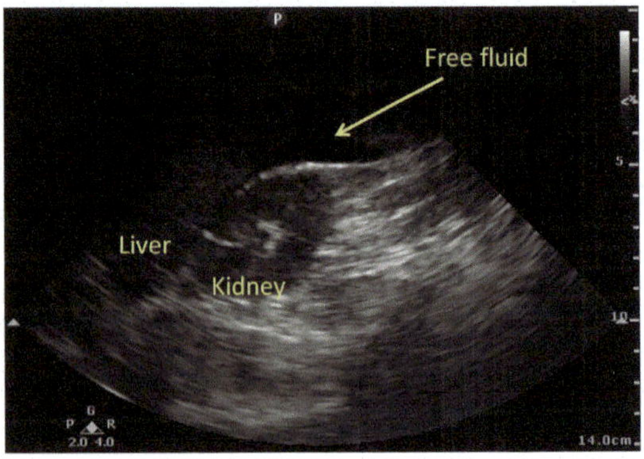

Fig. 37.69 RUQ FAST with a small amount of free fluid at the caudal tip of the liver

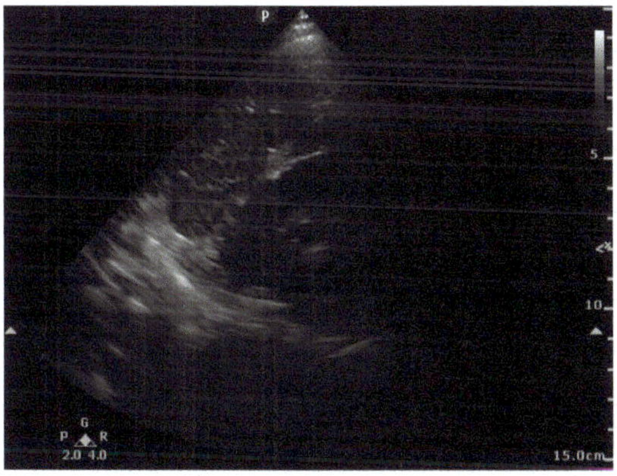

Fig. 37.70 Normal LUQ FAST

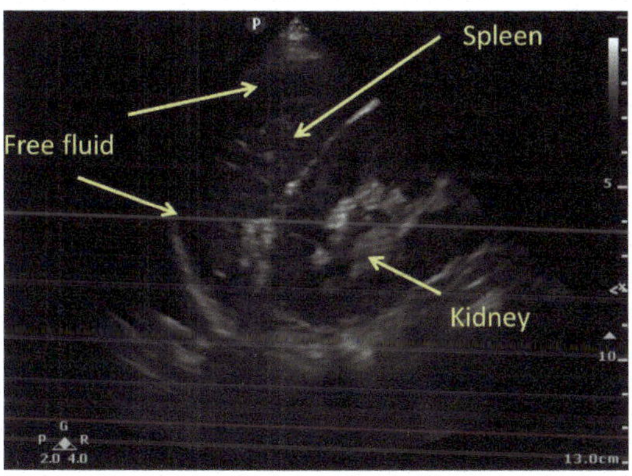

Fig. 37.71 Positive LUQ FAST with fluid above the spleen

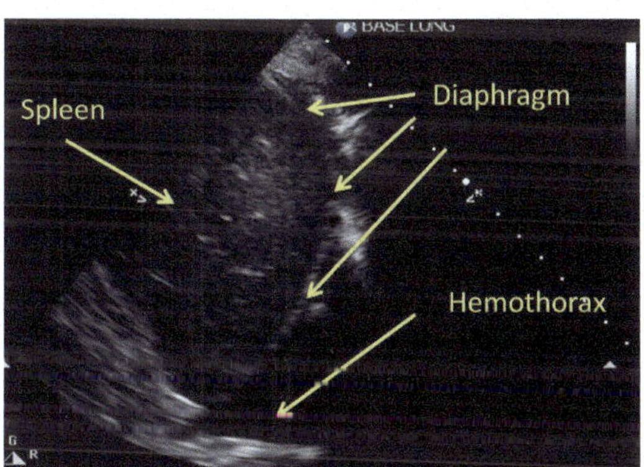

Fig. 37.72 LUQ FAST demonstrating hemothorax

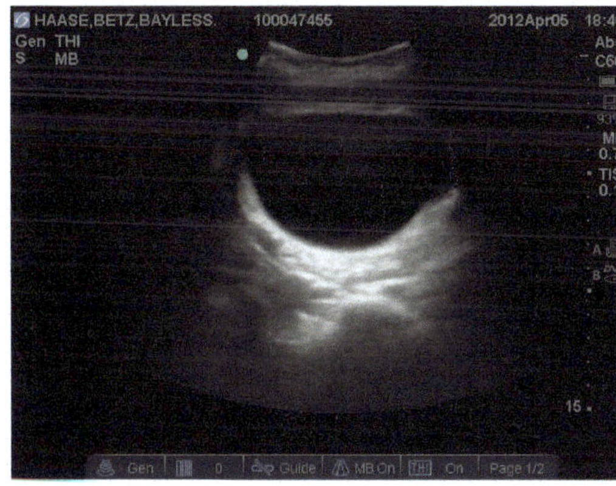

Fig. 37.73 Negative transverse view of the pelvis

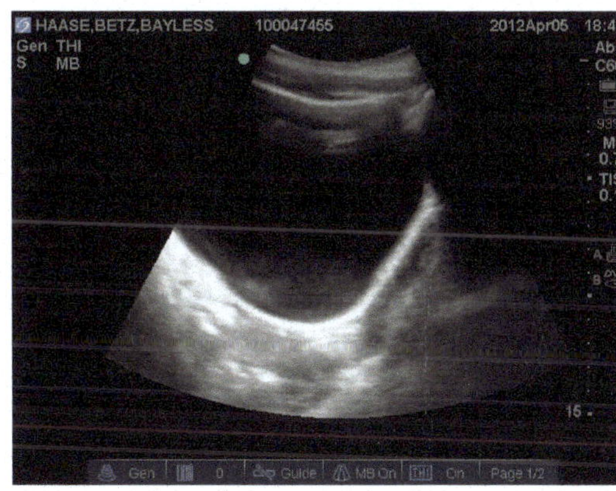

Fig. 37.74 Negative longitudinal view of the pelvis. The pubic symphysis is on the right of the image causing shadowing

marker pointed towards the patient's right and aiming inferiorly. Rotating the transducer 90° clockwise will obtain longitudinal views of pelvis. A full urinary bladder is useful as an acoustic window and may help to distinguish pelvic structures. In males, free fluid will appear posterior to the bladder, and in females, fluid will initially accumulate posterior to the uterus in the cul-de-sac, and as large amounts accumulate, fluid may be seen anterior to the uterus (Figs. 37.73, 37.74, and 37.75).

Pericardium On the FAST, pericardial fluid is typically assessed from the subxiphoid approach. The sonographer may have difficulty in obese patients or those with abdominal distension. Switching to a phased array (or cardiac) transducer may be helpful. Parasternal views should be attempted if subxiphoid views are inadequate or indeterminate (see section "Pericardial Effusion

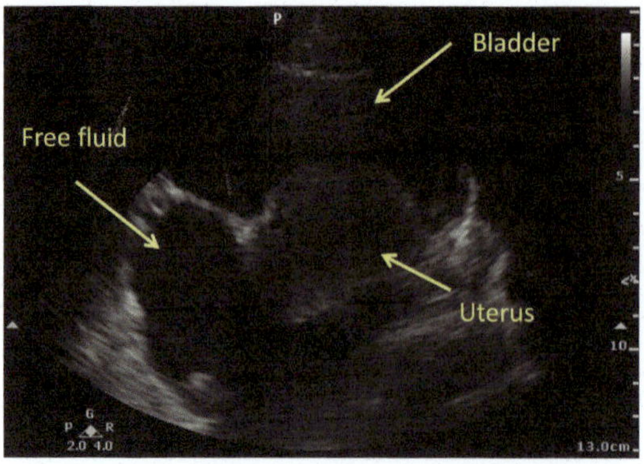

Fig. 37.75 Positive transverse view in a female. Free fluid initially accumulates posterior to the uterus

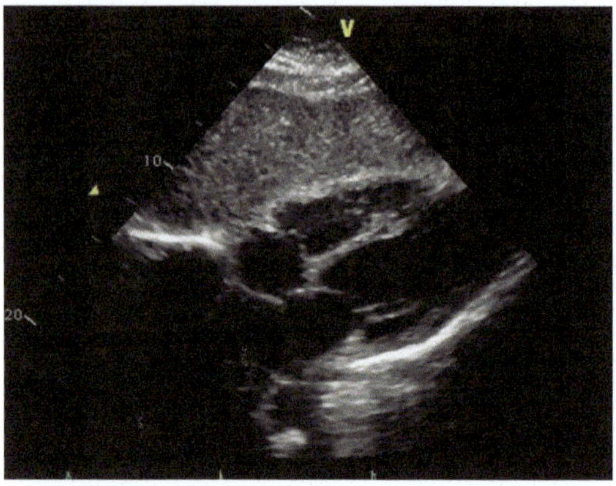

Fig. 37.76 Negative pericardial FAST

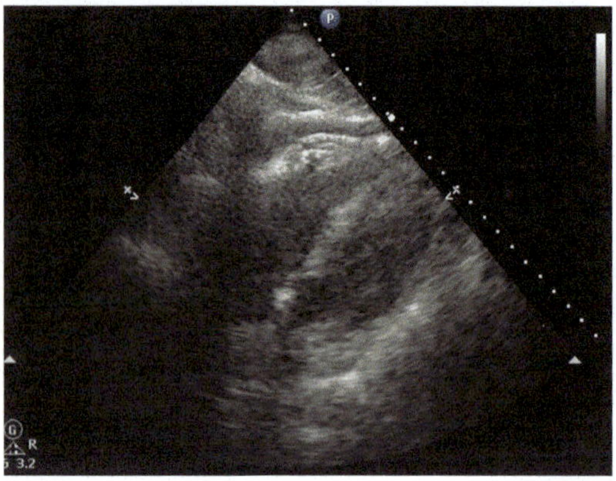

Fig. 37.77 Positive pericardial FAST

and Cardiac Tamponade" on pericardial effusion for further details regarding scanning technique) (Figs. 37.76 and 37.77).

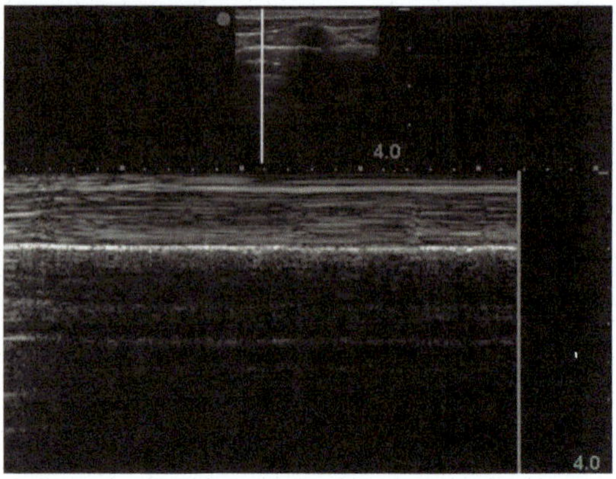

Fig. 37.78 Normal M-mode for pneumothorax

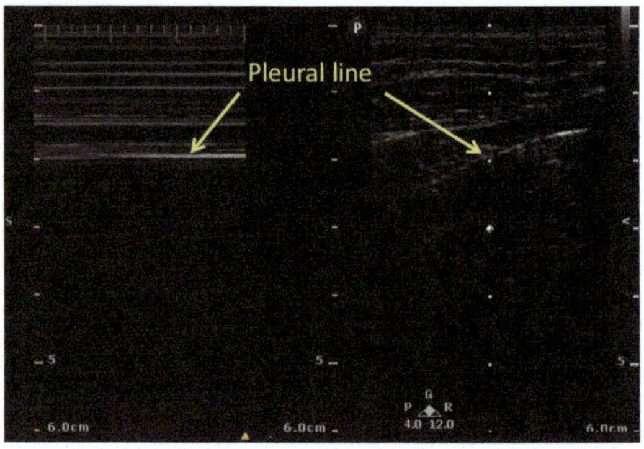

Fig. 37.79 EFAST of the thorax demonstrating pneumothorax on M-mode

Thorax Each hemothorax should be assessed for pneumothorax with both B-mode and M-mode. Since most patients will be supine, air typically accumulates in the anterior chest, making assessment of the lung via an anterior approach more sensitive. A complete thoracic exam would include multiple assessments on each side [130], though most trauma studies look at two sites on each hemithorax [125] (see section "Pneumothorax" on assessment of pneumothorax for further details regarding scanning technique) (Figs. 37.78 and 37.79).

In cases of penetrating chest trauma, many sonographers will assess the pericardium first, though there are no regulations dictating the order of the EFAST.

Supporting Literature

FAST

Bedside ultrasound is inferior to CT for the detection of any peritoneal free fluid or parenchymal injury of abdominal solid organs. However, recent studies suggest that sensitivity of the FAST in blunt trauma was 85% with specificity of 98%, giving an overall accuracy of 95% [131]. This study did not control for blood pressure. In hypotensive patients, the FAST may be 100% sensitive [121], making it a crucial test in bedside decision-making during trauma. Patients with a positive abdominal FAST and hypotension should undergo exploratory laparotomy [121, 132–134].

Ultrasound is unable to distinguish between different types of intra-abdominal fluid. CT scan may be able to distinguish simple fluid (i.e., ascites or urine) from blood using Hounsfield units, but all fluid appears anechoic on ultrasound. If clinical suspicion warrants, DPL or diagnostic peritoneal aspiration (DPA) will discern between different types of fluid.

The FAST is not a replacement for CT scan in patients with stable hemodynamics, because it is not effective at assessing retroperitoneal injuries or bleeding [135, 136], which may lead to a negative FAST in pelvic fractures. And similarly to CT scan, the FAST is unreliable in detecting hollow viscous injury without significant bleeding.

In penetrating chest trauma, the FAST exam is quite useful in helping surgeons with operative planning, and a positive pericardial FAST greatly predicts the need for the operating room [121, 137, 138]. In abdominal trauma, most patients with positive FAST should get exploratory laparotomy.

The role of the FAST has been criticizing in hemodynamically stable blunt trauma patients [139]. Again, a positive FAST greatly predicts the need for operative intervention [134], and in appropriate patients, observation may be able to replace CT scan as a second FAST improves accuracy from 92% to almost 97%. In this study, there was no significant hemoperitoneum in patients with negative FAST at 4 hours [140].

EFAST

Ultrasound sensitivity has been reported from approximately 50% [125] to as high as 98% [141, 142]. One must also consider the time spent on the thoracic portion of the EFAST (including the number of rib spaces assessed), the size of the pneumothorax, and whether or not the patient got a chest tube for the pneumothorax when considering the sensitivity of any given study. A recent meta-analysis suggests that ultrasound is 91% sensitive and 98% specific compared to supine AP chest x-ray, which was 50% sensitive and 99% specific [143].

Ultrasound for hemothorax may not be significantly better at detecting hemothorax than AP CXR [126, 144], but it is probably as sensitive, and may be quicker at identifying large hemothoraces in hemodynamically unstable patients.

Resuscitation Protocols

Hypoxia

Acute respiratory failure is encountered very frequently for any healthcare provider taking care of critically ill patients. The differential diagnosis of respiratory failure is broad, and one can use ultrasound to help rationalize diagnoses and treatment plans for patients. Lung ultrasound is becoming a valuable tool in critical care to help accurate bedside detection of thoracic disorders [145, 146]. We also know physical exam and chest radiography have limitations, resulting in need for more comprehensive exams that might delay diagnosis and treatment plans [147, 148]. Along with studies that show high interobserver agreement and equivalency to computed tomography in detecting most disorders, using lung ultrasound has been shown to save time and decrease the need for computed tomography [149–151].

In a study by Lichtenstein, an algorithm approach to evaluate the patient with respiratory failure ("BLUE" protocol), lung ultrasound found a correct diagnosis in 90.5% of cases. Using the previous signs discussed in this chapter, the clinician can use this algorithmic

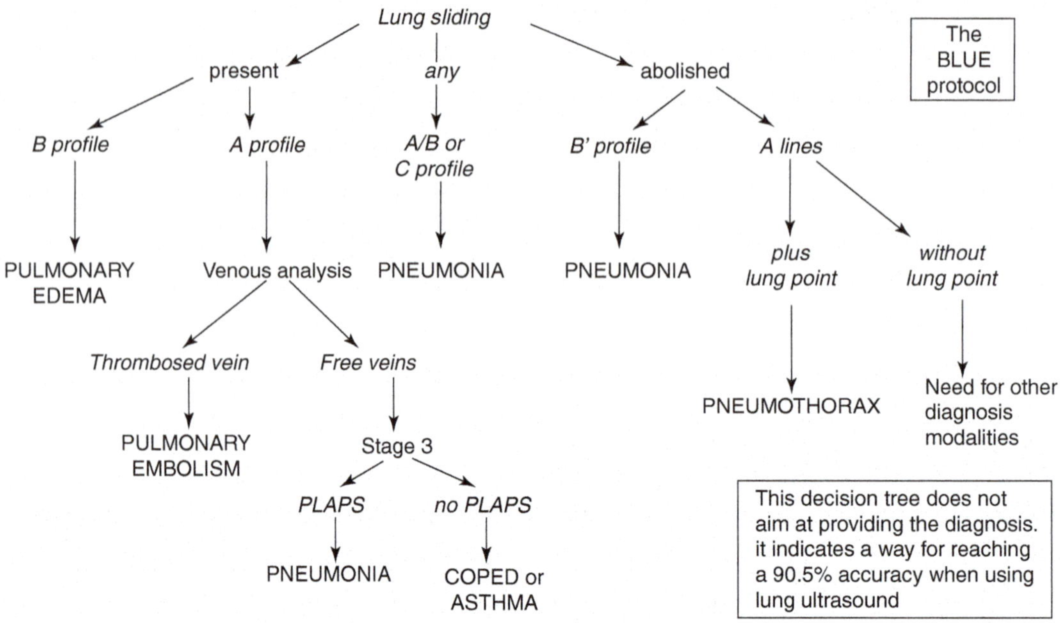

Fig. 37.80 Algorithm for BLUE protocol

approach to evaluate and help with diagnosis and treatment plans (Fig. 37.80). In this study it was useful to assign profiles to the different signs evaluated [152]:

- A profile = anterior predominant bilateral A lines associated with lung sliding (with possible focal B lines)
- A' profile = A profile with absent lung sliding
- B profile = anterior predominant bilateral B lines associated with lung sliding (with possible focalized A lines)
- B′ profile = B profile without lung sliding
- A/B profile = anterior predominant B lines on one side and predominant A lines on the other side
- C profile = anterior alveolar consolidations
- PLAPS profile = pleural effusion or consolidation in posterior exam

Pulmonary edema (cardiogenic): The B profile is seen. The transudate is pushed against gravity up to the anterior wall, with symmetrical patterns.

Chronic obstructive lung disease, asthma: The A profile is seen. These are bronchial disease and should give us a normal lung surface.

Pulmonary embolism: The A profile with lower extremity venous thrombosis is seen. This should not show us an interstitial change, and a normal anterior lung surface with addition of lower extremity ultrasound might help diagnose.

Pneumothorax: The A' profile is seen. Lung sliding is absent. No B lines, no lung pulse. A lung point should be searched for and if found can be sure pneumothorax is present (also can be mistaken with blebs).

Pneumonia: A/B profile, B′ profile, and C profile are the main ones seen. Due to many different types of pneumonias, the signs seen on lung ultrasound are various. The loss of lung sliding is due to inflammatory adherences due to exudate. They usually present with asymmetric patterns.

Pleural effusion: PLAPS point is seen with anechoic space in the midaxillary or posterior thorax regions.

Hypotension

The FAST has been used in trauma for decades, primarily focused at the trauma patient in shock [153].

However, only recently have ultrasound shock protocols been developed to assess medical causes of shock [154–170]. These are inherently more complex because of the many causes of medical shock. Many different ultrasound protocols for diagnosis and management of medical causes of shock currently exist, with some being more thorough than others. One of the more complete shock protocols is the rapid ultrasound in shock and hypotension (RUSH) exam [166, 167]. Regardless of the specific protocol, they all essentially combine a bedside ultrasound exam with a clinical picture to help better diagnose a cause of shock in real time. When choosing a shock protocol or developing one's own technique, the ultrasound exam should address all the causes of shock – obstructive, cardiogenic, hypovolemic/hemorrhagic, and septic/distributive [154].

RUSH: Rapid Ultrasound in Shock and Hypotension (Pump/Tank/Pipes) [166, 167]

- PUMP – What is the cardiac function?
  - Cardiac tamponade
  - LV hypokinesis
  - RV dilation, hypokinesis
- TANK – What is the fluid status and preload of the heart? Is the tank obstructed?
  - IVC and IJ collapsibility and fullness
  - Pneumothorax
- PIPES – Are the pipes leaking or bleeding? Are the pipes obstructed?
  - Hemothorax and abdominal FAST
  - AAA or aortic dissection
  - Lower extremity DVT

Shock protocols can always be abbreviated and adjusted based on clinical suspicions [154], but frequently patients have multiple factors contributing to their shock or hypotension. Spending the extra few moments performing a complete exam may help identify the septic patient with myocardial dysfunction that might benefit from the inotrope, or it may identify the postoperative patient with sepsis and acute RV failure from his pulmonary embolism.

In patients with cardiac arrest, PEA or asystolic arrest specifically, utilizing ultrasound in patients with cardiac arrest may be helpful by adding a few other pieces of information [170, 171]. Bedside ultrasound is also reliable for endotracheal tube placement during cardiac arrest [172]. Otherwise, a focused ultrasound shock exam should be performed in addition to clinical exam to rule out intervenable causes of cardiac arrest.

Critical Care Procedures: Ultrasound Guidance

Vascular Access

Over 5 million central venous catheters are placed in the United States in the internal jugular, subclavian, and femoral veins [173]. Ultrasound guidance for vascular access (venous and arterial) has been a landmark change in management of the critically ill patient over the last 10 years. Quality of care and reduction of complications has encouraged many organizations to publish documents making it standard of care to use ultrasound guidance in these procedures. Most of the evidence is for internal jugular vein for access [174]. Discussed below are general scanning techniques for the cannulation of vessel (arterial and venous) and afterwards with specific vessels that have growing literature supporting their use (subclavian vein, arterial access, peripheral vein, femoral vein).

Central Venous: Internal Jugular, Femoral, Subclavian

Probe Type Vascular (linear array) high frequency: 5–10 MhZ

Scanning Techniques The ultrasound should be used to identify the location of the vessel prior to the procedure and utilize external landmarks during the procedure itself (static technique) or use the ultrasound to visualize cannulation during the procedure (dynamic technique). The dynamic technique is the preferred technique. The vein and artery couple should be seen and clarification of a vein by its collapsibility should be obtained to confirm appropriate vascular structure and to confirm patency. Multiple points should be evaluated to make sure patency is not compromised more proximal to the entry site so that difficulty with wire placement will not occur due to clot. Once collapsible and appropriate structure for cannulation has been identified, follow sterile procedure precautions and place sterile ultrasound probe cover before proceeding with cannulation. The static view has the advantage in that the ultrasound transducer is not needed during the sterile portion of the procedure, but it does not allow for direct visual confirmation of the cannulation during the procedure. The dynamic technique allows for direct visualization throughout the procedure, but requires more experience in the technique and requires use of the transducer during the sterile portion of the procedure. The dynamic technique can be used in either the long axis or the short axis (Fig. 37.81). The short axis is easier for novice operators due to increased ability to see the artery and vein but has higher risk of posterior perforation if the needle tip is not visualized well. Once the short axis is used to find the vein, turning the probe 90° clockwise allows the operator to see the vein in long axis. In patients with short necks, it may be difficult to obtain the long-axis view and needle insertion in the limited space. The long-axis view allows for full visualization of the needle throughout the procedure and allows for better visualization and adjustment of needle depth. It is more technically difficult and key point is once a good section of the vein is obtained, the ultrasound probe should not be moved to find the hyperechoic needle; the needle trajectory should be adjusted into the ultrasound view. Make sure to visualize the vessel with the ultrasound such that you can see the greatest diameter of the vessel along the entire length of the ultrasound probe. Keep the ultrasound steady during the procedure and insert the needle at an angle at the lateral edge of the ultrasound probe. Using this technique, the clinician can visualize the entire length of the needle. Once the vein is cannulated, and wire introduced, the ultrasound can be used again to confirm wire placement into the vessel (preference is long axis). Using ultrasound to confirm guidewire placement can add an additional safety measure [175].

Supporting Literature The use of ultrasound to guide central venous access has been shown to reduce the failure rate, the risk of complications, and the number of attempts, as compared with the landmark technique, especially in the less experienced users or patients with more complex conditions [176, 177].

Ultrasound Guidance: Femoral Vein, Subclavian Vein, Arterial Access, Peripheral Veins

Femoral Vein There are several clinical situations when emergent femoral vein cannulation may be preferred. During cardiac or respiratory arrest, the femoral veins offer easy access and free of chest compressions. Coagulopathy can be a good site to use while anticoagulant agents are being reversed since this is an easily compressible site. It also eliminates the risk of pneumothorax in patients who have bilateral thoracic disease

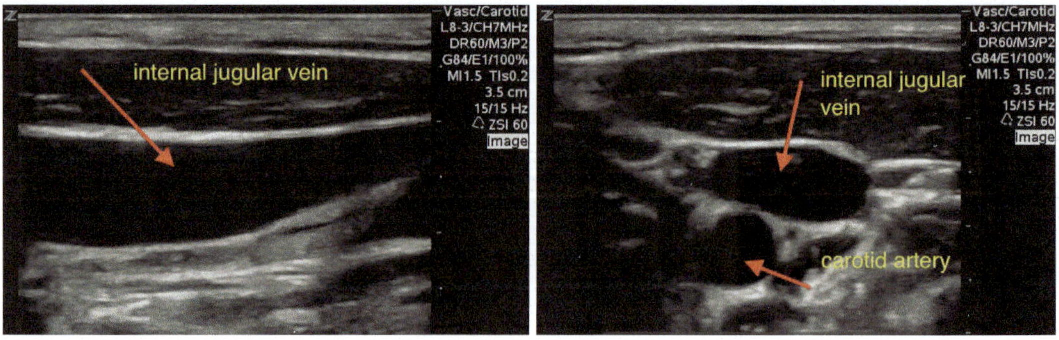

Fig. 37.81 Short- and long-axis view of internal jugular

processes. Unlike literature for internal jugular access, femoral vein ultrasound access support is scarce. A meta-analysis in 2011 showed that real-time ultrasound guidance for hemodialysis catheters decreased arterial punctures, risk of placement failure, and risk of failed first time access. This analysis however only included one study from India that showed improved first attempt success and decreased complications [178, 179]. As mentioned earlier, posterior wall penetration is common in short-axis view. In a study published by Blaivas and Adhikari in 2009, they showed a high incidence of posterior wall penetration and therefore recommendations in current literature are to use a long-axis view to guide central venous placement, even in the femoral region [180].

Subclavian Vein This is the site that has the most mechanical complications compared with internal jugular and femoral sites. Real-time ultrasound guidance has resulted in lower technical failures and faster access. However most of these studies have occurred evaluating the internal jugular site [181, 182]. In a recent study, the ultrasound technique was confirmed to decrease access time and number of attempts and reduction in complications such as arterial puncture, hematoma, pneumothorax, and hemothorax [183]. Scanning of the vessels prior to the procedure should be performed by obtaining appropriate infraclavicular views, and depth and caliber of the axillary vein and subclavian vein as well as patency should be evaluated. In anatomic terms, the axillary vein continues medially until it reaches the first rib when it becomes the subclavian vein. The probe marker can be placed towards the head of the patient and probe placed on the mid clavicle. The image seen should be the acoustic shadowing of the clavicle (Fig. 37.82). The probe can be moved laterally and the clinician will see the vein appear just below the clavicle. This is not easily found in every patient, but when it is gives opportunity to use ultrasound to cannulate the vessel. The probe can be moved a few more centimeters laterally and the vein and artery couple can be visualized. Once the axis is visualized in short axis, the probe can be turned

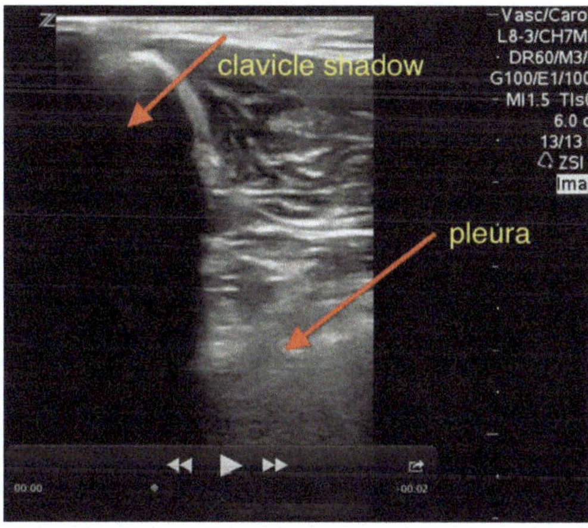

Fig. 37.82 Acoustic shadow of clavicle

90° clockwise to image the long axis of the vein (Fig. 37.83). Clinicians can use the acoustic shadow of the first thoracic rib and sternum to select as a site for access. The needle can be advanced slowly so that its trajectory is towards the lumen of the vein and purposefully directed towards the acoustic shadow of the thoracic rib underneath to minimize the risk of hitting the pleura.

Arterial Access Arterial access for hemodynamic monitoring has traditionally done by palpation techniques. Recently, ultrasound use has increased for access of sites such as radial, axillary, and femoral. The ultrasound techniques explained above for central venous catheterization can be used for arterial access, with increased success, decreased time to cannulation, and decreased risk of complications and should be considered as a first-line method of cannulation [184–186].

Peripheral Vein Access Peripheral vein cannulation using ultrasound has also grown over the past 10 years. Clinicians and nursing staff have started to use in increasing amounts in difficult venous access patients. In recent study by Gregg et al., it was shown that in critically ill patients, placement of peripheral vein ultrasound guided has reduced the amount of central line placements [187]. The methods used are similar to the central venous catheter technique explained

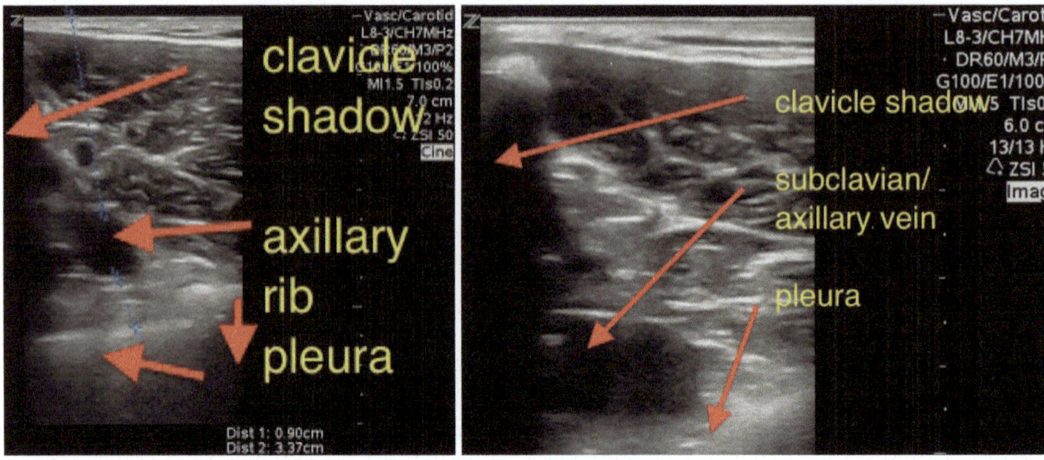

Fig. 37.83 Subclavian vein, axillary vein short, first rib relationship

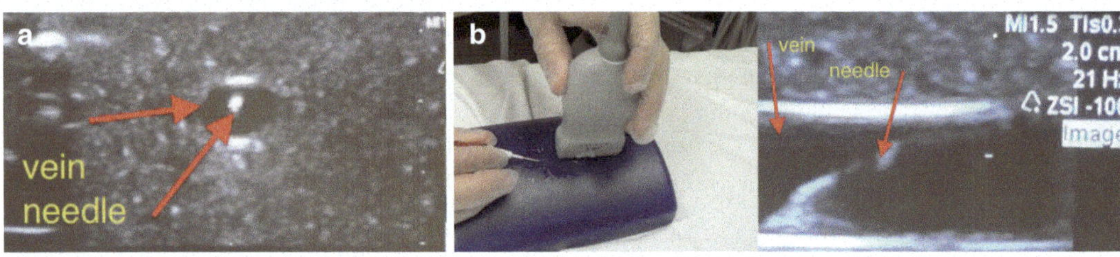

Fig. 37.84 (**a**) Bull's eye target view, (**b**) long-axis needle view

above. One significant difference is that in peripheral lines, the operator can follow the needle tip in the lumen of the vessel for longer distances. The author's success rate increased significantly for cannulation once the whole needle/catheter was advanced into the vessel and then needle removed. This can be done in short or long axis. Short axis seems to be easier since small movements of the ultrasound hand do not cause a loss of image and so is easier to start teaching novices with this technique. The technique involves obtaining a "bull's eye target"-type view with the needle tip in the center of the lumen (Fig. 37.84). Once this is achieved, after following the needle tip into the vessel from the skin surface, the needle and catheter combo is continuously advanced as the ultrasound probe is moved more proximally, always showing a "bull's eye target" view and adjusting the direction of the needle/catheter to remain in the center of the vessel. In order to remain in the vessel lumen, the operator usually has to get the needle/catheter combination parallel with the skin surface; otherwise the needle would puncture through the posterior wall.

Pericardiocentesis

Medical cardiac tamponade is a rare, but fatal, diagnosis that requires expeditious diagnosis and treatment. Most emergency and critical care physicians rarely perform emergent pericardiocentesis, and the prospect of performing one may cause anxiety, given that the complication rate is thought to be relatively high at 5% in elective pericardiocentesis and likely higher in emergent pericardiocentesis by inexperienced providers [188]. However, with the utilization of bedside ultrasound, the emergent pericardiocentesis can be performed efficiently and safely [189, 190].

Probe Type Cardiac (phased array) transducer: 2–5 MhZ

Indications

- Pericardial tamponade
- Relative: Consider in PEA cardiac arrest

Contraindications

- Absolute: None
- Relative: Anticoagulant or antiplatelet therapy, coagulopathy, thrombocytopenia, aortic dissection, or traumatic tamponade (can be considered if surgical therapy is not immediately available).

Procedure Technique Pericardiocentesis is a sterile procedure, and full barrier precautions should be used if time allows. However, given the true emergent nature of the procedure, this may not be possible. Skin prep and sterile gloves should always be used to help prevent infection. A pericardiocentesis kit may be available in your ED or ICU and may have all the necessary procedural equipment. Also, a central venous catheter kit will have the necessary equipment. A standard 18 g IV catheter or needle is unlikely long enough to drain an effusion, but an 18 g cutting or Quincke spinal needle would be sufficient.

The patient should be in the semirecumbent position, with the head of bed at 30–45°, if the clinical situation allows. Full barrier precautions should be used to create a sterile procedure, including chest prep, drapes, sterile gown and gloves, hat and mask, and sterile probe cover and gel.

There are three approaches to the emergency pericardiocentesis – subxiphoid, apical, and parasternal. The choice of approach should be based on which one allows for the largest pocket of fluid that is most accessible through a percutaneous approach. If cardiac tamponade does exist, the view obtained will not be an ideal view, demonstrating perfect cardiac anatomy. Note the depth of the fluid and use that as a guide when inserting the needle [189, 191].

First, from the subxiphoid approach, the needle should be inserted just below the xiphoid process at a 30–45° angle towards the left shoulder. Negative pressure should be held until pericardial fluid is aspirated. In this approach, the needle will likely pass through the liver and diaphragm into pericardial space to drain the effusive tamponade. While this approach should be used with ultrasound guidance, the subxiphoid view is the classic blind approach of choice. The needle tip should remain in view throughout the procedure by utilizing a longitudinal approach or following the needle tip in a transverse view [189, 191].

The apical approach can be attempted after the apical four-chamber view of the heart can be obtained on bedside echo. Once again, the transducer will be placed at the PMI and the effusion visualized. The needle will be inserted just inferior and lateral to the transducer, following the angle of the transducer towards the patient's right shoulder. Pericardiocentesis utilizing this approach has a higher risk of pneumothorax, but according to one review article, the apical four-chamber view provides the best approach in 80% of patients, although this was not in emergent situations [188, 192].

Last, a parasternal approach can be performed. Obtain an adequate parasternal long view, and the needle will be inserted almost perpendicular to the skin, following the angle of the transducer. His approach risks injury to the left internal mammary artery, which sits vertically in the anterior chest wall, 3–4 cm lateral to the sternal border [189, 193].

Regardless of approach, the general principles of the procedure remain the same – find the area with the largest fluid collection that is most accessible through a percutaneous approach. Needle insertion angle should follow that of the transducer when the initial view is obtained. After puncturing the skin, the needle tip should remain in view by using a longitudinal view or by following the needle tip in a transverse view [189, 191].

Confirmation of needle location is multifactorial. First, real-time confirmation with ultrasound is reliable, especially when confirmed with an agitated saline study. A small amount of agitated saline may be injected into the pericardial space, with care not to inject an air bolus, and confirmed with ultrasound by visualization of "bubbling" in the pericardium.

Classic methods of confirmation of pericardial versus intracardiac blood, such as assessment of clotting and EKG observation, are unreliable and more time-consuming than ultrasound confirmation.

Finally, the intensivist may choose to leave a catheter continuously drain the effusion. The remainder of the procedure is performed using Seldinger technique with a pericardiocentesis catheter, small pigtail catheter, or small gauge central venous catheter.

Complications Dysrhythmia, coronary vessel injury, myocardial injury, intercostal artery injury, and hemothorax likely have a similar incidence in all three approaches. LIMA injury is likely more common in a parasternal approach, liver and diaphragm injury more common in a subxiphoid approach, and pneumothorax more common in an apical approach. While this is a high-risk procedure with significant and fairly frequent complications, pericardial tamponade is a life-threatening and time-sensitive diagnosis, and pericardiocentesis is potentially lifesaving.

Thoracentesis

Probe Type Cardiac (phased array) or abdominal (curvilinear) probe: 2–5 MhZ; also can use the vascular (linear array) high-frequency 5–10 MhZ probe after appropriate location has been identified to better visualize the rib interspaces.

Scanning Techniques The critically ill patient most likely is in the supine position during thoracentesis for fluid analysis or chest tube placement. The patient's arms are usually placed superiorly over the head, or if more emergent move the upper arms more laterally to allow space to place the chest tube (Fig. 37.85). The author initially uses the curvilinear probe to identify the optimal site of entry for thoracentesis or thoracostomy tube placement and then switches to a high-frequency vascular probe to identify the rib spaces more clearly. The needle entry should be on the superior aspect of the rib to avoid any vascular injury. The probe marker is towards the patient's head or right side. See the scanning tips in section "Pleural Effusion" describing the best way to approach the space after identification of the diaphragm. Ultrasound use for guidance during thoracentesis and chest tube insertion has shown to increase success and safety, and international guidelines now recommend its mandatory use to guide all pleural drainage procedures [194–196]. Always identify the diaphragm. Hypoechoic fluid surrounding the liver or spleen can appear as a pleural effusion and must not be mistaken as such. In addition, lung tissue may mimic hepatic tissue in certain diseases such as dense consolidations termed "hepatization" of the lung. Proper probe positioning, clear identification of the diaphragm, subdiaphragmatic structures, and lung are crucial. This is a common error in novice operators due to the confusion of the hepatorenal or splenorenal recess for the diaphragm. Identifying the diaphragm can be technically difficult depending on patient position, size, and clinical condition. It may be useful to start below the diaphragm, identifying first the hepatorenal recess (liver and kidney view on FAST examination) and moving cephalad until you begin to see the lung and diaphragm. In addition as ribs change their orientation anatomically, the probe may need to be adjusted while still in the longitudinal axis. Moving the probe clockwise and counterclockwise may be of benefit to bring into view the lung, the diaphragm, and the subdiaphragmatic structures. Exudates, empyemas, and hemothoraces may appear more echogenic, unlike, for example, a transudative effusion that could be anechoic. Complex effusions can appear also as heterogeneous and echogenic. The consistency of the effusion can make identification technically difficult, as this can limit lung motion. Sometimes the operator may think there is no

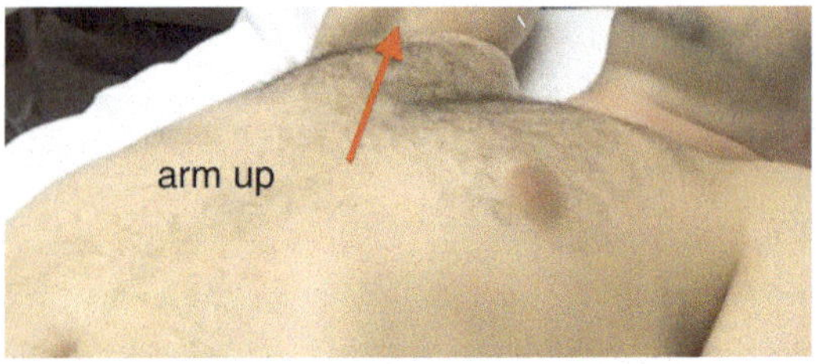

Fig. 37.85 Arm position for chest tube placement

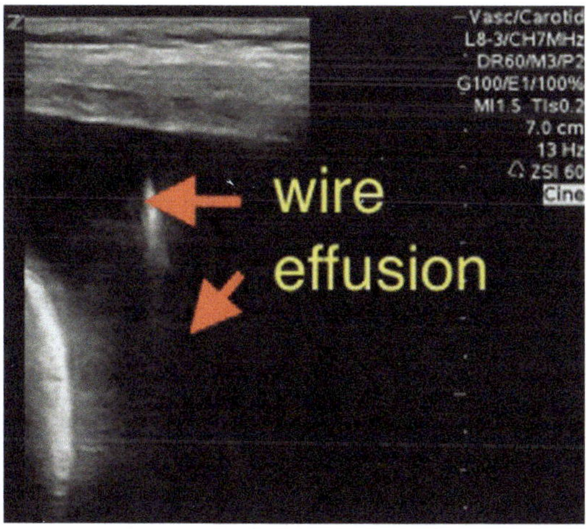

Fig. 37.86 Wire in pleural space

effusion when there is an echo-dense effusion. The lung may slide into the effusion during the respiratory cycle and can be problematic during needle insertion, causing pneumothorax or abnormal wire placement during performance of pigtail chest tube catheters. This is called a "curtain sign." Once the optimal site is visualized, the patient should not be moved and the procedure should be performed immediately. For the Seldinger technique of placement of chest tube or catheter placement for drainage of effusion, the clinician can use the ultrasound for wire confirmation in pleural effusion prior to dilation and placement of chest tube (Fig. 37.86).

Complications The complication of pneumothorax related to thoracentesis can occur with atmospheric air introduction with the catheter removal or aspiration of fluid, needle injury to the visceral pleura, permitting air into the alveoli, or rapid decrease in pleural pressure from aspiration resulting in visceral pleura rupture [197]. In the past there have been concerns of higher pneumothorax rates in mechanical ventilation, but a large study by Mayo et al. has shown that the risk of complication is no higher in patients requiring ventilation than in nonmechanically ventilated patients. It is important to note that the benefit of ultrasound use for site selection in decreasing complications such as pneumothorax occurs only when real-time or immediate pre-procedure marking occurs [198]. Another important complication is bleeding due to the neurovascular bundle at the inferior aspect of the rib on the subcostal groove. The variability in the course of the intercostal artery, especially in elderly patients, must be recognized. The collateral intercostal artery that usually runs on the superior border of the inferior rib can be lacerated during the procedure with the needle or during catheter insertion. Studies have shown that the intercostal artery is more exposed in the center of the interspace in positions more posteriorly on the chest wall [199–201].

Supporting Literature Thoracentesis may be needed to further classify a pleural effusion as an exudate or transudate. An anechoic effusion can be either transudate or exudate and can be differentiated through thoracentesis [202]. The optimal site to view a non-loculated pleural effusion is at the posterior axillary line above the diaphragm, but in the patient with a clinically significant pleural effusion, the midaxillary line may be an appropriate location to start. Estimation of the drainage amount has been reported in many studies, but has been shown to underestimate fluid quantity [203, 204]. Also clinical significance of fluid removal may depend on other physiological factors such as lung aeration prior to and after removal of fluid, work of breathing changes prior to and after removal, chest wall compliance, and hypodynamic cardiovascular state [205, 206].

Paracentesis

Intra-abdominal free fluid can be rapidly assessed with beside ultrasound. The etiology of ascites is most frequently due to liver disease, but other diseases include malignancy, heart failure, pancreatic disease, or renal failure. Not infrequently, intra-abdominal fluid is an iatrogenic process, secondary to aggressive fluid resuscitation in hypotensive, hypovolemic patients [207].

Diagnosis

Bedside paracentesis can be performed for both diagnostic and therapeutic reasons. In the ED or ICU, providers most frequently perform a diagnostic paracentesis on patients in whom spontaneous bacterial peritonitis (SBP) is suspected. In the ICU, therapeutic paracentesis may be performed in patients with tense ascites or in patients that have dyspnea, are difficult to ventilate, or have suspected abdominal compartment syndrome [208].

Physical exam may help in diagnosis of ascites, but is not sensitive. While CT may be the gold standard for diagnosis ascites, bedside ultrasonography is excellent in identifying patients with clinically significant intra-abdominal free fluid [209, 210].

Indications
- Diagnosis of ascites etiology or spontaneous bacterial peritonitis
- Fluid removal in patients with discomfort or pain, dyspnea, and abdominal compartment syndrome

Contraindications
- Absolute: None
- Relative: Coagulopathy, thrombocytopenia, anticoagulant or antiplatelet therapy, overlying cellulitis, or abscess

Materials
- Skin antiseptic, sterile gown, gloves and drapes, hat and mask, 18-gauge needle at least 1.5 inches long, sterile Luer-lock syringes, drainage bags, or containers
- Ultrasound machine with curvilinear transducer, sterile probe cover, and sterile gel
- If the patient is awake and alert, 1% or 2% lidocaine without epinephrine and a 25-gauge needle for local anesthesia
- A paracentesis kit may be available in your ED or ICU and may have all the necessary procedural equipment. Also, a central venous catheter kit will have the necessary equipment.

Procedure Technique The patient should be in the supine position, with the head of bed slightly elevated to 15–30°. This will help the ascites accumulate in the lower, more dependent portions of the abdominal cavity. The patient's bladder should also be empty, as not to misidentify urine in the bladder as ascites.

Identifying a pocket prior to skin sterilization and drape placement is recommended. It may be helpful to bump or boost a patient slightly on to one side if identification of a fluid pocket is not immediate.

Full barrier precautions should be used to create a sterile procedure, including chest prep, drapes, sterile gown and gloves, hat and mask, and sterile probe cover and gel.

Typically, fluid is located in either of the bilateral lower quadrants. The inferior epigastric arteries lie in the rectus muscle, and care to stay lateral to these structures is crucial. Ascites fluid will appear anechoic, and bowel loops will likely be visible, floating in the fluid. After identification of fluid, decrease the depth on the ultrasound machine, and use color Doppler to assure that there are no blood vessels in the abdominal wall that might be punctured [209, 210] (Figs. 37.87 and 37.88).

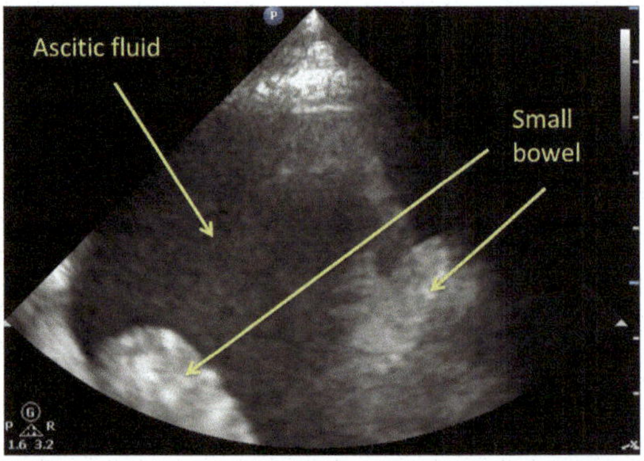

Fig. 37.87 A pocket of abdominal ascites with floating small bowel

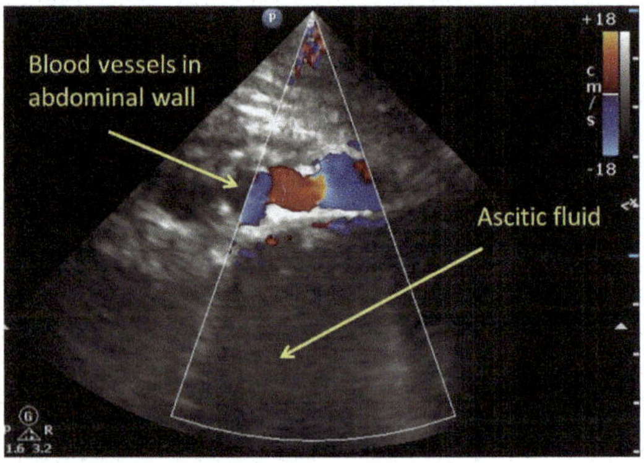

Fig. 37.88 Color Doppler demonstrating blood vessels over a pocket of ascites

Use of a Z-tract technique may help with leakage of ascites fluid after the procedure. Apply approximately 2 cm downward traction on the skin, puncture the skin, release traction, and then advance the needle through the remaining subcutaneous tissues and peritoneum. The skin and peritoneal puncture sites will not directly overlap, and post-procedural leakage of ascites may be reduced.

Finally, the intensivist may choose to leave a catheter continuously drain the ascites if the patient's hemodynamics will not tolerate large-volume paracentesis. The remainder of the procedure is performed using Seldinger technique with a pericardiocentesis catheter, small pigtail catheter, or small gauge central venous catheter.

Complications Small amounts of bleeding can be common after abdominal paracentesis, but significant bleeding is relatively uncommon, even in coagulopathic patients [211, 212]. Infection is uncommon if full barrier precautions are taken, and if a drainage catheter is left, it should be removed less than 72 hours after insertion due to increased infection rate [213]. Post-procedure ascites leakage can be mitigated by the Z-tract technique, though it does not eliminate the complication. Epigastric artery injury, bowel perforation, and bladder perforation are all significant complications that should be completely eliminated with the use of bedside ultrasound.

Supporting Literature Newer literature suggests that in large-volume paracentesis, wall suction can be used, reducing costs and time [214]. In hemodynamically unstable patients, or in large-volume therapeutic paracentesis, albumin replacement should be considered [215]. In patients with ascites and suspected SBP, consider albumin replacement as well [216].

References

Introduction

1. Lichtenstein D, Axler O. Intensive use of general ultrasound in the intensive care unit. Prospective study of 150 consecutive patients. Intensive Care Med. 1993;19:353–5.
2. Making health care safer: a critical analysis of patient safety practices. Rockville: Agency for Healthcare Research and Quality. (AHRQ publication no. 01-E058).
3. Nicolaou S, Talsky A, Khashoggi K, Venu V. Ultrasound-guided interventional radiology in critical care. Crit Care Med. 2007;35(Suppl):S186–97.
4. Fedson S, Neithardt G, Thomas P, Lickerman A, Radzienda M, DeCara JM, Lang RM, Spencer KT. Unsuspected clinically important findings detected with a small portable ultrasound device in patients admitted to a general medicine service. J Am Soc Echocardiogr. 2003;16:901–5.
5. Bossone E, DiGiovine B, Watts S, Marcovitz PA, Carey L, Watts C, Armstrong WF. Range and prevalence of cardiac abnormalities in patients hospitalized in a medical ICU. Chest. 2002;122:1370–6.

Training

6. Cholley BP, Vieillard-Baron A, Mebazaa A. Echocardiography in the ICU: time for widespread use! Intensive Care Med. 2005;32:9–10.
7. Mayse ML. Real-time ultrasonography— should this be available to every critical care physician? Crit Care Med. 2005;33:1231–8.
8. Duvall WL, Croft LB, Goldman ME. Can hand-carried ultrasound devices be extended for use by the noncardiology medical com- munity? Echocardiography. 2003;20:471–6.
9. Mayo PH, Beaulieu Y, Doelken P, Feller-Kopman D, Harrod C, Kaplan A, Oropello J, Vieillard-Baron A, Axler O, Lichtenstein D, Maury E, Slama M, Vignon P. American College of Chest Physicians/La Societe de Reanimation de Langue Francaise statement on competence in critical care ultrasonography. Chest. 2009;135:1050–60.
10. Eisen LA, Leung S, Gallagher AE, Kvetan V. Barriers to ultrasound training in critical care medicine fellowships: a survey of program directors. Crit Care Med. 2010;38:1978–83.
11. Rao S, van Holsbeeck L, Musial JL, et al. A pilot study of comprehensive ultra- sound education at the Wayne State University School of Medicine: a pioneer year review. J Ultrasound Med. 2008;27:745–9.
12. Carraccio C, Wolfsthal SD, Englander R, Ferentz K, Martin C. Shifting paradigms: from Flexner to competencies. Acad Med. 2002;77(5):361–7.
13. Wahidi MM, Silvestri GA, Coakley RD, et al. A prospective multicenter study of competency metrics and educational interventions in the learning of bronchoscopy among new pulmonary fellows. Chest. 2010;137(5):1040–9.
14. Liang BA, Mackey T. Quality and safety in medical care: what does the future hold? Arch Pathol Lab Med. 2011;135(11):1425–31.

Cardiac

15. Mayo PH, Beaulieu Y, Doelken P, Feller-Kopman D, Harrod C, Kaplan A, et al. American College of Chest Physicians/La Societe de Reanimation de Langue Francaise statement on competence in critical care ultrasonography. Chest. 2009;135:1050–60.
16. Perera P, Lobo V, Williams SR, Gharahbaghian L. Cardiac echocardiography. Crit Care Clin. 2014;30(1):47–92, v. https://doi.org/10.1016/j.ccc.2013.08.003. Review. PubMed PMID: 24295841.
17. Mark DG, Hayden GE, Ky B, Paszczuk A, Pugh M, Matthews S, et al. Hand-carried echocardiography for assessment of left ventricular filling and ejection fraction in the surgical intensive care unit. J Crit Care. 2009 Sep;24(3):470.e1-7. https://doi.org/10.1016/j.jcrc.2008.07.003. Epub 2009 Jan 17. PubMed PMID: 19327304.
18. Lang RM, Badano LP, Mor-Avi V, Afilalo J, Armstrong A, Ernande L, et al. Recommendations for cardiac chamber quantification by echocardiography in adults: an update from the American society of echocardiography and the European association of cardiovascular imaging. J Am Soc Echocardiogr. 2015 Jan;28(1):1-39.e14. https://doi.org/10.1016/j.echo.2014.10.003. PubMed PMID: 25559473.
19. Silverstein JR, Laffely NH, Rifkin RD. Quantitative estimation of left ventricular ejection fraction from mitral valve E-point to septal separation and comparison to magnetic resonance imaging. Am J Cardiol. 2006 Jan 1;97(1):137-40. Epub 2005 Nov 15. PubMed PMID: 16377299.
20. Secko MA, Lazar JM, Salciccioli LA, Stone MB. Can junior emergency physicians use E-point septal separation to accurately estimate left ventricular function in acutely dyspneic patients? Acad Emerg Med. 2011 Nov;18(11):1223-6. https://doi.org/10.1111/j.1553-2712.2011.01196.x. Epub 2011 Nov 1. PubMed PMID: 22044429.
21. McKaigney CJ, Krantz MJ, La Rocque CL, Hurst ND, Buchanan MS, Kendall JL. E-point septal separation: a bedside tool for emergency physician assessment of left ventricular ejection fraction. Am J Emerg Med. 2014 Jun;32(6):493-7. https://doi.org/10.1016/j.ajem.2014.01.045. Epub 2014 Feb 3. PubMed PMID: 24630604.
22. Weekes AJ, Reddy A, Lewis MR, Norton HJ. E-point septal separation compared to fractional shortening measurements of systolic function in emergency department patients: prospective randomized study. J Ultrasound Med. 2012 Dec;31(12):1891–7.

RV Function

23. Slama M, et al. Chapter 33: Evaluation of right ventricular function in the intensive care unit by echocardiography. In: Critical care ultrasound. 1st ed. Philadephia: Elsevier/Saunders; 2015. p. 179–84.
24. Kaplan A, Mayo PH. Chapter 11: Echocardiographic diagnosis and monitoring of right ventricular function. In: Critical care ultrasonography. 2nd ed. New York: McGraw-Hill; 2014. p. 115–26.
25. Armstrong WF, Ryan T. Chapter 8: Left and right atrium, and right ventricle. In: Feigenbaum's echocardiography. 7th ed. Philadelphia: Lippincott Williams & Wilkins; 2010. p. 203–15.
26. McConnell MV, Solomon SD, Rayan ME, Come PC, Goldhaber SZ, Lee RT. Regional right ventricular dysfunction detected by echocardiography in acute pulmonary embolism. Am J Cardiol. 1996;78(4):469–73. PubMed PMID: 8752195.
27. Rudski LG, Lai WW, Afilalo J, Hua L, Handschumacher MD, Chandrasekaran K, et al. Guidelines for the echocardiographic assessment of the right heart in adults: a report from the American Society of Echocardiography endorsed by the European Association of Echocardiography, a registered branch of the European Society of Cardiology, and the Canadian Society of Echocardiography. J Am Soc Echocardiogr. 2010;23(7):685–713; quiz 786-8. PubMed PMID: 20620859. https://doi.org/10.1016/j.echo.2010.05.010.
28. Lobo JL, Holley A, Tapson V, Moores L, Oribe M, Barrón M, Otero R, Nauffal D, Valle R, Monreal M, Yusen RD, Jiménez D, PROTECT and RIETE Investigators. Prognostic significance of tricuspid annular displacement in normotensive patients with acute symptomatic pulmonary embolism. J Thromb Haemost. 2014;12(7):1020–7. https://doi.org/10.1111/jth.12589. Epub 2014 June 19. PubMed PMID: 24766779.
29. Kopecna D, Briongos S, Castillo H, Moreno C, Recio M, Navas P, Lobo JL, Alonso-Gomez A, Obieta-Fresnedo I, Fernández-Golfin C, Zamorano JL, PROTECT Investigators. Interobserver reliability of echocardiography for prognostication of normotensive patients with pulmonary embolism. Cardiovasc Ultrasound. 2014;12:29. https://doi.org/10.1186/1476-7120-12-29. PubMed PMID: 25092465; PubMed Central PMCID: PMC4126908.
30. Jardin F, Dubourg O, Bourdarias JP. Echocardiographic pattern of acute cor pulmonale. Chest. 1997;111(1):209–17. Review. PubMed PMID: 8996019.
31. Frémont B, Pacouret G, Jacobi D, Puglisi R, Charbonnier B, de Labriolle A. Prognostic value of echocardiographic right/left ventricular end-diastolic diameter ratio in patients with acute pulmonary embolism: results from a monocenter registry of 1,416 patients. Chest. 2008;133(2):358–62. Epub 2007 Oct 20. PubMed PMID: 17951624.
32. Vieillard-Baron A, Charron C, Chergui K, Peyrouset O, Jardin F. Bedside echocardiographic evaluation of hemodynamics in sepsis: is a qualitative evaluation sufficient? Intensive Care Med. 2006;32(10):1547–52. Epub 2006 July 20. PubMed PMID: 16855828.

Pericardial Effusion and Cardiac Tamponade

33. Fitch MT, Nicks BA, Pariyadath M, McGinnis HD, Manthey DE. Videos in clinical medicine. Emergency pericardiocentesis. N Engl J Med. 2012;366(12):e17. https://doi.org/10.1056/NEJMvcm0907841. Review. PubMed PMID: 22435385.
34. Pepi M, Muratori M. Echocardiography in the diagnosis and management of pericardial disease. J Cardiovasc Med (Hagerstown). 2006;7(7):533–44. Review. PubMed PMID: 16801815.
35. Perera P, Lobo V, Williams SR, Gharahbaghian L. Cardiac echocardiography. Crit Care Clin. 2014;30(1):47–92, v. https://doi.org/10.1016/j.ccc.2013.08.003. Review. PubMed PMID: 24295841.
36. Lancellotti P, Price S, Edvardsen T, Cosyns B, Neskovic AN, Dulgheru R, et al. The use of echocardiography in acute cardiovascular care: recommendations of the European Association of Cardiovascular Imaging and the Acute Cardiovascular Care Association. Eur Heart J Acute Cardiovasc Care. 2015;4:3–5. pii: 2048872614549739. [Epub ahead of print]. PubMed PMID: 25378666.
37. Porter TR, Shillcutt SK, Adams MS, Desjardins G, Glas KE, Olson JJ, et al. Guidelines for the use of echocardiography as a monitor for therapeutic intervention in adults: a report from the American Society of Echocardiography. J Am Soc Echocardiogr. 2015;28(1):40–56. https://doi.org/10.1016/j.echo.2014.09.009. PubMed PMID: 25559474.
38. Nagdev A, Stone MB. Point-of-care ultrasound evaluation of pericardial effusions: does this patient have cardiac tamponade? Resuscitation. 2011;82(6):671–3. https://doi.org/10.1016/j.resuscitation.2011.02.004. Epub 2011 Mar 11. PubMed PMID: 21397379.

IVC Collapsibility and Echocardiographic Measures of Fluid Responsiveness

39. Prekker ME, Scott NL, Hart D, Sprenkle MD, Leatherman JW. Point-of-care ultrasound to estimate central venous pressure: a comparison of three techniques*. Crit Care Med. 2013;41(3):833–41.
40. Boyd JH, Forbes J, Nakada TA, et al. Fluid resuscitation in septic shock: a positive fluid balance and elevated central venous pressure are associated with increased mortality. Crit Care Med. 2011;39:259–65.
41. Rivers E, Nguyen B, Havstad S, Ressler J, Muzzin A, Knoblich B, Peterson E, Tomlanovich M, Early Goal-Directed Therapy Collaborative Group. Early goal-directed therapy in the treatment of severe sepsis and septic shock. N Engl J Med. 2001;345:1368–77.
42. Stawicki SP, Braslow BM, Panebianco NL, et al. Intensivist use of hand-carried ultrasonography to measure IVC collapsibility in estimating intravascular volume status: correlations with CVP. J Am Coll Surg. 2009;209:55–61.
43. Fields JM, Lee PA, Jenq KY, et al. The interrater reliability of inferior vena cava ultrasound by bedside clinician sonographers in emergency department patients. Acad Emerg Med. 2011;18:98–101.
44. Brennan JM, Blair JE, Goonewardena S, et al. Reappraisal of the use of inferior vena cava for estimating right atrial pressure. J Am Soc Echocardiogr. 2007;20:857–61.
45. Schefold JC, Storm C, Bercker S, et al. Inferior vena cava diameter correlates with invasive hemodynamic measures in mechanically ventilated intensive care unit patients with sepsis. J Emerg Med. 2010;38:632–7.
46. Bendjelid K, Romand JA, Walder B, et al. Correlation between measured inferior vena cava diameter and right atrial pressure depends on the echocardiographic method used in patients who are mechanically ventilated. J Am Soc Echocardiogr. 2002;15:944–9.
47. Marik PE, Baram M, Vahid B. Does central venous pressure predict fluid responsiveness? A systematic review of the literature and the tale of seven mares. Chest. 2008;134(1):172–8. https://doi.org/10.1378/chest.07-2331. Review. PubMed PMID: 18628220.
48. Nagdev AD, Merchant RC, Tirado-Gonzalez A, Sisson CA, Murphy MC. Emergency department bedside ultrasonographic measurement of the caval index for noninvasive determination of low central venous pressure. Ann Emerg Med. 2010;55(3):290–5. https://doi.org/10.1016/j.annemergmed.2009.04.021. Epub 2009 June 25. PubMed PMID: 19556029.
49. Stawicki SP, Adkins EJ, Eiferman DS, Evans DC, Ali NA, Njoku C, Lindsey DE, Cook CH, Balakrishnan JM, Valiaveedan S, Galwankar SC, Boulger CT, Springer AN, Bahner DP. Prospective evaluation of intravascular volume status in critically ill patients: does inferior vena cava collapsibility correlate with central venous pressure? J Trauma Acute Care Surg. 2014;76(4):956–63; discussion 963–4. PubMed PMID: 24662857. https://doi.org/10.1097/TA.0000000000000152.
50. Feissel M, Michard F, Faller JP, et al. The respiratory variation in inferior vena cava diameter as a guide to fluid therapy. Intensive Care Med. 2004;30:1834–7.
51. Barbier C, Loubières Y, Schmit C, Hayon J, Ricôme JL, Jardin F, Vieillard-Baron A. Respiratory changes in inferior vena cava diameter are helpful in predicting fluid responsiveness in ventilated septic patients. Intensive Care Med. 2004;30(9):1740–6. Epub 2004 Mar 18. PubMed PMID: 15034650.
52. Zhang Z, Xu X, Ye S, Xu L. Ultrasonographic measurement of the respiratory variation in the inferior vena cava diameter is predictive of fluid responsiveness in critically ill patients: systematic

review and meta-analysis. Ultrasound Med Biol. 2014;40(5):845–53. https://doi.org/10.1016/j.ultrasmedbio.2013.12.010. Epub 2014 Feb 2. Review. PubMed PMID: 24495437.
53. Kent A, Patil P, Davila V, Bailey JK, Jones C, Evans DC, Boulger CT, Adkins E, Balakrishnan JM, Valiyaveedan S, Galwankar SC, Bahner DP, Stawicki SP. Sonographic evaluation of intravascular volume status: can internal jugular or femoral vein collapsibility be used in the absence of IVC visualization? Ann Thorac Med. 2015;10(1):44–9. https://doi.org/10.4103/1817-1737.146872. PubMed PMID: 25593607; PubMed Central PMCID: PMC4286845.
54. Kent A, Bahner DP, Boulger CT, Eiferman DS, Adkins EJ, Evans DC, Springer AN, Balakrishnan JM, Valiyaveedan S, Galwankar SC, Njoku C, Lindsey DE, Yeager S, Roelant GJ, Stawicki SP. Sonographic evaluation of intravascular volume status in the surgical intensive care unit: a prospective comparison of subclavian vein and inferior vena cava collapsibility index. J Surg Res. 2013;184(1):561–6. https://doi.org/10.1016/j.jss.2013.05.040. Epub 2013 June 3. PubMed PMID: 23764308.
55. Mandeville JC, Colebourn CL. Can transthoracic echocardiography be used to predict fluid responsiveness in the critically ill patient? A systematic review. Crit Care Res Pract. 2012;2012:513480. https://doi.org/10.1155/2012/513480. Epub 2012 Feb 6. PubMed PMID: 22400109; PubMed Central PMCID: PMC3286892.
56. Ferrada P, Murthi S, Anand RJ, Bochicchio GV, Scalea T. Transthoracic focused rapid echocardiographic examination: real-time evaluation of fluid status in critically ill trauma patients. J Trauma. 2011;70(1):56–62; discussion 62–4. PubMed PMID: 21217482. https://doi.org/10.1097/TA.0b013e318207e6ee.

Vascular

57. U.S. Preventive Services Task Force. Screening for abdominal aortic aneurysm: recommendation statement. Ann Intern Med. 2005;142:198–202.
58. Thompson SG, Ashton HA, Gao L, Scott RA. Screening men for abdominal aortic aneurysm: 10 year mortality and cost effectiveness results from the randomised Multicentre Aneurysm Screening Study. BMJ. 2009;338:2307–18.
59. Knaut AL, Kendall JL, Patten R, Ray C. Ultrasonographic measurement of aortic diameter by emergency physicians approximates results obtained by computed tomography. J Emerg Med. 2005;28(2):119–26.
60. Tayal VS, Graf CD, Gibbs MA. Prospective study of accuracy and outcome of emergency ultrasound for abdominal aortic aneurysm over two years. Acad Emerg Med. 2003;10(8):867–71.
61. Dent B, Kendall RJ, Boyle AA, Atkinson PRT. Emergency ultrasound of the abdominal aorta by UK emergency physicians: a prospective cohort study. Emerg Med J. 2007;24(8):547–9.

Deep Vein Evaluation

62. Bernardi E, Camporese G, Büller HR, Siragusa S, Imberti D, Berchio A, Ghirarduzzi A, Verlato F, Anastasio R, Prati C, Piccioli A, Erasmus Study Group. Serial 2-point ultrasonography plus D-dimer vs whole- leg color-coded Doppler ultrasonography for diagnosing suspected symptomatic deep vein thrombosis: a randomized controlled trial. JAMA. 2008;300(14):1653–9.
63. Lensing AW, Doris CI, Mcgrath FP, et al. A comparison of compression ultrasound with color Doppler ultrasound for the diagnosis of symptomless postoperative deep vein thrombosis. Arch Intern Med. 1997;157(7):765–8.
64. Poppiti R, Papanicolaou G, Perese S, Weaver FA. Limited B-mode venous imaging versus complete color-flow duplex venous scanning for detection of proximal deep venous thrombosis. J Vasc Surg. 1995;22(5):553–7.
65. Ascani A, Radicchia S, Parise P, Nenci GG, Agnelli G. Distribution and occlusiveness of thrombi in patients with surveillance detected deep vein thrombosis after hip surgery. Thromb Haemost. 1996;75(2):239–41.
66. Labropoulos N, Waggoner T, Sammis W, Samali S, Pappas PJ. The effect of venous thrombus location and extent on the development of post-thrombotic signs and symptoms. J Vasc Surg. 2008;48(2):407–12.
67. Kory PD, Pellecchia CM, Shiloh AL, Mayo PH, DiBello C, Koenig S. Accuracy of ultrasonography performed by critical care physicians for the diagnosis of DVT. Chest J. 2011;139(3):538–42.
68. Stein PD, Henry JW. Prevalence of acute pulmonary embolism among patients in a general hospital and at autopsy. Chest. 1995;108(4):978–81.
69. Twigg SJ, McCrirrick A, Sanderson PM. A comparison of post mortem findings with post hoc estimated clinical diagnoses of patients who die in a United Kingdom intensive care unit. Intensive Care Med. 2001;27(4):706–10.
70. Williams MT, Aravindan N, Wallace MJ, Riedel BJCJ, Shaw ADS. Venous thromboembolism in the intensive care unit. Crit Care Clin. 2003;19(2):185–207.
71. Blaivas M, Lambert MJ, Harwood RA, Wood JP, Konicki J. Lower-extremity Doppler for deep venous thrombosis—can emergency physicians be accurate and fast? Acad Emerg Med. 2000;7(2):120–6.
72. Magazzini S, Vanni S, Toccafondi S, et al. Duplex ultrasound in the emergency department for the diagnostic management of clinically suspected deep vein thrombosis. Acad Emerg Med. 2007;14(3):216–20.

73. Jang T, Docherty M, Aubin C, Polites G. Resident-performed compression ultrasonography for the detection of proximal deep vein thrombosis: fast and accurate. Acad Emerg Med. 2004;11(3):319–22.
74. Tapson VF, Carroll BA, Davidson BL, Elliott CG, Fedullo PF, Hales CA, Hull RD, Hyers TM, Leeper KV Jr, Morris TA, Moser KM, American Thoracic Society. The diagnostic approach to acute venous thromboembolism. Clinical practice guideline. Am J Respir Crit Care Med. 1999;160(3):1043–66.

Lung

75. Volpicelli G, Elbarbary M, Blaivas M, Lichtenstein DA, Mathis G, Kirkpatrick AW, et al. International evidence-based recommendations for point-of-care lung ultrasound. Intensive Care Med. 2012;38(4):577–91.
76. Manno E, Navarra M, Faccio L, Motevallian M, Bertolaccini L, Mfochive A, Pesce M, Evangelista A. Deep impact of ultrasound in the intensive care unit: the ICU sound protocol. Anesthesiology. 2012;117(4):801–9.
77. Lichtenstein DA, Meziere GA. Relevance of lung ultrasound in the diagnosis of acute respiratory failure the BLUE protocol. Chest J. 2008;134(1):117–25.

Pneumothorax

78. Lichtenstein D, Meziere G, Biderman P, Gepner A. The "lung point": an ultrasound sign specific to pneumothorax. Intensive Care Med. 2000;26:1434–40.
79. de Moya MA, Seaver C, Spaniolas K, Inaba K, Nguyen M, Veltman Y, Shatz D, Alam HB, Pizano L. Occult pneumothorax in trauma patients: development of an objective scoring system. J Trauma. 2007;63:13–7.
80. Henry M, Arnold T, Harvey J, Pleural Diseases Group SoCCBTS. BTS guidelines for the management of spontaneous pneumothorax. Thorax. 2003;58(Suppl 2):ii39–52.
81. Lichtenstein DA, Lascols N, Prin S, Meziere G. The "lung pulse": an early ultrasound sign of complete atelectasis. Intensive Care Med. 2003;29:2187–92.
82. Volpicelli G. Sonographic diagnosis of pneumothorax. Intensive Care Med. 2011;37:224–32.
83. Lichtenstein DA, Meziere G, Lascols N, Biderman P, Courret JP, Gepner A, Goldstein I, Tenoudji-Cohen M. Ultrasound diagnosis of occult pneumothorax. Crit Care Med. 2005;33:1231–8.
84. Soldati G, Testa A, Sher S, Pignataro G, La Sala M, Silveri NG. Occult traumatic pneumothorax: diagnostic accuracy of lung ultrasonography in the emergency department. Chest. 2008;133:204–11.
85. Blaivas M, Lyon M, Duggal S. A prospective comparison of supine chest radiography and bedside ultrasound for the diagnosis of traumatic pneumothorax. Acad Emerg Med. 2005;12:844–9.
86. Rowan KR, Kirkpatrick AW, Liu D, Forkheim KE, Mayo JR, Nicolaou S. Traumatic pneumothorax detection with thoracic US: correlation with chest radiography and CT—initial experience. Radiology. 2002;225:210–4.
87. Zhang M, Liu ZH, Yang JX, Gan JX, Xu SW, You XD, Jiang GY. Rapid detection of pneumothorax by ultrasonography in patients with multiple trauma. Crit Care. 2006;10:R112.
88. Volpicelli G, Elbarbary M, Blaivas M, Lichtenstein DA, Mathis G, Kirkpatrick AW, Melniker L, Gargani L, Noble VE, Via G, Dean A, Tsung JW, Soldati G, Copetti R, Bouhemad B, Reissig A, Agricola E, Rouby JJ, Arbelot C, Liteplo A, Sargsyan A, Silva F, Hoppmann R, Breitkreutz R, Seibel A, Neri L, Storti E, Petrovic T, International Liaison Committee on Lung Ultrasound for International Consensus Conference on Lung Ultrasound. International evidence-based recommendations for point-of-care lung ultrasound. Intensive Care Med. 2012;38:577–91.

Pleural Effusion

89. Volpicelli G, Elbarbary M, Blaivas M, Lichtenstein DA, Mathis G, Kirkpatrick AW, Melniker L, Gargani L, Noble VE, Via G, Dean A, Tsung JW, Soldati G, Copetti R, Bouhemad B, Reissig A, Agricola E, Rouby JJ, Arbelot C, Liteplo A, Sargsyan A, Silva F, Hoppmann R, Breitkreutz R, Seibel A, Neri L, Storti E, Petrovic T, International Liaison Committee on Lung Ultrasound for International Consensus Conference on Lung Ultrasound. International evidence-based recommendations for point-of-care lung ultrasound. Intensive Care Med. 2012;38:577–91.
90. Balik M, Plasil P, Waldauf P, Pazout J, Fric M, Otahal M, Pachl J. Ultrasound estimation of volume of pleural fluid in me- chanically ventilated patients. Intensive Care Med. 2006;32:318–2.
91. Remerand F, Dellamonica J, Mao Z, Ferrari F, Bouhemad B, Jianxin Y, Arbelot C, Lu Q, Ichaï C, Rouby JJ. Multiplane ultrasound approach to quantify pleural effusion at the bedside. Intensive Care Med. 2010;36:656–4.
92. Doelken P, Abreu R, Sahn SA, Mayo PH. Effect of thoracentesis on respiratory mechanics and gas exchange in the patient receiving mechanical ventilation. Chest. 2006;130:1354–61.
93. Kopterides P, Lignos M, Papanikolaou S, Papadomichelakis E, Mentzelopoulos S, Armaganidis A, Panou F. Pleural effusion causing cardiac tamponade: report of two cases and review of literature. Heart Lung. 2006;35:66 7.
94. Kocijancic I, Vidmar K, Ivanovi-Herceg Z. Chest sonography versus lateral decubitus radiography

in the diagnosis of small pleural effusions. J Clin Ultrasound. 2003;31:69–74.
95. Lichtenstein D, Hulot JS, Rabiller A, Tostivint I, Meziere G. Feasibility and safety of ultrasound-aided thoracentesis in mechanically ventilated patients. Intensive Care Med. 1999;25:955–8.
96. Brooks A, Davies B, Smethhurst M, Connolly J. Emergency ultrasound in the acute assessment of haemothorax. Emerg Med J. 2004;21:44–6.
97. Chen HJ, Tu CY, Ling SJ, Chen W, Chiu KL, Hsia TC, Shih CM, Hsu WH. Sonographic appearances in transudative pleural effusions: not always an anechoic pattern. Ultrasound Med Biol. 2008;34:362–9.

Pneumonia or Lung Consolidation

98. Gehmacher O, Mathis G, Kopf A, Scheier M. Ultrasound imaging of pneumonia. Ultrasound Med Biol. 1995;21:1119–22.
99. Sperandeo M, Carnevale V, Muscarella S, Sperandeo G, Varriale A, Filabozzi P, Piattelli ML, D'Alessandro V, Copetti M, Pellegrini F, Dimitri L, Vendemiale G. Clinical application of transthoracic ultrasonography in in- patients with pneumonia. Eur J Clin Investig. 2011;41:1–7.
100. Parlamento S, Copetti R, Di Bartolomeo S. Evaluation of lung ultrasound for the diagnosis of pneumonia in the ED. Am J Emerg Med. 2009;27:379–84.
101. Lichtenstein D, Meziere G, Seitz J. The dynamic air bronchogram. A lung ultrasound sign of alveolar consolidation ruling out atelectasis. Chest. 2009;135:1421–5.
102. Volpicelli G, Elbarbary M, Blaivas M, Lichtenstein DA, Mathis G, Kirkpatrick AW, Melniker L, Gargani L, Noble VE, Via G, Dean A, Tsung JW, Soldati G, Copetti R, Bouhemad B, Reissig A, Agricola E, Rouby JJ, Arbelot C, Liteplo A, Sargsyan A, Silva F, Hoppmann R, Breitkreutz R, Seibel A, Neri L, Storti E, Petrovic T, International Liaison Committee on Lung Ultrasound for International Consensus Conference on Lung Ultrasound. International evidence-based recommendations for point-of-care lung ultrasound. Intensive Care Med. 2012;38:577–91.
103. Cortellaro F, Colombo S, Coen D, Duca PG. Lung ultrasound is an accurate diagnostic tool for the diagnosis of pneumonia in the emergency department. Emerg Med J. 2012;29:19–23.
104. Reissig A, Copetti R, Mathis G, Mempel C, Schuler A, Zechner P, Aliberti S, Neumann R, Kroegel C, Hoyer H. Lung ultrasound in the diagnosis and follow-up of community-acquired pneumonia: a prospective, multicenter, diagnostic accuracy study. Chest. 2012;142:965–72.
105. Lichtenstein D, Goldstein I, Mourgeon E, Cluzel P, Grenier P, Rouby JJ. Comparative diagnostic performances of auscultation, chest radiography, and lung ultrasonography in acute respiratory distress syndrome. Anesthesiology. 2004;100:9–15.
106. Lichtenstein DA, Lascols N, Meziere G, Gepner A. Ultrasound diagnosis of alveolar consolidation in the critically ill. Intensive Care Med. 2004;30:276–81.
107. Xirouchaki N, Magkanas E, Vaporidi K, Kondili E, Plataki M, Patrianakos A, Akoumianaki E, Georgopoulos D. Lung ultrasound in critically ill patients: comparison with bedside chest radiography. Intensive Care Med. 2011;37:1488–93.
108. Bedetti G, Gargani L, Corbisiero A, Frassi F, Poggianti E, Mottola G. Evaluation of ultra- sound lung comets by hand-held echocardiography. Cardiovasc Ultrasound. 2006;4:34.

Pulmonary Edema or Interstitial Syndrome

109. Reissig A, Copetti R. Lung ultrasound in community acquired pneumonia and in insterstitial lung diseases. Respiration. 2014;87:179–89.
110. Volpicelli G, Elbarbary M, Blaivas M, Lichtenstein DA, Mathis G, Kirkpatrick AW, Melniker L, Gargani L, Noble VE, Via G, Dean A, Tsung JW, Soldati G, Copetti R, Bouhemad B, Reissig A, Agricola E, Rouby JJ, Arbelot C, Liteplo A, Sargsyan A, Silva F, Hoppmann R, Breitkreutz R, Seibel A, Neri L, Storti E, Petrovic T, International Liaison Committee on Lung Ultrasound for International Consensus Conference on Lung Ultrasound. International evidence-based recommendations for point-of-care lung ultrasound. Intensive Care Med. 2012;38:577–91.
111. Mueller-Lenke N, Rudez J, Staub D, Laule-Kilian K, Klima T, Perruchoud AP, Mueller C. Use of chest radiography in the emergency diagnosis of acute congestive heart failure. Heart. 2006;92:695–6.
112. Gheorghiade M, Shin DD, Thomas TO, Brandimarte F, Fonarow GC, Abraham WT. Congestion is an important diagnostic and therapeutic target in heart failure. Rev Cardiovasc Med. 2006;7(Suppl 1):S12–24.
113. Prosen G, Klemen P, Strnad M, Grmec S. Combination of lung ultrasound (a comet-tail sign) and N-terminal pro-brain natriuretic peptide in differentiating acute heart failure from chronic obstructive pulmonary disease and asthma as cause of acute dyspnea in prehospital emergency setting. Crit Care. 2011;15:R114.
114. Cibinel GA, Casoli G, Elia F, Padoan M, Pivetta E, Lupia E, Goffi A. Diagnostic accuracy and reproducibility of pleural and lung ultrasound in discriminating cardiogenic causes of acute dyspnea in the Emergency Department. Intern Emerg Med. 2011;7:65–70.
115. Jambrik Z, Monti S, Coppola V, Agricola E, Mottola G, Miniati M, Picano E. Usefulness of ultrasound

lung comets as a nonradiologic sign of extravascular lung water. Am J Cardiol. 2004;93:1265–70.
116. Lichtenstein D, Meziere G, Biderman P, Gepner A, Barre O. The comet-tail artifact. An ultrasound sign of alveolar-interstitial syndrome. Am J Respir Crit Care Med. 1997;156:1640–6.
117. Agricola E, Bove T, Oppizzi M, Marino G, Zangrillo A, Margonato A, Picano E. 'Ultrasound comet-tail images': a marker of pulmonary edema: a comparative study with wedge pressure and extravascular lung water. Chest. 2005;127:1690–5.
118. Liteplo AS, Marill KA, Villen T, Miller RM, Murray AF, Croft PE, et al. Emergency thoracic ultrasound in the differentiation of the etiology of shortness of breath (ETUDES): sonographic B-lines and N-terminal pro-brain-type natriuretic peptide in diagnosing congestive heart failure. Acad Emerg Med. 2009;16:201–10.
119. Noble VE, Murray AF, Capp R, Sylvia-Reardon MH, Steele DJR, Liteplo A. Ultrasound assessment for extravascular lung water in patients undergoing hemodialysis. Chest. 2009;135:1433–9.

Abdomen

120. Rozycki GS, Shackford SR. Ultrasound, what every trauma surgeon should know. J Trauma. 1996;40:1–4.
121. Rozycki GS, Ballard RB, Feliciano DV, et al. Surgeon-performed ultrasound for the assessment of truncal injuries. lessons learned from 1540 patients. Ann Surg. 1998;228:557–67.
122. Chambers JA, Pilbrow WJ. Ultrasound in abdominal trauma. an alternative to peritoneal lavage. Arch Emerg Med. 1988;5:26–33.
123. Sisley AC, Rozycki GS, Ballard RB, Namias N, et al. Rapid detection of traumatic effusion using surgeon-performed ultrasonography. J Trauma. 1998;44:291–7.
124. Dulchavsky SA, Schwarz KL, Kirkpatrick AW, et al. Prospective evaluation of thoracic ultrasound in the detection of pneumothorax. J Trauma. 2001;50:201–5.
125. Kirkpatrick AW, Sirois M, Laupland KB, et al. Hand-held thoracic sonography for detecting post-traumatic pneumothoraces. the Extended Focused Assessment with Sonography for Trauma (EFAST). J Trauma. 2004;57:288–95.
126. Ma OJ, Mateer JR. Trauma ultrasound examination versus chest radiography in the detection of hemothorax. Ann Emerg Med. 1997;29(3):312–5.
127. ACEP Policy Statement. Emergency ultrasound guidelines. Approved October 2008. Accessed online acep.org on 26 Jan 2015.
128. American College of Surgeons Committee on Trauma. Advanced trauma life support (ATLS). 9th ed. Chicago: American College of Surgeons; 2012.
129. Abrams BJ, Sukumvanich P, Seibel R, et al. Ultrasound for the detection of intraperitoneal fluid: the role of Trendelenburg positioning. Am J Emerg Med. 1999;17(2):117–20.
130. Lichtenstein DA, Meziere GA. Relevance of lung ultrasound in the diagnosis of acute respiratory failure the BLUE protocol. Chest J. 2008;134(1):117–25.
131. Lee BC, Ormsby EL, McGahan JP, et al. The utility of sonography for the triage of blunt abdominal trauma patients to exploratory laparotomy. AJR Am J Roentgenol. 2007;188(2):415–21.
132. Wherrett LJ, Boulanger BR, McLellan BA, et al. Hypotension after blunt abdominal trauma: the role of emergent abdominal sonography in surgical triage. J Trauma. 1996;41(5):815–20.
133. Rose JS, Richards JR, Battistella F, et al. The fast is positive, now what? Derivation of a clinical decision rule to determine the need for therapeutic laparotomy in adults with blunt torso trauma and a positive trauma ultrasound. J Emerg Med. 2005;29(1):15–21.
134. Melniker L. The value of focused assessment with sonography in trauma examination for the need for operative intervention in blunt torso trauma: a rebuttal to "emergency ultrasound-based algorithms for diagnosing blunt abdominal trauma (review)", from the Cochrane Collaboration. Crit Ultrasound J. 2009;1:73–84.
135. Brown MA, Casola G, Sirlin CB, et al. Importance of evaluating organ parenchyma during screening abdominal ultrasonography after blunt trauma. J Ultrasound Med. 2001;20(6):577–83.
136. Ballard RB, Rozycki GS, Newman PG, et al. An algorithm to reduce the incidence of false-negative FAST examinations in patients at high risk for occult injury. Focused assessment for the sonographic examination of the trauma patient. J Am Coll Surg. 1999;189(2):145–50.
137. Plummer D, Brunette D, Asinger R, et al. Emergency department echocardiography improves outcome in penetrating cardiac injury. Ann Emerg Med. 1992;21(6):709–12.
138. Rozycki GS, Feliciano DV, Ochsner MG, et al. The role of ultrasound in patients with possible penetrating cardiac wounds: a prospective multicenter study. J Trauma. 1999;46(4):543–51.
139. Natarajan B, Gupta PK, Cemaj S, et al. FAST scan: is it worth doing in hemodynamically stable blunt trauma patients? Surgery. 2010;148(4):695–700.
140. Blackbourne LH, Soffer D, McKenney M, et al. Secondary ultrasound examination increases the sensitivity of the FAST exam in blunt trauma. J Trauma. 2004;57(5):934–8.
141. Blaivas M, Lyon M, Duggal S. A prospective comparison of supine chest radiography and bedside ultrasound for the diagnosis of traumatic pneumothorax. Acad Emerg Med. 2005;12(9):844–9.
142. Ianniello S, Di Giacomo V, Sessa B, Miele V. First-line sonographic diagnosis of pneumothorax in major trauma: accuracy of e-FAST and comparison with multidetector computed tomography. Radiol Med. 2014;119(9):674–80.

143. Alrajhi K, Woo MY, Vaillancourt C. Test characteristics of ultrasonography for the detection of pneumothorax: a systematic review and meta-analysis. Chest. 2012;141(3):703–8.
144. Abboud PA, Kendall J. Emergency department ultrasound for hemothorax after blunt traumatic injury. J Emerg Med. 2003;25(2):181–4.

Resuscitation Protocols

145. Irwin RS, Rippe JM. Intensive care medicine. 6th ed. Philadelphia: Lippincott Williams & Wilkins; 2008. p. 491–6.
146. Lichtenstein D, Meziere G. Ultrasound diagnosis of an acute dyspnea [abstract]. Crit Care. 2003;7(suppl):S93.
147. Greenbaum DM, Marschall KE. The value of routine daily chest X-rays in intubated patients in the medical intensive care unit. Crit Care Med. 1982;10:29–30.
148. Lichtenstein D, Goldstein G, Mourgeon E, et al. Comparative diagnostic performances of auscultation, chest radiography and lung ultrasonography in acute respiratory distress syndrome. Anesthesiology. 2004;100:9–15.
149. Brenner DJ, Elliston CD, Hall EJ, et al. Estimated risks of radiation-induced fatal cancer from pediatric CT. AJR Am J Roentgenol. 2001;176:289–96.
150. Berrington de Gonzales A, Darby S. Risk of cancer from diagnostic X-rays. Lancet. 2004;363:345–51.
151. Brenner DJ, Hall EJ. Computed tomography: an increasing source of radiation exposure. N Engl J Med. 2007;357:2277–84.
152. Lichtenstein DA, Meziere GA. Relevance of lung ultrasound in the diagnosis of acute respiratory failure: the BLUE protocol. Chest. 2008;134:117–25.

Hypotension

153. Scalea TM, Rodriguez A, Chiu WC, Brenneman FD, Fallon WF Jr, Kato K, McKenney MG, Nerlich ML, Ochsner MG, Yoshii H. Focused Assessment with Sonography for Trauma (FAST): results from an international consensus conference. J Trauma. 1999;46(3):466–72.
154. Seif D, Perera P, Mailhot T, Riley D, Mandavia D. Bedside ultrasound in resuscitation and the rapid ultrasound in shock protocol. Crit Care Res Pract. 2012;2012:503254. https://doi.org/10.1155/2012/503254. Epub 2012 Oct 24.
155. Jones AE, Tayal VS, Sullivan DM, Kline JA. Randomized, controlled trial of immediate versus delayed goal-directed ultrasound to identify the cause of nontraumatic hypotension in emergency department patients. Crit Care Med. 2004;32(8):1703–8. [PubMed].
156. Atkinson PRT, McAuley DJ, Kendall RJ, et al. Abdominal and Cardiac Evaluation with Sonography in Shock (ACES): an approach by emergency physicians for the use of ultrasound in patients with undifferentiated hypotension. Emerg Med J. 2009;26(2):87–91. [PubMed].
157. Boyd JH, Walley KR. The role of echocardiography in hemodynamic monitoring. Curr Opin Crit Care. 2009;15(3):239–43. [PubMed].
158. Lanctot YF, Valois M, Bealieu Y. EGLS: echo guided life support. An algorithmic approach to undifferentiated shock. Crit Ultrasound J. 2011;3:123–9.
159. Lichtenstein DA, Karakitsos D. Integrating ultrasound in the hemodynamic evaluation of acute circulatory failure (FALLS-the fluid administration limited by lung sonography protocol). J Crit Care. 2012;27(5):53.e11–533.e19. [PubMed].
160. Rozycki G, Oschner MG, Schmidt JA, et al. A prospective use of surgeon's performed ultrasound as the primary adjunct modality for injured patient assessment. J Trauma. 1995;39:879–85. [PubMed].
161. Kirkpatrick AW, Sirois M, Laupland KB, et al. Hand-held thoracic sonography for detecting post-traumatic pneumothoraces: the extended focused assessment with sonography for trauma (EFAST). J Trauma. 2004;57(2):288–95. [PubMed].
162. Breitkreutz R, Price S, Steiger HV, et al. Focused echocardiographic evaluation in life support and peri-resuscitation of emergency patients: a prospective trial. Resuscitation. 2010;81(11):1527–33. [PubMed].
163. Breitkreutz R, Walcher F, Seeger FH. Focused echocardiographic evaluation in resuscitation management: concept of an advanced life support-conformed algorithm. Crit Care Med. 2007;35(5, supplement):S150–61. [PubMed].
164. Ferrada P, Murthi S, Anand RJ, Bochicchio GV, Scalea T. Transthoracic focused rapid echocardiographic examination: real-time evaluation of fluid status in critically ill trauma patients. J Trauma. 2011;70(1):56–64. [PubMed].
165. Weingart SD, Duque D, Nelson B. Rapid ultrasound for shock and hypotension (RUSH-HIMAPP). 2009. http://emedhome.com/. Accessed: 6/25/2019.
166. Perera P, Mailhot T, Riley D, Mandavia D. The RUSH exam: rapid ultrasound in SHock in the evaluation of the critically Ill. Emerg Med Clin North Am. 2010;28(1):29–56. [PubMed].
167. Perera P, Mailhot T, Riley D, Mandavia D. The RUSH exam: rapid ultrasound in SHock in the evaluation of the critically ill patient. Ultrasound Clin. 2012;7(2):255–78.
168. Bahner DP. Trinity: a hypotensive ultrasound protocol. J Diagn Med Sonography. 2002;18(4):193–8.
169. Rose JS, Bair AE, Mandavia D, Kinser DJ. The UHP ultrasound protocol: a novel ultrasound approach to the empiric evaluation of the undifferentiated hypotensive patient. Am J Emerg Med. 2001;19(4):299–302. [PubMed].
170. Hernandez C, Shuler K, Hannan H, Sonyika C, Likourezos A, Marshall J. C.A.U.S.E.: cardiac arrest ultra-sound exam-A better approach to managing patients in primary non-arrhythmogenic cardiac

arrest. Resuscitation. 2008;76(2):198–206. Presence of cardiac contractility on bedside echo helps with prognosis.
171. Blyth L, Atkinson P, Gadd K, Lang E. Bedside focused echocardiography as predictor of survival in cardiac arrest patients: a systematic review. Acad Emerg Med. 2012;19(10):1119–26. https://doi.org/10.1111/j.1553-2712.2012.01456.x. Epub 2012 Oct 5. Review. PubMed PMID: 23039118.
172. Chou HC, Tseng WP, Wang CH, Ma MH, Wang HP, Huang PC, et al. Tracheal rapid ultrasound exam (T.R.U.E.) for confirming endotracheal tube placement during emergency intubation. Resuscitation. 2011;82(10):1279–84. https://doi.org/10.1016/j.resuscitation.2011.05.016. Epub 2011 June 1.

Critical Care Procedures

173. McGee DC, Gould MK. Preventing complications of central venous catheterization. N Engl J Med. 2003;348:1123–33.
174. Kumar A, Chuan A. Ultrasound guided vascular access: efficacy and safety. Best Pract Res Clin Anaesthesiol. 2009;23:299–311.
175. Stone MB, Nagdev A, Murphy MC, Sisson CA. Ultrasound detection of guidewire position during central venous catheterization. Am J Emerg Med. 2010;28:82–4.
176. Randolph AG, Cook DJ, Gonzales CA, Pribble CG. Ultrasound guidance for placement of central venous catheters: a meta-analysis of the literature. Crit Care Med. 1996;24:2053–8.
177. Hind D, Calvert N, McWilliams R, et al. Ultrasonic locating devices for central venous cannulation: meta-analysis. BMJ. 2003;327:361–8.
178. Rabindranath KS, Kumar E, Shail R, Vaux E. Use of real-time ultra- sound guidance for the placement of hemodialysis catheters: a systemic review and meta-analysis of randomized controlled trials. Am J Kidney Dis. 2011;58(6):964–70.
179. Prabhu MV, Juneja D, Gopal PB, et al. Ultrasound-guided femoral dialysis access placement: a single-center randomized trial. Clin Soc J Am Soc Nephrol. 2010;5:235–9.
180. Blaivas M, Adhikari S. An unseen danger: frequency of posterior vessel wall penetration by needles during attempts to place internal jugular vein central catheters using ultrasound guidance. Crit Care Med. 2009;37:2345–9.
181. Randolph AG, Cook DJ, Gonzales CA, et al. Ultrasound guidance for placement of central venous catheters: a meta-analysis of the literature. Crit Care Med. 1996;24:2053–8.
182. Karakitsos D, Labropoulos N, De Groot E, et al. Real-time ultrasound guided catheterization of the internal jugular vein; a prospective comparison to the landmark technique in critical care patients [ISRCTN61258470]. Crit Care. 2006;10:R162.
183. Fragou M, Gravvanis A, Dimitriou V, Papalois A, Kouraklis G, Karabinis A, et al. Real-time ultrasound-guided subclavian vein cannulation versus the landmark method in critical care patients: a prospective randomized study*. Crit Care Med. 2011;39(7):1607–12.
184. Shiver S, Blaivas M, Lyon M. A prospective comparison of ultrasound-guided and blindly placed radial arterial catheters. Acad Emerg Med. 2006;13(12):1275–9.
185. Levin PD, Sheinin O, Gozal Y. Use of ultrasound guidance in the insertion of radial artery catheters. Crit Care Med. 2003;31(2):481–4.
186. Shiloh AL, Savel RH, Paulin LM, Eisen LA. Ultrasound-guided catheterization of the radial artery: a systematic review and meta-analysis of randomized controlled trials. Chest J. 2011;139(3):524–9.
187. Gregg SC, Murthi SB, Sisley AC, Stein DM, Scalea TM. Ultrasound-guided peripheral intravenous access in the intensive care unit. J Crit Care. 2010;25(3):514–9.

Pericardiocentesis

188. Tsang TS, Enriquez-Sarano M, Freeman WK, Barnes ME, Sinak LJ, Gersh BJ, Bailey KR, Seward JB. Consecutive 1127 therapeutic echocardiographically guided pericardiocenteses: clinical profile, practice patterns, and outcomes spanning 21 years. Mayo Clin Proc. 2002;77(5):429–36. PubMed PMID: 12004992.
189. Nagdev A, Mantuani D. A novel in-plane technique for ultrasound-guided pericardiocentesis. Am J Emerg Med. 2013;31(9):1424.e5–9. https://doi.org/10.1016/j.ajem.2013.05.021. Epub 2013 July 1. PubMed PMID: 23809089.
190. Nagdev A, Stone MB. Point-of-care ultrasound evaluation of pericardial effusions: does this patient have cardiac tamponade? Resuscitation. 2011;82(6):671–3. https://doi.org/10.1016/j.resuscitation.2011.02.004. Epub 2011 Mar 11. PubMed PMID: 21397379.
191. Fitch MT, Nicks BA, Pariyadath M, McGinnis HD, Manthey DE. Videos in clinical medicine. Emergency pericardiocentesis. N Engl J Med. 2012;366(12):e17. https://doi.org/10.1056/NEJMvcm0907841. Review. PubMed PMID: 22435385.
192. Vayre F, Lardoux H, Pezzano M, Bourdarias JP, Dubourg O. Subxiphoid pericardiocentesis guided by contrast two-dimensional echocardiography in cardiac tamponade: experience of 110 consecutive patients. Eur J Echocardiogr. 2000;1(1):66–71. PubMed PMID: 12086218.
193. Tsang TS, Freeman WK, Barnes ME, Reeder GS, Packer DL, Seward JB. Rescue echocardiographically guided pericardiocentesis for cardiac perforation complicating catheter-based procedures. The Mayo Clinic experience. J Am Coll Cardiol. 1998;32(5):1345–50. PubMed PMID: 9809946.

Thoracentesis

194. Rahman NM, Singanayagam A, Davies HE, et al. Diagnostic accuracy, safety and utilisation of respiratory physician-delivered thoracic ultrasound. Thorax. 2010;65(5):449–53.
195. Diacon AH, Brutsche MH, Solèr M. Accuracy of pleural puncture sites: a prospective comparison of clinical examination with ultrasound. Chest. 2003;123(2):436–41.
196. Havelock T, Teoh R, Laws D, Gleeson F, BTS Pleural Disease Guideline Group. Pleural procedures and thoracic ultrasound: British Thoracic Society pleural disease guideline 2010. Thorax. 2010;65(suppl 2):i61–76.
197. Heidecker J, Huggins JT, Sahn SA, et al. Pathophysiology of pneumothorax following ultrasound-guided thoracentesis. Chest. 2006;130:1173–84.
198. Raptopoulos V, Davis LM, Lee G. Factors affecting the development of pneumothorax associated with thoracentesis. AJR Am J Roentgenol. 1991;156:917–20.
199. Rendina EA, Ciccone AM. The intercostal space. Thorac Surg Clin. 2007;17:491–501.
200. Yoneyama H, Arahata M, Temaru R, et al. Evaluation of the risk of intercostal artery laceration during thoracentesis in elderly patients by using 3D-CT angiography. Intern Med. 2010;49:289–92.
201. Salamonsen M, Ellis S, Paul E, et al. Thoracic ultrasound demonstrates variable location of the intercostal artery. Respiration. 2012;83:323–9.
202. Chen HJ, Tu CY, Ling SJ, Chen W, Chiu KL, Hsia TC, Shih CM, Hsu WH. Sonographic appearances in transudative pleural effusions: not always an anechoic pattern. Ultrasound Med Biol. 2008;34:362–9.
203. Balik M, Plasil P, Waldauf P, Pazout J, Fric M, Otahal M, Pachl J. Ultrasound estimation of volume of pleural fluid in mechanically ventilated patients. Intensive Care Med. 2006;32:318–2.
204. Remerand F, Dellamonica J, Mao Z, Ferrari F, Bouhemad B, Jianxin Y, Arbelot C, Lu Q, Ichaï C, Rouby JJ. Multiplane ultrasound approach to quantify pleural effusion at the bedside. Intensive Care Med. 2010;36:656–4.
205. Doelken P, Abreu R, Sahn SA, Mayo PH. Effect of thoracentesis on respiratory mechanics and gas exchange in the patient receiving mechanical ventilation. Chest. 2006;130:1354–61.
206. Kopterides P, Lignos M, Papanikolaou S, Papadomichelakis E, Mentzelopoulos S, Armaganidis A, Panou F. Pleural effusion causing cardiac tamponade: report of two cases and review of literature. Heart Lung. 2006;35:66–7.

Paracentesis

207. Runyon BA, AASLD Practice Guidelines Committee. Management of adult patients with ascites due to cirrhosis: an update. Hepatology. 2009;49(6):2087–107. https://doi.org/10.1002/hep.22853. PubMed PMID: 19475696.
208. Ginès P, Cárdenas A, Arroyo V, Rodés J. Management of cirrhosis and ascites. N Engl J Med. 2004;350(16):1646–54. Review. PubMed PMID: 15084697.
209. Hatch N, Wu TS, Barr L, Roque PJ. Advanced ultrasound procedures. Crit Care Clin. 2014;30(2):305–29, vi. https://doi.org/10.1016/j.ccc.2013.10.005. Epub 2013 Dec 4. Review. PubMed PMID: 24606778.
210. Thomsen TW, Shaffer RW, White B, Setnik GS. Videos in clinical medicine. Paracentesis. N Engl J Med. 2006;355(19):e21. Erratum in: N Engl J Med. 2007. 15;356(7):760. PubMed PMID: 17093242.
211. Pache I, Bilodeau M. Severe haemorrhage following abdominal paracentesis for ascites in patients with liver disease. Aliment Pharmacol Ther. 2005;21(5):525–9. PubMed PMID: 15740535.
212. McVay PA, Toy PT. Lack of increased bleeding after paracentesis and thoracentesis in patients with mild coagulation abnormalities. Transfusion. 1991;31(2):164–71. PubMed PMID: 1996485.
213. Nadir A, Van Thiel DH. Frequency of peritoneal infections among patients undergoing continuous paracentesis with an indwelling catheter. J Ayub Med Coll Abbottabad. 2010;22(1):37–41.
214. Konerman MA, Price J, Torres D, Li Z. Randomized, controlled pilot study comparing large-volume paracentesis using wall suction and traditional glass vacuum bottle methods. Ther Adv Gastroenterol. 2014;7(5):184–92. https://doi.org/10.1177/1756283X14532704. PubMed PMID: 25177365; PubMed Central PMCID: PMC4107699.
215. Kwok CS, Krupa L, Mahtani A, Kaye D, Rushbrook SM, Phillips MG, Gelson W. Albumin reduces paracentesis-induced circulatory dysfunction and reduces death and renal impairment among patients with cirrhosis and infection: a systematic review and meta-analysis. Biomed Res Int. 2013;2013:295153. https://doi.org/10.1155/2013/295153. Epub 2013 Oct 8. Review. PubMed PMID: 24222902; PubMed Central PMCID: PMC3816020.
216. Sort P, Navasa M, Arroyo V, Aldeguer X, Planas R, Ruiz-del-Arbol L, Castells L, Vargas V, Soriano G, Guevara M, Ginès P, Rodés J. Effect of intravenous albumin on renal impairment and mortality in patients with cirrhosis and spontaneous bacterial peritonitis. N Engl J Med. 1999;341(6):403–9. PubMed PMID: 10432325.

38 End-of-Life Care in the Emergency Department

Anton Travis Manasco and Brian T. Wessman

Introduction

Case vignette *Mrs. Smith is a 75-year old woman with metastatic squamous cell lung cancer who presents to the Emergency Department (ED) for cough, fevers, and chills. Her vital signs include oxygen saturation (SpO_2) on a nonrebreather mask of 88%, blood pressure of 100/50, pulse of 120, and temperature of 101.4F. A chest radiograph shows diffuse multifocal infiltrates. On chart review, it is discovered that this is her third visit to the hospital, having been discharged 3 days ago to a skilled nursing facility. She does not have a Physician's Orders for Life Sustaining Treatment or advanced directive. While calculating her weight-based antibiotic orders, you begin to ponder how to approach a discussion with this patient and her family in the ED setting.*

"Our ultimate goal, after all, is not a good death but a good life to the very end."
—Atul Gawande

A. T. Manasco
Anesthesiology – Critical Care Medicine, Washington University in St. Louis School of Medicine – Barnes Jewish Hospital, St. Louis, MO, USA

B. T. Wessman (✉)
Divisions of Critical Care Medicine and Emergency Medicine, Washington University in Saint Louis, School of Medicine, St. Louis, MO, USA
e-mail: brianwessman@wustl.edu

The role of the Emergency Provider (EP) is to appropriately diagnose and stabilize acute life-threatening injuries and illnesses. Despite good intentions and optimal medical therapies, some patients will not survive their ED course; others will die in the hospital, usually in the intensive care unit (ICU) days after admission. Medicare data shows that over one-third of patients who die receive medical care in the ED and ICU during their last 6 months of life [1]. Patients overwhelmingly prefer to die at home [2]. Unfortunately, studies show that 38% of people die in the hospital, specifically 22% occur in the ICU, often times while receiving maximum levels of care [3]. Since many of these patients are admitted through the ED, it is essential for an EP to be proficient with end-of-life (EOL) care.

The American Academy of Hospice and Palliative Medicine describes that the goal of Palliative Care (PC) is to "prevent and relieve suffering and to support the best possible quality of life for patients, facing life-threatening or debilitating illness, and their families, regardless of the stage of the disease or the need for other therapies [4]." PC is not the same as *hospice* care. Hospice care is a subset of PC focusing on patients with terminal illness and a predicted life expectancy of 6 months or less who forego therapeutic medical interventions in favor of comfort and quality of life.

In 2014, the American College of Emergency Physicians (ACEP), as part of the *Choosing*

© Springer Nature Switzerland AG 2020
J. R. Shiber, S. D. Weingart (eds.), *Emergency Department Critical Care*,
https://doi.org/10.1007/978-3-030-28794-8_38

Wisely campaign, recommended that EPs "(d)on't delay engaging palliative and hospice care services in the Emergency Department for patients likely to benefit." A recent study of ED-initiated PC in advanced cancer patients demonstrated improved quality of life (QOL) with no negative effect on survival [5]. Despite these recommendations and findings, only 18% of residents and medical students receive formal training in EOL care [6]. The goals of this chapter are to review medical ethics, discuss the concept of shared decision-making and goals of care, explore communication strategies for EPs, and examine the concept of medical futility.

Medical Ethics

The four pillars of medical ethics include *autonomy*, *beneficence*, *nonmaleficence*, and *justice* (*see* Box 38.1). Patients with decision-making capacity possess *autonomy*, the ability to make self-focused choices about their medical treatment. The patient may accept or reject any medical care and/or interventions according to their personal preferences and beliefs. The EP should fully explain, without bias, options for treatment and help patients make decisions that align with their own values. When the patient makes a decision, the EP, regardless of their personal preference or opinion, should honor it.

Beneficence is acting in the best interest of the patient. This could mean respecting a patient's prior stated wishes, written or verbal, regarding life-sustaining treatment or other medical interventions (dialysis, artificial nutrition, intubation, etc.).

Box 38.1 Four Traditional Pillars of Medical Ethics

1. Autonomy – The ability to determine self-focused decisions and actions.
2. Beneficence – Promoting what is best for the patient.
3. Nonmaleficence – Do no harm.
4. Justice – Using resources in an efficient, equitable manner. Patients should receive the same high-quality care.

Primum non nocere, meaning, "First, do no harm," is the basis of *nonmaleficence*. Many medical students are familiar with this principle from the Hippocratic Oath, a historical pledge taken by physicians. Procedures and medications all possess the possibility of both benefit and harm to the patient. EPs must weigh these harms with the patient's disease and care trajectory. If one intubates the patient with end-stage chronic obstructive pulmonary disease (COPD) and metastatic lung cancer, will they ever be liberated from the ventilator? Do intubation and mechanical ventilation align with the patient's values and wishes?

Justice refers to the equitable, fair treatment of all patients regardless of race, sex, color, creed, nationality, or socioeconomic status. Healthcare resources are limited. Every decision by the EP affects multiple other patients due to resource constraints. Medical actions will also impact the surrounding family members (i.e., emotional, financial, physical, etc.).

These four pillars serve as the foundation for ethical medical practice and decision-making. Returning to this solid ethical base will always help the EP when faced with a challenging EOL case [7].

Establishing Goals of Care

The ED is not the ideal setting for a GOC conversation. It is loud, chaotic, and frantic with little privacy. Interruptions are frequent. Providers regularly treat patients with minimal historical information. Acknowledging these limitations, it is the EP's duty to provide the best care possible to patients with terminal and chronic conditions. Many of these patients with chronic health conditions may benefit from early GOC discussions. The purpose of this conversation is to discuss realistic treatment options available and how they align with the patient's personal preferences regarding QOL [8]. This creates an "individualized roadmap" for future health care. Educating the patient and their family on the concept of *QUALITY of life* versus *the concept of QUANTITY of life* can be helpful to put future potential outcome pathways in perspective. Nonverbal components of communication are essential to the GOC conversation. Sitting down, making eye contact, turning off pagers/cell phone ringers, and showing empathy demonstrate compassion and respect to the patient and their family. Similar to the procedural skills of central venous cannulation or bronchoscopy, communication skills must be honed with practice. (*See* Box 38.2 *for a GOC discussion primer.*)

Some patients arrive to the ED with an advanced directive (AD), living will, appointed durable power of attorney (DPA), and/or a Provider Order for Life Sustaining Treatment (POLST) (*see* Box 38.3). A POLST is a physician-

Box 38.2 Goals of Care Discussion

1. Communicating prognosis
   (a) Answer two key questions: "What is wrong with patient? What will happen to him/her?"
   (b) Describe what could be the best and worst outcome for the patient.
   (c) Discuss the most likely scenario.
2. Eliciting patient values
   (a) "What is most important to you in your life right now?"
   (b) If the patient is unable to participate, discuss the decisions the patient makes, if present.
   (c) Consider any statements made by the patient regarding end-of-life care.
3. Using appropriate language
   (a) Avoid negative statements ("Do you want us to stop aggressive care?")
   (b) Avoid the phrase "do everything" when discussing curative versus palliative care.
4. Reconciling goals of care
   (a) Sometimes a time-limited trial of therapy is needed to elucidate the patient's course or facilitate decision-making.
   (b) Set a plan of action based on decisions.
   (c) Determine the time and location of a follow-up discussion, if applicable.
5. Recommending a care plan based on the established goals
   (a) Discontinue any medications or therapies not consistent with the GOC.

Adapted from Rosenberg M, Lamba S, Misra S. Palliative medicine and geriatric emergency care – challenges, opportunities, and basic principles. Clin Geriatr Med. 2013;29:1–29

Box 38.3 Important Goals of Care Definitions

1. Advanced Directive – Documents stating a patient's desire for future care in the event of serious illness or incapacity.
2. Physicians Order for Life-Sustaining Treatment (POLST) – A standardized form documenting a patient–physician discussion regarding a patient's desired future medical care and interventions.
3. Durable Power of Attorney – Designated individual acting as a surrogate or proxy for the patient; makes treatment decisions for an incapacitated patient.

signed document of a prior EOL discussion with the patient or their surrogate decision-maker. These documents state a patient's desires for care in certain medical situations (cardiopulmonary resuscitation (CPR), intubation, mechanical ventilation, artificial nutrition, etc.). If present, these documents should be honored, though subsequent discussions with the patient and/or their appointed decision should still remain part of the communication process.

Unfortunately, most patients arrive at the ED without any of the above documents. A 2017 systematic review reported that only 38% of patients with chronic illnesses and 33% of healthy adults complete any form of AD [9]. In the event of an absent AD, the provider should clarify GOC with the patient or a surrogate medical decision-maker. It is imperative that the EP offers accurate prognostic information while making clear the unpredictability of illnesses and the progression of disease. Prior to the discussion, a phone call to the primary care doctor, oncologist, or other involved physician may help clarify patient preferences and prognostic information.

Basic, evidence-based principles of EOL communication are shown in Box 38.4 [10]. When conducting a GOC conversation, remember to avoid negative phrases ("will *not do everything*," "will *not give* antibiotics for the infection"). Instead employ phrases that focus on the treatment and care you will offer to the patient: "WILL provide pain medications," "WILL ensure complete comfort." Use direct phrases such as "death" instead of "passing on" or other euphemistic phrases. Do not rush the family into a decision, but conduct the discussion from an information-sharing perspective. Usually, in the ED setting, patients and their family are suffering an acute change in condition, necessitating deliberation between the patient and/or their family members.

Box 38.4 Basic Principles for End-of-Life Communication

1. Be truthful regarding prognosis.
2. Do not delay discussions of end-of-life goals with patients.
3. Anxiety is normal for both patient and clinician during these discussions.
4. Patients have unique goals and desires about their care.
5. Encourage patient and family discussion on medical and nonmedical goals of care.

Adapted from Bernacki et al. [10]

Shared and Surrogate Decision-Making

The widespread adoption of shared decision-making (SDM) instituted a fundamental change in the practice of medicine. Instead of paternalistic physicians dictating the care plan for a patient and their family, the responsibility for patient care decisions is *shared* between the medical team and the patient/surrogate. Physicians provide medical expertise and experience and surrogates provide their personal knowledge of the patient [11]. Together, the two parties develop a patient-centered medical plan. SDM is characterized by active patient/surrogate involvement, a sharing of information between parties, consensus building, and agreement on which treatments to implement [12].

Studies have evaluated SDM in various disease processes, including pediatric lacerations and rehydration options, pediatric fever, and low-risk chest pain. A systematic review of SDM involving these disease processes showed improvement in patient knowledge and satisfaction with the explanation of their care [13].

In the event of incapacity, the patient needs a surrogate decision-maker. If the patient has an appointed DPA for Health Care, that individual should be used. In the majority of cases, there is no appointed surrogate. Many, but not all, states have a legal order of surrogacy (i.e., spouse or offspring). There are currently two types of default surrogate consent laws: (1) hierarchy surrogate consent laws and (2) consensus surrogate consent laws. In states with hierarchy surrogate consent laws, the decision falls to family members or offspring close with the patient. A few states have consensus statues requiring all "interested persons" come to a consensus to name a surrogate [14]. The EP should be familiar with their state laws when identifying a surrogate.

The surrogate's job is to act as the voice for the patient through the substituted judgment standard. They should decide what the patient would want, if they were present. The surrogate should not inject their own values and wishes when making medical decisions for the patient even if they have different values. Even with the best intentions, surrogate decision-makers have been found to follow patient treatment preferences only 68% of the time [15].

Withdrawing/Withholding Medical Treatment

Once the decision is made to allow natural death, how should the imminently dying patient be managed in the ED? If the patient or surrogate decides to pursue strictly comfort care, certain invasive or potential harmful medical treatments will need to be withdrawn. Focus should be placed on the comfort of the patient and the family. The patient should be moved to a private room, if possible, and offered all privacy measures available (corner area, curtains drawn) [16]. Many articles suggest relaxing visitor limitations if it does not interfere with the care of other ED patients.

Some patients will need prior interventions withdrawn. Consider a patient, not unlike the initial case vignette, arriving to the ED in a critically-ill unstable state. An acutely ill patient may be immediately intubated and started on vasopressors if they arrive without a documented AD. Later in their ED course, their family arrives and produces a signed DNR/DNI document. How does one proceed? What factors are associated with withdrawal of life-sustaining measures?

Usually, withdrawal of life support is equated to withdrawal of mechanical ventilation. However, other life supportive measures such as vasopressors, artificial nutrition, dialysis, and/or antibiotics also fall into this category. Prior to withdrawal, it is important to explain the dying process to the family. Thoroughly describe signs and symptoms such as "agonal" and noisy breathing from airway secretions ("death rattle"). Acknowledge the unpredictability of death; for example, consider saying, "It could be minutes to hours before your loved one dies, one is unable to predict the exact time frame." A spiritual care provider service, such as the hospital chaplain is a great resource to help guide and support the family.

Mechanical ventilation can be removed in one step or a graded fashion. There are no consensus guidelines for withdrawal of mechanical ventilation. Some providers argue that a terminal wean prolongs the dying process while others believe that it improves patient comfort. The authors of this chapter recommend following your hospital guidelines for terminal extubation. If no protocols exist, ensure that the patient is free of pain, using narcotics if necessary and discontinue the endotracheal tube while frequently reevaluating the patient for signs of dyspnea or discomfort [17].

Comfort measures include pain, delirium, and anxiety control (*see* Box 38.5). For pain, opioids are the preferred therapy. No evidence exists to support one pain regimen or opioid over another. Many providers and ICUs use opioid drips to control pain, allowing easy titration to patient symptoms. Benzodiazepines are the preferred treatment for anxiety and agitation. Similar to opioids, there is no evidence to support one agent over another. Attention to the patient's comfort is necessary when withdrawing life-sustaining treatment. Remember there is no maximum dose for medications when providing comfort care. There is ethical and legal consensus that although respiratory depression or hypotension may be a foreseeable consequence of these medications, if the intent is to relieve specific symptoms such as pain or dyspnea, it is essential to treat in adequate doses despite the possibility that death may be hastened. The concept of providing preemptive deep sedation to avoid patient suffering at the end-of-life is termed palliative sedation.

Box 38.5 Pharmacology of palliative sedation agents

Opioid	IV Push dose	Infusion dose	Half-life	Metabolism
Morphine	2–4 mg IV q1–2h	2–30 mg/h	3–4 h	Glucuronidation
Hydromorphone	0.2–0.6 mg IV q1–2 h	0.5–3 mg/h	2–3 h	Glucuronidation
Fentanyl	0.35–0.5 mcg/kg IV q0.5–1 h	0.7–10 mcg/kg/h	2–4 h	CYP3A4/5
Benzodiazepine				
Midazolam	0.01–0.05 mg/kg	0.02–0.1 mg/kg/h	3–11 h	Hepatic
Lorazepam	0.02–0.04 mg/kg (≤0.02	0.02–0.06 mg/kg q2-6h prn or 0.01–0.1 mg/kg/h. (≤ 10 mg/h)	8–15 h	Hepatic
Antipsychotic				
Haloperidol	0.5–10 mg	N/A	14–26 h	Hepatic
Anticholinergic Glycopyrrolate	0.2 mg SC Q4 h			

Adjunctive medications for comfort include antipsychotics (such as haloperidol) for symptoms of agitated delirium, and anticholinergics (such as glycopyrrolate or scopolamine) to decrease secretions.

Futility

"Futility" stems from the Latin word *futilis,* meaning leaky. The concept of futility originates from Greek mythology and the tale of the daughters of Danaus, who were condemned in the underworld to repeatedly fill a bathtub with leaky buckets. Schneiderman et al. defined futility as *quantitative* or *qualitative*. Quantitative futility is any intervention to produce an effect which "reasoning or experience suggest is highly improbable and cannot be systematically produced" with a 1% probability of improvement suggested. Qualitative futility is any therapy that does not change the patient's condition and/or complete dependence on intensive medical care [18].

Throughout the course of a career, EPs face numerous instances of presumed futility. For example, if our patient at the beginning of the chapter were to become asystolic, would cardiopulmonary resuscitation provide any benefit? Simon et al. described "bridge to nowhere" therapies in the ED when there is no survivable clinical endpoint. Examples include providing CPR on patients with metastatic cancer or imminent death from brain herniation, offering intubation on a patient unlikely to be liberated from the ventilator, or performing recurrent procedures or invasive interventions on chronically critically ill patients.

Regardless of the EP's personal views, it is essential to speak with the patient or their surrogate decision-maker about their personal preferences and values. Early and open communication can help align the medical treatment with the patient's personal GOC. Additionally, some patients and families may not reach a clear consensus in the ED, but the initiation of open and honest dialogue from the ED setting may help a family during future GOC discussions.

Conclusion

Let us return to Mrs. Smith from our case vignette at the start of the chapter. You join the family in the pre-identified ED family consultation room sit down, and ask open-ended questions about her life. You find out that prior to her cancer diagnosis, she gardened every day and retired 5 years ago from the public school system after more than 40 years as a science teacher. She has three living daughters, a husband, and multiple grandchildren. Her husband is the designated POA. There is no AD currently because the family was waiting for a time everyone could decide together. The daughters and husband note a precipitous decline over the past 2 months and acknowledge that Mrs. Smith would never want to be dependent on anyone for her care or live in a nursing home for a prolonged period of time. You state that intubation would likely not change her ultimate course but instead simply "prolong her dying process." The family and patient agree that CPR or intubation would not get Mrs. Smith the QOL she wishes. The patient is admitted to the medical floor, so loved ones may visit overnight. The next day, she is placed in inpatient hospice and dies with her family at her bedside.

Chapter Summary "CRITICAL POINTS"

1. Discuss end of life care with appropriate patients and families.
2. Early GOC conversations should focus around the patient and their wishes regarding medical treatment.
3. During a GOC discussion: (1) ask open-ended questions (2) make eye contact and (3) avoid negative terminology (i.e., "we will not…").
4. Identify if an AD is present or the patient has an appointed POA.
5. Use SDM when appropriate.
6. Opioids are the treatment of choice for pain and discomfort at the EOL.

References

1. Teno, J. Facts on Dying March 19, 2004. Center for Gerontology and Health Care Research, Brown University. 2006. http://www.chcr.brown.edu/dying/2001DATA.HTM
2. Loh AZ, Tan JS, Lyn TY, Krishna LK, Goh CR. Places of care at the end of life: what factors are associated with patients' and their family members' preference? Am J Hosp Palliat Care. 2016;33(7):669–77.
3. Angus DC, Barnato AE, Linde-Zwirble WT, Weissfeld LA, Watson RS, Rickert T, Rubenfeld GD. Use of intensive care at the end of life in the United States: an epidemiologic study. Crit Care Med. 2004;32:638–43.
4. American Academy of Hospice and Palliative Medicine (AAHPM). AAPHM home page. Available at: http://www.aahpm.org/about/college.html. Accessed 23 Aug 2017.
5. Grudzen C, Richardson L, Johnson P, Hu M, Wang B, Ortiz J, Kistler E, Chen A, Morrison S. Emergency-department –initiated palliative care in advanced cancer. A randomized control trial. JAMA Oncol. 2016;2(5):591–8.
6. Sullivan AM, Lakoma MD, Block SD. The status of medical education in end-of-life care: a national report. J Gen Intern Med. 2003;18:685–95.
7. American College of Emergency Physicians. Policy statement: code of ethics for emergency physicians. Approved January 2017.
8. Zieske M, Abbott J. Ethics seminar: the hospice patient in the ED: an ethical approach to understanding barriers and improving care. Acad Emerg Med. 2011;18(11):1201–7.
9. Yadav K, Gabler N, Cooney E, Kent S, Kim J, Herbst N, Mante A, Halpern S, Courtright K. Approximately one in three US adults completes any type of advance directive for end-of-life care. Health Aff. 2017;36(7):1244–51.
10. Bernacki RE, Block SD, for the American College of Physicians High Value Care Task Force. Communication about serious illness care goals: a review and synthesis of best practices. JAMA Intern Med. 2014;174(12):1994–2003. https://doi.org/10.1001/jamainternmed.2014.5271
11. Carlet J, Thijs LG, Antonelli M, Cassell J, Cox P, Hill N, Hinds C, Pimentel JM, Reinhart K, Thompson BT. Challenges in end-of-life care in the ICU. Statement of the 5th International Consensus Conference in Critical care: Brussels, Belgium, April 2003. Intensive Care Med. 2004;30:770–84.
12. Charles C, Whelan T, Gafni A. What do we mean by partnership in making decisions about treatment? BMJ. 1999;319:780–2.
13. Flynn D, Knoedler M, Hess E, Murad M, Erwin P, Montori V, Thomson R. Engaging patients in health care decisions in the emergency department through shared decision-making: a systematic review. Acad Emerg Med. 2012;19:959–67.
14. Wynn S. Decisions by surrogates: an overview of surrogate consent laws in the United States. Bifocal. 2014:36(1). Accessed on 9/5/2017 https://www.americanbar.org/publications/bifocal/vol_36/issue_1_october2014/default_surrogate_consent_statutes.html.
15. Shalowitz DI, Garrett-Mayer E, Wendler D. The accuracy of surrogate decision makers: a systematic review. Arch Intern Med. 2006;166(5):493–7. https://doi.org/10.1001/archinte.166.5.493.

16. Hunter JK, Dean T, Gowan J. Death with dignity: devising a withdrawal of treatment process. Br J Nurs. 2006;15(3):138–40.
17. Cook D, Rocker G, Marshall J, Sjokvist P, Dodek P, Griffith L, Freitag A, Varon J, Bradley C, Levy M, Finfer S, Hamielec C, McMullin J, Weaver B, Walter S, Guyatt G. Withdrawal of mechanical ventilation in anticipation of death in the intensive care unit. N Engl J Med. 2003;349:1123–32.
18. Schneiderman LJ, Jecker NS, Jonsen AR. Medical futility: its meaning and ethical implications. Ann Intern Med. 1990;112:949–54.

Index

© Springer Nature Switzerland AG 2020
J. R. Shiber, S. D. Weingart (eds.), *Emergency Department Critical Care*,
https://doi.org/10.1007/978-3-030-28794-8

B

O

P

Printed in Singapore by Markono Print Media Pte Ltd

Printed in Singapore by Markono Print Media Pte Ltd